SAVORING GOTHAM

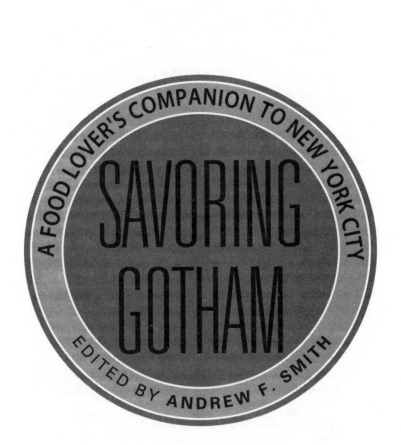

A FOOD LOVER'S COMPANION TO NEW YORK CITY

SAVORING GOTHAM

EDITED BY ANDREW F. SMITH

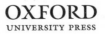

OXFORD
UNIVERSITY PRESS

OXFORD

UNIVERSITY PRESS

Oxford University Press is a department of the
University of Oxford. It furthers the University's objective
of excellence in research, scholarship, and education
by publishing worldwide.

Oxford   New York

Auckland   Cape Town   Dar es Salaam   Hong Kong   Karachi
Kuala Lumpur   Madrid   Melbourne   Mexico City   Nairobi
New Delhi   Shanghai   Taipei   Toronto

With offices in

Argentina   Austria   Brazil   Chile   Czech Republic   France   Greece
Guatemala   Hungary   Italy   Japan   Poland   Portugal   Singapore
South Korea   Switzerland   Thailand   Turkey   Ukraine   Vietnam

Oxford is a registered trademark of Oxford University Press
in the UK and certain other countries.

Published in the United States of America by
Oxford University Press
198 Madison Avenue, New York, NY 10016
www.oup.com

Library of Congress Cataloging-in-Publication Data
Smith, Andrew F., 1946-
Savoring Gotham : a food lover's companion to New York City / Andrew F Smith.
pages   cm
Includes bibliographical references and index.
ISBN 978-0-19-939702-0 (pbk. : acid-free paper) – ISBN 978-0-19-045465-4 (hardcover : acid-free paper)
1. Cooking—New York (State)—New York—History—Encyclopedias.   2. Restaurants—New York (State)—
New York—History—Encyclopedias.   3. New York (N.Y.)—History—Encyclopedias.   I. Title.
TX907.3.N72S65   2016
641.59747—dc23   2015018564

3 5 7 9 8 6 4 2

Printed in the United States of America
on acid-free paper

CONTENTS

Foreword vii

Introduction ix

Topical Outline of Entries xiii

Savoring Gotham: A Food Lover's Companion to New York City 1

Directory of Contributors 663

Bibliography 669

Index 675

FOREWORD

My father was from New York City, and he made very sure that we were from New York City too. I was born in Queens, and no one in my family ever mentioned the possibility of living anywhere else. Although we were an African American family living in a largely African American neighborhood, when we were kids, we did not eat quite like other Americans.

My mother cooked white rice with sugar and butter, a holdover from our southern ancestors. Other nights we ate our spaghetti with butter, pepper, and a shake of "Parmesan" cheese, a recipe I later saw in my many trips to northern Italy. One night would be chili con carne, the next night "rice and peas." Our neighbor, Mrs. Stafutti, would show up every Christmas with struffoli, a confection she referred to, somewhat less mellifluously, as "honey balls." My great-aunt Emma often brought over her homemade "chopped liver," and there was never even the slightest suggestion that it was Jewish in origin or that our neighbors had probably never heard of the dish. Then again, by my teens I had strong opinions about matzah ball soup and owned two yarmulkes—the "plain one" and the "fancy one"—for different styles of bar mitzvahs.

Aside from pizza, my favorite dish in the world was a concoction called "egg foo yong," a sort of deep-fried omelet of dubious Chinese ancestry, full of onions and swathed in a glassy brown cornstarch sauce. On the way home from school, waiting for the bus, I would pick up brown paper bags of hot zeppoli covered in powdered sugar. As the oil soaked through the bag in splotches, I would empty the bag before I got home. And on weekends, my father and I would gather our dogs—proud, funny German short-haired pointers—and take them into the fields of Long Island and Westchester, looking for pheasant, quail, and chukar partridge. When we returned triumphant, I would end up cleaning the still warm birds, and then my father, an advertising executive, would mount them in a flawless white wine and cream sauce. I never found out where he learned how to cook like that. Nor did I ever learn where he had met his hunting friends, gruff but friendly guys, a few of whom had lost fingers to the machinery of local canning plants.

We did not think we were strange. We were New Yorkers. When I graduated from junior high school, we put on suits and ate at the swanky Chateau Henri IV at the Hotel Alrae on East Sixty-Fourth Street, a haunt of movie stars and illicit lovers alike. My father wanted us to be suffused with the life of the city, and as much as that meant museums and the arts, it also meant food.

The world abounds with great cities, but when it comes to food, there has never been another like New York City. A century ago, people in their millions did not arrive from far-off foreign lands to make entirely new lives in London, Paris, Rome, Munich, Tokyo, or St. Petersburg. When I moved to London in 1983, London was almost entirely British. Yes, you could find good Indian and Pakistani food, and there was a thin smattering of Caribbean food around if you knew where to look. A few Jewish specialties were on the shelves of Golders Green. But London was British, and what you would largely find was English food, much of it gray. London has recovered nicely, but it is not Gotham. Even today, in a large city like Torino (Turin), Italy, home to 1.7 million people, you will find mostly Italian food—not even "Italian food" (a foreign construct that does not really exist) but Piemontese food. A great Thai restaurant will still be hard to find. More than a century ago, those millions, hailing from dozens of countries, began to stream into Gotham, and they made it the greatest food city on Earth.

In Lower Manhattan, in the late 1800s, you had choices. Was your family from Campania? Were you tired of Campanese food? All you had to do was take a walk, and you could visit parts of China or Germany. Make your way to Brooklyn, and you could eat in Norway and Russia and Sweden too. There were forty-eight breweries in Brooklyn alone, making 10 percent of all the beer in the country, and we had the most diverse beer culture in the world.

As the rest of the United States largely disappeared into the blandified world of highly engineered Frankenfood, a period from which the country is only now recovering, much of New York City held firm. Arthur Avenue did not hold truck with frozen "TV dinners." Fresh seafood still wriggled in baskets in Chinatown. We ate Ukrainian pirogies at 4:00 a.m. after the East Village clubs closed. There were still a half-dozen places in Red Hook, Brooklyn, where you could order the swift demise of a live chicken for dinner that night. Jamaican jerk seasoning bubbled in pots a few miles away.

It is true: the city has changed, and things have been lost. Only in the mid-1990s, as I got off the L train in Williamsburg every morning, I could smell the smoke. Lenny Liveri, down the block at Joe's Busy Corner, was smoking the freshly made mozzarella in a small box out on the sidewalk. By lunch, I would order that smoked mozzarella on a sandwich with prosciutto and pesto, while I listened to the little old Italian ladies verbally beat up the cowed, linebacker-sized Liveri brothers who were building epic sandwiches behind the counter. When the new bearded, tattooed kids started hectoring them for cappuccinos, in the afternoon, no less, the Liveris packed up and moved to New Jersey. They could not take it anymore—these kids. Joe's Busy. Those were the days.

But these are the days too: the days of the Latin American food at Red Hook ball fields, the days of the Arepa Lady, the days of deciding what region of Thailand you want to eat in tonight, the days of great cocktail bars and dozens of breweries. We always had everything, and we still do. Eating in New York City has never been better than it is today, and a lot of the best stuff is not even expensive.

One day, some years back, I drove from Cap-Martin, France, over the Alps, into La Morra, Piemonte, Italy, to eat lunch. Lunch was brilliant, of course, and I was back in Cap-Martin by nightfall. And I would still do that drive today. But in Gotham, you take such trips simply because you enjoy the journey. Here, at the center of the world, a universe of food is at your fingertips and always was. Between these pages are the many stories of our tables, millions strong, vaulting over centuries and into the future. Seek and ye shall find. Perhaps we New Yorkers *are* strange. Good thing, too.

Garrett Oliver

INTRODUCTION

Mention New York City food, and most people think of the white-hot restaurants of the moment, with their media-savvy celebrity chefs, glittering patrons, and sky-high prices. Upscale restaurants have long been an exciting part of the city's foodscape, but they are at one far end of the broad, colorful spectrum of New York eateries. Inhabiting the starry heights are temples of haute cuisine, such as Per Se and Le Bernardin; at the low end are hot dog carts and old-school Mexican taco trucks. In between, over the past three hundred years, have been all kinds of eating places: cafeterias, diners, luncheonettes, drugstore counters, fast-food chains, delis, cafes, coffee shops, juice bars, doughnut shops, ice cream parlors, cocktail lounges, dive bars, and corner sweet shops, not to mention theater snack bars, supermarket delis, farmers' markets, social club dining rooms, kiosks, and vending machines.

Today, New Yorkers have more than fifty thousand eating places to choose from. Of course, people eat most of their meals at home, prepared from ingredients purchased at the supermarket, corner grocery, fish market, butcher shop, or Greenmarket. (Less common items can easily be found at specialty food shops in ethnic neighborhoods like Chinatown, Little Italy, Spanish Harlem, Koreatown, and Little Odessa.) Or, if not inclined to cook, New Yorkers can pick up—or have delivered—food from a pizzeria, Chinese takeout shop, south Indian buffet, gluten-free bakery, sushi bar, or steakhouse.

The city's food scene is not limited to how and where New Yorkers—and visitors—get their daily sustenance. New York is home to culinary magazines, including *Food & Wine*, *Saveur*, *Food Arts*, and *Bon Appétit*. The city is also home to some of the nation's top culinary schools, such as the International Culinary Center and the Institute of Culinary Education, and influential organizations such as Slow Food USA, the James Beard Foundation, and the Culinary Historians of New York. The city's many renowned museums frequently mount food-related exhibits, whether at the Museum of Modern Art, the American Museum of Natural History, the Tenement Museum, or the fledgling Museum of Food and Drink. New York City's libraries have extensive culinary literature holdings, such as the New York Public Library's incredible menu collection, the Fales Library's fifty-five thousand cookbooks at New York University, and the New York Academy of Medicine Library's early medical and cookbook collection, including a copy of the ninth-century cookery manuscript attributed to the Roman gourmand Marcus Apicius.

Savoring Gotham weaves the full tapestry of the city's rich gastronomy: its culinary history and culture, beginning with the first inhabitants; profiles of influential people; the dishes, drinks, and food businesses that originated in the city; ethnic contributions to New York's foodways; and insights into the unique character of each borough and neighborhood.

My interest in New York's culinary life began in April 1991, when I realized that the Horn & Hardart automat at the corner of Forty-Second Street and Third Avenue was closing. Once a thriving chain of restaurants emblematic of New York City's hustle and bustle, the automats were distinguished by their unique mechanical food dispensers. The restaurant walls were lined with row on row of small windowed hatches behind which plates of food were displayed. The customer deposited one or more nickels into a slot, turned a knob, the little door popped open, and the food could be removed. Behind the wall, a worker slid in a replacement as soon as a dish was sold. It was a modern, efficient, and, to me, fascinating way to serve and enjoy a meal.

Some automats were open all night—just the thing for "the city that never sleeps." Their heyday was in the 1930s and 1940s, when tens of thousands of people visited them every day. By the 1980s, though, the few that remained were dingy and seedy. Even the poorest New Yorkers had long since deserted the once-novel mechanical food service in favor of cafeterias, coffee shops, delis, and fast-food chains. Still, the automat was one of those quintessential New York culinary landmarks, and I had visited several of them since arriving in the city in 1977. I was surprised that they should disappear with so little fanfare, without an audible murmur of public protest. As it turned out, the end of the automat was just one small facet in the city's ever-changing culinary kaleidoscope.

Over the past four centuries, thousands of books, dissertations, and academic studies and tens of thousands of newspaper and magazine articles have been written that touch on various aspects of the city's culinary life.

New York City started out as New Amsterdam, a small colonial village on the tip of Manhattan Island in a very big harbor. It was the administrative center for the Dutch colony of New Netherland, consisting of a few small settlements in parts of what are today the states of New Jersey, New York, Connecticut, and Pennsylvania. Other settlements were established in what are now the boroughs of Brooklyn, Queens, Staten Island, and the Bronx. The British acquired New Amsterdam in 1664 and renamed it New York. This village slowly expanded northward on the island, as did the other colonial communities on Long Island, on Staten Island, and in the Bronx. It was not until 1898 that Manhattan and the other four boroughs were united to create "Greater New York," which today has 8.3 million residents. Manhattan is the smallest borough (23 square miles), while Queens is the largest (109 square miles). Brooklyn has the largest population (2.6 million) and Staten Island the smallest (less than half a million). The Bronx is the only part of the city that is on the mainland. Historically, the city's food supply, cooking traditions, and diet have been closely linked with the surrounding hinterland. *Savoring Gotham*,

however, focuses only on the five boroughs that make up New York City today.

Three research challenges have confronted us in writing about New York City's culinary life. The first is the dearth of information about the years prior to about 1700. Little is known about the foodways of the Lenape, the Native American group who lived in the area when Europeans arrived, and few primary sources describing what the early Dutch colonists ate have survived. Neither is there much information about what was consumed in the city prior to the mid-eighteenth century.

The second research challenge is, conversely, the vast quantity of information dating from 1800 on. A superabundance of sources has survived in manuscripts, newspapers, magazines, books, autobiographies, diaries, letters, government reports, cookbooks, and television documentaries. Even so, the material does not always supply a truly inclusive view of New York's food culture; much of it was written by outsiders, visitors, and upper-class residents, and there are far fewer accounts of how working-class and poor New Yorkers cooked and ate. *Savoring Gotham* has tried to strike a balance between the highbrow and lowbrow aspects of the city's food scene, because both are important.

The final challenge was packing such a tremendous amount of information into encyclopedia form in a very limited space. *Savoring Gotham* has drawn on the expertise of researchers with a variety of interests, and it brings together the best scholarship on the subject. The 567 entries focus on every aspect of the city's food life:

* Beverages—from soda fountains to Manhattans to craft beers
* Biographies of important contributors to New York City's food and drink scene, including chefs, corporate leaders, critics, food writers, cookbook authors, restaurateurs, and others whom the editors considered influential in the city's culinary development
* Businesses and brands associated with the city, from Oreos to Snapple to Cronuts
* Education and culinary arts, including cooking schools and university food-studies departments and programs, such as the Institute for Culinary Education, the International Culinary Center, and New York University's Food Studies Department

* Contributions made to the city's culinary life by ethnic, religious, cultural, and racial groups, including African American, German American, Mexican American, Chinese American, and Jewish New Yorkers
* Food controversies, such as those related to the regulation of street vendors, restaurant grading, and the "ban" on oversized servings of soda
* Food services and retailing, including entries on King Kullen, food co-ops, and Zabar's
* Foods associated with New York City, such as bagels, hamburgers, and pizza
* Historical periods—chronological surveys that look at New York City's culinary history during different time periods, from the pre-Columbian era to the early twenty-first century
* Holidays, celebrations, and festivals, such as New Year's Day, Thanksgiving, and the West Indian Day parade
* Media and print, including newspapers, magazines, radio, television, and the Internet
* Museums, libraries, and historical sites, including Fraunces Tavern, the New York Public Library, and the Tenement Museum
* Neighborhoods and boroughs, including Manhattan, Brooklyn, the Bronx, Queens, and Staten Island
* Organizations and hunger programs, such as the James Beard Foundation, the New York Women's Culinary Alliance, and Meals on Wheels
* Restaurants and bars, including Delmonico's, the Grand Central Oyster Bar, and The Four Seasons
* Special topics, such as dieting programs, dumpster diving, and sex and food

The contributors have sought to write in clear language with a minimum of technical vocabulary. For the reader who wishes to pursue a topic in greater detail, a selective bibliography at the end of each article lists primary sources, the most important scholarly works in any language, and the most useful works in English.

To guide readers from one article to related discussions elsewhere in this work, end references appear at the end of many articles. There are cross-references within the body of some articles. Blind entries direct the user from an alternate form of an entry term to the entry itself. For example, the blind entry for "Horn & Hardart" tells the reader to look under "Automats." At the beginning of the volume, readers interested in finding all the articles on a particular subject may consult the topical outline, which shows how articles relate to one another and to the overall design of Savoring Gotham. At the end of the volume are a directory of contributors, a bibliography of useful works about New York City and its food and beverage history, and a comprehensive index that lists all the topics covered in Savoring Gotham, including those that are not headwords themselves.

Savoring Gotham is not intended to be comprehensive, and it does not include every possible topic. Because of the eclectic nature of New York City's gastronomy, Savoring Gotham covers a wide range of topics, but it can only scratch the surface of many of them. It is not intended as the final word on the city's culinary scene. Bibliographic resources are provided for most entries and in the appendix to help readers interested in knowing more about New York City food.

Many individuals could be singled out for their assistance in producing Savoring Gotham. I would particularly like to thank associate editor Cathy Kaufman and the area editors—Dr. Ari Ariel, Michael Krondl, Dr. Cindy Lobel, Kara Newman, Dr. Jonathan Deutsch, and Judith Weinraub—for their hundreds of hours of work on Savoring Gotham—designing and selecting entries, identifying and guiding authors, and reviewing and editing entries. I also want to thank advisory editor Cara de Silva for her assistance in identifying potential topics and writers, and Marty Levick and Meryle Evans for their help with the illustrations. I also thank the 174 writers who contributed entries.

On a personal note, I would like to thank Bonnie Slotnick, who commented on all of my entries and pointed out foolish mistakes of grammar as well as of content.

Finally, I thank the staff at Oxford University Press, especially Max Sinsheimer, my editor from Savoring Gotham's conception to its completion. Without his support and encouragement, we would never have made it to the finish line. Brad Rosenkrantz oversaw production efforts with professionalism and care. And Damon Zucca's support for the project throughout was crucial. It was a personal joy and professional pleasure to work with them all.

Andrew F. Smith
Editor-in-Chief

TOPICAL OUTLINE OF ENTRIES

Entries in the body of *Savoring Gotham* are organized alphabetically. This outline offers an overview of the book, with entries listed in the following categories:

Beverages
Biographies
Businesses and Brands
Education and Culinary Arts
Ethnicities and Immigrant
    Populations
Food Controversies and Regulation

Food Services and
    Retailing
Foods
Historical
Holidays, Celebrations, and
    Festivals
Media and Publishing

Museums, Libraries, and
    Historical Sites
Neighborhoods and Boroughs
Organizations and Hunger
    Programs
Restaurants and Bars
Special Topics

Beverages

Beer
Bloody Mary
Bronx Cocktail
Brooklyn Cocktail
Charlotte Russe
Cocktails
Coffee
Coffee Roasters
Cosmopolitan

Dr. Brown's Soda
Manhattan Cocktail
Manhattan Special
Martini
Mixology
No-Cal Soda
Old-Fashioned Cocktail
Queens Cocktail
Rum

Seltzer
Soda
Spirits
Tea
Water
Water, Bottled
Wine and Winemaking

Biographies

Allen, Ida Bailey
Barber, Dan
Bastianich, Lidia
Batali, Mario
Batterberry, Michael and Ariane
Baum, Joe
Beard, James
Benepe, Barry
Berry, Rynn
Bittman, Mark

Bloomberg, Michael
Bloomfield, April
Blot, Pierre
Borden, Gail
Bouley, David
Boulud, Daniel
Bourdain, Anthony
Brady, Diamond Jim
Brock, Carol
Cannon, Poppy

Chang, David
Child, Julia
Claiborne, Craig
Corson, Juliet
Cullen, Michael J.
De Gouy, Louis P.
DeGroff, Dale
Delmonico Brothers
De Voe, Thomas Farrington
Diat, Louis

Dufresne, Wylie
Fabricant, Florence
Feltman, Charles
Flay, Bobby
Franey, Pierre
Gold, Rozanne
Greene, Gael
Grimes, William
Hamilton, Dorothy Cann
Hamilton, Gabrielle
Hazan, Marcella
Hesser, Amanda
Hess, Karen and John L.
Hopper, Edward
Irving, Washington
Jones, Judith and Evan
Kump, Peter Clark
La Guardia, Fiorello
Lang, George
Lape, Bob
Lewis, Edna
Liebling, A. J.

Lucas, Dione
Lüchow, August Guido
MacAusland, Earle
Maccioni, Sirio
Macfadden, Bernarr
Mason, John L.
Meyer, Danny
Mitchell, Joseph
Moulton, Sara
Nestle, Marion
Nickerson, Jane
Nidetch, Jean
Nieporent, Drew
O'Neill, Molly
Paddleford, Clementine
Pépin, Jacques
Ranhofer, Charles
Ray, Rachael
Rector, Charles and George
Reichl, Ruth
Rodale, Jerome Irving
Runyon, Damon

Sailhac, Alain
Samuelsson, Marcus
Saunders, Audrey
Schwartz, Arthur
Sheraton, Mimi
Sinclair, Upton
Smilow, Rick
Sokolov, Raymond
Soltner, André
Soulé, Henri
Steingarten, Jeffrey
Thomas, Jerry
Toffenetti, Dario
Torres, Jacques
Trillin, Calvin
Tschirky, Oscar
Vongerichten, Jean-Georges
Waxman, Nach
Wechsberg, Joseph
Wolf, Clark
Woods, Sylvia
Zagat, Tim and Nina

Businesses and Brands

Breweries
Broadway Panhandler
Brooklyn Brewery
Chipwich
Chock full o'Nuts
Distilleries
Gulden's Mustard
Häagen-Dazs
Hellmann's Mayonnaise
Life Savers

Loft's Candy Stores
Microbreweries and Brewpubs
Momofuku Restaurant Group
Nabisco
Nathan's Famous
Oreos
Papaya King
Pepsi-Cola
Perrier
Reggie! Bar

Schaller & Weber
Snapple
Starbucks
Startups
Stella D'oro
Sugar Refining
Sweet'N Low
Tofutti
Tootsie Roll
Weight Watchers

Education and Culinary Arts

Astor Center
Careers through Culinary Arts
    Program (C-CAP)
City University of New York
Columbia University

Cooking Schools
Experimental Cuisine Collective
French Culinary Institute
Institute of Culinary Education
James Beard Awards

Natural Gourmet Institute
New School
New York Cooking School
New York University

Ethnicities and Immigrant Populations

African American
Arab Community
Armenian
Australian

Brazilian
Caribbean
Chinese Community
Colombian

Cuban
Dominican
Egyptian
Filipino

French
German
Greek
Hungarian
Indo-Caribbean
Irish
Italian
Jamaican

Japanese
Jewish
Korean
Mexican
Polish
Puerto Rican
Rastafari
Russian

Scandinavian
South and Central American
South Asian
Southeast Asian
Syrian and Lebanese
Thai
Ukrainian

Food Controversies and Regulation

Fast-Food Workers Strikes
Menu Labeling
Milk, Raw

Milk, Swill
Restaurant Letter Grading
Soda "Ban"

Street Vendors, Regulation of
Trans Fat Elimination

Food Services and Retailing

A&P
Appetizing Stores
Automats
Bakeries
Balducci's
Barney Greengrass
Beer Gardens
Bodegas
Butchers
Cafeterias
Caffe Reggio
Catering
Cheesemongers
Chelsea Market
Childs
Chop Suey Joints
Coffeehouses
Coffee Shops
D'Agostino
Dairy Stores
Dean & DeLuca
Delis, German

Delis, Jewish
Diners
Diners Club
Dylan's Candy Bar
Eataly
Essex Street Market
Fairway Market
Fast Food
Food Co-ops
Food Trucks
FreshDirect
Fulton Fish Market
Gourmet Garage
Great Performances
Greenmarkets
Gristedes
Grocery Stores
Groggeries
Hunts Point
Ice Cream Shops
Italian Ices
Kalustyan's

Key Food
King Kullen
Korean Taco
Lobster Palaces
Magnolia Bakery
Mrs. Stahl's Knishes
Murray's Cheese
New Amsterdam Market
Public Markets
Restaurant Associates
Restaurant Opportunity Center
Russ & Daughters
Schrafft's
Shake Shack
Stadium Food
Street Vendors
Supermarkets
Trader Joe's
Washington Market
Whole Foods
Yonah Schimmel Knish Bakery
Zabar's

Foods

Bagels
Baked Alaska
Bialys
Black and White Cookies
Bread
Candy
Cheesecake
Chestnuts

Chocolate, Craft
Cookies
Corned Beef Sandwich
Cream Cheese
Cronut
Cupcakes
Deep-Fried Twinkies
Dimsum

Doughnuts
Ebinger's Blackout Cake
Egg Creams
Eggs Benedict
Gum
Halva
Hamburgers
Hamburg Steak

Hot Dogs
Hummus
Ice Cream Sandwich
Kimchi
Knish
Lobster Newberg
Lox
Mallomars

Manhattan Clam Chowder
Matzah
New Year's Cakes
New York Strip Steak
Oysters
Pastrami
Pickles
Pizza

Pretzels
Reuben Sandwich
Smoked Fish
Steak Tartare
Sushi
Vichyssoise
Waldorf Salad
Zeppole

Historical

Algonquin Round Table
Antebellum Period
Boarding Houses
Bootleggers
Breadlines
Civil War
Colonial Dutch
Depression Food
Ellis Island Food (1892–1924)
English Colonial

Erie Canal
Gilded Age
Havemeyer Family
Late Twentieth Century
Niblo's Garden
Post–World War II (1945–1975)
Pre-Columbian
Prohibition
Soda Fountains
Speakeasies

Tea Party
Temperance Movement
Twenty-First Century
Victory Gardens
Women's Clubs
World's Fair (1939–1940)
World's Fair (1964–1965)
World War I
World War II

Holidays, Celebrations, and Festivals

Chanukah
Christmas
Dutch-Style New Year's Day
   Parties
Easter
Fancy Food Show
Fourth of July

New Year
New Year, Chinese
New York City Wine and Food
   Festival
Ninth Avenue Food Festival
NYC Food Film Festival
Passover

San Gennaro, Feast of
Smorgasburg
St. Patrick's Day
Street Fairs
Thanksgiving
West Indian Day Parade

Media and Publishing

Columbia University Press
Cookbooks
Cuisine
Culintro
Eater
Edible
Food52
Food & Wine
Food Arts
Food Network
Gourmet

Heritage Radio Network
Kitchen Arts and Letters
Knopf
Lucky Peach
Mad Men
Nation's Restaurant News
New Yorker
New York Magazine
New York Times
Oxford University Press
Radio

Random House
Rizzoli
Saveur
Scribner's
Sex and the City
Television
Television, Public
Theater and Food
Village Voice
Women's Magazines

Museums, Libraries, and Historical Sites

American Museum of Natural
   History

Cooper Hewitt, Smithsonian
   Design Museum

Fales Library
Fraunces Tavern

Museum Food
Museum of Chinese in America
  (MOCA)

Museum of Food and Drink
Museum of the City of New York
New York Academy of Medicine

New-York Historical Society
New York Public Library
Tenement Museum

Neighborhoods and Boroughs

Arthur Avenue
Astoria
Bay Ridge
Bedford-Stuyvesant
Bensonhurst
Brighton Beach
Bronx
Brooklyn
Bushwick
Curry Hill
Five Points
Greenwich Village
Harlem

Hell's Kitchen
High Line
Inwood
Jackson Heights
Jamaica (Queens)
Kleindeutschland
Koreatowns
Little India
Little Italy
Little Odessa
Little Syria
Lower East Side
Manhattan

Meatpacking District
Park Slope
Queens
Restaurant Row
Staten Island
Sunset Park
Times Square
Upper East Side
Upper West Side
Washington Heights
Williamsburg
Yorkville

Organizations and Hunger Programs

American Institute of Wine &
  Food
Citymeals-on-Wheels
Culinary Historians of New York
GrowNYC

Hunger Programs
James Beard Foundation
Les Dames d'Escoffier
New York Women's Culinary
  Alliance

Salvation Army
Slow Food
Street Vendor Project
Supplemental Nutrition
  Assistance Program (SNAP)

Restaurants and Bars

Aquavit
Astor House
Bars
Bickford's
Café Nicholson
Central Park Casino
Chalet Suisse
Clubs
Cocktail Lounges
Colony Club
Cotton Club
Delmonico's
Department Store Restaurants
Four Seasons
Gage & Tollner
Gay Bars
Gotham Bar and Grill
Grand Central Oyster Bar
Hotel Restaurants
Jack Dempsey's

Junior's Restaurant
Katz's Delicatessen
La Caravelle
Le Cirque
Le Pavillon
Lindy's
Lombardi's
Lutèce
Macy's
Maxwell's Plum
McSorley's Old Ale
  House
Menus
Nedick's
Nightclubs
Oyster Bars
P. J. Clarke's
Peter Luger's
Pizzerias
Plaza, The

Pop-Up Restaurants
Rainbow Room
Rao's
Restaurant Groups
Restaurant Reviewing
Restaurants
Restaurant Workers
Ritz-Carlton
Roberta's
Russian Tea Room
Saloons
Sardi's
Sherry's
Stonewall Inn
Stork Club
Sylvia's
Tavern on the Green
Taverns
Tearooms
"21" Club

Union Square Cafe
Veganism

Victor's Café
Waldorf, The

White Horse Tavern
Windows on the World

Special Topics

Advertising
America Eats Project
Beekeeping
Big Apple
Brunch
Business Lunch
Chefs
Chefs, Private
Commodity Exchanges
Community Supported
   Agriculture
Cries of New-York, The
Dumpster Diving
Falafel
Farm to Table

Fishing
Food Deserts
Fusion Food
Haute Cuisine
Ladies Who Lunch
Lunch
Modernist Cuisine
Movies
Novels
Organic Food
Paintings
Picnics
Power Breakfasts and Power
   Lunches
Prison Food

Railroad Dining
Raw Food
Restaurant Unions
Rooftop Garden
School Food
Sex and Food
Slang
Three-Martini Lunch
Urban Farming
Vending Machines
Vendy Awards
Walking Tours, Culinary

A&P

A&P dominated the grocery business in the United States for much of the twentieth century. It had a particularly large presence in New York City, home to its first stores. The firm made impressions across the country as part of a broader shift to mass retail in food. Despite its emphasis on standardized and scientific stores it was also a vital and highly personal space for many Americans, an important and familiar source of food.

New York City occupies a place of special importance in A&P's history. The coffee and tea wholesaler that became "The Great American Tea Company" and later "The Great Atlantic and Pacific Tea Company" (or A&P) opened on Front Street in 1860. When the owners, George Gilman and George Hartford, diversified into retail, they opened stores nearby. A&P was headquartered in New York's Graybar Building for much of its history, moving to Montvale, New Jersey, in 1974. The city and its suburbs were also home to the Hartford family, who operated the firm from its early days as a minor wholesaler through its heyday as the nation's largest retailer. Even as A&P fell on hard times in later years and disappeared from much of the country, the stores retained were on the East Coast and in New York City.

A&P grew quickly from the original five stores. By 1879, one hundred stores existed. These sold mostly coffee and tea, other dry groceries such as flour, and sometimes small selections of more perishable goods like eggs or butter. Like almost all stores, clerks retrieved and measured goods for customers. Smaller "economy stores," offering lower prices but more limited selection and almost no

services, followed in the early twentieth century; by 1930 the firm operated nearly sixteen thousand stores, most of them larger than the "economy stores" but still small by twenty-first-century standards. That year, A&P became the first retailer to have more than $1 billion in annual sales. It was the largest retailer and one of the largest corporations in the United States. The firm experienced losses during the early 1930s and World War II and, like many established chain store firms, was slow to shift into supermarkets, which featured huge varieties of goods and open shelving with very little clerical assistance. Nonetheless, the firm eventually embraced supermarkets and regained its profits and its dominance in the post–World War II years. By the early 1960s, A&P was "the goliath of the industry" according to one journalist.

A&P's dramatic success was based on several factors. Like many chain grocers, A&P emphasized its low prices. But low prices alone could not have caused any grocer's success (indeed, many grocers lost money by selling at prices too low for their costs). A&P, like other chains, employed a range of strategies. Detailed study of finances and record-keeping, carefully choosing locations, and controlling costs were all important. A&P was especially successful at controlling the amount it paid for goods—sometimes by exercising leverage with suppliers but also by producing some goods themselves. A&P had long sold coffee from its wholesaling business, but it expanded into baked goods, canned milk, and shelf-stable goods like peanut butter and hundreds of others. At its height, the firm even made the cans in which goods were sold and owned many of the trains and trucks on which they were

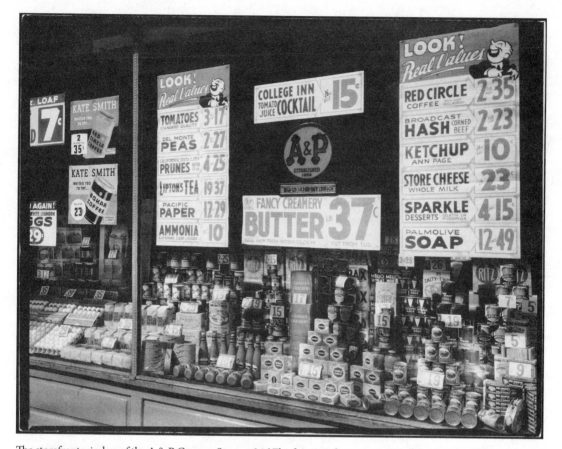

The storefront window of the A & P Grocery Store at 246 Third Avenue between East 20th and 21st Streets, on March 16, 1936. At the time, A & P was the most successful grocery store corporation. BERENICE ABBOTT. FEDERAL ART PROJECT / MUSEUM OF THE CITY OF NEW YORK

shipped. Its private brands, Eight O'Clock Coffee and Ann Page canned goods, became well known in their own right. (Eight O'Clock Coffee was later purchased by an outside company and continues to be sold in grocery stores.)

The store also relied on social convention, particularly around expectations of women. During its period of most dramatic expansion, A&P marketed heavily to middle- and upper-class women. Stores promised low prices but also "independence," understood as the "modern" practices of choosing goods off shelves and transporting them home themselves. The focus on women was epitomized by *Women's Day*, begun as a source for recipes, housekeeping advice, and a marketing vehicle in A&P stores in 1937 and later spun off as an independent magazine.

Hierarchies were reinforced—and challenged— in these stores. A&P remained a strong presence in poorer African American neighborhoods, in

distinction to other chain stores. However, it resisted hiring African American staff until pressured to do so by civil rights activists. And women, whatever their race, were rarely present as anything but customers or low-level clerks.

A&P also found itself at the center of numerous battles over the role of big business and the meaning of fairness in a new economy. Although the Justice Department asked that the firm be broken up into regional chains after it was found guilty of antitrust violations in 1949, in the end A&P simply limited its wholesale division to selling only to its own stores. Perhaps more importantly, it put more effort into its public and government relations. It happily enjoyed the embrace of big business by government in the 1950s.

The firm remained a family company through the middle of the twentieth century, closely managed first by George H. Hartford and then by his sons, John and

George L. Unlike many large chain grocery stores, its capital came largely from private sources rather than the stock market. The Hartford brothers set the course of the company during particularly dramatic shifts to self-service, supermarkets, manufacturing, and national expansion. But they also set day-to-day policy. Although division and store managers had significant authority, John Hartford was famous for intervening even over small matters, for example, when a manager set prices that were too high or too low or when employees' complaints seemed justified.

In later years, A&P struggled to hold down prices while maintaining its volume of sales. Analysts, rightly or wrongly, often blamed the firm's faltering in the latter half of the twentieth century on the death of the Hartford brothers (John in 1951 and George in 1955). Although A&P continued to experiment and expand and was an important presence in many Americans' lives, its business profile was shakier. The firm steadily lost profitability in the 1960s. In 1979, after decades of declining value on the stock market and declining profits, it was sold to the Tengelmann Group, a German conglomerate. It regained significant ground in the 1980s and 1990s, even purchasing other competing chains. However, the recession of 2008 made it impossible for the firm to keep up with its obligations. In 2010, with only four hundred A&P stores remaining, few of them operating under the A&P name, the firm filed for bankruptcy. It emerged in 2012 as it had started—a modest-sized, privately held corporation. Hundreds of stores operated by A&P nonetheless remain, many operating as "Pathmark," "The Food Emporium," or "Waldbaum's." Several are in New York City, connecting shoppers to a long history of neighborhood chain stores.

See also GROCERY STORES and SUPERMARKETS.

Anderson, Avis. A&P: The Story of the Great Atlantic and Pacific Tea Company. Mount Pleasant, S.C.: Arcadia, 2002.

Bowlby, Rachel. Carried Away: The Invention of Modern Shopping. New York: Columbia University Press, 2001.

Deutsch, Tracey. Building a Housewife's Paradise: Gender, Politics and American Grocery Stores in the Twentieth Century. Chapel Hill: University of North Carolina Press, 2010.

Levinson, Marc. The Great A&P and the Struggle for Small Business in America. New York: Hill and Wang, 2011.

Stanford, Karin L. "Reverend Jesse Jackson and the Rainbow/PUSH Coalition: Institutionalizing Economic Opportunity." In Black Political Organizations in the Post–Civil Rights Era, edited by Ollie A. Johnson III and Karin L. Stanford, pp. 150–169. New Brunswick, N.J.: Rutgers University Press, 2002.

Schragger, Richard. "The Anti–Chain Store Movement, Localist Ideology, and the Remnants of the Progressive Constitution, 1920–1940." Iowa Law Review 90 (March 2005): 1011.

Tracey Deutsch

Advertising

Modern advertisers, such as those portrayed in the television series Mad Men, about a fictional Madison Avenue advertising agency, are in the business of creating desires for products and services, especially nonessential or discretionary ones, through eye-catching, memorable, or even annoying imagery and sound. These slick, often manipulative ads are hallmarks of the post–World War II consumer culture, and New York City is home to many homegrown and international agencies that fashion campaigns to tempt us daily. But before there were such Mad Men, there were plenty of ways that New Yorkers advertised food and drink.

Before Mass Media: Street Cries and Newsworthy Statements

The cacophonous cries of street vendors and peddlers could be heard throughout city streets, from colonial days through the 1930s, when Mayor Fiorello La Guardia effectively removed peddlers from the streets of Lower Manhattan and Harlem and relocated them in public markets. See LA GUARDIA, FIORELLO. Designed to catch the ear of shoppers, especially those susceptible to a snack, many street cries were rhymes. One documented cry current from at least the 1820s went "Here's your nice Hot Corn! / Smoking Hot! Piping Hot! / Oh what beauties I have got? / Here's smoking hot Corn / With salt that is nigh / Only two pence an ear— / Oh pass me not by!" See CRIES OF NEW-YORK, THE.

More than one hundred years later, as noted by Terry Roth, writing for the Works Projects Administration, peddlers and their cries were being hounded off the streets, yet distinctive sounds could still be heard in different neighborhoods. In Harlem, market cries might be sung and delivered in syncopated rhythms, often with a southern lilt reflecting the influx of African Americans as part of the Great Migration, while immigrants from the West Indies advertised wares with a patois. On the Lower East

Side, cries could be heard "in the strange symphony of many foreign tongues," reflecting the mix of immigrants living in its teeming tenements. Faint echoes of the street cries are still heard in the pleas of vendors climbing stadium steps at New York's sports arenas, offering "Beer, here" and other refreshments.

For a tonier set, colonial newspapers carried advertisements for all sorts of products, including announcements of the arrival of ships bearing tea, coffee, chocolate, sugar, wine, spices, and other imports, as well as for seasonal produce, cakes, meat pies, tarts, sweet meats, pickles, pickled oysters, and many other products sold by city grocers and confectioners. Coffeehouses and taverns also advertised in newspapers. Samuel Fraunces, owner of the city's most famous colonial tavern, announced in 1770 that he would make home deliveries: "Dinners and Suppers dressed to send out, for Lodgers and others, who live at a convenient Distance." See FRAUNCES TAVERN. Several of New York's late eighteenth- and early nineteenth-century newspapers were called the *New York Commercial Advertiser* or a similar variation, showing the tight connection between news and commercial announcements.

But these advertisements had modest visceral impact as they were printed in the same typeface as the journals, visually indistinguishable from news stories. In 1856, the photographer Mathew Brady is credited with helping to invent modern print advertising when he advertised his services in the *New York Herald* using a distinctive and eye-catching font that jumped from the page.

From Small Trade Cards to Oversized Billboards and Icons of New York

Shortly after Brady's novel ad, advertising agencies emerged in the United States. Although a few advertising agencies had developed in Philadelphia in the 1850s to act as agents placing client-generated ads in newspapers, the technological development of chromolithography, a process where thousands of multicolor images could be printed in a single day, brought a new way of competing for consumers' attention. The possibilities of artistic expression as a means of capturing consumer attention changed the nascent industry from mere placement agents to one where agencies created content with talented graphic artists and copywriters.

A favorite medium was the trade card, polychrome art on the front of sturdy cardstock, with sales pitches or other information printed on the reverse. Restaurants, food manufacturers, and retailers were quick to join the Victorian fetish for trade cards. Like the toy in Cracker Jack, clever manufacturers used the inclusion of novel trade cards in packaged goods as a way of encouraging continuing purchases. In 1889, New York City's Arbuckle Brothers Coffee Company issued a series of trade cards depicting different states and territories in the United States: the cards had nothing to do with the quality of Arbuckle coffee, but the desire to collect a complete set spurred purchases. Restaurants were especially eager to issue trade cards, always with the address conspicuously displayed and decorated with photographs or drawings of the establishments. It is a practice still in vogue among many food businesses, although photography and thin, glossy postcard materials now often substitute for the satisfyingly thicker and more expensive rag cardboard on which the chromolithographs were printed.

Gotham has never shied away from extravagantly bold, electronic billboards, especially around Times Square, with its special tolerance for spectacle and gaudiness. Among the most arresting ads have been for A&P's Eight O'Clock Coffee, with a massive, steaming cup of coffee, erected in 1933, and Camel cigarettes in the 1940s, where a man blew gigantic steam "smoke rings," both designed by Douglas Leigh. Other striking New York City advertisements include the giant Pepsi-Cola sign in neon red. Originally located atop a Pepsi bottling plant, when the plant closed the sign was relocated to a park in Long Island City; the fate of the sign is unclear as there is a move afoot to deny the sign a landmark designation. The debate has stirred passions among New Yorkers who have long enjoyed its cheery glow. See PEPSI-COLA.

Among the most iconic of New York City's ads are those created by graphic artist Milton Glaser, who designed the "I ♥ NY" logo in 1977, since modified for a special September 11, 2001, commemorative. His designs for the Brooklyn Brewery and Windows on the World restaurant logos were only part of the entire communications and advertising package developed by Glaser's studio. Glaser's gastronomic credentials include being the cofounder, with Clay Felker, of *New York Magazine* and writing its original Underground Gourmet columns.

Glaser seems to fit the profile of the *Mad Men* team: his vivid use of color and late 1960s sensibility were saluted by the *Mad Men* creative team when he was commissioned to create images for the promotional materials for its final season.

See also MAD MEN.

"The Art of American Advertising: Advertising Products." Baker Library Historical Collections, Harvard Business School. http://www.library.hbs .edu/hc/artadv/advertising-products.html.
"Emergence of Advertising in America: EAA Timeline." Duke University Libraries, Digital Collections. http://library.duke.edu/digitalcollections/eaa/ timeline/#1850s.
Roth, Terry. "Research Report on Street Cries and Criers of New York." Works Projects Administration, Federal Writers' Project. New York, November 3, 1938. http://lcweb2.loc.gov/mss/wpalh2/23/ 2306/23060109/23060109.pdf.
Walker, Alissa. "*Mad Men*–Era Legend Milton Glaser Designed the New Posters for *Mad Men*." Gizmodo, March 7, 2014. http://gizmodo.com/mad-men-era-legend-milton-glaser-designed-the-new-poste-1538459506.
Whitaker, Jan. "Victorian Trade Cards." Restaurant-ing through History, February 8, 2015. http://restaurant-ingthroughhistory.com/tag/victorian-trade-cards.

Cathy K. Kaufman

African American

New York City has had a culinary presence from people of African descent since its beginnings in the seventeenth century. Through the Dutch, Africans of Angolan origin were present in New Netherland from the start, and many more would arrive after the British claimed the area as New York. Little evidence exists from this period suggesting that there was an African influence on early Anglo-Dutch cuisine in New York. The Atlantic Creoles who initially arrived were already familiar with Western cuisine through the cultural flow of the slave trade and the Atlantic world. Whatever their cuisine was beyond the standards of johnnycake, samp, and preserved pork, early African New Yorkers certainly found ways to create edible semblances of home with what they had available to them.

Arriving from the end of the seventeenth through the mid-eighteenth century was a far more influential group of Africans and Afri-Creoles from the British West Indies, Senegambia, Ghana, and other parts of West Africa. The Negroes Burial Ground, now known as the African Burial Ground, bears witness not only to this group but also to the relatively malnutrition-delayed bone development and large-scale food insecurity faced by New York's newly arrived enslaved workforce. These conditions amid other forms of brutality led to slave resistance, evidenced most notably by the 1712 slave rebellion and the 1741 slave conspiracy. Nevertheless, Africans from this period, especially those with connections to the Caribbean, brought hot peppers, peanuts, turtle feasts, and dishes and flavors from the Afro-Caribbean to the north.

Much of the food that supplied New York was grown by enslaved laborers. By the mid-eighteenth century, New York City proper had an urban enslaved population second only to Charleston, South Carolina. From the Hudson Valley, New Jersey, Long Island, and Staten Island came wheat, rye, corn, orchard fruit, and garden vegetables. Through the end of slavery in New York in 1827, enslaved people brought not only crops and flour to the city markets but also marketed vegetables grown on their own separate patches; gathered berries, fruits, and walnuts; and brought wild resources like game, oysters, clams, eels, and other seafood to Sunday markets much like those farther south. These markets formed an early and important form of an underground economy that on occasion also included the leftovers prepared by black cooks from New York's wealthiest households. See PUBLIC MARKETS.

Enslaved and free blacks were not only food producers but also food preparers and proprietors of food businesses in colonial and antebellum New York. Oystering and oyster houses, along with ice cream makers, bakers, and a few other food professions offered significant paths to entrepreneurship for African Americans. Taking advantage of these rare opportunities, oystermen like Thomas Downing served the likes of Charles Dickens down on Broad Street such dishes as turkey stuffed with oysters, oyster pie, and fish with oyster sauce. His son continued the family dynasty, turning his culinary gifts into a family franchise.

Over the course of the nineteenth century, as slavery waned, refugees and migrants from Haiti and Jamaica and freedom seekers from the Chesapeake region of Maryland and Virginia poured into the city. More black cooks worked for taverns, hotels, and restaurants, bringing the seafood, corn, and chicken dishes of the Tidewater to great New York restaurants. Haitians and West Indians merged with African American families as in other northern cities, making way for catering businesses that endured among both white and black high society. Black cooks were particularly valuable in the rise of the great New York restaurant. Delmonico's, Gage and Tollner, and many other prominent New York eateries depended on black culinary skill for their success. One of the many who became adept at this work was Edna Lewis, who worked as both partner and head of Café Nicholson, serving the mid-twentieth century's leading bohemian clientele. See DELMONICO'S; GAGE & TOLLNER; CAFÉ NICHOLSON; and LEWIS, EDNA.

The Great Migration (1910–1945) brought a third wave of black southern food north to New York City, and by way of Ellis Island came black immigrants from the West Indies. The new black New Yorkers came from the southeastern seaboard—South Carolina, Georgia, Florida. Black West Indians came from Barbados, Jamaica, Trinidad, Tobago, and St. Vincent. It bears noting that black Latinos from Puerto Rico, Cuba, and other locales also arrived and settled in adjacent communities. The soul food restaurant culture that developed outside of the South in storefront eateries and clubs flourished in Harlem. Harlem was home to pigs' feet, chitlins, collards, sweet potatoes, peanuts, and sugarcane from Georgia side by side with sugarcane from Jamaica, yams, salt fish, tannier root, cassava, and christophene. Unique to New York food culture was the mixing of old and new African American styles of cooking—drawn from the North and South combined with Afro-Caribbean and Afro-Latino foodways as black communities coalesced. Rent parties, jazz clubs, mega-churches, and other community institutions helped forge a new and vibrant expression of black food in the Americas. See CARIBBEAN; HARLEM; and SOUL FOOD.

The Great Depression saw African American communities in New York suffer, but African American foodways flourished despite the immense poverty thanks to soup kitchens and the mission restaurants of Father Divine, offering a bounty of traditional southern soul food fare. What was true in 1928 remained true up to World War II; in the words of John Walker Harrington, "Harlem is the cosmopolis of colored culture, of gaiety, of art, and the capital of Negro cookery. Harlem's visitors come from the southern United States, the West Indies, from South America and even from Africa. In what it eats, Harlem shows itself less a locality than an international rallying point. It is heaven where food had the odd psychology, where viands solace the mind as well as feed the body" (Harrington, 1928). Tillie's Chicken Shack, famous for its fried chicken, and the Sugar Cane were popular with Harlem's black community, while the Cotton Club and Connie's Inn became culinary embassies to whites looking to be thrilled and entertained with a taste of the exotic; and eventually these establishments opened their doors to a select black clientele. See COTTON CLUB and DEPRESSION FOOD.

New York's African American restaurants spanned from institutions associated with migrants and nightlife to community eateries where black dignity was assured during the transitional years of the civil rights movement, which turned such institutions into places where important meetings could take place that changed history. Today, African American foodways have found great expression in contemporary institutions like The Cecil, led by J. J. Johnson, drawing on African American, African, West Indian, Brazilian, and Asian influences and receiving high honors for its Diasporic approach to cuisine, and Red Rooster, led by Marcus Samuelsson, with an expanded notion of the foods that the Harlem community has to offer from the South to Senegal, Ethiopia, the West Indies, and Europe. More traditional eateries include the late Sylvia Woods's Sylvia's Harlem Restaurant, Amy Ruth's founded by Carl Redding, and the Darden sisters' Miss Mamie's Spoonbread Too and Miss Maude's Spoonbread Too. The latter three emphasize traditional southern soul food with distinct regional differences. See SAMUELSSON, MARCUS and SYLVIA'S.

New York's African American foodways were not limited to soul food, however. Many men and women created great cuisine inside and outside of southern food, soul food, and the heritage of the African Diaspora. Chief among these was the legacy of Patrick Clark, who opened his first restaurant in 1980 in what would become Tribeca. Clark was known for his mastery of French haute cuisine but branched out into American regional cuisine with a base of solid French techniques. Clark said famously, "I consider myself a chef. The press has considered me a prominent Black chef" (Harris, 2011, p. 230). Before he died in 1998 he briefly headed the kitchen at Tavern on the Green. Since Patrick Clark, many black chefs have distinguished themselves in sushi, modernist cuisine, and other areas considered atypical for African American chefs. See TAVERN ON THE GREEN.

Black community life and culinary culture expanded beyond Manhattan over sixty years to the Bronx, Brooklyn, and Queens and traveled up the Hudson. There had always been black communities in the outer boroughs, like Weeksville in Brooklyn, and vestiges of early slavery that supplied food to New York; but gentrification and white flight created multiple inner-city neighborhoods where black New York created hip-hop, spoken-word poetry, breakdancing, and political and cultural movements like Afrocentrism that flourished despite poverty, crime, and despair. As elements of city life declined, African Americans unfortunately caught the brunt of food insecurity, the growing landscape of food deserts, and became dependent on fast food and small bodegas for their daily bread. Counter to these trends has emerged a culture of community gardens, food and holistic health movements based on religious movements and political ideologies, and a recommitment to traditional foods and organic eating.

Berlin, Ira, and Leslie M. Harris, eds. *Slavery in New York*. New York: New Press, 2005.

Harrington, John Walker. "Food That Tempts Harlem's Palate," *New York Times*. July 15, 1928.

Harris, Jessica B. *High on the Hog: A Culinary Journey from Africa to America*. New York: Bloomsbury, 2011.

Lobel, Cindy R. *Urban Appetites: Food and Culture in Nineteenth-Century New York*. Chicago: University of Chicago Press, 2014.

Opie, Frederick Douglass. *Hog & Hominy: Soul Food from Africa to America*. New York: Columbia University Press, 2008.

Michael Twitty

Algonquin Round Table

The Algonquin Round Table was a distinguished group of New York writers who met for lunch at the Algonquin Hotel (59 West Forty-Fourth Street) in Manhattan. The hotel had opened in 1902, and Frank Case served as its manager (and later owner). Alexander Woollcott (1887–1943), the *New York Times* drama critic, reportedly liked the Algonquin's apple pie, so he often dined at the hotel, usually with two friends, Heywood Broun, the novelist, and Franklin Pierce Adams, the newspaper columnist. They were sometimes joined by other writers.

When the United States entered World War I, Woollcott volunteered as a medical orderly but ended up on the staff of *Stars & Stripes*, the newspaper of the American Expeditionary Forces. Upon his return to New York, in June 1919, the theatrical agents John Peter Toohey and Murdoch Pemberton invited a group of New York literati—journalists, writers, critics, actors, and publishers—to honor him with a luncheon at the Algonquin Hotel. Woollcott had such a good time that he suggested that the group meet regularly for lunch.

They first met in the hotel's main restaurant, The Rose Room. The conversation was lively, and as the group increased in size, guests moved chairs from other tables, causing a traffic problem for other guests and staff. Case moved them to the smaller Pergola Room (the now defunct Oak Room) and seated them at a long rectangular table. But the group continued to grow, so Case moved them back to The Rose Room, this time seating them at a round table in the corner. The group continued to lunch together at the Algonquin for the next ten years. Core members of the Algonquin Round Table included George S. Kaufman, Dorothy Parker, Harold Ross, Robert E. Sherwood, John Peter Toohey, Harpo Marx, and Alexander Woollcott. Visiting writers and other luminaries often attended. The group's witticisms and wisecracks often appeared in the members' newspaper and magazine columns.

The informal group gradually fell apart about a decade after it started, but the Round Table was not forgotten. Frank Case's *Feeding the Lions: An Algonquin Cookbook* (1942) featured comments from the famous—Dorothy Parker, Robert Benchley, and the like—on their favorite dishes. Dozens of other books and hundreds of articles have been written about what was reportedly said—and sometimes even the food got a mention.

The Algonquin Hotel is still open. When it was remodeled in 1998, The Rose Room was removed. Today, a replica of the original Round Table can be found in the Round Table Room, which features "retro" dishes inspired by Case's *Feeding the Lions*.

Case, Frank. *Feeding the Lions: An Algonquin Cookbook*. New York: Greystone, 1942.

Harriman, Margaret Case. *The Vicious Circle: The Story of the Algonquin Round Table*. New York: Rinehart, 1951.

Andrew F. Smith

Allen, Ida Bailey

Born in Danielson, Connecticut, the granddaughter of a sea captain, Ida Bailey Allen (1885–1973) made a name for herself in New York as an authority on contemporary home cooking. She began her professional life with a degree in dietetics from the New York Metropolitan Hospital but quickly moved on to food journalism and cookbook writing.

Allen's career spanned sixty years and included work as a food editor for *Good Housekeeping* as well as a host of a popular radio cooking show. Allen's focus was always on the practical and the affordable as well as on current trends. Although the *New York Times* included her recipe for Boston baked beans in her obituary, Allen was not tied to tradition but rather built from it to serve the needs of contemporary cooks.

Some of her earliest books responded to the crisis of World War I by helping home cooks to substitute for three staples of the American diet in the early twentieth century: meat, wheat, and sugar. See WORLD WAR I. In her 1918 *Mrs. Allen's Book of Wheat Substitutes* she exhibited the forthrightness and encouraging tone that would endear millions of readers to her books and listeners to her radio show. The first attempts at wheatlessness "that came from my conservation experiment kitchen, looked rather sad and dejected." With some further research, however, she had solved all problems and now "every woman who is patriotic and who has applied her splendid American brain power to her personal food problems is equipped to meet the situation."

Allen became the food editor for the *New York American* in 1924 and was among the first women to host a regularly scheduled culinary radio program, beginning in 1928. She later became a food columnist for *Good Housekeeping Magazine*. She also continued to produce cookbooks in most of the major food trends. She wrote for corporate sponsors with great success. Her *When You Entertain*, written for Coca-Cola in 1932, sold almost four hundred thousand copies when it was first offered.

In later years, Allen acknowledged the shrinking American family with her *Cookbook for Two*, as well as the impact of Julia Child with *Gastronomique: A Cookbook for Gourmets*. The last of her cookbooks to be published was *Best Loved Recipes of the American People*, published in 1973 shortly after her death. During her lifetime, she sold an estimated 20 million copies of her books.

Allen, Ida Bailey. *Mrs. Allen's Book of Wheat Substitutes*. Boston: Small, Maynard, 1918.
"Ida Bailey Allen, Cookbook Author; Home Economist, 88, Dies—50 Books Sold 20 Million." *New York Times*, July 17, 1973.
Neuhaus, Jessamyn. *Manly Meals and Mom's Home Cooking: Cookbooks and Gender in Modern America*. Baltimore: Johns Hopkins University Press, 2003.

Megan Elias

America Eats Project

During the Great Depression, many writers and journalists found themselves unemployed and hungry. To provide them with work and regular paychecks, in 1935 the administration of Franklin D. Roosevelt started the Federal Writers' Project, which was part of the Works Progress Administration. Between 1935 and 1940, the Federal Writers' Project's major program was the American Guide series, a collection of guidebooks to all fifty states. This was the brainchild of Katharine Amend Kellock, an editor who planned the series to reintroduce Americans to the history, culture, architecture, geology, and so on of their native land.

As the American Guides wound down, the Federal Writers' Project realized it needed new projects to employ its writers. Kellock came up with the idea for *America Eats*, a one-volume compendium of traditional American cookery. This book would focus on group eating as an important American social institution as opposed to the "mass production of food stuffs and partly cooked foods and introduction of numerous technological devices that lessen labor of preparation but lower quality of the product." The book, which was divided into sections on the Northeast, South, Middle West, Far West, and Southwest, would particularly focus on church suppers, clambakes, political barbecues, cemetery cleaning picnics, and other traditional culinary gatherings. The book's chief editor was New Orleans writer Lyle Saxon, while the Federal Writers' Project's New Jersey office was given charge of the Northeast Eats section, including New York City.

After the project was announced, the Washington office of the Federal Writers' Project instructed writers to send to their editors notes on local "foods, food customs, development of various dishes, usual and unusual group gatherings of the past and present whose primary concern was eating and food." The editor in the New Jersey office asked New York City's writers to focus on "the influence of foreign foods and mass cooking on the eating customs of the region." Specifically, the editor requested descriptions of foreign group meals, particularly Jewish seders; private group meals in public restaurants that hearkened back to the old "beefsteak dinners"; hotel banquets; and drugstore lunches. They were also told to collect information on well-known restaurants such as Delmonico's and Rector's and the famous dishes they introduced.

New York City's Municipal Archive now holds the local records for the Federal Writers' Project's *America Eats* project. They include the initial proposal and twelve short articles for the book. These cover the Passover seder, Jewish hors d'oeuvres, literary teas, automat restaurants, drugstore lunches, soda fountain and luncheonette slang, the Grand Central Oyster Bar's oyster stew, McSorley's Tavern, Gallagher's steakhouse, hotel banquets, famous hotel dishes, and an apocryphal tale of the "first cocktail." They also contain a chapter called "Dining Abroad in New York," covering the city's many varieties of foreign restaurants, originally written for a project titled "Oddities of New York." Allan Ross MacDougall, writer of *The Gourmet's Almanac* (1930), was one of the local authors; the rest were various editors, playwrights, and others without an obvious background in food writing. Arthur Zipser, a coauthor of the Passover seder article, was also an organizer for the Communist Party, an affiliation shared by many Federal Writers' Project writers.

The deadline for all the *America Eats* materials was the end of December 1941. On December 7, however, the Japanese bombed Pearl Harbor, leading the United States to declare war against the Axis powers. Most work on existing writing projects ground to a halt as the Works Progress Administration turned to publications supporting the war effort. The Federal Writers' Project offices in New York emptied out, and in May 1942 Kellock lost her job in Washington. The Federal Writers' Project officially closed its doors in 1943, and all its records were divided among the Library of Congress, the National Archives, and various local government repositories. The New York City *America Eats* files are mixed among the Municipal Archives files for *Feeding the City*, another local project. Never published, *Feeding the City* covers the city's food system, including transportation, inspection, markets, stores, restaurants, eating at home, and all the major foodstuffs. It provides a detailed portrait of how New Yorkers were fed circa 1940.

See also BREADLINES and DEPRESSION FOOD.

America Eats. Files, records of the Federal Writers' Project, Work Projects Administration, Reel 153, New York City Municipal Archives, New York.

Kurlansky, Mark. *The Food of a Younger Land*. New York: Riverhead, 2009.

Penkower, Monty N. *The Federal Writer's Project: A Study in Government Patronage of the Arts*. Urbana: University of Illinois Press, 1977.

Willard, Pat. *America Eats! On the Road with the WPA*. New York: Bloomsbury, 2008.

Andrew Coe

American Institute of Wine & Food

Founded by beloved food personality and cookbook author Julia Child and famed California wine producers and marketing geniuses Robert Mondavi and Richard Graff, in partnership with other members of the American food and beverage community, the American Institute of Wine & Food (AIWF) has worked to advance the understanding, appreciation, and quality of what people eat and drink since 1981. The New York chapter is one of many around the United States, each with a slightly different take on the original mission. This individualism permits each chapter to best serve its local community based on challenges and needs within the area.

In New York, the AIWF brings together food professionals and enthusiasts through publications (*Savor This*, a quarterly online magazine detailing developments of each chapter) and programs (including professional development workshops and tasting events). What sets this organization apart is its openness to non–food industry members. Anyone interested in expanding his or her knowledge and palate is welcome to join what has, at times, been an incredibly elite group of food and industry professionals. To this day, the mission remains open, inclusive, and welcoming.

Collaborations with New York–area colleges, culinary schools, and universities allow for ongoing educational opportunities, from wine, cheese, and oil tastings to demonstrations and networking events. These programs create opportunities for members to stay current in dining trends while maintaining their commitment to heritage and tradition.

The AIWF has a rich history of scholarship and educational opportunity for all ages. The most notable is the Days of Taste scholarship program, wherein all of the AIWF chapters come together to raise money to provide food appreciation, access, and education for middle school–aged learners around the country. Local leaders organize fundraising events, seminars, and workshops that support the development of members, students, and their community.

The New York chapter is undertaking a campaign to revitalize and return to the original mission, including returning scholarships to the forefront. The initial drive is a Culinary Sabbatical Scholarship program, which funds a year-long sabbatical to one back-of-house employee per year.

American Institute of Wine & Food website: http://www.aiwf.org.

Alexandra Olsen

American Museum of Natural History

One of the preeminent museums in New York City, and one of the oldest in the entire country, the American Museum of Natural History has been attracting visitors since it was founded in 1869. An enormous building facing the west side of Central Park from Seventy-Seventh to Eighty-First Streets, the museum is one of the city's most popular destinations, attracting tourists, school groups, the general public, and people particularly interested in the natural history of the planet, its cultures and species, as well as the cosmos. Visitors to the museum can enter through its main doors on Central Park West or through a side entrance on West Eighty-First Street that leads directly into the Rose Center for Earth and Space, a vast exhibit exploring the 13 billion–year history of the cosmos.

The museum's forty-five exhibition halls are dedicated to different areas that make up its collections, such as biodiversity; human biology and evolution; meteorites; gems and minerals; ocean life; peoples

from all over the world including Asia, Africa, South and Central America; Native Americans from the Northwest coast; North American and African mammals; and birds of the world. Particularly popular destinations are the Hall of Ocean Life, which contains a 21,000-pound model of a blue whale; the Butterfly Conservatory in the Hall of Oceanic Birds; and the Hayden Planetarium.

Over the years, the museum has had special exhibits that have explored food both from an anthropological perspective as well as current-day trends. The first food exhibit was the 1917 Food Values and Economies Exhibition, which was created during World War I and had a dual purpose: practical education and supporting the war through food conservation. At the time, because of bad crops, wheat was in short supply, but there was a surplus of corn, which Americans were not used to eating. The exhibit featured many ways to consume corn, such as adding cornmeal to cakes and breads. Professor Graham Lusk, who worked as an adviser on the exhibit, noted that "corn bread became the bread of every patriotic citizen." The exhibition was praised by the U.S. Department of Education as well as the Department of Agriculture. Details of the exhibit have been studied and even copied by museums and food educators around the country. It traveled to schools and events around New York City and was on view in the gallery of the concourse of Grand Central Station in the spring of 1918.

In recent years, the museum mounted a specifically agriculture- and food-centered exhibit titled *Our Global Kitchen: Food, Nature, Culture*, which aimed to answer essential questions, such as the following: How does food reflect and influence culture and identity? How does what we eat affect the planet? And what is the role of food in human health? Visitors to the exhibit discovered how what they choose to eat helps shape the planet. They were also able to taste seasonal food, prepare a virtual meal, take a look at food-related artifacts housed at the museum, and peek into imagined dining rooms of famous historical figures.

Hungry visitors have had various dining options over the years. Today Café on One is located in the Grand Gallery and caters to adult appetites. The Starlight Café, near the Hayden Planetarium, has a menu that is more child friendly. The Powerhouse, which overlooks the Arthur Ross Terrace and the Rose Center for Earth and Space, accommodates up to six hundred guests for banquets, events, and receptions.

See also COOPER HEWITT, SMITHSONIAN DESIGN MUSEUM; MUSEUM FOOD; MUSEUM OF CHINESE IN AMERICA (MOCA); MUSEUM OF FOOD AND DRINK; MUSEUM OF THE CITY OF NEW YORK; and TENEMENT MUSEUM.

American Museum Journal 17 (May 1917).
Delson, Roberta Marx. "OVER HERE: The American Museum of Natural History during World War I." *Natural History Magazine* 122, no. 1 (February 2014).

Tracey Ceurvels

Ansel, Dominique

See CRONUT.

Antebellum Period

In the four decades before the Civil War (1820–1860) New Yorkers had access to a varied diet, though its quantity and quality differed according to social class. Not surprisingly, the wealthiest New Yorkers enjoyed more variety and abundance of foodstuffs, while the poorest had a meager subsistence.

Seasonality determined availability even for the wealthiest. The summer months were most bountiful. Fresh fruits and vegetables were available from local farms including berries, stone fruits, lettuces, apples, pears, and melons. In the colder months, the markets stocked root vegetables. Meat was available year-round, and New Yorkers, even those of modest means, enjoyed a protein-heavy diet, with beef being the most predominant meat on their tables. Indeed, during the early antebellum period, the ready availability of meat, a rare treat for European laborers, became an indicator of mobility for prospective immigrant workers.

In addition to beef, New Yorkers ate large amounts of pork, as well as mutton and lamb in lesser amounts. They also had access to a variety of fresh game and, of course, fish and shellfish from local waters. They supplemented their protein-rich diet with grains (especially corn and wheat) and dairy products including milk, butter, and cheese. In this era before refrigeration, food preservation, such as pickling, drying, and salting, as well as laying in hearty provisions for the winter months, was an important

ritual, especially for families of means who had both the available cash to lay out for advance provisions and the cellar space to store them.

Public Markets

Antebellum New Yorkers got most of their fresh food from six major public markets, the Washington and Fulton Markets being the largest among them. These markets, meant to service the local neighborhood, were supplied by local butchers, hunters, fishermen, and farmers from Long Island, New Jersey, Staten Island, and Westchester who arrived via ferry to sell fresh fruits, vegetables, and dairy products from their farms. The markets were highly regulated by the city to protect the public health as well as to shield fee-paying market vendors from unfair competition. While the public markets provided the bulk of fresh foods, retail and wholesale grocers, peddlers, and hucksters supplemented them. See PUBLIC MARKETS; WASHINGTON MARKET; and FULTON FISH MARKET.

Peddlers and Hucksters

Street peddlers and hucksters sold goods throughout the streets of New York that they scavenged or bought from market vendors late in the day. Antebellum hucksters were almost entirely poor women, often widows, who had few other avenues to support themselves and their families. The city allowed them to sell goods outside of the markets (and after market hours were over), recognizing that they could become wards of the city without this meager means of self-support. Hucksters and peddlers sold all manner of foodstuffs—strawberries, clams, walnuts, and hot corn—often accompanied by a "street cry" or call. Late nineteenth-century New Yorkers nostalgically recalled the street cries of the food vendors of early national (1790–1830) and antebellum (1830–1860) New York. See CRIES OF NEW-YORK, THE and STREET VENDORS.

Grocers and Private Food Shops

Grocers had existed alongside the public markets since the colonial period, offering mainly dry goods and preserved food items (teas, spices, salt fish, jellies, canned oysters, etc.) to their customers. During the antebellum period, groceries began to branch out

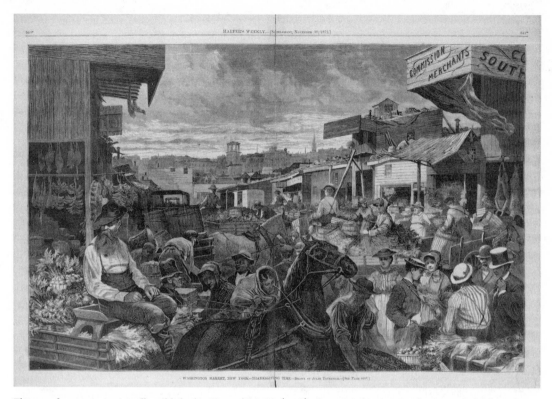

This wood engraving, originally published in *Harper's Weekly* (v. 16), shows Washington Market around Thanksgiving in 1872. Washington Market was the largest public market of the antebellum period in New York. LIBRARY OF CONGRESS

and offer goods traditionally dominated by the public markets—fresh produce, meats, and dairy products. In some cases (meat, for example), selling outside of the markets was illegal thanks to regulations aimed at protecting the licensed butchers who paid fees to the city for the privilege of maintaining a license and leasing a stall within one of the public markets. But beginning early in the antebellum period, the city loosened its stance toward the public markets, shifting from the patrician oversight of the eighteenth century to the more laissez-faire attitudes of the nineteenth century.

Leaders of the increasingly corrupt city government came to see the public markets more as a way to line their pockets through kickbacks and graft rather than a public good worthy of protecting. Even a virtuous city government would have had difficulty keeping up with the rapid growth of the city and its expanding food supply, aided by technological and transportation developments like canals, steamboats, and railroads, which extended from the hinterlands of New York City all the way to the Mid-

west and the Deep South. With the exception of Harlem Market, the city did not sponsor the building of any new public markets after 1830. See ERIE CANAL.

Thus, even as the city grew geographically and most residents lived above Fourteenth Street, there were no public markets to serve the newer residential neighborhoods. The city thus endorsed a loophole in the market laws allowing private shops to service emerging neighborhoods where no public market existed.

In 1843, the city government made official what had become custom—it deregulated the public markets and allowed private food shops to sell fresh foods, competing directly with the public market vendors. Retail food shops proliferated throughout the city, and by the Civil War most New Yorkers got their food from neighborhood retail shops rather than the public markets. The public markets, meanwhile, took on a more wholesale function, serving local shops and restaurants as well as a national market. In addition to private grocers and butchers, a host of other specialized food shops emerged during the antebellum period including confectioners, bakers, poulterers, pastry shops, and ice creameries.

Ice and Cookstoves

Meanwhile, novel technologies contributed to changes in food storage and preparation in the antebellum period. New, patented forms of ice production, for example, allowed for the development of the commercial ice industry beginning late in the 1820s. During the antebellum period, the bulk of commercial ice in New York City was used by businesses (grocers, butchers, brewers, hotels, and restaurants), but commercial ice delivery to New York's residences began during this period as well. By 1860, many New Yorkers had iceboxes in their homes, for which they received regular ice delivery.

Likewise, use of the coal-fired cookstove expanded during the antebellum period, replacing wood-fired open hearths. By the 1850s most New Yorkers were acquiring cookstoves. Cookstoves required instruction in their use, and many home cooks were flummoxed by the technology. But once mastered, the cookstove allowed for different kinds of preparations and accelerated a move away from the one-pot meals of the colonial period toward more complex kinds of cooking. Home cooks (including servants; even middle-class homes usually employed a few servants, including a cook) were aided by a plethora of cookbooks—over 160 new titles were issued during the first half of the nineteenth century. New York City was the center of antebellum cookbook publishing. See COOKBOOKS.

Rise of Restaurants

One of the most important developments on the food landscape of antebellum New York City was the rise of restaurants. While taverns and inns had existed since the colonial period, freestanding restaurants, which served hot meals on demand, were unheard of until the nineteenth century. The 1810 city directory listed five freestanding victualing houses. By the 1830s there were hundreds of restaurants in New York City. See RESTAURANTS.

The earliest restaurants arose to cater to the business crowd. As the city expanded geographically in the antebellum period, more New Yorkers commuted to their jobs from the edges of Manhattan or new suburbs like Brooklyn Heights. Sixpenny houses (which charged sixpence for a main dish) opened in the business districts to cater to the needs of these businessmen. Among the most famous of the sixpenny refectories were Sweet's and Sweeney's. These establishments were known for their fast pace and unappetizing food. They also became emblematic—and encouraging of—the hustle-and-bustle business culture of the growing metropolis.

Of course, the short-order houses were not the only restaurants on the antebellum dining scene. This period also saw the opening of one of the most famous restaurants in New York's history, Delmonico's. Opened in 1830 by Swiss brothers Peter and John Delmonico, the restaurant introduced the business lunch and fine dining to the United States. Caterer to New York's (and America's) economic and political elite, Delmonico's remained the ne plus ultra of New York and American dining until the early twentieth century. See DELMONICO'S.

By the mid-nineteenth century, New York City's restaurant scene was in full bloom. Over five thousand public dining options existed in the city, from the splendor of Delmonico's to the all-night cake and coffee shop to the oyster cart on the street. Specialized restaurants catered to various groups of New Yorkers, including the theater crowd, newsboys, southern travelers, and the black elite. And as immigrants arrived in New York City in large numbers in the 1830s and 1840s, new cuisines were introduced to the city's culinary landscape. Of particular note were the German restaurants and beer gardens that opened beginning in the 1830s, serving up sausages, hamburger, sauerkraut, and pretzels. Restaurants also emerged to cater specifically to the ladies' trade, Thompson's and Taylor's being the most famous ladies' restaurants. Except in these spaces (where men were prohibited unless escorted by a lady) ladies still could not dine out without escort and maintain respectability. See BEER GARDENS and GERMAN.

Nineteenth-century New York was known for its oysters and had dozens of establishments that specialized in shucking and preparing them. These oyster cellars or saloons ranged from the opulent to the barebones, and some had a very seedy reputation. Even some fancy oyster saloons were considered salacious, offering private boxes where assignations were made with prostitutes. Oyster cellars held late hours and offered the bivalves in various preparations, shucked raw but also cooked in oyster pie or made into a sauce and served over fish. Many oyster cellars offered an all-you-can-eat plan, known as the "Canal Street Plan," in recognition of the concentration of oyster cellars along that street. See OYSTER BAR and OYSTERS.

The most famous oysterman in antebellum New York City was Thomas Downing, who ran a respectable oyster house on Broad and Wall Streets in the heart of the city's financial district. Downing was one of many African American migrants to New York in the early nineteenth century who made a living from food service. Downing became one of the most respected and wealthiest black men in antebellum New York; other African Americans also made relative fortunes through food service (as waiters, caterers, and cooks). Indeed, the majority of antebellum food service professionals were African Americans and Irish immigrants, but unlike Downing, most of them scraped by on a meager subsistence. See AFRICAN AMERICAN.

See also CIVIL WAR.

Lobel, Cindy R. *Urban Appetites: Food and Culture in Nineteenth Century New York.* Chicago: University of Chicago Press, 2014.

Cindy R. Lobel

Appetizing Stores

The neighborhoods of New York City were once notable for commercial centers containing specialty food shops catering to local ethnic populations. There would be a bakery, a butcher shop, a fresh fish store, and a fruit and vegetable stand. If it was a Jewish enclave in one of the five boroughs of New York City, there would also be a delicatessen and an appetizing store. These were mom-and-pop shops often founded by immigrants. Family members acted as employees. The family name was on the sign above the door, assuring customers that a member of the family was on hand, behind the counter. This is the way business was done.

The *Oxford English Dictionary* defines "appetizing" as "Exciting a desire or longing, especially for food; stimulating or whetting the appetite." But "appetizing" as in "appetizing store" is best defined by what it is not. It is not a delicatessen, though many people today confuse the two. The traditional delica-

tessens specialized in smoked, salted, or pickled meat products—corned beef, pastrami, salami, tongue, and frankfurters—and the accompaniments—pickles, sauerkraut, French fries, mustard, ketchup, and relish. The traditional appetizing stores specialized in smoked, salted, and pickled fish products—whitefish, salmon, carp, mackerel, and herring—and everything that went along—butter, cream cheese, sour cream (i.e., dairy items). Since Jewish dietary laws proscribe the mixing of meat and dairy products, the delicatessen and the appetizing store became two parallel worlds in the universe of Jewish food.

The universe of Jewish food in New York City began on the Lower East Side, with the largest wave of Eastern European Jewish immigrants arriving between 1880 and 1923. By the 1930s there were twenty to thirty delicatessens on the Lower East Side and an equal number of appetizing shops. Many of the first-generation appetizing store owners had transitioned from selling herring out of pushcarts or large wooden barrels in stalls. Then, in small shops requiring little capital outlay they could expand their offerings to other types of preserved fish, appetizers, and canned goods.

Smoked fish and herring items were traditionally eaten with large chunks of rye or pumpernickel bread slathered with butter. By the 1930s bagels and bialys became the bread of choice for the fish and cream cheese, the method of holding it all together. At about the same time, some enterprising appetizing store owner, no one knows who, added a sweets department to the store; and soon almost all followed suit. Dried fruits and nuts, halvah, hard candies, and chocolates provided a counterpoint to the salty, smoky, and pickled tastes of the fish side. As the Jews became more affluent, the Sunday brunch featuring smoked fish and sweets became a tradition; and the local appetizing stores provided not only the ingredients but a meeting place for the neighborhood.

As many Jews of the Lower East Side neighborhood became more assimilated and less religious, the appetizing stores followed suit, selling items that were not "strictly kosher," like sturgeon, and opening on Saturdays. Some stayed open all day Saturday; others opened after sundown to abide by their religion and then to capture the late-night business of theater-goers leaving the Yiddish theaters that lined Second Avenue.

As the Jews moved out of the neighborhood—this pattern was most rapid following World War II—

their delicatessens and appetizing stores followed, first to the outer boroughs and then to the suburbs. Repeal of the Sunday blue laws was the death knell to the Lower East Side as a bargain shopping district. The former residents who had relocated to the suburbs could now shop near home on Sundays—in malls, department stores, and supermarkets, with free and easy parking. By the 1960s the Lower East Side demographic had changed as other immigrant groups had moved in. For the most part the first- and second-generation Jewish appetizing store owners did not want their children in the business. Standing behind a fish counter ten to twelve hours a day six days a week was just hard work with little financial return. The Jewish customer base and the Jewish labor pool could no longer sustain the many appetizing stores of the Lower East Side.

The appetizing stores of the outer boroughs and suburbs did not fare well either. Supermarkets were installing appetizing counters. Fewer people were taking up the trade of slicing lox, preferring to sit behind a desk or in front of a computer. Then technology made packaging possible: presliced smoked salmon in vacuum-sealed pouches, pickled herring in jars, frozen bagels. The freestanding, family-owned and -operated appetizing store had seen its day. It would be consumed into the new shopping patterns of big-box, big-glitz, one-stop-shopping, gourmet supermarkets.

The few appetizing stores that survive today have held on to their traditions while adapting to changing tastes and ways of doing business. Where the original appetizing stores sold only salt-cured belly lox and mild smoked "nova," there is now an array of smoked salmons from around the world. Where the herring sold was north Atlantic salt brine herring doled out from large wooden barrels and wrapped in day-old newspaper or pickled herring smothered in onions and sour cream sauce, there is now herring in curry, mustard and dill, or lemon and ginger. Canned salmon, tuna, and sardines have been replaced on the shelves by Italian olive oils, French mustards, and Spanish anchovies. Where business was done strictly across a counter, it can now be done across cyberspace. Those true appetizing stores that exist today do so by being able to adapt: extending the line of products, shipping their wares throughout the country, training the help in the art of slicing, and the fierce—often generational—loyalty of their customers

intent on maintaining a relationship and keeping a culture.

See also BARNEY GREENGRASS; JEWISH; LOWER EAST SIDE; RUSS & DAUGHTERS; and SMOKED FISH.

Diner, Hasia R. *Hungering for America: Italian, Irish, and Jewish Foodways in the Age of Migration.* Cambridge, Mass.: Harvard University Press, 2001.
Durham, T. R. "Salt, Smoke, and History." *Gastronomica* (Winter 2001): 78–82.
Federman, Mark Russ. *Russ & Daughters: Reflections and Recipes from the House That Herring Built.* New York: Schocken, 2013.
Marks, Gil. "Lox." In *Encyclopedia of Jewish Food,* pp. 369–371. Hoboken, N.J.: John Wiley, 2010.
Ziegelman, Jane. *97 Orchard: An Edible History of Five Immigrant Families in One New York Tenement.* New York: HarperCollins, 2010.

Mark Russ Federman

Aquavit

Named after the traditional Scandinavian liquor, typically flavored with caraway seeds and fennel, Aquavit is a restaurant that was opened in 1987 by owner Håkan Swahn, in a former Rockefeller townhouse across the street from the Museum of Modern Art in midtown Manhattan. Aquavit received a three-star review by Ruth Reichl in the *New York Times* in 1995, with Marcus Samuelsson as executive chef. At just twenty-four years old, Samuelsson was the youngest chef to receive the coveted trio of *Times* stars.

In December 1998, Swahn and Samuelsson opened the first Aquavit outpost beyond New York, in Minneapolis. The Midwestern location was chosen for its large Scandinavian population as well as its then bustling culinary scene. It shuttered in 2003.

The New York original moved one block east in 2005. Five years later, Samuelsson formally parted ways with Aquavit, and Marcus Jernmark succeeded him as executive chef. Jernmark had been Aquavit's executive sous-chef previously, following a stint as head chef at the Swedish Consulate. Aquavit maintained its three-star rating from the *New York Times*—thanks to Reichl's 1995 write-up and William Grimes's 2001 review—until 2010, when Sam Sifton knocked off a star.

In April 2014, the restaurant's former pastry chef, Emma Bengtsson, succeeded Jernmark as executive chef. Six months later, Aquavit scored two Michelin stars, making Bengtsson one of just two female chefs to earn a pair of Michelin stars: "Bengtsson, who was previously pastry chef at Aquavit, is continuing the good work of her predecessor, Marcus Jernmark, in producing fare that's leaner, more focused, and more Swedish than Samuelsson's" (Sutton, 2014).

See also SAMUELSSON, MARCUS and SCANDINAVIAN.

Lee, Felicia R. "In the Kitchen with: Marcus Samuelsson; From Africa to Sweden to Aquavit." *New York Times*, July 10, 1996.

Nelson, Rick. "Aquavit: New Fancy Swedish Restaurant Comes to Downtown Minneapolis." *Star Tribune*, December 3, 1998.

Sutton, Ryan. "New Chef Breathes New Life into Scandinavian Stalwart Aquavit." Eater, October 21, 2014. http://ny.eater.com/2014/10/21/7026973/aquavit-restaurant-review-emma-bengston.

Tishgart, Sierra. "Aquavit Chef Emma Bengtsson on Reluctantly Taking Over the Kitchen and Winning 2 Michelin Stars." Grub Street, October 9, 2014. http://www.grubstreet.com/2014/10/aquavit-michelin-star.html.

Alexandra Ilyashov

Arab Community

The Arab American community in New York City is as diverse as the food it prepares and serves. While Arabs living in the United States can trace their ancestry to any of the twenty-two countries of the Arab world, the majority of Arabs living in New York are of Lebanese, Syrian, Egyptian, Yemeni, and Palestinian heritage; but the community also includes thousands of people from Morocco, Iraq, Sudan, and other countries.

The Arab American population of New York City is estimated at ninety thousand people, according to the U.S. Census Bureau's American Community Survey, though the number is likely much higher given the historical census undercounting of Arab Americans. Like the national Arab American community, the New York community is both Christian and Muslim. A unique feature of the New York community, particularly in Brooklyn, is the sizeable Jewish community that traces its heritage to Syria and other Arab countries. Arabs of all nationalities and religions have been running ethnic grocery stores, restaurants, bakeries, butcher shops, and confectionaries for more than a century.

Hundreds of Arab and Arab American grocery stores, restaurants, cafes, and food trucks can be found throughout the city. There is a vast diversity of Arab food offerings in New York, especially compared to other large Arab American communities. For example, in metropolitan Detroit, the region with the highest concentration of Arab Americans in the country, the majority of restaurants serve Levantine-inspired food (from Syria, Lebanon, Palestine, and Jordan), regardless of the nationality of their owners. In New York, restaurants offer a wider variety of cuisines, including Moroccan, Egyptian, Sudanese, Yemeni, Iraqi, and, of course, Levantine.

Historical Foundations

The Arab American community began in the 1880s in Lower Manhattan, on and around Washington Street, in an enclave known as Little Syria. See LITTLE SYRIA. As in other Arab immigrant communities, some of the first businesses to open were restaurants and grocery stores. These establishments were a main cultural link for the early émigrés. Most of the early Arab restaurants in New York City were intended mainly for an immigrant clientele. The signage, menus, and advertising (if any) were typically in Arabic. The cafes were also spaces, mainly for men, to gather, smoke *argileh* (hookah), play backgammon, and converse.

In the early 1900s, some Syrian-owned restaurants began attracting non-Arab customers, mostly adventurous writers, researchers, and "bohemians" who ventured to the heavily immigrant area of Lower Manhattan to sample ethnic cuisines. Eventually, Syrian-owned restaurants, with their wonderful foods, inviting décor, and genuine hospitality, became institutions in Lower Manhattan and along Atlantic Avenue in Brooklyn, which developed alongside Little Syria and became a bedroom community for many of the merchants in Lower Manhattan. As immigration from the Arab world began to diversify after World War II and Little Syria became just a collection of memories displaced for construction of the Brooklyn–Battery Tunnel, Yemeni, Sudanese, Egyptian, and Palestinian restaurants captured the success of the early Syrian and Lebanese establishments. See SYRIAN AND LEBANESE. Along with the third- and fourth-generation Syrian and Lebanese restaurant and grocery store owners, new immigrant entrepreneurs continued to make Brooklyn an Arab

American stronghold. New York is also home to a large and diverse Muslim community, and many of the Arab-owned restaurants and food carts serve halal foods. "Halal" refers to the religious proscriptions governing the production and consumption of food, similar to kosher rules within Judaism. Besides the prohibition against pork, for meat to be halal it must come from an animal slaughtered by a Muslim who invokes the name of God, slits the animal's throat, and drains the blood. The absence of alcohol at many Arab-owned establishments is also related to Muslim religious proscriptions. Halal food served by Arab Americans has become so popular in New York, among Muslims and non-Muslims alike, that in 2014 an Egyptian-owned food cart, Halal Guys, signed a deal to franchise and open locations across the United States, Europe, and the Middle East.

Arab and Arab American Cuisine

Arab cuisine is difficult to define because of the diversity of Arab Americans. From Morocco to Egypt to Lebanon, differences in geography, climate, and location along historic trade routes, along with the influences of European colonialism, are reflected in the vast array of foods available at grocery stores and restaurants. However, there are some commonalities. Lamb is more prevalent than beef, with a near total lack of pork because of Islamic proscriptions against it. Even restaurants owned by Arab Christians in New York will not typically offer pork products because of its absence in the Arab world.

Many traditional dishes are combinations of meat and rice and are meant to be eaten communally using hands or bread instead of utensils. The bread is usually flat and round. Desserts rely heavily on nuts (pistachios, almonds, and walnuts) and fruits (dates), and Levantine cuisine is famous for *baqlawa* (baklava) and *knafeh* (a sweet cheese dessert). Coffee and tea are prevalent and offer a distinctive element to a traditional Arab meal. Turkish coffee, sometimes referred to as "Arabic coffee," is brewed in an *ibriq* (coffee pot) without a filter; and the finely ground coffee is mixed with ground cardamom to give it its distinctive flavor. Moroccan tea is famous for its inclusion of fresh mint, and Yemeni tea is heavily spiced with cloves.

The most distinguishing feature of Arab cuisine is not the food but the role of hospitality, a central feature of Arab and Arab American households and restaurants. Visitors are greeted with a welcoming *ahlan wa sahlan*, which is part of an older, longer saying that essentially means, "You are among family, so take it easy." Food and drink are main features of hospitality. Large amounts of food are prepared, and guests are encouraged, even against protest, to eat multiple helpings. Coffee and tea, especially when served at the conclusion of a meal, encourage guests to stay, relax, and enjoy more conversation.

Benson, Kathleen, and Philip M. Kayal, eds. *A Community of Many Worlds: Arab Americans in New York City*. New York: Museum of the City of New York; Syracuse, N.Y.: Syracuse University Press, 2002.

Lockwood, William, and Yvonne Lockwood. "Continuity and Adaptation in Arab American Foodways." In *Arab Detroit: From Margin to Mainstream*, edited by Nabeel Abraham and Andrew Shryock, pp. 515–549. Detroit: Wayne State University Press, 2000.

Orfalea, Gregory. *The Arab Americans: A History*. Northampton, Mass.: Olive Branch, 2006.

Staub, Shalom. *Yemenis in New York City: The Folklore of Ethnicity*. Philadelphia: Balch Institute Press, 1989.

Matthew Jaber Stiffler

Armenian

Armenians originate from central and eastern Anatolia, a region which has historically been at the crossroads of the Roman, Persian, Russian, and Ottoman Empires. Their distinct ethnic and later Christian minority status ensured cultural cohesion for over three thousand years, with some influence from their hosts and neighbors.

While migration and displacement were not uncommon for this community, in the 1890s, Armenians began arriving in New York in significant numbers as a result of increasing Christian persecution in the Ottoman Empire, culminating in the 1915–1923 Genocide, which "cleansed" modern-day Turkey of its Christian minorities. Some 1.5 million Armenians were killed or died of starvation to the extent that the phrase "Eat your food—think of the starving Armenians" became common in American households.

Armenians settled on the east side of Manhattan between Twenty-Third and Thirty-Fourth Streets in Murray Hill in a neighborhood that became known as "Little Armenia." Several family-run Armenian restaurants began opening, introducing New Yorkers for the first time to foods that were common to the Armenian diet, such as stuffed vegetables, kebabs, and rice pilaf. They also introduced Armenian coffee, ground fresh and served strong, bitter, and in tiny cups. The restaurants which were upscale and elegant became quite famous, such as Arakel's, and nationally recognized, such as the Golden Horn, promoting immigrant food as gourmet and exotic. Other restaurants, such as the Balkan, Dardanelles, and Ararat, also familiarized New Yorkers to hearty, homemade Armenian–Anatolian cuisine, but in a more relaxed atmosphere.

The second wave of Armenian immigration in the mid-1960s brought diaspora Armenians from Egypt, Lebanon, Iran, Russia, and elsewhere. By this period, shops in Little Armenia promoted an additional layer of Armenian cuisine to New York, specializing in rare spices and foods imported from the Middle East that could not be found elsewhere. Stores like Kahayan's and Kalustyan's carried imported caviar, stuffed grape leaves, bulgar wheat, dried spices like ground sumac berry, pomegranate syrup, nuts, dried fruit, and other staples of Armenian cuisine. These shops attracted native New Yorkers who had returned home from World War II with an interest in "ethnic" and "foreign" food. Kalustyan's (Lexington Avenue near Twenty-Seventh Street) remains open and is quite famous for its very large herb, spice, and tea collection among other international items. See KALUSTYAN'S.

As New York's original Armenians became more successful, they left Little Armenia for more upscale areas, such as Washington Heights, Queens, Brooklyn, and New Jersey, joining Armenian communities from the Mediterranean and former Soviet republics. The upscale Armenian restaurants of Manhattan closed, while more modest restaurants and bakery/grocery stores opened in the outer boroughs, which remain open today.

Baruir's Coffee (40-07 Queens Boulevard, Sunnyside, Queens) opened in 1966. It is a family-run business of the Romanian-Armenian Nersesian coffee roasting family, who import high quality coffee beans and roast and ground them on-site.

Sevan Restaurant & Catering (216-07 Horace Harding Expressway, Oakland Gardens, Queens), also family run, began as a grocery store and expanded to include a bakery, catering, and a restaurant. Their products reflect the Russian, Middle Eastern, and Anatolian influences on Armenian cuisine, and include quintessentially Armenian items such as rose petal jam, quince jam, sea buckthorn berry juice, wild cherry juice, and sweet sunflower *halva*. See HALVA. Sevan also carries and serves classic Armenian foods like *soujouk* (spicy sausage) and *tahn,* the national yogurt drink, much like the "kefir" that has become quite mainstream.

Nearby, Mt. Ararat Bakery (220-16 Horace Harding Expressway, Oakland Gardens, Queens) is known for its homemade, Persian-influenced Armenian foods and bakery items, such as *barbari,* a large, oval flat bread.

Brooklyn Bread House (1718 Jerome Avenue, Sheepshead Bay, Brooklyn) specializes in Caucasus-influenced Armenian lavash (flatbread), Georgian breads, and other foods typical of modern-day Armenia, like gata cakes.

Across the river in Manhattan, the recently opened upscale Almayass Armenian–Lebanese restaurant (24 East Twenty-First Street) is quite different from its peers. In New York and through its many branches around the world, the trendy and chic Almayass is rebranding Armenian cuisine as healthy, refined, and exquisite, to be enjoyed in a fine dining setting by both Armenians and non-Armenians alike. It is internationally managed and staffed by Armenians from Lebanon, Cyprus, Iraq, Syria, and the United States. The menu is a mix of Lebanese and Armenian, traditional and fusion dishes, such as lentil and bulgar wheat kufte, and spicy Armenian sausage topped with quail egg. Almayass is reshaping how New Yorkers think about Armenians and their food, and evolving and expanding the repertoire of Armenian dishes.

Patel, Bhavna. "Little Armenia, New York." *The Armenite,* March 17, 2014. http://thearmenite.com/2014/03/little-armenia-new-york-bhavna-patel.

Vartanian, Hrag. "Tracking Armenians in New York." *AGBU Magazine,* April 1, 2002. http://agbu.org/news-item/tracking-armenians-in-new-york.

Aren Seferian

Arthur Avenue

Arthur Avenue is a street in the Belmont neighborhood of the Bronx and the heart of the borough's Little Italy. The food and cultural venues of Arthur Avenue spill beyond the avenue itself to surrounding streets, particularly East 187th Street. The center of a thriving Italian neighborhood from the early to mid-twentieth century, Arthur Avenue is today a vibrant heritage center of Italian and Italian American food and culture. See BRONX; ITALIAN; and LITTLE ITALY.

Among the most famous and long-standing businesses on Arthur Avenue are Italian pastry shops Artuso, Egidio, Madonia Bakery, and DeLillo's; the third-generation Addeo Bakery, which offers crusty Italian bread wrapped in paper and string; Terranova bakery; Randazzo's and Cosenza's fish markets, the latter of which sells clams on the half shell freshly shucked at a cart on the sidewalk; Calabria sausage shop; Tino's deli; Borgatti's pasta, where fresh pasta is rolled, cut, filled, and sold; Calandra formaggio; and Casa della Mozzarella, thought by many to offer the best fresh mozzarella (made daily on the premises) in the city. Also notable is Teitel's deli, a Jewish-owned shop that sells Italian delicacies (the religion of its owners signaled by the Star of David embedded in the sidewalk at the entrance to the store). Jacob and Morris Teitel, Austrian Jewish immigrants, opened the store in 1915, moving to the Bronx from the Lower East Side and catering to the needs of their mostly Italian neighbors. Today, Jacob's son and grandsons run the shop.

Arthur Avenue also has a number of restaurants that draw both locals and tourists, including Domenick's and the Michelin-recommended Tra di Noi. While many of the above-mentioned businesses have been operating on Arthur Avenue for nearly a century, newer food businesses have opened on the avenue in recent years, including Roberto's restaurant, Zero Otto Nove, and the Arthur Avenue Trattoria.

The centerpiece of Arthur Avenue is the Arthur Avenue Retail Market, opened in 1940 as one of a series of indoor markets sponsored by then-mayor Fiorello La Guardia in an effort to regulate and concentrate the many street peddlers in the immigrant wards of the city. See LA GUARDIA, FIORELLO. Today, the retail market contains old and revered stalwarts like Mike's Deli, owned and operated by David Greco, whose Italian immigrant father Mike established the business in 1951. The affable Greco is both a culinary centerpiece of the retail market and an ambassador for Arthur Avenue. He offers mozzarella demonstrations from his deli counter and has participated in televised culinary competitions such as *Chopped* and *Throwdown with Bobby Flay*. Newer businesses in the retail market include the Bronx Beer Hall, a sixty-seat bar opened in 2013 that showcases local Bronx breweries. The retail market also hosts several green grocers, butchers, delis, pork stores, pastry shops, and other fresh-food vendors

as well as housewares shops and a cigar maker. See PUBLIC MARKETS.

While primarily an Italian heritage site, today Arthur Avenue is also at the center of a growing immigrant neighborhood, dominated by immigrants from the Balkans, particularly Albania. The Albanian presence can be seen in the ubiquitous red, double-headed-eagle flags as well as pizza places that sell the Balkan specialty *burek*, a pizza-sized flaky-doughed pastry packed with cheese, spinach, and other savory fillings. The recent wave of Mexican immigration to the Bronx is also making a mark on Arthur Avenue and the surrounding neighborhood.

Crowley, Chris. "The Ultimate Guide to Buying Italian Ingredients on Arthur Avenue." Serious Eats, May 28, 2014. http://www.seriouseats.com/2014/05/ultimate-shopping-guide-arthur-avenue-little-italy-bronx.html.

Cindy R. Lobel

Astor Center

Astor Center is a wine education and event rental space at the corner of Lafayette and Fourth Streets. When Edwin Fisher, then the owner of Astor Wines and Spirits, purchased the historic DeVinne Press Building in 1982, he had no plans to create Astor Center, the carefully considered and innovative space for education and events devoted to passionate consumers of drink and food. Ed Fisher entered the liquor retailing business after World War II and eventually purchased Astor Liquors, then located in leased space at the corner of Lafayette and Eighth Streets. Astor's focus on non-mass-produced offerings was a natural fit with the eclectic, anti-elitist spirit of its Greenwich Village neighbors. See GREENWICH VILLAGE.

Ed's son, Andrew, started working at Astor Liquors in 1971 after graduating from Johns Hopkins and, as he puts it, "completing three days of law school." The younger Fisher was a wine aficionado at a time when Americans' interest in wine—and in artisanal offerings—was just emerging. Andrew recognized that Astor's proven ability to identify and feature high-quality, less well-known offerings from smaller spirits producers could also be applied to the wine category. In 1980, reflecting the new mix of revenues and products, the store name was changed to Astor Wines and Spirits. In terms of revenues per square foot, the store had become one of the largest wine retailers in the nation.

By the early 2000s, however, Astor was running out of room. As a renter at Lafayette and Eighth Streets, the store had only limited flexibility to expand its sales floor and embrace the tastings, education, and other events that were becoming part of wine aficionados' desired experience.

Moreover, Astor's chief wine buyer, reacting to consumer demand, was requesting that more temperature-controlled product be displayed on the sales floor and more temperature-controlled storage be made available in the back of the house. In 2005, an offer for the space from a national drugstore chain provided Andrew Fisher with the incentive to move to the DeVinne building.

Fisher also realized that he now had the opportunity to expand far beyond retail. From 1980 to 2000, the wine market boom had expanded to embrace consumers who were interested in wine not only as a beverage but as a window into other cultures, their cuisines, and the challenges facing artisanal producers around the world. Moreover, New York City had become the hub of a growing food media industry, including cookbooks, magazines, a cable television network devoted to food and cooking, and the marketing firms focused on building and serving foodies' passions. New Yorkers wanted to talk about, explore, learn about, and submerge themselves in food and wine–related classes, discussions, lectures, and more.

Against this cultural backdrop, Fisher decided to move beyond simply developing an expanded store with new areas for tastings and information. He would also use the vacant floor above the retail space to offer a forum for expanded discussion and experience. This space, separate from the retail store, was christened "Astor Center." The design eventually featured four parts: the Study, a thirty-six-seat classroom for wine tastings and food demonstrations; the Kitchen, designed both for hands-on classes and as a full-service, professional catering kitchen for events; the Gallery, an open space for large events; and the Lounge, with a long mahogany bar and ready utility connectors for easy customization. Throughout, the spaces include state-of-the-art audiovisual capabilities that allow interactions with teachers and students, as well as many purpose-built features for wine and spirits tastings. For audiences dedicated to mastering and celebrating artisanship, the historically landmarked DeVinne interiors were maintained, including soaring arched ceilings, original brick and wooden floors, and other architectural details.

The new store opened in 2006, and construction on Astor Center was completed in 2007. Preopening presentations from culinary luminaries such as Harold McGee, Fergus Henderson, and Ariane Daguin culminated in an opening gala announcing Astor Center's "eat, drink, think" purposes to New York's unique mix of professional and recreational enthusiasts. In the ensuing years, Astor Center has featured an ongoing stream of thought leaders, experts, and celebrities at tastings, classes, demonstrations, launch parties, and other events, prompting *Saveur* magazine's 2010 Top 100 List to pronounce it "the ultimate culinary cultural center." In subsequent years, the center's focus has narrowed to events and classes primarily devoted to wine and spirits.

Astor Center website: http://www.astorcenternyc.com.

Doug Duda

Astor House

New York's Astor House was America's largest and most luxurious hotel when it opened in 1836. Its dining rooms, under the direction of a French chef, served *la haute cuisine française*. Guests praised the fare as "excellent French cookery."

The palatial Astor House was constructed by German immigrant John Jacob Astor (1763–1848), who had made his first fortune in the fur trade, his second in the tea trade with China, and his third in Manhattan real estate. He purchased property on Broadway at Vesey Street in downtown Manhattan, and here he spent $600,000 building a block-square, five-story hotel illuminated with the new gaslight. He initially called it the Park Hotel, but when it proved a financial success he changed its name to Astor House. It was New York's first luxury hotel, complete with gas lighting, individual room keys, and water pumped to upper floors. It was where famous visitors to New York City stayed.

When Astor House opened, guests paid three dollars per week for room and full board. Its bar was one of the largest in the city, offering a prodigious free lunch for anyone who bought a drink. But as well-to-do foreign visitors discovered the hotel, prices began to climb. The dining room's bill of fare was large and varied; a new menu was printed—in French—every day. The staff was highly organized

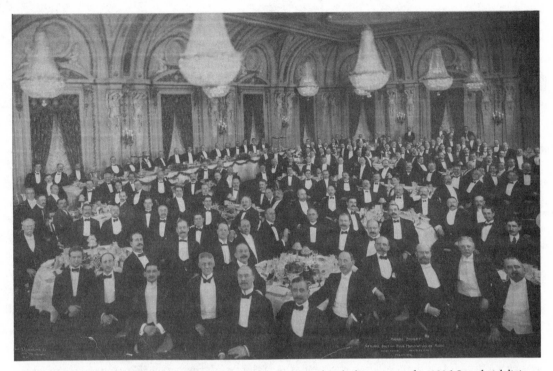

The Astor House was known as America's largest and most luxurious hotel when it opened in 1836. Its palatial dining rooms frequently hosted gatherings of politicians and businessman, as evidenced in this photo of an annual banquet held by the National Boot and Shoe Manufacturers' Association, February 23, 1906. LIBRARY OF CONGRESS

and efficient: a British officer who visited in the late 1830s concluded that the waiters must have been drilled regularly to perform in such a highly organized manner. The hotel operated on the American plan, where meals were included with the price of lodgings and served family style at set times of day.

European guests were astonished by the hotel's massive breakfasts, which included three types of pancakes, eggs, ham, sausages, oysters, fish, chicken, steak, pork, and several kinds of biscuits and breads along with coffee, tea, and chocolate. In the late nineteenth century the hotel's rotunda quickly became the city's most popular luncheon venue, and its dining rooms hosted the city's most exclusive gatherings of political, cultural, and business luminaries.

By the 1870s, however, the Astor Hotel was considered outdated and run-down. Newer hotels uptown, such as the Metropolitan Hotel and the St. Nicholas Hotel, had lured away its fashionable customers. The hotel was partly demolished in 1913 and 1926.

See also HOTEL RESTAURANTS.

Kaplan, Justin. *When the Astors Owned New York: Blue Bloods and Grand Hotels in a Gilded Age*. New York: Viking, 2006.

Andrew F. Smith

Astoria

Astoria, a neighborhood in northwestern Queens, is a draw for people seeking diverse cuisines as well as for residents who appreciate its lower rents and fifteen-minute commute to Manhattan. Visitors from other boroughs and beyond appreciate its broad range of ethnic cuisines, from Egyptian to Korean to the more established Italian and Greek. This mini melting pot bubbles over with markets and eateries catering to its population of immigrants from China, the Philippines, India, eastern and southern Europe, Central and South America, and all over the world.

You could not always get Czech beer, French pastries, Chilean empanadas, thin-crust authentic Italian pizza, or even fresh baklava in Astoria. Dutch explorer Adrian Block is said to have been the first white man to set eyes on the area, in 1614. Forty years later Englishman William Hallett took control of the land after paying the natives a few kettles, coats, beads, and a blanket for the fifteen hundred acres. Then, Hallett's Cove stayed mostly undeveloped for 185 years until in 1839 fur trader Stephen A. Halsey developed the area as a settlement and renamed it "Astoria" after his rich fellow trader John Jacob Astor, in hopes of financial backing. Until 1870 it was a separate village, settled in part by German farmers and furniture makers; then it became part of Long Island City and in 1898 incorporated as part of New York City. By the turn of the twentieth century Irish and Italian immigrants fleeing Manhattan tenements settled there.

The first Greeks arrived in 1927, yet Astoria remained mostly Italian until 1965 when the Hart-Celler Immigration Bill opened the country's borders to many more immigrants, including thousands of Greeks, mostly professionals from Athens but also people from other parts of Greece as well as from Cyprus. By the 1990s a little less than half the population of Astoria was Greek. Other groups also moved in, bringing their own ethnic markets, cafes, and restaurants. A significant Middle Eastern population lived around Steinway Street, and immigrants have arrived from many parts of south and east Asia as well. Then, in the mid-1990s began an influx of young professional Manhattanites, lured by Astoria's proximity to Manhattan and its more affordable rents.

The food scene reflects the neighborhood's remarkable melting pot nature. There are Italian pork stores, Japanese sushi houses, Colombian rotisserie chicken restaurants, cheap Thai spots, modern fusion bistros, and Greek steak or seafood houses. The Czech and Slovak Bohemian Hall and Beer Garden on Twenty-Fourth Avenue is the oldest such establishment in the city. Many popular bars draw locals and people from other boroughs for live music or drinks with friends. Food and drink spots cluster on streets near the subway stops: Ditmars Boulevard between Thirty-First and Thirty-Fifth Streets, Thirtieth Avenue between Thirty-First and Thirty-Seventh Streets, and Broadway between Twenty-Ninth and Thirty-Sixth Streets.

Yet in many ways Astoria remains essentially Greek, with a surfeit of casual places to satisfy the appetite. Many offer a warm welcome at the door, simple décor dotted with mementos of the old country, and an assortment of inexpensive, regional Greek specialties like eggplant or garlic-potato dip, grilled octopus, and whole fish or lamb, much of it simply made and often with ample fresh lemon, herbs, and fruity olive oil. Taverna Kyclades on Ditmars is an example of a still popular classic, as was Uncle George's, which closed in 2013 after more than thirty years.

Restaurants and bakeries sell confections like flaky, custardy, not-too-sweet *galactoboureko*, and sweet fried *loukoumades* dusted with sugar. Residents can find the fixings to cook their supper from Astoria's seafood markets, butcher shops, fruit and vegetable stands, shops full of Greek wines, and markets like the grand Titan on Thirty-First Street. The biggest Greek food store in the country, which author Molly O'Neill called "the A&P of Astoria," Titan offers eight or nine varieties of feta cheese alone. Many locals prefer shopping this way rather than at the Costco on Vernon Boulevard. To visitor and resident alike it is the Greek culture that appeals: families strolling around and greeting neighbors, stopping for coffee and pastries, late dinners of good simple food and music, a warmth with rich traditions that the temples of haute cuisine in Manhattan just cannot match.

See also GREEK and QUEENS.

Astoria website: http://www.astoria.org.
"Halsey, Stephen Alling [1798–1875]—American Entrepreneur." My Celebrity Relations. Rootsweb. freepages.history.rootsweb.com/~dav4is/people/HALS546.htm.
Leeds, Mark. *Ethnic New York: A Complete Guide to the Many Faces & Cultures of New York.* 2d ed. New York: Passport, 1997.
O'Neill, Molly. *The New York Cookbook.* New York: Workman, 1992.
Roleke, John. "Eating in Astoria, Queens: Restaurants, Cafes, Bakeries, and Markets." http://queens.about.com/od/eatingout/a/eating_astoria.htm.

Jennifer Brizzi

Australian

Australian cuisine is similar to modern American cuisine: a mélange of global flavors that rely on simple, bright, and fresh ingredients. The growing number of Australian restaurants in New York have menus that reflect Australian's love for meat and seafood. Instead of faithfully reproducing dishes from Down

Under, they focus on creating an ambience that captures a laid-back antipodean spirit. This Australian version of hospitality was first introduced to New Yorkers in 1999 by Eight Mile Creek in Nolita. The restaurant closed, but not before it helped establish Nolita as Little Australia.

Today Nolita contains a number of other Australian restaurants, like Ruby's Café, Public, The Musket Room, and Two Hands, that continue the tradition. Other Australian restaurants in Manhattan include Burke & Wills, Flinders Lane, Dudley's, Van Diemen's Café and Bar, and the aptly named The Australian. So far Brooklyn contains Sheep Station, Northern Territory, Milk Bar, and Sunshine Co., while Queens has The Thirsty Koala.

With so many authentic options, it would be unfortunate if New Yorkers associated Australian food only with the Outback Steakhouse, a kitschy pastiche of Australiana where nothing on the menu comes close to resembling authentic Australian cuisine. It even lacks the benefit of being Australian-owned.

Iconic Foods

Ingredients like barramundi (a sweet, mild tasting fish similar to sea bass), shrimp, Australian lamb, and kangaroo are easily found on menus in New York's Australian restaurants. Chances are menus will also include an Aussie-style hamburger "with-the-lot," which includes bacon, a fried egg, and pickled beets, in addition to the American traditional deluxe hamburger upgrade of lettuce, tomato, onion, and cheese. See HAMBURGER.

For dessert the Aussie favorite is pavlova: a baked meringue, crisp on the outside with a soft marshmallow center, topped with whipped cream and seasonal fresh fruit, berries, or passion fruit pulp. Treats like lamingtons (vanilla sponge cake with a strawberry jam layer, dunked in chocolate syrup, and covered in coconut) are invariably featured.

Australia's two most iconic foods are the meat pie and Vegemite. The meat pie, a one-handed fast-food staple at the footy (Australian Rules Football), typically contains chunks of beef and gravy encased in flaky pastry. For more than ten years DUB Pies have been serving this fast-food snack from locations in Brooklyn, including a food truck. See FOOD TRUCKS. In Manhattan "the great Aussie bite" can be had at Tuck Shop at its locations in the East Village and Chelsea Market. See CHELSEA MARKET.

Vegemite is a black, salty, strong-smelling paste that Australian children enjoy as American children might enjoy peanut butter. It is spread on toast, crackers, and sandwiches. Made famous worldwide with the help of the 1981 Men at Work song "Down Under," it was previously difficult to find and stocked only in specialty grocers like Myers of Keswick, a traditional British grocery store in New York. Today, Vegemite can be easily found in larger grocery stores like Fairway Market. See FAIRWAY MARKET.

Coffee Culture

Post–World War II immigration brought hundreds of thousands of Europeans to Australia to start a new life. They imported their love of coffee and a supporting café culture. A benefit of this influx is that almost any establishment serving food in Australia can produce a flat white (a layer of steamed-milk microfoam poured over a double shot of espresso that was created in Australia) proficiently extracted from a gleaming professional espresso machine. Americans may be shocked to discover that the McDonald's Café concept was actually conceived and launched in Australia.

While New York easily satisfied Australians' appetite for diverse ethnic foods, it used to be that finding coffee that matched the strength and quality of what Australians were used to at home required an expedition. This is no longer the case. A new class of work visa (E-3) available only to Australians has seen the number of Australians living in New York quadruple from five thousand in 2005 to twenty thousand in 2011. As a result, Australian-style cafés are opening up all over the city. From smaller outfits like Little Collins, Brunswick, Bluebird Coffee Shop, and Bluestone Lane to fast-growing chains like Toby's Estate and Café Grumpy, entrepreneurial Australians are educating and caffeinating New Yorkers on great coffee. See COFFEE SHOPS.

Baird, Saxon. "What's the Deal with All These Australians in NYC?" Gothamist, June 9, 2014. http://gothamist.com/2014/06/09/australians_everywhere.php.
Clayton, Liz. "Is All New York Coffee Secretly Australian?" Serious Eats, November 6, 2013. http://drinks.seriouseats.com/2013/11/new-york-australian-coffee-trend-flat-white-nyc-brooklyn.html.
Embassy of the United States. "Additional E3 Information." http://canberra.usembassy.gov/e3visa/additional.html.

Munro, Ian. "Big Apple Embraces Little Australia." *The Age*, September 8, 2007.
Strand, Oliver. "Australian Cafes Arrive in New York." *New York Times*, July 29, 2014.

Domenic Venuto

Automats

Automats were restaurants that vended food through mechanical dispensers, their contents visible through a little glass door. To buy the food, customers placed coins in a slot and turned a knob, which opened the door. Workers behind the wall replaced food items as they were removed. Automats did not require waiters—just attendants to make change for customers and the staff behind the wall. Automats were especially popular in New York City during the first half of the twentieth century.

The world's first automat was Quisisana, which opened in Berlin in 1895 and was followed by outlets in other European cities. In 1898 a salesperson for the maker of Quisisana's automated system arrived in America in search of customers. He approached Joseph Horn and Frank Hardart, owners of a small chain of quick-service lunchrooms in Philadelphia. The salesperson's pitch intrigued Hardart, an immigrant from Bavaria, and in 1901 he visited Quisisana's operation in Berlin. Upon his return, he convinced his partner to buy the equipment, and in June 1902 Horn and Hardart established America's first automat in Philadelphia. It proved a success, and the partners proceeded to open more of them.

New York City's first automat was opened in December 1902 by a restaurateur named James Harcombe, who spent $75,000 on its lavish interior decoration. He advertised it as "Europe's Unique Electric Self-serving Device for Lunches and Beverages. No Waiting. No Tipping. Open Evenings Until Midnight." Prices ranged from a nickel to a quarter. To compete with full-service restaurants, the automat offered a wide assortment of items, including lobster à la Newberg, beer, wine, and cocktails. Despite widespread promotion, the public did not flock to this novel eating place, and it closed around 1907.

Horn & Hardart's successful Philadelphia chain expanded into New York City in 1912, and within a few years, there were fifteen automats in the city. September 1922 brought the company's first combination automat–cafeteria, which they touted as the city's largest restaurant. Soon most of New York's

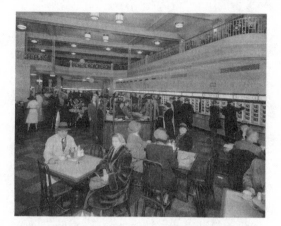

A Horn & Hardart automat on 1165 Sixth Avenue in January 1969. Automats were precursors to fast-food restaurants, where diners in a hurry dropped nickels into slots to unlock their premade meal of choice. ROBERT F. BYRNES AUTOMAT COLLECTION, MANUSCRIPTS AND ARCHIVES DIVISION, NEW YORK PUBLIC LIBRARY/ ASTOR, LENOX, AND TILDEN FOUNDATIONS

automats included cafeterias, which allowed wide menu choices. In order to maintain its high-quality standards, the company opened a central commissary that supplied all of its operations in the city. Horn & Hardart did well during the 1920s but really came into its own during the Depression. During the company's heyday in the 1930s, a single Horn & Hardart outlet served on average ten thousand customers daily. In 1933, the company took the unusual step of hiring a classically trained chef, Francis Bourdon, who had worked at top restaurants in Europe and America. Bourdon ran the Horn & Hardart commissary for the next thirty-five years, developing new recipes and assuring uniform quality throughout the chain. His credentials also added some prestige to what was perceived as a working-class restaurant.

After World War II, Horn & Hardart expanded, growing to fifty outlets in New York City by 1950, but by this time most had been converted into cafeterias, the little glass cabinets of food and the small-change prices becoming a thing of the past. Then the chain began a downhill slide, caused by a combination of factors, including a new city tax on prepared food: the required additional pennies could not be put into the nickel slots. As Horn & Hardart began losing money on its popular (and excellent) coffee, it raised the price to a dime a cup. But when they began to water down the coffee and skimp on the quality of their food, the end was near. Fast-food establishments, the latest novelty, lured away automat customers; within four decades most of them were closed, many converted into Burger King outlets. The last automat in New York City closed in April 1991.

Automats are gone, but the fascination with them has lingered. New Yorkers were reintroduced to the real, original automat through a show at the Museum of the City of New York in 2002 and again when the "Lunch Hour" exhibition opened at the New York Public Library in the fall of 2012. On display was a panel of shiny glass-and-chrome automat food compartments (alas, empty), presenting visitors the rare opportunity to see what the equipment looked like from the back. For many visitors with fond memories of automats, it was the high point of the exhibition. See MUSEUM OF THE CITY OF NEW YORK and NEW YORK PUBLIC LIBRARY.

Bromell, Nicolas. "The Automat: Preparing the Way for Fast Food." *New York History* 81, no. 3 (July 2000): 300–312.

Diehl, Lorraine B., and Marianne Hardart. *Automat: The History, Recipes, and Allure of Horn & Hardart's Masterpiece.* New York: Clarkson Potter, 2002.

Freeland, David. *Automats, Taxi Dances, and Vaudeville: Excavating Manhattan's Lost Places of Leisure.* New York: New York University Press, 2009.

Andrew F. Smith

Bagels

Ed Levine, New York City food connoisseur and chronicler of New York food markets and ethnic delicacies, wrote in the *New York Times*, "no city... is so closely identified with a breadstuff as New York is with the bagel" (Levine, 2003, p. 1). But while bagels are perhaps most widely associated with New York City, they originally came from Eastern Europe.

According to folklore, seventeenth-century Polish king Jan Sobieski defied a 1496 ruling that permitted only the Krakow Bakers Guild to bake all white and parboiled bread, thus allowing Jews (non–guild members) to bake as well. A baker, grateful to King Sobieski for protecting Austria from invading Turks, created a roll in the shape of a riding stirrup. Bakers named the roll a *beugel*, Austrian for "stirrup," to commemorate both the heroic act and the king's horseback-riding hobby. The legend itself may be suspect, but the bagel's popularity continued throughout the seventeenth and eighteenth centuries in Eastern Europe and particularly within the Jewish community, now able to prepare their own breads according to dietary laws.

Although not ritualistically Jewish, once in the United States, bagels remained associated with the Jewish community during the late nineteenth and early twentieth centuries as Jews quickly established bakeries in New York, boasting seventy on the Lower East Side by 1900. In 1907, to address dangerous and unjust labor practices and wages, producers formed the International Beigel Bakers' Union, employing strict membership rules. Three hundred bagel bakers joined Local 338 and set forth criteria and standards for handmade bagel production as well as membership guidelines that passed down from fathers to sons, ensuring that the bagel craft remained within a small isolated group. Bagel production necessitated both extensive skill and physical labor. To achieve union membership, bakers' sons apprenticed for several months before earning their labor cards. All Local 338 members were male and Jewish and spoke Yiddish. Within eight years of the union's formation, they signed contracts with thirty-six New York bakeries.

Early bagels, as defined by Local 338, were two to three ounces in weight, rolled out by hand, and prepared with high-gluten flour, malt, water, and yeast to create a chewy crust that became hard within a few hours. Because of their perishable nature, bakeries delivered them throughout the day, stringing them together in five-dozen batches. Bagel production included two groups: bench men, who both kneaded the dough and boiled the bagels, and oven men, who baked the bagels and completed the process.

As New York's bagel consumption and demand increased over the decades, so did Local 338's strength. Countless times from 1948 to 1953, and again in 1962, labor disputes between Local 338 and the Bagel Bakers Association resulted in widespread strikes and bagel shortages that the *New York Times* deemed "Bagel Famine." Negotiations over wages for bench men and oven men, paid holidays, sick days, and pension plan contributions continually pitted Local 338 workers against the bagel bakeries, with subsequent strikes lasting weeks and months.

Although Local 338 achieved great gains for its members, it lost favor in the 1960s. Bakeries suffered

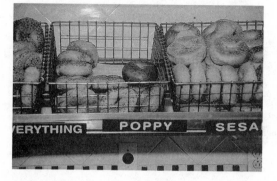

An assortment of bagels on display at La Bagel Delight in Brooklyn. PHOTO BY JOE ZARBA

huge economic losses, with countless strikes, competition from non-union bagel shops, frozen bagels entering the market, and greater mechanized production all contributing to weakening Local 338's power. The Thompson Bagel machine, invented by a Canadian, automated bagel production, negating the value of artisan union workers. The situation for union bakers weakened further when Lender's Bagels in New Haven, Connecticut, employing the Thompson machine, began saturating the market with commercialized bagels, producing 300 dozen in the same time as it took two bench men to prepare 125 dozen by hand.

The Lender family recognized the Jewish bagels' mass appeal to other immigrant groups. In 1956, Lender's introduced a freezer to their production, enabling them to mass-produce bagels, freeze them for ease, and deliver them thawed to consumer retailers. When they added polyethylene bags, Lender's Bagels became more stable with a prolonged shelf life.

Mass-produced, mechanized bagels with a longer shelf life allowed Americans across the country to enjoy bagels originally consumed by New York City Jews, then New Yorkers in general. Featured in supermarkets next to Wonder Bread or in freezer cases next to Pepperidge Farm, New York–style bagels became America's new convenience food during the mid-twentieth century. Jewish assimilation to the suburbs and increased acceptance of Jewish culture post–World War II helped forge bagel enthusiasm. Some national supermarket chains, however, did not market bagels as Jewish but instead situated them alongside all sandwich breads and rolls as just another American option. In the mid-twentieth century, bagels transformed from Jewish bread to standard American breakfast fare.

Blueberries, raisins, and cinnamon became as ubiquitous as onion, garlic, and poppy. The bastion of middle America, *Family Circle* magazine, featured a bagel recipe in the 1950s. Lender's Bagels sold across the country, and Kraft's aggressive advertising campaign showcasing Philadelphia Cream Cheese alongside bagels helped make bagels America's bread. Back in New York City, *Time* magazine wrote about a 1951 Broadway comedy *Bagels and Yox*, securing "bagel" as a household word.

Whether consumed hot from a New York bagel bakery or defrosted from a Lender's bag purchased elsewhere, bagel association remained with New York City. However, as bagels moved beyond New York, consumption and characteristics evolved as well. By the mid-1980s Americans consumed an average of one bagel monthly, and by 1993 the bagel per capita consumption statistic doubled to a bagel every other week. The once two- to three-ounce handcrafted bagel became "supersized," with an average bagel weighing seven ounces.

During that late 1990s, New Yorkers embraced artisan bagels versus mass-produced ones that were unrecognizable from the unique chewy, boiled bread a century earlier. Several handcrafted bakeries opened in Brooklyn, Manhattan, and Queens and adopted old-style bagel production. Food-savvy New Yorkers clamored for bagels smaller in size, individually hand-rolled, and with a reverence for traditional toppings and fillings.

New York City's Jewish artisan bagel has thus come full circle. Local 338's commitment to distinct practices, recipes, procedures, ingredients, and craft, though temporarily challenged through industrialized food methods, are enjoying a renaissance of both time-honored traditions and Jewish cultural association.

See also BAKERIES; BIALYS; CREAM CHEESE; DELIS, JEWISH; and JEWISH.

Balinska, Maria. *The Bagel: The Surprising History of a Modest Bread.* New Haven, Conn.: Yale University Press, 2008.

Berg, Jennifer S. "From Pushcart Peddlers to New York Take-Out: New York City's Iconic Foods of Jewish Origin, 1920–2005." PhD diss., New York University, 2006.

Levine, Ed. "Was Life Better When Bagels Were Smaller?" *New York Times,* December 31, 2003.

Mariani, John F. *The Dictionary of American Food and Drink.* New York: Hearst, 1994.

Jennifer Schiff Berg

Baked Alaska

Baked Alaska is an igloo-shaped dessert made by topping a round piece of sponge cake with ice cream that is covered with uncooked meringue. It is then browned in a hot oven.

The concept of serving ice cream with cake dates back to the Renaissance. Throughout the years, earlier versions of what is now known as baked Alaska were known as omelet *á la norvégienne*, omelet surprise, and *glace au four*, a French term meaning that ice cream is enclosed in something hot such as pastry dough, which is how they were made in the past. The current version of baked Alaska is topped with meringue.

This dessert of varying textures and temperatures was not known as baked Alaska until French chef de cuisine Charles Ranhofer of Delmonico's in Lower Manhattan coined the name. In his cookbook *The Epicurean* (1894), Ranhofer explains that the dessert was named to honor and commemorate the United States' purchase of Alaska on October 18, 1867. George Sala, an English journalist who dined at Delmonico's during the 1880s, said, "The Alaska is a baked ice…the nucleus or core of the entremet is an ice cream."

Kept frozen until serving time, baked Alaska is placed in the oven for a few moments to brown the meringue. When the dessert made a comeback in the 1990s, in such restaurants as Union Square Café, pastry chefs began using blowtorches to create the same effect. Today it is not easy to find in New York restaurants, but many recipes can be found online from chefs and food personalities, including Martha Stewart and Alton Brown. Dessert lovers can celebrate this decadent dessert on February 1: National Baked Alaska Day.

See also DELMONICO'S and RANHOFER, CHARLES.

O'Neill, Molly. *New York Cookbook*. New York: Workman, 1992.
Ranhofer, Charles. *The Epicurean*. New York: R. Ranhofer, 1893.

Tracey Ceurvels

Bakeries

Bakeries producing and selling bread or pastry, or more typically both, have been a city fixture since the beginnings of European settlement. More than most Americans, New Yorkers, ever short of time and space, have long depended on the local baker to provide their daily bread, pie, or sweet pastry.

From New Amsterdam to New York

The Europeans who settled around what is now New York Harbor tried as best as they could to maintain their old-world food ways. Here, as in Europe, bread was the single largest source of calories and was typically baked by professionals. In New Amsterdam, the bakers made a variety of baked goods, including white and dark bread as well as cakes and gingerbread. By 1684 twenty-four bakers practiced their craft in the city. Given bread's pivotal role in the diet, governments had every interest in regulating the baker's trade. As in Europe, the size, composition, and price of bread were fixed by the colonial rulers, though given the continuous stream of often repetitive regulation, it is clear that the

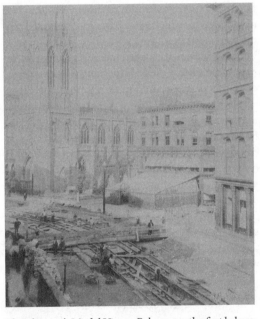

Fleischmann's Model Vienna Bakery was the first bakery business in New York to have the capability to produce bread and other baked goods on a mass scale. It is also credited with isolating the strain of yeast that made mass production of bread possible. PHOTOGRAPHY COLLECTION, MIRIAM AND IRA D. WALLACH DIVISION OF ART, PRINTS AND PHOTOGRAPHS, THE NEW YORK PUBLIC LIBRARY, ASTOR, LENOX, AND TILDEN FOUNDATIONS

authorities were often unsuccessful. And Europeans were not the bakers' only customers. The Lenape natives had apparently acquired a taste for white bread and cake and were willing to pay a premium for it, purportedly leaving little or none for the settlers. In 1649, to rein in the bakers' "greed and desire for greater profits," the director general and council forbade the bakers from selling white bread or cakes to anyone at all, native or immigrant, on pain of a massive fine of fifty Carolusgilders. A decade later, the authorities were still trying to keep the native population from easy access to the bakers' cakes.

When the city traded hands from the Dutch to the English, the bakery industry initially received no less government scrutiny. Following the Revolution, prices, weights, and even shape continued to be controlled; bakers were required to stamp their bread so that its source could be identified; and when it seemed that grain merchants and bakers were colluding to raise prices, the city's chamber of commerce sent in the police. The attempt to control prices was soon abandoned, though in most other respects the neighborhood bakery remained much the same until after the Civil War.

However, not all bakers limited their market to New York. Bread (in the form of hardtack or ship's biscuit) was exported to the Caribbean and other British colonies by at least the mid-eighteenth century, planting the seeds for the city's eventual industrial-scale baking industry. In the nineteenth century, some of the ship's biscuit bakeries transitioned to making crackers. The cracker trade, unlike bread making, was heavily automated early on. The needed capital investment encouraged the industry to consolidate into ever fewer large firms. It was as a result of this sort of merger of multiple biscuit companies that the National Biscuit Company (later Nabisco) was created in 1898. See NABISCO.

Bakers and Bakeries

Bakers did not command much respect. Most nineteenth-century Americans considered homemade bread not only safer but actually morally superior. Yet as cities like New York became increasingly packed, homemade bread became impractical for most households and impossible for many. The cost of fuel and lack of ovens gave the working class no choice but to depend for their daily bread on the neighborhood baker. As the cities exploded—by a factor of more than eight in the half-century before 1900—the number of bakeries kept pace. In 1850 the census reported 2,027 bakeries in all the United States; by century's end, New York City alone had more than double that number. According to a 1924 study by J. Walter Thomson, whereas in 1850 only some 10 percent of bread was store-bought, by 1900 it was closer to 25 percent.

In the mid-nineteenth century, many of New York's bakeries were both retail and wholesale operations, selling bread, cakes, and pies to restaurants, hotels, and grocery stores as well as to retail customers. As in Europe, customers could pay a baker to cook their homemade pastries in the professional oven. According to Virginia Penny, author of *The Employment of Women: A Cyclopaedia of Woman's Work* (1863), women generally attended to the counters of New York bread bakeries, while the arduous work of bread making was relegated to men, mostly Germans in her day. Confectioners, by contrast, did employ women to bake cakes and cookies, as well as a wide variety of confectionery. At the time, New York also had four large bakeries dedicated solely to pie. Here, a woman might earn some five or six dollars a month (with room and board) preparing the fruit and rolling out pastry. Men generally made that per week.

The baker's lot was never easy, and by the late 1800s working conditions in New York bakeries were often appalling. Thousands were situated in low-ceilinged cellars with inadequate light and ventilation. Most tenement cellar bakeries were not even fireproofed. Workdays ranged from thirteen to eighteen hours, or even longer on Saturdays. In an attempt to ameliorate their lives, the bakers sought to unionize; and after some twenty years of struggle, bakers' unions, mostly organized along ethnic lines (the Bohemian Bakers, the Hebrew Bakers, and so on), eventually convinced the legislature to act. Yet the laws intended to regulate minimum sanitation and working conditions had only limited effect as attested to by numerous reports and attempts to improve enforcement. In 1915, new cellar bakeries were finally outlawed altogether, though over three thousand of these remained in 1924.

The neighborhood bakeries eventually saw their demise not so much at the hand of the labor regulators and health inspectors but rather by the changing demographic and retail environment of New York City. With the coming of the subways, the crammed tenements of Lower Manhattan were abandoned for brighter pastures in the outer boroughs, denuding the bakers of their customers. Local bakers could not compete with large bakery concerns such as Hecker's or Fleischmann's, which could produce bread more cheaply, hygienically, and often under better working conditions than the mom-and-pop bakeries. Increasingly, the bread sold at the rapidly multiplying chain grocery stores was the standardized, "hygienic" product of the large commercial bread factories.

The Baking Industry

Whereas mechanization had allowed cracker bakeries to expand and consolidate early, bread and pastry baking was a relatively old-fashioned business until late in the nineteenth century. It was not until new yeast strains were isolated and ovens allowing continuous production invented that the age-old staple was embraced by the age of progress. Fleischmann's, which relocated to New York after gaining fame for its yeast at the 1876 Philadelphia Exhibition, had every intention of making the neighborhood baker obsolete. In the 1880s from their Vienna Model Bakery, located next door to Grace Church on Lower Broadway, and another nearby plant, the company produced twelve thousand to fifteen thousand loaves of their signature bread daily. See BREADLINES. Thirty years on, the company (since 1911 part of the national General Baking Company) boasted massive bakeries on Duane Street, on East Eighty-First Street, and in the Bronx. By this point the city's largest operation, Ward's Bakery (also part of the same "trust") produced some half-million loaves a day at its Brooklyn and Bronx bread factories.

Bagels and Cannoli

Each wave of immigrants, unaccustomed to, if not baffled by, commercial American bread, has opened up its own bakeries, catering to its own people and other curious New Yorkers. Italian bakeries originally sold breads and cookies of specific regions, but with subsequent generations a repertoire of New York–style "Italian" baking developed. Today, a pastry shop such as Manhattan's Veniero's (established 1894) stocks Sicilian cannoli, Neapolitan *sfogliatelle*, and New York cheesecake. Early Jewish bakeries specialized in Eastern European–style breads and pastries, developing a specifically New York style of "Jewish" rye bread, bagels, rugelach, and *hamantaschen*. Currently, the city's largest kosher bakery is Zaro's, established in the Bronx in 1927 by Joseph Zaro and expanded by his descendants into some dozen branches today. It too has diversified, selling everything from seeded pumpernickel to *pain au chocolat*. Specialized Jewish bakeries dedicated to making matzo used to be scattered across the Lower East Side; today, a few remain in Brooklyn.

As the city's population has diversified since 1965, there has been an explosion of ethnic bakeries. Chinese bun shops, Mexican *panaderias* stacked with *pan dulce*, Polish bakeries featuring giant loaves of rye bread and poppy seed cake, and storefronts selling lavash, pita, and any other number of flatbreads can be encountered across the five boroughs. International bakery chains have also succeeded in gaining a foothold in the city, from Belgium's Pain Quotidian and France's Maison Kayser to Korea's Paris Baguette.

The Artisanal Revival

Beginning in the 1980s and in part inspired by artisanal bread bakers in California and France, New York bakers began to try to emulate the slow-risen loaves they had encountered on their travels. Eli Zabar was perhaps the first to rise to the challenge at his culinary boutique E.A.T., when in 1985 his bakers started producing French-style sourdough bread for sale to local restaurants. In Long Island City, Tom Cat Bakery followed suit with a crusty and personable baguette in 1987. Amy Scherber started baking a wide array of breads and pastries in her Hell's Kitchen outpost of Amy's Bread in 1992. Two years later Sullivan Bakery's Jim Lahey began to sell rustic, Italian-style breads and pizzas out of a tiny storefront in Soho. The idea of small-batch, artisanal baking has since been extended to pies, cupcakes, doughnuts, as well as a wide variety of gluten-free, vegan, and other niche products. Today, whether Native American, Dutch, or Brooklyn hipster, all are now welcome to partake of the city bakeries' cornucopia.

See also BREAD.

Bobrow-Strain, Aaron. *White Bread*. Boston: Beacon, 2013.

Fernow, Berthold, and E. B. O'Callaghan. *The Records of New Amsterdam from 1653 to 1674 Anno Domini*. New York: Knickerbocker, 1897.

Kummer, Corby. "The Best of Bread." *New York Magazine,* 14 April 1997, 49–50.

Panschar, William G., and Charles C. Slater. *Baking in America.* Evanston, Ill.: Northwestern University Press, 1956.

Michael Krondl

Balducci's

Balducci's was a family-owned gourmet market specializing in Italian products. Louis Balducci, an Italian immigrant from Puglia, began selling bananas from a cart in Greenpoint in 1915. By 1917 he operated a produce stand there, which he moved to Greenwich Village in 1947. At the time, the neighborhood was heavily Italian, and Balducci's gained a reputation for an abundant supply of high-quality and hard-to-find produce.

Balducci's moved to a new location, on Sixth Avenue near Ninth Street, in 1972, and it was in this spot that it became one of the foremost gourmet grocers in New York City. Balducci's continued to innovate in its produce section, importing exotic fruits and vegetables. But it also expanded its offerings, adding a bakery; a butcher section stocked with all kind of meats, including a wide selection of Italian salamis and sausages; and a cheese shop with more than two hundred varieties, including Italian specialties like *mozzarella di bufala* and ricotta. Soon, Balducci's added a prepared food section and became a popular place for locals to pick up lunch or dinner.

By the 1980s, Balducci's was one of several popular gourmet grocery stores in New York. But the store's success and good reputation spurred competition. A crowded gourmet market, combined with intense and publicized fighting between Louis and Maria Balducci's three children, Andy, Charles, and Grace, started to chip away at the business. Andy had left Balducci's in the 1950s to work at his father-in-law's granite business. When he returned fifteen years later, he had ambitious plans to expand the company. He orchestrated the move to the new location, and he formed a new corporation. This new corporation was the source of the tension. The contract gave Andy and his wife a 51 percent share of the business, with the 49 percent share going to his sister Grace and her husband, Joe Doria.

Different family members argue about the details and the motivation, but Louis and Maria, the founders of Balducci's, and their oldest son, Charles, had no ownership in the new business. Charles and Louis sued Andy for a share of the corporation; Grace and Joe, chafing under Andy's management, decamped to start their own store, suing Andy for a fair buyout of their share of the corporation. Andy sued them to prevent their use of the Balducci name, and subpoenaed his mother in that lawsuit. Charles and Andy got into a fistfight outside the courtroom about what Charles said was disrespectful treatment of their mother. Grace's Marketplace opened on the Upper East Side in 1985 and moved to a larger location on Second Avenue in 2013.

By the late 1990s, Balducci's reputation had begun to falter; in part, its offerings had begun to seem less special and less worth the price in the face of so many other gourmet grocers in the city. The Balducci family sold the business to Sutton Place Gourmet in 1999, and its flagship store in the Village closed in 2003. A new Balducci's location opened on the Upper West Side in 2003, but as a result of a combination of internal troubles, a saturated gourmet market, and the economic downturn that followed the recession of 2008, that location closed in 2009. Joe Doria and Andy Balducci began doing some wholesale distributing at the Ninth Avenue store in the 1980s. In 1991, Kevin Murphy, Andy's son-in-law, established Baldor Specialty Foods as a separate company, which continues to operate in New York and New England.

Today Balducci's still has stores in Connecticut, Virginia, Maryland, and Westchester but has been unable to reassert itself in New York City, which boasts a thriving and variegated gourmet market scene that Balducci's helped create.

See also GROCERY STORES; ITALIAN; and SUPERMARKETS.

Anderson, Susan Heller. "Louis Balducci, Grocer, Dies at 89 after Years as Chefs' Inspiration." *New York Times,* August 13, 1988.

Buckley, Cara. "Balducci's Makes a Quiet Exit from Manhattan." *New York Times,* April 27, 2009.

Burros, Marian. "Balducci's: A House Divided Stands in Name Only." *New York Times,* June 28, 2000.

Costikyan, Barbara. "The Joy of Shops." *New York Magazine,* December 23, 1991.

Hewitt, Jean. "Now, Prosciutto Is Sold with the Melon." *New York Times,* April 22, 1972.

Mariani, John F. *How Italian Food Conquered the World.* New York: Palgrave Macmillan, 2011.

Katie Uva

Barber, Dan

Dan Barber (b. 1969) is an award-winning chef and influential activist. Born in New York City, he graduated from the prestigious Dalton School and Tufts University. After college, Barber moved to California, where he first tasted life in the kitchen, working at Alice Waters's Chez Panisse. He returned to New York to attend the French Culinary Institute, after which he spent nearly two years in apprenticeships in France, including a year-long stint in Paris's Michelin two-starred restaurant Michel Rostang. See FRENCH CULINARY INSTITUTE.

He returned to New York, working at the acclaimed restaurant Bouley and then opening a catering company. In May 2000, with his brother David, he opened Blue Hill Restaurant in Greenwich Village, which has been called a "farm-to-table" restaurant, although Barber prefers the term "sustainable." See FARM TO TABLE. Barber's rigorous training led to immediate recognition and success. In 2002, *Food & Wine* honored him as one of the country's best new chefs. The James Beard Foundation named Barber "Best Chef in New York City" in 2006 and "Chef of the Year" in 2009. See JAMES BEARD AWARDS. That year, *Time* magazine called him one of the world's "100 Most Influential People."

The *Time* magazine accolade was based on Barber's second restaurant-cum-educational center, Blue Hill at Stone Barns Center for Food and Agriculture, located in Potanico Hills, 30 miles northwest of Manhattan. Stone Barns is a 3,500-acre estate owned by David Rockefeller, an early and frequent patron of Blue Hill; Rockefeller wanted to find a good use for the stone dairy located on an 80-acre portion of the estate, one that could justify the investment in preserving the buildings. Developing a center for agricultural education and a restaurant proved the answer, and the complex opened in 2004. The center's mission is to "create a healthy and sustainable food system that benefits us all," and it hosts more than one hundred thousand visitors each year.

Barber is a member of the advisory board of the Harvard Medical School's Center for Global and Environment Health and a member of President Barack Obama's Council on Fitness, Sports, and Nutrition. He is the author of *The Third Plate: Field Notes on the Future of Food* (2014), which details his philosophy of the interrelationships among farming, cooking, and eating responsibly and sustainably. More than "organic" and "farm-to-table," Barber sees the essential future of food as one of "an integrated system of vegetable, grain, and livestock production" that includes the responsibility of the cook in choosing what to prepare for dinner.

Aronica, Molly. "Chef Bios: Dan Barber." The Daily Meal, December 6, 2010. http://www.thedailymeal .com/chef-bios-dan-barber.
Barber, Dan. *The Third Plate: Field Notes on the Future of Food.* New York: Penguin, 2014.
Blue Hill website: http://www.bluehillfarm.com/food/ blue-hill-new-york.
McBride, Anne E. "Interview with Dan Barber." Institute of Culinary Education, September 2007. http://www.ice .edu/press/the-ice-interviews/interview-with-dan-barber.

Cathy K. Kaufman

Bar Cars

See RAILROAD DINING.

Barney Greengrass

The iconic Upper West Side appetizing store that also boasts an off-to-the-side dining room that seemingly has not changed since the 1950s, Barney Greengrass is a third-generation-owned mecca of smoked fish and the foods that pair with it—bagels, bialys, borscht, and the like. The store and restaurant, which still sees lines out the door for weekend brunch and a brisk dining and take-away business all week long, proudly carries the tag line "The Sturgeon King," a title bestowed by Groucho Marx in a condolence card sent to second-generation owner Moe Greengrass when his father Barney died. Marx wrote, "He may not have ruled any kings or written any symphonies but he did a monumental job with sturgeon."

It was sturgeon, and other fish, that Barney and his family members started selling in Harlem, around 113th Street and St. Nicholas Avenue, in 1908 (they relocated to the current Amsterdam Avenue location in 1929). Harlem was a Jewish neighborhood back then, and Greengrass's grandfather, Barney, was one of ten children who lived there. Many of the siblings worked in the business alongside Barney, and when the current Greengrass took over multiple uncles were still involved.

The family involvement kept the focus tightly on selling the best fish they could, unlike other neighborhood appetizing stores which have diversified. As Greengrass says, "We are not selling pots and pans, we are focused on one area primarily." Greengrass jokes about being the generation that runs things into the ground, but he is carrying on tradition by keeping his store and restaurant streamlined. By design, the deli still looks very much the same as it did decades ago. The floor is new, but it is the same pattern it has been for generations. The showcase in which the smoked fish and its accoutrements rest is encased in white porcelain enamel. What is now just a mirror used to be the icebox, in which blocks of ice were stored, keeping everything cold and fresh. Today, the case is refrigerated using modern technology—electricity and motorization—but in Moe's day he would remind his staff, "Close the icebox."

The unwillingness to change is not strictly for sentimental reasons. Keeping the status quo pleases both Hollywood and other patrons from around the globe who flock there en masse. The shop and restaurant have an impressive broadcast resume, having appeared regularly in episodes of *Law & Order* and *30 Rock* and in such movies as Woody Allen's *Deconstructing Harry* and Tom Hanks's *Extremely Loud and Incredibly Close*.

Traditions at Barney Greengrass endure. Greengrass concludes, "They call me when they are coming into the world and going out. I'm the first call after the grandparents."

See also DELIS, JEWISH and UPPER WEST SIDE.

Steintrager, Megan O. "Top Chefs Share Their 'Bucket List' Restaurants." *Gourmet Live*, September 12, 2012.
Witchel, Alex. "Counterintelligence; The Comfort of Sturgeon." *New York Times*, September 23, 2001.

Francine Cohen

Bars

Bars have not always been just about the cocktails. In the beginning, they were about community. The earliest places in which people congregated to drink were inns, like the King's Head Inn in southern England, which dates back to the thirteenth century. Different from taverns, because they offered lodging as well as food and drink, these early establishments were a welcoming place for weary travelers (and their horses) to rest and recharge. Taverns, on the other hand, which advertised their existence via outside signage that used branches and leaves as a symbol that wine was available, were drinking houses often found in the center of town. Colonial settlers in New York continued British traditions in the New World, gathering at inns and taverns to drink local beer, ale, and cider, as well as imported wine and spirits when available. See TAVERNS.

The Industrial Revolution of the nineteenth century had an impact on the way people lived and socialized, and the liquor industry, as well as bars, were the great beneficiaries of this sea change. With factories luring people into cities, restaurants without lodging became a destination; and the communal traditions carried by the immigrants melded together in pubs and taprooms. Often these establishments offered food and music as well as drink and became gathering places where working men of the neighborhood would discuss politics and local news. Many of these taprooms were affiliated with local breweries, and beer and ale were the featured alcoholic beverages, although whiskey or other liquors might be available.

As boarding houses morphed into "hotels" at the turn of the nineteenth century, one of the hallmarks of the grand hotel was that in addition to offering room and board, it offered facilities for banquets, dances, and other public entertainments—including drinking. Compared to humble beer-fueled pubs and taprooms, these fancy hotels often had extensive bars and wine cellars, including vintages of fine Madeira, port, and sherry. See BOARDING HOUSES.

Many of these hotels also had bartenders overseeing those well-stocked bars, developing and serving cocktails. Professor Jerry Thomas, for example, presided over the bar at the Metropolitan Hotel until 1859, where he was said to have a repertory of at least one hundred and fifty cocktails, shrubs, punches, cobblers, juleps, smashes, and "eye-openers." Many of his original drinks, such as the Blue Blazer, a hot whiskey drink—noted because its dramatic presentation involved setting the drink aflame and pouring the blue-flamed libation between two silver mugs—and the Tom and Jerry, an egg nog–like rum punch, continue to be classic cocktails today. See THOMAS, JERRY.

By the late 1850s, many of these barrooms and hotel bars were referred to as "saloons." Despite the Wild West connotation of the word today, it was more of a broad term for a wide range of bars at the time, from a neighborhood spot to a tony hotel bar. "Saloons" were generally considered refuges for men only, and many offered free lunch spreads. These spreads ranged from Spartan to expansive but had in common that they were laden with salty, thirst-inducing foods. The free lunches and saloon culture faded away when Prohibition roared in during the 1920s, replaced by furtive but more egalitarian speakeasies. After Prohibition's repeal in 1933, those speakeasies disappeared and public drinking in bars and restaurants returned. See PROHIBITION; SALOONS; and SPEAKEASIES.

Cocktails remain a point of New York pride. Indeed, a New York publication, *The Balance, and Columbian Repository*, was in 1806 the site of the first instance of the term "cocktail," defined as a "stimulating liquor, composed of spirits of any kind, sugar, water and bitters—it is vulgarly called a bittered sling." The number of New York City–themed cocktails—the Manhattan, the Bronx Cocktail—also attests to the importance of cocktails in New York and national bar culture, as well as important drinks that claim New York as a point of provenance, from the classic martini to the new classic cosmopolitan. See MANHATTAN COCKTAIL; MARTINI; and COSMOPOLITAN.

The birth of bellwether drinks is not all that New York bars have contributed to the fabric of the city; as gathering places from the moment of their inception, monumental events have happened in bars, making them important historic landmarks. George Washington bade farewell to his troops at Fraunces Tavern, the gay rights movement experienced a monumental shift with the Stonewall riots in 1969, and women's rights improved in the 1970s when McSorley's, with its dark and light beers served alongside sleeves of crackers and sliced onion and cheese, finally admitted women into the bar. See FRAUNCES TAVERN; MCSORLEY'S OLD ALE HOUSE; and STONEWALL INN. Craft cocktails may be on the rise, but even those looking for a shot and a beer and a simple conversation with the bartender about those Knicks or the stock market can easily find a multitude of New York City bars to call their own.

Batterberry, Michael, and Ariane Batterberry. *On The Town in New York: The Landmark History of Eating, Drinking, and Entertainments from the American Revolution to the Food Revolution*. New York and London: Routledge, 1999.

Kosmas, Jason, and Dushan Zaric. *Speakeasy: Classic Cocktails Reimagined, from New York's Employees Only Bar*. Berkeley, Calif.: Ten Speed Press, 2010.

Francine Cohen

Bastianich, Lidia

Lidia Bastianich (b. 1947) is a highly successful New York restaurateur, the author of nine popular cookbooks, and an Emmy award–winning figure on public television. She is an active presence at her website lidiasitaly.com; a blogger; a businesswoman; a purveyor of her own line of pastas, sauces, and cookware; and, with her son Joseph, the founder of the Azienda Agricola Bastianich winery in northeast Italy. Her restaurants include her northern Italian flagship Felidia on East Fifty-Eighth Street in Manhattan, which she opened with her then-husband Felice in 1981; the more casual Becco in New York's theater district, which her son Joseph (her partner in the enterprise) opened in 1993; Del Posto, an upscale 2010 restaurant in Chelsea, where her partners are her son Joseph and the well-known chef Mario Batali; Lidia's Italy in Kansas City (1999, again with her son); and Lidia's Italy in Pittsburgh (2000).

Lidia Matticchio Bastianich was born on February 21, 1947, in Pula in the Friuli Venezia Giulia region of Italy, the northeast part of the country that bordered on Austria to the north, Slovenia to the east, and the Adriatic to the south. After World War II, when Italy was forced to give up part of its territories, her birthplace was given to the then-newly formed Yugoslavia, displacing 350,000 ethnic Italians, her family among them. Lidia often stayed with her grandparents in the countryside, where they lived and ate according to the seasons—growing their own vegetables, harvesting their olives and grapes in the fall, and taking their homegrown wheat to the local mill when they needed flour.

In 1956, her parents, Erminina and Vittorio Matticchio, decided to emigrate, first by getting to Trieste, where they lived in a refugee camp, and in 1958, with the help of the Catholic Charities, to the United States. Lidia never saw her grandmother again. The family eventually settled in New York, where Lidia, who spoke the best English in the family, was essential to helping them get established. She always worked—part-time when she was still in school and full-time after she graduated.

On her sixteenth birthday, she was introduced to her future husband, Felice Bastianich, also an Italian immigrant. They married in 1966 and had two children, Joseph, born in 1968, and Tanya, in 1971. That same year, the couple opened Bonavia, a thirty-seat Italian American restaurant in Forest Hills, Queens.

Its success led to a larger restaurant in Queens, the Villa Secondo, where Bastianich's cooking began to attract attention.

In 1981, the family took a financial plunge, selling those restaurants and buying a brownstone building in Manhattan near the Fifty-Ninth Street Bridge, where, after extensive renovations, they opened Felidia. With Lidia as the chef for twelve years, the restaurant featured the northern Italian food of her childhood and attracted the attention of the culinary world, including James Beard and Julia Child, as well as a three-star rating from the *New York Times*.

In 1993 Child asked Bastianich to appear on her television program *Cooking with Master Chefs*, where Bastianich's comfort with the format eventually led to her own television career, which has flourished ever since. Her series on public television includes *Lidia's Italian-American Kitchen*, *Lidia's Family Table*, *Lidia's Italy*, and *Lidia's Italy in America*. At the end of each program, Lidia invites her family to the table to eat (*Tutti a tavola a mangiare*) and share the meal she has just cooked.

Lidia has written nine cookbooks, the first *La Cucina de Lidia* (1990), with Jay Jacobs, and some with her daughter Tanya Bastianich Manuali. The books include *Lidia's Italian Table* (1998), *Lidia's Italian American Kitchen* (2001), *Lidia's Family Table* (2004), *Lidia's Italy* (2007), *Lidia Cooks from the Heart of Italy* (2009), *Lidia's Italy in America* (2011), *Lidia's Favorite Recipes* (2012), *and Lidia's Commonsense Italian Cooking* (2013). She has also written two children's books: *Nonna Tell Me a Story: Lidia's Christmas Kitchen* (2010) and *Nonna's Birthday Surprise* (2013). Her television production company, Tavola Productions, created an animated children's special for public television: "Nonna Tell Me a Story: Lidia's Christmas Kitchen." Her books characteristically combine recipes, culinary history, and recollections of how the foods fit into Italian lives, Italian American lives, and in particular her own family's life.

Family has been a continuous thread in Bastianich's career, although she and Felice divorced in 1997 after disagreements about the direction of the business and the toll that the rapid expansion took on their personal lives. Her mother, children, and grandchildren sometimes appear on her television programs, which are shot in her own home. She co-owns several Manhattan restaurants (Becco, Esca, and Del Posto) with her son and chef Mario Batali

and has an ownership interest (with the Italian company Farinetti) in Eataly, launched in 2010. See BATALI, MARIO and EATALY. Other commercial ventures include a line of cookware and a travel company, Esperienze Italiane, the latter in partnership with her daughter. She still lives in Queens, with her mother.

Bastianich, Lidia. Oral history. In "Voices from the Food Revolution: People Who Changed the Way Americans Eat," New York University Fales Library and Special Collections, New York, 2009.
Lidia's Italy (website). http://www.lidiasitaly.com

Judith Weinraub

Batali, Mario

Mario Batali (b. 1960), with a style all his own (including the idea that orange Crocs and shorts can be worn everywhere), is a multitalented red-haired ball of energy, an American so well versed in Italian regional cooking that New Yorkers can enjoy his special brand of cuisine in all ten of his New York City restaurants. Born and raised in Seattle, Batali combed the United States and Europe for culinary inspiration. After stints in New Jersey, Spain, France, England, and Italy, he made it back to the United States and New York City to settle down, giving millions of New Yorkers and TV viewers worldwide an understanding of the best regional cooking of Italy.

In 1993, Batali, along with his business partner, Steven Crane, opened a restaurant called Po on Cornelia Street in New York's Greenwich Village. The menu at this small Italian trattoria was made up of regional Italian specialties, something Batali had spent three years perfecting in Italy. His love affair with Crocs also began at Po when his wife bought him his first pair as an opening gift. The orange color was his attempt to be visible in a city where everyone seems to wear black. After seven years that saw him blossom as a restaurateur and chef, both in the kitchen and on TV, and saw Cornelia Street become the "restaurant row" of Greenwich Village, Batali exited Po to more fully concentrate his energies on new ventures.

In 1998 Batali and new business partner Joe Bastianich opened Babbo Ristorante e Enoteca on Waverly Place. Their commitment to the great Italian traditions of hospitality and quality soon garnered the restaurant three stars from *New York Times* restaurant critic Ruth Reichl. The James Beard Foundation named Babbo the "Best New Restaurant of 1998." Their collaboration continued with a string of hit restaurants that opened in New York and elsewhere over the next twelve years.

In 2002 Batali won the James Beard Foundation's "Best Chef: New York City" award, and in 2005 it awarded him the designation "Outstanding Chef of the Year." In 2008 it crowned him "Best Restaurateur," after which he was named to the Culinary Hall of Fame.

In part, Batali's fame is driven by his mastery of social media and digital marketing as much as his culinary skills. The Batali team offers a YouTube channel; TV shows on Food Network, ABC, PBS, and Hulu; e-mails of recipes and videos; and a website with more food prep videos, all promoted across a broad spectrum of social media platforms. From 1997 to 2008 Batali regularly appeared on the Food Network in the shows *Iron Chef* and *Molto Mario*, among others. He hosted a culinary travel show focused on Spain for PBS. In 2011 he became cohost of the daytime TV show *The Chew* on ABC. Through it all, videos of his cooking techniques and recipe preparation appeared on YouTube and on his personal website. *The High Road with Mario Batali* is a Hulu channel show that began in June 2014, with each episode featuring conversations with interesting personalities on journeys around New York City. While there may be food in the show, it is more about experiencing little-sung places and events, with a different celebrity guest each week, than it is a culinary tour.

Batali is an active supporter of the Food Bank for New York City, which is the city's major hunger-relief organization. Since the mid-1980s it has provided hunger assistance in the form of meals, food stamps, tax assistance, dietary education, and increased awareness of food poverty through its network of more than one thousand charities and schools citywide. In 2003 Batali joined its board of directors. Since 2005 he and his wife, Susan, have co-chaired the Food Bank's Can-Do Awards Dinner. He also founded and chairs the Food Bank's Culinary Council, which is made up of top chefs and food industry leaders joined in the fight to end hunger.

Bill Buford, an editor at the *New Yorker* magazine, used his growing interest in food and Batali's passion for Italian cooking to secure an assignment for a magazine article on him. Then, in 2005 Buford quit his position for a career-changing full-time job in the kitchen at Babbo under "iron chef" Batali. That experience led to his book *Heat*. According to Anthony Bourdain, *Heat* "is a long overdue portrait of the real Mario Batali" who "is finally revealed for the Falstaffian, larger than life, mercurial, frighteningly intelligent chef/entrepreneur he really is."

Batali is the author of ten cookbooks, including the James Beard Award–winning *Molto Italiano: 327 Simple Italian Recipes* (2005). *America Farm to Table: Simple, Delicious Recipes Celebrating Local Farmers* was published in 2014.

Besides his TV shows, restaurants, cookbooks, and even a brief interest in a wine shop, Batali has other culinary interests. Eataly is a megastore chain encompassing everything Italian that is part open market, part grocery store, and part food court. It features restaurants, wine shops, and artisanal food distributors that fill the 50,000-square-foot space. The New York City Eataly, which is partly owned by Batali, opened in 2010 to positive reviews and weeks of customers lining up outside waiting for the chance to experience it.

Batali resides in New York City's Greenwich Village with his wife Susi Cahn (her parents own Coach Dairy Goat Farm in Dutchess County) and two sons, Leo and Benno. The boys also have their own cookbook, *The Batali Brothers Cookbook*. The original handmade version was a birthday gift for their father, which was picked up by his publisher.

See also BASTIANICH, LIDIA and EATALY.

Bourdain, Anthony. Review of *Heat*. http://www .amazon.com/Heat-Amateur-Cook-Professional-Kitchen-ebook/dp/B000GCFVUQ.
Buford, Bill. *HEAT: An Amateur Cook in a Professional Kitchen*. New York: Random House, 2013.
Mario Batali (website). http://www.mariobatali.com.

Richard Frisbie

Bathtub Gin

See DISTILLERIES.

Batterberry, Michael and Ariane

Longtime New Yorkers Michael and Ariane Batterberry created two groundbreaking national food magazines: *Food & Wine* in 1978 and *Food Arts* in

1988. They also cowrote the first serious book to examine the history of eating and drinking in America, *On The Town in New York* (1973, revised in 1999). Together they helped shape the way Americans think about cooking, chefs, and restaurants.

Their backgrounds were different, but both Batterberrys developed an appreciation for good food early on. Each had family cooks, and each had been exposed to much more than basic American cooking. Michael Batterberry was born in 1932 to American parents in England, where his father represented Procter & Gamble. Family travels to Belgium and France for his father's job introduced him to European food, and trips back and forth to the United States on ocean liners gave him an appreciation for fine service. When he was seven and a half, the family returned to the United States, living in Cincinnati, in Kentucky where his grandmother lived, and eventually in Greenwich, Connecticut, and New York City. Ariane Ruskin was born in 1935 on the Upper East Side of Manhattan. Her parents loved good food, and in an era when people dressed up to eat out, she accompanied them to fine restaurants like Le Pavillon and The Colony Club at an early age. See LE PAVILLON and COLONY CLUB. A graduate of Barnard and a former graduate student at Cambridge University, she had also written a survey of the history of art for young people.

At the age of twenty, Michael Batterberry left New York with his family to move to Venezuela for his father's job. While based there, he also spent time traveling with friends to Haiti and European hot spots like Rome and Madrid, where he cooked, learned local cuisines, painted, did some interior design, and occasionally performed in cabarets. When he returned to New York, he continued to paint and write and even tried his hand at designing store windows. Batterberry met Ariane Ruskin at a party. In 1968, the couple married.

Although initially the Batterberrys wrote separately, they decided to work together over several years to write what became *On The Town in New York: The Landmark History of Eating, Drinking, and Entertainments from the American Revolution to the Food Revolution* (1973). The book traced developments in eating and drinking establishments—the restaurants, the chefs, the clientele, the menus, the trends—from the taverns of the late eighteenth century to the pleasure gardens of the early nineteenth century through the post–World War II years and the beginnings of the American food revolution. Twenty-five years later they released a revised and updated edition.

In 1978, when American interest in food, chefs, and cooking had spread far beyond French restaurants and traditional home cooking, the Batterberrys came up with a new magazine, *Food & Wine*. Published with backing from Playboy Club founder Hugh Hefner, the publication celebrated regional cuisines and the fine chefs who were emerging and developing a following all over the country—people like Paul Prudhomme, Alice Waters, and Jasper White. Two years later, when their investors wanted their money back for other projects, the couple left *Food & Wine* and eventually set up Batterberry Associates, which took on different kinds of food, film, television, and publishing projects, several of them for Time, Inc.

In 1988, they created *Food Arts*, an entirely new kind of glossy trade magazine for chefs and people in the food and hospitality industries. Michael Batterberry was the editor and Ariane Batterberry the publisher, an arrangement that continued after Marvin Shanken bought the magazine from them two years later. *Food Arts* was unusual. It focused not only on trends and people in the fine dining industry, including articles accompanied by fine photography and often recipes, but also on subjects that Michael Batterberry thought people in the industry should know about. These subjects included trends that would become important but had not quite emerged yet: food history, the congressional farm bills, female chefs, and immigrant farmers. One of its popular features was its Silver Spoon awards, a monthly column that highlighted the achievements of individuals throughout the food industry and its supporters.

Michael Batterberry died in 2010. Ariane Batterberry stayed at the magazine until September 2014, when, after twenty-five years, *Food Arts* ceased publication.

See also FOOD & WINE and FOOD ARTS.

Batterberry, Michael, and Ariane Batterberry. *On The Town in New York: The Landmark History of Eating, Drinking, and Entertainments from the American Revolution to the Food Revolution.* Rev. ed. New York and London: Routledge, 1999.

Batterberry, Michael, and Ariane Batterberry. *Voices from the Food Revolution: People Who Changed the Way Americans Eat.* Fales Library and Special

Collections, New York University. http://dlib.nyu.edu/beard/content/welcome-voices-food-revolution.

Judith Weinraub

Baum, Joe

Joseph H. Baum (1920–1998) was "the most important restaurateur of the twentieth century," according to food critic Craig Claiborne. The theatrical wizard of food and hospitality created more than sixty-five restaurants in his lifetime, including five of New York's three-star restaurants and two of the world's largest-grossing and most dramatic restaurants—the Rainbow Room atop Rockefeller Center (1987–2000), Windows on the World (1976) (and indeed all of the restaurants at the World Trade Center complex), and the re-creation of Windows on the World (1996), which included "The Greatest Bar on Earth." Another major triumph of his career included the three-star restaurant Aurora. See RAINBOW ROOM and WINDOWS ON THE WORLD.

Born in 1920 in Saratoga Springs, New York, Baum began working in his parents' hotel at age fourteen, then went to Cornell University, to the U.S. Navy, and on to make culinary history. Baum revolutionized restaurants. He stopped "doing the Continental" and broke from the European model, turning instead to thematic dining concepts based on sensuality, theatrical design, and culinary discovery.

As an executive of the firm Restaurant Associates in the 1950s and 1960s and president from 1963 to 1970, Baum redesigned or created dozens of New York's iconic dining spots, including The Hawaiian Room, Zum Zum, Charlie O's, Fonda del Sol, Tower Suite, and even a high-end restaurant famous for flambé in Newark airport called The Newarker. He introduced the city to two new types of restaurants that he called by their *forms*, trattoria and brasserie; and he masterminded the outlandish Forum of the Twelve Caesars, where pheasant was served on a soldier's shield and wine buckets, made from glittering warriors' helmets, reflected the obsessively designed lighting. The menu's preamble, *Cenabis Bene...Apud Me* (You will dine well at my table), was the essence of Baum. His restaurants exemplified his larger-than-life style with a new kind of casualness set in the midst of high-minded design and high-end cuisine. His prescient menu at the Four Seasons, created in 1959, was peppered with Baum's sensibility: "Our field greens are selected each morning and will vary daily." Farmer's Sprouts with Bacon, Beets with Rosemary, and Braised Lettuce with Marrow and Almonds were among the sixteen side dishes offered. More than half a century later, the Four Seasons restaurant still sparkles with seasonal, local ingredients and feels modern in the exuberant mode he established. See FOUR SEASONS.

Baum formed his own company in 1971 with partners Michael Whiteman, founding editor of *Nation's Restaurant News*, and Dennis Sweeney. See NATION'S RESTAURANT NEWS. It lives on today as the international consulting company Baum + Whiteman. Hired by the Port Authority, their first project was the creation of twenty-two restaurants at the World Trade Center, including the Big Kitchen (the world's first food court), the three-star Market Bar & Dining Rooms, Cellar in the Sky, and the legendary Windows on the World. Also included was the Hors d'Oeuvrerie, opening in 1976 on the 107th floor. There, Baum merged small plates of sushi, quesadillas, *bündnerfleisch* (an air-dried beef), and Thai spring rolls on a single menu that foretold the ultrarelaxed "grazing" craze. This concept would reappear at Rainbow in 1987 as "Cocktails and Little Meals" and ignite America's cocktail revolution.

With culinary luminaries James Beard, Barbara Kafka, Jacques Pépin, Albert Cumin, and Rozanne Gold, Baum developed numerous innovative concepts and menus that still reverberate today. He was the first restaurateur to hire world-famous architects and artists, including Hugh Hardy, Warren Platner, and Milton Glaser, to implement his ideas. Baum received the industry's most prestigious awards, including the Escoffier Medal and the James Beard Lifetime Achievement Award. Baum died in 1998. His influence on New York City restaurants lives on through Baum + Whiteman, and through a newer generation of chefs, restaurateurs, and New Yorkers who continue to eat and drink his dreams.

See RESTAURANT ASSOCIATES and RESTAURANTS.

Greene, Gael. "Remembering Joe Baum." *New York Magazine*, October 26, 1998.
Grimes, William. *Appetite City: A Culinary History of New York*. New York: North Point, 2009.
Matsumoto, Nancy. "Tastemaker: The Legacy of Joe Baum." *Edible Manhattan*, July–August 2010.

Rozanne Gold

Bay Ridge

Bay Ridge is a neighborhood located in the southwest corner of Brooklyn. See BROOKLYN. Successive immigrant populations have called Bay Ridge home and have helped to create a diverse and interesting culinary landscape in the neighborhood.

Bay Ridge was far removed from New York City throughout the eighteenth and early nineteenth centuries. But with the consolidation of the five boroughs in 1898 and the development of transportation lines into the area, Bay Ridge began to develop as a middle-class suburb of Manhattan. Since then, Bay Ridge has drawn generations of immigrant homeowners, including Scandinavians, Italians, and Greeks in the early twentieth century and Southern European and Middle Eastern immigrants since the mid-twentieth century. Each of these groups has left its mark on the food landscape of Bay Ridge. More recent immigrant groups, including East Asians and Russians, are sure to add to the culinary diversity of the neighborhood.

Bay Ridge's main commercial strips run along Third Avenue and Fifth Avenue, and each is lined with restaurants and stores, including a host of halal butchers and specialty food shops selling Arabic, Greek, Italian, and other delicacies. Among the most famous of these shops are The Family Store on Third Avenue and the half-century-old Leske's Bakery, A&S Greek Deli and Butcher, and spice and provisions shop Balady on Fifth Avenue (which rivals the venerable Sahadi's on Brooklyn's Atlantic Avenue). See ARAB COMMUNITY; GREEK; and ITALIAN. Famous Bay Ridge restaurants include the Italian restaurant Gino's (established 1964) and chef Rawia Bishara's Tanoreen (established 1998), the highest-rated Middle-Eastern restaurant in the 2014 Zagat Guide. While few Scandinavians remain in Bay Ridge, the neighborhood's history as "Little Norway" is recalled by the annual Norwegian Day Parade (established in 1951). Nordic Delicacies, which opened in 1987 and sold Norwegian meatballs, herring salad, and lingonberry jelly to residents and visitors, closed in early 2015. See SCANDINAVIAN and SYRIAN AND LEBANESE.

Bay Ridge has an active nightlife with sports bars, Irish pubs, hookah lounges, and nightclubs lining Third and Fifth Avenues. One of these clubs, 2001 Odyssey Disco (closed 2006), was the home away from home of disco champ Tony Manero in the movie *Saturday Night Fever*, which took place in Bay Ridge.

While the neighborhood maintains an old-school, small-town feel and counts among its residents many third-generation Bay Ridgers, the area is not immune to the real estate boom overtaking much of Brooklyn. Rents and home prices in Bay Ridge are rising and newcomers to the neighborhood include not only working- and middle-class immigrants but also young professionals and families from other parts of Brooklyn and Manhattan. Bay Ridge's food scene is reflecting these recent changes with farm-to-table restaurants such as Petit Oven and Brooklyn Beet Company, along with the Owl's Head Wine Bar, A.L.C. Italian Grocery, Robicelli's Bakery, the Lock Yard beer garden, Ho'Brah taco shop, and Zito's Sandwich Shoppe. Many of these businesses are owned and operated by native Bay Ridgers who have returned to the neighborhood after living elsewhere in the city and opened food businesses to cater to the "new Bay Ridge." Bay Ridge also has two community-supported agriculture farms, a weekly greenmarket, and a burgeoning food co-op. See COMMUNITY SUPPORTED AGRICULTURE; GREENMARKETS; and FOOD CO-OPS.

Bay Ridge has spawned two national chains. Sbarro began as an Italian grocery in Bay Ridge in the mid-twentieth century, and Boulder Creek Steakhouse originated in Bay Ridge as well.

Falkowitz, Max. "A Tour of Bay Ridge with Allison Robicelli." Serious Eats, August 15, 2013. http://newyork.seriouseats.com/2013/08/allison-robicelli-tour-bay-ridge-where-to-eat.html.

Hanson, Barbara. "Find the Classic Bay Ridge at Nordic Delicacies." Serious Eats, August 21, 2008. http://newyork.seriouseats.com/2008/08/nordic-delicacies-in-bay-ridge-scandinavian-brooklyn-new-york-city-nyc.html.

Reiss, Marcia. *Bay Ridge Fort Hamilton Guide*. Brooklyn, N.Y.: Brooklyn Historical Society, 2003.

Cindy R. Lobel

Beard, James

James Beard (1903–1985), often referred to as the "Dean of American Cookery" and the "Father of American Gastronomy," was a cookbook author, teacher, and cultural icon who helped bring approachable, seasonal cooking into the American kitchen.

Author of over twenty cookbooks, many of which remain in print today, Beard rose to prominence during the postwar boom, championing American cooking in the age of French haute cuisine and paving the way for the food revolution of the 1970s and 1980s through his writing and his cooking schools.

Born on May 5, 1903 in Portland, Oregon, Beard arrived at an astonishing fourteen pounds, foreshadowing both his imposing adult physique (six feet four, over three hundred pounds) as well as the outsized imprint he would make on the American culinary world. He gained an early appreciation for food and the kitchen from his mother, Elizabeth Beard, an English immigrant who owned a hotel in Portland prior to marriage and who during Beard's childhood ran a boarding house out of their home.

Elizabeth had traveled extensively in her youth, a passion she would pass on to her son, along with a sophisticated palate and a flair for the dramatic. Beard's father, John, an employee at the local Customs House, was more of a distant figure in his son's life but is credited with teaching him about foraging, fishing, and outdoor cooking, skills that Beard later incorporated into his classes and books.

Beard's fascination with food first blossomed during trips to the Lewis and Clark Exposition of 1905, where at age three he was mesmerized by a demonstration of the manufacture of Triscuit crackers. His formative years were also influenced by Jue-Let, the Chinese cook Elizabeth employed in the boarding house kitchen, who looked after the young James and launched Beard's lifelong interest in Asian cultures, seen later in his home decorating and fashion aesthetic (he was often photographed in one of many custom-made kimonos). It also manifested itself in his personal brand of cooking, which emphasized stir-fries just as much as sloppy joes.

The introduction of exotic cuisines from his mother and Jue-Let intermingled with the lessons from his summers in coastal Gearhart, Oregon, where the family had a vacation home. Those trips spent fishing, clamming, gathering wild produce, and cooking with the results were some of Beard's fondest memories. He would carry this duality with him throughout his life. Despite the sophisticated tastes developed by his well-traveled mother and his own admitted ardor for French cuisine above all else, Beard always held onto his roots in the Pacific Northwest, returning to the Oregon coast throughout his life

and later establishing a cooking school in Seaside, Oregon.

Beard studied briefly at Reed College, where he was active in student government and theater, participating in operas and winning a prize in a Halloween costume contest for his appearance in full drag. He was expelled in 1923; Reed claimed it was because of poor scholastic performance, but Beard maintained it was because of his homosexuality. He then traveled to Europe to study voice and theater for two years, before returning to the United States and settling in New York City to pursue an acting career.

Unfortunately, stage roles for someone of Beard's size and stature were limited, and he soon turned his full attention to food. In 1935, with siblings Bill Rhode and Irma Rhode, he opened Hors d'Oeuvre, Inc., a small food shop and catering service. Located on New York's tony Upper East Side, the company appealed to the neighborhood's wealthy clientele and sought to revamp the current offerings of American party appetizers. Beard used lessons gleaned from this period to publish his first cookbook, *Hors d'Oeuvre & Canapés* (1940), which he wrote in just six weeks. He followed up in 1942 with *Cook It Outdoors*, the first tome dedicated to open-air cooking, which in classic Beard fashion included over a dozen recipes for hamburgers, ranging from the traditional ground meat patty to the "Baghdad burger" with eggplant and barbecue sauce.

Beard's writing career and business were interrupted by the eruption of World War II. After a brief stint in the cryptography division, Beard moved to the United Seamen's Service, where he spent the rest of the war setting up canteens for soldiers in Puerto Rico, Rio de Janeiro, and Panama.

After the war, luxury industries like fashion, travel, and food were feeding off of the availability of disposable income and television was exploding into the cultural consciousness. This proved a perfect fit for Beard's penchant for performance. He returned to New York in 1945 and shortly afterward appeared on some of NBC's earliest programming as the cooking expert on the daytime "magazine show" *Radio City Matinee* in 1946 (retitled *For You & Yours* when it moved to prime time) and later as the host of one of the first televised cooking shows, *Elsie Presents James Beard in "I Love to Eat,"* in 1947.

With the publication of his exhaustive, illustrated love letter to home cooking, *The Fireside Cookbook*, in 1949, Beard was considered "America's fore-most culinary authority." The 1950s saw his writing career expand even further afield as he contributed articles and columns to *Woman's Day*, *Gourmet* (edited by his old partner Bill Rhode), and *House & Garden*. In his cookbooks and articles he presented an approachable, vernacular voice that made space for a more conversational tone in food writing as a genre. This also allowed Beard to communicate without pretension the vast knowledge of world cuisines accumulated in his travels, leading to regional American recipes made of seasonal ingredients accented with French techniques. He was also employed by Restaurant Associates as a consultant to food producers and restaurateurs and even found time to manage Chez Lucky Pierre, a short-order beach restaurant in Nantucket. See RESTAURANT ASSOCIATES.

It was there on Nantucket that Beard met André Surmain, then owner of the New York City restaurant Lutèce. Surmain would help Beard establish the James Beard Cooking School in 1955. Originally located in Surmain's own drawing room, the school eventually moved to Beard's first house on West Tenth Street in Greenwich Village; he and the cooking school later moved to 167 West Twelfth Street. Beard continued to conduct classes for the next thirty years at both his New York and Seaside, Oregon, schools, as well as across the country at women's clubs, civic groups, and other cooking schools.

Despite coauthoring a budget-based cookbook, *How to Eat Better for Less Money* (1954), Beard struggled to manage his own finances. As a result, throughout his life he sought out endorsements and commercial opportunities to support himself, unintentionally becoming a pioneer of the sponsorships commonly seen in the food world today. Some of his major corporate partnerships included consulting on boil-in-bag technology for Green Giant, helping Pillsbury create refrigerated crescent rolls, and writing a cookbook to introduce Americans to the Cuisinart food processor. There was one type of endorsement Beard continually resisted, however: he refused to write any sort of "diet" cookbook, considering them fleeting fads.

Beard's innumerable contributions to the culture of food in America continued in his later life. Beard counted the elite of the food world—M. F. K. Fisher, Craig Claiborne, Alice B. Toklas, and Marion Cunningham—among his inner circle, and in the 1960s he became close with Julia Child, introducing her to the New York food scene and helping to promote *Mastering the Art of French Cooking*. See CHILD, JULIA.

Health issues plagued Beard as he aged, and despite his earlier resistance to trendy diets, in the early 1970s he was forced to go on a severe low-calorie, no-salt diet. This led to the publication of *The New James Beard* in 1981, a cookbook of recipes that followed his new dietary restrictions. It was during this period that he moved to his last house at 167 West Twelfth Street, today the home of the James Beard Foundation. The James Beard Cooking School continued there until his death, although Beard hired other staff to teach the classes as his health declined.

In 1978 Beard was given *Le Médaille d'Ordre du Mérite Argicole* by the French Consulate, a testament to his lifelong devotion to Gallic culture and cuisine and a prize he valued more than any Oscar dreamt of in his youth. He spent his final years as he had the bulk of his career—writing, teaching, and traveling—and was crowned "King of Food" by *Cuisine Magazine* in 1983. He was set to be the honorary chair at the International Association of Cooking Professionals conference in Seattle in March 1985 but died just before, on January 21, 1985. Today, Beard's legacy lives on through the James Beard Foundation, which continues in his spirit by celebrating, nurturing, and honoring America's diverse culinary heritage.

See also JAMES BEARD AWARDS; JAMES BEARD FOUNDATION; and TELEVISION.

Beard, James. *Delights and Prejudices*. New York: Collier, 1964.
Fussell, Betty. "James Beard, American Icon." *Beard House Magazine* 17, no. 1 (2003): 77–78.
James Beard Foundation. "About James Beard." http://www.jamesbeard.org/about/james-beard.
Jones, Evan. *Epicurean Delight: The Life and Times of James Beard*. New York: Knopf, 1990.
Polan, Dana. "James Beard's Early TV Work: A Report on Research." *Gastronomica: The Journal of Food and Culture* 10, no. 3 (2010): 23–33.

Maggie E. Borden

Bedford-Stuyvesant

If you talked about a "food scene" in Brooklyn's Bedford-Stuyvesant neighborhood as recently as the 1990s, you were probably referencing corner bodega sandwiches, fried chicken restaurants, or maybe the occasional Jamaican roti spot. Nowadays, when people talk about the neighborhood made famous by hip-hop artists and Spike Lee's movie *Do the Right Thing*, it sounds like they are talking about a trendy strip of the West Village.

The neighborhood, once mostly known for its beautiful Victorian brownstones but also its high rate of crime and riots in the 1960s, is now a destination for hot dining spots like Black Swan, a European-centric gastropub serving jerk pork chops and steak and chips platters along with a hearty selection of craft beers. Stop by the small bakery SCRATCH-bread in the mornings, and you will find a line of people waiting outside for vanilla bean shortbread and orange currant scones. The owner, Matt Tilden, was so passionate about the project that he tattooed the SCRATCHbread logo onto his left forearm, before he even opened the business.

The neighborhood—bordered on the west by Clinton Hill, on the east by Bushwick, with Williamsburg to the north and Crown Heights to the south—has emerged as a popular place to live for young people priced out of other areas. Naturally, coffee shops, trendy restaurants, and gastropubs have followed. A YouTube video of seventeen-year-old Notorious B.I.G., the late rapper behind hits like "Juicy" and "Big Poppa" (who claimed the neighborhood as his home even though he was technically from neighboring Clinton Hill) shows him free-style rapping on the street with a large group of other black teens; now the spot is home to Do or Dine, a trendy restaurant that opened in 2011, selling foie gras doughnuts and twenty-eight-dollar New Zealand duck breast. That doughnut, by the way, comes from nearby Dough, which *New York Magazine*'s Grub Street blog rated the best in the country in 2014. See DOUGHNUTS.

Like a lot of New York history, it started with the Dutch, who established a farming community on the land in the seventeenth century. See COLONIAL DUTCH. The neighborhood's black population began to boom in the 1950s when people settled there after being locked out of many white residential areas. Eventually that attracted other black immigrants and their cuisines that still influence the neighborhood. See CARIBBEAN. For instance, the A&A Bake and Doubles Shop on Nostrand Avenue has been a neighborhood staple for years, serving up its famous doubles (chickpea sandwiches in fried bread) and even accepting Trinidadian currency. Senegalese and West African dishes serving up okra stew and sorrel are still easily found in long-standing eateries.

Now that Bed-Stuy is changing again, long-time residents are wary of intense gentrification but are also celebrating a successful rebirth. The Bedford Hill Coffee Bar hosts readings before diverse crowds over espresso drinks; across the street, the bar One Last Shag features frozen cocktails and bumping dance parties almost every weekend. The folks behind the craft beer–loving Brooklyn chain that includes Bar Great Harry and Mission Dolores opened Glorietta Baldy in 2013, offering tasty brews and pin-ball in a no-frills setting. The old neighborhood spots are getting new life too: beloved dive bar Tip Top Bar and Grill still slings cheap drinks and hot jams on the jukebox; an old Salvation Army building has become home to Crazy Legs, a roller disco that is keeping New York's roller-skating tradition alive.

See also BROOKLYN; BUSHWICK; and WILLIAMSBURG.

Echanove, Matias. "Bed-Stuy on the Move: Demographic Trends and Economic Development in the Heart of Brooklyn." M.S. thesis, Columbia University, 2003.

Tim Donnelly

Beekeeping

New Yorkers have played an important role in the development of the commercial honey industry, beginning in the mid-1800s. By this point, honey-bees were prevalent everywhere in the eastern part of the country. Around this time, Moses Quinby, a New Yorker, became the first documented person to make a living solely on the production and sale of honey. Quinby inspired other beekeepers in his area to join him, making the Catskill region of New York the first commercial center of honey production (Oertel, 1980, p. 5).

New York's climate and landscape continue to make it ideal for honey production. Variety in the flowers, and even the seasons, means variety in the tastes and flavors of the honey produced. Ross Ber, a Queens beekeeper of twelve years and producer of Berz Beez Honey, elaborates that what makes New York State amazing is that you will find the same diversity of plants in the north of the state that you will find in the east, west, or south. This means that honey collected from the Niagara Falls region of New York could taste the same as honey collected within the five boroughs of New York City.

What a bee eats is what determines the taste of its honey; therefore, within the state of New York, the season in which the honey is collected will impact the taste more so than the location of the hives. Ber, for example, sells four types of honey: spring, summer, fall, as well as a buckwheat honey. The taste of the seasonal honeys reflects what is in season at that time of year. Springtime dandelions, clovers, and forsythias yield a honey fragrant, light in color, and tangy in flavor. As the seasons progress, the flowers get darker and more vibrant in color, while at the same time becoming less fragrant. Accordingly, Ber's summer honey is floral in taste, midtoned in color, and semifragrant, while his fall honey is dark in color, robust in flavor, but lacking aroma.

Although New York City enjoys the same lush diversity of flora as the rest of the state, it can also provide some interesting obstacles for a would-be honey producer. Bees are extremely resourceful, and if they cannot find a sufficient natural source of sugar within the three-mile fly zone radius of their hive, they will make use of whatever source of sugar they do find. Ber recounts story after story of city apiarists who have learned this lesson all too well. There was, for example, the purple honey sourced from the Manischewitz kosher wine plant, the red honey found in hives by the maraschino cherry factory, and even the green honey derived from a faulty vat of green coloring at the M&M candy factory. Unfortunately, none of the resulting honeys tasted very good, and more importantly, the human-made sugars were terrible for the health of the bees.

Finding the right location to maintain a beehive within the five boroughs has been tricky for other reasons as well. In 1999, under Mayor Rudolph Giuliani, the city's Department of Health and Mental Hygiene passed a law that prohibited wild animals (including honeybees) from being kept by New York City residents. In 2010, after much lobbying by Gotham's bee and honey enthusiasts, the bees were given a pass by the city council. Ber confided that people had found loopholes to the ban, either by having historical and environmental societies house their hives or by just keeping them on their own property and hoping for the best.

The bill restoring the rights of city residents to keep hives came with the provision that all managed hives should be registered with the Department of Health and Mental Hygiene. According to the *New York Times*, in June 2012, 141 people had registered 182 hives with the Department of Health and Mental Hygiene since the ban was lifted; but those figures only cover the people who were willing to register their hives. The article estimated that the actual number of hives could be as many as four hundred.

Because of the lack of space, the city's honey producers find all sorts of creative spots to locate their hives. According to the *New York Times*, hives were stashed on the roof of the Waldorf Astoria Hotel as well as at the Whitney Museum of Art in its former Upper East Side location. With the advent of "green" roofs, bees have found homes atop some of Manhattan's tallest skyscrapers. In 2013, the Durst Organization imported some one hundred thousand bees to populate its vegetation-covered roofs in midtown Manhattan, including the fifty-one-story One Bryant Park. See ROOFTOP GARDEN.

Most of the city's producers are small. The largest of the city's producers operate around thirty to fifty hives, which is minimal when compared to the tens of thousands of hives managed by producers with hives in multiple states. Because of the space limitations, larger producers in the city are likely to use multiple locations and share these with other apiarists. Ber, for example, is just one of several apiarists with hives in Alley Pond Park in Queens. These small-scale operations provide many benefits for the consumer.

A producer like Ber can keep his operation natural, avoiding chemicals and antibiotics without the same threat of loss that a larger producer would have. Illnesses spread quickly through hives in close proximity to one another. Although not all small-scale producers keep their operations natural, they at least have the option to, and many in New York City exercise that option. Another benefit to keeping things small-scale is that honey is considered a farm product, so it falls under the jurisdiction of the U.S. Department of Agriculture, which means that a producer would have to sell about fifty thousand dollars worth of honey before the agency's rules would begin to apply. No small-scale producer is going to sell that much. Meanwhile, the revenue from a small-scale operation is enough to cover the start-up and annual operating costs and still make a reasonable profit.

In an age where "small," "local," and "all natural" are marketable buzzwords and a growing agricultural movement is pushing for a return to a more localized system, the demand for hyperlocal honey has grown. The city has also seen an explosion of farmers' markets, health food stores, and specialty markets since the mid-1990s, many of which sell honey from these local, small-scale producers. This means that the possibilities for profit continue to grow.

Bono, Pat. "The Big New York State Honey Harvest: Empire State Honey Producers Association, New York's State Beekeeping Organization." September 12, 2013. http://www.prweb.com/releases/2013/9/prweb11111626.htm.

Horn, Tammy. *Bees in America: How the Honey Bee Shaped a Nation.* Lexington: University Press of Kentucky, 2005.

Oertel, Everett. "History of Beekeeping in the United States." In *Beekeeping in the United States*, pp. 2–9. Agriculture Handbook 335. Washington, D.C.: U.S. Department of Agriculture, 1980.

Satow, Julie. "Worker Bees on a Rooftop, Ignoring Urban Pleasures." *New York Times*, August 6, 2013.

Michele Louis

Beer

From the first settling of what is now Manhattan island until the present, beer has been an industry vital to the social, political, and commercial interests of New Yorkers. Although potable water was available, beer was the beverage of choice from the early seventeenth century through the late eighteenth century. It was considered the drink of moderation when compared to rum, the city's early spirit of choice. See RUM.

Among the first buildings constructed in New Amsterdam in 1612 was a brewery housed in a log structure, home to Jean Vigne, the first white child born in the colony. Vigne would survive to become a brewer and prominent citizen of the colony. By 1629, there were only 350 people in the settlement, but the West Indies Company constructed another brewery just outside the fortification on a path that became known as "Brewers Street." Vigne was the brewer. When the English seized control of New Amsterdam in 1664, renaming it New York, there were at least ten breweries serving a population of only sixteen hundred people. Prominent brewing families exerted considerable influence on New York's government for generations.

In 1748, a visiting Swede noted in his journal that, "there is no good water to be met with in the town itself; but at a little distance there is a large spring of water, which the inhabitants take their tea, and for the uses of the kitchen." Author and historian Stanley Baron records in *Brewed in America* (1962, p. 71) that "Until the ordinary water was proven to be wholesome and pure, the people of New York would go on drinking manufactured beverages, preferably those with some alcoholic content." A historian of 1756 reported that the common drinks were "beer, cider, (and) weak punch and Madeira wine. Beer in particular was used in large-scale celebrations."

During the early nineteenth century, beer production in New York declined, in part because of the deteriorating quality of the city's water. City brewers complained to the city government about the inadequate water supply. This concern, and others, encouraged the city to embark on a massive project to bring water to Manhattan from upstate via the Croton Aqueduct. With the completion of the Croton Aqueduct in 1842, the city's brewing industry took off. The explosion of the popularity of pale, yellow, crystal, effervescent "lager" beer in the mid-1800s was the result of a major influx of German immigrants and a high point for the brewing industry in New York City. See GERMAN and WATER.

Brooklyn and Manhattan became two of the major brewing centers of the country. In 1898 Brooklyn had forty-eight working breweries. In 1920 there were still at least thirty-nine major commercial brewing enterprises in New York and Brooklyn. Some of the most popular were S. Liebmann's Sons, Piel Bros., F. & M. Schaefer Brewing, John F. Trommer, Ebling Brewing, Hell Gate Brewery, Jacob Hoffman Brewing, Oriental Brewery, John Eichler Brewing, Valentine Loewer's Gambrinus Brewing, Jacob Ruppert, and Kips Bay Brewing.

Anti-German sentiment during World War I was a major factor in Congress passing the Eighteenth Amendment and the Volstead law that outlawed the manufacture, sale, and importation of alcoholic beverages. When Prohibition began in 1920 most of New York's breweries closed, though they revived when Prohibition ended in 1933. But anti-German sentiment again played a role in closing a number of breweries during World War II. See PROHIBITION; WORLD WAR I; and WORLD WAR II.

The growth of nationally distributed beers, the influence of mass media advertising, and the ease of transporting product over the interstate highway system set the stage for the development of mega-breweries with international business connections. As late as 1960 Brooklyn was still brewing 10 percent of the beer manufactured in this country, but by 1969 only four breweries operated in New York City, and soon there were none. The first to go were Piel Brothers and Joseph Schlitz Brewing in 1973. Brooklyn lost its last remaining breweries in 1976 when both F. & M. Schaefer and Rheingold closed their doors.

What is now known as the microbrewing, or craft brewing, movement began in 1976 with a single brewery in California called New Albion Brewing. It took nearly ten years for the movement to reach New York City, when the Manhattan Brewing Company began producing beer in 1984. Microbreweries and brewpubs in New York City today are spread over all five boroughs of the city.

The "beer scene" in New York City has again begun to catch the imagination of beer drinkers, bartenders, restaurateurs, and chefs. There are over 159 beer bars (restaurant, pubs, bars, and taverns that take pride in the quality and variety of beers served) scattered among the five boroughs of New York City and over a dozen breweries currently in operation. They vary from a five-gallon operation on Coney Island to the Brooklyn Brewery, which brewed approximately 260,000 barrels of beer in 2014 (though a significant percentage of that total was brewed on contract in upstate Utica by F. X. Matt Brewing). Each of these breweries produces at least three different styles of beer, resulting in over sixty made-in-New York choices for beer drinkers.

New York City brewers created the New York City Brewers Guild to interface with the breweries with relation to legislation and taxation. The guild also sponsors New York City Beer Week each February. A recent trend that has developed among restaurants is to have one of the city breweries produce a beer especially for that restaurant. New York City may not be beer nirvana, but it can again be considered a beer destination.

See also BROOKLYN BREWERY; BREWERIES; and MICROBREWERIES AND BREWPUBS.

Baron, Stanley. *Brewed in America*. Boston: Little Brown, 1962.
Oliver, Garrett, ed. *The Oxford Companion to Beer*. New York: Oxford University Press, 2012.
United States Brewers Foundation. *Brewers Almanac*. Frankfort, Ky.: United States Brewers Foundation, 1960.
Valentine, David T. *History of the City of New York*. New York: Putnam, 1853.
Western Brewer, ed. *100 Years of Brewing: A Complete History of the Progress Made in the Art, Science and Industry of Brewing in the World, Particularly during the Nineteenth Century*. Chicago: H. S. Rich, 1903.

                                                Peter LaFrance

Beer Gardens

German immigrants, who made up a large portion of the workforce that powered New York City in the nineteenth century, brought the *biergarten* (beer garden) tradition to New York. Compared to Irish immigrants, who preferred the saloons where no women were allowed, the Germans preferred venues where the entire family was welcomed, fed, and entertained. This preference took shape in the German tradition of the *biergarten* where, under shady trees near the town square and close at hand to a brewery, families enjoyed eating and drinking together.

In *America Walks into a Bar* (2011), Christine Sismondo describes the classic New York City beer garden as "well lit and relatively quiet and orderly," although "the term 'beer garden' is slightly misleading; there was rarely any garden involved and was really just a large hall with tables for people to sit at. Occasionally, there might have been a large mural or some natural scenery but, where budgets were tight, the artwork was a luxury."

Beer gardens were in large part responsible for the introduction of lager beer to the United States. Lager had its origins in Bavaria and what is now the Czech Republic. It was served in glassware that showed off attributes that ale could not compete with: it was crystal clear, pale gold, frothy, and served chilled. Most German immigrants demanded lager when they visited beer gardens, and as Germans migrated west and as rail transport and industrial refrigeration advanced, the style soon flourished throughout nineteenth-century America. Today, it is the most popular beer style worldwide.

One of the earliest, and most popular, beer gardens was Castle Garden at the Battery on the southern tip of Manhattan Island. But two of the most famous beer gardens were the Volks Garten and the Atlantic Garden. The Atlantic Garden, established by William Kramer in 1858 at what is now 50 Bowery, faced the Volks Garten (231 and 233 Bowery) until the Volks Garten was destroyed by a fire in 1895. Germans especially patronized the Atlantic Garden, which featured a restaurant, several bars, a bowling alley, a shooting gallery, billiard tables, and a theater, where "variety" acts and music concerts were performed.

To soak up all that beer, the kitchens turned out old-country fare like schnitzel and wursts. Entertainment was also part of the appeal. Many of these gardens hosted shooting galleries, bowling alleys, and live classical music. Some charged admission because certain patrons would come simply for the tunes and the atmosphere but would abstain from eating and drinking.

Although there are no venues that can compare to the most famous New York beer gardens from the 1900s, a number of modern-day beer gardens give a taste of the classic, pre-Prohibition era of American beer gardens. For example, Astoria's Bohemian Hall and Beer Garden (29–19 Twenty-Fourth Avenue) is the oldest existing beer garden in New York City and has perhaps the grandest scale. Completed in 1919, the beer garden at Bohemian Hall is associated with the Bohemian Citizens' Benevolent Society and officially seats eight hundred, though it often entertains more during festivals. On a smaller scale, venues such as Guastavino's, Hallo Berlin, and Zum Schneider, all in Manhattan, offer beer, German-style food, and a sense of the ambiance of the *biergartens* of Bavaria.

See also BEER and GERMAN.

Amell, Robert. "In and Around the Bowery Theatre." *Manhattan Unlocked* (blog), March 12, 2011. http:// manhattanunlocked.blogspot.com/2011/03/ in-and-around-bowery-theatre.html. Quotes a *New York Times* article of 1910.

Koegel, John. *Music in German Immigrant Theater: New York City, 1840–1940*. Rochester, N.Y.: Boydell & Brewer, 2009.

Sismondo, Christine. *America Walks into a Bar*. New York: Oxford University Press, 2011.

Peter LaFrance

Benepe, Barry

Barry Benepe (b. 1928), architect, urban planner, and cofounder of Greenmarket, the groundbreaking farmers' market, helped pilot New York City toward the pedestrian-friendly, neighborhood-preserving, fresh-produce-consuming urban environment it is today. Benepe was born in New York City to a family that managed to remain relatively wealthy through the Great Depression. As a result, his education was privileged, attending a series of all-boys schools and academies, eventually matriculating to Williams, an all-men's college in the Berkshires that has since become co-ed.

Benepe's coming-of-age summers were spent on the family farm in Princess Anne County on the eastern shore of Maryland, where he was deeply involved in harvesting, handling, loading, and shipping food to local buyers. His father's insistence upon making the farm self-sufficient taught Benepe both the value of hard work and the cash value of food.

From Williams he attended Cooper Union and then MIT before graduating to entry-level jobs with various architectural firms in New York City. Benepe worked for the Housing and Planning Board, preparing plans for the West Side Renewal Area. At that time he wrote *Pedestrian in the City*, the blueprint for a pedestrian-friendly urban environment. He then became the director of planning in Newburgh, New York. It was here, seduced by its extraordinarily visible nineteenth-century architecture, that he initiated one of the first state-designated historic districts in New York State.

When he returned to Manhattan in 1970, he had already been an architect, an urban planner, and a preservationist, with a rural farming background. He was invited by his mentor and friend Bob Weinberg to join the planning firm Hancock, Little, Calvert. When Weinberg died, the partners moved to Toronto and Benepe took over the New York City office on Fortieth Street on his own. His increasing importance in his field gained him the nomination as a fellow of the American Institute of Architects in 1975. His multifaceted background, coupled with his ability to navigate through the government bureaucracy acquired during his early years in New York, served him well during his nearly quarter-century with Greenmarket.

In 1976 Benepe hired Bob Lewis as his sole employee but considered him more of a colleague. Both were talented planners who wanted to put their ideas about farmland conservation to practical use. They sought to address the loss of farmland in the regions surrounding the city and the lack of availability of fresh locally grown food in New York City's retail supermarkets.

When the *New York Times* reported that 35 percent of the shoppers in a Syracuse farmers' market went on to shop downtown, Benepe and Lewis realized that their farmers' market was a draw that benefited nearby businesses. Encouraged by that realization, they set out to implement a similar plan in New York City. See HESS, KAREN AND JOHN L.

Together, they obtained the sponsorship of the Council on the Environment of New York City, whose board was composed of city agency heads and presidents of corporations interested in improving the urban environment. It was then that "Greenmarket" was registered as their title because too many retail grocers were using the name "farmers' market" when no farmers were present and no local produce was being sold.

The first Greenmarket opened in 1976 with twelve farmers. Its location—a city-owned vacant lot south of the entrance to the Fifty-Ninth Street Bridge, just a block from Bloomingdale's and Alexander's—made it an instant success. Extensive coverage on the nightly news of the three metropolitan television stations also helped deliver customers and more farmers.

That year they opened two more Greenmarkets. One of them was in Union Square, at the nexus of Gramercy Park, Greenwich Village, and the burgeoning Flat Iron District. Originally a bust, within a few years the market became wildly successful as the area drug dealers gradually departed, stimulating the economic resurgence and higher property values of these neighborhoods. That original Greenmarket's success prompted other communities to seek their own Greenmarkets.

Today there are fifty-three market sites, some of which are seasonal, most of which are year-round, with several open two or more days a week. Union Square, by far the most productive, runs four days a week.

In 1977 Bob Lewis invited author John McPhee to work at a Greenmarket in Harlem and write about it for *The New Yorker* magazine. McPhee's article, "Giving Good Weight," attracted nationwide attention and eventually was incorporated in McPhee's book of the same name. He exhibited an uncanny ability to place the reader in a Greenmarket, feeling the different rhythms and hearing the speech patterns of the customers in each neighborhood, ethnicity by ethnicity. McPhee's "dirty fingernails" account of the hardscrabble life of Greenmarket farmers, the amazing produce they brought into the city before dawn every day, and their engagement with customers became national news.

From Greenmarket's beginning it was apparent it could not support itself, and other funds needed to be found. Richard Pough, head of the America the Beautiful Fund, who was trying to stem the loss of farms to suburban development, gave Benepe and Lewis eight hundred dollars to find nonprofit sponsors for Greenmarket. Then the J. M. Kaplan Fund said it would match anything they raised. With the farmers' rents covering about one-third of the expense, other funds and agencies opened their coffers so that Greenmarket's costs were covered.

From its inception, Greenmarket was one of three programs run under the auspices of the Council on the Environment, which eventually renamed itself GrowNYC. See GROWNYC. The city continued to support Greenmarket through the administration of five mayors. Current Greenmarket director Michael Hurwitz is "incredibly optimistic" that Mayor Bill de Blasio understands the role "infrastructure plays in creating an efficient and accessible food system." Even former parks commissioner Henry Stern, who famously said, "We are not running a fruit and vegetable stand in Union Square," came around eventually. In fact, he selected Barry's son, Adrian Benepe, as his Manhattan borough commissioner. Adrian later replaced Stern as parks commissioner under Mayor Michael Bloomberg.

In 2000 Barry Benepe retired as Greenmarket director and as a planning consultant. While continuing their same responsibilities, the Greenmarket staff became employees of the Council on the Environment. A new director, Nina Planck, was appointed. She was replaced six months later by Michael Hurwitz.

See also GREENMARKETS.

"Interview with Michael Hurwitz, Director, Greenmarket Program." New York City Food Policy Center. http://nycfoodpolicy.org/interview-michael-hurwitz-director-greenmarket-program/.
McPhee, John. *Giving Good Weight*. New York: Farrar, Straus and Giroux, 1979.
Minichiello, Michael D. "West Village Original: Barry Benepe." *WestView News*, October 2012.
Smith, Peter. "Talking with New York City Greenmarket Co-founder Barry Benepe." *GOOD*, April 24, 2010.

Richard Frisbie

Bensonhurst

Bensonhurst is a large neighborhood in southwestern Brooklyn. In the twentieth century, its population was mostly Italian American. Although the area's demographics have shifted significantly since the 1990s, Italian American food remains the culinary centerpiece. See ITALIAN.

Named for Arthur W. Benson, who divided the area into lots in the 1830s, "Bensonhurst-by-the-Sea" came to prominence in the 1880s after the developer James Lynch transformed 350 acres into an enclave of one thousand villas. Access to Bensonhurst was improved by the inauguration of the West End Line, an elevated line above Eighty-Sixth Street, in 1916. Jews from the Lower East Side, many Sephardic, were able to leave that area's crowded and unsanitary conditions for the open spaces of Bensonhurst and other neighborhoods throughout Brooklyn.

Italian Americans, the ethnic group most commonly associated with Bensonhurst, have a rich history here, particularly after World War II, when thousands of Italians sought new lives in this neighborhood. Since about 1990, however, many Italian Americans have left, replaced by members of other ethnic groups. In the 2010 Census, 36 percent of Bensonhurst residents identified as Chinese; Latinos, southeast Europeans, and Russian Jews have also increased in number, bringing diversity to the gastronomic scene in southwest Brooklyn.

Despite this change, Italian eateries continue to dominate the image of Bensonhurst in the popular mind, as they did in 1977, when John Travolta purchased two slices at Lenny's Pizza on Eighty-Sixth Street in the opening scene of *Saturday Night Fever*. L&B Spumoni Gardens (founded 1939) is consistently ranked among the top pizzerias in the city, while Pastosa Ravioli (founded 1966), purveyor of high-end pasta, is now in its third generation of ownership in the Ajello family. One seeking the prosciutto bread at Il Fornaretto (founded 1927) must go early in the day, lest it sell out.

Those wishing for more than bread have multiple options. Ordering at Lioni Italian Heroes (founded 1980) can be a difficult task; the menu lists over 150 sandwiches, all named for famous Italian Americans. One can also hear the famous cry "Thank you, subway!" after leaving a tip at John's Deli (founded 1968), once used to thank a customer for covering the five-cent fare home.

When it is time for dessert, the popular choice is Villabate Alba Pasticerria (founded 1979), which offers Sicilian sweets, including a chocolate mousse cannoli sponge cake. With the influx of other ethnic groups has come a host of new options, including Net Cost, a local chain specializing in Russian and Ukrainian food, and Bamboo Pavilion, a popular Sichuan restaurant.

But the soul of Bensonhurst remains Italian; the Festa di Santa Rosalia, an annual event since the 1940s, serves as its anchor. The ten-day celebration, which ends the day before Labor Day, honors the patron saint of Palermo; nearly one hundred local vendors line Eighteenth Avenue (Cristoforo Colombo Boulevard) each evening, offering traditional Italian food. The neighborhood's dwindling Italian population, however, has caused some concern over the future of the event. The 2011 installment was canceled because of a permit dispute, a disappointment that was almost repeated in 2013. The event's organizers have discussed hiring a private contractor to run future editions, as has been the case for the Feast of San Gennaro in Manhattan's Little Italy since the late 1990s.

See also BROOKLYN and STREET FAIRS.

Merlis, Brian. *Brooklyn's Bensonhurst, Bath Beach, and New Utrecht Communities: A Photographic History*. With Lee A. Rosenzweig. Brooklyn, N.Y.: Israelowitz, 2007.
Walsh, Kevin. "86th Street in Bensonhurst." Forgotten N.Y. http://forgotten-ny.com/2011/12/86th-street-in-bensonhurst/.

Keith Williams

Berry, Rynn

Rynn Berry (1945–2014) was one of New York City's most famous vegetarians; he eventually became a vegan and a raw foodist. Born in Hawaii, Berry lived much of his early life in Florida. In the 1970s he came to New York, where he studied literature, archaeology, and classics at Columbia University. He became a vegetarian while in college, a raw foodist in 1994, and a vegan in 1996.

For his first book, *The Vegetarians* (1979), Berry interviewed fourteen famous men and women, including Isaac Bashevis Singer, Dick Gregory, and Dennis Weaver, about why they became vegetarians. Berry's second book, *Famous Vegetarians and Their Favorite Recipes* (1989), offered biographical vignettes of prominent vegetarians "from Buddha to the Beatles." In his third book, *Food for the Gods: Vegetarianism & the World's Religions* (1998), Berry wrote about vegetarianism in spiritual practices, including Buddhism, Catholicism, Hinduism, Islam, and Judaism. His fourth book, *Hitler: Neither Vegetarian nor Animal Lover* (1998), explored the myth that Adolf Hitler and other highly placed Nazis were vegetarians. He contributed articles and chapters to many books, including *Becoming Raw: The Essential Guide to Raw Vegan Diets* (2010). He was a frequent speaker on vegetarianism, veganism, and raw foodism in the United States, Brazil, and other countries. He was frequently interviewed on these subjects for newspapers and magazines. At the time of his death (he collapsed while jogging in Prospect Park, Brooklyn), Berry was working on *Fruits of Tantalus: A History of Vegan Rawfoodism and the Origins of Cooking.*

Rynn Berry frequently dined at New York City's vegetarian restaurants and contributed reviews to *The Vegan Guide to New York City*, first published in 1994. He coauthored annual editions beginning in 2002.

See also RAW FOOD and VEGANISM.

Berry, Rynn. *The Vegetarians*. Brookline, Mass.: Autumn, 1979.

Berry, Rynn. *Famous Vegetarians and Their Favorite Recipes: Lives and Lore from Buddha to the Beatles.* Bradford, Mass.: Pythagorean, 1993.

Andrew F. Smith

Bialys

While Sunday morning bagels and lox are a New York staple, bialys, the bagel's distant cousin, do not come close in either name recognition or popularity. Both round breads hail from Poland (although the bagel's history is less factually known). Similarly, in New York they are both traditionally breakfast or brunch foods associated with New York's Jewish food culture—but here end the similarities.

Bialys, the shortened Yiddish term for the more accurate *bialystoker kuchen*, hail from the northeast Polish (but under Russian occupation) town of Bialystok and in many ways can be seen as a metaphor for the precarious Eastern European Jewish immigrant experience. Round and approximately 6 inches in diameter, the individual roll known as *cebularz* in Poland was traditionally consumed by the five thousand Ashkenazi Jews living in Bialystok before the onset of World War II. Most of the Jewish population died during World War II—many during the infamous 1941 burning of Bialystok's synagogue or later in concentration camps. Those who survived World War II immigrated to New York City, leaving just a handful of Jews behind.

The once ubiquitous bread eaten by Jews throughout Bialystok, a city that was 50 percent Jewish prior to World War II, was now firmly transplanted to New York and is barely seen today in its original hometown. Mimi Sheraton in her thorough history, *The Bialy Eaters: The Story of a Bread and a Lost World*, states that following the decimation of Bialystok's Jewish community, bialys there became a thing of the past. The only bialys available there today are at a recently opened bakery, fittingly named New York Bagels.

Early immigrants in the 1920s from Bialystok who left Europe before World War II brought bialys to New York City's Lower East Side. Most bakers joined the Local 3 of the Bakery and Confectionary International Workers Union, while bakery owners joined the Bialy Bakers Association. The bialy union was a distinctly different union from that of the bagel bakers in that bakers could only apprentice and join one union that specifically prepared one type of bread. The popularity of bialys paled in comparison to that of bagels from the beginning. Bagels were consumed throughout Poland and had widespread appeal in Europe and among the Jewish immigrant population in New York. Bialys, on the other hand, came from just one area in Poland and had a narrow following. Because of this, far fewer bialy

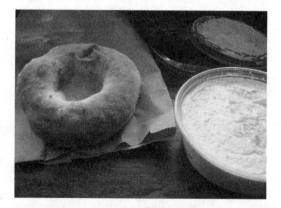

Like bagels, bialys are made from yeast-based dough, but they are not boiled before they are baked. The center indentation is not a complete hole, as in a bagel, but rather a depressed circle meant to hold traditional savory fillings of chopped onions, poppy seeds, or garlic.
ERNESTO ANDRADE

bakeries opened in New York compared to bagel bakeries.

Kossar's, rumored to be the oldest continually operating bialy bakery in the United States, opened in 1936 near the Bialystoker Synagogue, which along with the Bialystoker Center Home for the Aged served as the immigrant community's cultural and religious center. Although Kossar's ownership changed through the years, it remains the original and most sought-after bakery preparing New York bialys. In the 1950s, at the height of bialy popularity, Kossar's shared bialy production with several other bialy bakeries situated mostly on the Lower East Side. Local folklore suggests that a huge fire in the 1950s that burned down the original Kossar's may have been set by competing bialy bakeries involved in a union dispute with Kossar's. The bakery was quickly rebuilt at its current location, 367 Grand Street.

New York bialys prepared at Kossar's and elsewhere are similar in taste and texture to the bread developed by Jewish bakers in Bialystok yet somewhat smaller in size. Like the bagel, it is a yeast-based dough, but it is not boiled before it is baked. The center indentation is not a complete hole, as in a bagel, but rather a depressed circle meant to hold traditional savory fillings of chopped onions, poppy seeds, or garlic. Because the bialy is not boiled, it has a very short shelf life of a few hours, making shipping problematic. This may be one crucial reason that bialys primarily remained in New York City.

Bialy production is basic, employing just a few ingredients: high-gluten flour, water, yeast, and salt. They require more yeast than bagels and do not include malt and sugar—used to create the bagel's shiny, golden crust. After kneading the bialy dough into balls, referred to as *tagelach*, bakers hand-shape the bialys; rub the chopped onion, garlic, or poppy seeds into the well; and bake directly in 500°F brick ovens. Bialys, with their short shelf life, must be consumed within a few hours after baking. Although most New Yorkers slice a bialy lengthwise, as they would a bagel, bialy bakers and aficionadas claim that fillings should be spread across either the top or bottom and never sliced.

As with many artisan foods making a comeback in New York, bialys are gaining in popularity. Seen as an "endangered" culinary artifact, New Yorkers want to save this almost lost bread.

See also BAGELS; DELIS, JEWISH; and JEWISH.

Sheraton, Mimi. *The Bialy Eaters: The Story of a Bread and a Lost World*. New York: Broadway, 2000.

Jennifer Schiff Berg

Bickford's

Bickford's is a family-style restaurant chain established in 1921 that had an important presence in New York City from its founding until the 1970s. While established in New England, Bickford's was ubiquitous in New York City from the 1920s forward. Beginning as self-service lunch counters, a competitor to automat giant Horn & Hardart, the chain expanded into a full-service lunchroom and cafeteria. See AUTOMATS. Bickford's offered convenient early morning and late evening hours and inexpensive but quality food, featuring popular items such as cheesecake, apple pie, and rice pudding. They were located throughout the boroughs and could be found near train stations, subway stops, and other hubs.

In the 1960s, Bickford's was a New York institution. A 1964 guidebook described breakfast at Bickford's as "an old New York custom," singling out the chain for its convenience, "speedy-service," and modest prices. At Bickford's, the guide noted, "a torrent of traffic is sustained for a generous span of hours with patrons who live so many different lives on so many different shifts." Among those patrons were Beat authors Jack Kerouac and Allen Ginsberg, who mentions Bickford's in a line in his masterpiece poem "Howl."

In 1960, there were forty-eight Bickford's in New York City. But with rising costs and the city's decline in the 1970s, the chain suffered. In the subsequent decades, that number dwindled, to forty-two in 1970 and only two in 1982, the year that the last Bickford's in the city closed. The brand lived on outside of the city however, and today Bickford's exists as a chain of pancake houses throughout New England.

See also COFFEE SHOPS and LUNCH.

"Breakfast at Bickford's." *New York Times*, December 10, 2000.

Cindy R. Lobel

Big Apple

New York City's nickname "The Big Apple" is best understood as a multistage development. During the 1870s, Big Red Delicious apples were developed in Iowa, greatly increasing the already considerable importance of apples in popular consciousness. This in turn led to the colloquialism "big apple," meaning "big shot" and "the big time." Neither meaning is current anymore, but both are attested in the early twentieth century.

By the 1920s, the meaning "the big time" was applied to the New York City horse racing tracks. Two columns by *Morning Telegraph* turf reporter John J. Fitz Gerald, published on February 18, 1924, and December 1, 1926, are key for clarifying his important role in this development. They differ slightly in detail, though both involve Fitz Gerald overhearing a conversation of two or three stable hands in New Orleans. In the 1924 account there are just two. In the 1926 account a boy from an adjoining barn called over to two other stable hands, "Where are you shipping after the meeting?" And the reply came, "Why we ain't no bullring stable; we's goin' to 'the big apple'" ("bull" was a derogatory term for a horse). Clearly, the stable hand meant he was going to the big time in horse racing. This conversation occurred January 13 or 14, 1920, and the two stable hands were African Americans—"dusky" as described in the 1924 column. They therefore deserve mention in any compilation of African American contributions to the English language.

Fitz Gerald was certain they were referring to the New York City racetracks. He liked the sound of it and adopted "The Big Apple" as a sobriquet for the New York City racetracks in his newspaper columns. Over a period of several years the sobriquet won acceptance, and in 1926 Fitz Gerald described it as "his phrase." Recognition came in 1997 when Fitz Gerald's last residence, at Broadway and West Fifty-Fourth Street in Manhattan, was honored with a "Big Apple Corner" street sign.

In the 1930s "The Big Apple" (and usually, for short, "the Apple") was picked up by black jazz musicians to refer to New York City in general (and Harlem in particular) as the place where the greatest jazz in the world was being played. "The Big Apple" had retained overtones of "the big time," and this may have facilitated the transfer of the term to jazz (New York City as the big time in jazz).

A bar called "The Big Apple," at Seventh Avenue and West 135th Street in Harlem, existed briefly from 1934. An iconic upside-down apple at the entrance remained until 2006, when a Popeye's fast-food restaurant took over the space and the façade was destroyed. A "Big Apple" dance craze—started by white college students who picked up the dance from the black patrons of Fat Sam's Big Apple nightclub (Charleston, S.C.) in 1937—became the hit of Harlem, especially the Savoy, that year.

The phrase "Big Apple" has been used in many food and drink names. The annual Big Apple Barbecue Block Party began in 2003. Johnny Rocket's introduced a "Big Apple Shake" in 2005. And, upon entering the Manhattan market for the first time in 2014, Dairy Queen introduced a "Big Apple Blizzard." "The Big Apple" (a drink with apple jack brandy) dates from 1938, "Big Apple Martini" (or "Big Apple-tini") is from 2000, "Big Apple Mojito" (suggested by Bacardi's Big Apple Rum) is from 2005, and a "Big Apple" sake cocktail was introduced in 2013.

Starting in 1971 Charles Gillett (president, New York Convention and Visitors Bureau) revived "The Big Apple" as part of a public relations campaign on behalf of New York City. Its acceptance exceeded all his expectations. Also, a colleague at the Visitors Bureau later wrote that Gillett had already been planning his campaign in 1963; Gillett told him,

> "Well, Gilbert, if I ever get to run this place, I'm going to start a campaign based on"—and here he gestured with both hands to indicate a banner headline in the air over his desk—"New York: The Big Apple."
> "The Big Apple?" I asked. "Why?"
>
> "It's an old jazz musicians' nickname for New York. They used to call it that because New York is where they'd get the best-paying jobs." (Cohen and Popik, 2011, p. 92)

See also SLANG.

Big Apple Barbecue Block Party website: http://www .bigapplebbq.org.
Cohen, Gerald Leonard, and Barry A. Popik. *Origin of New York City's Nickname "The Big Apple,"* 2d ed. Frankfurt am Main: Peter Lang, 2011.
Popik, Barry. The Big Apple (website). http://www .barrypopik.com.

Gerald Cohen and Barry Popik

Bittman, Mark

Few celebrity chefs would describe themselves as merely "adequate," but Mark Bittman, author of *How* to Cook Everything and more than a dozen other books on food, is no mere chef. Equal parts cook, activist, and journalist, Bittman has mediated the realms of food preparation and food policy for the New York Times's readership for nearly two decades, first through his singular "Minimalist" column and later as an op-ed contributor. He has since appeared with Mario Batali and others as part of PBS's Spain ...On the Road Again, the Today show, and Chopped. (He's also a sometime guest on National Public Radio's Wait Wait...Don't Tell Me.).

A New York City native (he graduated from Stuyvesant High School), Bittman went to college in Massachusetts and began his food writing career in Connecticut as a contributor to the New Haven Advocate. From small-town, alternative weeklies Bittman eventually graduated to the New York Times, where he penned nearly seven hundred iterations of the Minimalist column for the paper's Dining section. Though the Minimalist has famously made its exit, Bittman remains with the Times and considers the promotion of home cooking to be his "life's work."

In 1997, the Minimalist launched, declaring every day to be "a red pepper day." This focus on fresh foods, prepared unfussily and elegantly, came to define the column, which alternated its weekly attentions between technique and ingredients. At a time when gourmet food was still a largely rarefied affair—something that well-heeled Americans were prepared to pay handsomely for—Bittman's column illustrated that sophisticated dishes could be prepared simply, without the aid of white tablecloth restaurants and formal culinary training. (One interviewer called him "about as pretentious as a potato.") Through the Minimalist, Americans became acquainted with the joys of scallops ("nature's original fast food," Bittman proclaimed), the virtues of steamed lamb ("Steam Dinner, Add Morocco"), and the power of their own existing kitchen implements ("The Boring Old Broiler Turns Out to Be a Superstar"). Like most serious cooks, Bittman eschews the plethora of expensive gadgets on the market in favor of a few well-made implements, creatively utilized.

This emphasis on quality over formality continued with How to Cook Everything, now in its tenth edition. In each volume, Bittman concerns himself with presenting efficient, accurate information in a concise manner—taking the encyclopedic approach of How to Cook Everything's thematic pred-

ecessor, Erma Rombauer's Joy of Cooking, and excerpting its effusiveness. The series has expanded to include a supplemental digital app, and several varying print volumes and eBooks on the How to Cook Everything theme, including "The Basics," "Thanksgiving," "Christmas," "Vegetarian," and "Summer," with the latest addition to the brand being How to Cook Everything Quickly.

Bittman published a number of books as the Minimalist as well—The Minimalist Cooks at Home, The Minimalist Entertains, The Minimalist Cooks Dinner, and The Mini Minimalist. Another book, Fish, was published shortly after How to Cook Everything's first edition and describes how to select and prepare more than seventy species of fish. Many of the original featured species are now extinct.

In this respect, Bittman is at the forefront of the food movement's current trends toward locavorism and sustainability. Bittman began his career as a community organizer in Boston, Massachusetts, and that activist past remains a key component of his career now. During a TED Talk, he linked meat consumption and the widespread adoption of a Western diet to climate change, then drew parallels between climate change and the nuclear threat, calling it "a holocaust of a different kind."

This social awareness and commitment to sustainability guide Bittman's writing on food policy and dietary recommendations. In Vegan Before 6—a self-described "flexitarian" diet that Bittman initially developed to aid his own weight loss—Bittman advises his readers that meat should be "a garnish, not a centerpiece," for reasons related to personal health—and sustainability. In Food Matters, Bittman connects readers' food choices to greater global consequences and lays out a path for sustainable eating that goes beyond TED Talk buzzwords.

Bittman is wary of sounding didactic when grappling with the big issues surrounding the future of food, and his distinctly New York acerbity marks a final defining quality. "Make all the jokes about cow farts you want," he quips to one TED Talk audience. In an op-ed discussing the future of fast food, Bittman explains a particularly New Agey name for a California chain of vegan restaurants ("Lyfe" stands for "love your food everyday"), then adds a parenthetical aside for the benefit of his New York readers: "I know, but please keep reading." Sarcastic, affable, and no-bull, Mark Bittman is the quintessential New Yorker.

Bittman, Mark. "The Minimalist Makes His Exit." *New York Times*, January 25, 2011.
"Mark Bittman: Food Writer." TED, May 2008. https://www.ted.com/speakers/mark_bittman.
Marshall, Jane P. "For Cookbook King Mark Bittman, Less Is More." *Houston Chronicle*, June 18, 2003.
Wegman, Jesse. "The Making of the Minimalist." *New York Observer*, November 25, 2008.

Alexis Zanghi

Black and White Cookies

The iconic New York black and white cookies are made of butter (or shortening), sugar, eggs, flour (both cake and all purpose), sometimes milk, vanilla and lemon extracts, maybe orange, with a frosting of confectioner's sugar, water, bitter chocolate, and a bit of corn syrup. Black and whites are much bigger than a cookie ought to be and, obviously, half black and half white, though color variations can occasionally be seen.

The confection's origin is a bit of a mystery. Some maintain that it may be related to the half-moon of upstate New York and New England. Hemstrought's, a Utica bakery, started selling the half-moon in the early 1900s. This had a chocolate or vanilla cake foundation, with the white part of the icing a buttercream and the chocolate half a fudge, both frostings rich and fluffy. Whether the half-moon was the inspiration for the black and white or not, the New York treat is invariably made with a white cake base, never chocolate, with a subtle hint of lemon flavor; and the light and dark icing halves are a smooth, glossy fondant rather than the fluffy frosting of the half-moon.

Another theory of origin points to the German *Amerikaner*, which is usually frosted all in white, and that German Jewish immigrants may have brought it to the United States in the early twentieth century and begat our own black and white. Glaser's Bake Shop in Yorkville offered a "black and white cookie" when its Bavarian owners opened it in 1902.

Or it may have been here first and was later brought to Germany by American soldiers after World War II, and thus dubbed *Amerikaner* because Germany already had an entirely different cookie they called black and white. Or both could be true, the cookie going full circle. A less plausible premise is that the name *Amerikaner* is short for *Ammoniakaner*, for the ammonium bicarbonate, a

precursor to baking powder, used for leavening in their cookies.

Wherever they come from, black and whites are now a New York City icon. Their fame spread when they starred in a *Seinfeld* episode called "The Dinner Party" in early 1994. "The key to eating a black and white cookie, Elaine, is you want to get some black and some white in each bite," Seinfeld explained to his friend as they waited in line at a bakery for chocolate babka. "Nothing mixes better than vanilla and chocolate. And yet, still, somehow racial harmony eludes us. If people would only look to the cookie. All our problems would be solved." Despite Seinfeld getting a stomachache after eating it, interest in black and whites increased nationwide after the show aired. Fourteen years later, on the campaign trail in Miami, President Barack Obama called it a "unity cookie." See TELEVISION.

Although recipes abound, the best sources for black and whites seem to be certain busy city bakeries, places most known for their doughnuts, bagels, or wedding cakes. Today, many city delis carry questionable plastic-wrapped versions, but there is better to be found. In 2014, the *Times* former food critic Molly O'Neill compared this deli version to a superior black and white sold at Zabar's, noting it was "what pâté is to chopped liver." Most acclaimed were those from the 113-year-old Glaser's Bake Shop and the less orthodox William Greenberg's, which jazzed things up by making the chocolate part mocha and offering a red velvet version plus a rainbow of color choices for the fondant. Now that knowledge of black and whites has spread, you can get mini-approximations at Starbucks and Entenmann's countrywide.

See also COOKIES.

Grimes, William. "'Look to the Cookie': An Ode in Black and White." *New York Times*, May 13, 1998.
Johnson, Sasha. "Obama: McCain Is 'Running Out of Time' and 'Making Stuff Up.'" CNN, October 21, 2008. http://politicalticker.blogs.cnn.com/2008/10/21/obama-mccain-is-running-out-of-time-and-making-stuff-up/.
McGavin, Jennifer. "Amerikaner—Cake-Like Cookies Frosted on the Bottom." About.com. http://germanfood.about.com/od/baking/r/Amerikaner_Cookies.htm.
O'Neill, Molly. *The New York Cookbook*. New York: Workman, 1992.
Schwartz, Arthur. *Arthur Schwartz's New York City Food*. New York: Stewart, Tabori & Chang, 2004.

Wallace, Siobhan. "NYC's 5 Best Black & White Cookies." CBS New York, January 30, 2013. http://newyork.cbslocal.com/top-lists/nycs-5-best-black-white-cookies/.

Jennifer Brizzi

Bloody Mary

The Bloody Mary cocktail—tomato juice, vodka, Tabasco sauce, and spices—is widely credited to bartender Fernand (Pete) Petiot, around 1920. But the saga of the drink spans two continents and several decades.

Most likely, the earliest iteration of the Bloody Mary in Paris coincided with the end of World War I, when tomato juice in cans began to arrive from the United States. According to historian Jeffrey Pogash, who has chronicled in great detail the evolution of the drink, prior to that Frank Meier, barman at the Ritz Bar in Paris, created a drink called a tomato juice cocktail, made with crushed fresh tomatoes but not vodka.

At Harry's Bar in Paris, Pete Petiot took Meier's recipe for the "cocktail" and added vodka, and the Bloody Mary was born. The origins of the drink's name are unclear, but according to one story, it was named for a frequent customer by the name of Mary, who on several occasions waited at the bar with a tomato juice cocktail in hand for a man who never came.

The drink was popularized when Petiot moved to the United States after Prohibition ended and became head bartender at the St. Regis Hotel, then owned by the Astor family. The drink was renamed the red snapper as the "bloody" name was considered too gruesome for high-society clientele. The first version of the cocktail served in the King Cole Room at the St. Regis was made with gin instead of vodka, Pogash says, as vodka was hard to come by in early post-Prohibition years. However, vodka was widely available by the 1940s and likely was a standard part of the snapper by then.

Petiot also is credited with adding Tabasco sauce and spices to the tomato juice mixture when he arrived at the St. Regis, completing the drink's transformation. The now traditional celery stalk garnish was added in the 1960s, according to Pogash, and was the idea of a patron of the famed Pump Room in the Ambassador East Hotel in Chicago.

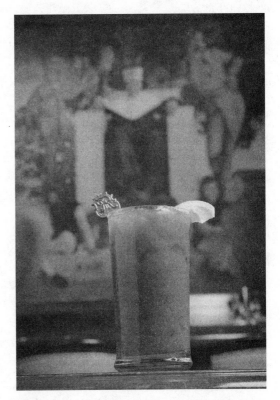

The Bloody Mary was originally a French drink; it was renamed the "red snapper" to better appeal to high-society patrons of the King Cole Bar at the St. Regis Hotel, where it was first served in America after Prohibition ended. COURTESY OF THE ST. REGIS HOTEL

Although some stories point to comedian George Jessel as the creator of the drink in 1939, that claim has been discredited. Jessel was featured in an advertising campaign for a vodka brand that made it appear as though he created the drink.

See also COCKTAILS and MIXOLOGY.

Pogash, Jeffrey M. *Bloody Mary*. Newburgh, N.Y.: Thornwillow, 2011.

Kara Newman

Bloomberg, Michael

New York City's 108th mayor, Michael Bloomberg held office from 2002 to 2013. He is best known for his unprecedented term extension in 2009, his shifting political affiliations, and his strong stances on health issues such as smoking, cycling, sugar and soda portion limitations, calorie labeling, and trans fat consumption in New York City. Some have accused him of creating an overprotective "nanny state," while others have supported the health initiatives and programs introduced during his tenure.

Born in 1942 in Massachusetts, Bloomberg had a long entrepreneurial career. He is the founder and largest shareholder of Bloomberg LP, a global financial data and media company and creator of the Bloomberg terminal, a specialized computer, information service, and trading platform utilized widely in the financial industry. Bloomberg LP was also one of the first companies to offer free food for employees, to encourage healthier diets, promote professional mingling, and keep productivity high.

The Bloomberg administration worked to bring higher-quality produce and healthy items into low-income areas. Programs included the Healthy Bodega Initiative to introduce healthful fruits and vegetables as well as promotional support to grocers, the Green Carts bill in support of mobile produce vendors, and the Health Bucks Program, which provided coupons to eligible individuals specifically to encourage produce purchases in farmers' markets.

On the sports and recreation front, Bloomberg dedicated $111 million in funding for playground improvements in all five boroughs, proclaiming, often, that all New Yorkers should have access to parks. He restructured roads and public spaces to incorporate bike paths and introduced expansive programs to encourage community composting.

New York was one of the first cities to enforce calorie labeling in fast-food and chain restaurants (those with more than fifteen locations or branches) in an effort to encourage consumers to make healthier menu choices and slow the consumption of highly caloric food items that contribute to obesity and its attendant health consequences. The administration also banned the use and sale of products containing trans fat.

Bloomberg's most controversial initiative was his campaign to reduce sugar consumption by eliminating the sale of sodas and sugary drinks in portion sizes over sixteen ounces. The regulation, enacted by the New York City Board of Health, was challenged by beverage trade industry groups as overreaching its jurisdictional authority. Critics also noted that the cap was not equal across the board in its restrictions in that restaurants and movie theaters were required to comply, while supermarkets

and some convenience stores were not. The industry also launched a vigorous public relations campaign against the proposed cap, making it unpopular with many New Yorkers. The cap was successfully challenged in the New York State courts, with the highest court ruling in June 2014 that such policy initiatives were reserved to the legislature.

Bloomberg's philanthropic efforts have won awards in the areas of health, community building, leadership, and physical activity development in New York City.

See also MENU LABELING and SODA "BAN".

Colvin, Jill. "New York Soda Ban Approved: Board of Health OKs Limiting Sale of Large-Sized, Sugary Drinks." HuffingtonPost.com, September 13, 2012. http://www.huffingtonpost.com/2012/09/13/new-york-approves-soda-ban-big-sugary-drinks_n_1880868.html.
Department of Mental Health and Hygiene, and Center for Economic Opportunity. *New York City Healthy Bodegas Initiative: 2010 Report.* http://www.nyc.gov/html/doh/downloads/pdf/cdp/healthy-bodegas-rpt2010.pdf.
Mike Bloomberg.com (website). http://www.mikebloomberg.com.
"New York's Calorie Counting." *The Economist*, July 28, 2011. http://www.economist.com/blogs/babbage/2011/07/menu-labelling.
"Playground Improvements Planned for NYC Children." http://www.activeliving.org/node/677.

Alexandra Olsen

Bloomfield, April

April Bloomfield (b. 1974) is a British-born chef and partner in several New York City restaurants, including the Spotted Pig and the Breslin Bar and Dining Room. Born in Birmingham, she worked at several restaurants, including London's River Café and Alice Waters's Chez Panisse in Berkeley, California, before moving to New York in 2003 to become the executive chef (and part owner) of the Spotted Pig, a gastropub in the West Village launched by music industry executive Ken Friedman. Their second joint venture, the John Dory Oyster Bar, a seafood restaurant in Chelsea, opened in 2008 but closed the following year, only to be reopened at a new location in 2010. Their third venture was the Breslin Bar and Dining Room in the Ace Hotel in midtown

Manhattan. In December 2012 Bloomfield and Friedman opened Salvation Taco, a taqueria, inside the budget Pod Hotel 39 on East Thirty-Ninth Street.

Two of April Bloomfield's restaurants, the Spotted Pig and the Breslin, hold a Michelin star. She has appeared on several television programs, including *Iron Chef America*; and she was the focus of the six-part second season of the PBS series *The Mind of a Chef*. In 2012 Bloomfield published her first cookbook, *A Girl and Her Pig*, coauthored with J. J. Goode; her second book, *A Girl and Her Greens: Hearty Meals from the Garden*, also with J. J. Goode, was published in 2015.

See also RESTAURANTS.

Goode, J. J., and April Bloomfield. *A Girl and Her Pig: Recipes and Stories*. New York: Ecco, 2012.
The Mind of a Chef, Season 2. DVD. Boston: PBS, 2013.

Andrew F. Smith

Blot, Pierre

Pierre Blot (ca. 1818–1874), a French political refugee, came to New York City around 1855 and quickly saw the need for a cooking school. He was unable to speak English proficiently, so while he worked on the language he taught French in New York schools and to some of New York's leading families. Within a decade, he was ready to publish his first book in English, *What to Eat, and How to Cook It*, which the *New York Times* praised highly. It is a large and systematic cookbook, which thoroughly captured the imagination of New Yorkers as numerous publications began to trumpet his activities.

With the book a success, Blot opened his New York Cooking Academy in 1865, at 90 Fourth Avenue; it was the first cooking school in New York. The *Times* began a series of lengthy and almost idolatrous articles on Blot and his work, praising him as "a benevolent missionary of civilization."

By early the next year the academy had moved to 896 Broadway, and Blot was offering a new series of courses. The *Times* continued its high praise, describing the twenty lessons and warning "all who wish to join the class just formed had better make early application, as each lecture is invaluable" (January 11, 1866). Blot's successes in New York induced him to establish a branch of his academy in Brooklyn, and in 1866 he took his show on the road,

giving a series of fourteen lectures in Mercantile Hall in Boston. Newspapers throughout New England and New York enthusiastically chronicled Blot's travels and activities.

Between May 1866 and February 1872, Blot wrote a series of articles for *The Galaxy*, an influential literary magazine of the day. His articles were one of the *The Galaxy*'s most popular series. When his second major book, *Hand-Book of Practical Cookery*, was published in November 1867, the *Times* called Blot "the eminent gastronomist and founder of the New York Cooking Academy, whose name has become a household word. . . . The book ought to be in the hands of every housekeeper in the land."

In later years disillusionment set in, on both sides. On March 9, 1871, the *Times* reported that Blot was beginning a new series of lectures at Cooper Institute, in which he opined that "there is no country where there is as much dyspepsia as America, because our people pay but little attention to food and eat too much meat for the exercise they take."

Even while Blot's most successful articles were being published in *The Galaxy*, some were beginning to question his work. His last article for *The Galaxy* (May 1872) was a diatribe, with much sexist twaddle and some negative views of the American housewife. Clearly, Blot had fallen out of favor with the public and the press. When he died in Jersey City, New Jersey, on August 26, 1874, the *Times* did not even bother to publish his obituary. He is buried in the Bayview–New York Bay Cemetery in Jersey City.

Pierre Blot's name appears in a few books on American culinary history, usually as the founder of the first French cooking school in New York. But his true legacy needs further elucidation.

See also COOKING SCHOOLS and FRENCH.

Blot, Pierre. *Hand-Book of Practical Cookery, for Ladies and Professional Cooks*. New York: Appleton, 1867. Reprinted 1973, 2001.
Blot, Pierre. *Professor Blot's Lectures on Cookery: The Substance of His "Immensely Popular" Course of Lectures Delivered in Mercantile Hall, and Reported with Great Care*. Boston: Loring, 1866.
Blot, Pierre. *What to Eat, and How to Cook It*. New York: Appleton, 1863.
Longone, Jan. "Pierre Blot." In *Culinary Bibliographies*, edited by Alice Arndt, pp. 70–73. Houston, Tex.: YES Press, 2006.

Longone, Jan. "Professor Blot and the First French Cooking School in New York, Part 1." *Gastronomica* 1, no. 2 (Spring 2001): 65–71.

Longone, Jan. "Professor Blot and the First French Cooking School in New York, Part 2." *Gastronomica* 1, no. 3 (Summer 2001): 53–59.

Janice Bluestein Longone

Blue Hill

See BARBER, DAN.

Boarding Houses

While they had offered an alternative to long-term travelers and transients of the colonial period, boarding houses became an entrenched institution in nineteenth-century New York. During the 1800s, the city's population grew from about sixty thousand at the start of the century to eight hundred thousand in 1860, reaching three million when the five boroughs were consolidated into Greater New York in 1898. This unprecedented demographic growth exacerbated an already existing housing shortage, which in turn made owning a home in New York astronomically expensive. In the 1850s, Walt Whitman estimated that three-quarters of all adult New Yorkers "boarded out." This figure was exaggerated, but the number of boarding house residents was nonetheless significant: about one-third to one-half of nineteenth-century urbanites either boarded in someone's home or took in boarders to their homes.

Boarding houses were especially popular among clerks, usually native-born young men who migrated to New York City from rural areas within the United States to seek their financial fortunes in the city. They served as agents, scriveners, bookkeepers, salespeople, and apprentices in the city's growing commercial sector. A clerk's job offered entry into the middle class for many young, rural men who in previous generations would have taken over their family's small-town businesses or farms.

Boarding houses covered a range, from the elite to the downtrodden. In 1857, English-born New Yorker Thomas Butler Gunn described them in his book *The Physiology of New York Boarding-Houses*. Among the almost thirty different kinds of boarding houses that Gunn described were "The Fashionable Boarding-House Where You Don't Get Enough to Eat," "The Dirty Boarding-House," "The Vegetarian Boarding-House," and the "Hand-to-Mouth Boarding-House." Certain boarding houses catered to particular immigrant groups, to middle-class families, to women, and to men traveling away from their families and staying in New York for an extended period of time. There also were boarding houses for those who subscribed to particular tastes and lifestyles, for example, temperance and vegetarian boarding houses.

Providing meals was a central part of the boarding house keeper's role. Boarding house residents gathered for three family-style meals a day (breakfast at 6:00 a.m., lunch—then called dinner—at noon, and supper or tea at 5:00 p.m.). Mainstays in most boarding houses included beef, cabbage, potatoes, cakes, and pies. Fruits and vegetables were a rare treat. Boarders were summoned to the table by the sound of a gong, and those who missed the scheduled meal had to fend for themselves. Of course, residents could choose to dine out—and many did so for dinner since they worked too far away from their boarding houses to return for the midday meal. But few exercised this option very frequently as meals were included in the price of lodging.

Those who wrote about boarding house meals described them as hectic affairs. Up to three dozen individuals rushed into the dining room after the bell was sounded and, if the descriptions are to be believed, fought over the food, which was never served in sufficient amounts to suit the crowd. It is from these catch-as-catch-can meals that the term "boarding house reach" emerged as hapless boarders grabbed whatever they could before the food ran out.

Boarding houses were much disparaged by nineteenth-century social critics, in part because they were not considered proper homes. This situation was damning in an age when middle-class arbiters placed an intensely high value on the domestic realm. Observers argued that boarding houses encouraged promiscuity by mixing unrelated men and women under the same roof. They complained that they were not well kept, that the structures were rickety, and that the accommodations were dirty. They derided the "boarding house keeper," invariably a woman, for her obsession with economy over quality of accommodations. And the first thing that suffered from her parsimoniousness, at least according to these accounts, was the food. Critics (and boarders themselves) complained that there was never enough food and that quality suffered in favor of economy. Boarding house keepers also were accused of adulterating the food to make it stretch from one meal to another—for example, adding extra salt to the butter or watering down the milk.

At the city's public markets too, boarding house keepers were depicted as stingy bargain hunters, arriving at the end of market hours when the cheapest—and poorest-quality—goods were available. Journalist Junius Henri Browne described "the cheap boarding-house keeper" as "resolved on buying much for little," including "leather steaks, highly perfumed butter, limed eggs, green fruit and unsavory vegetables."

Of course, boarding house keepers were responsible not only for buying and serving food but also for cooking it in their home kitchens. These jobs were among the myriad tasks involved with running a boarding house. Historian Wendy Gamber suggests that boarding house food may have suffered from the split attention of the boarding house keeper. For example, she posits that "boarding house beef," was by definition dried out because the cook also had to maintain the rest of the house, leaving little time for basting roasts. Likewise, the lack of chickens on boarding house tables, much lamented by residents and observers, may have been the result of not the cost but the labor-intensive nature of preparing and cooking poultry.

Despite accounts of the stinginess of boarding house living, elite boarding houses did exist. These genteel houses, which catered to men and families of means, offered the best the market had to offer. The tables of these establishments had more in common with the city's luxury hotels than the boarding houses in the immigrant wards of the city.

Boarding houses faded out in the twentieth century as population growth slowed down and apartment living became more of a norm. The factors that brought them about, however—a perennial housing shortage, exorbitant housing costs, and a constant influx of newcomers to the city—still very much characterize New York today.

See also HOTEL RESTAURANTS.

Browne, Junius Henri. *The Great Metropolis: A Mirror of New York*. Hartford, Conn.: American, 1868.
Gamber, Wendy. *The Boardinghouse in Nineteenth-Century America*. Baltimore: Johns Hopkins University Press, 2007.
Gunn, Thomas Butler. *The Physiology of New York Boarding-Houses*. Edited by David Faflik. New Brunswick, N.J.: Rutgers University Press, 2008.

Cindy R. Lobel

Bodegas

Bodegas, small neighborhood grocery stores, are icons of New York City's Latino communities. The name comes from a Spanish word for warehouse, and bodegas serve the same purpose as old-time general stores. The city's first bodegas were opened by Puerto Rican immigrants who began arriving in New York after World War I. See PUERTO RICAN. By 1928 several bodegas, typically identified by their yellow and red signs, had opened in East Harlem. More than just corner grocery stores, they served as meeting places for neighbors for whom Spanish was the common language.

Bodegas sold groceries that reminded their customers of their homeland. They supplied staples, such as bread, flour, and beans, as well as produce unfamiliar to most non-Hispanic New Yorkers, including *plátanos* (plantains), avocados, cassava (a starchy root vegetable), and *calabaza*, a winter squash. Packaged foods such as *habichuelas* (pigeon peas), garbanzos (chickpeas), and *sofrito* (a seasoning base for savory dishes) were also sold at bodegas. Goya Foods, a distributor founded in Manhattan in 1936, provided many of these. In addition, bodegas offered Spanish-language newspapers and picture books, tobacco products, beer, and sundries—and they extended credit to their customers. By 1957, Puerto Ricans owned about four thousand bodegas in New York City. See GROCERY STORES.

When the United States changed its immigration laws in 1965, Dominicans began arriving in force, opening bodegas in neighborhoods where they settled, mainly Washington Heights and the Bronx. By 1991 Dominicans owned 80 percent of the estimated nine thousand bodegas in New York City. Many sold imported Dominican foods and beverages, such as Presidente beer and *dulce de coco* (coconut fudge). See DOMINICAN. When other Spanish-speaking groups, such as Mexicans, Salvadorans, and Hondurans, arrived in New York City, they too opened bodegas. Today, bodegas sell a wider variety of foods, such as *canario* beans, from Peru; *dulce de leche* (a caramel spread used in desserts); *chivo* (goat meat); and fresh, canned, and dried chiles.

Although their prices are higher than those at su-permarkets, bodegas offer convenience and com-munity—the neighborliness and trust that can only be found in small, local stores. Bodegas generate rela-tively small profits for their owners, most of whom work twelve to fourteen hours a day, seven days a week. The Bodega Association of the United States was formed out of conversations that began in 1997 to address common problems, such as crime. By 2014, the association had seven thousand members; it is headquartered in Washington Heights. According to the association, there are an estimated 16,500 bode-gas in the city; 85 percent are owned by Latinos.

Bodega Association of the United States. "New York City Bodega Owners Survey." http://www.newgeography .com/files/Bodegas%20Surverv%20%20Results.pdf.
Krohn-Hansen, Christian. *Making New York: Dominican Small Business, Politics, and Everyday Life.* Philadel-phia: University of Pennsylvania Press, 2014.

Andrew F. Smith

Bootleggers

When men wore high-top boots, a man could hide an object, such as a knife or a flask, in his bootleg. This became a popular method for smuggling small items, and the smuggler was called a "bootlegger."

Countless Americans smuggled illegal liquor in cars, trucks, boats, and railcars during Prohibition (1920–1933). Although these liquor traffickers hauled payloads far too big for a bootleg, they were called bootleggers. America's big cities, including New York, had heavily armed bootleg gangs that de-livered booze to the marketplace. The *New York Times* identified gangsters Dutch Schultz, Owney Madden, and Waxy Gordon as "the big three of the bootlegging era" in Gotham.

Dutch Schultz was born Arthur Flegenheimer in 1901 in Manhattan's Yorkville area, where his father eked out a living in a livery stable. After his father de-serted the family, Schultz became a roofer's helper, a pool hustler, and a petty thief. In Prohibition's early days, he drove a beer wagon for a clan of small-time bootleggers in the Bronx. An ambitious young man, he wanted to be more than a driver. He partnered with a friend to distribute beer and operate a speakeasy. A rival gang killed his partner, but Schultz did not flinch. He outfought his enemies and added illegal gam-bling and a protection racket to his criminal ventures.

Selling illegal beer was Schultz's core business. In-itially, he bought beer from illicit breweries in New Jersey, but transporting it to New York was risky and expensive. To reduce his overhead, he began buying beer from mob-owned breweries in Manhattan and Yonkers. Then he bought an illegal brewery on Chicken Island in Yonkers and made most of the beer he sold. His fleet of delivery trucks rumbled through the streets before dawn, taking suds to his "beer drops" where bootleggers would pick up their loads. A busy drop in Mott Haven was called "the Tins" because it had rows of gleaming metal garages.

Owney Madden was born in Leeds, England, in 1892. After his father died, his mother immigrated to New York City and later sent for her children. The family lived in a tenement in Hell's Kitchen, where Madden joined the notorious Gopher Gang. A born leader and gutsy fighter, he soon took con-trol of the gang. In 1915 he was accused of ordering two Gophers to kill a rival gangster, and the jury found him guilty. He served time in prison, was pa-roled, and returned to gangland.

Madden teamed up with accomplices to steal liquor stored in bonded warehouses and private wine cellars. He also used his underworld connec-tions to become a kingpin in a syndicate that sold liquor in Manhattan, Brooklyn, the Bronx, and Long Island. He bought a legal cereal beverage plant in Manhattan and converted it to an illegal brewery. His beer, branded Madden's Number One, became the city's bestselling suds. Alone or with partners, he owned several speakeasies, including the upscale Royal Box on West Fifty-Sixth Street and the famous Cotton Club in Harlem. See COTTON CLUB.

Waxy Gordon, born in Manhattan in 1888, had a criminal career that lasted more than five decades. He graduated from purse-snatcher to master pick-pocket to drug pusher, trafficking in cocaine and other narcotics in Philadelphia and New York. When Prohibition began, he diversified, adding illegal liquor to his product mix.

With financial backing from a notorious gambler, Gordon began rum-running on a grand scale. His ships picked up liquor cargos in Great Britain, The Bahamas, and Nova Scotia. After the booze was brought ashore on Long Island, bootleggers distrib-uted it. Despite occasional raids and arrests, Gor-don's operation ran smoothly and made millions of dollars. In the late 1920s, Gordon felt threatened by both law enforcement and other mob bosses in

New York. He moved his headquarters to New Jersey and, with two partners, operated illegal breweries in several states.

Gotham's beer barons thrived in the 1920s, but the tide turned against them in the 1930s. The Great Depression ended the party of the century. Americans were disgusted with the crime and corruption spawned by Prohibition. In 1933 Waxy Gordon was convicted of tax fraud and sent to prison. Owney Madden went to prison for parole violations in 1932. When he was released, law enforcement turned up the heat in Gotham. He moved to Hot Springs, Arkansas, where he married the postmaster's daughter and reigned as a rural vice lord. A mob hitman, probably on orders from Mafia boss Lucky Luciano, killed Dutch Schultz in 1935.

See also BEER; PROHIBITION; and SPIRITS.

"Began as Street Hoodlum." *New York Times*, November 29, 1934.
Funderburg, J. Anne. *Bootleggers and Beer Barons of the Prohibition Era*. Jefferson, N.C.: McFarland, 2014.
Lawson, Ellen NicKenzie. *Smugglers, Bootleggers, and Scofflaws: Prohibition and New York City*. Albany: State University of New York Press, 2013.

J. Anne Funderburg

Borden, Gail

Gail Borden Jr. (1801–1874) was an entrepreneur who perfected the process of condensing and canning milk; he founded what would become the Borden Company. Born in Norwich, New York, Borden spent his early life in the Midwest and Texas, engaged in teaching, surveying, selling real estate on Galveston Island, and publishing a newspaper. In 1848 he invented a process for combining dehydrated meat and flour to create meat "biscuits" that he alleged would keep indefinitely and believed would be useful to explorers, settlers, and the military. Two years later he moved to Brooklyn, New York, to promote his product; but there was little demand for it, and the endeavor collapsed.

Continuing with his inventing career, in 1856 Borden patented a method of preserving milk by adding sugar, heating it until it was reduced to a creamy consistency, and vacuum-canning it. In 1858 he launched the New York Condensed Milk Company in Connecticut, and after a few false starts, the product began to catch on. Just as Borden began

shipping condensed milk to New York City, *Leslie's Illustrated Newspaper* launched a revolting exposé of the "swill milk trade"—the city's distilleries kept dairy cows in filthy conditions, fed them on distillery waste, adulterated their milk in various ways, and then sold it to the public as "pure country milk." In the wake of this series of articles, which went on for months, Borden's canned milk found a ready market as panicked New Yorkers eagerly snapped it up. Encouraged by early sales figures, Borden optimistically began construction on several plants. These new factories came on line just as the Civil War began in April 1861.

Beginning in the fall of 1861, the commissary department of the Union Army began purchasing Borden's condensed milk to supply the troops. Once the military contracts came through, the future of Borden's enterprise was assured. Contracts also came from Sanitary Commissions, which had been set up in northern cities to nurse sick and wounded soldiers back to health.

In 1871 Gail Borden retired and turned over administration of the company to his sons. He returned to Texas, where he started several small businesses. He died three years later; his body was returned by train to New York, where it is buried in Woodlawn Cemetery in the Bronx. The New York Condensed Milk Company thrived through the late nineteenth century; in 1899 the name was changed to the Borden Company. In the twentieth century, the company diversified into a wide range of foods as well as products such as Elmer's glue and Krazy Glue. By the turn of the millennium the conglomerate was restructured and sold to various international players, including the Mexico-based Grupo Lala.

See also CIVIL WAR and MILK, SWILL.

Comfort, Harold W. *Gail Borden and His Heritage since 1857*. New York: Newcomen Society in North America, 1953.
Frantz, Joe B. *Gail Borden, Dairyman to a Nation*. Norman: University of Oklahoma Press, 1951.

Andrew F. Smith

Born, Samuel

See BROOKLYN and CANDY.

Bouley, David

Critically acclaimed chef and downtown Manhattan culinary stalwart David Bouley was born in 1953 and hails from Storrs, Connecticut. His formative food exposure occurred at his French grandparents' farm in Rhode Island, as well as at restaurants in Sante Fe and Cape Cod. He qualified for a French passport thanks to his French ancestry and studied art at the Sorbonne after leaving the University of Connecticut, where he was studying business. Post-Sorbonne, Bouley realized that cooking was his true passion and found a job in 1977 with chef Roger Verge. He also worked under Joel Robuchon, Paul Bocuse, Fredy Giradet, and Gaston Lenotre in France and Switzerland. Bouley arrived in New York in 1980, working at Le Cirque, Le Perigord, and La Côte Basque. He then headed west to be sous chef in Verge's San Francisco eatery Sutter 500.

In 1985, Bouley paired up with Drew Nieporent to open Montrachet in TriBeCa. Montrachet netted a three-star review in the *New York Times*. Two years later, the chef's eponymous French-inflected establishment, Bouley, opened. The restaurant earned a sacred four-star review from the *New York Times* in 1990: "David Bouley's rapid zeal for fresh regional ingredients, his cerebral approach to textures and flavors, and his obvious delight in wowing customers make this one of the most exciting restaurants in New York City," then-critic Bryan Miller wrote.

The James Beard Foundation named it "best restaurant" in 1991. Another pivotal moment for Montrachet was its superb 29 out of 30 rating by Zagat in 1994, 1995, and 1996. The chef wanted his culinary prowess to be devoured by a wider clientele than his four-starred fine dining hit allowed, so he shocked loyal diners and critics by closing Bouley in 1996. In 1997, he debuted Bouley Bakery, offering wholesale breads plus a retail bakery, café, and restaurant. An expansion followed two years later.

The chef kept things very local for his next project but explored a different pocket of Europe with the opening of Danube on Hudson Street in 1999. The *New York Times* gave the Viennese restaurant three stars. A year later, the James Beard Foundation nominated the eatery for its Best Restaurant in the United States award, in addition to naming Bouley Outstanding Chef of the Year. After 9/11, Bouley Bakery transformed into a base of operations in tandem with the Red Cross, prepping over 1 million meals for relief workers.

In 2003, Bouley continued to dabble with Eastern European cuisine—as he had done with Vienna's culinary traditions with Danube—via his first cookbook, *East of Paris*. Two years later, the celebrated chef added to his cluster of TriBeCa projects with a three-story corner space housing a bakery, restaurant, and market. The restaurant, Upstairs, boasted an open kitchen, cooking demos, and sushi chefs Tadeo Makami and Isao Yamada rolling up masterpieces. In 2006, a loft space nearby debuted, featuring Bouley cooking demonstrations, a library, and event venue.

In 2008, Bouley's flagship reopened in a new space twelve years after the original shuttered. In the original location, Bouley Bakery and Market debuted. "In an era when the trend in restaurants is toward sleek minimalism, Bouley is a thrilling blast from the gaudy past, a reminder of how much pleasure can be had just from being tucked into such opulent chambers and attended with such formal manners," Frank Bruni wrote of the relocated restaurant in 2009, maintaining its three-star rating.

Brushstroke opened in the old Danube space in April 2011, created in tandem with the Tsuji Culinary Institute and focused on Kyoto's *kaiseki* methods of healthful, seasonal cooking. A more intimate, personal piece of Bouley became available in late 2011 with Chef's Pass, a private dining room that can accommodate eight to twelve diners.

Bouley, David (website). http://www.davidbouley.com/bouley-main/david-bouley/.

Bruni, Frank. "Boyley Quietly Uproots, Conjuring a French Countryside." *New York Times*, March 24, 2009.

Conley, Kevin. "Haute Health Food." *Town & Country*, January 22, 2013.

DeLucia, Matt. "David Bouley, Refocused on Cooking." *Restaurant Insider*, December 2005.

MacVean, Mary. "N.Y. Chef Blends Vision with Hard Work as Recipe for Top U.S. Rating." *Los Angeles Times*, June 14, 1992.

Miller, Bryan. "Restaurants." *New York Times*, August 3, 1990.

Wohl, Kit. *The James Beard Foundation's Best of the Best: A 25th Anniversary Celebration of America's Outstanding Chefs.* San Francisco: Chronicle, 2011.

Alexandra Ilyashov

Boulud, Daniel

Daniel Boulud (b. 1955) grew up in a small village outside Lyons. His first job was an apprenticeship in Lyons' Gerard Nandron at age fourteen, "peeling carrots and potatoes." He then apprenticed at L'Auberge du Pont de Collonges, helmed by Paul Bocuse, who ultimately became a key mentor to Boulud: "He took me under his wing, and over the years we developed a close bond. Today I consider him my guiding shepherd, a spiritual father." He honed his culinary chops as a cook in the three-Michelin-starred kitchens of Georges Blanc's La Mere Blanc in Vonnas, Roger Vergé's Moulin de Mougins in Mougins, and Michel Guerard's Les Prés d'Eugénie in Eugénie-les-Bains.

After a stay in Denmark, Boulud arrived in the United States in 1981. From 1984 to 1986, Boulud served as executive chef at Le Regence at the Plaza Athénée Hotel. Boulud arrived at Le Cirque in 1986; within a year, he helped the iconic restaurant earn its fourth star in the *New York Times*.

In May 1993, Boulud opened Daniel in the Surrey Hotel. "My goal is not to be number one. It is to be one of the best French restaurants in New York and maybe *the* best French restaurant in New York. I want to grow. Who knows—maybe in a couple of years I may want to change the whole thing and turn it upside down," Boulud told journalist Leslie Brenner in 1996. Two years later, he closed Daniel and opened up Café Boulud in its place. He went on to reopen Daniel in January 1999, at a $10 million cost, ambitiously aiming to serve upward of four hundred diners nightly.

Weeks after the restaurant's reopening, *Times* critic Ruth Reichl gave a promising sneak peek in the Diner's Journal column: "How's the food? Do you really need to ask? If you were a fan of Daniel, you know what to expect: first-rate French food from a talented chef at the peak of his powers." Daniel went on to a three-star review from Reichl's successor, William Grimes. Other early accolades for the restaurant included four-star reviews from the *Daily News* and *New York Observer* and a nod as one of the top ten restaurants globally by the *International Herald Tribune*.

In 2001, db Bistro Moderne opened its doors. The chef dabbled in brats and beer—and a downtown locale—with the 2009 opening of DBGB Kitchen and Bar on the Bowery. Boulud Sud opened in 2011, serving up Mediterranean fare; the same year, casual cafe and takeout spot Épicerie Boulud rolled out.

See also FRENCH.

Boulud, Daniel (website). http://www.danielboulud .com/about-daniel-boulud/.
Boulud, Daniel, and Sylvie Bigar. *Daniel: My French Cuisine.* New York: Grand Central Life & Style, 2013.
Brenner, Leslie. *The Fourth Star: Dispatches from Inside Daniel Boulud's Celebrated New York Restaurant.* New York: Clarkson Potter, 2002.

Alexandra Ilyashov

Bourdain, Anthony

Anthony Bourdain (b. 1956) may not have helmed the kitchen of a New York City restaurant in quite a while and may be as well known for his transcontinental eating and "bad boy of cuisine" reputation as he is for putting out perfectly cooked steaks, yet despite this he remains the poster child for classic New York chefs who make a name for themselves outside the kitchen. The brash New York native, who mostly grew up in Leonia, New Jersey, where he graduated from Dwight Englewood High, had a bad case of food-driven wanderlust from an early age. Family trips to France to visit his father's side of the family sparked his interest in what was, to him at the time, exotic cuisine. After two years as an undergraduate at Vassar College, when he worked in seafood restaurants in Provincetown, Massachusetts, Bourdain dropped out and enrolled in the Culinary Institute of America. He hit his stride in New York City kitchens after graduating from the Culinary Institute of America in 1978, passing through Supper Club, Sullivan's, and One Fifth. But it was in his 1998 role as executive chef at Brasserie Les Halles that he first earned name recognition.

In 2000 Bourdain published a memoir, *Kitchen Confidential*, the expansion of an article he had penned for the *New Yorker*. The article and book pulled back the curtain on the underbelly of sweaty, hot, close-quartered restaurant kitchens. Bourdains explosively popular book was followed up with others—*A Cook's Tour* and *Nasty Bits*, a Les Halles cookbook, and some mystery novels as well. Television was next.

Bourdain's *A Cook's Tour* was the first travel show to air on the Food Network in 2002. What he may be best known for is *No Reservations*, a program that ran from 2005 to 2012 on The Travel Channel, and *Parts Unknown* on CNN. Another show, *The Layover*, condenses his food and travel experiences into easily digestible city visits, but it is the longer-format shows that allow Bourdain to do what he clearly loves best: to share the heart of a country with his audience. In an interview with Blogsofwar.com during which he shares a story about breaking bread with former Vietcong in the Mekong Delta he says, "Everything, particularly something as intimate as a meal, is a reflection of both a place's history and its present political and military circumstances."

Bourdain is the head of a book imprint for Ecco Books, where he curates an eclectic list of titles by authors who have compelling firsthand stories to tell. His latest project is an effort to build a street food destination in New York in the style of the hawker centers of Asia he loves so much.

See also CHEFS and TELEVISION.

Grant, Drew. "Anthony Bourdain to Open World Market in New York." *New York Observer*, January 9, 2014.

Morabito, Greg. "Anthony Bourdain Is Planning a Massive NYC Food Market." Eater NY, January 9, 2014. http://ny.eater.com/2014/1/9/6299755/anthony-bourdain-is-planning-a-massive-nyc-food-market.

Francine Cohen

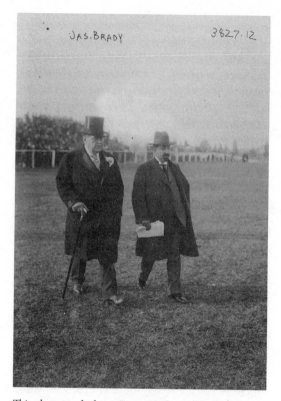

This photograph shows James Buchanan Brady (*left*; 1856–1917), also known as Diamond Jim Brady, most likely at the opening event of the 1916 racing season. LIBRARY OF CONGRESS

Brady, Diamond Jim

"Diamond Jim" Brady was a larger-than-life businessman who became synonymous with the excesses of Gilded Age New York, especially in regard to food. James Buchanan Brady was born in 1856 in New York City. Through a combination of earnings (he sold railroad equipment to the large rail lines) and playing the stock market, he worked his way up from modest means to millionaire status. His nickname came from his love of precious gems, with which he was generally adorned. Brady was a fixture on New York's Gilded Age dining scene, often with his frequent and longtime companion Lillian Russell.

Tales of Brady's feats of gluttony have become legend. In *Appetite City*, his culinary history of New York, William Grimes describes Brady as "a Paul Bunyan of the dinner table." Brady was purported to eat enough food daily to sate dozens of diners. His biographer H. Paul Jeffers (2001, pp. 2–3) offered the following descriptions of a standard Brady day: "A typical lunch consisted of two lobsters, deviled crabs, clams, oysters, and beef. He finished with several whole pies." For dinner, "a couple of dozen oysters, six crabs, and bowls of green turtle soup," followed by a main course of "two whole ducks, six or seven lobsters, a sirloin steak, two servings of terrapin, and a variety of vegetables." And for dessert, "pastries and perhaps a five-pound box of candy." Brady was purported to begin his meals four inches from the table's edge, only declaring himself finished when his stomach reached it. Another Brady legend is that he offered doctors at Johns Hopkins University $100,000 worth of gold to give him a second stomach. George Rector, whose restaurant Brady frequented, described him as "the best twenty-five customers I ever had." When he died at the age of sixty-one, Brady's stomach was said to be six times the size of a normal man's. See RECTOR, CHARLES AND GEORGE.

Such stories about Brady's overeating are, clearly, apocryphal. In a 2008 *New York Times* article, David Kamp compellingly traces the legends back to their roots, showing Brady to be a big eater but not quite the glutton that history has portrayed him to be.

Nonetheless, Brady's legend is emblematic of the culinary excesses of his age. See GILDED AGE.

Grimes, William. *Appetite City: A Culinary History of New York.* New York: North Point, 2009.

Jeffers, H. Paul. *Diamond Brady: Prince of the Gilded Age.* Hoboken, N.J.: Wiley, 2001.

Kamp, David. "Whether True or False, a Real Stretch." *New York Times,* December 30, 2008.

Cindy R. Lobel

Brazilian

Brazilian cuisine and the appreciation of it have been defined through a gustatory, racial, and religious lens predicated by northeastern Brazil's colonial history. Brazilian or Luso-Brazilian food in America began with the arrival to New Amsterdam of twenty-three Sephardic Jews seeking religious freedom after the Portuguese had recaptured the Dutch colony of Recife (in the northeastern state of Pernambuco) in 1654. Asserting their Jewishness was of utmost importance since most had had to live as *conversos* to escape the Inquisition's torturers. While their diet of vegetables, beans, pulses, fish, and meat appears to have had many similarities to the Catholic Portuguese diet of the time, they also maintained kosher dietary laws and conducted ritual slaughter with a *shochet* (ritual butcher) and *mashgiach* (an inspector for *kashrut/kosher* religious culinary practice). During this period kosher meat was not imported to the colonies. Some residents possessed viticultural knowledge, though evidence of its application is not forthcoming. They exchanged cultural traditions with recent Ashkenazi immigrants, obstructing a clear line of culinary influence to the New Amsterdam colony.

Following the Portuguese colonial domination of the sugar trade, New Yorkers were most likely to encounter Brazil through its commodity exports of coal, cacao, citrus juice, poultry, and coffee. Between 1830 and 1964 coffee was the country's main export. During this period Brazil sold between 30 percent and 64 percent of the world market in coffee and nearly 80 percent of the coffee sold in the United States. Coffee was sold and packaged as Folgers, Buttercup, and Maxwell House, among other brands. See COFFEE. By midcentury chefs discovered and coveted Brazil's wild teal and Muscovy duck breeds. The latter proved to be excellent for foie gras production.

Popular entertainer Carmen Miranda, the "Chiquita Banana Girl" or the "Lady with the Tutti-Frutti Hat," was an icon of Brazilian culture whose immense displays of tropical fruits as headdress recalling colonial culture and tropical fecundity contributed to an ongoing fascination with Brazil as an exotic locale. Miranda bolstered the recent "good neighbor" policy, inserting food and agricultural exports such as coffee as a metaphor of goodwill. Miranda arrived in New York two weeks after the 1939 World's Fair opened. See WORLD'S FAIR (1939–1940). From the deck of the SS *Uruguay* she addressed a phalanx of journalists:

> I say monee, monee, monee...I say twenty words of English. I say yes and no. I say hot dog! I say turkey sandwich and I say grapefruit...I know tomato juice, apple pie and thank you...De American men is like potatoes. (Shaw, 2010, p. 287)

Miranda's Creole caricature and Baiana costumes complemented the Brazilian pavilion's "native entertainment" and local foods associated with slave cuisines: *vatapá* and *feijoada,* adjacent to the lavish tropical fruit displays and the modern coffee bar that served one hundred coffees per minute.

The United States and Brazil had had an amicable and deeply interconnected relationship dating back to the "good neighbor" program initiated in 1933 during Franklin D. Roosevelt's New Deal, exposing a cadre of government workers and entrepreneurs to Brazilian food and culture. In 1940 the Brazilian Consulate left the Financial District to move to Rockefeller Center in Midtown. In 1974 it moved within the neighborhood before settling on the corner of West Forty-Sixth and Avenue of the Americas in 1999.

Between 1940 and 1980, Brazil's economy had a steady annual growth rate of 7 percent and a real gross domestic product of 4 percent per person per year, largely supported by exports of products such as rubber and coffee. Since the so-called miracle economy was so stable, there were not many incentives for Brazilians to emigrate until the rise of the 1964 dictatorship. The ensuing economic downturn in the early 1970s fostered a major exodus of primarily middle- and upper-middle-income Brazilians seeking political and economic freedom. Initially, immigrants were predominantly a small percentage of the economically stable Brazilians of European descent who emigrated to the United States among other countries (Seigel, 2009, pp. 13–66).

Working-class Brazilians followed until quotas were established, forcing asylum seekers to either overstay their visas or enter the country illegally. Legendary New York restaurateur Joe Baum opened La Fonda del Sol, the first Pan-Latino restaurant, at the end of 1960. *Feijoada Carioca* was the Saturday night special; this dish became foundational on most menus. See BAUM, JOE. Shortly thereafter a few restaurants appeared on the New York landscape, beginning with Casa Brasil on the garden floor of Dona Helma Dellorto's brownstone at 405 East Eighty-Fifth Street in 1963. Casa Brasil set the initial tone for Brazilian dining in New York. By 1970 retail shops, restaurants, and expatriates had gravitated to West Forty-Fifth and Forty-Sixth Streets near the Brazilian Consulate, becoming the anchor for a restaurant row named "Little Brazil" that ran west from Fifth Avenue to Seventh Avenue along Forty-Sixth Street.

Based on *New York Times* restaurant reviews, 1960–1984 appears to have been the first watershed moment for Brazilian restaurants and cuisine in New York City. In 1979 Mimi Sheraton's roundup of thirteen Brazilian establishments provided a clear view of the state and status of Brazilian cuisine within the New York dining scene. Key establishments such as Casa Brasil, the Brazilian Coffee Restaurant, and Cabana Carioca received multiple reviews during this period to better gauge the dining scene. Bryan Miller wrote another key survey in 1984, and more journalists and Americans traveled to Brazil to write about the cuisine in the country in the early 1980s.

Data from the 1980 U.S. Census reveal that 67 percent of the Brazilian men and 65 percent of the Brazilian women arrived between 1965 and 1980. These and later increases were direct results of the 1965 Immigration and Naturalization Act, which opened the doors of this country to immigrants from South America and other formerly restricted places for the first time. The 1975–1980 era witnessed the greatest movement as 32 percent of all Brazilian men and 27 percent of all Brazilian women present in 1980 entered at that time as the Brazilian economic crisis took root. During the 1980s and 1990s the Brazilian community diversified by moving to Astoria, Queens, the historic Portuguese neighborhood of Ironbound near Newark's Penn Station, Westchester and Rockland Counties, and northwestern Connecticut. Prior to the consulate's relocation to East Forty-First Street, Little Brazil had lost its gloss and many of its tenants to escalat-

ing real estate prices. The network of Brazilian restaurants and food stores and the scope of the cuisine expanded throughout the city and the nation. Regional population centers began shifting between New York, Florida, Massachusetts, and other locales. Ironbound's Luso-American newspaper continues to unite all of the regional Brazilian American communities.

Concurrently the Nuevo Latino movement arose, reinventing and rebranding Latin cuisine from a subsistence cuisine, based upon iconic national dishes, to one that is cosmopolitan, exotic, and reflective of greater access to heritage ingredients and marketing to new and sophisticated clientele. The 1990s saw the rise of Rodizio restaurants, all-you-can-eat Brazilian steakhouses, and Churrasco, southern Brazilian barbeque restaurants.

Diner, Hasia R. *The Jews of the United States, 1654 to 2000*. Berkeley: University of California Press, 2004.

Ribemboim, José Alexandre. *Senhores de Engenho: Judeus em Pernambuco Colonial, 1542–1654*. Recife, Brazil: 20-20 Comunicação e Editora, 1995.

Seigel, Micol. *Uneven Encounters: Making Race and Nation in Brazil and the United States*. Durham, N.C.: Duke University Press, 2009.

Shaw, Lisa. "The Celebritisation of Carmen Miranda in New York, 1939–41." *Celebrity Studies* 1, no. 3 (2010): 286–302.

Tota, Antônio Pedro. *The Seduction of Brazil: The Americanization of Brazil during World War II*. Translated by Lorena B. Ellis. Austin: University of Texas Press, Teresa Lozano Long Institute of Latin American Studies, 2009. See especially "Brazil for the Americans" (pp. 59–79) and "Conclusion" (pp. 111–120).

Wiznitzer, Arnold. *Jews in Colonial Brazil*. New York: Columbia University Press, 1960.

Scott Alves Barton

Bread

Before the arrival of Europeans, the Lenape Indians who occupied the lands at the mouth of the Hudson River consumed bread made from ground corn. Often mixed with berries and seeds, the corn dough was flattened into cakes and cooked on hot stones or placed directly on glowing embers. See PRE-COLUMBIAN.

Leavened bread arrived with Dutch settlers, who brought with them barrels of grain for making into bread and for planting. By 1628, Manhattan Island was home to a number of farms growing wheat, rye, and buckwheat. In 1631, the first windmill was constructed for processing grain, and two years later the Dutch West India Company opened a bakery on Pearl Street. Most bread consumed in New Amsterdam was produced by housewives at home, as it would be for at least the next two centuries. See COLONIAL DUTCH.

During the colonial era, bread was a staple, usually baked in wheat, rye, and white (the most expensive) loaves, weighing two, four, and eight pounds. It was not cheap; a day's pay for a seventeenth-century worker could buy five pounds of bread (versus at least 30 pounds today). The grain was grown in Brooklyn, New Jersey, or upstate near Kingston. The wheat was then shipped to Manhattan, which under British rule became the flour milling and trading center for the western hemisphere. Citizens often accused bakers of being more interested in earning a profit than making affordable bread for the city. In 1649, the city government adopted the first assize, or ordinance, on bread. Depending on the era, these regulations forbade the export of bread and flour, made bakers stamp each loaf with their initials, and insured that no adulterants were added to the loaves. In years of large wheat crops, bakers often petitioned to have the assize eased so that they could earn greater profits.

By the mid-eighteenth century, the Middle Atlantic eclipsed New York as the center of wheat growing and flour milling. In 1776, the city was home to only twelve bakeries, serving a population of twenty-five thousand. The 1825 opening of the Erie Canal proved a huge boost to New York, which quickly resumed its place at the center of the flour industry. As western wheat poured into the city, new mills and bakeries specializing in ship's biscuit (a dry, hard, and therefore long-lasting bread suited for long voyages) opened up along the waterfront. One of the largest in the trade was George Hecker & Company, which operated a bread bakery on Rutgers Street and a large mill on Cherry Street. Despite the growth of the trade, the quality of the loaves eaten in nineteenth-century New York often left much to be desired. Citizens complained of bread that had poor texture and a sour aftertaste that caused stomach woes. As a result of cutthroat competition, bakers mixed their product with old or rotten flour that had been laced with alum and other chemicals to make it look white and appealing. Conflicting claims about bread and nutrition made it hard to decide which loaf to buy. Many believed that white bread made from bolted, or sifted, flour was the best because it was less likely to be sour and therefore

indigestible. A minority followed the health regimen of Sylvester Graham, who espoused loaves made from unsifted wheat flour rich in bran.

In 1876, New Yorkers were ecstatic when Louis Fleischmann opened his Vienna Model Bakery at Broadway and Tenth Street. Fresh from his success at that year's Centennial Exhibition, Fleischmann sold Vienna-style loaves and Kaiser rolls made from white flour, milk, water, salt, and his own patent yeast. These breads were light, white, and aromatic, and his café was crowded morning and night. Fleischmann was part of a wave of German-speaking bakers who came to dominate the baking trade. After 1880, they were joined by immigrant artisans from Eastern Europe, Italy, France, Scandinavia, Syria, and other countries. Jewish and Italian bakers found spaces for their ovens in tenement basements, where they turned out huge wheels of Italian bread and dark, heavy, and sour Eastern European ryes. French bakers produced loaves for both their compatriots and many restaurants. Immigrant housewives also baked bread at home to save money and retain a connection to their native culinary culture.

According to a city business census, New York was home to 2,489 bakeries in 1900, the vast majority of them two- or three-person, coal-fired operations housed in cellars. Bakery workers frequently slept in these filthy, poorly ventilated spaces and often came down with fatal lung diseases. The city passed strict bakery regulations that forced many to close. This provided an opening for new wholesale bakeries that boasted of their "scientific" and "hygienic" facilities and sold their loaves wrapped in waxed paper. During World War I, the U.S. Food Administration told housewives to stop baking bread because their homemade product was less nutritious and more wasteful than industrial loaves. The number of small ethnic bakeries dropped, while modern wholesale bakeries opened around the boroughs, most producing a limited roster of white, milk, wheat, light rye, and raisin pan loaves. The largest was the Consolidated Baking Company, home of Wonder Bread.

The dominance of industrial loaves continued well after World War II. During the 1970s, however, gourmets and young followers of the counterculture began to rebel against sterile, puffy, "plastic" bread. They had tasted loaves with more texture, flavor, and "soul" in the city's surviving ethnic bakeries and on trips to Europe and decided to teach themselves the trade. One of the first was Eli Zabar, whose sour-dough ficelles became the rage. See ZABAR'S. Artisan bakeries such as Ecce Panis, Tom Cat, Sullivan Street, Balthazar, and Amy's followed, offering their versions of French, Italian, and Jewish loaves. At the same time, eased immigration restrictions brought new immigrants from Eastern Europe, the West Indies, Mexico, China, and other countries who opened their own bakeries.

Today, sales of supermarket bread are down, partially because of concerns over gluten and carbohydrate consumption, while many New Yorkers eat their bread in the form of fast-food hamburger rolls and sandwiches. Though a few venerable ethnic bakeries have been forced to close because of high rents, others have found a strong base in outer borough ethnic communities. Artisan bakeries continue to thrive. Some have grown into large wholesale operations, while others still make small batches of bread in wood-fired ovens and sell them at farmers' markets and other venues. Many now bake with heirloom varieties of wheat that are again being grown in upstate New York.

See also BAKERIES.

Blumenthal, David. *Parsons Bread Book*. New York: Harper & Row, 1974.
Panschar, William G. *Baking in America*. Evanston, Ill.: Northwestern University Press, 1956.
Teague, Walter Dorwin. *Flour for Man's Bread, a History of Milling*. Edited by John Storck. Minneapolis: University of Minnesota Press, 1952.

Andrew Coe

Breadlines

A form of charity traditional to New York, breadlines once provided the city's poorest residents with simple, on-the-spot nourishment. Initially, that meant bread, or an unadorned roll, though breadline fare would grow more elaborate over time. The first breadlines were patronized by a rough-and-tumble transient population. In the 1930s, their customer base expanded broadly but not broadly enough to include significant numbers of women. Today, breadlines are mainly associated with the plight of the unemployed during the Great Depression.

While they served similar functions, breadlines and soup kitchens evolved separately. By the mid-nineteenth century, wealthy New Yorkers could fulfill their sense of civic responsibility by sponsoring "soup houses," public dining rooms which served soup or stew to needy men, women, and children. The wealthy were also known to pay for church-based bread distributions, but the city's first breadline, strictly speaking, dates to the winter of 1896. In a story well known to New Yorkers of the period, a baker named Louis Fleischmann was working at his bakery on Broadway and Tenth Street late one night when he noticed a group of vagrants warming themselves over a vent in the sidewalk. Fleischmann took pity on the men, presenting each with a loaf of bread. The men returned the following night and the one after that, their numbers quickly growing into the hundreds.

While Fleischmann's line carried on for decades, in 1902 the breadline found a second home at the Bowery Mission. By the start of the twentieth century, the Bowery had become the winter retreat for a drifting population of seasonal workers. Here, the men lived frugally, turning to the breadlines when their money ran out. Waiting for the breadline kitchens to open, "breadliners" were required to queue up on the sidewalk, often standing for hours in severe weather, their wintery suffering the subject of the Stephen Crane short story "The Men in the Storm." The men's reward was a midnight portion of bread and coffee, euphemistically referred to as a "breakfast promenade." The Bowery Mission breadline operated between Thanksgiving and Easter to accommodate the winter influx of farmhands, ditch diggers, and the like. On a busy night it could feed a crowd of twenty-five hundred.

Growing apprehension over urban poverty at the turn of the twentieth century fueled public fascination with the breadlines. However, the breadlines were also subjects of heated sociological debate. Defended, on the one hand, as safety nets for the destitute, on the other hand, they were condemned for rewarding idleness. Between 1902 and 1929 assorted Bowery breadlines opened and closed in accordance with demand, attendance spiking in 1919 with the sudden rise in unemployment after World War I.

In March 1930, New Yorkers were surprised—and even annoyed—to find that a breadline had opened in a church on East Twenty-Ninth Street just off fashionable Fifth Avenue. Over the next eighteen months, as unemployment continued to climb, the number of breadlines proliferated. By 1931 the official count was eighty-two. Breadline sponsors ranged from churches to debutante societies. No longer reserved for drifters and drunks, with the arrival of the Great Depression, breadlines became an important defense in the city's fight against starvation. Those at risk belonged to the

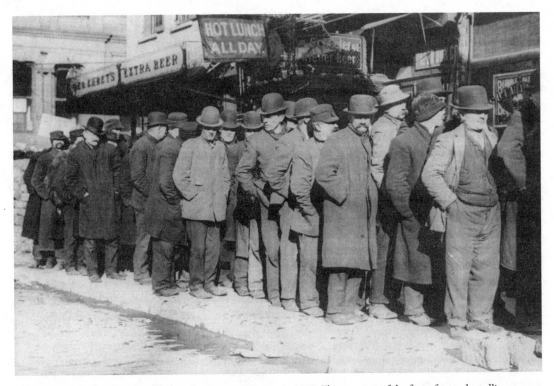

Men waiting for bread in a breadline at the Bowery Mission in 1910. This was one of the first of many breadlines in New York City. Now, there is only one regular breadline left, at the St. Francis of Assisi Church. LIBRARY OF CONGRESS

growing ranks of the new poor, men and women who had worked all their adult lives but who suddenly found themselves dependent on charity for survival. (In New York, the breadlines' importance as a food provider was due in part to a nineteenth-century statute which forbade the city from giving charitable assistance outside of an institutional setting, such as an orphanage or hospital, thus consigning food distribution to private charities.)

At their busiest, the New York breadlines could collectively serve up to eighty thousand meals in a single day. From the bread and coffee stations of old, breadlines had evolved into grand-scale public cafeterias. The mainstays of the breadline kitchen were beef, bread, and coffee. For breakfast at the YMCA, a man could expect a cup of coffee, three slices of bread, and a bowl of steaming oatmeal. For lunch, there was stew. Meals at the Municipal Lodging House alternated between beef and mutton stew, franks and beans, and on Fridays clam chowder, every entrée served with coffee and a half-pound of sliced bread.

Once again, the breadlines had their supporters and detractors. While a sympathetic public rallied behind them, city officials believed they were magnets for tramps from around the country. The breadlines' most vehement critics, however, were social workers. Convinced that the breadlines were detrimental to the morale of those being fed, they called for them to be abolished. Before 1931 was over, the Department of Welfare had closed down most of the city's breadlines, directing the hungry to the Municipal Lodge House, which ran a separate dining room for women and children.

Today, the sole survivor of New York's many Depression-era breadlines is run by the Franciscan friars of the St. Francis of Assisi Church on West Thirty-First Street in Manhattan.

See also BREAD; DEPRESSION FOOD; and HUNGER PROGRAMS.

Bremer, William W. *Depression Winters: New York Social Workers and the New Deal*. Philadelphia: Temple University Press, 1984.

Giamo, Benedict. *On the Bowery: Confronting Homelessness in American Society*. Iowa City: University of Iowa Press, 1989.

Martindale, James K. "Bowery Dines as It Votes, Repeating on Free Coffee." *New York Evening Post*, November 7, 1931.

Owen, Russell. "The Army of the Unemployed Has Drawn Strange Recruits." *New York Times*, November 16, 1930.

Jane Ziegelman

Breweries

Dutchman Peter Minuit purchased the island of what is now Manhattan from Native Americans in 1626 and named it New Amsterdam. In 1629, there were only 350 people in the settlement. "About three years later, however, the West India Company saw fit to build a brewery not far from the Fort, on the street which became known afterwards as Brewers Street," writes Stanley Baron in his book *Brewed in America*. This first brewery was a log house. It was among several structures inside the fort erected by the first Dutch colonist. The log cabin brewery was the birthplace of the first white child born in Manhattan, Jean Vigne, who became the first brewer born in America.

As the nation expanded westward, a major German migration resulted in the settling of the Midwest. Before the turn of the seventeenth century, the city of Brooklyn was, along with Manhattan, one of the brewing centers of the country. In the early 1800s New York State could boast that it was able to supply the nation with most of the hops used by the nation's brewers, and by the 1880s it was home to 405 breweries. When Brooklyn was annexed by the city of New York in 1898, there were forty-eight working breweries in that combined city.

Immigrants dominated particular trades by virtue of special skills. German brewers brought something called "lager" beer with them. Previously, the beers brewed by New York City brewers were English-style top-fermented ales, porters, and stouts. The brews were best brewed and consumed in the fall and winter months. In the warmer seasons these styles had a very limited shelf life.

All of this changed dramatically with the arrival of Frederick and Maximilian Schaefer, immigrants from Prussia, who brought over some bottom-fermenting yeast and began producing German "lager" at a brewery on Fourth Avenue between Fiftieth and Fifty-First streets. Lagers were more highly carbonated, lighter, less intoxicating, and less bitter. By the 1850s New York had gone mad for lager. The Schaefers' competition launched

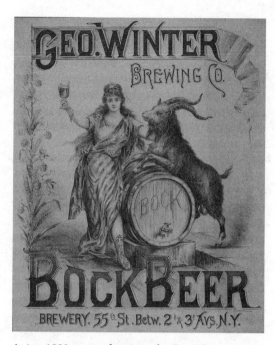

A circa 1900 poster advertising the Geo. Winter Brewing Co., which served bock beer, a style of beer that commonly was stronger, with a higher gravity level and alcohol level, than other beers. LIBRARY OF CONGRESS

operations in Williamsburg, Bushwick, and the Bronx. By 1860 forty-six breweries were in operation, mostly consisting of a brewmaster and five or ten workers.

The number of breweries in New York City, including Brooklyn, in 1920 numbered at least thirty-nine major commercial enterprises. Some of the most popular were S. Liebmann's Sons, Piel Bros., F. & M. Schaefer Brewing, John F. Trommer, Ebling Brewing, Hell Gate Brewery, Jacob Hoffman Brewing, Oriental Brewery, John Eichler Brewing, Valentine Loewer's Gambrinus Brewing, Jacob Ruppert, and Kips Bay Brewing. By 1969 there were only four breweries operating in New York City.

F. & M. Schaefer Brewing (1916–1976)

The Schaefer brothers, Frederick and Maximilian, introduced New York to "lager" beer. At the time, beers were top-fermenting types, such as ale, porter, and "common" or still beer. All were heavy, cloudy, bitter, and completely lacking in sparkle. They were consumed at room temperature a few days after fermentation was completed.

The new "lager" beer, however, was made with a different type of yeast, which worked at low temperatures and settled to the bottom after completion of fermentation. It also required a lengthy period of secondary fermentation, during which the brew was kept in cold storage—which is the meaning of the word "lager" in German. It was in this "lagering" period that the beer clarified and developed its lighter body and, unlike the beers of the time, possessed a sparkling quality and clarity. Lager beer was served cold. New Yorkers liked Schaefer Lager Beer so much that in 1845 the Schaefer brothers found it necessary to move their brewery to larger quarters.

In 1971 Schaefer made a move that would eventually cause the closure of the Schaefer brewery in Brooklyn. That was the year that Schaefer decided to build a new, ultramodern brewery just outside of Allentown, Pennsylvania. This brewery opened in 1972. It was one of the most modern and efficient breweries in the world. In 1974 that brewery expanded, and in 1975 it added even more capacity, reaching 5 million barrels. In 1976 Schaefer announced the closing of the Brooklyn plant. This announcement, only one week after Rheingold disclosed its plans to also shut down in Brooklyn, left Brooklyn and New York City without a brewery.

Piel Brothers (1933–1973)

In 1883 the brothers Michael, Gottfried, and Wilhelm Piel founded a typically German brewery in East New York. The enterprise prospered, and the partnership became a corporation in 1898, an established business of national reputation. The popular demand for the products of the plant—a typical German beer was then a novelty in the American brewing industry—necessitated enlarged facilities. The plant represented a new achievement in brewing construction. Michael retired from active management as the technical head of the corporation in 1900, devoting his last years to the acquisition of German paintings of hunting scenes.

In the 1950s, Piels hired the Young & Rubicam ad agency to develop their advertising campaign. The result was the marketing team of "Bert" and "Harry" Piel, the pitchmen for the brewery. Voices were provided by the comedians Bob Elliott and Ray Goulding (known as Bob and Ray on the comedy circuit). The first Bert and Harry commercials aired in December 1955 and ran until 1960.

Piels was turning into a Brooklyn brewing giant, buying up the competition that included Trommer's beer in Bushwick, Brooklyn. However, in 1955 local competitors Ballantine as well as Schaefer and Ruppert, in addition to Piels, were facing an influx of national brands such as Schlitz, Pabst, and Budweiser. In 1963 management decided to sell the company to Associated Brewing Company of Detroit, Michigan.

In the 1970s, F. & M. Schaefer Brewing, another Brooklyn-based brewer, bought the rights to the Piel Brothers brands and continued to brew it at its Brooklyn and Allentown, Pennsylvania, plants. Schaefer was subsequently bought out by the Stroh Brewery Company of Detroit, Michigan. Under Stroh's, Piels sales stabilized for a time. However, Stroh's succumbed to marketing pressure from industry giants Anheuser-Busch and Miller and threw in the towel after 149 years in business. On September 20, 1973, the Piel Brothers plant in East New York was closed down after ninety years of operation.

Joseph Schlitz Brewing (1949–1973)

In 1949 Schlitz began its national expansion when it purchased the brewery formerly owned by George Ehert, at 193 Melrose Street, in Brooklyn, New York. This was the beginning of the growth of Schlitz breweries throughout the country.

However, in the 1960s Schlitz, faced with the competition of Anheuser-Busch and Miller as well as rising operating costs, decided to adjust its brewing process and cut quality standards. The resulting public relations fiasco resulted in millions of cases of beer being removed from the market for quality reasons.

Nevertheless, Schlitz continued to make acquisitions and expand the market. This was the death knell for the Brooklyn brewery. In a move to increase its influence through expansion of production, Schlitz opened a new state-of-the-art brewery in North Carolina. The Winston-Salem rail facilities and cheaper labor made it less expensive to brew in North Carolina and ship the beer 500 miles to New York than it was to brew in New York itself. The Brooklyn brewery shipped its last batch of beer in March 1973.

Rheingold Breweries (1964–1976)

One of the first New York City "lager" brewers, Philip Liebmann developed a dry lager beer with a European character that soon became one of the most popular lager beers brewed in New York. Rheingold Beer, founded in 1883, claimed 35 percent of the state's beer market from 1950 to 1960. In 1883, at a brewery dinner following a performance at the Metropolitan Opera, the musical conductor declared the beer served at the event was "Rhine Gold." The name was adopted and continued to be used.

From 1941 to 1964, the election of a new Miss Rheingold was designed to sell Rheingold Beer. At the height of the campaign there were thirty-five thousand boxes displayed at the end of aisles, atop crates of Rheingold beer, and on bar tops—always with pictures of the six finalists framing the box. At its peak, the campaign cost $8 million a year—the equivalent of $60 million today.

Miss Rheingold was the perfect girl next door. "A friendly, warm, nice girl," according to celebrity judge Tony Randall. "Clean-cut All-American," according to Emily Banks, Miss Rheingold 1960. "Clean, lovely, graceful." It all ended in 1964. By the mid-1960s, no business could advertise its brand with just demure, smiling white women.

For over thirty years, from the 1950s through the 1970s, Rheingold Beer was the most popular New York City brew. But by 1976, as a local brewery, it could no longer compete with nationwide companies such as Anheuser-Busch, Miller, and Schlitz and closed its brewery.

Rise of the Microbreweries

What is now known as microbrewing started in 1969 with a single brewery in California. It took almost ten years for New York City to have its first microbrewery. The first wave of microbreweries, with the exception of Brooklyn Brewery, were all situated on the island of Manhattan. Real estate, building codes, labor, and inexperience were the seeds of failure for those first brave microbrewery pioneers.

Microbreweries in New York City today have the advantage over their predecessors in that there is a cadre of brewers who have experience and are at least familiar with the development of business planning. They are also spread out over all five boroughs of the city. See MICROBREWERIES AND BREWPUBS.

See also BEER and BROOKLYN BREWERY.

Burrows, Edwin G., and Mike Wallace. *Gotham: A History of New York City to 1898*. New York: Oxford University Press, 1999.

Oliver, Garrett, ed. *The Oxford Companion to Beer*. New York: Oxford University Press, 2011.

Van Wiereen, Dale P. *American Breweries II*. West Point, Pa.: Eastern Coast Brewiania Association, 1995.

Baron, Stanley Wade. *Brewed in America: A History of Beer and Ale in the United States*. Boston: Little, Brown, 1962.

Peter LaFrance

Brighton Beach

Located on the very southernmost part of Brooklyn, near Coney Island, Brighton Beach was once an English settlement of little farms known as Gravesend. In 1868, entrepreneur William A. Engeman envisioned the area as a beach resort like that of Brighton, England. He built roads to the area, a pier for steamboats, the Brighton Beach Bathing Pavilion, and the Ocean Hotel. Vaudeville theaters sprang up, as well as a race track and the famous boardwalk.

For a few decades, Brighton Beach was a playground for the wealthy, vacationers, and tourists. However, as is common in New York, the neighborhood eventually evolved into something quite different. An influx of Eastern European Jews escaping from World War II Europe in the 1930s, 1940s, and 1950s changed the character of the neighborhood, and it has since come to be known as "Little Odessa," or "Little Russia." More Russians came in the 1970s with the relaxation of Russian immigration rules, and so the neighborhood came to be filled with Eastern European shops, restaurants, and bars. Although the area was hit hard by Hurricane Sandy in 2012—the boardwalk covered in sand and many businesses damaged and shut down—the restaurants and stores of Brighton Beach have rebounded, and a rich Soviet culinary culture still thrives today. Signs are in Cyrillic, conversations are rarely in English, and foods may be totally unfamiliar to those who are not of Eastern European descent. For those new to this world, Brighton Beach is a place to experience culture shock and exciting new culinary discoveries, while those familiar with Eastern European cuisine can satisfy their cravings.

In Brighton Beach, one can find rare and elusive specialties from countries like Russia, Georgia, Ukraine, Uzbekistan, and Turkey. One can even feast on Uighur cuisine—a hybrid of Chinese, Russian, Indian, Arab, and Turkish cooking.

An exciting array of foods can be found within Brighton Beach restaurants, bazaars, buffets, delis, grocery stores, and nightclubs, including a variety of dumplings (Ukrainian *vareniki*, Siberian *pelmeni*, and Uzbek *manti*), Georgian cheese bread (*khachapuri*), all kinds of smoked fish and meats, Turkish grape molasses (*pekmez*), chicken Kiev, honey pepper vodka, borscht, caviar, Georgian mineral water, Russian sour cream cake (*smetannik*), and *tkmali* sauce (a kind of Georgian ketchup made with red or green sour plums).

Restaurants

Brighton Beach's proximity to the water means that many restaurants offer boardwalk dining, including Volna, where the Black Sea may not feel so distant eating *khachapuri* and Russian imported crawfish, or Tatiana Restaurant, featuring composed seafood salads, caviar, and beef Stroganoff. Other well-known restaurants in the area include Café Glechik, known for authentic Ukrainian food; Café Kashkar, known for its Uighur specialties like *lagman*; Varenichnaya, where one can sample a variety of Eastern European dumplings; Elza Fancy Food, which serves Korean-Uzbek-Russian fusion food; Beyti Turkish Kabob, source of a variety of skewered meats (including *kofte*, lamb Adana, and *yogurtlu* kebabs); and Gambrinus Seafood Café, a pirate-themed beer hall which serves classic Russian food alongside sushi.

For those looking to take things home or have a picnic on the beach, Brighton Beach's avenues and streets are lined with bakeries, bazaars, buffets, delis, and shops where one can buy food by the pound and vodka by the gram (100 grams equals a double shot).

Bakeries

Dense breads like Russian "grey bread" can be found at Brighton Bazaar, while airy Georgian-style baguettes (*shoti*) are found at Toné Café, named for the round clay oven used to bake them. Bakery La Brioche Café is known for delectable Russian pastries like brioche filled with rose petal jam and layered caramel cake, while Güllüoglu is best for baklava and Turkish coffee.

Markets

The buffet or salad bar is a common feature in many Brighton Beach food stores. Although this kind of presentation is often unappealing with American food, in Brighton Beach, buffet foods are of high quality and inexpensive. Take Gastronom Arkadia, which features a well-known buffet filled with blintzes, stuffed pancakes, pigs' feet, beef tongue, kasha, and *tvarog* (farmers' cheese mixed with sour cream), or Brighton Bazaar, with its exciting salad bar featuring sautéed chicken livers, roasted sturgeon, and Uzbek carrot salad. Food Heaven is Brighton Beach's fancy food emporium where one can find delicacies such as Ukrainian *salo* (a kind of cured lardo), and Vintage Food Corporation offers goods from Turkey, including a large assortment of dried fruits and nuts. Gold Label Deli is known for its cakes, candies, cheeses, and *pirozhki*. Ocean Wine and Liquor has varieties of vodka unavailable anywhere else.

Nightclubs

The quintessential Brighton Beach nightlife experience includes dancing, vodka, and decadent banquet dining. The most reputable restaurants-cum-nightclubs in Brighton Beach are Tatiana Restaurant and Nightclub, Primorski Restaurant, and National Restaurant. After dining upstairs at Tatiana, venture downstairs late at night, when the restaurant transforms into a nightclub. One can enjoy live music at Primorski Restaurant, which also specializes in the Georgian dish *chakrapuli* (braised veal) and *solyanka* (a sweet and sour soup with shredded lamb and coriander), while National Restaurant's banquet menu features Bavarian roast meat, Russian pancakes, hot smoked sturgeon, and "Monastery salad," accompanied by a gaudy stage show with singing, dancing, and spectacular costumes.

See also BROOKLYN; LITTLE ODESSA; and RUSSIAN.

Alperson, Myra. "Brighton Beach." In *Nosh New York: The Food Lover's Guide to New York City's Most Delicious Neighborhoods*, pp. 107–118. New York: St. Martin's Griffin, 2003.

Amand, Lisa. "A Year after Sandy, Brighton Beach Struggles to Get Back on Feet." *Jewish Daily Forward*, October 26, 2013.

Coe, Andrew. "Where to Find Shoti, the 'Georgian Baguette,' in South Brooklyn." Serious Eats: New York, September 18, 2013. http://newyork .seriouseats.com/2013/09/best-georgian-bread-shoti-brooklyn-brighton-beach-sheepshead-bay.html.

Falkowitz, Max. "Russian Pastries on a Budget at Bakery La Brioche." Serious Eats: New York, August 27, 2013. http://newyork.seriouseats.com/2013/08/

russian-pastries-on-a-budget-at-la-brioche-cafe-
bakery-brighton-beach.html.
Kusnyer, Laura. "Must-See Brighton Beach: 13 Great
Things to See and Do." Nycgo.com, January 1, 2010.
http://www.nycgo.com/slideshows/must-see-
brighton-beach.
"Our Brooklyn: Brighton Beach." Brooklyn Public
Library. http://www.bklynlibrary.org/ourbrooklyn/
brightonbeach/.
Pado, Fran. "An Air of Russia and Ocean Breezes." *New
York Times*, June 26, 2010.
Sietsema, Robert. "Sietsema Immerses Himself in
Brighton Beach." Eater NY, August 12, 2013. http://
ny.eater.com/maps/sietsema-immerses-himself-in-
brighton-beach.
Von Bremzen, Anya. "In a World of Tasty Meat-Filled
Starches." *New York Magazine*, April 12, 2009.

Mackensie Griffin

Broadway Panhandler

Broadway Panhandler: A Cook's Best Resource is a family-owned, gourmet cookware store in Lower Manhattan. One of the first stores of its kind in New York City, Broadway Panhandler opened in 1976, but its roots date back to the late 1930s.

Owner Norman Kornbleuth came up with the idea for Broadway Panhandler in the 1970s while working for his father, Harry, a Polish immigrant who had opened up a wholesale store on the Bowery in 1939 that supplied the U.S. Navy with large wooden bowls. The father's business, Anchor Equipment Company, expanded to provide cookware to hospitals, restaurants, schools, correctional facilities, and well-known people in the culinary world, including American chef and food writer James Beard, who, in the 1970s, along with Calphalon inventor Ron Kasperzak, inspired Norman Kornbleuth to sell restaurant-style kitchen and cookware for home use. See BEARD, JAMES.

Kornbleuth said his earliest memories were of visits to his father's store, where he would play with the appliances, using large mixing bowls as a rocking horse or hiding in huge stockpots. Having spent most of his life surrounded by kitchenware, Kornbleuth followed in his father's footsteps and opened up Broadway Panhandler in 1976 with his wife, Babette. While Norman's father's business was wholesale, Norman decided to sell commercial-quality items to consumers, including chefs and home cooks at his store, which stood on Broadway

and Spring Street in SoHo. Its name was a play on words based on the panhandlers who populated the Bowery where his father's business was located, plus the fact that they were going to sell pans.

In 1995 the store moved from Broadway to nearby Broome Street, and then in 2006 it moved to its current location on East Eighth Street between Broadway and University Place. The store is well stocked with pots, pans, cutlery, tableware, small kitchen appliances, knives, coffee and tea accessories, bakeware, and cake decorating tools—just about anything a customer might need for cooking, baking, and entertaining, including high-end brands such as Le Creuset, Wusthof, Bourgeat, Lodge, All-Clad, and Mosser crystal. The staff includes food service professionals knowledgeable about how each item works. In-store services include cooking demonstrations, knife sharpening, and private shopping.

Kornbleuth, Norman. "A Personal Note from Norman."
http://www.broadwaypanhandler.com/note_from_
owner.aspx.
Matsumoto, Nancy. "It's All Cutting Edge at This Kitchen
Tool Mecca." *Edible Manhattan*, November 4, 2010.

Tracey Ceurvels

Brock, Carol

Carol Brock (b. 1923) founded Les Dames d'Escoffier, an exclusive philanthropic society of professional women, in 1976 to support the careers of women working in food, fine beverage, and hospitality. Having grown up in Queens with a father who had been a butcher for a time and a mother with excellent baking skills, Brock was no stranger to the culinary world. She attended Queens College, receiving her bachelor's degree in home economics in 1944, and married soon after. But the homemaker's life was not for her.

Brock started her career in food journalism in 1944 as the "hostess editor" at *Good Housekeeping* magazine. After twenty-three years there, she left for a nearly three-year stint as a food editor at *Parents* magazine. In 1970, she moved to the *New York Daily News* as food reporter, responsible for the Sunday magazine section, a position she held until 1985. She developed recipes for food photographs, conducted interviews, and wrote articles on the New York food scene. A highlight of that period was when she hosted chef and food writer James Beard at her home. See BEARD, JAMES.

In 1985, she focused on her home borough, Queens, where she reviewed restaurants for thirteen years for the *TimesLedger*. The only time Brock missed work in all those years of journalism was to give birth to her three sons.

The Feminist Movement

It was during her time at the *Daily News* that she became acutely aware of the inequality of opportunities for women versus men in professional roles in the food world and the inequities in hiring, pay, and educational opportunities. Brock learned of a Boston women's group, Les Dames des Amis d'Escoffier Society, which was formed in response to the all-male fine dining association Les Amis d'Escoffier Society. Les Dames des Amis is an all-women dining association which, like the male group, raises money for the Escoffier Foundation for culinary education. Brock was inspired by the idea of a women-only food and wine society but felt the need for something greater than a charity group. That need was for culinary professional women to help other women who were working to get established in the culinary world.

In 1973, Brock received a charter from the New York chapter of Les Amis d'Escoffier Society to form the ladies chapter of New York. She put together a task force of influential female food professionals: Mary Lyons, marketing and communications director, Foods and Wines from France; Elayne Kleeman, creator of the first U.S. wine auction at Heublein; Helene Bennett, executive director, Wine and Food Society; Beverly Barbour, an international education, marketing, and public relations professional; and Ella Elvin, food editor, *New York Daily News*.

Birth of an Organization

Over the next three years the women worked to form what they felt would be a supportive organization to help overcome the enormous gender barriers in their industry, and Les Dames d'Escoffier, New York, was born. Now there are more than thirteen hundred members in twenty-seven chapters across the United States and Canada. Les Dames offers grants and scholarships (almost $4 million to date), mentoring, and community service programs. All of that grew from Brock's desire to give women their due. "I wasn't thinking women's lib," she said. "I didn't want to turn the world upside down. I wanted to do it in a ladylike way."

See also LES DAMES D'ESCOFFIER.

Duke, Nathan. "Food Celebrities' Book Dedicated to Douglaston Resident." *Times Ledger*, November 28, 2008. http://www.timesledger.com/stories/2008/48/whitestone_times_newsmygcwnp11262008.html.

Hindman, Susan. "Silver Star Carol Brock." Silver Planet, February 28, 2009. http://www.silverplanet.com/lifestyles/silver-stars/silver-star-carol-brock/49256#.VNE1SylN3Hg.

Smith, Katherine Newell. "Les Dames d'Escoffier International—A History." http://www.ldei.org/index.php?com=aboutus&c=history.

Linda Pelaccio

Bronx

The Bronx is the northernmost borough of New York City and the only one on the North American mainland. It occupies an area of 42 square miles, and with nearly 1.4 million inhabitants, it is the third most densely populated county in the country. Long home to the Weckquasgeek and Siwanoy Indians, the first European settlers arrived in 1639, when Jonas Bronck established a farmstead at what is now 132nd Street and Lincoln Avenue. Through the seventeenth and eighteenth centuries, the Bronx was a collection of small towns and large manors. Farming was the chief means of livelihood: grains, fruits, vegetables, and livestock, as well as dairy products. Fish and game were also abundant, with the Bronx River being the only freshwater river in New York City.

During the mid-nineteenth century, European immigrants began populating the area, creating numerous discrete ethnic enclaves replete with street vendors and small, family-owned shops and restaurants. Thousands of Irish immigrants came to the Bronx as laborers in the 1840s, fleeing severe famine in Ireland, and settled in the neighborhoods of Highbridge, Wakefield, and Woodlawn, where Irish butchers, pubs, and eateries, such as Mary's Celtic Kitchen on Katonah Avenue, still abound. With railroad expansion, the Bronx also became an attractive residential option for wealthy industrialists and financiers, who could now live in the country but still commute to work in the city. See IRISH.

Breweries

Following the failed 1848 revolution in Germany, thousands of Germans fled to the United States; many of them settled in Unionport (now Castle Hill), Melrose, and Morrisania, becoming shopkeepers, saloon owners, and brewers. German American beer brewing flourished in the Bronx from the middle of the nineteenth century to the first decades of the twentieth century, with numerous breweries operating in Melrose and Morrisania, including the American Brewing Co., Kuntz's, Northside, Mayer's, Eichler's, Rivinius, Haffen, and Hupfel Breweries. The largest was Ebling, on East 156th Street and St. Ann's Avenue. Some breweries also built dance halls that operated as cultural and social centers, as well as outlets for beer. See GERMAN; BEER; BREWERIES; and BEER GARDENS.

The brewing industry in the Bronx largely collapsed with Prohibition. Only Ebling, Mayer, and Eichel continued brewing operations after 1933; by the 1960s all the Bronx breweries were gone. Since the turn of the twenty-first century, however, the borough has seen something of a revival of the industry, with several Bronx-based companies selling beer: the Bronx Brewery was founded in 2009, followed by the Jonas Bronck Beer Company and the City Island Beer Company in 2011. The first company to actually start brewing beer in the Bronx recently was the Gun Hill Brewery, which began operations in its Williamsbridge facility in March 2014.

First Immigration Boom (1890–1930)

By the latter half of the nineteenth century, it was generally assumed that the towns on the mainland would be absorbed by the rapidly expanding New York City; the process of annexation began in 1874 and ended in 1898 with the Greater New York Charter creating the borough of the Bronx. Throughout this period, the area was also industrializing, manufacturing an array of products in its iron foundries, timber mills, ice houses, commercial kilns, and paint, carpet, and piano factories. These industries, along with the extension of elevated and subway lines into

the Bronx, drew newer immigrants (predominantly central and Eastern European Jews as well as Yugoslavians, Armenians, and Italians) into the area, attracted by jobs and spacious, affordable, modern housing. See JEWISH and ITALIAN.

With the tremendous influx of people, the economy of the Bronx also grew. While grocery stores, candy shops, vegetable stands, butcher shops, delicatessens, hand laundries, tailors, and hardware stores were common to most neighborhoods, the largest shopping district in the early part of the twentieth century was an area called the Hub, at East 149th Street and Third Avenue. In addition to boutiques and department stores—including Alexander's, which opened in 1928—there were movie palaces, vaudeville houses, and even the Bronx Opera House. There were also several fine dining establishments; some, such as the High Mandarin on Third Avenue and 149th Street and the Bronx Tea Garden by the Prospect Avenue subway station, offered Chinese cuisine. Later, Fordham Road, by the Grand Concourse, would eclipse the Hub as the Bronx's premier shopping district. Dominated by the Loew's Paradise Theatre and an Alexander's branch that opened in 1938, the area offered a panoply of culinary delights: Bronxites who grew up in the 1950s and 1960s fondly recall eating at the Chinese Casino near Fordham Road and stopping for pastries and cakes at Sutter's Bakery on the Concourse. Ice cream parlors were in particular abundance, with Schrafft's and Krum's Ice Cream and Candy Shop on the Concourse and a Jahn's Ice Cream Parlor—famous for its "kitchen sink sundaes"—on Kingsbridge Road. (The original Jahn's opened in Mott Haven in 1897.) See ICE CREAM SHOPS.

Many of the southern Italian immigrants who came to the Bronx at the turn of the twentieth century settled in Belmont and found work as builders and landscapers for the nearby New York Botanical Gardens (1891) and Bronx Zoo (1899), creating what would come to be known as the "Little Italy" of the Bronx. The area has since condensed to the blocks surrounding Arthur Avenue and its retail market, a Works Progress Administration project that was part of Mayor Fiorello La Guardia's citywide campaign to eliminate pushcarts. Some of the specialty stores there have been family-owned and operated for the better part of a century. Restaurants serving Italian American food—many at least fifty years old—include neighborhood standards like Mario's, Dominick's, and Roberto's. Alex and Henry's, a steakhouse on 161st Street, was a favorite for the lawyers and judges of the County Courthouse as well as a popular spot for Yankee fans. Stella d'Oro, a maker of Italian cookies and breadsticks, had its factory bakery in Kingsbridge, and the smell of freshly baked cookies permeated the neighborhood from 1931 to 2009. See ARTHUR AVENUE; LA GUARDIA, FIORELLO; and STELLA D'ORO.

While the commercial identity of Arthur Avenue remains Italian, the ethnic composition of the neighborhood has been undergoing a subtle transformation. Albanians, who began settling around Fordham Road and Pelham Parkway in the 1960s and 1970s, have taken over some of the pizzerias and restaurants (Tony & Tina's, Kulla), serving Albanian fare such as *burek* (savory baked pastries filled with cheese, vegetables, or meat wrapped in a phyllo-like dough) and *hurmaxhik* with *kajmak* (grilled beef patties stuffed with a fermented cream similar to crème fraîche; some stuff the patties with mozzarella). Some local stores have also begun to carry Albanian products and halal meat.

German and Hungarian Jews initially settled in Kingsbridge, Riverdale, Tremont, and Mount Eden in the 1840s and later populated the art deco buildings lining the Grand Concourse. The Jewish population in the Bronx reached its height in the 1930s. Synagogues and schools were built, and kosher stores proliferated. For a time, Jewish commercial life centered on Bathgate Avenue, although many establishments all over the Bronx became destinations, especially the delicatessens: Schweller's and Epstein Brothers on Jerome Avenue; Mos Kov's on Mount Eden Avenue; Mount Eden Deli, 167th Street Deli, and Fried's on West Burnside Avenue; and Spiegel's Hungarian Restaurant on East 167th Street. Both Loeser's (1960) and Liebman's (1953) in Riverdale are still open today. Moishe's Appetizing and Supermarket provided lox, dairy goods, chopped salads, bread, bagels, and bialys; and, of course, there were open-air stalls that sold pickles. See APPETIZING STORES; DELIS, GERMAN; DELIS, JEWISH; and PICKLES.

The Great Depression marked the end of a period of tremendous growth and expansion for the Bronx. After World War II the population began to shift, with longtime residents and returning GIs leaving older housing in the southern neighborhoods for private homes in the northern Bronx and the surrounding suburbs. Approximately 170,000 people, mostly African American and Puerto Rican, displaced by urban renewal (slum clearance) programs in Manhattan, moved into Hunts Point, Melrose, Morrisania, and Tremont, thereby dramatically changing the demographics of the southern Bronx. The citywide economic crisis of the 1970s was particularly disastrous for the Bronx; a period of rampant arson devastated the physical landscape of huge swaths of the borough, and the southern Bronx became a national symbol of urban blight.

New Immigrants

As a result of the cooperative efforts of grassroots organizations, community groups, and local government, the Bronx began to reemerge and grow again in the 1990s and early 2000s. Recent arrivals from the Caribbean and West Indies settled along the Grand Concourse and throughout the northeast Bronx. At The Good Dine Restaurant in Williamsbridge and Jackie's West Indian Bakery, diners can feast on oxtail, red peas, tripe and beans, spinners (dumplings), curry chicken or curry goat, and spicy pepper shrimp. Royal Caribbean Bakery, one of the largest Jamaican food companies in New York, was founded in Edenwald by Jamaican immigrants Vincent and Jeanette HoSang in 1978. It produces and distributes a wide variety of Jamaican specialties, including hard dough bread, spice buns, coco bread, pastries, *bulla*, black fruit cakes, and, of course, beef, chicken, and vegetable patties. See CARIBBEAN.

Hispanics constitute 53 percent of the current population, predominantly Puerto Rican and Dominican; two well-established Puerto Rican restaurants are 188 Restaurant in Fordham and El Nuevo Bohio in Tremont. The Mexican population is rapidly rising, especially in the Belmont–Fordham–Bedford Park area. This can be seen in the restaurants along Arthur Avenue, where many workers are Mexican and restaurants such as Estrellita Poblana 3 have begun to dot the Italian landscape. Other Mexican restaurants, such as Taqueria Tlaxcalli in Parkchester and Carnitas El Atoradero in Mott Haven, have received praise for their authenticity from a variety of food blogs and the *New York Times*. Many Dominicans settled along the Grand Concourse, and their food, subtly different from its Latinate Caribbean neighbors, is well represented at restaurants like Molino Rojo (Melrose) and Nano Billiards (Morrisania). See PUERTO RICAN; DOMINICAN; and MEXICAN.

The Bronx has welcomed other populations as well: Cambodians (Fordham), Pakistanis and Bengalis (Parkchester), Greeks and Russians (Riverdale), Ecuadorians (Morris Heights and Highbridge), Hondurans (Mott Haven), and Koreans (Bedford Park). There is also a growing population of West Africans, particularly from Ghana and Nigeria, throughout the central Bronx. West African cuisine can be sampled at Bate and Patina African Kitchen in Morrisania, Papaya on the Concourse, Sankofa on Webster Avenue, and Saloum in Williamsbridge, all serving stews of goat or fish, *mafe* (peanut stew), and *fufu* (thick paste made from plantain and cassava). Many Garifuna—Caribs who descend from West and central African, Island Carib, and Arawak people—also live in Mott Haven and celebrate their culture with traditional foods such as *carneada* (grilled steak with *chismil*—a raw sauce of bell peppers, tomatoes, cilantro, and white onion, obviously related to *pico de gallo*—and pickled onions, jalapeno, and cabbage), *judutu* (plantain and coconut soup with fish), *betata* (sweet potato cake), and *dabuledu* (coconut-ginger crisp).

The vibrancy of the current food culture in the Bronx is perhaps best represented by the Baron Ambrosia, the flamboyant alter ego of Justin Fornal, whose adventures on public-access television explore ethnic enclaves and cuisines, celebrating the diversity of the borough. A theatrical and passionate eater, the Baron has starred in, written, directed, and edited all episodes of *Underbelly NYC* and *Bronx Flavor*, while his season on the Cooking Channel show *The Culinary Adventures of Baron Ambrosia* took him farther afield.

There are some enclaves in the Bronx that seemed to have changed little over time. City Island, for instance, has retained the character of a New England fishing and clamming village. The restaurants along City Island Avenue serve mostly seafood, featuring shrimp, lobster, and clams. Across Pelham Bay is Orchard Beach, a beach created by Robert Moses that housed the Orchard Beach Pavilion, a place where bathers could once purchase food from a variety of eateries, from counter to white cloth service.

Food Access: Issues and Community Initiatives

In the 1930s, in an effort to address sanitary problems associated with street vendors, Mayor La Guardia began a campaign to eliminate pushcarts. Part of his program involved expanding the Bronx Terminal Market—originally built in 1917 along the Harlem River between 149th and 152nd Streets in Mott Haven—by adding ten buildings to the original warehouse. For a time, it became the city's main wholesale distributor of ethnic foods; but after a decline in the 1990s, the market was reconstituted as a shopping mall. Much of its business had been taken away by the new Hunts Point Terminal Market, which was opened by the city in 1967 to replace the Washington Wholesale Market in Manhattan. See HUNTS POINT.

The Hunts Point Market, while the largest produce market in the world, is situated in one of the poorest congressional districts in the country. Although none of the Bronx technically qualifies as a "food desert" according to the U.S. Department of Agriculture's definition, residents still have limited access to high-quality produce. Access is a question of both physical proximity to fresh foods (many local markets do not have quality produce) and affordability: according to 2004 census data, 50 percent of households in the Bronx are eligible for food stamps and, for many, the choice of ubiquitous fast food over quality produce is an economic one. The high concentration of poverty and the lack of healthy food options have led to endemic health problems in the borough, particularly high levels of obesity and diet-related diseases. See FOOD DESERTS.

Several local, community-based initiatives are trying to give residents access to quality produce and food products. In Morrisania, the Women's Housing and Economic Development Corporation (WHEDco) provides technical assistance to local residents interested in becoming Green Cart produce vendors (250 certified in 2014) and runs a commercial incubator kitchen for local, small food businesses (168 food entrepreneurs used the space in 2014).

Tanya Fields, a Bronx mother and executive director of the BLK ProjeK, a nonprofit group committed to pursuing food justice and economic development opportunities for underserved women of color, introduced the South Bronx Mobile Market in 2013 to provide organic produce to local residents on a community supported agriculture model, complemented with portioned bulk grocery purchases. See COMMUNITY SUPPORTED AGRICULTURE.

The New York City government is also involved in changing what food is available in the Bronx: the Department of Health Green Cart program licenses vendors of mobile carts to provide fresh produce directly to neighborhoods where access is limited. Ten out of the Bronx's twelve precincts are involved. Also, City Farms Markets, a network of community-run farmers' markets, opened a market in Mott Haven in 2014. The number of vendors tripled in the first year, evidence of the unrelenting evolution of the Bronx.

Badillo, David A. "New Immigrants in the Bronx: Redefining a Cityscape." *Bronx County Historical Society Journal* 44, nos. 1–2 (Spring/Fall 2007): 19–37.

Bronx County Historical Society website: http:// www .bronxhistoricalsociety.org.

Samtur, Stephen M., and Martin A. Jackson. *The Bronx: Lost, Found, and Remembered, 1935–1975.* Scarsdale, N.Y.: Back in the Bronx, 1999.

Ultan, Lloyd. *The Beautiful Bronx (1920–1950).* New York: Harmony, 1979.

Ultan, Lloyd, and Gary Hermalyn. *The Bronx: It Was Only Yesterday, 1935–1965.* Bronx, N.Y.: Bronx County Historical Society, 1992.

Lisa DeLange and Alan Houston

Bronx Cocktail

As with many classic cocktails, the Bronx cocktail has multiple possible origin stories. But the version that receives the widest circulation is the tale of Johnny Solon, a bartender at the original Waldorf Astoria Hotel—not the one that stands today on Park Avenue but the one that occupied the current Fifth Avenue site of the Empire State Building.

Solon's story appears on page 41 of *The Old Waldorf-Astoria Bar Book* (1934) by Albert Stevens Crockett, a historian of the venerable hotel. Solon was an unusual man in that he was a teetotaling bartender. Though he never drank, he was noted for his talent in creating new cocktails on the spot. When a waiter dared Solon to create something new, he mixed gin, sweet and dry vermouth, and orange juice and handed it to the waiter, who first sipped it and then swallowed the rest in one gulp. Duly impressed, the waiter asked Solon what it was called. Solon replied that it was the Bronx cocktail, saying he had been to the Bronx Zoo the previous day and had seen many wild animals. He then noted, "Customers used to tell me of the strange animals they saw after a lot of mixed drinks," and he named his new cocktail in honor of the animals. In this story, then, the drink is named not for the borough but for the zoo that bears its name.

Cocktail history being what it is, though, other bartenders have claimed the drink over the years, including several, of course, in the Bronx and, oddly enough, one in Philadelphia. Most notably, a Hoffman House bartender named William F. Mulhall claimed to create it in the 1880s. No one knows the truth.

One thing that is known about the Bronx is that it is certainly a pre-Prohibition cocktail. The earliest references to the drink show up around 1905. The ingredients are as mentioned in Johnny Solon's tale: gin, sweet vermouth, dry vermouth, and orange juice. In a manner of speaking, the drink is essentially a perfect martini (that is, one made with both types of vermouth) with the addition of orange juice. By 1912, the drink was already popular enough to inspire a silent short film, called *The Bronx Cocktail*. Film historians seem to know little about this picture, except that it was released alongside a comedy short called *A Bad Tangle*. In a 1914 telegram to his girlfriend, F. Scott Fitzgerald—then a college sophomore—recounts a train ride with a friend of his, in which Fitzgerald drank three Bronx cocktails. By the 1930s, the Bronx was one of the most popular cocktails in the United States. A 1934 volume called *Burke's Complete Cocktail & Drinking Recipes*, by Harman Burney Burke, lists the ten most popular cocktails in the country. The Bronx is third, after the martini and the Manhattan.

Perhaps the most famous media reference to the Bronx appears in the 1934 film *The Thin Man*. The movie starts with the main character, William Powell's Nick Charles, instructing a group of bartenders on how to mix various classics. Powell's opening line in the film is, "The important thing is the rhythm. Always have rhythm in your shaking. Now a Manhattan you shake to foxtrot time, a Bronx to two-step time, a dry Martini you always shake to waltz time."

Though such drinks as the martini and the Manhattan remain as popular today as they ever were, the Bronx is nearly unknown today, and no one seems quite sure why. The drinks historian Ted Haigh attributes the cocktail's decline to the popularity of packaged orange juice, which he says makes the drink taste awful. Haigh suggests using fresh-squeezed juice for this drink.

See also MANHATTAN COCKTAIL; MARTINI; and MIXOLOGY.

Felten, Eric. *How's Your Drink? Cocktails, Culture, and the Art of Drinking Well*. Chicago: Surrey, 2007.
Grimes, William. *Straight Up or On the Rocks: A Cultural History of American Drink*. New York: Simon & Schuster, 1993.
Haigh, Ted. *Vintage Spirits and Forgotten Cocktails: From the Alamagoozlum to the Zombie and Beyond: 100 Rediscovered Recipes and the Stories Behind Them*. Beverly, Mass.: Quarry, 2009.

Michael Dietsch

Brooklyn

Brooklyn: the name conjures specific cuisine flavors on the tongue and shouts a brand of time-tested foods that you will see mimicked across the world. New York City's largest borough by population, with 2.6 million people, Brooklyn's name is attached to a bevy of classic dishes: Brooklyn bagels, legendary cheesecake from Junior's diner, egg creams, and a handful of pizzerias that are gladiators in the fiercely competitive coliseum of "best New York City pizza" (which makes them also up for best pizza in the world, as any loyal Brooklynite will tell you). Beyond its pizza-and-bagels roots, Brooklyn is a diverse landscape of food: the old standards are complemented by imports from pockets of ethnic neighborhoods with foods that immigrants have brought from all over the world, including Polish bakeries, Russian seafood restaurants, and Jamaican *roti* shops. On top of that, the modern food movement has given Brooklyn the reputation for being the home for all things artisanal and farm-to-table.

The Dutch

Back before "Brooklyn" was a brand, before it was associated with hip-hop, skinny jeans, or Pabst Blue Ribbon beer, before the intense foodie movement included everything from locally produced honey to artisanal mayonnaise, it was Breuckelen. That's what the Dutch named it when they first settled a part of western Long Island near the East River—what is present-day Brooklyn Heights and Dumbo—in the seventeenth century, borrowing a name from the Holland town of Breukelen. See COLONIAL DUTCH.

For the first 250 years after those settlers arrived, the area that is now known as Flatbush was a town of farms. Those farmers planted various crops through the end of the eighteenth century, including wheat, rye, oats, barley, corn, and other grains, transported by cart to the East River to be sold across the river in Manhattan. The farms involved a lot of slave labor until the state legislature ended slavery in 1827.

When the Erie Canal opened in 1825, it allowed cheaper grain from the Midwest to be transported to New York, so the farmers changed crops. They cultivated market gardens growing cabbage, turnips, potatoes, and other fruits and vegetables. Through the end of the nineteenth century, Kings County (home to Brooklyn) was one of the largest providers of produce in the country, according to the Brooklyn Historical Society. The canal also meant the shipyards in Red Hook became key destinations for ships. Grain, livestock, and produce were stored there before being shipped off to other destinations or used locally. See ERIE CANAL.

Revolutionary War

Brooklyn was a crossroads of the Revolutionary War, though things looked bleak for the colonials for a while. The British captured the city in 1776 and held it for seven years. Some soldiers who were captured by British forces were imprisoned in decommissioned ships anchored off the coast, but others were held in old churches and sugar refineries. The makeshift holding facilities were overcrowded and lacked clean water. Thousands died from the disease-ridden conditions and lack of medical care. In honor of the Battle of Brooklyn, the first battle after the signing of the Declaration of Independence, the Old Stone House in Park Slope hosts an annual Revolutionary Fare event offering up dishes from the era of the battle: corned ham, coleslaw, biscuits, and pies.

Born in Brooklyn

Brooklyn has always been an epicenter of creativity, which is why many common foods today got their start as Brooklyn inventions. In 1910, Samuel Born invented a "Born Sucker Machine," which automatically stuffed sticks into lollipops, changing the way the treats were sold. He opened a shop in Brooklyn in 1923, with a sign that declared the fresh candy "Just

Born." The company later moved to Pennsylvania and started a marshmallow forming process; its signature product, marshmallow chicks called Peeps, would become an Easter candy tradition. See CANDY.

The artificial sweetener Sweet'n Low was created in the borough in 1957. It started when Benjamin Eisenstadt, the man already credited with the idea of putting sugar in packets, created an artificial saccharine-based sweetener at the request of a drug company. The company changed its mind, so he decided to produce it himself as a low-calorie sugar alternative. It is still produced in the same Brooklyn factory today, pumping out one million pink packets a day. See SWEET'N LOW.

Regular sugar had a home there even before that. The Domino Sugar factory was built in 1856 by the Havemeyer family as the first of the dozens of sugar refineries that helped New York become an industrial port city. By the end of the Civil War, the factory had become the largest sugar refinery in the world, churning out 3 million pounds of sugar every day. The 90,000-square-foot building on the Williamsburg waterfront was finally razed in 2014 to make way for new development. Shortly before its destruction, the empty building housed an installation by New York–based artist Kara Walker of a giant sphinx called "A Subtlety"—a sculpture made from sugar—raising issues of race, slavery, and sex. See SUGAR REFINING.

You can trace the all-American hot dog back to a German immigrant in Brooklyn: Charles Feltman is said to have been the first to serve sausage on a bun in 1871, from his pushcart set up near Coney Island's amusements. The ten-cent specialties became known as "hot dogs" by the 1890s, and he expanded his service into a full restaurant. See FELTMAN, CHARLES.

Though several people get credit for it, the famous New York egg cream is surely a Brooklyn invention. The nonalcoholic drinks, made of milk and chocolate syrup frothed with carbonated water (but no actual egg), were popular treats at soda fountains in the 1920s. It was usually made with Fox's U-Bet Chocolate Syrup, which was invented by Brooklynites Herman and Ida Fox in 1895. See EGG CREAMS.

Ethnic Enclaves

Even as gentrification has reshaped the borough, some neighborhoods remain stark ethnic enclaves

that feel like stepping into different worlds. Head to Brighton Beach to find Russian men sipping vodka at Tatiana on the boardwalk, red-sauce Italian restaurants are ample in Bensonhurst, parts of south Williamsburg are home to insular Hasidic communities with their kosher restaurants, Sunset Park has its own Chinatown along Fifth Avenue, and parts of Bushwick are known for excellent tortillerias and Mexican tacos. See JEWISH; RUSSIAN; ITALIAN; CHINESE COMMUNITY; and MEXICAN. The large Caribbean population in Crown Heights celebrates each Labor Day with the West Indian Day Parade, where you can find vendors selling doubles (chickpea sandwiches on fried bread) and *roti* along the Eastern Parkway parade route. See WEST INDIAN DAY PARADE.

Resurgence

Brooklyn was associated with crime and poverty for decades through much of the late twentieth century, but it started to bounce back as a cheaper alternative to Manhattan in the 1980s and 1990s. One of the earliest stalwarts to champion the Brooklyn name was Brooklyn Brewery, which opened in 1988. The borough was once a beer paradise, home to forty-eight breweries; but the last old-line one, Rheingold, closed its doors in 1976. When Steve Hindy first tried to sell his new beer, no restaurants or bars wanted to carry a beer with the down-at-heel "Brooklyn" name. "Truck drivers would not come in after dark because of the crime," Hindy said in an interview. Now, not only is the Williamsburg brewery a staple across the city but it opened an outpost in Stockholm, and its beer can be found from Israel to El Salvador. See BREWERIES and BROOKLYN BREWERY.

The next era of new Brooklyn began in 2012, when, after a long political fight, the new Barclays Center arena opened on part of what was an old train yard. With the help of Jay-Z (who owned a tiny fraction of the team), the New Jersey Nets relocated to Brooklyn, making them the first professional sports team in the borough since the Dodgers. The state-of-the-art arena included an outpost of Jay-Z's 40/40 Club and swapped out typical stadium food for many of Brooklyn's famed food options: Fatty 'Cue barbecue, Junior's restaurant (home to that famous cheesecake), Nathan's hot dogs, and Habana Outpost, a Cuban eatery from nearby Fort Greene. See JUNIOR'S and NATHAN'S FAMOUS.

Rooftop farms have sprung up, bringing greenery to the often gray cityscape. Brooklyn Grange, opened in 2010, is the world's largest rooftop farm, according to *National Geographic*. It covers 2.5 acres of two separate buildings, producing more than fifty thousand pounds of organically grown produce each year. Much of it is sold to local restaurants or through its own farmers' market. See ROOFTOP GARDEN.

A long way from its gritty roots, Brooklyn has become a brand, with the name popping up in fashionable contexts from Dubai to Paris, where *New York Times* reporter Julia Moskin wrote in 2012 that "très Brooklyn" was being used as a haute compliment: "Among young Parisians, there is currently no greater praise for cuisine than 'très Brooklyn,' a term that signifies a particularly cool combination of informality, creativity and quality."

See also BAY RIDGE; BEDFORD-STUYVESANT; BENSONHURST; BRIGHTON BEACH; BUSHWICK; LITTLE ODESSA; PARK SLOPE; SUNSET PARK; and WILLIAMSBURG.

Anderson, Will. *The Breweries of Brooklyn: An Informal History of a Great Industry in a Great City*. Croton Falls, N.Y.: Anderson, 1976.

Benardo, Leonard, and Jennifer Weiss. *Brooklyn by Name: How the Neighborhoods, Streets, Parks, Bridges and More Got Their Names*. New York: New York University Press, 2006.

Miller, Mark J. "A Farm Grows in Brooklyn—On the Roof." *National Geographic*, April 2014. http://news .nationalgeographic.com/news/2014/04/140429-farming-rooftop-gardening-brooklyn-grange-vegetables-science-food/.

Montrose, Morris. "Walkabout: Brooklyn and the Erie Canal, Part 2." *Brownstoner*, October 4, 2012. http://www.brownstoner.com/blog/2012/10/walkabout-brooklyn-and-the-erie-canal-part-2/.

Moskin, Julia. "Food Trucks in Paris? U.S. Cuisine Finds Open Minds, and Mouths. *New York Times*, June 3, 2012.

Smith, Andrew F. *New York City: A Food Biography*. Lanham, Md.: Rowman & Littlefield, 2013.

Thompson, Nato. "CreativeTime Presents Kara Walker: Curatorial Statement." http://creativetime.org/projects/karawalker/curatorial-statement/.

Tim Donnelly

Brooklyn Brewery

Founded in 1988 by Steve Hindy, a former war correspondent for the Associated Press, and Tom Potter, a banker, the Brooklyn Brewery brought locally made and marketed beer back to a borough that had once been a brewing powerhouse. With $500,000 in startup capital raised from family and friends, Hindy—a newspaperman—had sought to call the business the Brooklyn Eagle Brewery, a nod to the historic afternoon paper.

Among the first things the duo did was contact and eventually convince legendary graphic designer Milton Glaser to create a logo that would give their fledgling venture an instant identity. Glaser convinced them to drop the word "eagle" from the business name, allowing the borough of Brooklyn to be the focus. Glaser waived his usual fees in exchange for an equity stake in the brewery. To this day, Glaser designs every label produced by the brewery and receives a regularly delivered fresh supply of beer to his office.

Rather than building a traditional brewery at the onset, Hindy and Potter contracted the F. X. Matt Brewery in Utica, New York, to brew the flagship Brooklyn lager. For the recipe, the partners contracted William M. Moeller, a fourth-generation brewmaster who, according to the brewery, pored over brewing logs kept by his grandfather, who had brewed in Brooklyn at the turn of the twentieth century. The result, the brewery says, was an all-malt lager beer with a tangy aroma created by "dry-hopping," an age-old technique of adding hops during the maturation process to create a robust aroma.

The pair began selling and delivering beer. Their first account was Teddy's, a Williamsburg bar run by longtime neighborhood activist Felice Kirby and her husband in the old Peter Doelger's Extra Beer pub.

Eventually the company was ready for a brewery of its own, and in 1994 Garrett Oliver was hired as brewmaster. During his first meeting with Hindy, Oliver, a former president of the New York City Homebrewer's Guild, brewer at the now closed Manhattan Brewing, and rock band manager, discussed a recipe that would eventually become Brooklyn Black Chocolate Stout. Oliver is also the author of several books, served as editor of the *Oxford Companion to Beer*, and received the 2014 James Beard Award for Outstanding Wine, Beer, or Spirits Professional. The new brewery was officially opened on May 28, 1996, with a ribbon cutting by Mayor Rudy Giuliani.

In 2003 Potter retired and sold his shares to the Ottaway family, longtime friends and early investors. He would later start the New York Distilling

Company. In 2014, Eric Ottaway was named chief executive officer and his brother Robin, president. That same year the brewery and Carlsberg opened a joint venture, Nya Carnegie, a brewery and tasting room in Stockholm, Sweden. Also in 2014 Brooklyn donated a microbrewery to the Culinary Institute of America, and Oliver is developing a brewing curriculum for the CIA to familiarize students with the brewing process and produce beers for the school's restaurants. In 2014 the brewery shipped 252,000 barrels of beer, with one barrel representing 31.5 gallons.

See also BEER; BREWERIES; and BROOKLYN.

Beer Marketer's Insights 6, no. 7 (2015).
Brooklyn Brewery website: http://www.brooklynbrewery.com.
Hindy, Steve. *The Craft Beer Revolution: How a Band of Microbrewers Is Transforming the World's Favorite Drink.* New York: Palgrave Macmillan, 2014.
Oliver, Garrett. *The Brewmaster's Table: Discovering the Pleasures of Real Beer with Real Food.* New York: Ecco, 2005.
Oliver, Garrett, ed. *The Oxford Companion to Beer.* New York: Oxford University Press, 2011.

John Holl

Brooklyn Cocktail

The Brooklyn cocktail is a variation on the Manhattan. See MANHATTAN COCKTAIL. The latter drink is a blend of American whiskey (either rye or bourbon), sweet vermouth, and Angostura bitters. The Brooklyn is not much more than a dry Manhattan, with dry vermouth replacing the sweet. It also originally called for a dash of maraschino liqueur (a cherry-based liqueur) and a small amount of Amer Picon (a bitter liqueur produced in Europe, which is still relatively hard to find in the United States; as a result, most modern bartenders either use other bitter liqueurs in place of Amer Picon or craft their own re-creation of Amer Picon).

The Brooklyn cocktail was first described in print in 1908, in J. A. Grohusko's *Jack's Manual*, a book aimed at innkeepers, bartenders, and restaurateurs. Grohusko's recipe called for equal parts rye whiskey and Italian (sweet) vermouth, plus maraschino liqueur and Amer Picon bitters. In short, the first printed Brooklyn recipe was a barely modified Manhattan. By 1914, the vermouth had changed. Jacques Straub's *Drinks* offers a recipe identical to Grohus-

ko's, except that it calls for French (dry) vermouth in place of the sweet Italian type. Though the proportions changed over time, this recipe has stuck: rye whiskey, dry vermouth, maraschino, and Amer Picon.

The Brooklyn gave rise in the early 2000s to several variations, all named for various Brooklyn neighborhoods, usually modifying the sweet vermouth but keeping most other ingredients intact. This trend started in 2004 at the neo-speakeasy Milk & Honey, where bartender Vincenzo Errico created a drink called the Red Hook, which uses a bittersweet vermouth called Punt e Mes in place of dry French vermouth. Similarly, the Greenpoint uses the herbal liqueur yellow Chartreuse along with a bit of sweet vermouth, while the Bensonhurst calls for Cynar, an Italian bitter liqueur that has artichoke as an ingredient. Other variants have arisen, named for other Brooklyn neighborhoods, including the Cobble Hill, the Carroll Gardens, and the Bushwick.

Grohusko, J. A. *Jack's Manual: A Treatise on the Care and Handling of Wines and Liquors, Storing, Binning, and Serving; Recipes for Fancy Mixed Drinks and When and How to Serve.* New York: E. V. Brokaw, 1908.
Hepburn, Jay. "Exploring the Borough." *Oh Gosh!* (blog), February 23, 2010. http://ohgo.sh/archive/brooklyn-cocktail-variations-red-hook-greenpoint-bensonhurst-recipe/.

Michael Dietsch

Brooklyn Flea

See SMORGASBURG.

Brunch

The word "brunch"—a meal that combines breakfast and lunch—originated in England during the late nineteenth century. It was a leisurely meal, served in the early afternoon after a late Saturday night out. Brunch did not become a New York City culinary experience until the early 1930s, when Chef Werner Haechler offered it in the dining room at the Hotel Lombardy, on East Fifty-Sixth Street in Manhattan. Also called the "tally-ho lunch" or the "hunt lunch," it was served as a buffet from noon until 4:00 p.m. on Sundays; the price was $1.25. Typical brunch items

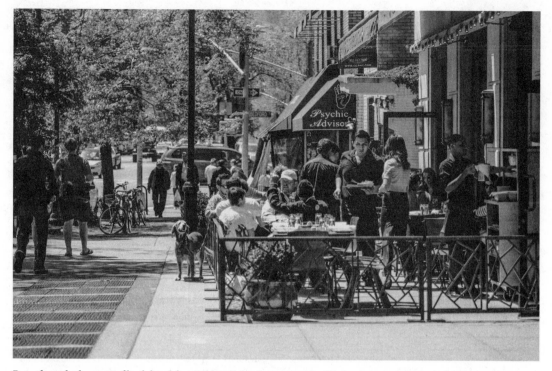

Brunch, with elements of both breakfast and lunch, has become a New York institution, particularly after 1960 as incomes rose and Sunday church attendance fell. MICHELE URSINO

at the Lombardy included fruit juices, scrambled eggs and bacon, rolls, brioches, croissants, toast, and coffee. There was also a substantial main dish, such as kidney stew, sausage cakes, codfish cakes, fried oysters, shrimp, hash, or tomato salad. Chef Haechler would ask diners about their favorite Sunday dishes and then feature them at future brunches. The cost of the meal included a drink, such as a whiskey sour, and free entertainment: music, performances, and dancing.

Although the idea of brunch was catching on, not everyone was happy with the word. James Beard, for instance, complained about it; he preferred "late lunch." See BEARD, JAMES. Restaurateur George Rector despised the word—until he ate at Lombardy's: "René is maitre d'hotel at the Lombardy, and he loves brunch. He caresses the word. 'Brrhrhrrunch,' he says, happily rolling the r's deep in his throat in a manner to excite the envy of any French instructor" (Rector, 1939, p. 247). See RECTOR, CHARLES AND GEORGE.

Although leisure time was a scarce commodity during World War II, brunch reemerged during the 1950s with new juice-and-vodka drinks tailor-made

for the meal: the Bloody Mary (tomato juice and vodka), the apple-knocker (apple juice and vodka), the screwdriver (orange juice and vodka), and the bulldozer (beef bouillon and vodka). See BLOODY MARY. Other popular brunch drinks were champagne, mimosas (champagne and orange juice), brandy Alexanders, and even mint juleps. During the late 1930s alcohol could not be served in New York City restaurants before 1:00 p.m., so brunch service usually began at that hour. When the law was changed, brunch started earlier.

During the 1950s Saturday became a second brunch day, and some restaurants even served it on weekdays. With the exception of large hotels, most restaurants gave up the buffet and served orders to tables. Standard brunch menus included traditional breakfast dishes, such as eggs, French toast, pancakes, hash browns, and bacon; but they also included dishes more commonly eaten for lunch. In 1958, Craig Claiborne, the New York Times food writer, recommended this menu for an Easter brunch: eggs Benedict, kedgeree, baked kippered herring, and smothered shad roe.

Beginning around 1960, as incomes rose and Sunday church attendance fell, brunch became even more popular. Ethnic foods found a wider audience. For instance, bagels with cream cheese and lox, which had long been a Sunday morning tradition among Jewish New Yorkers, was enjoyed by New Yorkers of all ethnicities. Chinese, Mexican, and other ethnic restaurants served brunch. Restaurants all over the city offered brunch, but in the 1970s *New York Times* writer Mimi Sheraton identified newly chic SoHo as "Brunchville."

Sunday brunch remains an important New York culinary tradition. The Lombardy Hotel, where the New York brunch began, is still open but, ironically, it no longer serves Sunday brunch.

See also BAGELS; CREAM CHEESE; EGGS BENEDICT; and LOX.

Lahman, DeDe, Neil Kleinberg, and Michael Harlan Turkell. *Clinton St. Baking Company Cookbook: Breakfast, Brunch & Beyond from New York's Favorite Neighborhood Restaurant.* New York: Little, Brown, 2010.
Rector, George. *Dining in New York with Rector.* New York: Prentice-Hall, 1939.
Sheraton, Mimi. "A Savory Guide to the Town's Best Brunches." *New York Times,* March 18, 1977, 56.
Ternikar, Farha. *Brunch: A History.* London: Rowman & Littlefield, 2014.

Andrew F. Smith

Burns, Jabez

See COFFEE ROASTERS.

Bushwick

Bushwick, a neighborhood in North Brooklyn, has developed from farmland to a center of food industry in the nineteenth century to a symbol of urban blight in the late twentieth century to its current position as a burgeoning artist and hipster community with a lively and active local food scene. The long-established taquerias remain along with new destinations for food lovers. Bushwick is known for its creative residents, who brought new life to this once-industrial neighborhood. Now upscale restaurants exist on otherwise desolate-looking blocks. When Williamsburg restaurant space became just as expensive as or surpassed that in Manhattan, a modest number of restaurants opened in Bushwick. These restaurants helped Bushwick rise as a neighborhood worth the trip for a unique dining experience.

From a bucolic area in the seventeenth century, Bushwick began to industrialize by the 1830s. Drawing immigrant German workers, Bushwick became a major center for brewing in the nineteenth century, housing such famous German breweries as Piels, Schaefer's, and Schlitz. It soon became populated with Italian American communities. In the early twentieth century, the Bushwick breweries supplied almost 10 percent of pilsner beer sold in the United States. These family-run breweries dominated the area and helped it develop into an industrial center. See BREWERIES.

By the era of Prohibition, Bushwick was becoming an industrial slum, aided by the criminal syndicates that took advantage of antiliquor legislation to gain a powerful foothold in New York's underworld. See PROHIBITION. In the mid-twentieth century, most of the breweries had closed down or left New York. With few jobs, poor and abandoned housing, and neglect by the city government, Bushwick disintegrated into a low-income area with high rates of poverty and crime. During the 1977 blackout, looting and riots broke out around the city but were especially concentrated in Bushwick, which became a symbol of this urban unrest. The blackout completed the cycle of devastation in the neighborhood. Rather than rebuild damaged properties, many remaining Bushwick residents fled the city. In the 1980s, Knickerbocker Avenue was notorious for drug activity and crime.

In the early twenty-first century, Bushwick began a recovery. Newer immigrants from the Caribbean and Latin America have helped to revitalize the neighborhood's economy. The Bushwick Initiative, a city program aimed at improving housing and fostering commercial activity, has improved the quality of life for Bushwick residents. And Bushwick has become a magnet for artists and young professionals seeking affordable housing and studio spaces. The first artists transformed industrial buildings seemingly overnight into artist studios. Bushwick Open Studios, an annual event, draws people from other neighborhoods.

Today, Bushwick has a reputation as a trendy, hip neighborhood, characterized by its gritty atmosphere. In *Frommer's NYC Free & Dirt Cheap*, Ethan Wolff (2007) wrote, "Bushwick's blend of young, arty energy and rundown streets is about as close as you can get to the East Village in the 1980s. (There's even an offshoot of the original Life Cafe immortalized in *Rent*.)" Bushwick also has a thriving local food scene.

The linchpin of the Bushwick food revolution was Roberta's. This pizza restaurant revitalized interest from people throughout the city. Even locals are willing to endure the wait for pizzas, covered with unconventional ingredients such as Brussels sprouts and honey and burnished to perfection. Short of raising their own livestock, much of the work is done on the premises. Roberta's has become more of a compound than a restaurant. Out back, the garden is the source of the Brussels sprouts on the pizza. The bees housed on the rooftop make the honey. Roberta's also offers a line of frozen pizzas and takeout, sold from a space next door. See ROBERTA'S.

Other notable restaurants abound, including Northeast Kingdom (for seasonal vegetables and countrified charm), Tortilleria Mexicana Los Hermanos (a long-standing Mexican joint inside a tortilla factory), Momo Sushi Shack (a hidden sushi gem), Dear Bushwick (for homemade classics), and Boona Cafe (large-format, shareable Ethiopian fare). Next door to Roberta's is Blanca, an expensive tasting counter. Former *New York Times* restaurant critic Pete Wells characterized Blanca as a restaurant "where the abundance of courses is Roman, the structure of the meal is Italian, the rigorous minimalism of the cooking is Japanese and the easy and improbable grace with which it all hangs together is unmistakably American" (Wells, 2012). At $185 per person, it is by far the priciest restaurant in Bushwick. In 2010, the literary zine *Bushwick Review*, published haiku restaurant reviews written by the Village Voice's restaurant critic, Zachary Feldman. He wrote about the most popular restaurants in Bushwick: Roberta's, Momo Sushi Shack, and Tortilleria Mexicana Los Hermanos. This demonstrated how the artist community embraced the neighborhoood's cluster of popular restaurants new and old.

Once the rebuilding was under way, The Heritage Radio Network, a nonprofit Internet radio station about food, started webcasting its broadcasts out of a studio in the lot next to Roberta's. It was hyperlocal and hyperniche, and listeners from around the world tuned in. One of the first shows was *Urban Foragers*, a meandering dialogue hosted by Jori Jayne Emde and Zakary Pelaccio. The hosts were obsessive explainers of all things edible, with a focus on environmentally conscious food. Industry professionals gave brief, to-the-point reviews of restaurant experiences; and they also discussed restaurant reviews. Today, Heritage Radio Network hosts *The Main Course, Eat Your Words, Eating Disorder, Inside School Food, Roberta's Radio, Cooking Issues, Taste Matters*, and *Food Talk with Mike Colameco* (former chef and food personality). Their show *All in the Industry* hosts "insider" personalities to give their take on food by supplying quick answers to a series of predetermined questions. The founder of Heritage Radio Network, Patrick Martins, is also the coauthor of *The Carnivore's Manifesto: Eating Well, Eating Responsibly and Eating Meat*, and he created Heritage Foods USA. He is an advocate for eating sustainably. See HERITAGE RADIO NETWORK.

See also BROOKLYN.

"Bushwick History." *The Food Communities of NYC* (blog). http://macaulay.cuny.edu/eportfolios/lobel11neighborhoods/bushwick/bushwick-history/.
Heritage Radio Network website: http://www.heritageradionetwork.org.
Malanga, Steven. "The Death and Life of Bushwick." *City Journal* (Spring 2008). http://www.city-journal.org/2008/18_2_bushwick.html.
Thilman, James. "Photo Tour of Bushwick in Brooklyn, New York City." *TimeOut New York*, September 18, 2012.
Wells, Pete. "A Tiny Stage Full of Song in Bushwick." *New York Times*. October 16, 2012.
Wolff, Ethan. *Frommer's NYC Free & Dirt Cheap*. 2d ed. Hoboken, N.J.: Wiley, 2007.

Ashley Hoffman

Business Lunch

Mealtime—particularly lunch, in the middle of a workday—is at the center of many a business negotiation. Historians of American dietary patterns demonstrate how industrialization and urbanization interrupted the practice of families dining together in the middle of the day. Then as now, laborers bound by the work clock's regimentation were often limited to brief lunch periods of thirty minutes or less. They lunched on comestibles brought from home or hastily purchased at a lunch cart or counter. Those with the pocketbook and work schedule to support it, however, dined out, enjoying lunch at a more leisurely pace. More than a break for respite and nourishment, the business lunch emerged as a pivotal time—and the restaurant a powerful place—to share ideas and conduct business.

These negotiations took place prominently and with great luxury in New York City. In fact, the noon meal stands out so decidedly in the city's history that it inspired a recent exhibition by the New York Public Library, which ran from June 2012 through February 2013 and can still be viewed online. *Lunch Hour NYC* contends that on the busy streets of New York City lunch attained a newfound sense of modernity. See NEW YORK PUBLIC LIBRARY. Decidedly modern ideas were hatched at a number of notable New York restaurants and watering holes, including many specific to certain industries. For example, with its prime location in the financial district, Delmonico's sophisticated offerings supported business lunches from at least the 1830s. See DELMONICO'S. At the Algonquin Hotel, critics, essayists, playwrights, and editors gathered around what came to be called the Round Table, sharing conversations that led to the founding of the *New Yorker* in 1925. See ALGONQUIN ROUND TABLE. Against a backdrop of the caricatures that decorated the walls, theater critics, columnists, and press agents lunched at Sardi's, which opened in 1927. See SARDI'S. Starting in 1959, the most famed and fortunate rubbed shoulders at the Four Seasons, where the prices on the menu towered as high as the egos. See FOUR SEASONS.

Pertaining to meals both within and outside of New York City, Roland Barthes writes of business lunches as evidence of the duality within the modern culinary condition. Often structured around set, commercialized menus, business lunches also adhere to a more traditional commitment to leisurely timing and a dedication to long and meaningful conversation. As such, business lunches retain "the mythical conciliatory power of conviviality," albeit to facilitate the desires of business. Such sentiment surely fed the creation of the term "power lunch," which first appeared in *Esquire* in 1979, inspired by the goings-on at the Four Seasons' Grill Room. As both a business ritual and a cultural custom, lunching together, especially in New York City, continues to provide opportunity for networking and connecting, developing personal relationships and building community, sharing ideas and gathering information—as well as hammering out deals and forging the future.

See also POWER BREAKFASTS AND POWER LUNCHES.

Barthes, Roland. "Toward a Psychosociology of Contemporary Food Consumption." In *Food and Culture: A Reader*, edited by Carole Counihan and Penny Van Esterik, pp. 23–30. New York: Routledge, 2013.
New York Public Library. "Power Lunch." *Lunch Hour NYC*. http://exhibitions.nypl.org/lunchhour/exhibits/show/lunchhour/power.

Emily J. H. Contois

Butchers

The Northeast was a utopia of wildlife during early colonial periods. Markets began selling meat and fowl as early as the late 1600s. With the innovation of railways and waterways, it became significantly easier to transport food to the island of Manhattan. Meat, as opposed to livestock, was transported in much larger quantities once modern refrigeration techniques were invented. "Railways and refrigeration transformed meatpacking from a local and seasonal small business enterprise into an industry that distributed its product year-round and nationwide" (Stull and Broadway, 2004, p. 39).

Markets became more prevalent and sold increasingly exotic wares throughout the 1800s, most commonly along the East River. The quality of the product varied depending on the time of day and what was available, but customers built relationships with the skilled butchers who had an in-depth knowledge about the animals and their origins. Becoming a butcher was a profession and livelihood, often requiring long apprenticeships and training.

The importance of the butcher declined beginning in 1908 as a result of the invention of the conveyor belt system. New York City was introduced to the industrialization of butchering by way of assembly lines and mechanized slaughterhouses, eliminating the need for skilled butchers in lieu of low-wage laborers. The meat industry was later significantly affected by the economic boom, technological innovations, and the major cultural shift that came about at the end of World War II. Modern home refrigeration systems were perfected, ensuring that meat could last for weeks instead of mere days. Chemicals and hormones were introduced to young animals to speed up the maturation process. Next, a company called DuPont took the concept of cellophane wrapping and applied it to meat packaging. The thin plastic wrapping material sealed the meat, locking in its "freshness" by protecting it from bacteria and oxygen—hence the birth of a marketing scheme. Meat became instantly more appealing simply because of its plastic casing. Shopping became more of an impersonal experience. Production was outsourced great distances from the Northeast to unskilled laborers in factories, and the food was laden with chemicals. The industry rose to meet the demands of the public, but it did so with consequences.

Shopping to feed one's family was originally a tradition rooted in social interaction with a value placed on quality and origin of product as well as on the integrity and skill of those who produce and distribute. Because of industrialization and consumer demand, the meat industry has since morphed into a business of mass production based upon convenience and accessibility. The social experience of knowing one's local butcher and his product and of interacting with him during the process of choosing one's meal has been lost with the frenetic pace and desire for convenience of modern life. However, increased incidences of food-borne illnesses, diseases from food additives, and negative environmental impacts of the current meat industry have led many people to question this business model. Consumers are increasingly opting for alternative routes of procurement that harken back to traditional butchering practices. The time is ripe for the resurgence of the specialty butcher.

Although Manhattan is still a city primarily driven by convenience, price, and speed, many consumers who have the means and flexibility have adopted emerging trends in food culture. "Distance traveled," "organic," "grass-fed," and "hormone-free" are newer terms used to describe basic practices of the 1900s and earlier. More Americans have come full circle and are getting back to the traditional roots of butcher shops. Not only do health and safety create motivation for consumers to shop through local vendors, but the explosion of "foodie culture" since the mid-1990s has also opened the door for niche and artisanal purveyors to expand their businesses.

When opening the now famed franchise Shake Shack, Danny Meyer asked specialty butcher Pat LeFrieda to create a mix for his burgers. See SHAKE SHACK. This subtle change on the recipe of a classic burger opened the door for creativity and innovation from simply altering a recipe to experimenting with different cuts of meat. Suddenly, as Florence Fabricant (2011) explains, butcher shops, "once a vestige, are opening in many New York neighborhoods where buying meat has often been reduced to staring down a sea of plastic-wrapped foam trays." Taking a stroll to the neighborhood butcher or through a local market is now a pastime. One can talk to experienced butchers about everything from the farm a cow was raised on to the health benefits of eating bison. Unusual cuts not often found in grocery stores are commonplace in the butcher shop, and they are sold proudly by young men who not only dismembered the carcasses themselves but also offer classes for interested New Yorkers to learn how to do the same. The famed Williamsburg butcher shop Meat Hook does just that.

Butchers also offer services to increase convenience, such as deboning or grinding in-store. The experience can be customized. Customers can buy alternative cuts of meat at cheaper prices while attaining better service and a superior product. "They want to talk to the butcher. They want the down-home touch," explains *New York Times* writer Marian Burros (1983). There is now a shift in consumer demand, away from the mysterious, prepackaged, and mass-produced meat toward fresh, unique cuts of meat, sold à la carte by trained and knowledgeable professionals. The company Dickson's Farmstand Meats takes pride in butchering all its animal products from its upstate New York farms in-house at its Chelsea Market outpost. Similarly, Heritage Meat operates out of the Essex Street market, offers "break-down demos" on whole animal butchering, and lists the breed of each animal on what it sells. There are also shops, such as Fleisher's of Kingston, that proudly sell only locally sourced, sustainable, hormone- and antibiotic-free meat. Additionally, the shop offers a comprehensive three-month butchering apprenticeship program as well as shorter "butchery 101" classes.

The industrialization of the meat industry produced amazing innovations and proved that humans have the ability to meet the changing demands for survival. However, these developments came at the cost of public health. Additionally, the development of the meat industry damaged the traditional institution of shopping for one's food. The personal connection with a meal as well as between the customer and distributor was lost. Today, consumers are beginning to realize the worth of small businesses that provide quality products by trained professionals. The power of consumer demand to elicit change in "foodie culture" has enacted a shift back toward traditional roots, favoring the specialty butcher.

Burros, Marian. "Supermarkets Enter the Age of Specialty Foods." *New York Times*, April 6, 1983.
Fabricant, Florence. "The Lost Art of Buying from a Butcher." *New York Times*, November 1, 2011.
Shulman, Robin. *Eat the City: A Tale of the Fishers, Trappers, Hunters, Foragers, Slaughterers, Butchers, Farmers, Poultry Minders, Sugar Refiners, Cane Cutters, Beekeepers, Winemakers, and Brewers Who Built New York.* New York: Crown, 2012.
Stull, Donald D., and Michael J. Broadway. *Slaughterhouse Blues.* 2d ed. Belmont, Calif.: Thomson/Wadsworth, 2004.
Wasserman, Suzanne, dir. *Meat Hooked.* DVD. New York: Phizmonger Pictures, 2012.

Kristina Mellegard

Butler Grocery Stores

See GROCERY STORES.

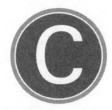

Café Nicholson

Café Nicholson, a tiny, notably eccentric restaurant located at 323 East Fifty-Eighth Street in Manhattan, opened in 1949 with chef Edna Lewis at its helm, attracting society types and artists for more than a half-century. Johnny Nicholson, a window dresser and antiques dealer, found inspiration in Café Greco, a coffeehouse in Rome, and aimed to replicate it with his eponymous café, described by writer John T. Edge in his retrospective of the restaurant as a sort of "bohemian supper club set in the back courtyard of an antique store." It originally opened on East Fifty-Seventh Street, moving to the Fifty-Eighth Street location after a couple of years—a former artists' studio, nearly hidden at the edge of the entrance to the upper roadway of the Queensboro Bridge.

The restaurant served as a launching pad for Edna Lewis, a Virginia native and African American chef noted for her role in preserving traditional southern foods and preparations. In the late 1940s, female chefs were few and far between and black female chefs were a rarity, yet Edna Lewis became well known and beloved for her simple but delicious cooking—roast chicken, chocolate soufflé—which attracted celebrities such as Tennessee Williams, Truman Capote, Richard Avedon, Gloria Vanderbilt, Marlene Dietrich, and Diana Vreeland. Lewis stayed with the restaurant until 1954.

The restaurant also was famed for its hushed, "butler-like" service and willfully eclectic décor, which Nicholson once termed "fin de siecle Caribbean of Cuba style." One press report called it "Spanish-Portuguese belle époque," and another described it as "a turn-of-the century Parisian pleasure palace."

Café Nicholson's idiosyncratic hours also were a point of legend. From 1978 to 1981 the restaurant was open only during the fall and spring. A 1986 Zagat review warned that the "romantic hideaway" was open "when Mr. Nicholson is in the mood, i.e., not often."

Nicholson sold the restaurant in 1999 to chef Patrick Woodside, who dropped "Café" from the name. It did not last long; in 2000, Nicholson closed its doors for good.

See also LEWIS, EDNA.

Burros, Marian. "An Innovator in Café Décor and in Food." *New York Times*, March 10, 1982.
Edge, John. "Debts of Pleasure." *Oxford American*, September 16, 2013.
Edna Lewis Foundation website: http://www .ednalewisfoundation.org.
Grimes, William. "Restaurants; Curiouser and Curiouser, Chapter 2." *New York Times*, June 21, 2000.

Kara Newman

Café Royal

See RESTAURANTS.

Cafés

See COFFEEHOUSES.

Café Society

See STORK CLUB and "21" CLUB.

Cafeterias

Self-service restaurants, called "cafeterias," were a novelty in New York City in the 1880s. The first on the scene was the Exchange Buffet, which opened its doors across the street from the New York Stock Exchange on September 4, 1885. It catered to busy stockbrokers and other financial district workers, almost exclusively men, who did not have the luxury of a leisurely lunch hour. Customers at the Exchange Buffet picked up their selections—sandwiches, salads, perhaps a slice of cake, and tea, coffee, or milk—from a buffet along the wall. They carried the full plates and cups as best they could to tall counters, where they ate standing up. Each customer bused his own dishes, tallied his own bill, and then told the cashier what he owed. This self-service operation based on the honor system was surprisingly successful, and over the next few years the Exchange Buffet opened thirty-five more cafeterias in Manhattan, Brooklyn, and Newark, New Jersey.

The crowds surging around these cafeterias inspired others to open quick, casual lunch places. In 1889, William and Samuel Child opened their first lunchroom on the main floor of the Merchants Hotel. Cleanliness was a keynote of the operation, and workers wore pristine white aprons and caps. Unlike the Exchange Buffet, the lunchroom catered mainly to women. In 1898 the Childs introduced trays—so that their customers did not have to juggle dishes. By 1925 the Childs brothers had expanded their successful restaurant into a national chain—one of America's first—with more than one hundred outlets.

The Horn & Hardart automat, created by Joseph Horn and German-born Frank Hardart, was a new twist on the cafeteria: its walls were lined with row upon row of little glass doors, displaying dishes of food behind them. When customers selected what they wanted, deposited one (or several) nickels into a slot, and turned a knob, the little door popped open, allowing the customer to remove the food. Behind the wall, workers replaced the dishes with fresh ones as necessary. Beverages were dispensed from wall spouts concealed in fanciful lion or dolphin heads. Philadelphia-based Horn & Hardart expanded its operation to New York City in 1912 and within a few years operated fifteen automats in the city. In September 1922, the company opened a combination automat–cafeteria, which it claimed was the largest restaurant in the city, with the capacity to feed ten thousand New Yorkers daily. Most automats included or converted entirely to cafeterias in the 1930s.

The key to success for a cafeteria was the scale of the operation. It required a larger investment, more kitchen space, and a bigger dining room for a greater volume of customers than other restaurants did. Cafeterias were widely adopted in factories as a means of feeding workers efficiently. The New York Young Men's Christian Association (YMCA) opened its first cafeteria in 1916. New York City schools soon opened cafeterias for their students. By 1929 the city had 786 cafeterias.

Charities opened cafeterias for the poor. In the extremely cold winter of 1902, many New Yorkers were out of work. The vegetarian health guru Bernarr Macfadden ran a cafeteria for the unemployed at City Hall Park. Although customers paid just a penny per course, its cafeteria actually made a profit. The New York's Young Women's Christian Association (YWCA) opened a cafeteria in 1916. When the Depression hit, beginning in 1931, cafeteria-style "penny restaurants" opened around the city. Macfadden, the pioneer in this, set up a cafeteria-style operation that served "cracked wheat, Scotch oatmeal, lima bean soup, green pea soup, soaked prunes, seeded raisins, whole wheat bread, butter, raisin coffee and cereal coffee." Each dish cost one cent. Macfadden said he charged for the food so that unemployed workers would not feel that they were accepting a handout.

Macfadden's penny restaurants served fifteen hundred to three thousand customers every day. As at the Exchange Buffets, there were no chairs—just counters where customers ate standing up. In the depths of the Depression, Macfadden's cafeterias served an estimated eleven thousand New Yorkers a day. The Salvation Army offered meals for a nickel. Diners were given a tray of food—typically something like corned beef and cabbage, potatoes, coffee, stewed prunes, and bread. Unlike Macfadden's restaurants, the Salvation Army's had tables and chairs. They invited men and women of all ages to share a meal, regardless of "race, creed, or color."

Other cafeterias catered to particular groups. The Garden Cafeteria, next door to the *Jewish Daily Forward* newspaper office on bustling East Broadway, was a partly self-service kosher vegetarian restaurant. It catered to immigrant Yiddish intellectuals, reporters, actors, poets, artists, and writers; Isaac

Bashevis Singer dubbed them "cafeteria-niks." The Hudson Cafeteria, in the Hudson Hotel on West Fifty-Eighth Street, was a popular destination for midtown shoppers.

The Exchange Buffet went bankrupt in 1963, but cafeterias still serve hundreds of thousands of New Yorkers every day, especially in institutional settings, such as schools, government offices, museums, military installations, and prisons, such as Rikers Island.

See also AUTOMATS; CHILDS; DEPRESSION FOOD; JEWISH; MACFADDEN, BERNARR; RESTAURANTS; and SALVATION ARMY.

Batterberry, Michael, and Ariane Batterberry. *On the Town in New York: The Landmark History of Eating and Entertainments from the American Revolution to the Food Revolution.* New York and London: Routledge, 1999.

Grimes, William. *Appetite City: A Culinary History of New York.* New York: North Point, 2009.

Schadt, Mabel E. *Cafeteria Recipes Arranged in Three Proportions for Use in Cafeteria, Tea Rooms, Schools and Institutions.* New York: Woman's Press, 1926.

Andrew F. Smith

Caffè Reggio

Caffè Reggio, on MacDougal Street between Houston and West Fourth Streets, was once a western satellite of Little Italy. As recently as the 1970s, now vanished coffeehouses with names like Borgia and Figaro anchored the intersection of Bleecker and MacDougal Streets. But walk north toward West Third Street and your eye will light upon the brilliant emerald awning and storefront of Caffè Reggio at 119 MacDougal. Although it may not be the oldest Italian coffeehouse in New York (Ferrara's on Grand Street makes that boast), it is surely the most atmospheric.

Opened in 1927, an antique, coal-powered espresso maker presides majestically over the room. Embellished with brass gargoyles and surmounted by a striding angel, it was one of the first espresso machines ever made and dates to 1902. Domenico Parisi, original owner, purchased the device for the princely sum of $1,000. He claimed that his was the first espresso machine in the United States. Its novelty attracted the attention of food writers such as Clementine Paddleford, who wrote in the *Herald*

Tribune in 1945 about the machine's complicated workings, including Parisi's decision to temporarily close the caffè when he was briefly hospitalized for surgery, rather than trust the machine to another's touch. See PADDLEFORD, CLEMENTINE. The caffè, purchased by the Cavallacci family in 1955 and still owned by Fabrizio Cavallacci, now brews its *espressi* and *cappuccini* from a modern chrome machine using updated, more foolproof technology.

The caffè boasts other Italian treasures. One can sit on an elaborately carved wooden bench that was once purportedly owned by the Medici family of Florence while gazing at a painting attributed to the school of Caravaggio, dating to the seventeenth century. Generations of cigarette smoke deposited by members of the Beat Generation, who flocked to the caffè for endless smokes and poetry readings, lend a blackened patina to the woodwork. Its romantically tatty setting has served as a location for movies such as *The Godfather: Part II, Serpico, Next Stop Greenwich Village,* and *Inside Llewyn Davis.* Famous patrons have included Jack Kerouac, Bob Dylan, John Huston, Elvis Presley, Al Pacino, Umberto Eco, and, more recently, Sean Lennon.

See also COFFEEHOUSES and LITTLE ITALY.

Caffè Reggio website: http://www.caffereggio.com.

Cathy K. Kaufman

Candy

From colonial days, candy making has been an important part of New York City's culinary life. Using imported sugar and molasses, colonists made various types of confections, such as marzipan cakes, comfits, cinnamon letters (made from sugar gum paste), and sugar-coated fruits and nuts.

When sugar began to be refined in New York City during the early eighteenth century, candy making became more economical. By midcentury, even the poor could occasionally enjoy sweets made from molasses or raw sugar. Commercial candy making was established in the city by the late eighteenth century. A French nobleman, Auguste Louis de Singeron, a refugee from the French Revolution, set up shop selling confectionery and pastries on Pine Street in the 1790s. He had been eking out a living as a French teacher, but having perfected a recipe for molasses candy, he branched out to other sweets, including marzipan, plum puddings, and New Year's cookies. Singeron became known for the quality of his products and the elegance of his displays. Later he moved his shop to William Street and then to Broadway. By the 1830s, many small shops selling molasses candy, taffy, stick candy, pulled candy, and other sweets operated in Manhattan.

In the mid-nineteenth century the price of sugar had begun to drop sharply, allowing candy makers to expand their business. High-end candy chocolatiers produced filled chocolates, chocolate bars, and other luxury items. Confectioners also made small sugar sculptures, such as Fourth of July flags, Easter lilies, and hatchets (for George Washington's birthday). For parties, the guests' names could be added to the sugar sculptures, making them edible place cards. For the more common trade, city manufacturers turned out penny candies including peppermints, licorice, chocolate drops, taffy, red hots, horehound drops (made with the herb *Marrubium vulgare*, which was believed to aid in digestion and soothe sore throats), and other hard candies. These were displayed in large glass bowls or jars in many shops. Larger stores had candy counters where customers could purchase a wide variety of sweets. Cheap candy was also sold by street vendors and by kiosk operators. When the city subway opened in 1904, passengers found coin-operated chewing gum and candy machines on the platforms. Penny candy all but disappeared in the 1920s, only to return during the Depression, when cheap candy was a luxury that New Yorkers with even a little money could afford.

At the turn of the twentieth century, between the penny-candy business and the luxury chocolate trade was a middle range of sweet shops, run by women who had begun by making candy at home and then opened small stores, which they could do without much equipment or capital. One such woman was Mary Elizabeth Evans of Syracuse, New York. Her candy-making career (begun in 1900, when she was fifteen years old) was such a success that by 1904 several elite New York City clubs and hotels were selling her products. Less than ten years later, with her mother and sister as her partners, she opened a candy store on Fifth Avenue in midtown Manhattan, close to all the finest department stores. Soon the shop became the Mary Elizabeth Tearoom, offering sandwiches and cakes as well as candy; and Evans later opened branches in Boston and Newport,

Rhode Island. The last of the Mary Elizabeth Tearooms, on East Thirty-Seventh Street, closed in 1985.

Other New Yorkers opened small candy shops that expanded into larger businesses. Leo Hirschfeld, an immigrant from Austria, opened a Brooklyn candy store in 1896. One of his products was a small, log-shaped, chewy chocolate caramel, which he called a "Tootsie Roll." When the Tootsie Roll went into commercial production, it was the first penny candy to be individually wrapped. See TOOTSIE ROLL.

Samuel Born, a Russian Jew who immigrated to New York in 1910, invented the "Born Sucker Machine," which automatically inserted sticks into lollipops, thereby revolutionizing their manufacture. In 1917 he opened a retail store in Brooklyn, advertising his candies as "Just Born" (i.e., freshly made), and in 1923 started his own manufacturing company with the same name. Today, Just Born, headquartered in Pennsylvania, is most famous for its marshmallow Easter candies, called Peeps.

Yet another iconic candy was launched by Edward Noble, owner of the Mint Products Company of New York. In 1913 he acquired the rights to manufacture Life Savers, ring-shaped mints. Noble packaged stacks of the candies in foil and sold them for a nickel a roll. See LIFE SAVERS.

A major player on New York City's candy scene was Thomas Loft, a second-generation candy maker. He opened a candy shop in Manhattan in 1860 and developed it into a chain that became famous for its chocolates. It remained part of New York City life for 130 years. See LOFT'S CANDY STORES. Another very popular chain of chocolate shops was Barricini, founded in 1931, which at one time had 250 outlets in the New York metropolitan area. Its main rival was Barton's, founded by Viennese émigré Stephen Klein as Barton's Salon du Chocolat in 1938. By 1952 there were fifty Barton's Bonbonnières in New York, with the chocolates being manufactured in Brooklyn. Loft's and Barricini merged in 1970; but over the next two decades the business declined, and by 1990 all the retail stores had closed.

Other homegrown chocolate emporia continue to dot the city: Li-Lac Chocolates, founded in the West Village in 1923 by Greek immigrant George Demetrious, is a local institution; its signature color pastel boxes cradle chocolate mints, butter crunch pralines, and truffles. Kee's Chocolates, founded in SoHo in 2002 by Macao native Kee Ling Tong, fuses Asian flavors and spices into award-winning truffles, while Jacques Torres Chocolates, founded in 2000 in Brooklyn's Dumbo, sells truffles and chocolate bars, among other confections, in nine New York City establishments. See TORRES, JACQUES.

Various branded candies celebrating famous New Yorkers have been released occasionally. The prime example is the Reggie! Bar, which celebrated Reggie Jackson of the Yankees, one of the city's most popular baseball players in the 1970s. It was manufactured by Standard Brands, a New York–based corporation; the candy bar disappeared after a few years, but it made a short encore appearance in 1993. See REGGIE! BAR.

Although weight-conscious, health-conscious New Yorkers are less likely to indulge these days, New York City still boasts quite a few candy stores, such as Economy Candy on Rivington Street, founded in 1937; Philip's Candy, which opened on the Coney Island boardwalk in 1916 and is now on Staten Island; Williams Candy Shop, founded in Coney Island in 1940; and relative newcomer Dylan's Candy Bar (owned by Dylan Lauren, the daughter of fashion designer Ralph Lauren). See DYLAN'S CANDY BAR.

Following 2000, the city has seen a candy revival, with shops catering to children and increasingly adults. Shops such as Dylan's Candy Bar peddle a vast array of mass-market and nostalgic treats in two New York locations as well as other national outposts, while Sockerbit in the West Village sells purely Swedish candies. The candy revival has also led New Yorkers to concoct a huge variety of newfangled artisanally produced candies, from Brooklyn's Salty Road Taffy in flavors that include salted mango lassi and bergamot to Dosha Pops, which peddles lollipops supposedly based on Ayurvedic principles.

Candy Professor website: http://candyprofessor.com.
Grimes, William. *Appetite City: A Culinary History of New York*. New York: North Point, 2009.

Andrew F. Smith

Cannon, Poppy

Poppy Cannon was a cookbook writer and food editor known as the "Can-Opener Queen" because of her expertise with prepared and packaged foods. At various times she was the food editor of *Mademoiselle*, *Town & Country*, *House Beautiful*, and *Ladies' Home Journal*. Her *Can Opener Cook Book*, first printed in 1951, was a bestseller.

Cannon deemed the can opener a "magic wand when put in the hands of the brave young women who were engaged in frying as well as bringing home the bacon." Cannon did not present recipes made with processed foods as simple or unsophisticated. She instead positioned their use as a sign of modernity, as a woman's way of asserting her independence from drudgery by allowing her time to dispose of arduous cooking tasks and instead focus on innovation and creativity in the kitchen.

Cannon's life, surprisingly tumultuous, was spent primarily in New York City. Born Lillian Gruskin in South Africa to Lithuanian Jews, she moved to the United States as a young child. She graduated from Vassar and married four times. Her last marriage, in 1949, was to Walter White, an African American who was executive secretary of the National Association for the Advancement of Colored People (NAACP). White came under tremendous criticism, and his position at the NAACP was jeopardized by accusations that marriage to a white woman was harmful to the organization's cause. Claudius Charles Philippe (the longtime maître d'hôtel of the Waldorf Astoria) accused his former wife Cannon of being an unfit mother to their daughter because of the controversy surrounding the interracial marriage. He threatened a custody suit and denounced Cannon for exposing their child to the then very public scandal.

In 1975 Poppy Cannon died in a fall from the twenty-third-floor balcony of her Park Avenue apartment. She was sixty-nine years old. Whether she fell or jumped is still a subject of some ambiguity. Oddly, Cannon's son, Jon Alf Askland (from her second marriage), had fallen from a balcony at the age of thirty a few years earlier.

Cannon's contemporary, James Beard, reportedly was "horrified" by her style of cooking, yet a fresh look at big sellers like *The Can Opener Cook Book* and *The Bride's Cookbook* reveals that her work was relatively progressive. She did not emphasize that a dutiful wife should act as a type of hostess to her husband every day, and she did not lecture that good food could help "keep" a man or "tame" him, both common themes of cookbooks of the 1950s.

It is true that the popularity of processed food brought an eventual backlash, with women eventually making ever more convoluted and inconvenient combinations from an armory of packages. In retrospect, however, Cannon's particular message was one of nonconformity. A decade before the women's revolution, she wrote recipes for women who worked outside the home. She promoted packaged food as worldly and presumed readers would be glad to have short-cuts to prepare cassoulet and lobster thermidor. She assumed that her reading audience knew who Auguste Escoffier was, quoted Shakespeare in her recipe for apples and cheese, and edited a sophisticated and clever cookbook for Alice B. Toklas.

Poppy Cannon's charm lay in her boldness. Here was a writer who quoted Escoffier while instructing readers to make chicken soufflé with cream of chicken soup. She was shameless in her recommendation of processed foods but genuine in her desire that readers should be empowered, not intimidated, by cooking.

Cunningham, George, and H. Dean. *Guide to the Walter Francis White and Poppy Cannon Papers*. Beinecke Rare Book and Manuscript Library, Yale University Library, 1973. http://drs.library.yale.edu/fedora/get/beinecke:wfwhite/PDF.

Fisher, Carol. *A History of the American Cookbook*. Jefferson, N.C.: McFarland, 2006.

Inness, Sherrie A. *Secret Ingredients: Race, Gender, and Class at the Dinner Table*. New York: Palgrave Macmillan, 2005.

Claire Stewart

Careers through Culinary Arts Program (C-CAP)

The Careers through Culinary Arts Program (C-CAP) was founded in New York City in 1990 by culinary educator and cookbook author Richard Grausman to provide a glimmer of taste, flavor, and cooking to youth within the public schools. Recognizing a need, the program quickly expanded to seven locations nationwide, providing support to inner-city culinary high school students and teachers. C-CAP organizes and coordinates classroom visits, donations of sponsor-partner ingredients, professional development for teachers, and celebrated competitions for scholarships to postsecondary culinary schools valued in the millions of dollars each year.

C-CAP offers both college advising and job training and is one of the only resources in which high school students can obtain specific advice on a career in the culinary field, including assistance applying for financial aid and loans (an effort to combat rising debt concerns for young people). Students undergo internal training on soft skills, such as timeliness, phone etiquette, professional attire, attitude, and trouble-shooting employment mishaps, as well as hard skills, transferring their kitchen mentality from one of school to work, including production, problem solving, culinary math, safety, and sanitation. Students who complete the training are referred to multiweek paid internships in professional kitchens within their city. Throughout these internships, students receive personal support that allows them to learn, grow, and make the most of the experience.

With an ongoing drive for expansion and a mission statement that supports students and alumni indefinitely, this organization's industry connectivity provides enrichment and support to teachers, students, and schools as it prepares young people for lives and careers in the culinary arts.

Careers through Culinary Arts Program (C-CAP) website: http://www.ccapinc.org.

Alexandra Olsen

Caribbean

In New York City, English, Spanish, French, Dutch, Kreyol, and various Creole speakers represent the Caribbean. The Caribbean as an entity, through cultural and historical ties and geographic proximity, includes the countries of Belize, Guyana, Suriname, Bermuda, El Salvador, parts of Panama, and the coastal islands of Central America as well as islands in the Caribbean Sea. These groups have brought with them their respective social, cultural, economic, and political traditions that tend to share common historical origins in European colonialism and enslavement but are quite distinctive nonetheless.

Migration from the Caribbean to New York City has unfortunate origins in the transatlantic slave trade, and the history is a fairly long one. New York was the largest slaveholding state in the North (the region was not exempt from active participation in chattel slavery) and imported enslaved Africans directly from Africa, the southern United States, Jamaica (which was, for hundreds of years, a slaving center in the Caribbean where West Africans were bought and sold and often the first stop in the New World for most kidnapped West Africans before being dispersed to North, South, or Central America or other areas in the Caribbean), Barbados, and other small islands. These people toiled as domestics, including in kitchens, where they brought their own knowledge of cooking and food traditions with them, unwittingly helping to shape the palates of New York's elite as well as offering their contributions to the city's diverse culinary culture. After emancipation, a long period of voluntary migration began with Caribbean migrants from English-, Spanish-, French-, Dutch-, Kreyol-, and Creole-speaking islands arriving and settling in New York, enriching the city's cultural landscape by leaving their marks on just about every aspect of city life.

After emancipation, Caribbean immigrants settled throughout the city, beginning with a large and vibrant community in Harlem where they mixed with the African American population. From the late 1800s through the 1940s most settlers, generally skilled and educated and often businesspeople, settled there, founding the first grocery stores, restaurants, and bakeries catering to the Caribbean population. The majority of these people of Caribbean descent settling in West Harlem came from primarily English-speaking islands including Jamaica, Barbados, and Antigua, while settlement of East or Spanish Harlem (also known as El Barrio), primarily by Puerto Ricans and eventually Dominicans, began in the 1940s. White Cubans, having traditionally been better educated and more financially stable, immigrated to the city before the Cuban Revolution.

As immigration progressed the people fanned out to other boroughs, choosing to settle in Brooklyn, Queens, and the Bronx in greater numbers. Dominicans and other Spanish-speaking Caribbean immigrants tended to stay in Manhattan, which is where you can find the Cuban restaurant Floridita, on 127th Street near the Hudson River and its original 125th Street location, and multiple locations of Malecon in Washington Heights and El Nuevo Caridad, both Dominican, dotting the neighborhoods of East and West Harlem.

The central Brooklyn neighborhoods of Crown Heights, Flatbush, and Bedford-Stuyvesant are vibrant centers of Caribbean life where one can easily find Jamaican, Trinidadian, and Haitian restaurants and bakeries to stop in for patties (spicy, baked Jamaican stuffed pastries filled with chicken, beef, tofu, or vegetable mixtures), doubles (filling sandwiches from Trinidad consisting of fried bread filled with spicy chickpeas and drizzled with hot sauce), dishes such as taso et bananes pesées (fried goat with sweet plantains from Haiti), and other various dishes and varieties of bread and baked goods from all over the Ca-

ribbean. Immigrants from every island and area of the Caribbean, from Panama and Dominica to St. Kitts and Nevis and Curaçao, are represented, making Brooklyn grocery stores a great place to go to stock up on plentiful, affordable, hard-to-find, high-quality spices, dry goods, and produce used across the Caribbean. Though clustering in the Lefferts Gardens and Bedford-Stuyvesant areas, Puerto Ricans and Dominicans are scattered across Brooklyn, and access to "Spanish food" is a possibility for and an expectation of New Yorkers citywide.

The southeastern Queens neighborhood of Jamaica is still a Jamaican enclave. The area surrounding the Jamaica Center Mall, in particular, is dotted with mom-and-pop Caribbean restaurants and chains like the ubiquitous Jamaican-owned Golden Krust seen throughout the city. Just southwest in Ozone Park and Richmond Hill Indo-Caribbean immigrants (West Indians of south Asian descent) cluster, hailing from across the Caribbean, notably Trinidad and Jamaica. Little Trinidad is also located in Richmond Hill. In these areas, restaurants serve standards of pan-Caribbean cuisine along with a lesson on the diversity within Caribbean cultures. Here it is made clear that western African and southern Asian flavors and techniques dominate the Caribbean cooking of many islands of the region.

In the Bronx Latin Caribbean immigrants have also shaped the culinary landscape. Puerto Ricans moved into the area from El Barrio in Harlem as new waves of people began to arrive in the city from the island in the 1960s. Small family-owned restaurants offer specialties such as mofongo, arroz con gandules, and lechón, while food trucks and carts sell frituras, which are various fried meats, and snacks such as cuchifrito (fried pig ears and other parts, generally offal), alcapurrias (starchy balls of dough made from tubers and stuffed with seasoned ground beef), pastelillos (Puerto Rican–style empanadas filled with anything from quince paste to seasoned pork), and soups and stew such as mondongo and sancocho.

While centered mostly in upper Manhattan in Washington Heights and Inwood, Dominicans add to the Latin Caribbean mix of the Bronx. Jamaicans and non-Spanish-speaking Caribbean immigrants also live throughout the borough in large numbers. Golden Krust and Royal Caribbean Bakery, two of the largest and best-known West Indian bakery and restaurant chains, are based in the Bronx, founded by Jamaican immigrants in the 1960s and 1970s, respectively.

Very likely without realizing it, New Yorkers now consider Caribbean food to be an integral part of their culinary landscape. Walking into bodegas anywhere in Astoria, the Upper West Side, or Sunset Park one would be hard pressed not to find Jamaican patties as a "to-go" option in the deli case. Chinese restaurants run by people with no ties to the Caribbean offer "fried bananas" alongside their crab Rangoon and egg rolls, and a preponderance of New Yorkers expect that their neighborhood will have a great "Spanish restaurant," often meaning Dominican or Puerto Rican. In Harlem fancy Caribbean fusion restaurants dominate the culinary scene, and every large grocery store chain in the city has at least one aisle dedicated to any product needed to stock a Caribbean pantry. Just try opening your average New Yorker's kitchen cabinet thinking you will not find a container of adobo seasoning salt or packets of *sazón*.

The city continues to see a steady influx of immigrants from the Caribbean, settling all over, so Caribbean food (and culture) is mainstream, as New York as bagels and lox and pastrami sandwiches.

See also CUBAN; DOMINICAN; JAMAICAN; and PUERTO RICAN.

Floridita website: http://harlemsfloridita.com.
Golden Krust Caribbean Bakery and Grill website: http://www.goldenkrustbakery.com.
Henker, Holger. *The West Indian Americans*. Westport, Conn.: Greenwood, 2001.
Malecon website: http://maleconrestaurants.com.
Royal Caribbean Bakery website: http://www.royalcaribbeanbakery.com.
Schomburg Center for Research in Black Culture. "Caribbean Migration." In Motion: The African American Migration Experience. http://www.inmotionaame.org/migrations/landing.cfm?migration=10.

Rachel Monet Finn

Carnegie Deli

See DELIS, JEWISH.

Catering

Caterers are culinary professionals who provide meals in private homes or other venues for special occasions. They have long been part of the urban fabric. Ancient Greeks would go to the agora to hire a *mageiros*, a "cook-sacrificer," who would slaughter, butcher, and roast an animal for sacrifice; the meats would be consumed as part of the ceremony. The guild of French *traiteurs* in pre-Revolutionary Paris had the exclusive monopoly to provide full dinners to wealthy Parisians in their homes. In New York City, early catering was an offshoot from the kitchens of taverns and other eateries. In the latter eighteenth century, Fraunces Tavern, known for the excellence of its cooking, delivered meals to those nearby. See FRAUNCES TAVERN. The convenience and cachet of hiring meals from expert cooks grew in the nineteenth century.

Catering was an important—and rare—business opportunity for New York's African American population in the nineteenth century. Thomas Downing, who owned and ran one of New York's best oyster cellars, also acted as a caterer to New York's elite; an 1856 advertisement from Downing claimed that his boned turkeys and pickled oysters would not only save ladies money but make "their guests, if they have any taste, go into ecstacies [*sic*]." Downing regularly catered dinners for one-time mayor Philip Hone and catered the famous 1842 Boz Ball in honor of Charles Dickens. Many other African Americans, including several women, also had catering businesses, among them Cornelia Gomez and Katie Ferguson. See AFRICAN AMERICAN.

Catering soon became more than the mere provision of delicious food; it required the caterer to create an elegant aura through supplying the china, silverware, crystal, and other rental accouterments of a festive banquet. Edward Clark, an African American jeweler and "public waiter," as caterers were called in the mid-nineteenth century, was reported to have an extensive inventory of silver service items used in his highly profitable catering business. In addition to their economic success, these African Americans were highly respected members of New York society and politically active in the abolitionist movement. By the late nineteenth century, however, the ownership of many of New York's catering businesses was changing and immigrants, especially Italians, were becoming dominant in the industry.

After World War II, a new audience for catering emerged: the business meeting and convention. Major hotels created catering departments to address these specific needs, among them the Waldorf Astoria. In 1958, the National Association for Catering and Events was founded in New York City to promote professionalism and good relations among the catering managers; it now has more than forty chapters nationwide and launched, in 1986, an examination and certification process for the catering executives.

Catering halls, complete with in-house culinary and waitstaff that can serve hundreds of guests, dot the city as special venues to celebrate life's great transitions, including bar and bat mitzvahs, *quinceañeras*, birthday parties, weddings, anniversaries, and retirements. Museums, libraries, and other public buildings also cash in on the market for high-end events, and independent caterers are now ready to create any fantasy for a special event. With a caterer from an "approved" list, one can stage an over-the-top celebration, such as a dinner at the Metropolitan Museum of Art's Temple of Dendur, where great pyramids of salmon mousse rest on deserts of couscous. Many of New York's caterers have also published cookbooks. The popular *Silver Palate* cookbooks were offshoots from the catering company of the same name; society caterer Abigail Kirsch, who specializes in weddings, has extended the brand with "bride and groom" cookbooks.

"BizBash Venue Coverage in New York." BizBash. http://www.bizbash.com/new-york/venues.

Harmon, J. H., Jr. "The Negro as Local Businessman." *Journal of Negro History* 14, no. 2 (1929): 116–155.

Hewitt, John H. "Mr. Downing and His Oyster House: The Life and Good Works of an African-American Entrepreneur." *American Visions* 9, no. 3 (1994): 22.

Walker, Juliet E. K. *The History of Black Business in America: Capitalism, Race, Entrepreneurship.* Vol. 1: *To 1865.* 2d ed. Chapel Hill: University of North Carolina Press, 2009.

Cathy K. Kaufman

Cel-Ray

See DR. BROWN'S SODA and SELTZER.

Central American

See SOUTH AND CENTRAL AMERICAN.

Central Park Casino

In 1864, the Central Park Casino began as a stone cottage, located on East Drive and Seventy-Second Street. The quaint building, designed by Calvert Vaux, was originally used as the Ladies' Refreshment Lounge, where "unaccompanied ladies could relax during their excursions around the park and enjoy refreshments at decent prices, free of any threat to their propriety" (Broyles, 2013). The establishment would open its doors to both sexes twenty years later and assume the name the Casino; however, the name was intended to invoke the Italian translation of "little house," not a place to gamble. It was where well-to-do diners could get a steak for seventy-five cents, paired with a glass of wine, that could be enjoyed either inside the building or on the outdoor seating terrace, under the trees, or in the sun.

As the *New York Times* wryly observed in June 1929, the Casino had never been noted for catering to the poor, but instead as "a place for the fashionable and fastidious." Accordingly, that same unforgiving year of the Stock Market crash, the Casino would be transformed into the place for socialites, politicians, and entertainers during the height of the Jazz Age. Mayor James "Jimmy" Walker (aka Gentleman Jimmy or Beau James) spent $500,000 to renovate the building. Walker would hire noted hotelier Sidney Solomon to execute the project. Solomon intended to make the old drab casino into a new "outstanding restaurant"; he saw the project as "not just a renovation" but "something that has never before existed so perfectly in the world."

Of course, such bold perfection came at a price, and it was one that reinforced the economic disparities and inequities of the Roaring Twenties and subsequent Depression. While the city's starving masses waited in long breadlines for little food, rich and powerfully corrupt society types dined on oysters and steaks and drank illegal Prohibition booze. Solomon and Walker's new improved Casino delighted those fortunate enough to enjoy it. They could have their cars parked by a valet in a parking lot large enough to hold three hundred automobiles. The dining facilities held room for six hundred elite patrons. The once quaint little cottage in the park was now a premier dance spot in the city. Mayor Walker himself could be found many evenings dancing and socializing in the spectacular black-glass ballroom with his young mistress, Broadway actress Betty Compton. The laughs and smiles from those inside the Casino were far removed from the poverty and hardship that gripped the rest of the city.

Eventually, the playground for the rich became a symbol of decadence and corruption. The New Deal would usher in reformist politicians like Mayor Fiorello La Guardia, who would ultimately task his Parks Commissioner, Robert Moses, to demolish the Casino and replace it with the Rumsey Playground for children. See LA GUARDIA, FIORELLO. Today, the site is a public space, used for large outdoor concerts. It is where Central Park's Summer Stage is located.

See also GILDED AGE; PROHIBITION; and WOMEN'S CLUBS.

Broyles, Susan. "The Central Park Casino." *Museum of the City of New York* (blog), September 10, 2013. http://mcnyblog.org/author/sbroyles/page/2/.

Kessner, Thomas. *Fiorello H. La Guardia and the Making of Modern New York.* New York: Penguin. 1991.

"Brilliant Throng Opens Park Casino." *New York Times,* June 5, 1929.

Nicholas Allanach

Chalet Suisse

The Chalet Suisse was one of New York City's most popular restaurants during its heyday from the 1950s through the 1970s. It introduced New Yorkers to many Swiss foods and dishes, the most popular of which was fondue.

The restaurant opened on West Fifty-Second Street during the 1920s and was initially managed (and later owned) by Alfred and Clara Baertschi, immigrants from Switzerland. Konrad Egli, the restaurant's chef and later owner, innovated with many traditional Swiss dishes. He is credited with introducing New Yorkers to the classic *fondue neuchateloise*—a pot of molten Gruyère and Emmental cheese flavored with a touch of garlic, white wine, and a little kirsch, a cherry liqueur. The simmering fondue is served with pieces of bread to be skewered on long forks and dipped into the cheese. Egli hired Erwin Herger, a chef from Lausanne, in 1952. Two years later, Egli arranged for Herger to demonstrate the preparation of fondue on the just-launched NBC television program *Tonight with Steve Allen*.

Patrons at the Chalet Suisse were charmed by this novel, convivial way to dine, so Egli experimented with other dishes that could be enjoyed from a communal pot. He came up with *fondue bourguignonne* in 1956. For this dish, a pot of bubbling oil was brought to the table, and guests lowered strips of beef into the oil, cooking the meat to taste. A variety of savory sauces accompanied the fondue. Chefs at Chalet Suisse later extended this concept to include other meats and seafood.

In 1966 Chalet Suisse moved to 6 East Forty-Eighth Street—just one block from the Swiss Center, which housed the Swiss National Tourist Office, SwissAir, and other Swiss businesses. Beverly Allen of Allen Associates, a public relations firm responsible for promoting the Swiss chocolate brand Toblerone in America, brainstormed with Egli about new ways to promote the product. Egli came up with *fondue au chocolat*—a pot of melted Toblerone chocolate blended with heavy cream and kirsch. The intended dippers in this case were cubes of plain cake. Egli introduced his creation at the Chalet Suisse in 1966.

A few savory fondue recipes had been published in American cookbooks, newspapers, and magazines in the previous decades; but the sweet chocolate fondue introduced by Chalet Suisse ignited a firestorm. Within five years of its introduction, more than a score of fondue cookbooks had been published. Fondue pots proliferated in kitchenware stores, becoming de rigueur as wedding gifts; and fondue parties became a craze throughout America.

Chalet Suisse was praised by many prominent culinarians, including Mimi Sheraton and William Grimes, both of the *New York Times*. In 1980 Sheraton reported that the Chalet Suisse was a "charmer that still glows with warmth and hospitality.... The setting is operetta Swiss chalet, complete with dark wood beams, rough plaster walls, black wrought iron and waitresses in folkloric costumes, a combination that would be considered corny if newly created, but altogether felicitous as a longstanding tradition." She described the fare as "delicious, solid, countrified food presented attractively."

Dietmar Schlüter had joined the restaurant's staff in the early 1960s; he took over from Erwin Herger in 1975 and remained at the restaurant until it closed in 1988. In 2007, Schlüter published *Chalet Suisse: Fondue, Veal and More*, the only cookbook to emerge from one of New York's most beloved restaurants.

See also RESTAURANTS.

Schlüter, Dietmar. *Chalet Suisse: Fondue, Veal and More.* BookSurge, 2007.

Sheraton, Mimi. "Delicious, Solid, Countrified Swiss." *New York Times*, December 19, 1980, p. 30.

Andrew F. Smith

Chang, David

David Chang (b. 1977) grew up in suburban Virginia, the youngest of four children of Korean immigrants. His father had worked his way up from washing dishes to owning several restaurants and later a golf shop. Chang's culinary stirrings, though, came during a semester abroad in London during college, when he discovered Wagamama, run by chef Alan Yau. Chang attended the French Culinary Institute and worked at Tom Colicchio's Craft and Jean-Georges Vongerichten's Mercer Kitchen. Chang's penchant for noodles brought him to Tokyo for eight months, living in a homeless men's shelter sans rent and working at a ramen shop. He then cooked at the Tokyo Park Hyatt as well as at an izakaya.

Back in New York, Chang attempted to get a job at Chipotle as he'd considered opening an Asian burrito restaurant someday. "They wouldn't hire me ... they knew what I was up to," Chang told *New York* (Patronite and Raisfeld, 2007). He then dabbled in fine French cuisine at Café Boulud as a line cook but was unhappy with the dining culture. "I want to cook for real people who want to eat. When I worked at Café Boulud, I hated making food for East Siders. I hate their air of superiority. I hate investment bankers," Chang told *GQ* (Richman, 2007).

Momofuku Noodle Bar opened in August 2004. The name means "lucky peach" in Japanese and is also the first name of instant ramen's inventor, Momofuku Ando. Chang spent a week apprenticing at ramen spot Rai Rai Ken before opening up his own shop. The eatery had a quiet start—the odd, tightly edited menu did not gain a following immediately. Chang weathered a dicey beginning to take in $500,000 in Noodle Bar's first year and $1 million in its second year in business.

In August 2006 Chang opened Momofuku Ssäm Bar, offering Korean-inflected burritos. Despite buzz from Noodle Bar's success, the first nine months were again rocky. A separate late-night menu proved popular but perplexingly different from the daytime offerings.

The most upscale outpost in Chang's mini-empire, Momofuku Ko, opened in March 2008. Eight months later, the first location of Momofuku Milk Bar debuted. Helmed by Christina Tosi, the tiny spot translated Chang's wacky style to desserts, including crack pie and cereal milk soft-serve ice cream. There are now five locations in Manhattan and Brooklyn.

Chang released his first cookbook, *Momofuku*, in 2009, which quickly made the *New York Times* bestseller list. He then unveiled a quarterly food magazine, *Lucky Peach*, with Peter Meehan, published by McSweeney's, in summer 2011. See LUCKY PEACH.

A few months later, Chang opened his first overseas operation, Momofuku Seiōbo, in Sydney, Australia. In April 2012, Chang expanded to equally unfamiliar territory, midtown Manhattan, with Má Pêche. Chang then experimented with libations with the January 2012 unveiling of Booker & Dax, where the chef and French Culinary Institute director of technology Dave Arnold created high-concept cocktails utilizing liquid nitrogen, hot pokers, and rotary evaporators.

Chang was featured on the debut season of *Mind of a Chef* in 2012, an Anthony Bourdain–produced PBS show. See BOURDAIN, ANTHONY. In June 2015, Chang unveiled his first fast-food venture, Fuku, which serves a streamlined menu of spicy, fried chicken sandwiches in the East Village space that housed Momofuku's first-ever iteration.

See also MOMOFUKU RESTAURANT GROUP.

David Chang bio. http://momofuku.com/wp-content/files_mf/davidchangbio.pdf.

Henry, Michele. "Inside Momofuku Toronto's Tumultuous First Year." *Toronto Star*, January 31, 2014.

Patronite, Rob, and Robin Raisfeld. "The I Chang." *New York*, January 22, 2007.

Richman, Alan. "Year of the Pig." *GQ*, November 2007.

Alexandra Ilyashov

Chanukah

Chanukah, also spelled Hanukah and Hanukkah, is the Jewish "festival of lights" commemorating the Maccabean revolt against the Seleucid king Antiochus IV. According to Jewish tradition, the king outlawed many Jewish rites and defiled the Jewish Temple in Jerusalem in an effort to more fully Hellenize Judaea. Judah the Maccabee, of the priestly Hasmonean family, led an uprising and in 164 B.C.E. took the Temple. The Maccabees lit the sanctuary lamp, which was to burn continuously, but could only find enough oil to last one day. Miraculously the lamp burned for eight days, until they could secure more oil. Thus, Chanukah lasts for eight days and is commemorated by the lighting of a candelabrum called a Chanukah menorah (often shortened to "menorah") or a *hanukiyyah*. The Chanukah menorah has nine branches, eight to represent the days of the holiday and one used to light the others.

Chanukah is not mentioned in the Bible and has traditionally been a holiday of minor importance in the Jewish calendar. In the United States, however, Chanukah took on greater significance. Unlike other Jewish holidays, Chanukah is unbridled by religious restrictions. (For example, work is permitted during Chanukah.) This made the festival particularly adaptable to the American Jewish experience. Likewise, Chanukah's importance was amplified in the United States because it occurs during the Christmas season.

Chanukah has certainly been celebrated in New York since the middle of the nineteenth century, when American Jewish leaders increasingly used the story of the Maccabees to debate how Judaism should be preserved or reformed in the United States. Then, from 1881 to 1924, a massive wave of migration brought more than 2 million Jews from Europe to the United States. Many of these immigrants were Yiddish speakers from Eastern Europe. A large majority of them arrived in New York and settled, at least temporarily, on the Lower East Side. These newcomers would again alter the way Chanukah was celebrated. They placed less emphasis on the holiday's role in religious reform and more on gift giving and other forms of pleasure.

Chanukah celebrations included food, though not necessarily in a prominent role. Early American Jewish cookbooks did not always include Chanukah recipes, even when they provided specific recipes for other holidays. As late as 1959, the *New York Times* would write, "There is much less tradition about foods for Hanukkah than for most other Jewish holidays. Several persons, asked what they remembered about the foods they ate for Hanukkah when they were young, had only the haziest recollections." Some European Chanukah foods fell out of favor or were transformed in the United States. In a 1957 *Times* piece, Craig Claiborne listed roast goose among the "traditional foods" for the holiday. In parts of Europe, of course, Jews had raised geese and used their fat much like Chris-

tians used lard. The fattened geese were slaughtered at Chanukah time.

Both *Times* articles do, however, mention potato pancakes. Eastern European immigrants commonly ate latkes (pancakes) during Chanukah, made from grated potato, potato flour, or buckwheat. Although these would have traditionally been cooked in *schmaltz* (rendered poultry fat), in the United States this was replaced by Crisco or vegetable oil. Other American adaptations were made; Aunt Jemima marketed its pancake flour as great for latkes.

Symbolically, dairy foods are associated with Chanukah. According to folklore, during the Maccabean revolt, a Jewish woman entered an Assyrian general's tent and fed him salty cheese, which made him so thirsty that he consumed large amounts of wine. When he fell asleep, she killed him. Dairy is now eaten in her honor.

Most often, however, Chanukah is associated with fried foods, symbolizing the oil used to light the Temple candelabrum. In addition to latkes, doughnuts and other kinds of fried dough are very common. Jelly doughnuts are typical in the United States and in Israel, where they are called *sufganiyot*. Likewise, Sephardic and Middle Eastern Jews prepare doughnut-like fritters called *burmuelos* in Ladino and *zalabiyah* in Arabic.

See also JEWISH and LOWER EAST SIDE.

Ashton, Dianne. *Hanukkah in America: A History*. New York: New York University Press, 2013.
Claiborne, Craig. "Setting a Traditional Table for Festival of Hanukkah." *New York Times*, December 12, 1957.
Cooper, John. *Eat and Be Satisfied: A Social History of Jewish Food*. Northvale, N.J.: Jason Aronson, 1993.
"Food: Feast of Lights." *New York Times*, December 23 1959.

Ari Ariel

Charlotte Russe

The charlotte russe, a whipped cream–topped cake in a push-up cardboard wrapping, is synonymous with 1950s New York City, where youngsters knew it as a nickel treat available at bakeries and candy stores. The roots of the delicacy can be traced to the famed French chef Marie-Antonin Carême, who invented it in the early nineteenth century while working in the kitchen of England's prince regent. In England at the end of the eighteenth century a charlotte was a kind of bread pudding filled with baked apples. Before being baked, it resembled an Elizabethan trifle or layered custard. The dessert was likely named after Queen Charlotte, wife of King George III. Carême originally distinguished his concoction by calling it *Charlotte à la parisienne*. The dessert's name is said to have acquired the "russe" suffix when table service in France switched to Russian style, *service à la russe*, at a banquet held in honor of Tsar Alexander I.

Joel Barlow's late eighteenth-century poem "Hasty Pudding" introduced the baked version of the dessert: "The Charlotte brown, within whose crusty sides a belly soft the pulpy apple hides." This fruit-filled charlotte made its way to the United States—as documented in *The Virginia House-wife* in 1824—as did its sister pastry, filled with Bavarian cream.

The confection that captivated the eyes, stomachs, and after-school longings of children of 1950s and 1960s New York City was a humbler variety, sometimes called a "charley roose." The portable, push-up dessert consisted of a circle of sponge cake topped with a towering heap of whipped cream (chocolate sprinkles optional) crowned with a maraschino cherry. The cake was surrounded by stiff cardboard and sat on a circle of cardboard atop a stick. After licking away the whipped cream, eager eaters pushed up on the cardboard base to gain access to the cake.

The charlotte russe was a cool-weather treat that can still be found in the occasional bakery vitrine—one was spotted in Jamaica, Queens, as recently as 2005. In its heyday, the snack enjoyed popularity throughout the boroughs of New York City, but the authors of *The Brooklyn Cookbook* remember the candy-store delicacy distinctly as "Brooklyn ambrosia."

Barlow, Joel. "The Hasty-Pudding: A Poem, in Three Cantos." New London, Conn.: Charles Holt, 1797.
Randolph, Mary. *The Virginia House-wife.* Columbia: University of South Carolina Press, 1984. Facsimile reprint of 1824 edition with historical notes and commentary by Karen Hess.
Stallworth, Lyn, and Rod Kennedy Jr. *The Brooklyn Cookbook.* New York: Knopf, 1994.

Laura Silver

Cheesecake

One of the most iconic New York foods to find its way into the mainstream American diet is "Jewish-style" cheesecake. New Yorkers had been familiar with cheesecakes since colonial times. Early recipes called for fresh curds, or perhaps for cream thick-

ened with eggs, to make a thick custard. The cheesecakes baked in New York City's early days were similar to those eaten elsewhere in America (and in Western Europe, where the recipes originated). Later immigrants to New York—Germans and Italians among them—brought their own recipes, made with ricotta, cottage cheese, or farmer's cheese; the filling was most often baked in a pastry crust. Some of these cheesecakes continue to be sold in New York today.

It was in the early twentieth century that a different type of cheesecake appeared in New York City's bakeries and restaurants. The ingredients were simple: cream cheese, eggs, sugar, vanilla, and, sometimes, heavy cream or sour cream. Smooth, creamy, and dense, it was made with Philadelphia Cream Cheese, a recent arrival on the market. Despite its name, Philadelphia Cream Cheese was first manufactured in South Edmeston, New York; by 1903 the trademark was owned by the Phenix Cheese Company. A similar cream cheese was later made by Isaac Breakstone, an immigrant Russian Jew. (Both companies were later purchased by Kraft, which popularized the cheese throughout America.) See KRAFT.

Breakstone marketed his cream cheese in bulk to Jewish restaurateurs, such as Arnold Reuben, owner of the Turf Restaurant, at Forty-Ninth Street and Broadway. See REUBEN SANDWICH. Reuben served a widely admired cheesecake using Breakstone cream cheese. He claimed to have created the cake himself around 1928. Over the next ten years, the cake became so renowned that Reuben began shipping it to other places in the United States and around the world. The shipping charges were often four times the cost of the cake, but his customers—many of them, no doubt, homesick New Yorkers—were willing to pay the price. Other city restaurants were by then touting their own versions of New York–style cheesecake, and Reuben later complained that his recipe was stolen by others, specifically Leo Lindemann.

Lindemann was a German-Jewish immigrant who opened a restaurant he called Lindy's, near Times Square, in 1921. By 1948 Lindy's had become famous for its velvety cream cheese–based cheesecake, served plain or with a sweet fruit topping. The cake had a cookie-like crust, and the filling was flavored with citrus zest. Lindy's cheesecake received a nod in the Broadway musical *Guys and Dolls*, where it was referred to as "Mindy's cheesecake." Today Lindy's cheesecake is a trademark of Lindy's Food Products of New York.

The next cheesecake to capture the hearts of New Yorkers was from Junior's, a Brooklyn restaurant established in 1950 by Harry Rosen, who was born on the Lower East Side. Rosen worked with a Danish baker named Eigel Peterson to develop a distinctive version of the classic cheesecake. Junior's cheesecake, a little lighter and less sweet than Lindy's, had a thin layer of sponge cake as a base and was flavored with vanilla. Today, Junior's sells cheesecakes in myriad flavors and sizes; *Junior's Cheesecake Cookbook*, published in 2007, contains recipes for fifty of them. Although its original location closed in 2014 to make way for a condominium tower, the owners hope to reopen the restaurant, much as it was, in the new building. Junior's also has a restaurant in Times Square and an outlet in Grand Central Terminal.

Sylvia Balser Hirsch, a Texan transplanted to New York, began her professional baking career preparing desserts for a barbecue restaurant her husband had opened in the city. The restaurant did not last long, but by then Hirsch's cheesecakes were the talk of the city. Using the trade name "Miss Grimble," she opened a bakery and cafe on the Upper West Side and began supplying New York's upscale restaurants and gourmet shops with a distinctive vanilla cheesecake (and a range of other desserts) with a cookie-crumb crust.

Today, cheesecake is served in many of the city's restaurants and bakeries. It has become a signature dessert at most of New York City's venerable steakhouses, including The Old Homestead (founded in 1868), Peter Luger's (1887), and Keen's (1885). (Perhaps it is seen as the most appropriate finale for a high-fat, high-cholesterol meal.) Many of the cheesecakes served in restaurants are made by S&S Cheesecake, founded in the 1960s. Although its name is not as familiar as that of other cheesecakes, many New Yorkers who have sampled a slice consider it the city's best and make the trip to the S&S factory in the Bronx to buy a whole cake.

Plain cheesecake is the classic, but many prefer it with a sweetened fruit topping (often cherry, strawberry, or pineapple). The cake itself also comes in a range of flavors, with chocolate, mocha, chocolate chip, and pumpkin among the most popular. New variations are constantly appearing. In addition to Lindy's and Junior's, other popular cheesecake makers include Eileen's Special Cheesecake (opened in 1974) and a newcomer, Two Little Red Hens Bakery.

See also CREAM CHEESE; JEWISH; JUNIOR'S; and LINDY'S.

Fabricant, Florence, ed. *The New York Times Dessert Cookbook*. New York: St. Martin's, 2006.
Hirsch, Sylvia Balser. *Miss Grimble Presents Delicious Desserts*. New York: Macmillan, 1983.
Reynolds, Joey, and Myra Chanin. *The Ultimate Cheesecake Cookbook*. New York: St. Martin's, 2001.
Rosen, Alan, and Beth Allen. *Junior's Cheesecake Cookbook: 50 To-Die-for Recipes for New York–Style Cheesecake*. Newtown, Conn.: Taunton, 2007.
Segreto, John J. *Cheesecake Madness*. New York: Simon & Schuster, 1981.

Andrew F. Smith

Cheesemongers

Cheese has been an important food in New York since colonial times. The Dutch introduced dairy cows into Manhattan in 1625, and cheese was sold in farmers' markets by 1656. Cheese was also imported from Europe, but in order to protect the local cheese industry, import duties were enacted. Cheese was served at breakfast and dinner.

As Manhattan's population increased, the dairy industry moved upstate; but cheese remained an important part of New Yorkers' diet. By the mid-nineteenth century, shops specializing in domestic and imported cheeses were common in New York.

By the early nineteenth century, many stores sold domestic and imported cheeses. Cheese plates were commonly served in New York restaurants by the mid-nineteenth century. Cheese importers, traders, and retailers formed the Butter and Cheese Exchange in 1873. It fostered trade, tried to prevent the adulteration of cheese, and promoted the profession. (It later expanded its membership and was renamed the New York Mercantile Exchange.) See COMMODITY EXCHANGES.

A cheesemonger's responsibilities include the purchasing, storing, maintaining, and selling of an array of cheese varietals, as well as educating consumers about them. By the mid-twentieth century, cheeses sold in New York included American cheeses such as brick cheese, Colby, Monterey Jack, and Teleme and Italian imported selections such as Parmiggiano-Reggiano and Asiago. Authentic European and American artisan collections became available in the retail market from the mid- to late twentieth century as a result of individual mongers' ambitions in the industry.

Greenwich Village, celebrated for its rich Italian food history, housed Murray Greenberg's cheese shop called Murray's, which sold predominantly butter, eggs, and large blocks of cheese from 1940 until the 1990s. Rob Kaufelt bought the store from the second owner, Louis Tudda, in 1991 and soon began to travel throughout the United States and Europe in order to introduce new cheeses into the marketplace. Since 2004, he has expanded operations, including the installation of numerous cheese caves that store over one hundred different kinds of cheese and a selection of cheese education classes for the inquisitive customer.

Steven Jenkins, the first employee of the gourmet food shop Dean & DeLuca in SoHo in 1977, developed an expansive cheese counter after an inspirational visit to the Rungis wholesale cheese market in Paris. In 1980, he took over the cheese counter at Fairway Market and became the first French-certified master cheesemonger in North America, an award given by the Guilde de St. Uguzon in France. In 1988, he left Fairway to improve the cheese department at Balducci's, returning to Fairway in later years. See DEAN & DELUCA; BALDUCCI'S; and FAIRWAY MARKET. Olga Dominguez, the manager of Zabar's cheese counter since 1979, grew the department to a staff of over twenty-five people and nine hundred cheeses by 2008 by focusing on imports and building long-lasting relationships with her clientele. See ZABAR'S.

Since the early 2000s, specialty cheese shops have created a niche market for themselves in New York City. Notable additions include the Bedford Cheese Shop in Williamsburg, followed by its sister shop in Gramercy Park, Saxelby Cheesemongers in Essex Market, Lucy's Whey in Chelsea Market, and Beecher's Handmade Cheese in the Flatiron District. In addition to sales, Beecher's, the sibling of the store in Pike's Place Market, Seattle, is bringing back cheesemaking to New York, purchasing milk from dairies south of Albany and making the cheeses in view of customers in its glassed-in Manhattan kitchens. The cheeses are aged in its subterranean cave, adjacent to a cellar wine bar.

Manhattan cheesemongers have made the industry of sourcing, selling, and maintaining cheese an art, a story, a spectacle, and a marketing strategy, rather than simply a basic domestic chore and ration of early North America.

Hess, Diane C. "Grocer Finds Experienced Staff Pays." *Crains New York*, June 29, 2008.
"The 9 Best Cheese Shops in NYC." Gothamist, September 4, 2013. http://gothamist.com/2013/09/04/the_best_cheese_shops_in_nyc.php.
Paxson, Heather. "Cheese Cultures: Transforming America's Tastes and Traditions." *Gastronomica: The Journal of Critical Food Studies* 10, no. 4 (2010): 35–47.
Wharton, Rachel. "Murray's Cheese." *Edible Manhattan*, March 6, 2012.

Jessica Sennett

Chefs

In the nineteenth century and the first half of the twentieth century, in New York City, as in the European tradition, teenage boys apprenticed to chefs. As originally codified by August Escoffier, it was not unusual for these apprenticeships to last for a decade or more, as budding chefs learned the craft and developed sufficient skills to advance to roles of increasing responsibility on the kitchen brigade line.

While many New York City restaurants that opened in the mid- to late 1800s (Old Homestead, Keens Chop House, Peter Luger's) based their menus on all-American grilled steaks and oyster bars and thrived, the more refined menus offered at restaurants such as Delmonico's and Gage & Tollner and the premier hotels of New York City, such as the Waldorf, later the Waldorf Astoria, came from kitchens led and staffed by European men. (The Waldorf Astoria hired their first female chef, Leslie Revsin, in 1972, in the entry position of "kitchen man.") See DELMONICO'S; PETER LUGER'S; and WALDORF, THE.

These large-scale kitchens offered multicourse, complex menus requiring significant skill at the higher levels, based on many hours of unskilled or semi-skilled labor. The all-male commercial kitchen hierarchy moved from unskilled prep and washing stations to, with increasing skills, garde manger, entremettier, rotisseur, saucier, poissonier, sous, and, ultimately, executive chef. Many low-skill positions were available, and training under European chefs was prized employment, providing learning opportunities for the immigrant populations flooding into urban areas, especially New York City.

The chefs formed professional and burial societies to take care of themselves as they aged. The American

Culinary Federation was founded in 1929 in New York City, joining three earlier organizations: the Société Culinaire Philanthropique (1865), the Vatel Club (1913), and the Chefs de Cuisine Association of America (1916), which all started in New York City.

African American men were permitted limited opportunities in commercial kitchens. They found culinary work on the railroad, as caterers and bakers in private homes, and in small businesses. Some worked in military or religious facilities, taverns, or local ethnic restaurants but were excluded from the elite European kitchens. See AFRICAN AMERICAN.

Women were generally not permitted to enter the finer establishments, unless escorted by a man. Some women, including African Americans and ethnic minorities, were able to work in and own casual food counters, pubs and taverns, lunchrooms, tea shops, and bakeries and could find work as caterers or household cooks; but they were not offered the respectful title "chef."

Escoffier's brigade system continued as the main training option for upscale culinary work until the GI Bill offered veterans returning from World War II financial assistance. This allowed them to attend culinary programs at the Culinary Institute of America (originally in New Haven, Connecticut, then relocated to Hyde Park, New York, in 1946) and a few local community colleges where "home economics" programs tracked women for different careers but provided some men with culinary and nutrition training. See COOKING SCHOOLS.

In the late 1950s, as more women sought higher education and entered and remained in the workforce, American eating habits began to change. This coincided with major advances in food packaging, shipping, storing, and manufacturing convenience products. New equipment, expanded refrigeration, freezers, and microwaves, which became standard in homes, increased the variety of ingredients available for purchase, while travel, television, and other media increased exposure to different cultures and raised expectations of "what's for dinner." New restaurants began to offer Italian, Chinese, and other ethnic cuisines in casual settings; and fast-food establishments emerged in increasing numbers. In the 1960s, countering the proliferating packaged products and even faster fast food, home cooks began to watch Julia Child to learn French cooking techniques. These same consumers began to reconsider local ingredients, vegetarianism, and "alternative" diets. Mean-

while, the French chefs continued to control "fine dining" in New York City.

In France, the "nouvelle cuisine" of the 1970s spawned the "new American cuisine." As classically trained chefs lightened up on sauces, aspics, and terrines and began to highlight fine, fresh ingredients and locally sourced products, the American response incorporated a wide range of international products and ethnic foods. The media noticed, reviewed restaurants, and published recipes, which drove broader curiosity about cuisines, ingredients, and cooking techniques from around the world. The innovators began to take food out of restaurants, hotels, and homes and into museums, gardens, and other open spaces, to serve the fashion industry, incorporating Mediterranean (especially Italian), Indian, and Asian flavors. Fusion cuisine became mainstream on American menus; the training to become a chef changed.

Women took leadership roles in the new ventures. Catering, bakeries, food styling, recipe development, the burgeoning TV channel Food Network, and employment as private chefs extended opportunities well beyond tearooms and family dinner. As they began to claim more places in the culinary schools, women also opened more culinary schools (some 1,700 throughout the United States); and their efforts increased access to the training that was needed for work in the expanding variety of commercial kitchens.

One school owner and former James Beard student, Peter Kump, created a celebrity chef star system through the James Beard Foundation, seeking to recognize the value of American ingredients and cooking, as Beard had urged throughout his writing and teaching career. See KUMP, PETER CLARK.

It was no longer necessary to apprentice for a decade to gain entry and promotion to lead a kitchen. In 1976, the position of executive chef moved from a "service" status to a "professional" classification in the U.S. Department of Labor's *Dictionary of Occupational Titles*. By the 1980s, people working at food styling, creating specialty food products, and sourcing artisanal products all contributed to an exploding food scene. The new businesses emerged in response to the changing marketplace, and in turn, these businesses hired many more educated young people with culinary, artistic, and entrepreneurial skills, which continues to extend the ways chefs are employed.

When food sourcing became global, New Yorkers expected all-season availability, and identifying the best ingredients was paramount, without regard for the true costs of shipping, environmental damage, and fair labor concerns. Creating trends became part of the life of chefs as they claimed celebrity and lucrative fees well beyond chefs' salaries. Everyone had a shot at becoming a star chef, with or without education or formal training. Publicity, platforms for writing, blogging, and public relations campaigns have now become part of the work of chefs.

Moving into the twenty-first century, we see a return to farmers' markets and concern about sustainable agriculture, local farming, and animal husbandry taking front page in media stories along with the discovery of new products, new mixology, nutrition, molecular gastronomy, and health and obesity concerns. Each aspect offers specialized work for those with culinary interests, well beyond the hot line of a traditional kitchen establishment. Multiple schools, internships at all kinds of establishments, opportunity centers for food enterprise, food trucks, farmers' markets, and tax breaks for opening manufacturing operations in economic development centers all contribute to the plethora of options available to those who seek to become chefs in Gotham.

See also FRENCH.

Culinary Institute of America. *Remarkable Service*. 2d ed. Hoboken, N.J.: Wiley, 2009.

Escoffier, August. *The Complete Guide to the Art of Modern Cookery*. Translated by H. L. Cracknell and R. J. Kaufmann. New York: Mayflower, 1979. English translation of *Le Guide Culinaire*, first published in 1903.

Grimes, William. *Appetite City: A Culinary History of New York*. New York: North Point, 2009.

Lovegren, Sylvia. *Fashionable Food: Seven Decades of Food Fads*. Chicago: University of Chicago Press, 1995.

Mariani, John F. *America Eats Out*. New York: William Morrow, 1991.

Pépin, Jacques. *The Apprentice: My Life in the Kitchen*. New York: Houghton Mifflin, 2003.

Carol Durst-Wertheim

Chefs, Private

The wealthy of New York City have always had household staff, and the role of a private chef has long been unique. When the grand mansions of Fifth Avenue were first built, and before hotels were considered respectable venues, sprawling households needed sizeable staff so that their owners could maintain social position. The household chef focused exclusively on catering to the tastes of the family and their guests, cooking for banquets and balls held in their mansions. The chef supervised the cooks, who primarily prepared meals for the children and staff. The modern rich of New York City now generally reside in penthouses and apartments yet still require staff to keep their residences humming.

Affluent families now seek chefs with a pedigree. It is common to hire headhunters to procure cooks who have worked at particular high-profile restaurants, making their employment on par with the acquisition of valued artwork or furnishings. These "name-brand" chefs can command a high salary, work desirable hours, and receive a benefit package—all impossible in small restaurants.

Private chefs are often live-in, pay no rent, and have access to expense accounts and the same luxurious pantry they enjoyed in the public sector. They often travel with their employers, cooking in their summer homes (typically in the Hamptons or Martha's Vineyard).

The sporadic use of a personal chef (distinguished from a private chef, who works exclusively for one client) is also on the rise, and organizations such as the American Personal & Private Chef Association helps to match expert cooks to employers in the New York area. The use of on-demand apps (in which a chef can be ordered with the same ease as calling a cab) may eventually change the pastiche of having one's "own" chef tucked away in the kitchen. Placement agencies, however, continue to be a trusted source for finding elite labor. They vet employees, perform background checks, and often require "gag" orders, in which personnel agree never to speak to a reporter or write a "tell-all" book.

Home to thousands of laudable chefs, New York City hosts a broad labor market, and competition is ferocious for the best-paid and most secure household positions. Having once attained a position, the novelty of being "on call" may wane and the temperament of a pampered boss may no longer be charming. And then there will be a new wave of chefs eager to take their place.

See also CHEFS.

"Food Timeline FAQs: Professional Food Service...." FoodTimeline Library. http://www.foodtimeline .org/restaurants.html.

Hyman, Gwen. "The Taste of Fame: Chefs, Diners, Celebrity, Class." *Gastronomica: The Journal of Food and Culture* 8, no. 3 (Summer 2008): 43–52.

"New York Personal Chefs Listings." American Personal & Private Chef Association. http://newyork.personalchef.com.

Claire Stewart

Chelsea Market

Chelsea Market, between Ninth and Tenth Avenues and Fifteenth and Sixteenth Streets, is an indoor food hall housed in the former National Biscuit Factory (Nabisco), where treats like the Oreo cookie were invented. See OREOS and NABISCO. Over 22,000 people walk through the stripped-down brick walls every day to visit more than thirty-five vendors, ranging from gourmet food shops, top-notch restaurants, kitchen supply shops, and bookstores to anything food related in between. As one of the most highly trafficked and written-about destinations in New York City, Chelsea Market counts 6 million national and international visitors annually, and many New Yorkers use it as their everyday market.

Chelsea Market's motto, "Building community through food," extends to the area around the market, which has long been a vital part of New York City's food hub. In its early days, in the late nineteenth century, Nabisco took advantage of butchers' lard from the nearby Meatpacking District. See MEATPACKING DISTRICT. As the bakery grew, it acquired the entire tract between Fifteenth and Sixteenth Streets, from Ninth to Tenth Avenue, with the meatpacking industry growing alongside it. To support this vital food production, railroads were built at street level along Tenth Avenue, but by the mid-1930s it was deemed too dangerous to operate trains at street level, so the tracks were elevated, thus creating the High Line. See HIGH LINE.

As new technologies developed in the late 1950s, the vertical ovens at the bakery became outdated, and Nabisco moved its plant to New Jersey, where ample space was more conducive to the assembly line operation that was by then necessary to sustain production. A growing majority of the wholesale butchers moved to Hunts Point, the city's newest central market. See HUNTS POINT. Food transportation was also evolving; rail cars were no longer an efficient means of transport and were replaced by small delivery trucks, followed by larger trucks and, finally, international jets. The last food delivery by rail to the Meatpacking District was in 1980.

In the 1990s, Irwin B. Cohen, a prominent investor, organized a syndicate to buy the principal National Biscuit buildings, from Ninth to Eleventh Avenues and Fifteenth to Sixteenth Streets. He reinvented the complex by renting the upper floors to emerging tech companies, and on the ground floor he transformed the bakery's open-air loading dock into a long interior concourse of food stores. The well-appointed modern building with a strong link to New York's culinary past was the perfect outlet for innovative food companies to sell their products. Original tenants like Manhattan Fruit Exchange, Bowery Kitchen Supply, Amy's Bread, and Sarabeth's Bakery helped make the market a resource for both home cooks and professionals.

The blend of history and modern times is also evident in the market's décor and further contributes to its unique character. If you look closely, you'll notice existing elements like steel plates, lamps, rails, grilles, and assorted found objects throughout the market. Sculptor Mark Mennin has a strong presence in the market; his large-scale carvings of New York granite can be found in the middle of the market in the angular industrial waterfall feature he helped design, and on the façades of both Avenue entrances. More recently, the interior walls of the market serve as a rotating art gallery featuring photography collections.

Other tenants tucked inside this culinary architectural wonderland include Buon Italia, purveyor of fine imported Italian food products, from cheeses to cured meats; The Lobster Place, a seafood emporium; Italian import Rana Pasta, serving sit-down modern Italian cuisine, as well as a fresh pasta takeout operation; cold-pressed juice and vegetarian and vegan eats retailer LOLO Organics; and an outpost of Corkbuzz wine studio. The variety of vendors and types of products also speaks to the global scope of the market's offering: Australian meat pies from Tuck Shop, French crêpes from Bar Suzette, authentic Mexican tacos from Los Tacos No. 1, and Cambodian-style sandwiches from Num Pang.

The market also provides office space for media companies like Food Network and its production studio and test kitchen, MLB.com, local cable station NY1, and Oxygen Network. It counts among its neighbors Google and the High Line, which was converted into a popular elevated urban park built on the reclaimed railroad tracks of yesteryear.

"Chelsea Market, The Highline, & the Meatpacking District." Foods of New York Tours. http://www.foodsofny.com/chelseamarket.php.

Phillips, Michael, with Rick Rodgers. Chelsea Market Cookbook: 100 Recipes from New York's Premier

Indoor Food Hall. New York: Stewart, Tabori & Chang, 2013.

Wong, Sharon. "Traces of Chelsea Market's Industrial Past in the Meatpacking District." Untapped Cities, May 23, 2013. http://untappedcities.com/2013/05/23/chelsea-market/.

Layla Khoury-Hanold

Chestnuts

In 1828, a Frenchman began selling chestnuts at the corner of Broadway and Duane Street, bringing a touch of Paris (where roasted chestnuts had long been sold) to the city. When he died he had become an institution; his passing was noted in the papers.

This first chestnut vendor sold the large Spanish or possibly French variety of chestnut. If native New York chestnuts were ever used, this would have ended in the years following 1904, when an Asian fungus was detected in Central Park and, by 1912, had destroyed all those in the city and begun to move to other states. In later years, Italian chestnuts have been used, and the street price is a function of their cost.

By the late nineteenth century, such vendors were a familiar sight. By then, they were typically Italian. Cecil B. Demille (1881–1959) recalled, "When I was a little boy in New York, there used to be Italian chestnut vendors on the street corners in the wintertime. The chestnuts cost a nickel a bag. They roasted them right there and sold them hot out of the roaster, and you'd hold the bag to keep your hands warm while you ate the chestnuts" (Birchard, 2009, p. 48). This was also a time of anti-Italian sentiment, and these vendors, often unlicensed, were subject to harassment, as when a group of them had their carts confiscated in 1891.

Over time, changing taste has hurt the trade. As late as 1958, sales of chestnuts began in the fall. By the 1990s, they were a winter specialty. Now they are primarily sold around Christmas. See CHRISTMAS. In 2010, vendors complained that sales had become uncertain and unprofitable and were increasingly limited to tourist areas. As a European import, chestnuts can be costly. What is more, says an advocate for the vendors, "It's nostalgic street food. I think it smells better than it tastes" (Bultman and Siemazko, 2010).

See also STREET VENDORS.

Birchard, Robert S. *Cecil B. DeMille's Hollywood.* Lexington: University Press of Kentucky, 2009.

Bultman, Matthew, and Corky Siemazko. "Chestnut Tradition Is Toast! Few N.Y.C. Vendors Offer Treat." *NY Daily News,* December 10, 2010.

Haswell, Charles Haynes. *Reminiscences of an Octogenarian of the City of New York: (1816 to 1860).* New York: Harper, 1896.

Kaufman, Michael T. "New Yorkers Bask in Christmas Warmth." *New York Times,* December 26, 1988.

Jim Chevallier

Chewing Gum

See GUM.

Child, Julia

Julia Child (1912–2004) was a highly regarded chef, author, and television host. Her groundbreaking 1961 book *Mastering the Art of French Cooking* transformed the way generations of Americans cook.

Julia Carolyn McWilliams was born in Pasadena, California, on August 15, 1912. After graduating from Smith College in 1934, she moved to New York City, where she worked as a copywriter in the advertising department of the upscale furniture and rugs store W. & J. Sloane. She later transferred to the Los Angeles branch but was soon fired. In 1941, at the onset of World War II, she moved to Washington, D.C., and decided to join either the Women's Army Corps or the U.S. Navy's WAVES (Women Accepted for Volunteer Emergency Service). But at 6 feet 2 inches she was considered too tall, so instead, in the early 1940s she joined the Office of Strategic Services, a newly formed government intelligent agency, as a typist. In 1944 the OSS promoted her to research assistant and sent her to Ceylon, where she met Paul Cushing Child. During their off hours the couple explored local cuisine at local restaurants. They returned to the United States and were married on September 1, 1946.

Paul, who had lived in Paris, was known for his sophisticated palate. In 1948, the Childs returned to France when Paul was assigned by the U.S. Foreign Service to be an exhibits officer. While in France, Paul introduced his wife to the art of fine cuisine, and one meal in particular inspired Julia, so much so that she spoke about it often. This meal, which included oysters, sole meunière, and wine that they shared together at LaCouronne in Rouen, became for her a revelation. In 1949, when Child was thirty-seven, she enrolled at the prestigious Le Cordon Bleu in Paris, where her love of French cuisine blossomed.

After studying at Le Cordon Bleu, Child studied with several master chefs. Around the same time, Child joined a cooking club, Le Cercle des Gourmettes. A fellow club member, Simone Beck, was writing a cookbook together with a friend, Louisette Bertholle, about French food for an American audience. Child joined them in writing a cookbook and in creating a cooking school for Americans in Paris called L'École des Trois Gourmandes. The three friends spent ten years writing the cookbook, during which time Child moved to Cambridge, Massachusetts, where she created, tested, and wrote recipes for the book. Child, Beck, and Bertholle ended up signing a contract with Houghton Mifflin, which later rejected the manuscript, saying it seemed too much like an encyclopedia. Child shopped the book around, and in 1960 it landed on the desk of Judith Jones, a young editor at Knopf in New York City who published *Mastering the Art of French Cooking* when no other publishing houses were interested. Child and Jones became lifelong friends. This monumental cookbook, published in 1961, was 726 pages long. It became a bestseller and catapulted Child's career. Writing about the cookbook, Craig Claiborne said in the *New York Times* that it "may be the finest volume on French cooking ever published in English."

In 1963, the cookbook's success resulted in her notable television show *The French Chef* on WGBH (Boston's PBS member station) when Child was 50. This groundbreaking show was a huge success and was televised on PBS for ten years, even garnering an Emmy and a Peabody Award. Child, ever cheerful and enthusiastic about cooking French food, was extremely popular with her audience, so much so that she starred in a variety of other shows in the 1970s and 1980s, including *Julia Child & Company* and *Dinner at Julia's*. In the 1990s, Child starred in *Baking with Julia* and *Julia Child and Jacques Pépin Cooking at Home*.

The popularity of *Mastering the Art of French Cooking*, as well as Child's televisions shows, inspired many Americans to master every recipe. In 2002, Julie Powell, a young woman living in Queens, decided to cook her way throughout the book and to blog about the experience. The blog turned into a book, which subsequently inspired a movie starring Meryl Streep as Julia Child called *Julie & Julia*.

Although Child lived in Cambridge, Massachusetts, for many years, she often traveled to New York City and maintained friendships there, including with James Beard, a New Yorker, cookbook author, teacher, and television host. When Beard died in 1985, Child spearheaded the campaign to preserve his home in Greenwich Village as a community meeting place, as it was during Beard's life. Today the James Beard House is a highly regarded foundation that celebrates, nurtures, and honors America's diverse culinary heritage through programs that educate and inspire. See JAMES BEARD FOUNDATION.

Julia Child died on August 13, 2004, in Montecito, California, two days before her ninety-second birthday.

See also JONES, JUDITH AND EVAN.

Barr, Luke. *Provence, 1970: MFK Fisher, Julia Child, James Beard, and the Reinvention of American Taste*. New York: Clarkson Potter, 2013.
Central Intelligence Agency. "A Look Back…Julia Child: Life before French Cuisine." 2008. https://www.cia .gov/news-information/featured-story-archive/2007-featured-story-archive/julia-child.html.
Child, Julia, with Alex Prud'homme. *My Life in France*. New York: Knopf, 2006.
Grimes, William. "Julia Child's Memoir of When Cuisine Was French for Scary." *New York Times*, April 8, 2006.
James Beard Foundation website: http://www .jamesbeard.org/about.

Tracey Ceurvels

Childs

Established in 1889 in New York City, Childs was a lunchroom chain that was very popular throughout the northeastern United States in the 1920s and 1930s. At the height of its business, Childs operated over one hundred locations in thirty-two cities.

Childs was one of a group of restaurants that sought to both standardize and sanitize the experience of public dining during the nascent years of restaurant development in the United States. At a time when a sector of inexpensive restaurants in New York were known as "cheap and nasty," Childs tried to offer good food in a hygienic environment to New Yorkers of modest means. The management placed an emphasis on cleanliness, showcasing the restaurant's white tile walls and floors, spotless porcelain countertops, and the starched, white, nurse-like uniforms of its female servers. In addition to pioneering the use of female servers (instead of

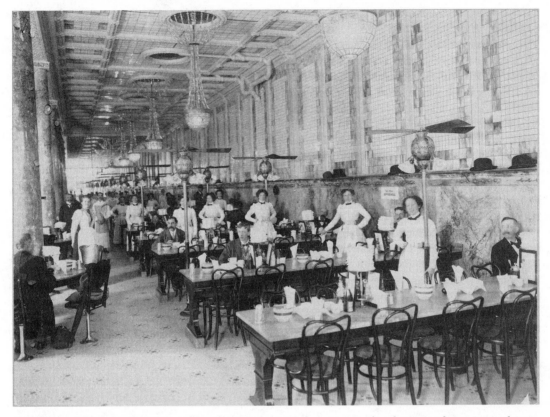

Childs was notable for its devotion to sanitary conditions as a chain restaurant. This photo was taken in 1900, when it already had more than five locations, which would grow to thirty-two over the next three decades. MUSEUM OF THE CITY OF NEW YORK

waiters), Childs experimented with other novel forms of service, including self-service along cafeteria-style tray lines. They were known for featuring their pancake production in the front window of the restaurant. Childs also hired notable architects to design its restaurants, including William van Alen (who designed the Chrysler Building) and famed New York architectural firm McKim, Mead, and White.

The first Childs was opened by brothers Samuel and William Childs in 1889 in Lower Manhattan, in the Merchants' Hotel on Cortlandt Street. Revolted by the restaurants they experienced on an extended trip to North Dakota, the Childs brothers returned to New York convinced, as William later put it, "that clean, good restaurants were a needed thing." By 1894, the restaurant had expanded to five locations; a few years later, the brothers incorporated the business, taking on investors (including employees who owned one-quarter of the company's stock), and began a period of aggressive expansion. By 1925, they operated

over one hundred locations throughout the Northeast (including a famous one on Coney Island, whose landmark building is still extant) and served 50 million meals per year. The restaurant's dairy-heavy menu included such dishes as creamed oysters, corned beef hash, graham crackers and milk, corned beef sandwiches, and famed butter cakes (akin to English muffins, cooked on a griddle) and pancakes. The Childs family operated a dairy farm in New Jersey, for many years the restaurants' sole dairy provider.

In the 1920s, the Childs chain experienced some difficulties. Samuel Childs died in 1925, and his brother William made some questionable business decisions, including stripping the menu of almost all meat dishes in favor of vegetarian options. This move reflected William's increasing concern about the health properties of food and his (incorrect) assumption that customers would prefer lighter fare. In the face of falling stock prices and rapidly declining sales, Childs shareholders insisted that William restore the menu (which he did), and in 1928 they removed him from the presidency.

While Childs scored a concession at the 1939 World's Fair, the 1930s were difficult years for the chain. See WORLD'S FAIR (1939–1940). Childs continued to lose money through the 1930s, eventually filing for bankruptcy in 1943. While the chain emerged from bankruptcy in 1947 and continued to operate through the 1950s, Childs never managed to regain its hold against competitors such as Horn & Hardart's. See AUTOMATS. In 1961, the Riese Organization acquired the Childs chain and within a decade had replaced the Childs restaurants with other properties.

Batterberry, Michael, and Arianne Batterberry. *On the Town in New York: The Landmark History of Eating, Drinking, and Entertainments from the American Revolution to the Food Revolution*. New York: Routledge, 1999.

Gray, Christopher. "Streetscapes: The Childs Building; Fast Food, Then and Now, on Stylish Fifth Avenue." *New York Times*, November 6, 1988.

Grimes, William. *Appetite City: A Culinary History of New York*. New York: North Point, 2009.

Cindy R. Lobel

Chinese Community

Only scant traces of a Chinese community existed in New York until the 1870s, when anti-Chinese violence in the far West caused thousands to seek safety in Midwestern and East Coast cities. Though bilingual researchers with roots in the community are now starting to document Manhattan Chinatown's history, early published accounts were by whites who did not know Chinese. They suggest that in the mid-1870s a merchant named Wo Kee moved from a tiny Chinese settlement on the East River to the vicinity of Mott Street. Several other merchants soon managed to buy properties nearby, making Mott Street a byword for "Chinatown."

Accurate population statistics are elusive since new arrivals often lived on the wrong side of the law. The 1882 Chinese Exclusion Act and other attempts to bar Chinese manual laborers from the United States drove many into a shadowy undocumented status. A newspaper estimate of about five hundred people in 1873, and official census figures showing 747 in 1880, 2,048 in 1890, and 6,321 in 1900, roughly indicate the growth of Chinatown and other clusters of settlement. The real totals were probably at least three times greater.

The community during this time was almost wholly male. Most owned or worked in small laundries, often located in neighborhoods close to a white clientele. Chinese residents came to Chinatown on Sundays to buy food in neighborhood stores and eat in large restaurants or snack shops serving Cantonese food to fellow countrymen. (Nearly all were from Toisan District in southern Guangdong Province.) An 1898 account estimates the number of "restaurant keepers and pastry makers" at forty-five.

Drastic changes occurred after 1896, when the prominent Chinese statesman Li Hongzhang (Li Hong Chung) made an extravagantly publicized visit to the United States. Inexperienced white diners invaded Chinatown restaurants hoping to sample something like the food that newspapers reported Li's cooks to be preparing at the Waldorf Astoria Hotel. Scenting opportunity, Mott Street eateries created America's first ethnic culinary fad by devising versions of Cantonese dishes adroitly tailored to American preferences that the Chinese had seen firsthand while working as house servants or camp cooks in the far West.

For two or three generations, a made-up cuisine served to non-Chinese patrons amid "Oriental" atmospheric flourishes was the mainstay of Chinatown restaurants such as the Chinese Rathskeller, Lee's, and Port Arthur. Its star attraction was "chop suey." See CHOP SUEY JOINTS. English speakers appear to have picked up this garbled phrase from the Cantonese *chow tsap sui*, meaning "stir-fried this-and-that," unwittingly leaving out the most important word—chow, for "stir-frying," a method at which Cantonese cooks were considered peerless. The new cuisine regularly paired bland batter-fried morsels with equally bland, somewhat sweetish brown sauces or very sugary sweet-and-sour ones. (Chinese patrons expected meals cooked to quite different standards.)

The popularity of "chop suey" cuisine with both white and black American diners encouraged a shift from laundries to restaurants as the community's chief source of employment. As the economic base of Chinatown shrank between about 1910 and 1940, many Chinese restaurants appeared in the Manhattan theater district, Harlem, and the outer boroughs. Depending on the location, they sometimes featured dancing and nightclub-style entertainment. A 1939 survey estimated the number of New York City Chinese restaurants at 248, with 111 in Manhattan and 82 in Brooklyn. See HARLEM and AFRICAN AMERICAN.

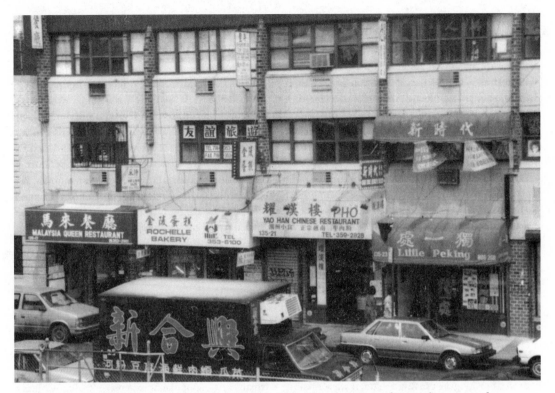

A row of Asian food providers on Fortieth Road, Flushing, 1990. Chinese cuisines often vary by region and are influenced by nearby countries. Malaysian-Chinese, Vietnamese-Chinese, Hunanese, Sichuanese, Dongbei (the former "Manchuria"), and the varied styles of Jiangnan cuisines are all popular in Flushing and elsewhere throughout the city. QUEENS HISTORICAL SOCIETY

During America's Cold War alliance with Chiang Kai-Shek's exiled Nationalist regime on Taiwan, wealthy Mandarin-speaking diplomats, military attaches, and businessmen arrived on the social scene with cooks highly trained in versions of Chinese cuisine unfamiliar to Americans. Some of these employees eventually launched ambitious, stylish restaurants aimed at affluent white customers. Several VIP wives followed suit. Leading American food writers quickly hailed the smart new establishments as models of "authentic" Chinese cuisine, while dismissing chop suey as a shoddy Cantonese peasant creation.

Non-Chinese patrons often preferred to dine conveniently in their own neighborhoods, and Cantonese Americans in Chinatown understandably disliked renting restaurant space to interloping Mandarin speakers. For an interval before more opportunities opened up in Chinatown, the chief new restaurants were located in mid-Manhattan and along upper Broadway. Some had mainland-born chefs with links to the last generation of imperial palace cooks. In the 1960s and 1970s Shun Lee Dynasty, Shanghai Cafe, the Hunam, Uncle Tai's Hunan Yuan, Peng's, and other regionally focused restaurants introduced white New Yorkers to new dishes including Sichuan-style sesame noodles, Shanghai soup dumplings, scallion pancakes, potstickers, and (in a syrupy bastardized version) General Tso's chicken. Peking duck became nearly commonplace. Meanwhile, the China Institute in America, a cultural institution on Manhattan's East Side, had opened a new age of culinary education in 1955 by offering Chinese cooking classes. The program's continuing success under Grace Zia Chu and Florence Lin encouraged an unprecedented interest in Chinese home cooking for non-Chinese Americans.

As in chop suey days, successful restaurateurs needed a fan base in the white (sometimes black) community. That situation changed after 1968, when a 1965 immigration-reform law went into effect. Chinese-born people were now free to enter the country and apply for citizenship on the same basis as anybody else. Within a few years, Chinatown was receiving new arrivals from Taiwan and Hong Kong along with ethnic Chinese fleeing hostility in many parts of Southeast Asia. After the early 1980s, newly established diplomatic relations between the United States and the People's Republic of China, together with relaxed Chinese emigration policies, brought to the United States a rising tide of mainlanders from various regions.

Census figures for New York City residents of Chinese origin grew nearly tenfold between 1970 and 2011, from 37,348 to 350,231. The real increase certainly was much greater, thanks to an enormous undocumented flow of people smuggled in from Fujian Province (historically, a hotbed of crime) by "snakeheads." The groups with the greatest economic impact were entrepreneurs and professionals from the Far Eastern "little tigers" (postwar economic powerhouses) Taiwan, Hong Kong, and Singapore.

Top-notch seafood restaurants and Hong Kong–style dimsum palaces started appearing in Manhattan's Chinatown during the mid-1970s. A little later, East Broadway and Eldridge Street acquired dozens of Fujianese restaurants serving many kinds of soup and dishes made with the region's special red wine lees. At Flushing in northern Queens, a Korean–Indian–Chinese enclave close to the last station of the number 7 subway line suddenly expanded into the city's biggest, most affluent Chinatown. A lesser Queens colony later formed in Elmhurst. In south Brooklyn, many newly arriving Chinese (with a large Fujianese contingent) settled in Sunset Park. Each of these settlements has branched into nearby neighborhoods or produced smaller satellite communities, so that today it is hard to calculate the number of actual New York Chinatowns. See SUNSET PARK.

All the new enclaves, but especially Flushing, contain Chinese of diverse Far Eastern origins, together with restaurants supported by these clienteles. Non-Chinese patrons and mainstream restaurant critics seldom play major roles in the success of such eateries. A few, however, have courted non-Chinese fans, and a large sprinkling of elegant Sichuan-style restaurants has grown up in midtown Manhattan.

Among the cuisines that command large followings (aside from Fujianese and Taiwanese) are Malaysian-Chinese, Vietnamese-Chinese, Hunanese, Sichuanese, Dongbei (the former "Manchuria"), and the varied styles of "Jiangnan" (a general term for Shanghai and neighboring areas south of the Yangtze River).

Immigrants from Shaanxi, Xinjiang, and other western and northern provinces have introduced Muslim culinary traditions; recently arrived Cantonese have infused new blood into that cooking style.

Fish markets, produce stores, and herbal remedy shops abound in the New York Chinatowns. Investors from the "little tigers" and, more recently, the mainland have opened ambitious emporiums—notably, branches of the international Hong Kong Supermarket chain—stocked with enormous arrays of Chinese ingredients. They have also founded several Flushing shopping malls containing food courts that are star attractions in their own right, with assorted food stalls serving short-order specialties of different regions: Lanzhou-style hand-swung noodles, kebabs of anything from lamb morsels to chicken innards, many kinds of handmade dumplings, various stuffed flatbreads, or hot pots with ingredients selected by customers.

After the 1959 communist revolution, a few thousand people from Cuba's small Chinese community (originally composed of sugar-plantation laborers and merchants) relocated to New York, founding a smattering of popular, inexpensive "Cuban-Chinese" restaurants. More recently, Chinese from Lima (mostly descendants of Peruvian plantation and railroad workers) have also brought chifas, or restaurants specializing in their hybridized versions of stir-fried rice, noodles, and pork, to a few Queens neighborhoods. Meanwhile, emigrants from a Chinese colony in Calcutta have started New York restaurants serving dishes like "gobi Manchurian" (spiced batter-fried florets of cauliflower) and stir-fried paneer (in place of tofu). A successful franchise called Chinese Mirch is popularizing this fare among a larger audience.

Because the Internet has made possible instant exchanges between home cooks, restaurant goers, and chefs everywhere on earth, people in all the city's Chinese communities can effortlessly follow trends in China, the Far East, and elsewhere. Much "fusion" cooking and experimentation is occurring at all levels, from dumpling shops to luxury restaurants. Non-Chinese diners revel in the inventive Chinese-inspired offerings of such mainstream Manhattan pacesetters as Mission Chinese, Momofuku, and Red Farm. It is little exaggeration to say that some acquaintance with Chinese culinary techniques and regional schools is now mandatory for the city's aspiring chefs, no matter what their own areas of specialization.

See also MUSEUM OF CHINESE IN AMERICA (MOCA).

Chen, Yong. *Chop Suey, USA: The Story of Chinese Food in America*. New York: Columbia University Press, 2014.

Coe, Andrew. *Chop Suey: A Cultural History of Chinese Food in the United States*. New York: Oxford University Press, 2009.

Guest, Kenneth J. "From Mott Street to East Broadway: Fuzhounese Immigrants and the Revitalization of New York's Chinatown." In *Chinatowns around the World: Gilded Ghetto, Ethnopolis, and Cultural Diaspora*, edited by Bernard P. Wong and Tan Chee-Beng, pp. 35–54. Leiden, The Netherlands, and Boston: Brill, 2013.

Anne Mendelson

Chipwich

The Chipwich is an ice cream sandwich made from vanilla ice cream between two chocolate chip cookies, with the sides rolled in additional miniature chocolate chips. The product was developed by New Yorker Richard LaMotta (1942–2010) in 1981, based on his experience as the owner-operator of the Sweet Tooth ice cream parlor in Englewood, New Jersey, in the 1970s and experimentation in his Brooklyn home. LaMotta began selling his Chipwiches for one dollar each via street vendors in New York City in the spring of 1982, quickly building a team of sixty vendors.

Later in the 1980s, LaMotta moved to a more traditional distribution method, through the frozen food aisle of the grocery store. His plants in Queens, New York, and Lodi, New Jersey, manufactured over two hundred thousand units per day. In 2002, Cool-Brands International, a leading ice cream and frozen novelty manufacturer, bought Chipwich. By then the company had sold over one billion units. Chipwich was later sold to Nestle in 2007. Nestle stopped production of the product within a couple of years of purchasing the brand. Speculation is that they bought Chipwich to reduce competition with its own Nestle Toll House Chocolate Chip Cookie Sandwich, a story that angers nostalgic fans of the iconic treat.

LaMotta died of a heart attack in 2010, having, in his words, devoted "twenty pounds of my life to Chipwiches."

See also ICE CREAM SANDWICH.

"Dividends: War of the Chocolate Chips." *Time*, September 28, 1981.

Hevesi, Dennis. "Richard LaMotta, Creator of Chipwich Ice Cream Sandwich, Dies at 67." *New York Times*, May 16, 2010, A23.

Jonathan Deutsch

Chock full o'Nuts

Chock full o'Nuts was a chain of coffee shops that thrived during the Great Depression, serving wholesome lunches to legions of New Yorkers. It was launched by a Russian immigrant, William Black (1898–1983), who had opened a shelled-nut stand in a basement in Times Square in 1926. That business was successful, and by 1932 Black had opened eighteen additional nut shops around the city.

During the Depression, Black converted his nut shops into inexpensive cafés where a nickel would buy a cup of quality coffee and a "nutted cheese" sandwich—cream cheese with chopped walnuts on lightly toasted whole wheat raisin bread (he would later switch this to a dense, dark date-nut bread). Over time Black added other sandwich options, including lobster salad and liverwurst, as well as grilled hot dogs, split-pea soup, doughnuts, coffee cake, and pie. But the most popular item remained the "nutted cheese." By the 1960s there were more than thirty Chock full o'Nuts outlets in Manhattan and Brooklyn. In 1962 Craig Claiborne, the *New York Times* food critic, sang the praises of the familiar coffee shops, calling them "first-class establishments.... They are neat as a whistle and the sandwiches and pastries are of a high order." Indeed, the company boasted that the food served in its shops was "untouched by human hands."

In 1953, Black began selling Chock full o'Nuts–brand ground coffee in supermarkets. He advertised extensively in print and on the radio, where a memorable jingle extolled the "heavenly coffee—better coffee a Rockefeller's money can't buy." (The boss's wife, cabaret singer Page Morton Black, was the voice behind that commercial.) When the Rockefeller family complained, the words were changed to "better coffee a millionaire's money can't buy." Chock full o'Nuts became New York City's most popular brand of coffee.

Black scored another promotional coup by hiring Jackie Robinson, recently retired from his glory days with the Brooklyn Dodgers, as vice president in charge of personnel; Robinson was also appointed to the company's board of directors. At that time, aside from management, many Chock full o'Nuts employees were African American. The Chock full o'Nuts chain eventually expanded to more than 125 outlets but began to downsize during the 1970s, when competing national brands took over the market share in New York. When William Black died in 1983, there were only twenty-five shops still open, and by decade's end there were none. The coffee brand survived by advertising itself as New York's coffee. The brand is now owned by an Italian coffee company, Massimo Zanetti Beverage Group USA.

In 2010 Chock full o'Nuts attempted a revival, opening a coffee shop on Twenty-Third Street and announcing plans for as many as fifty more outlets. But the new outlet lasted only about two years at that location.

See also COFFEE SHOPS.

Claiborne, Craig. "1960s: Haute Cuisine in America." *New York Times*, January 1, 1970, p. 27.
Pendergrast, Mark. *Uncommon Grounds: The History of Coffee and How It Transformed Our World*. 2d ed. New York: Basic Books, 2010.

Andrew F. Smith

Chocolate, Craft

Craft chocolate, or what is also often called "bean-to-bar" chocolate, is made by producers who source their own cacao beans, roasting and grinding the ingredients themselves before making them into bars or other end products. While cacao, the main ingredient in chocolate, can only be sourced from equatorial regions, chocolate became a staple in Western diets centuries ago. First brought to Europe by explorers in the 1500s, who initially encountered cacao as the bitter drink revered by the Mayans and Aztecs, this "food of the gods" became a luxury good in the Western world by the end of the century. Until the 1800s, it was consumed primarily as a beverage that was mixed by hand, after which advances in technology and the increasing availability of sugar spawned the modern chocolate bar. Quickly the production of solid milk chocolate became mechanized, and the demand was so high that new sources for cacao were sought. For the next century, the goal of cacao producers was high yield, no matter the toll it took on the land or the workers. And the mass-produced chocolate changed as well, with a low cacao content and a high percentage of additives such as milk and sugar.

This interest in bean-to-bar chocolate rose in America around the same time that the handmade food movement took hold in the first decade of the new millennium. While there had been a small handful of bean-to-bar makers in the country previously, the vast majority of chocolate was made from lower-quality cacao sourced mainly from Africa, where the intensive planting of cacao deteriorated the farmland and many workers were unpaid or severely underpaid. The modern craft chocolate makers recognized the harm the mass production of chocolate caused and sought to source higher-quality cacao and harvest it in a way that was more socially and environmentally responsible. This led to a new breed of chocolate makers becoming more involved with the growing of multiple varieties of cacao and in a number of regions where the climate could affect the flavor, often emphasizing single-origin cacao and the resulting nuances of flavor. Amid a push toward organic cacao production, the growing number of bean-to-bar chocolate makers created mission statements concerning their own intent for how their cacao is sourced, including higher wages for the workers and attention to lowering the environmental impact.

Mast Brothers Chocolate, located in the Williamsburg neighborhood of Brooklyn, was among the bean-to-bar chocolate makers who set up shop in the early 2000s. Part of the community credited as among the first wave of the new artisanal food revolution in the city, the owners were inspired to experiment with making chocolate bars from scratch as they saw chocolate as a popular food but one that was largely unavailable in its more simple form. One goal of these new craft chocolate makers was to take the idea of terroir—or the expression of flavor from the way the raw ingredients were grown and initially handled, most often spoken about regarding wine or coffee—and apply it to chocolate.

As Mast Brothers Chocolate grew in the following years, it became known for its distinctive packaging, designed after vintage wallpaper found in a shop in Manhattan, as well as dedication to educating consumers about the process of making chocolate and the possibilities of flavor from carefully sourced beans. To this end it has a production facility in Brooklyn that is open to viewing by the public, and the owners publicly support sustainable cacao sourcing, going so far as to sail beans from the Caribbean to New York City, in part to show that this once-common, environmentally friendly form of transporting raw materials is still possible. Today it is one of the best-known bean-to-bar chocolate makers in the country.

Cacao Prieto is another New York–based bean-to-bar chocolate maker, and it sources its cacao from its own farm in the Dominican Republic, which is then produced into chocolate at its factory in Brooklyn. Committed to combining a modern approach to preserving the tradition of chocolate, Cacao Prieto is one of only a few chocolate companies that can claim to be completely vertically integrated, from farm to bar. It also produces a line of chocolate-making machinery, inspired by hundred-year-old technology sold under its sister company, Brooklyn Cacao. It also uses cacao to make a line of spirits that feature hand-roasted, -cracked, and -winnowed cacao.

Other New York–based craft chocolate makers include Nunu Chocolate, which features single-origin Colombian cacao from a sustainable farm, and raw chocolate makers Raaka Chocolate and Fine and Raw Chocolate, both of which make chocolate without roasting the raw cacao. All of these chocolate makers are located in Brooklyn.

As with other industries that have seen an increased interest in handmade and traditional production methods, the bean-to-bar chocolate makers in New York City focus on taking a modern approach to a classic food, bringing a sensibility that supports both workers' rights and environmental sustainability. They also offer an elevated flavor palate with few additives and a high cacao percentage to help modern consumers rethink their relationship with a familiar food.

See also STARTUPS.

Off, Carol. *Bitter Chocolate*. New York: New Press. 2008.
Coe, Sophie D., and Michael D. Coe. *The True History of Chocolate*. 2d ed. London: Thames & Hudson, 2007.

Suzanne Cope

Chop Suey Joints

A chop suey joint is a restaurant specializing in chop suey and other Chinese American specialties. Chop suey was first discovered by New Yorkers during the mid-1880s in Manhattan's Chinatown. As non-Chinese began to crowd into their restaurants, chefs began to replace more "exotic" ingredients, such as chicken gizzards and dried seafood, with easily identifiable meats, onion, celery, bean sprouts, and

the like. In 1896, the taste for the dish spread from the city's Bohemian crowd to the larger population when Li Hongzhang, China's de facto foreign minister, visited New York, setting off a fad for all things Chinese, including the food.

Seeing their chance, Chinese restaurateurs began opening the first eateries outside of Chinatown. Called "chop sueys" or "chop suey joints," these restaurants focused on a limited menu of dishes whose recipes had been tailored to non-Chinese tastes: chop suey, chow mein, and *yat gaw mein* (a noodle soup often topped with shredded chicken). For less adventurous eaters, they also offered ham sandwiches, tomato soup, and other American dishes. Within a few years, the city was home to over one hundred chop sueys, ranging from small side-street joints to sprawling eateries in the theater district. Decorated with colored lanterns and Chinese tapestries, they were usually open until the wee hours of the morning, drawing the city's raffish set after an evening's entertainment. Unlike most other restaurants, they did not discriminate against African Americans and welcomed Jews, helping them to gain a devoted following among those populations.

Chop suey joints remained a popular part of the city's dining scene for most of the twentieth century. Over the decades, they gradually lost their exotic ambience, becoming comfortable neighborhood restaurants known for their rows of padded booths and menus featuring familiar dishes such as chop suey, egg foo young, roast pork, and egg rolls. They were often run by Chinese American families, with the mother behind the cash register, the father in the kitchen, and the children waiting on tables after school.

Although chop suey is still served in New York, the city's old-time chop suey joints have all but disappeared. Among the last in Manhattan was the East Village's Jade Mountain, which closed in 2007.

See CHINESE COMMUNITY.

Coe, Andrew. *Chop Suey: A Cultural History of Chinese Food in the United States*. New York: Oxford University Press, 2009.

Andrew Coe

Christmas

As a religious holiday, Christmas reverentially celebrates the birth of Christ on December 25; as a secular holiday, the long Christmas season, stretching from late November to early January, boisterously combats the darkest, shortest days of winter. These two aspects of Christmas annually collide in what pundits call "the war on Christmas," where cultural debates over what, and how much, religious iconography can form part of the public observances. This battle is nothing new. Versions have been fought for centuries, including on the streets of New York, and the battle even touches the foods and drinks we associate with Christmas. And although New York City contributed no distinctive culinary traditions to Christmas (except for Jews passing the day at Chinese restaurants), it nonetheless played a central role in shaping the culture of the modern Christmas.

The first widespread religious celebrations of Christmas on December 25 likely date to the fourth century, when Christianity was supplanting paganism as the official religion of the Roman Empire. Lacking specific biblical authority identifying when Christ was born, church elders proposed dates in March, April, May, and November. It is often thought that December 25 was selected to coincide with, and thus to substitute for, Saturnalia and the Mithraic feasting of the pagan calendar. This legislated date would fuel religious fires centuries later, when the Puritans during the English Civil War called Christmas a "popish" invention. Many of the early colonists (in Massachusetts) were Puritan Dissenters who brought their antagonism to Christmas to American shores. While English colonists in New Amsterdam were not as dour about holidays as the Puritans, there is no evidence of any enthusiasm for Christmas.

Nor do popular histories of the Dutch colonists in seventeenth-century New Amsterdam make any mention of Christmas, but they do claim that the Dutch celebrated Saint Nicholas's feast day on December 6. Saint Nicholas's hagiography included giving gifts of money or sweets to children, and the only evidence that New Amsterdamers observed Saint Nicholas's Day is that the government back in Amsterdam issued a decree to quash public disorder (if any) by banning public assemblies at the holiday with "any kind of candy, eatables or other merchandise." Whether these assemblies were a problem seems unlikely as records show that in 1643 there were eighteen different languages in Manhattan spoken by a mere five hundred colonists, which included French Huguenots, Flems, Walloons, Germans, and a few Jews, in addition to the Dutch and some English. Adding to the cultural

and linguistic cacophony was the Algonquian spoken by the area's Native Americans and the several languages spoken by enslaved Africans from Angola. To the extent that anyone celebrated Christmas, there was no uniformity in observances, nor was it an important holiday. When New Amsterdam became New York in 1664, English cultural influences—via the Anglicans—increased.

Anglicans largely ignored Christmas in the colonial period and in the Revolution's immediate aftermath; it was not until the first several decades of the nineteenth century that Christmas began to take its distinctive shape in New York City through a remarkable, concerted effort to invent ancient traditions. The cultural solutions created in New York acted as a balm to raw ethnic and socioeconomic tensions caused by a rapidly increasing immigrant population, seasonal labor dislocations, and changing notions of family relationships. These forces soon influenced Christmas celebrations throughout the country.

Part of the problem arose from the strong strain of anti-Catholicism and anti-Irish immigration that permeated parts of New York in the early nineteenth century. In 1806, riots broke out after Catholic worshippers were attacked by Protestants as they left Christmas masses at Saint Peter's Church on Barclay and Church Streets, hearkening back to English colonists' earlier accusations of "popery."

"Frolickings," a European folk tradition, were also becoming part of public life in American cities, especially New York and Philadelphia, where masked revelers roamed the streets, firing guns, banging on doors, and demanding food and drink. The old carol lyrics, "now bring us some figgy pudding...we won't go until we get some," took on ominous meaning. By the 1820s, these frolics turned to rancor as laborers, seasonally unemployed with the onset of winter, pounded on the doors of wealthy townhouses in the newly developed tony neighborhoods of Greenwich Village and Chelsea and protested in the streets. Newspaper editorials demanded that action be taken to quell this undesirable Christmas tradition.

New York's cultural elite responded, taking advantage of preexisting Dutch culinary traditions to make Christmas more of a family holiday. John Pintard, founder of the New-York Historical Society in 1804, made Saint Nicholas the society's patron saint, implying a long relationship between the city and the saint. In 1808, Washington Irving, a member of the society, wrote about an old New Year's tradition of cookies impressed with the image of "St. Nicholas, vulgarly called Sancte Claus [sic]" in his satirical periodical *Salmagundi*. These cookies, eaten at both Christmas and New Year's, were already well known and popular: recipes for stamped "Christmas cookeys" appear in the second edition of Amelia Simmons's *American Cookery*, published in Albany, New York, in 1796, and records show that such cookies were sold in Manhattan pastry shops. The next year, Irving's *Knickerbocker History of New York* contained multiple references to "Sancte Claus" and his gifts of oranges, almonds, raisins, waffles, doughnuts, and "Crullers and Oley-Cooks fresh from the pot." In 1823, Chelsea resident Clement Clarke Moore wrote his famous poem "A Visit from Saint Nicholas," with its "visions of sugar-plums [candied nuts, spices, and dried fruits]" that would fill children's Christmas stockings.

This domestic, idealized Christmas quickly became a dominant trope as editorials lauded the focus on the family and, especially, children. Sugary treats were a taken-for-granted meme for Christmas celebrations. In 1838, Philip Hone, briefly mayor of New York, critiqued an ostentatious dinner party where the table was "covered with confectionary and gew-gaws, [and] looked like one of the shops down Broadway in the Christmas holidays." At the same time, a fine roasted bird was becoming the iconic centerpiece of Christmas dinner. Hone's diary for Christmas Day, 1842, merrily asked where enough turkeys, geese, ducks, and chickens could be found to satisfy the New Yorkers strolling about on the brilliant Christmas morning. Hone's question anticipated the repast found in Charles Dickens's *A Christmas Carol*, published in England in December 1843 and syndicated in New York City a few weeks later. For at least the next fifty years, the roast bird, potatoes, and plum pudding of Dickens's novella would be found on tables in New York City and, indeed, through America; it continues to be de rigueur in some households.

By the early twentieth century, Christmas menus published in the *New York Times* offered alternatives to the traditional roast bird, including a mock wild duck or mock rabbit (both based on flank steak), Spanish beefsteak, or veal curry. The choices offered in Charlotte Turgeon's *Cooking for Christmas*, published in New York in 1950, added roast

suckling pig, crown roast of pork, and a Yule ham to the requisite birds. She also included the traditional dishes of plum pudding, mincemeat pies, and fruitcakes, recipes that would have brought caustic accusations of "popish idolatry" in previous centuries because the spices evoked the gifts of the Magi.

Nowadays, newspapers such as the *Times* publish recipes for "the ultimate Christmas dinner," mixing tradition with innovation and reflecting the ethnicity found in New York: among the recommended dishes in 2013 was a spicy Thai squid with chilies and cilantro, claimed to be perfect for Christmas Eve.

See also DUTCH-STYLE NEW YEAR'S DAY PARTIES.

Chandler, Adam. "Why American Jews Eat Chinese Food on Christmas." TheAtlantic.com, December 23, 2014. http://www.theatlantic.com/national/archive/2014/12/why-american-jews-eat-chinese-food-on-christmas/384011/.
Jones, Charles W. "Knickerbocker Santa Claus." *New York Historical Society Quarterly* 38, no. 4 (1954): 357–383.
Kaufman, Cathy K. "The Ideal Christmas Dinner." *Gastronomica* 4, no. 4 (2004): 17–24.
Nissenbaum, Stephen. *The Battle for Christmas*. New York: Vintage, 1995.

Cathy K. Kaufman

Citarella

See GROCERY STORES.

City Harvest

See HUNGER PROGRAMS.

Citymeals-on-Wheels

Citymeals-on-Wheels is one of the largest meals-on-wheels programs in the United States, delivering 2 million meals to eighteen thousand homebound elderly New Yorkers each year. Food luminaries Gael Greene and James Beard founded the organization in 1981 after learning that many homebound elderly New Yorkers who relied upon city agencies to provide weekday meals had nothing to eat on weekends and holidays when city budget funding did not stretch to seven days a week. They rallied the restaurant community and raised private donations to supplement the government-funded weekday meal delivery program.

In 1981 the plight of hungry homebound New Yorkers was chronicled in the *New York Times*. Greene and Beard both independently read this story and were appalled. As Greene recalls, "It was outrageous! I couldn't live with the delicious excess of my life knowing someone next door to me was an invisible prisoner." After a brief phone conversation during which they shared their disgust at the situation, they decided to do something about it, and the idea for Citymeals-on-Wheels was born. They began reaching out to their colleagues in the food world to solicit financial support to keep food on the tables of these homebound elderly.

The reception from the food community was strong; that from the corporate world was less so. Many of Beard's and Greene's colleagues had been touched by the same story. Their first efforts raised over $30,000 in just a few days, enough to bring a Christmas meal to six thousand elderly neighbors.

Greene was emphatic that the funds raised be used to provide meals, rather than for administrative costs. Janet Sainer, the commissioner of New York City's Department for the Aging, assured Greene that administrative funds were in place and that monies raised by Greene and friends would go directly to the delivery of meals. There was some discussion about the legalities of how the commission accepted the money, and Sainer conferred with Mayor Ed Koch, who said "Take their money."

Decades later Citymeals-on-Wheels continues to serve homebound elderly, with every mayor since Koch continuing to be supportive of the program. What started as a grassroots fundraising effort that fed six thousand people has swelled to delivery of over 40 million meals according to Beth Shapiro, who is only the second executive director the organization has had after taking over from Marcia Stein in 2011. Having served that many meals over the years is impressive, as is the fact that the organization has raised more money every year than the year before.

This fundraising is, in great part, thanks to the commitment of chefs, like Jonathan Waxman and Larry Forgione, who were there from the very beginning when the plan was to make the spring fundraiser a birthday bash for James Beard; but since he died a few months prior, they turned it into a tribute and corralled their fellow chefs to get involved. Giving their fellow chefs only the direction to come and cook whatever they wanted, Edna Lewis turned up with a ham and two other chefs prepared suckling pig. Somehow they and the other thirty-seven participating chefs coinhabited the kitchen of Nick Valenti's Patina restaurant in Rockefeller Center with his staff still operating there.

Though chef support remains high—Daniel Boulud is currently co-chair—and a cadre of supportive young professionals grows more involved every day, the business of delivering a healthy meal to an elderly neighbor does not slow down. Citymeals-on-Wheels now delivers eighteen thousand meals annually. However, the fast-rising number of senior citizens in New York raises concern. By the 2020s it is estimated that seniors will outnumber children for the first time in New York City's history, shifting the culture in some ways. With the average age of recipients in their eighties, this will, as executive director Beth Shapiro says, "tax this city, not just Citymeals, if we don't prepare. That will take more fundraising but also an understanding of who these people are, where they are and the diversity that's reflective of the city." Taking care of these people and enabling them to remain in the familiar homes and neighborhood settings in which they are comfortable is only possible if a simple meal comes to the door every day.

See also HUNGER PROGRAMS.

Shulman, Robin. "Poorest Feel Downturn as Donations Fall." *Washington Post*, October 5, 2008.
Turner, Kathleen. "NYC Chefs Rally for Citymeals-on-Wheels." *Gotham*, May 2013.

Francine Cohen

City University of New York

The City University of New York (CUNY) serves over 250,000 degree-seeking students at its twenty-four campuses and nearly 250,000 students through a variety of nondegree adult, continuing education, and professional development programs. A number of undergraduate, graduate, and nondegree programs support the study of food through the lens of culinary arts, hospitality, public health and nutrition, and other disciplines. Moreover, with the food-service sector's sustained growth and an increased awareness of the role of food and its intersections with various aspects of our lives, there are efforts to establish additional programs to support the study of food at CUNY.

For students interested in working in the food-service industry as line cooks, dining room managers, or pastry chefs and in other careers that involve preparing and serving food, CUNY offers several options. At Kingsborough Community College, one of CUNY's seven community colleges, students can earn associate's degrees in culinary arts, where the majority of classes are hands-on and taught in the college's commercial-grade kitchens. Kingsborough's hospitality degree program prepares students for careers in food and beverage management, with an emphasis on marketing, sales, purchasing, and operations. Kingsborough Community College also offers a number of nondegree workforce training and professional development opportunities, as well as a certificate in culinary arts designed for students who have already earned a college degree in another field. A kitchen incubator, the Kitchen Ventures Incubator Program, supports food entrepreneurs. The New York City College of Technology, a four-year CUNY college, offers a bachelor's degree in hospitality management that combines hands-on culinary arts training with business and management courses. LaGuardia Community College offers an associate's degree in food-service management, with an emphasis on production management and nutrition, preparing students for careers in institutional food.

There are many opportunities to learn about food and its intersections with public health, policy, epidemiology, and nutrition. The CUNY School of Public Health offers bachelor's, master's, and doctoral degrees; a number of faculty members' research is focused on food policy, food-related illnesses, and nutrition. Two-year and four-year colleges offer degrees in community health, public health, food service management, and nutrition, preparing students for careers as registered dieticians, community food advocates, and food policy researchers, for example.

Although the university supports the study of food in several ways, it does not have a food studies degree program. The Graduate Center, CUNY's PhD-granting institution, offers a concentration in food studies for students who choose to focus their re-

search on the social and cultural aspects of food. Hostos Community College has developed an associate's degree in food studies, with an emphasis on social justice and public health. Numerous faculty across the university conduct research on food, integrating their research into courses and supporting graduate-level research on food-related topics.

Other entities have been established to support student and faculty interest in food. The CUNY Foodways Seminar was founded by two CUNY faculty members, Annie Hauck-Lawson and Jonathan Deutsch, with the goal of creating a forum for interdisciplinary research in food studies. It was the first CUNY-based effort to identify and support faculty and graduate students interested in food-related topics. The CUNY Food Policy Seminar meets once a month in the fall and spring semesters. Participants are an interdisciplinary group of faculty from within and outside of CUNY, graduate students, and individuals associated with nonacademic institutions. The seminar fosters discussion, hosts speakers, and sponsors events, in addition to sponsoring original research and publication on policy issues. Kingsborough Community College's Farm Faculty Interest Group convenes faculty interested in integrating food with existing curricula and supporting the development of grants to support research and programs focused on food and farming.

Urban agriculture is generating interest across New York City as a strategy for increasing food security, building community, driving economic development, and mitigating the environmental impacts of industrialized food systems. Many of CUNY's campuses have limited space with which to support urban agriculture. Nonetheless, several campuses are farming on-site. For example, Brooklyn College raises tilapia in a recirculating farm overseen by the Aquatic Research and Environmental Assessment Lab; Lehman College has a campus community garden where herbs and other produce are grown for use in nutrition classes; and Kingsborough Community College's high-production, organic farm raises produce that is used by the Culinary Arts program and distributed through the college's food pantry.

Food insecurity at CUNY is high. A 2011 study by the Campaign for a Healthy CUNY suggested that 40 percent of undergraduates experienced food insecurity in the previous twelve months. Colleges have responded in various ways: partnering with organizations such as Single Stop USA that screen students for benefits eligibility, issuing vouchers for free meals on campus, establishing food pantries, and encouraging students to advocate for food security.

City University of New York website: http://www .cuny.edu.

Freudenberg, Nicholas, Luis Manzo, Hollie Jones, et al. "Food Insecurity at CUNY: Results from a Survey of CUNY Undergraduate Students." The Campaign for a Health CUNY. April 2011. http://www.gc.cuny.edu/ CUNY_GC/media/CUNY-Graduate-Center/PDF/ Centers/Center%20for%20Human%20 Environments/cunyfoodinsecurity.pdf.

New York City Food Policy Center at Hunter College, City University of New York School of Public Health. "Jobs for a Healthier Diet and a Stronger Economy: Opportunities for Creating New Good Food Jobs in New York City." August 2013. nycfoodpolicy.org/ wp-content/uploads/2013/05/jobs_wholereport .pdf.

Babette Audant

Civil War

During the Civil War (1861–1865), New York City businesses flourished as government contracts poured in and trade prospered. Factories manufacturing military hardware and shipyards constructing or refitting ships boomed. Canneries, such as Gail Borden's New York Condensed Milk Company, thrived as contracts were let for canned goods to help feed the military. Jobs were readily available and incomes for well-to-do New Yorkers greatly increased during the war. Food and alcoholic beverages were plentiful in the city throughout the war, and the city's prosperity meant that its restaurants and saloons stayed busy. The working class, however, suffered, as salaries did not keep pace with high inflation during the war. Food prices doubled and tripled during the war, while salaries increased at an estimated 12 percent.

When European crops (especially in England) failed in 1860 and 1861, wheat was transported into New York City by rail from the Midwest and shipped right out to Europe. The city was also the receiving point for cattle from the Midwest. Illinois alone shipped more than two thousand head of cattle to New York, where they were processed in the city's two hundred slaughterhouses. In 1864 more than 1 million animals were butchered in New York.

New York women played important roles throughout the Civil War. They joined Sanitary Commissions, which helped wounded soldiers and their families. The city's women, including wives of the city's well-to-do, organized two sanitary fairs to raise money for the U.S. Sanitary Commission, the predecessor of the Red Cross. The Brooklyn fair was held on vacant lots belonging to the Brooklyn Academy of Music in February 1864. Its New England Kitchen offered frugal fare, such as chowder; but Knickerbocker Hall, the fair's more upscale dining room, served food from the city's best restaurants (including green turtle soup).

The Metropolitan Sanitary Fair, held in Manhattan, ran for twenty days in April 1864. Its main building was on Sixth Avenue between Fourteenth and Fifteenth Streets. An estimated 350,000 visitors each paid one dollar for admission to view the exhibits. The children's department sold ice cream and soda. For more serious dining there was the fair's restaurant, where thirty thousand oysters were consumed on the first day. An alternative was the Knickerbocker Kitchen, a reconstructed eighteenth-century Dutch farmhouse complete with colonial antiques. It was staffed by women in colonial garb who traced their ancestry to the original Dutch settlers in New Amsterdam. See COLONIAL DUTCH. The kitchen served a light menu of coffee, doughnuts, crullers, waffles, ham, pickles, headcheese, and spiced beef. The restaurant grossed $12,000 and the fair took in $1.3 million.

As the city's millionaires multiplied, they typically dined at luxurious restaurants, such as Maison Dorée and Delmonico's, enjoying the best food available. See DELMONICO'S. The wealthy, most of whom had avoided the draft by paying a substitute, formed the Union League Club in 1863 to support the war effort. In 1864 the Union League Club, whose members numbered among the city's elite, launched a major effort to give Union soldiers and sailors a turkey dinner on Thanksgiving in 1864. See THANKSGIVING.

When the Civil War ended in 1865, New York was America's manufacturing, banking, and culinary capital, with the majority of the nation's finest restaurants. Immigrants from abroad poured into the city after the war, as did professional chefs from France; some took jobs as cooks and servants in private homes, schools, and hotels. The Gilded Age, a

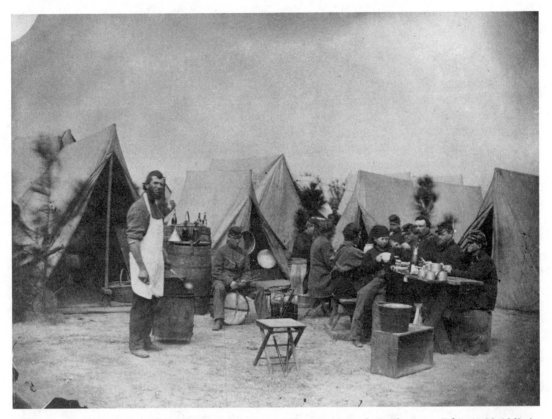

Soldiers at a table eating, along with a cook and drummer, at Hilton Head, South Carolina, circa February 28, 1862. As soldiers were often far from home and unable to gather fresh food, canned goods would be sent to them so that they could cook on the go. LIBRARY OF CONGRESS

great era in New York City food, was about to commence. See GILDED AGE.

McKay, Ernest A. *The Civil War and New York City*. Syracuse, N.Y.: Syracuse University Press, 1990.

Miller, Richard F., ed. *States at War*. Vol. 2: *A Reference Guide for New York in the Civil War*. Hanover, N.H.: University Press of New England, 2014.

Morgan, Bill. *The Civil War Lover's Guide to New York City*. El Dorado Hills, Calif.: Savas Beatie, 2013.

Smith, Andrew F. *Starving the South: How the North Won the Civil War*. New York: St. Martin's, 2011.

Spann, Edward K. *Gotham at War: New York City, 1860–1865*. Wilmington, Del.: Scholarly Resources, 2002.

Andrew F. Smith

Claiborne, Craig

As food editor of the *New York Times*, Craig Claiborne brought worldliness, new excitement, and new standards to New York City's restaurants and home kitchens at a low point in the city's gastronomic history. See NEW YORK TIMES. It was 1957. Grilled ham steak with pineapple rings reigned on mainstream restaurant menus. Young homemakers were succumbing to the temptations of frozen dinners. Curried whatever with "condiments" was the ultimate in elegant dinner party fare. Home economists and socialite wannabes were still running most newspaper food pages. Then, the *New York Times* gave a thirty-seven-year-old man the job of food editor, making him the first male newspaper food editor in the country.

Claiborne was well prepared. He grew up in a boarding house in Mississippi, eating his mother's southern cooking. He had a University of Missouri journalism degree. He had spent years as an officer in the Navy, in communications, then wined and dined clients as a public relations man in Chicago. Crowning all this, he was a graduate of a top Swiss hotel school, an education in classic French cuisine and dining room service that he got courtesy of the GI Bill.

In 1954, after graduation from L'Ecole Hôtelière in Lausanne, Switzerland, he came to New York to be a food writer. "Not without guile," as he pointed out in his sometimes shocking autobiography, *A Feast Made for Laughter*, he made a point of meeting Jane Nickerson, who was then the food editor at the *Times*. See NICKERSON, JANE.

Claiborne always talked about his insecurity, but he somehow found the muster to phone Nickerson and ask her if she was interested in writing a story about a young American who had studied French cuisine in Switzerland—himself. He took her to lunch at The Colony. She wrote the story.

The story got him a job at *Gourmet* magazine as a receptionist and answering the mail. He did eventually graduate to a writing post but was dismayed that his work did not always get a byline. So he was eager to move on when word got to him in 1957 that Nickerson had decided to leave the *Times*. She had two small children and a happy marriage to a man who was making his fortune in Florida. She wanted to devote herself to her family. Claiborne called her, took her to lunch, this time at 21 Club, and told her he was interested in the job. She did not hold out much hope because, as she told him, no one had ever heard of a man being a food editor. See "21" CLUB.

Claiborne went through the usual series of interviews at the *Times*, but it seems to have been Turner Catledge, the managing editor, who was ultimately responsible for his hiring. Catledge was another drawling boy from Mississippi, and he and Claiborne bonded.

Claiborne brought exactitude to the *New York Times* recipes and unquenchable culinary curiosity to the job. He interviewed and wrote about great home cooks and the world's most accomplished chefs with the same interest and respect. If you were a cooking teacher or cookbook writer, a story by Craig Claiborne in the *New York Times* would establish your career. And he blew the horn in America for some of the century's top French chefs—Paul Bocuse, the Troisgros brothers, Michel Guérard—whom he would invite to his specially designed kitchen in East Hampton to cook and be interviewed for the *Times*. Here was a man who admitted he could not pass up a hot dog on the street and at the same time could, with authority, critique the haute-est of French meals. He loved to travel, and he loved it when he found genuine cooking from other cultures in New York.

In 1959, he was approached to write a book based on the *New York Times* recipe archive, not just from his time but also from Jane Nickerson's day. Strangely, the *New York Times* gave Claiborne the right to use its name on a cookbook without asking for any of the proceeds from publication. No one could have predicted that the cookbook would become a huge bestseller and make its sole copyright owner, Craig Claiborne, a rich man.

A few years after joining the *Times*, Claiborne also became its restaurant critic and created the model for serious restaurant criticism. Before Claiborne, reviewers were guests of the house, received free meals, and were more cheerleaders than critics. Claiborne changed this by going anonymously so that he could have the same experience as the general public. He dined with several friends so that he could try many dishes in each course. And he returned several times to check on a restaurant's consistency. He always paid the bill, so he would not be beholden to the management. His ratings balanced the food quality and cooking, the décor, the service, and the "value," to produce a no-star to four-star review.

Just before he started reviewing restaurants, in late 1959, Claiborne wrote a feature on Henri Soulé, the great restaurateur who owned Le Pavillon, then the best French restaurant in the city. See SOULÉ, HENRI and LE PAVILLON. In the kitchen of Le Pavillon, Claiborne met Pierre Franey, Soulé's chef. They were to remain nearly lifelong friends and professional collaborators. They even lived next door to each other in East Hampton. See FRANEY, PIERRE.

In fact, Claiborne left his post as food editor of the *Times* in 1970 to write a newsletter with Franey. The business did not work out, and Claiborne went back to the *Times* in 1974, to write the Sunday magazine column with Franey, to ghostwrite Franey's 60-Minute Gourmet column in the weekly food section, and to write several books together.

In 1975, Claiborne had no idea he was going to invoke the wrath of the pope when he bid $300 for dinner anywhere, at any price, during a public television auction. He won, and he and Franey flew to Paris, on the tab of American Express, for a thirty-one-course meal at an obscure restaurant called Chez Denis. It cost $4,000, although most of it was for wine, which no one at the time seemed to want to point out.

It also was not a good meal. The best Claiborne ever said of it was that it was amazing that he did not "really feel that stuffed." Nevertheless, the *Times* reported that it got "nearly a thousand" angry letters. Claiborne never hid his homosexuality from his friends and associates. Wags who did not know them gossiped that Claiborne and Franey were a couple. Those who did know Claiborne knew that Henry Creel was his lover during his early years in New York. With Claiborne's guidance and with a forward by Claiborne, Creel even wrote a cookbook in 1976, *Cooking for One Is Fun* (Times Books). In later years, Claiborne had "a gentleman friend," as he called him, who was a doctor in Atlanta.

It was not that he publicly confessed his homosexuality in his autobiography that set New York abuzz in 1982. It was that he told of his incestuous relationship with his father. This public display embarrassed and infuriated Franey. It was the end of their friendship.

Claiborne died January 22, 2000. He was 79 years old. He had been frail for a long time but continued to go out, nearly to the end, often by himself, to restaurants not far from his New York apartment in The Osborne on West Fifty-Seventh Street.

Claiborne, Craig. *A Feast Made for Laughter.* Garden City, N.Y.: Doubleday, 1982.

Fussell, Betty Harper. *Masters of American Cookery: M.F.K. Fisher, James Andrew Beard, Raymond Craig Claiborne, Julia McWilliams Child.* Lincoln: University of Nebraska Press, 2005.

McNamee, Thomas. *The Man Who Changed the Way We Eat: Craig Claiborne and the American Food Renaissance.* New York: Free Press, 2012.

Arthur Schwartz

Clark, Patrick

See AFRICAN AMERICAN.

Clubs

New York clubs are thought of as old-money venues with generally WASP membership rosters, reading rooms furnished with huge upholstered chairs, and a pervading atmosphere of privilege, decorum, and quiet. Dining rooms for club members and their guests are a given. Men's clubs predominate, although the women-only Colony Club on the Upper East Side has been around since 1903. See COLONY CLUB. Some clubs are so private that their websites

reveal little about what goes on behind their massive doors, and everyday details like menus are not mentioned, although a few boast fine dining and catering and promote themselves as venues for weddings and banquets.

Typically these clubs have not been known for their food, which tends toward safe, conservative offerings served on white tablecloths—and tables far enough apart for private conversations. But recently, serious chefs have been hired, fresh fruits and vegetables have been emphasized, and current restaurant trends, although certainly not prominent, are visible at some venues.

Many of these traditional clubs were founded in the nineteenth century. The oldest, the Union Club on Park Avenue and East Sixty-Ninth Street, was founded in 1836. In 1863 during the Civil War, abolitionist members of the Union Club broke away and founded the Union League, now on East Thirty-Seventh Street in Murray Hill.

Founded in 1847, the Century Association, on West Forty-Third Street, boasts authors, artists, and serious "amateurs" of similar inclinations. It is now one of the largest private clubs. The Harmonie Club was founded in 1852 by a group of six German Jewish men and thirty or forty of their friends and acquaintances. Its original activities featured song recitals and declamatory contests, although it celebrated its tenth anniversary with a banquet and ball attended by more than 150 members. Now located at 4 East Sixtieth Street, the club no longer requires German descent for membership. Italian heritage is celebrated in the Tiro a Segno, founded in 1890, on Greenwich Village's MacDougal Street.

Other prominent social clubs founded in the nineteenth century include the Knickerbocker Club (1871) and the University Club (1856). The hightoned Metropolitan Club, now at 1 East Sixtieth Street, was founded in 1891. Original members included Cornelius Vanderbilt and J. Pierpont Morgan. Women's clubs include the Colony Club on Park Avenue and Sixty-Second Street and the Cosmopolitan Club on a genteel block on East Sixty-Sixth Street. Not too fashion-forward, not too conservative, and with menus to match, the Colony Club has an impeccably trained executive chef and an extensive wine list. The Cosmopolitan Club (for "women of accomplishment") has a dining room with a fully canopied outdoor space that is popular for entertaining. Other women's clubs include the intentionally small Belizean Grove on East Eighty-Ninth Street for influential women in the military, financial, and diplomatic worlds, and Soho House, a multicity club for women in creative fields.

Wealth, personal achievement, and social standing are, of course, not the only measures of desirability for membership in certain clubs. Graduates of some of the country's toniest universities can continue their connection with the schools by belonging to, among others, the Harvard Club (founded in 1865) on West Forty-Fourth Street, the Yale Club (founded in 1897) at 50 Vanderbilt Avenue near Grand Central Station, and the Princeton Club (founded 1899) at 15 West Forty-Third Street. These university-related clubs frequently allow limited memberships to graduates of other top-drawer schools and are often affiliated with other clubs around the country.

In recent years clubs have been organized around different principles, such as the Brooklyn Edible Social Club, a former culinary collective on DeKalb Avenue in Brooklyn, which has turned into the Brooklyn Sandwich Society. Others are clubs whose members have achieved success through financial acumen and celebrity. Some of these more contemporary clubs stage special food-focused dinners for their members at restaurants, public venues, and other available spaces. One of these is Parlor, a club in the Meatpacking District whose client list comes from the worlds of fashion, arts and entertainment, finance, as well as top tech and insurance companies. Parlor features up-to-the-minute cuisine and a new menu every week. The Core Club (2005), on East Fifty-Fifth Street, proudly focuses on the top 1 percent, costing many thousands of dollars to join, with an equally high annual membership fee.

See also WOMEN'S CLUBS.

Smith, Andrew F. *New York City: A Food Biography.* Lanham, Md.: AltaMira, 2014.

Judith Weinraub

Cocktail Lounges

The upscale cocktail lounge had its heyday in mid-twentieth century Manhattan, bridging the divide between Prohibition-era speakeasies and modern-day cocktail bars. Although the definition of the cocktail lounge is fluid, spanning hotel bars, airport bars, "martini bars," and even 1960s- and 1970s-era

singles bars, what all have in common is an upscale clientele and, of course, lots of alcohol, particularly cocktails—which served to lubricate the social activity taking place within these public spaces.

These lounges exist in striking contrast to the taverns and saloons of the 1800s and very early 1900s, which functioned as centers of community for many working-class and immigrant groups, as well as places to purchase alcohol. See SALOONS and TAVERNS. During these same years, bars within upscale hotels and elite private clubs also served plenty of cocktails and spirits, catering to a wealthier group.

When Prohibition went into effect in 1920, saloons were widely shuttered, while hotel bars and the like were converted into ice cream parlors or other milder entertainments. During this era, spanning until the repeal of Prohibition in 1933, drinking moved to speakeasies or cocktail parties held in private homes, the latter a trend that continued well into the Depression-era 1930s as a practical, economical way to entertain. Alcohol consumption did not go away; it merely moved underground. Indeed, many famed cocktail lounges started and thrived during Prohibition, such as the glamorous, celebrity-studded Stork Club and 21 Club. See PROHIBITION; STORK CLUB; and "21" CLUB.

In the years following Prohibition, consumption of alcoholic drinks swiftly moved back into the public sphere. According to Andrew Barr's *Drink: A Social History*, in the years immediately following repeal a whopping nine-tenths of alcoholic drinks were consumed in bars and restaurants, and this was despite measures taken to stem public drinking, such as abolition of the word "saloon" in many states; other states restricted sale of spirits "by the drink" to hotels, restaurants, and clubs where meals were served.

Of course, this did not mean that the speakeasy had been completely forgotten. Indeed, the mid-century cocktail lounge often invoked nostalgia for the naughty thrill of the speakeasies, serving martinis and other classic cocktails in a swanky setting that also nodded to customers' rising appetite for Hollywood-style glamor in the 1940s and 1950s. Cocktail lounges were often a favored setting in films and patronized by movie stars and society types, and many offered entertainment (creating some overlap with nightclubs and jazz clubs).

As the 1960s and 1970s brought the sexual revolution, the dimly lit cocktail lounge also became synonymous with the thriving singles scene at bars like Maxwell's Plum. See MAXWELL'S PLUM. In general, the potent drinks of this period were of little culinary note, and the thriving nightlife was of paramount importance.

Cocktail lounges continue to exist today. A distinction should be drawn, however, between lounges and the highly drink-centric cocktail bars that have grown and flourished in the past two decades.

See also COCKTAILS.

Barr, Andrew. *Drink: A Social History of America*. New York: Carroll & Graf, 1999.

Kara Newman

Cocktails

New Yorkers have long had a thirst for cocktails. Although most records show the earliest colonial Americans drinking locally made products such as hard cider, beer, and ale, it was not long before many New Yorkers developed a taste for spirits. According to Michael and Ariane Batterberry's *On The Town in New York*, before the American Revolution there was a tavern for every forty-five residents (man, woman, and child) in the city. Fortified wine—port, Madeira, and sherry—was common, as were brandy, gin, and rum.

And, of course, there were cocktails, which often ran to the rich and heavy: purl, a medicated malt liquor in which wormwood and aromatics were combined, and posset, a similar drink to which milk was added, were commonly found. Mixed punches and "sangaree" were available year-round; grogs, eggnogs, and syllabubs (cider enriched with sugar, spices, milk, and cream) were cold-weather specialties.

Social gatherings took place in taverns, private homes, and restaurants. Coffeehouses also filled in gaps, selling ale and cider as well as liqueurs. By the early 1800s, hotels began to take shape as grand public spaces for hosting banquets and other entertainments, often accompanied by wine and liquor, though not necessarily cocktails—at least not yet. By the mid-1800s, this began to dramatically change. At the Metropolitan Hotel, "Professor" Jerry Thomas presided behind the bar until 1859. See THOMAS, JERRY. Thomas is widely regarded as the forefather of mixology, creating cocktails, making cocktail bitters, and even publishing the country's first authoritative manual on the art of imbibing, *Bartenders Guide: How To Mix Drinks*. A first-rate bartender of one of the great hotels of the nineteenth century was expected to maintain a working repertory of at least 150 cocktails—shrubs, slings, punches, cobblers, juleps, smashes, flips, and nogs. The Waldorf Astoria claimed to have 490 different drinks available. It is also worth noting that refrigeration was still hard to come by in the nineteenth century, and outside of the winter months, ice for cocktails was considered a luxury for the rich.

Meanwhile, in the saloons, poorer New Yorkers were less likely to be sipping cooling cocktails. Some might have taken to rock and rye—rye whiskey sweetened with rock candy, horehound, or fruit peels—but many more took their beer or spirits straight.

Women generally were not welcome at either the decadent hotel bars or the gritty saloons. By the early 1900s, suffragettes had begun to march for women's rights, and the "drys" were slowly gaining traction with the temperance movement, which by the 1920s gave way to full-on prohibition of alcohol. See PROHIBITION and TEMPERANCE MOVEMENT. New York's golden age of cocktails had drawn to a close.

Although alcohol consumption continued underground in speakeasies like 21 Club, good-quality alcohol was expensive and hard to obtain. See "21" CLUB. Some mixed drinks were created to help disguise the taste of local moonshine or adulterated liquor, but altogether few cocktails were invented during the Prohibition era, and a great many bartenders decamped for Europe or elsewhere to continue their craft.

After the repeal of Prohibition in 1933, cocktails had a slow comeback. In cocktail lounges in hotels and nightclubs, New Yorkers relearned how to drink in public. Speakeasies had been coed, and the tradition of men and women drinking together in public spaces continued into the 1940s, 1950s, and beyond. Strong, spirituous drinks—what we now consider classics—were often the order of the day: gin-based martinis, whiskey-based old-fashioneds and Manhattans, and vodka-based Bloody Mary's. See BLOODY MARY; MANHATTAN COCKTAIL; MARTINI; and OLD-FASHIONED COCKTAIL. As tiki culture began to drift in from the West Coast, New Yorkers also developed a taste for these rum-based and many other sweeter cocktails. In the 1970s and 1980s, cocktails took a back seat to the burgeoning wine culture among sophisticated New Yorkers as Italian and French cuisines grew in stature.

Luckily for today's New Yorkers, cocktail culture found a second golden age in the twenty-first century. Driven by a confluence of interest in culinary culture, which extended to beverages, an artisan drinks renaissance spearheaded by influential bartenders such as Dale DeGroff and the availability of once obscure spirits and other ingredients for making better-quality and historically accurate cocktails, the numbers of bars and bartenders in New York City have expanded rapidly. See DEGROFF, DALE. Amid this second golden age for cocktails, New York has become a cocktail mecca once again.

See also COCKTAIL LOUNGES and MIXOLOGY.

Batterberry, Michael, and Ariane Batterberry. *On the Town in New York: The Landmark History of Eating, Drinking, and Entertainments from the American Revolution to the Food Revolution.* New York: Routledge, 1999.

Thomas, Jerry. *Bartenders Guide: How to Mix Drinks.* New York: Dick & Fitzgerald, 1862.

Wondrich, David. *Punch: The Delights (and Dangers) of the Flowing Bowl.* New York: Penguin, 2010.

Warren Bobrow

Coffee

The writer Simone de Beauvoir said, "There is something in the New York air that makes sleep useless," a quote that evolved into "the city that never sleeps." As such, a caffeinated cup of coffee is a popular beverage—and has been since the seventeenth century. All around New York City there is a place to buy a cup of coffee for every taste and budget, from local bodegas to national chains, from quaint cafés to corner diners.

The coffee shops of early New York were called "coffeehouses" and became, like the coffeehouses in London, Paris, and other European capital cities, hubs for business, politics, and social life. Coffeehouses were a particularly important aspect of early New York City life. They were a place where, unlike their European counterparts, colonists held trials and citizens could convene and voice their complaints.

One of the first known coffeehouses opened in 1696. The King's Arms, which sat on a lot on Broadway between Trinity Church and what is now Cedar Street, was two stories high and had an observatory on the roof where visitors would sit and sip their coffee. The King's Arms was the only coffeehouse

for many years. Soon thereafter many others opened up in Lower Manhattan, including The Exchange, The Merchants, and The Tontine. In addition to coffee, wine and other beverages were served, lubricating numerous business exchanges.

In 1793, the first coffee roaster opened on Pearl Street and sold beans, wholesale, to taverns and hotels. Farther north, Niblo's Garden, which sold coffee, ice cream, and beverages, opened on Broadway and Prince Street in 1828. Many coffee-related artifacts from old New York, including a coffee pot, a coffee roaster, and a spice grinder, are on exhibit at the Van Cortlandt House Museum.

In 1926, Chock full o'Nuts opened as a nut shop on the corner of Broadway and Forty-Third Street. In 1931, owner William Black opened a shop in the Empire State Building, which sold nuts and later coffee for over forty-five years. After the Depression, Black felt that shelled nuts were a luxury he no longer wanted to sell, so he turned his chain of Chock full o'Nuts into coffee shops, where a sandwich and a cup of coffee cost a nickel. In 1953 he startled the coffee trade by coming out with his own brand, Chock full o'Nuts, building the vacuum-packed yellow and black cans into a successful supermarket brand. Driven in part by a catchy radio jingle and new advertisements that promoted the "coffee break," Chock full o'Nuts became New York City's most popular brand of coffee by 1955. See CHOCK FULL O'NUTS.

New Yorkers love to take their coffee to go, often grabbing a cup and heading into a taxi or onto the subway on their way to work. The Anthora, a paper coffee cup, seen all over the city, became a symbol for coffee; by 1994 sales of the cup reached 500 million. Bearing the words "We are happy to serve you," in all capital letters and in a font that looks like ancient Greek letters, the Anthora cup is an ode to the many Greek-owned diners and coffee shops around New York City. Designed by Leslie Buck of the Sherri Cup Company in 1963, this coffee cup was deemed by a *New York Times* writer to be "the most successful cup in history." The Museum of Modern Art sells a ceramic version designed by Graham Hill.

In 1994, the first Starbucks opened, on Broadway and West Eighty-Seventh Street on the Upper West Side. It changed the way New Yorkers enjoyed coffee. Now they could sit in comfortable seats and linger over a tall, grande, or venti cup. As of 2014 there were over 250 Starbucks located in all the boroughs, with nearly 200 in Manhattan. See STARBUCKS. With the advent of Starbucks, coffee shops and stores became increasingly popular from the mid-1990s to the early 2000s—and coffee became a beverage to take seriously. Gourmet stores like Dean & DeLuca, Zabar's, Fairway, and Citarella sold wide varieties of coffee beans, even hiring coffee experts to travel the world in search of beans to sell to New Yorkers. Coffee shops became a popular destination, for either a cup or a bag of beans to take home and brew. Café Lalo on the Upper West Side, which became popular because of its appearance in the Nora Ephron movie *You've Got Mail*, opened in 1988 and was a popular place to get coffee and dessert before and after the theater or movies.

Other coffee shops and roasteries have opened and continue to open around the city, including Abraço, Blue Bottle, Brooklyn Roasting Company, Budin, Café Grumpy, Ground Support, Kings Coffee, Little Collins, Nespresso, Ninth Street Espresso, Parlor Coffee, Pushcart Coffee, The Queens Rickshaw, Steeplechase Coffee Shop, and Whynot Coffee and Wine. These shops offer cozy atmospheres, cappuccinos made on expensive espresso machines, stellar beans, unique blends, and more to attract customers in search of one of New York City's most popular beverages.

See also COFFEEHOUSES and COFFEE ROASTERS.

Chock full o'Nuts website: http://www .chockfullonuts.com.

Hemler, Allison. "Coffee Chronicles: Coffee's History in America, a Short Primer." Serious Eats, November 24, 2009. http://newyork.seriouseats.com/2009/11/coffee-chronicles-coffee-in-america-new-amsterdam-market-starbucks.html.

Pendergrast, Mark. *Uncommon Grounds: The History of Coffee and How It Transformed Our World.* New York: Basic Books, 2010.

Ukers, William K. "History of Coffee in Old New York." In *All About Coffee*. New York: Tea & Coffee Trade Journal Co., 1935.

Tracey Ceurvels

Coffeehouses

Coffeehouses have existed in New York City for more than three hundred years. They have no single definition as they have performed dramatically different roles over those centuries, serving as hubs for commercial and political activity, clubhouses for men from various ethnic groups, bohemian and counterculture cafés, and, most recently, hipster offices. Coffeehouses differ from coffee shops, which started in the late nineteenth century as venues for ladies and office workers to grab a light bite, and from coffee bars, a recent addition to New York's gourmet scene.

New York's earliest coffeehouses were patterned after their British counterparts as places where men gathered to conduct business, learn news, and debate politics. Food and beverages, including the alcoholic drinks traditional in tavern culture, were available, yet refreshments were not central to coffeehouse culture; they were, first and foremost, places of public assembly.

Gotham's first coffeehouse was the King's Arms, located on Broadway near the Trinity Church graveyard. Constructed by John Hutchins in 1696, it boasted booths that could be screened off with green curtains for private business dealings and balconies from which merchants could watch ships entering the harbor. The atmosphere was loud and frenetic, as it was the venue for commodities and real estate auctions, stock trading, and magistrate's hearings.

Soon coffeehouses would move eastward, to what would become known as the Coffeehouse Slip at the foot of Wall Street, where merchant ships docked to unload passengers and cargo; the cargo often included slaves and indentured servants who would be put up for auction at the open-air Merchant's Exchange, located at Broad and Water Streets. By 1729 a coffeehouse served the Merchant's Exchange, and when it erected an enclosed structure in 1754, it built the Exchange Coffee Room above the trading floor.

The most important of the pre–Revolutionary War coffeehouses was the Merchant's Coffee House, located on the southeast corner of Wall and Water Streets and opening no later than 1750. Although frequented by New York's business elite for auctions and commercial transactions, by the 1770s, the Merchant's was in financial trouble. Writing in the October 19, 1775, *New York Journal*, an editorialist blamed the difficulties on the many men who used its space and amenities but, stingily, bought no coffee. In spite of the red ink, the Merchant's was the site of galvanizing political speeches and activity in the early days of the American Revolution until its owner, Cornelius Bradford, temporarily fled during the British occupation of New York City.

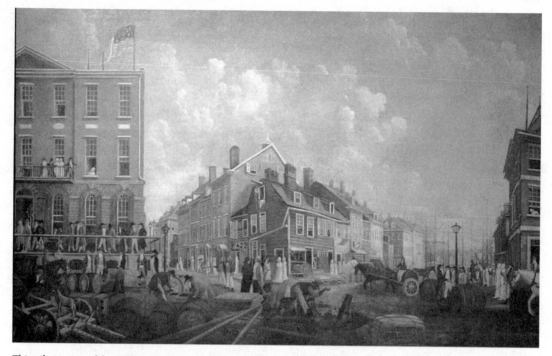

This oil painting of the Tontine Coffee House, by Francis Guy (1760–1820), was created circa 1797. Early coffeehouses were, first and foremost, places of public assembly. NEW-YORK HISTORICAL SOCIETY. PURCHASE, THE LOUIS DURR FUND, 1907

After the Revolution, coffeehouses took a leading role in establishing New York as the nation's financial center. Bradford used his proximity to the harbor in the repatriated Merchant's to maintain records of arriving mercantile ships, which were then published in newspapers, and he started a registry of merchants that evolved into the city's first business directory. The Bank of New York also was founded there in 1784. Tontine's, located cater-cornered from the Merchant's, was born out of the 1792 Buttonwood Agreement. Reached, according to legend, under a buttonwood tree, twenty-four stockbrokers created what is now known as the New York Stock Exchange. Named after the Neapolitan banker Lorenzo di Tonti, it opened in 1793, with trading and auctions by day and balls and gambling at night. Tontine's was the city's financial heart until 1817, when the stockbrokers drafted new organizational documents and decamped to a dedicated building at 40 Wall Street.

With the increasingly sophisticated business development, much of the raison d'être of the coffeehouses was lost. Tontine's became a tavern in 1826 as New Yorkers separated business from pleasure,

sipping their coffee at the new pleasure gardens that were opening north of Wall Street.

Coffeehouses would reemerge to serve a different audience in the late nineteenth century. Mediterranean immigrants, especially Italians and Syrians, imported their coffeehouse culture. Little Italy's Ferrara's, established in 1892, claims to be the oldest Italian coffeehouse in New York; many others would be scattered in the next decades in neighborhoods with Italian populations. Similarly, Little Syria was famous for its strong coffee and sweet pastries. Both the Italian and Syrian coffeehouses were male bastions for recent immigrants; their respectable women might enter briefly to purchase sweets for home consumption but not to socialize in public. An exception was made for the occasional uptown, fully Americanized woman with a yen for bohemian adventure. She might patronize Syrian coffeehouses, where she was treated with "Chesterfieldian politeness."

Changing mores after World War I brought more women into mixed-gender public entertainments, and by the 1950s the Italian coffeehouses of Greenwich Village became gathering spots for poets and musicians of the Beat Generation. Poetry readings often took on a counterculture, political message, and Village coffeehouses were shut down temporarily in police raids on the thin pretense that these entertainments were in violation of cabaret laws. Poetry slams, readings, and other artsy events can still be found; some have been tamed as book readings in the Starbucks cafes nestled in Barnes and Noble bookstores.

The newest addition to the coffee scene are small chains and one-off shops; priding themselves on carefully prepared drinks, these establishments satisfy both the harried office worker, who dashes in for a quick jolt, and the serious aficionado, who can discourse with the barista over roasts, grinds, and single-sourced beans. The numbers of open laptops and group discussions at some of these spots suggest often impromptu office space, indicating that New Yorkers have come full circle in the way they use their coffeehouses.

See also CAFFÈ REGGIO; COFFEE; COFFEE SHOPS; LITTLE ITALY; LITTLE SYRIA; and NIBLO'S GARDEN.

Ellis, Markham. *The Coffee-House: A Cultural History.* London: Phoenix, 2005.
Kane, Daniel. *All Poets Welcome: The Lower East Side Poetry Scene in the 1960s.* Berkeley: University of California Press, 2003.
Serratore, Angela. "Little Syria." *Paris Review*, September 17, 2013.
Strand, Oliver. "Where to Find Serious Coffee in New York? Everywhere!" *New York Times*, May 6, 2014.
Ukers, William. *All About Coffee.* New York: Tea & Coffee Trade Journal Co., 1922.

Cathy K. Kaufman

Coffee Roasters

In the seventeenth century, New Yorkers who could afford luxuries drank coffee made from imported beans, but it did not become an important beverage until the early nineteenth century, when coffee beans were imported from the Caribbean and, later, from Brazil. Until the late 1860s, green coffee beans were roasted by the consumer, at home, or at a coffeehouse or restaurant for serving there. Once roasted, the beans were ground as required. Coffee roasting was an art because roasting beans in a wood or other solid-fuel oven was a tricky process. Coffee beans that scorched were ruined, while underroasted beans failed to develop their full flavor. Home-roasted

coffee beans often produced an acrid brew that needed milk, cream, or sugar to make it palatable.

The first successful commercial coffee roaster was invented in 1864 by Jabez Burns, who came to New York from London in 1845 and found employment with coffee and spice merchants. Experimenting with more reliable methods for roasting coffee beans, he realized that the key was not to allow the beans to rest directly on a hot surface, where they could quickly scorch. Burns devised a screw-like device to keep the beans moving as they roasted. Establishing himself as Jabez Burns & Sons, he began to manufacture the improved coffee roaster. It was too bulky and expensive for home use, but it was ideal for large-scale coffee-roasting operations.

Burns founded his coffee roaster business at about the same time that America's first paper bag factory opened in New York City. Coffee could be roasted and then sold in paper bags at retail. These two inventions revolutionized the sale of coffee in America.

See also COFFEE and COFFEE SHOPS.

Pendergrast, Mark. *Uncommon Grounds: The History of Coffee and How It Transformed Our World.* New York: Basic Books, 2010.
Smith, Andrew F. *Drinking History: Fifteen Turning Points in the Making of American Beverages.* New York: Columbia University Press, 2012.
Ukers, William H. *All About Coffee*, 2d ed. New York: Tea & Coffee Trade Journal Co., 1935.

Andrew F. Smith

Coffee Shops

Coffee shops historically were inexpensive corner restaurants that catered to workers. They were distinct from coffeehouses, which catered to the well-to-do during the seventeenth to the nineteenth centuries. See COFFEEHOUSES. Understandable confusion abounds: much of popular press nowadays uses the term "coffee shop" to denote the modern descendants of coffeehouses—upscale spots that focus on preparing gourmet coffee- and espresso-based drinks. Meanwhile, just a small number of traditional coffee shops remain in New York, such as the Red Flame at Sixth Avenue and Forty-Fourth Street, which grandiosely calls itself a diner/coffeehouse.

Coffee shops emerged during the late nineteenth century when New York zoning laws forced vendors with carts off the streets. Jewish, Greek, and later Italian vendors opened small restaurants in neighborhoods; these establishments served as meeting places for local immigrants. By 1913 at least two hundred of these working-class restaurants served customers on Seventh Avenue alone.

Unlike coffeehouses, which sold mainly coffee, tea, and alcoholic beverages, coffee shops had full menus. They acquired their name from their promise to refill customers' coffee cups at no extra charge. New York City–based Chock full o'Nuts was among the best known of the coffee shop chains. See CHOCK FULL O'NUTS.

Coffee shops were also known for the large portions that they served, particularly giant breakfasts, sandwiches, and sugary desserts. Their busiest meals were (and are) breakfast and lunch. They emerged as a distinct type of eatery during Prohibition (1920–1933), when workers were deprived of free lunches at saloons and bars. During the Depression, coffee shops' low-cost menus continued to attract customers. Many lunch counters transformed themselves into coffee shops by installing padded stools with upholstered backs with Formica-topped tables. Edward Hopper's painting *Nighthawks* (1941–1942), complete with coffee urns in the background ready to replenish cups, was inspired by a coffee shop on Greenwich Avenue.

Coffee shops continued to thrive until the 1960s, when chain restaurants began to take trade away. In 1994 Starbucks opened its first outlet in New York City, and they too took business away from city coffee shops. See STARBUCKS. Coffee shops are not as plentiful as they once were, but a dwindling number of independent coffee shops have survived. Grungy city coffee shops have frequently appeared in films and on television, and recently trendy retro coffee shops have opened. Dining at a coffee shop remains a classic New York experience.

See also COFFEE.

Barnard, Anne. "Hold the Home Fries. Forever." *New York Times*, July 3, 2014.

Smith, Andrew F. *New York City: A Food Biography.* Lanham, Md.: AltaMira, 2014.

Andrew F. Smith

Colameco, Mike

See TELEVISION and TELEVISION, PUBLIC.

Colombian

Colombian cuisine can be found in Colombian restaurants and bakeries, primarily in Jackson Heights in an area known as "Little Colombia." The big influx of Colombians into New York came during the 1990s, when Colombians accounted for over 40 percent of the population of the area, according to census data. The area most heavily populated by Colombians and referred to as "Little Colombia" is Northern Boulevard from around Eightieth Street east to the border of Corona on Junction Boulevard. A large number of the immigrants opened businesses, many of which are restaurants and bakeries. As New York City and its boroughs became more heterogeneous and the different cultural pockets began to mix, Colombians also set up shop in Manhattan and other areas, where the food is also represented today. However, the best and most authentic Colombian eats are still found within Jackson Heights. See JACKSON HEIGHTS.

Colombian food is very regional as a result of the country's dramatically varied topography and, consequently, climate. This leads to great diversity in especially fruit. New York Colombian restaurants and bakeries tend to feature a selection of the best-known dishes of each region, introducing them as "Colombian" rather than making regional distinctions.

Most of the bakeries in New York feature *pandebonos*, a cheese roll made of yucca starch and Colombian white cheese, sporting a chewy texture with cheese pockets and a hint of sweetness. Traditionally from the South Pacific coast of the country, it is the most commonly known item within the New York bakeries. *Arepas*, white or yellow corn patties, which vary in thickness and sweetness depending on the region of origin, are also ubiquitous. They are usually served with cheese or as a side to pork products such as fried pork belly (*chicharrones*), chorizo, or blood sausage (*morcilla*).

For the heartier meals, the *plato montañero*, also known as *bandeja paisa*, is the common dish from the coffee-growing region. It features beef (panfried, ground, or braised), white rice, kidney beans, *chicharrón*, chorizo, fried sweet plantains, *arepa*, and a fried egg. *Ajiaco*, chicken soup with three different varieties of potatoes and the Colombian herb *guasca*, is the representative from the capital city of Bogotá and a specialty of the Colombian restaurants in the area. Other items vary depending on the menu and the origin of the owners of the restaurant.

Whatever the dish, it is best paired with Colombian beer or a tropical juice. Juices range from soursop (*guanabana*) to blackberry (*mora*), mango, passion fruit, and *lulo*, a typical fruit that is orange on the outside and kiwi green on the inside, of a similar texture to the passion fruit, and citrusy and floral in taste. These can be enjoyed also as a juice (fruit blended with water) or a shake (with milk). These beverages, along with the traditional coffee or hot chocolate, can be found in both bakeries and restaurants in the city.

See also SOUTH AND CENTRAL AMERICAN.

Kasinitz, Philip, John Mollenkopf, and Mary C. Waters. "Becoming American/Becoming New Yorkers: Immigrant Incorporation in a Majority Minority City." *International Migration Review* 36, no. 4 (2002): 1020–1036.
Kugel, S. (2008). "A Fruit Shake, Then Shaking to the Beat of Cumbia." *New York Times*, June 15, 2008.

Vivian Liberman

Colonial Dutch

When you eat some coleslaw with your sandwich or nibble on a cookie with your coffee or tea, you do not think about a Dutch connection to these seemingly so American foodstuffs. Yet there is, and it started early in the seventeenth century when the Dutch East India Company hired Englishman Henry Hudson to find a northerly passage to the Orient. In his travels Hudson explored the coast of North America and sailed up the river that would later be named for him. He called the area he found "a beautiful and fruitful place" in his report to the company. Others followed him, and as early as 1614 a small fort was built near present-day Albany. By 1621, the Dutch West India Company was founded with exclusive trading rights in the Western Hemisphere. Settlement took place from that point on, and the Dutch colony lasted seven decades until the final English takeover in 1674. The Dutch cultural and culinary influences have lasted until this day.

The settlers, who came to the vast colony of New Netherland, wedged between New England and Virginia, brought not only their seeds for herbs and vegetables, tree stock for fruit trees, and farm animals but also their well-established and well-documented diet and customs. The common meal pattern consisted of breakfast, a midday dinner, if necessary an afternoon snack, and a meal before going to bed. Bread was the mainstay of the diet. Breakfast was mainly bread with butter or cheese and a thick soup of root vegetables and greens. The midday meal consisted of bread, a one-pot dish of meat and vegetables, more meat or fish as available, and perhaps fruits or vegetables; but it also could be nothing more than porridge and bread. Since the midday meal might be as early as 10:00 a.m., for those who worked the land or were otherwise engaged in physical labor an afternoon snack of bread and onions, butter, or cheese was in order. Wealthy families might serve a small afternoon repast of wine and fruit, as we can see in many a painting of the period. The evening meal would be nothing more than bread and porridge or leftovers from the main meal.

Beer, a nutritious drink made from grain, was the common beverage for all meals. Affluent families often drank wine, which was imported from France and Germany. Tea and coffee did not become popular until the second half of the seventeenth century. See BEER; COFFEE; and TEA.

In the Netherlands, a country without the vast forests we know here, a town's bakers owned a central oven, stoked with reeds and later turf, and baked the daily bread. Since bread was such an important item in the daily diet, its preparation was carefully regulated by local governments. We know that a similar practice was in effect in New Amsterdam. Approximately twelve thousand documents remain from the Dutch period, 65 percent of which so far have been translated by the New Netherland Research Center in Albany, and they contain many ordinances regarding bread and beer. See BAKERIES and BREAD.

Bakers were responsible for the daily bread, and they also baked sweet bread, pastries, and *koekjes* (cookies), of which the Dutch are so fond. These sweet baked goods were even used for trading with Native Americans. Waffles, wafers, *olie-koecken* (forerunners of the doughnut), and pancakes were made at home. See DOUGHNUTS.

Settlers of New Netherland duplicated life in the homeland in the new country. From a 1655 book by Adriaen van der Donck, who wrote it to entice his fellow countrymen to come and settle the new colony, we know that they succeeded. He noted that the European vegetables and fruits "thrive well" and marveled at the abundant fish and other seafood, such as oysters; fowl, particularly carrier pigeons; and other wildlife readily available. While trade with Native Americans was one of the main reasons for the settlement, trade in the Atlantic was equally as important and ultimately more so. The merchants who formed the Dutch West India Company therefore expected the colony not only to be self-sufficient but also to supply the ships engaged in this Atlantic trade; for example, the oysters Van der Donck mentioned would be layered with sawdust in small kegs for trade in the West Indies.

Toward the end of the eighteenth century church services ceased to be held in Dutch, but although descendants might have forgotten their native tongue, they continued to prepare the foods they were used to, particularly for holidays and special occasions, such as births or funerals. Pancakes, waffles, *olie-koecken*, pretzels, coleslaw (from the Dutch *koolsla* or cabbage salad), and above all *koekjes*, the word easily adapted in American English as "cookies," are some of the items that were brought to America by the Dutch almost four hundred years ago.

See also COOKIES and DUTCH-STYLE NEW YEAR'S DAY PARTIES.

Rose, Peter G. *The Sensible Cook: Dutch Foodways in the Old and the New World.* Syracuse, N.Y.: Syracuse University Press, 1998. First published 1989.
Van der Donck, Adriaen. *A Description of New Netherland.* Edited by Charles T. Gehring and William A. Starna. Translated by Diederik Willem Goedhuys. Lincoln: University of Nebraska Press, 2008.

Peter G. Rose

Colony Club

The elite Colony Club traces its roots back to 1900 when five women meeting at the exclusive resort town of Newport, Rhode Island, spoke about creating a club in New York City to provide a space for women to relax, socialize, and exercise. Officially organized three years later, one of the club's founding members was Anne Morgan, J. P. Morgan's daughter, and its first president was Florence J. Harriman, who served until 1917. One of the founders' top priorities was to build a clubhouse that rivaled those created by men's organizations. With $400,000, the women purchased property at Thirtieth Street and Madison Avenue and selected famed architect Stanford White to build their clubhouse, which had a range of features: a "parking room" for small dogs, a ballroom, a swimming pool, a restaurant, dining rooms, and a gymnasium with a track. Elsie de Wolfe decorated it, and the clubhouse opened in March 1907. The original initiation fee was a steep $150, and there was a $100 annual fee for members. Lunch was available at the clubhouse for $1.25, dinner for $2.00, and a light breakfast for thirty to fifty cents.

By January 1907, the Colony Club claimed nearly seven hundred resident members, and in 1910 it had a waiting list of two hundred. The membership's growth along with changes in Murray Hill—the neighborhood was shifting from a residential to a more commercial district—led the Colony Club to decide to relocate in 1913. At Park Avenue and Sixty-Second Street, Colonists (as members are called) built a new, thirteen-story clubhouse that included a gymnasium, a swimming pool, guest rooms, and a library. The clubhouse's third floor was designed with two main dining rooms, and its kitchen facilities, which included fifteen iceboxes, were said to equal those of nearby hotels. It opened in 1915.

At the clubhouses, Colonists attended lectures on everything from literature to politics; held dances, dinners, and debuts; and took special pride in caring for Colony Club employees. Many events there revolved around fine food. In 1952, for instance, Queen Juliana of the Netherlands welcomed the United Nations Security Council for a dinner that included imported Dutch cheeses.

Despite their upper-class status, Colonists invited strikers in to share their stories during the 1909 shirtwaist strike and raised $5,000 to support the labor protest. Women's right to vote also became a subject debated at the Colony Club in the early twentieth century. During World Wars I and II, the gym shifted from a space for physical exercise to a venue from which to support the home front. In the mid-twentieth century, Colonists decided to permit husbands to stay overnight with their wives at the clubhouse.

The Colony Club remains an exclusive space in Manhattan for women. In 2007, the Park Avenue clubhouse even hosted a reception in memory of Brooke Astor following her funeral service.

See also CLUBS and WOMEN'S CLUBS.

"Colony Club Builds an Elaborate Home." *New York Times*, August 8, 1915.
Cox, Anne F. *The History of the Colony Club, 1903–1984.* New York: Colony Club, 1984.

Lauren C. Santangelo

Columbia University

Columbia University was founded in 1754 as King's College. It is the oldest institution of higher learning in New York State and the fifth oldest in the United States. Beginning in a modest building adjoining Trinity Church in Lower Manhattan, the college grew throughout the remainder of the eighteenth century and into the nineteenth century to include its renowned medical school as well as its schools of engineering and, in the early twentieth century, of journalism. Following a move to Midtown, the college relocated to its present site in Morningside Heights with its stately modern campus, designed by the famed turn-of-the-century architectural firm McKim, Mead and White. Renamed Columbia University in 1896, the institution celebrated its bicentennial in 2014.

The Center for Food and Environment at Teachers College houses the university's leading center for food and nutrition studies. Faculty members of world renown lead a curriculum focusing on education, research, and policy change that ranges from childhood obesity to food system sustainability. The Center for Food and Environment was begun in the 1970s as an initiative to pioneer a new vision of local, sustainable food systems. Since its inception, one of the center's objectives has been to educate children in New York City schools through its programs, including EarthFriends, established in the 1970s to educate children and families about the connections among health, personal behavior, and the environment, and Cookshop, established in the 1990s to connect local schoolchildren with area farms. The 1990s brought funding for the establishment of the Linking Food and the Environment (LiFE) curriculum to further help children understand the connectivity of food and environment.

Columbia University also houses the Earth Institute, under the direction of Professor Jeffery D. Sachs. The institute comprises more than thirty research centers and nearly one thousand staff and students working to lead the world to solutions in sustainability. Recent work has focused on issues of food security, environmental quality, and land use in Latin America, the Caribbean, and Africa.

Columbia University Press, now part of the university, publishes an extensive list of books on food and culture including *Food: A Cultural History*, edited by Jean-Louis Flandrin and Massimo Montanari; *Gastropolis: Food and New York City*, edited by Annie Hauck-Lawson and Jonathan Deutsch; *Creamy and Crunchy: An Informal History of Peanut Butter, An All-American Food* by Jon Krampner; and *Kitchen Mysteries: Revealing the Science of Food* by Hervé This.

The Columbia University faculty has included a number of noted academics specializing in food and culture. Marion Franco Chevalier Professor of French and Comparative Literature Albert Sonnenfeld, known as the "West Side Guru of Gastronomy," retired in 2004. He had edited a series for Columbia University Press titled "Arts of the Table: Perspectives on Culinary History." Joan Dye Gussow was the Mary Swartz Rose Professor Emeritus of Nutrition and Education at Teachers College and formerly head of the Nutrition Education Department. Noted as an early proponent of the "eat locally, think globally" movement and a longtime analyst and critic of U.S. food systems, Gussow's work includes her classic *The Feeding Web: Issues in Nutritional Ecology*, *This Organic Life: Confessions of an Urban Homesteader*, and *Growing Older*. Priscilla Parkhurst Ferguson has been a professor of sociology at Columbia since 1998. Her work, focused largely on French culture, has included *Accounting for Taste: The Triumph of French Cuisine* and *Word of Mouth: What We Talk about When We Talk about Food*.

Columbia students and faculty can find a wide range of American and international cuisine on campus in the spacious, modern dining room at the Faculty House overlooking Morningside Park. Student life at Columbia offers many opportunities for graduates and undergraduates to expand their experience of food and culture. Columbia's Maison Française, a campus social organization focused on cultivating French language and culture, sponsors receptions, cafe events, and dinners. The Columbia Business School alumni association hosts the Gourmet Club with regular outings and get-togethers that provide networking opportunities, as well as the opportunity to learn about and enjoy good food.

Columbia's Bartending Agency and School of Mixology is renowned for training both professional and amateur bartenders since its inception in 1965. Teachers are practicing professional bartenders who are all graduates of the program, as well as Columbia University students. The student-run bartending school emphasizes creativity as well as responsibility, and all bartenders are certified under a nationally recognized safety program.

See also COLUMBIA UNIVERSITY PRESS.

Columbia Bartending School website: http://columbiabartending.com.
Columbia Teachers College website/blog: http://www.tc.columbia.edu.
Columbia University website: http://www.columbia.edu.
Earth Institute, Columbia University website: http://earth.columbia.edu.

Carl Raymond

Columbia University Press

Since the mid-1990s, "food studies" has moved from a marginalized, amateurish pursuit to a legitimate academic topic of inquiry. Columbia University Press has been integral to this transition. Two series in particular—Arts and Traditions of the Table: Perspectives on Culinary History, and European Perspectives: A Series in Social Thought and Cultural Criticism—have provided a respectable platform for scholars to write books blending specific culinary concerns with larger historical, cultural, and scientific trends. A defining feature of these collective studies is the assumption that the most basic aspects of material life—such as food and drink—not only are often overlooked by scholars but yield insights that are fundamental to a better understanding of the human place in the natural world.

Several general questions underscore Columbia University Press's ample attention to culinary topics. First, how do eating and drinking habits shape the process of adaptation to new geographical environments? James McWilliams's *A Revolution in Eating* (2007) explores the role of food in fostering a unique North American identity among a panoply of European cultures in the eighteenth century. Carlo Petrini's *Slow Food: The Case For Taste* (2004) goes local, exploring the cultural politics of restricting the migration of ingredients and culinary traditions, making a case that food traditions thrive best when they are sheltered from globalizing forces. Second, what is the molecular and chemical foundation of taste and texture? In other words, why do we experience food the way that we do? Hervé This's *Molecular Gastronomy* (2008) and *Kitchen Mysteries* (2010) investigate the hidden chemistry of cooking, elucidating everything from the proper way to poach an egg to the neurobiological basis of experiencing flavor. Third, how do food traditions intersect with spiritual and philosophical traditions? Benjamin E. Zeller et al.'s edited volume *Religion, Food, and Eating in North America* (2014) looks into the ways that a variety of culinary traditions—Jewish, Christian, Muslim, and Buddhist—shape religious belief in a variety of North American settings, including southern Appalachia and the Caribbean. Similarly, *Food and Faith in Christian Culture* (2011), edited by Ken Albala and Trudy Eden, reveals the numerous ways that Christians throughout the world have used food to enhance faith.

The press has also dedicated a notably large number of titles to the culinary traditions of particular regions. Annie Hauck-Lawson's and Jonathan Deutsch's *Gastropolis: Food and New York City* (2010) documents the city's deep culinary heritage, with a special emphasis on immigration and assimilation. David Gentilcore's *Pomodoro! A History of the Tomato in Italy* (2010) describes the incorporation of a New World ingredient into an Old World cuisine. Colin Spencer's *British Food* (2003) delineates the fall and rise of British food over several hundred years. Finally, Yong Chen's *Chop Suey, USA* (2014) explores the emergence of Chinese food on American soil, highlighting the entrepreneurial aspect of this food's rise to prominence.

Considered together, the food studies titles published by Columbia University Press confirm that this is an interdisciplinary and deeply scholarly endeavor that has only just begun to capture the imagination of scholars and their students. Several other university presses—most notably the University of California Press and the University of North Carolina Press—have followed Columbia University Press's lead in ushering food studies into the academic canon.

See also COLUMBIA UNIVERSITY.

Sonnenfeld, Albert. Arts and Traditions of the Table: Perspectives on Culinary History. Columbia University Press. http://cup.columbia.edu/series/arts-and-traditions-of-the-table-perspectives-on-culinary-history. This website shows the individual titles in the series.

James McWilliams

Commodity Exchanges

Commodity exchanges and the agricultural commodity contracts that trade on those exchanges have long played a key role in regulating food prices in New York and elsewhere in the United States. New York's position as a densely populated port city and financial center meant its commodities markets were particularly influential, especially in the late 1800s. A number of key commodities contracts also originated trading on New York's exchanges. However, because of its proximity to farms and ranches in the Midwest, Chicago's commodities markets became the most important and powerful in the United States, and the majority of commodities trades now execute there.

The New York Produce Exchange

The New York Produce Exchange had several antecedents, making it the oldest of all the exchanges that make up modern trading organizations. In fact, its earliest participants were the Dutch burghers of Nieuw Amsterdam who gathered to trade essential commodities such as grain and provisions. By 1658 the small group of farmers trading these products had moved from Bowling Green to what is now Broad Street, and it was called the Broadway Shambles Market. In 1754 the outdoor trading was at Broad and Water Streets, and the market was known as the Royal Exchange.

The Royal Exchange gave way to the Merchants Exchange on Wall Street, and by 1840 it moved to Broad and South Streets. Soon after, the trading was moved to a warehouse, and the Corn Exchange was born. However, the Corn Exchange was not terribly successful. The warehouse was deemed unsuitable for trading, and a few merchants monopolized trading. In 1861, those not in the group formed the New York Commercial Association and built a trading floor and office building at 39 Whitehall Street. Eventually, the New York Commercial Association became the New York Produce Exchange, a name it would retain for nearly a century.

What traded at the Produce Exchange? Not just produce. The *New York Times* listed among the products traded on its opening day flour, corn, barley, oats, "provisions" (including pork, beef, butter, cheese, and "country mess"), hops, and whisky.

By the 1920s, the Produce Exchange, now located at 2 Broadway, off Battery Place, had also become a world market for corn, wheat, barley, and oats; and it was a chaotic, noisy hub. In his 1972 book *Run-Through*, John Houseman, then an aspiring young trader, said the floor "looked, sounded, and smelled like something between a railroad terminal, a midway and a monkey house." Prices arrived by Morse code, which clerks would hurriedly transcribe on a blackboard.

Butter and Egg Exchanges

The venerable New York Produce Exchange also spawned the now defunct Butter and Cheese Exchange of New York, when dairy merchants split off in 1872. With the addition of eggs, it became the Butter, Cheese, and Egg Exchange, and by 1882, the organization was renamed yet again, to the New York Mercantile Exchange, as trade broadened to include dried fruits, canned goods, and poultry.

New York's Tribeca neighborhood was once the butter, cheese, and egg section of the city, populated by middlemen who would bring in barrels full of eggs from local farms, cushioned by oats, and sell to New York's stores, restaurants, and hotels. However, the old egg men began to recede after their produce counterparts on the other side of Greenwich Street were moved to Hunts Point in the Bronx in 1967. Meanwhile, the rise of huge distribution networks—supermarkets and industrial farms—changed the way business was conducted in a sweeping way, and one by one New York's butter and egg men left Lower Manhattan behind. See HUNTS POINT.

Coffee, Sugar, and Cocoa Exchanges

While the products behind many other agricultural commodities (grain, dairy products, etc.) were harvested or made relatively nearby, others were shipped in from distant ports: notably coffee, sugar, and cocoa. As the center of shipping activity, New York also became the center of trading activity for these products, although coffee exchanges also sprung up in other port cities, notably in Baltimore (1884) and New Orleans (1903).

However, New York was where most of the action centralized as exchanges began, splintered, merged, and eventually became the New York Board of Trade and, finally, the InterContinental Exchange, which remains the primary U.S. market for coffee, sugar, and cocoa trading today. Of the mighty triumvirate that would one day compose the Coffee, Sugar, and Cocoa Exchange, the New York Coffee Exchange was established first, in 1882.

While tea played a critical role in the Old World—from both an economic and a culinary standpoint—in the New World coffee was king. Britain was the hub for importing and trading tea (which has traded briefly on U.S. exchanges), but with its proximity to coffee-growing countries in Central and South America, coffee played a key role in the early American diet. See COFFEE and TEA.

Throughout the first half of the 1800s the American taste for coffee swelled, particularly after the War of 1812, which temporarily shut off access to tea just when all things French, including coffee drinking, were stylish. By that time Brazilian coffee was closer and cheaper.

Prior to the Civil War, New Orleans had been the major point of entry for coffee in the United States. By the end of the war, New York had become the hub of the American coffee trade.

Europeans drank (and traded in) coffee, of course. But by the 1870s, coffee had become downright indispensable to Americans, who consumed six times as much as most Europeans. Coffee had become big business in America, and businessmen needed to find a way to protect those interests. Modeling itself on the already existing Chicago Board of Trade and the New York Cotton Exchange, the New York Coffee Exchange was incorporated on December 7, 1881.

Meanwhile, exchanges trading cane sugar and beet sugar futures operated in London and Hamburg and had been since the 1890s. When World War I closed the European sugar exchanges down, on December 16, 1914, the Coffee Exchange expanded its facilities to include sugar and changed its name on October 1, 1916, establishing the New York Coffee and Sugar Exchange.

As the New York Coffee and Sugar Exchange gathered steam, it was not until later that a need for trading in cocoa was established. But in 1925 the New York Cocoa Exchange was created, as an "adjunct" of the New York Coffee and Sugar Exchange. In January 1926 the name was changed briefly to the Cocoa and Rubber Exchange of America, Inc. Six months later, it was switched back to the New York Cocoa Exchange, Inc.

Immediately, the New York exchange became the preeminent marketplace for setting cocoa prices. Within three years trading volume outpaced the combined volume of the two next largest cocoa exchanges, in London and Liverpool. The cocoa exchange would continue to operate separately for several decades,

eventually merging into the New York Coffee and Sugar Exchange on September 28, 1979, creating the Coffee, Sugar, and Cocoa Exchange.

In 1998, the New York Board of Trade became the parent company of both the New York Cotton Exchange (which also included frozen orange juice contracts) and the Coffee, Sugar, and Cocoa Exchange. And on September 14, 2006, the Intercontinental Exchange agreed to become the parent company of the New York Board of Trade, a transaction completed on January 12, 2007.

Houseman, John. *Run-Through: A Memoir*. New York: Simon and Schuster, 1972.

Lambert, Emily. *The Futures: The Rise of the Speculator and the Origins of the World's Biggest Markets*. New York: Basic Books, 2011.

Newman, Kara. *The Secret Financial Life of Food: From Commodities Markets to Supermarkets*. New York: Columbia University Press, 2013.

Pendergrast, Mark. *Uncommon Grounds: The History of Coffee and How It Transformed Our World*. New York: Basic Books, 1999.

Kara Newman

Community Supported Agriculture

Community supported agriculture (CSA) is a network of locally based programs that connect farmers directly with consumers. The concept originated in Europe and Japan in the 1960s and appeared in the United States two decades later. It was championed as farmers and community members working together as partners to create a local food system, where consumers share the risk with farmers and enjoy the benefits. Connecting a face and a name to a farm and ensuring organic and fresh produce foster a heightened sense of locavorism in a society that prides itself on procuring delicacies regardless of the season. It has become hip to eschew mainstream grocery chains in favor of supporting local farmers, and as increasing numbers of chefs are labeling their restaurants "farm-to-table," patrons are following suit in droves. See FARM TO TABLE. Community-supported agricultural ventures give us a chance to actively participate in the production of our food.

Traditionally, farmers offer shares of their harvest to the public who sign up to receive fresh produce that varies with the season, which is then picked up from a designated location. Along with paying a fee, members of a CSA may also work directly at the farm or help with administration. Members interact with those responsible for growing their food, instead of simply preparing meals from store-bought ingredients with sketchy origins.

The desire to connect more deeply with what we eat has become a widespread ideal, famously skewered on the well-known television show *Portlandia*. However, the basic tenets of CSA have existed for many years, even before the cosmopolitan citizens of New York City embraced them. In the 1960s, Swiss and possibly German farmers partnered with consumers to create a support system for sustainable and safe agriculture. Likewise, in 1965 Japanese mothers started a project called *Teikei*, which philosophically translates to "food with the farmer's face on it." As Robyn Van En (1995, p. 29) writes, "farmers agreed to provide produce if multiple families made a commitment to support the farm.... Clubs operating under the *teikei* concept in Japan today serve thousands of people sharing the harvest of hundreds of farmers."

Most researchers agree that the first CSA farms in the United States were established in 1986. Van En and collaborators at Indian Line Farm in South Egremont, Massachusetts, offered the first vegetable shares, while Trauger Groh, Lincoln Geiger, and Anthony Graham founded Temple-Wilton Community Farm in Wilton, New Hampshire. In 1990, Jean-Paul Courtens founded Roxbury Farm in Claverack, New York, on the principles of biodynamic farming and anthroposophy. In 1991, Roxbury became the first farm to distribute shares in New York City, from a stall in the renowned Union Square Greenmarket; and in 2000, it moved to Kinderhook, New York. See GREENMARKETS. Roxbury Farm still operates today, delivering to sites in the Capital Region in upstate New York, Westchester, Harlem, and the Upper West Side, as well as its own North Farm location in Columbia County.

In 1996, Courtens partnered with Just Food to help establish six more CSA sites. Founded in 1995 to help increase and support sustainable food models, Just Food is an eminent organization in the world of CSA. It operates approximately 110 CSAs serving the New York City area, and according to the 2013 FoodWorks report update, "initiatives have been growing rapidly throughout the City, with the City Council leading by example and running its own CSA for the workplace" (Weiss, 2013, p. 7).

Typically, farmers and members work together to ensure that shares are successfully harvested and delivered. In New York City, Just Food uses a "shared-management" model in which a farmer grows and delivers the product, while members are responsible for organization, distribution, and administration. In CSAs outside of the city, members often volunteer directly at the farm. Roles change depending on the size and type of the farm share; the three most common types are sole proprietorship single farms, partnerships and multifarm cooperatives, and limited liability corporations. Partnerships and cooperatives are able to offer a greater variety of goods than sole proprietorship farms, and many offer a selection beyond produce, including eggs, meat, and flowers. Some even offer a choice between a meat-specific or dairy-specific share. However, the more farms involved, the more complicated coordination can become and the further it strays from *teikei* and the single farm origination. Those interested in joining or starting a CSA should decide which type is right for them before applying, as well as noting the length of harvest; most run from June to November, but a few do offer winter shares.

Through Just Food, anyone can apply to start a CSA, but a core group of about ten members is recommended to ensure adequate leadership and support. Upon approval, applicants are matched with an appropriate farm. Small groups sharing a collective passion and interest in providing fresh food to their communities have founded several of Just Food's CSAs. Some are motivated by social justice causes, such as Sixth Street Community Center, which aims to educate youth about sustainable agriculture, expand food accessibility, and strengthen food safety laws. Others focus on opportunities for low-income members, such as Prince George and Project Harmony/Kitchen Table, which accept payment via electronic benefits transfer.

Because of the short attention span of the everyday consumer and the increasing ease of food accessibility, CSAs must find new ways to survive and thrive. A new group of CSA businesses has recently emerged that utilize Internet technology and merge the farm share model with modern hipster sensibilities. These include the food delivery system Quinciple, the San Francisco transplant Good Eggs, and farm share subscriptions that are beginning to incorporate diverse and specialized ingredients to set them apart from the crowd. To persist, CSA must adapt to the current mindset of the consumer and be as available and visible as possible.

See also URBAN FARMING.

Farnsworth, R. L., Sarahelen R. Thompson, Kathleen A. Drury, et al. "Community Supported Agriculture: Filling a Niche Market." *Journal of Food Distribution Research* 27, no. 1 (1996): 90–98.

Martinez, Steve, Michael Hand, Michelle Da Pra, et al. *Local Food Systems: Concepts, Impacts, and Issues.* Economic Research Report 97. Washington, D.C.: U.S. Department of Agriculture, Economic Research Service, 2010.

McFadden, Steven. "The History of Community Supported Agriculture, Part II: CSA's World of Possibilities." Rodale Institute, 2003. http://newfarm.rodaleinstitute.org/features/0204/csa2/part2.shtml.

Van En, Robyn. "Eating for Your Community: A Report from the Founder of Community Supported Agriculture." *A Good Harvest (In Context)* 42 (Fall 1995): 29.

Weiss, Alissa. *FoodWorks: A Vision to Improve NYC's Food System. Accomplishments and New Ideas.* New York: New York City Council, 2013.

Woods, Timothy, Matt Ernst, Stan Ernst, et al. "2009 Survey of Community Supported Agriculture Producers." University of Kentucky College of Agriculture Collaborative Extension Service, 2009. http://www.uky.edu/Ag/CCD/csareport.pdf.

Emma Becker

Coney Island

See BROOKLYN; FELTMAN, CHARLES; and HOT DOGS.

Cookbooks

For all the fame New York has achieved as a culinary capital, it has not been the subject of cookbooks for very long. Known as a restaurant city since the late nineteenth century, the city did not have the reputation for home cooking that travelers ascribed generally to the South and to New England. New York was where one went to dine *out*.

The earliest cookbook to focus on New York City home cooking is Maria Lo Pinto's *New York Cookbook*, published in 1952. As she noted herself, despite the city's great fame, "no one had thought of collecting its history of food into the covers of one book" (p. 8). Since "Food in New York, the center of cosmopolitan eating, is a big business... why not write about it?" (p. 9).

Lo Pinto used immigration as her organizing theme for the *New York Cookbook*, mapping immigrant groups to particular neighborhoods and beginning with a brief historical chapter that allowed her to include some Native American, Dutch, English, and Scottish dishes. The ethnic neighborhoods of Lo Pinto's time included Scandinavians in Sunset Park and Bay Ridge (*stegt gaas*), Syrians and Armenians in Brooklyn Heights (Persian chicken stew), Jews in Brownsville and Brighton (fish Shapiro), and Cuban "Harlemites" (*pescado a la Aguacate*). The melting pot sections of the book were followed by an "all American" chapter that included dishes reflecting trends of the era such as meatloaf and "health slaw." Lo Pinto's book concluded with a list of New York restaurants considered notable and arranged by ethnicity.

Lo Pinto reinforced the idea of New York as an important restaurant city that could offer a wide diversity of flavors, from the Eighty-Sixth Street Brauhaus, where there were not only "good Bavarian dishes" but also yodeling, to the Chinese Rathskeller, The Ebony Lounge in Harlem, and Lundy's famous seafood palace in Sheepshead Bay, Brooklyn.

In 1972, when Bobbs-Merrill published *All Around the Town*, focus had settled again on New York as a restaurant city, though the authors followed Lo Pinto's lead in dividing the book along lines of ethnicity. Like Lo Pinto, they also offered brief summaries of ethnic neighborhoods—who lived where—before offering recipes associated with particular restaurants. Authors Ceil Dyer and Rosalind Cole, both professional food writers, singled out New York for its "wonderful independence" and the rich diversity of its eating places and markets: "There are Latin markets where akee and plantains are as common as potatoes and peas... and if one is in need of soybean curd, wooden ear, ginger root, rice wine, or a sauce made from plums, a telephone call will bring it to your door" (p. 14).

Ethnic diversity was easy to find in New York, Dyer and Cole noted, while any "mainstream" cuisine was not: "Would you believe it, we only ran into trouble when we searched out real American food!" Identifying the 21 Club, The Coach House, and The Forum of the 12 Caesar's among others as "American," the authors discovered that these establishments "were run by people of diverse backgrounds... the owner was of Italian descent, the chef was from Puerto Rico and the captain was French." See "21" CLUB.

In 1961, the *New York Times* published its first significant cookbook, edited by Craig Claiborne, the restaurant reviewer and food editor who had made both "ethnic" foods and American food respectable to the upper-middle-class readers who had previously considered only French food to be really fine dining. The book reflected Claiborne's confident and joyous eclecticism. Claiborne's biographer, Thomas McNamee, re-created the kind of conversation he often overheard or participated in after the book came out: "I must get your recipe.— It's in the *Times* cookbook—you do have it?—I've barely scratched the surface.—I know what you mean" (p. 94). Claiborne's book was implicitly a representation of the cosmopolitan food ways of the city. See CLAIBORNE, CRAIG.

Like Lo Pinto, the few other cookbook writers who took New York City as theme emphasized New York's diversity, dividing their books by restaurant or ethnicity, rather than by meal or substance, both more traditional divisions for cookbooks. Famous fashion designer Bill Blass and his writing partner, Joan G. Hauser, for example, gave each of twenty-one restaurants (including "21") its own chapter and provided a few recipes from each. The book, one in a national series, was titled *Dining In—Manhattan.* Hauser wrote that in Manhattan "dining has always been an invitation to adventure," while Blass celebrated the great variety of options for dining out. Blass called the book "a rather eclectic list of the places I like...one man's choice for the exciting event of 'Dining In—Manhattan'" (p. ix)

In a similar vein, Molly O'Neil published the very successful *New York Cookbook*, which combined home recipes of New Yorkers with recipes from well-known restaurants. Organized idiosyncratically around such topics as noshes, noodles, greens, "significant culinary events," and birds, O'Neil's book strove to capture the diffuse energy of the city. O'Neil, like Dyer and Cole before her, credited New Yorkers with a special attitude toward food: "New Yorkers bring the same sort of obsessive drive to their cooking that they bring to every other aspect of their daily life...a certain kind of ornery perfectionism, a combative and indefatigable connoisseurship" (p. xi). Like a giant community cookbook, *New York Cookbook* is full of recipes attributed to individuals who are not known beyond its covers, as O'Neil and her intrepid helpers followed tantalizing leads such as "Angela Palladino makes the best meatballs,

but I haven't seen her in years." The meatballs are on page 293. See O'NEILL, MOLLY.

When Amanda Hesser produced *The Essential New York Times Cookbook* in 2012, she was adamant about *not* updating Claiborne's 1961 classic. That book was still in print and still in use, but it was also very specific to a moment in time: ten years of Claiborne's career as a writer for the *New York Times.* Hesser, instead, produced a compendium of favorite recipes from the newspaper's entire history. Less focused on culinary quirks and characters of the city, Hesser's book is more of a testament to changing food fashions in the Anglo-American world. See HESSER, AMANDA.

Since the 1990s, New York City cooking has largely been represented by cookbooks produced by famous chefs from famous restaurants like Gramercy Tavern and Prune. Brooklyn now has more than one cookbook of its own.

In 2012, Emily Brooks challenged readers' assumption that the city is purely a consumer and not also a producer of fine fresh food. With visits to beekeepers in the Bronx and a fish farm at Brooklyn College as well as more predictably agricultural spots in Orange and Westchester Counties, Brooks exhorts her readers not only to see the city as a site for farming but to "get dirty" by growing food in the city however we can. Like O'Neill, Brooks associates her recipes with individuals, giving the big city the feel of a small-town potluck.

Blass, Bill, and Joan G. Hauser. *Dining In—Manhattan.* Mercer Island, Wash.: Peanut Butter Pub., 1983.

Brooks, Emily. *New York City Farmer & Feast: Harvesting Local Bounty.* Guilford, Conn.: Globe Pequot, 2012.

Claiborne, Craig. *The New York Times Cookbook.* New York: Harper, 1961.

Dyer, Ceil, and Rosalind Cole. *All Around the Town.* Indianapolis, Ind.: Bobbs-Merrill, 1972.

Hesser, Amanda. *The Essential New York Times Cookbook.* New York: Norton, 2012.

Lo Pinto, Maria. *New York Cookbook.* New York: Wynn, 1952.

McNamee, Thomas. *The Man Who Changed the Way We Eat: Craig Claiborne and the American Food Renaissance.* New York: Free Press, 2012.

O'Neil, Molly. *New York Cookbook.* New York: Workman, 1992.

Megan Elias

Cookbook Stores

See KITCHEN ARTS AND LETTERS and RIZZOLI.

Cookies

Cookies (or biscuits) have been a popular item on the New York culinary scene since colonial times. The word "cookie" (sometimes "cooky") is derived from the Dutch *koeptje* or *koekje*, meaning a small cake. Although it was the seventeenth-century Dutch settlers who brought the item over from the old country, the first located use of the English word "cookie" in New York City did not occur until 1786. Washington Irving popularized the word in *Salmagundi* (1808): "Those notable cakes, hight [called] new-year-cookies" were "impressed on one side with the honest burly countenance of the illustrious Rip [Irving's beloved character, Rip Van Winkle]; and on the other with that of the noted St. Nicholas, vulgarly called Santa Claus.... These cakes are to this time given on the first of January to all visitors, together with a glass of cherry-bounce, or raspberry-brandy."

During the nineteenth century, New Year's cookies or cakes (also called Christmas or New York cookies in some cookbooks) were commonly enjoyed at Christmas and on New Year's Day. Recipes for stamped Christmas "cookeys" appear in Amelia Simmons's *American Cookery* (1796). New Year's or New York cakes or cookies were described in publications beginning in at least 1837 when Eliza Leslie included a recipe for "New York cookies" in her *Directions for Cookery. The Improved Housewife* (1844) by A. L. Webster includes New Year's cookies flavored with caraway and nutmeg; the stiff dough is rolled out and cut into shapes before baking. When, in 1857, Eliza Leslie reprised her recipe for New-Year's cake in *Miss Leslie's New Cook Book*, she noted, "The bakers in New York ornament these cakes, with devices or pictures raised by a wooden stamp. They are good plain cakes for children." The carved wooden stamp or mold, like the caraway flavoring, is a traditional Dutch feature.

During the nineteenth century, carved rolling pins or *springerle* boards (flat molds) were used to stamp cookies with images of animals, flowers, and other decorative designs. Cookie cutters formed the dough into fanciful shapes. Cookies were most often made in home kitchens, but they were also produced by bakeries. The era of the commercial cookie began in 1898, when the Manhattan-based National Biscuit Company (later renamed Nabisco) began producing the Graham cracker. Although made with the type of wholewheat flour endorsed by dietary reformer Sylvester Graham, these cookies also con-

tained plenty of sugar and would probably not have found favor with Graham. See NABISCO.

Animal crackers, small cookies in the shape of animals, were commercially baked and sold in Brooklyn and Manhattan by the late nineteenth century. P. T. Barnum was a popular showman and circus organizer, whose name was well remembered after his death in 1891. In 1902 Nabisco capitalized on his name by introducing Barnum's Animal Crackers, which were promoted throughout the United States. Shaped and stamped to depict zoo animals, the cookies were packed in a small box resembling a circus wagon, with a string handle attached at the top.

When Nabisco introduced the Oreo cookie in 1912, it quickly became America's bestselling cookie (which it still is). See OREOS. Nabisco's most iconic New York cookie, however, was the Mallomar, a plain round cookie topped with a dome of marshmallow and coated in dark chocolate. These were first made in 1913, at the same bakeries where Oreos were produced. Because the chocolate coating melts in warm temperatures, Mallomars are made and sold only in the autumn and winter; 70 percent of the total production is snapped up by New Yorkers. See MALLOMARS.

Another iconic New York cookie is the black and white (elsewhere called half-moons or harlequins), which is typically sold in bakeries and delis. It is a large, somewhat soft, chewy vanilla cookie frosted half-and-half with chocolate and vanilla icings. It was popularized outside New York by an episode of the *Seinfeld* TV series, "The Dinner Party," in 1994. Jerry Seinfeld's character muses to his friend, "Look, Elaine, the black and white cookie. I love the black and white—two races of flavor living side by side in harmony." See BLACK AND WHITE COOKIES.

New York bakeries turn out cookies in thousands of shapes, sizes, textures, and flavors. Neighborhood Italian bakeries specialize in *biscotti* of all kinds; Jewish bakeries sell *kichlach* and *hamentaschen*. Glaze-lacquered almond cookies lure tourists into bakeshops in Chinatown. The Greek bakeries of Astoria, Queens, offer *kourabiedes*, and Middle Eastern bakeshops make *maamoul* filled with dates or nuts. News of a superior new chocolate-chip cookie will always bring crowds—and controversy. Cookies are destined to remain a permanent part of New York's culinary culture.

See also CHRISTMAS.

Cahn, William. *Out of the Cracker Barrel: From Animal Crackers to ZuZu's.* New York: Simon and Schuster, 1969.

Panschar, William G. *Baking in America.* Evanston, Ill.: Northwestern University Press, 1956.

Andrew F. Smith

Cooking Schools

During the mid-nineteenth century, increasing numbers of well-to-do New Yorkers began to hire domestic help to assist with cooking, cleaning, and laundry—usually young immigrant girls, many fresh off the boat from Ireland. But few of these novice servants were able to prepare the meals that their employers were accustomed to—traditional American home cooking, with perhaps a few fancier French dishes for entertaining. Pierre Blot, a Frenchman who came to New York about 1855, came up with a solution: with financial assistance from a daughter of the railroad magnate Commodore Cornelius Vanderbilt, in 1865 Blot opened the Culinary Academy of Design on Fourth Avenue, America's first French cooking school. It mainly catered to wealthy women, who brought their cooks with them for training, and lasted only a few years; but Blot's *Handbook of Practical Cookery, for Ladies and Professional Cooks,* published in 1867, provided a template for the curriculum of an up-to-date cooking school. See BLOT, PIERRE.

Cooking schools experienced a resurgence after the Civil War as the middle-class population of New York swelled along with the need for domestics and restaurant cooks. During the 1860s, a German immigrant, Gesine Lemcke, opened the Greater New York Cooking School on East Forty-Second Street, with a second branch in Brooklyn. Her aim was to train cooks, butlers, and waitresses. When Lemcke died in 1904, her daughter became the principal, and the school continued to operate until 1934.

In 1873 the nation went into an economic recession that continued for several years. Many immigrants lost their jobs, and new employment was hard to find. Juliet Corson, a thirty-two-year-old librarian at the Working Women's Library in New York, began teaching cookery classes in hopes that her students might find work as domestics. Corson's cooking courses attracted the attention of middle- and upper-class women, and she decided to launch her own cooking school. See CORSON, JULIET.

In November 1876 Corson opened the New York Cooking School, with a sliding-scale tuition that made it affordable for women from every walk of life. The school offered a series of twelve lessons. Based on her lectures and experiences, Corson wrote *The Cooking Manual of Practical Directions for Economical Every-Day Cookery* (1877), which presented her culinary philosophy—to make "the most wholesome and palatable dishes at the least possible cost." Corson's cooking school and lectures were so successful that she received inquiries from women in other cities about how to start and manage a cooking school. She published *Cooking School Text Book and Housekeepers' Guide* (1879), which became the textbook for other cooking schools in places like Boston and Philadelphia. Corson's efforts—and those of home economics professionals—led to the teaching of cookery in New York City's public schools. See NEW YORK COOKING SCHOOL.

The twentieth century saw the establishment of other culinary schools in New York. Maria Matilda Ericsson Hammond's Swedish, French, American Cooking School on East Forty-Sixth Street was likely attended by Swedish immigrants looking for work as cooks.

In 1942 a school was launched by Dione Lucas, an Englishwoman born in Italy and brought up in France. She had attended Le Cordon Bleu in Paris and opened a restaurant and cooking school in London just before the outbreak of World War II. When the war began, Lucas immigrated to New

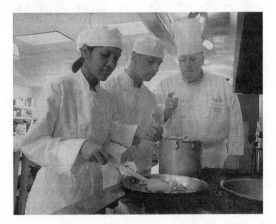

The Institute of Culinary Education offers over 1,700 classes a year to thousands of food professionals and amateurs. INSTITUTE OF CULINARY EDUCATION

York, where she opened the cooking school at her restaurant, Le Petit Cordon Bleu, in Manhattan. It offered lessons for five dollars apiece and "a course of forty-eight lessons for $192." Lucas later changed the school's name to the Gourmet Cooking School, and she continued to run it at various locations, including restaurants where she cooked. See LUCAS, DIONE.

Another culinary school was opened by caterer and cookbook author James Beard in his townhouse on West Tenth Street and later on West Twelfth Street. The school closed in the mid-1980s, but the Tenth Street townhouse is now home to the James Beard Foundation. See BEARD, JAMES and JAMES BEARD FOUNDATION.

There were at least sixteen cooking schools or programs operating in New York City during the 1960s. They included Diana Kennedy's Mexican Cooking School, Madame Grace Chu's Chinese Cooking Classes, the Gourmet Cooking School, Michael Field's Cooking School, the Maurice Moore-Betty Cooking School, and Helen Worth's Cooking School, which according to Worth, offered culinary classes "taught as an art based on a science." By the mid-1970s New York City had forty-five different cooking schools and programs, including one at the New School for Social Research with a faculty that featured big-name instructors such as Madhur Jaffrey and Jacques Pépin.

Most of these schools died with their founders, but some survived. Peter Kump's New York Cooking School, founded in 1975, was sold and later renamed the Institute for Culinary Education in 2001. See KUMP, PETER CLARK. The Natural Gourmet Cooking School, which teaches professional cooking with a basis in nutrition, was founded by Annemarie Colbin in 1977. De Gustibus Cooking School was launched at Macy's in 1980 by Arlene Feltman Sailhac. The French Culinary Institute in SoHo was founded by Dorothy Cann Hamilton in 1984. It later added an Italian cuisine program, then a Spanish program, and restyled itself the International Culinary Center. See HAMILTON, DOROTHY CANN.

See also FRENCH CULINARY INSTITUTE; INSTITUTE OF CULINARY EDUCATION; NEW SCHOOL; and SMILOW, RICK.

"Cooking Schools in the City: It's [sic] Mouth-Watering Array." New York Times, September 6, 1975.

Andrew F. Smith

Cookstoves

See ANTEBELLUM PERIOD.

Cooper Hewitt, Smithsonian Design Museum

The Cooper-Hewitt, Smithsonian Design Museum, a branch of the Smithsonian Institution and the only museum in the nation devoted exclusively to historic and contemporary design, was established in 1897 by three Hewitt sisters, granddaughters of industrialist Peter Cooper. The sisters' collecting passion started in childhood when they made scrapbooks preserving ephemera, including an 1877 menu handwritten in French. Such culinary artifacts remain integral to the Cooper-Hewitt, now housed at the former Andrew Carnegie mansion on Fifth Avenue in Manhattan. Visitors can explore the breakfast room where the steel magnate sated his taste for oatmeal, dine in the museum's contemporary café, and advance their understanding of design across thirty centuries of creativity represented by the collection's 217,000-plus objects. The museum offers a master's program in the history of decorative arts and design and honors excellence, innovation, and lasting achievement with National Design Awards (a 2014 award was conferred on an ice cream scoop).

Exhibitions have targeted specific artifacts—*Silver Mustard Pots from the Colman Collection*—and diffuse themes—*Packaging the New: Design and the American Consumer*, a 1994 show that re-created a 1950s supermarket, explored obsolescence through abandoned toasters, and brought back a groovy 1960s Formica kitchen with a horizontal eye-level refrigerator and freezer. The Cooper-Hewitt's most thorough culinary exhibition was *Feeding Desire: Design and the Tools of the Table, 1500–2005*, a tracing of the development of Western civilization through knives, spoons, and forks.

The national design collection also preserves a 1940 aluminum, steel, and rubber "Streamliner" meat slicer; a 1981 fabric sidewall depicting junk food; Tibor Kalman's map of Restaurant Florent; a 1943 U.S. Office of War Information poster trumpeting "Food is a weapon—don't waste it"; and stellar examples of quotidian artifacts like matchbooks, cookbooks, and product labels. The museum's most important culinary artifact, a French Empire *surtout de table*, is over 10½ feet long and 2½ feet tall. The hand-engraved ormolu and cut and silver-mirrored glass centerpiece includes candelabra, eight-tiered cake servers, fruit baskets, tazza, and ten female figures. It was probably a present from Napoleon to his adopted son Eugène de Beauharnais.

The building received landmark status in 1974, and in 1976 reopened as the Cooper-Hewitt, National Design Museum, Smithsonian Institution. It was renamed the Cooper-Hewitt, Smithsonian Design Museum in 2014.

See also MUSEUM FOOD.

Coffin, Sarah D., Ellen Lupton, Darra Goldstein, et al. *Feeding Desire: Design and the Tools of the Table, 1500–2005*. New York: Assouline, 2006.

Harley Spiller

Corned Beef Sandwich

The corned beef sandwich, preferably eaten at Katz's on the Lower East Side or the Carnegie Deli, is arguably the quintessential delicatessen sandwich of New York City. See KATZ'S DELICATESSEN. The fatty red meat is kept hot in a steam tray and should rightly be cut by hand for each order. It is typically piled so high on rye bread that it can scarcely fit in the human mouth. Mustard is the appropriate condiment, and requests for mayonnaise would be met with sharp opprobrium. A kosher dill pickle is also requisite. With a can of Dr. Brown's Cel-Ray soda, this is a classic meal. Only the foolhardy or those with prodigious appetites would dare to order sides like a knish, *kishkas* (stuffed derma—i.e., beef intestine stuffed with crumbs and chicken fat), or chopped liver. The Reuben is another matter, comprised of corned beef with Swiss cheese, sauerkraut, and Russian dressing and grilled until melted. Strictly speaking, it is not kosher but arguably is the apotheosis of corned beef nonetheless.

The term "corned beef" is said to derive from the British practice of using coarse salt or "corns" or kernels to cure the meat. The term was already in common usage in the early seventeenth century, and Richard Burton uses the term in his *Anatomy of Melancholy*, published in 1621. "Beef, a strong and hearty meat (cold in the first degree, dry in the second, saith *Gal. l. 3. c. 1. de alim. fac.*) is condemned by him and all succeeding Authors, to breed gross melancholy blood: good for such as are sound, and of a strong constitution, for labouring men if ordered aright, corned, young, of an ox (for all gelded meats in every species are held best), or if old, such as have been tired out with labour, are preferred."

There is no doubt that corned beef was also known among the early colonists in America. How it came to be associated with Jewish delis is a matter of pure speculation, and it may be that it is mostly a New World phenomenon when kosher butchers of Eastern European Ashkenazic origin started curing beef, which may be an extension of the koshering process that involves salting to remove the blood. Pastrami, on the other hand, has clear Romanian origins.

Today corned beef is usually made from brisket or belly, cured from roughly a week to a month in a "dry cure," laden historically with a little saltpeter (potassium nitrate) but now more often with sodium nitrite and spices such as coriander, pepper, mustard seeds, garlic, and bay leaves. The nitrite makes the meat firm and gives it an unmistakable texture and the signature red color. It also prevents botulism. Commercial corned beef is usually cured much quicker by injection of brine, and it is sometimes turned red with food coloring. Corned beef can be made without nitrates, but the color is an unappealing gray, and it tends to shred when cut, more like a pot roast.

The cured meat is then gently boiled until tender and kept hot until slicing. Proper corned beef is not a mass-produced cold cut sliced by a machine at the supermarket delicatessen counter, nor is it even faintly similar to the canned product, also known as "bully beef," which was produced largely in Uruguay and supplied the British navy and its colonies in the nineteenth and early twentieth centuries. Pastrami, though a cousin, differs in that it is covered in crushed pepper and spices and smoked. Tongue is cured much the same way as corned beef, and any self-respecting deli carries it.

Perhaps the strangest fate of corned beef is its association with the Irish and St. Patrick's Day. See IRISH and ST. PATRICK'S DAY. Corned beef is seldom eaten in Ireland today. It may have been served as a substitute for bacon and cabbage among Irish American immigrants. It is believed that they purchased corned beef from Jewish butchers in New York because it was readily available and fairly inexpensive. It is true that great quantities of salt beef were produced in Ireland in the eighteenth century, especially in the city of Cork, most of it for export for the British navy. Historically the Irish did eat corned beef on holidays, but for the most part cattle were kept for milk, cheese, and butter. So it may well be that the tradition is more of a borrowing by Irish Americans from their Jewish neighbors in New York City.

Today the fate of the Jewish deli is in jeopardy. While a few well-established emporia serve eager tourists in large, somewhat Disneyfied surroundings, the small hole-in-the-wall, mom-and-pop delicatessen serving home-cured corned beef is becoming a rarity. Some aficionados insist that only a truly kosher establishment should be trusted. Cheap, industrially manufactured substitutes may appease outsiders, but a true New Yorker is adamant about the real thing.

See also DELIS, JEWISH.

Lebewohl, Sharon, Rena Bulkin, and Jack Lebewohl. *The 2nd Ave Deli Cookbook*. New York: Villard, 1999.

Mac Con Iomaire, Máirtín, and Pádraig Óg Gallagher. "Irish Corned Beef: A Culinary History." *Journal of Culinary Science and Technology* 9, no. 1 (2011): 27–43.

Parker, Milton, and Allyn Freeman. *How to Feed Friends and Influence People: The Carnegie Deli…A Giant Sandwich, a Little Deli, a Huge Success*. Hoboken, N.J.: Wiley, 2004.

Sax, David. *Save the Deli: In Search of Perfect Pastrami, Crusty Rye, and the Heart of Jewish Delicatessen*. New York: Houghton Mifflin Harcourt, 2009.

Ken Albala

Corson, Juliet

Juliet Corson (1841–1897) was born in Roxbury, Massachusetts. When she was six, her family moved to New York City, where she lived for the rest of her life. While working as a librarian, Corson became concerned about the plight of the city's poor, especially the women. She volunteered as secretary to the Women's Educational and Industrial Society of New York, whose purpose was to offer free vocational training for unemployed working-class women. Corson was asked to give cooking classes (despite her lack of culinary experience or knowledge); the hope was to help students find jobs as domestics. Corson studied contemporary cookbooks and began giving cooking classes in her home. In 1875 she began submitting articles on cookery to newspa-

pers and magazines and lecturing at various venues around the city. In November 1876 she opened the New York Cooking School, with a sliding-scale tuition that made it affordable for women from every walk of life.

In 1877 the nation was in the midst of an economic depression; unemployment hit 14 percent. Railroad executives cut wages, leading railroad workers to strike, paralyzing the nation. Corson prepared a pamphlet, *Fifteen Cent Dinners for Workingmen's Families* (1877), to help the wives of those on strike and out of work "to make savory and nutritious meals" and not "tasteless or sodden messes," which "sends the man to the liquor shop for consolation." When she could not find a commercial publisher for it, Corson printed fifty thousand copies at her own expense, noting that the pamphlet was "published for free circulation only." *Fifteen Cent Dinners* received widespread acclaim, and the recipes were republished in newspapers and magazines across the country. Corson subsequently published *Twenty-five Cent Dinners for Families of Six* (1878), *Meals for the Million* (1882), and *Family Living on $500 a Year* (1888)—all of which were widely distributed.

Corson's fame spread throughout the United States, and she was asked to lecture all over the country. Based on these lectures, Corson wrote *The Cooking Manual of Practical Directions for Economical Every-Day Cookery*, which presented her culinary philosophy—to make "the most wholesome and palatable dishes at the least possible cost." Corson's cooking school and lectures achieved such renown that she received inquiries from many cities, including Philadelphia and Boston, on how to run a cooking school. She published *The Cooking School Text Book and Housekeepers' Guide to Cookery and Kitchen Management* (1879), which became the text for many schools in the United States and Europe. It supplied materials for three different levels of cooking courses—"Artisans," "Plain Cooks," and "Ladies"—and included an appendix titled "Dietary for Schools," a thorough introduction to the nutritional needs of children and adolescents. Copies of the "Dietary" were reprinted by the U.S. Secretary of the Interior and sent to schools around the country.

In 1879, *Harper's* magazine proclaimed Corson "the benefactor of the working classes, for she teaches them how to make two dishes where formerly they made but one; and the friend of women, for she has shown them the way to a useful and honorable profession." Her efforts—and those of other home economics professionals—led to the teaching of cookery in New York City's public schools. Juliet Corson died in 1897, at the age of 56, and is buried in Green-Wood Cemetery, in Brooklyn.

See also COOKBOOKS; COOKING SCHOOLS; and NEW YORK COOKING SCHOOL.

Corson, Juliet. *Cooking School Text Book and Housekeepers' Guide*. New York: Orange Judd, 1879.
Corson, Juliet. *Fifteen Cent Dinners for Workingmen's Families: Fifteen Cent Dinners for Families of Six*. New York: Printed by author, 1877.
Fryatt, F. E. "The New York Cooking School." *Harper's New Monthly Magazine* 60 (December 1879): 22–29.
Shapiro, Laura. *Perfection Salad: Women and Cooking at the Turn of the Century*. New York: Farrar, Straus and Giroux, 1986.

Andrew F. Smith

Cosmopolitan

Like many cocktails, it is difficult to pinpoint the exact date and place of birth of the frothy pink Cosmopolitan. Some say a drink of the same name existed in San Francisco; others credit Cheryl Cook, a Miami bartender nicknamed "The Martini Queen of South Beach," who claimed to have invented the drink in the mid-1980s. Regardless of where it started, the Cosmo undoubtedly was perfected and popularized in New York.

In his 2003 book *Cosmopolitan: A Bartender's Life*, Toby Cecchini insists, "I did not invent the Cosmopolitan" but concedes that he might have "reinvented" the drink in 1988, while he worked at Odeon in Tribeca. "I did invent what you think of as the drink, the version everyone means when they order it, last decade's instantly understood signifier of crass, table-hopping New York privilege."

Cecchini says an Odeon coworker showed him a drink she knew about from San Francisco: "It was called the Cosmopolitan and she made it with vodka, Rose's Lime, and grenadine. It looked pretty but tasted awful: jarring and artificially sweet and just wrong." He subbed in Absolut Citron, then newly introduced, "for no particular reason other than that it was the new, cool thing at the moment," plus fresh lime juice, Cointreau orange liqueur, and "just

enough cranberry juice to give it a demure pink blush."

Farther uptown, at the Rainbow Room, bartender Dale Degroff perfected a slightly different version (his version calls for less orange liqueur and lime juice and more cranberry compared to Cecchini's recipe) and officially placed it on the menu in 1996. He had first tried a variation at Fog City Diner in San Francisco, he says in his book *The Essential Cocktail*, and notes that he did not invent the drink but did "popularize a version…which became something of the standard." See DEGROFF, DALE.

The drink was widely popularized as the tipple of choice among fashionable Carrie Bradshaw and her friends in the HBO series *Sex and the City* (1998–2004). The characters were frequently shown ordering and sipping the pink cocktail from martini glasses. See SEX AND THE CITY.

See also COCKTAILS.

Cecchini, Toby. *Cosmopolitan: A Bartender's Life*. New York: Broadway, 2003.
Degroff, Dale. *The Essential Cocktail: The Art of Mixing Perfect Drinks*. New York: Clarkson Potter, 2010.

Kara Newman

Cotton Club

The Cotton Club was a popular nightclub in Harlem from 1923 to 1935. Located on 142nd Street and Lenox Avenue, the club was known for its live dance and music performances as well as for its restrictive door policy, which allowed entry only to white patrons even though the entertainers were almost entirely African American.

When the Cotton Club opened, Harlem was emerging as the black mecca of the United States. Between 1920 and 1930, two hundred thousand black newcomers moved to Harlem from the American South as well as the Caribbean islands. While its developers intended Harlem to be a middle- and upper-class white neighborhood, when African Americans began to settle in the area, most whites moved out. In 1920, 30 percent of Harlem's population was African American; by 1930, that number had increased to 70 percent. Harlem became the center of a tremendous flowering of African American arts and culture during the 1920s, known as the Harlem Renaissance. A celebration of African American

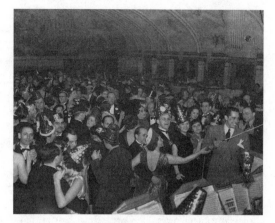

New Year's Ball at the Cotton Club, 1937. The Cotton Club was known for its live music and dance – and for only allowing white patrons in the door, despite the fact that the entertainers were almost entirely African American.

music and performance was part of this movement. Harlem also became an important entertainment center during this time. White folks from downtown flooded into the neighborhood seeking a release in the clubs and restaurants of Harlem.

Like many of these clubs, the Cotton Club offered an exotic environment—and a patronizing, stereotypical depiction of black life—to its white patrons. The club's décor aimed to depict a "stylish plantation environment." The stage shows at the Cotton Club were lavish musical revues showcasing musicians, dancers, comedians, and variety acts. Featuring scantily clad dancers dancing to a jungle beat, these shows perpetuated white-held myths about the exoticism and sensuality of African American women. Perhaps the most famous of the Cotton Club dancers was the legendary singer and dancer Lena Horne. See NIGHTCLUBS.

Duke Ellington led the house band at the Cotton Club from 1927 to 1930 and beyond. Other legendary performers at the club included Cab Calloway, Ethel Waters, Fletcher Henderson, Bill "Bojangles" Robinson, Count Basie, Louis Armstrong, Billie Holliday, Stepin Fetchit, and the Nicholas Brothers. The club illustrates the challenge faced by African American performers who were forced to balance the need to earn a living and to practice their craft with the limited, often demeaning roles available to them.

Much of the Cotton Club's heyday occurred during Prohibition. Liquor flowed freely at the club,

as it did at many hot spots in Harlem. Indeed, the club's owner, Owney Madden, was a bootlegger and gangster who used the venue to sell his beer and liquor. Once Prohibition ended, the drinks menu was published and included such "fancy mixed drinks" as sloe gin rickey, silver fizz, sherry flip, and whiskey sour. The club also offered an extensive list of champagnes, wines, liquors, and liqueurs. For supper, diners at the Cotton Club could enjoy such delicacies as lobster, capon, and roast lamb; an assortment of tea sandwiches (imported caviar, tongue, roast beef, cream cheese, and jelly); and, interestingly, a number of Chinese dishes including chicken chow mein, chop suey, fried rice, and "moo goo guy pan." See BOOTLEGGERS; COCKTAILS; and PROHIBITION.

The Harlem riots of 1935, sparked by complaints about police brutality and unfair hiring practices in Harlem, led the Cotton Club to close. It reopened in 1936 in the midtown Theater District, where it operated until 1940. A contemporary jazz club called the Cotton Club is located on West 125th Street in today's Harlem. It is unaffiliated with the original club except by name.

See also HARLEM.

Haskins, James. *The Cotton Club*. New York: New American Library, 1977.
Lewis, David Levering. *When Harlem Was in Vogue*. New York: Penguin, 1997. First published 1989.
Winter, Elizabeth. "Cotton Club of Harlem (1923–)." BlackPast.org. http://www.blackpast.org/aah/cotton-club-harlem-1923.

Cindy R. Lobel

Cream Cheese

Spread on crackers for hors d'oeuvres, shmeared on bagels for brunch, or used as cheesecake filling for dessert, cream cheese is the most ubiquitous soft cheese in America. Though centuries old, its modern development took place in New York when, in 1875, Joseph Park and John Tilford, the founders of Park & Tilford grocery stores, went looking for a new cheese. Their high-end stores on Broadway and on Sixth Avenue, carrying fancy domestic and imported goods, had been selling French cheeses that had become popular in New York restaurants and hotels: Brie, Camembert, and Neufchâtel. Now, they sought an even richer and more delicate cheese. Park and Tilford approached William Lawrence (1842–1911), a farmer and cheesemaker from Chester, New York, some 65 miles north of the city, who had been supplying them with Neufchâtel. Lawrence's Neufchâtel was made by curdling whole milk, squeezing out the whey, adding salt, and forming it into a cylinder, the signature form of Neufchâtel. Now, Lawrence added cream to the curds, creating a cheese with a higher milk fat content (about 6 percent), resulting in a richer taste. He called his product "cream cheese."

Lawrence's name for his cheese was not original, nor was his recipe. "Cream cheeses" made from curdled milk or cream, such as Stilton, had been known in England since the early 1700s, and the English colonialists brought along the recipes for making them to America. By the early 1800s, Philadelphia had gained a reputation for these fine cream cheeses. Returning New Yorkers came home from visits there with stories of these culinary delights, but since the cheeses were a perishable product, they could not survive the trip (by horse or stagecoach) up to New York City. The advent of steamship service shortened the journey, and thus, by 1847 cream cheeses could be found, in small quantities, in New York City markets. Lawrence's real contribution—due to small, economical steam engines that mechanized dairy product production in the 1870s—was to mass-produce, for the first time, these cream cheeses. Railroad lines and commercial ice production allowed him to ship increasing amounts of these perishable cheeses to New York City.

Cream cheese found a wider audience when, by 1880, Lawrence was approached by a cheese distributor, Alvah Lewis Reynolds (1853–1919), a New York City native, who offered to deliver the cream cheeses to a wider number of New York City grocers. Reynolds's skills, however, were not just in distribution but in advertising as well. Rather than pack the cheeses into boxes that had Lawrence's brand (a cow) stenciled on the side, Reynolds suggested that each cheese be wrapped in foil, upon which would be imprinted a brand name. He proposed calling it "Philadelphia Cream Cheese," based on Philadelphia's reputation for fine dairy products. He painted the name on the side of his first wagon and on each of the fifteen wagons he had in operation by 1890. Reynolds advertised the cream cheese in theater programs, hotel bulletins, and streetcars.

When Reynolds sold his Philadelphia brand to Phenix Cheese Corporation (later merged with Kraft)

in 1903, there was an established market for cream cheese in New York City. In addition to Philadelphia, a number of competing cream cheese brands could be found: Clover, Double Cream, Eagle, Manhattan, Mohican, Nabob, Star, White Rose, and World. Cream cheese, however, continued to be an expensive product. In 1889, Muenster sold for thirteen cents a pound, Parmesan for twenty-three cents, while cream cheese was thirty cents a pound. In 1903, the St. Denis Hotel on Broadway and Eleventh Street concluded its multicourse Thanksgiving dinner with an offering of Roquefort, Camembert, or Philadelphia Cream Cheese. Into the early 1920s, ladies' journals and newspaper columns devoted to home entertaining touted the use of cream cheese for fancy social gatherings.

Cream cheese would become more affordable and ubiquitous with the introduction of Downsville Cream Cheese in 1923 by Breakstone Brothers Dairy. Joseph (1859–1930) and Isaac (1864–1945) Breakstone, two Jewish immigrants from Lithuania, opened a wholesale dairy business on Jay Street and on First Avenue in 1897. They distributed sweet (unsalted) butter shipped from the Midwest to Lower East Side grocers, together with pot cheese, milk, sour cream, and eggs purchased from New York farmers and creameries. By 1906 they had purchased a number of creameries, becoming one of the largest dairy manufacturers and distributors in New York City.

In 1923, Breakstone Brothers created Downsville Cream Cheese, an exceedingly rich cheese containing 33 percent milk fat. Moreover, due to new advances in dairy manufacturing, the shelf life of this cream cheese was extended and it was more economical to produce, resulting in a low-cost cheese that would keep well. Cream cheese thus became affordable for the average consumer. In addition, bakers were quick to seize on its rich taste and full-bodied consistency. Cheesecakes, made with Downsville Cream Cheese, began to find their way onto the menus of New York City restaurants. See CHEESECAKE.

Forty-five years after its start as a fancy cheese, cream cheese was now, truly, an integral part of New York City foodways.

See also BAGELS and LOX.

"Breakstone" File. Research Library, National Museum of American Jewish History, Philadelphia, Pa.

International Cheese Company v. Phenix Cheese Company. Supreme Court, Otsego County, N.Y. (1906).

Lawrence et al. v. P. E. Sharpless Co. U.S. Circuit Court, Eastern District PA, DC 637 (1912).

Marx, J. " 'The Days Had Come of Curds and Cream': The Origins and Development of Cream Cheese in America, 1870–1880." *Food, Culture & Society* 15, no. 2 (2012): 177–195.

Jeffrey A. Marx

Cries of New-York, The

Street vendors selling food and household goods were a vital part of urban commerce from the earliest days of New Amsterdam. Their cries, called out to attract buyers, were part of the everyday tapestry of city sounds. In 1808 Samuel Wood published a small children's book titled *The Cries of New-York*. Its illustrations were taken from *The Cries of London*, originally published in 1778, but the content of the New York book was original. It presented twenty-six different street vendors and their cries, as well as a two-page discussion about each item sold, sometimes with a description of how it was prepared. The book went through several printings and revisions, and additional cries were added. The 1830 edition included fifteen original illustrations of New York street vendors—children and adults, whites and African Americans.

Some illustrations depicted street vendors in their wagons or pushing barrows, others on foot going door to door. Those depicted in the books sold strawberries, cherries, oranges, limes and lemons, "fine pines" (pineapples), baked pears, "water-milyons," onions, radishes, white and sweet potatoes, rusks, tea, "mint-wa-ter," milk, "butter mil-leck," "hot muffins," "hot, spic'd, gin-ger bread," oysters, clams, and "hot corn." Wood wrote that corn was widely sold in the fall, boiled in the husks while green; sprinkled with salt supplied by the vendor, the hot corn made for "very pleasant eating."

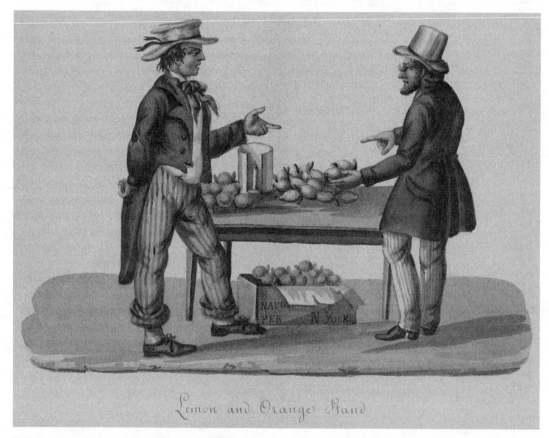

"The Lemon and Orange Stand" (1840–1844), from a series of watercolor paintings depicting street vendors by Nicolino Calyo titled "Street Cries of New York." The series was a tribute to Samuel Wood's children's book *The Cries of New-York*. MUSEUM OF THE CITY OF NEW YORK

The Cries of New-York was arguably the first children's book and the first picture book published in America. Copies of early editions can be found at the New York Public Library. See NEW YORK PUBLIC LIBRARY.

See also STREET VENDORS.

The Cries of New-York. New York: S. Wood, 1808.
The Cries of New-York; Illustrated by Fifteen Original Designs. New York: S. King, 1830.

Andrew F. Smith

Cronut

The Cronut is the 2013 invention of pastry chef Dominique Ansel. The name is trademarked and the recipe is proprietary, but it involves a croissant-style dough that is fried and filled with a flavored cream before being glazed. The confection is produced in only one flavor, which is changed monthly. Production is limited to 350 per day, and each pastry sells for $5 (pretax) at Ansel's eponymous bakery at 189 Spring Street. In the year following its introduction it was the luxury "it" pastry for New Yorkers and tourists alike, who would line up to purchase one or two (the bakery's imposed maximum) every morning. The website reassures that "if you arrive prior to 7:00 a.m. on a week day, you have a great chance of getting the Cronut™ pastry." The shop opens at 8:00 a.m.

The Cronut's sizzling popularity was ignited by a brilliant social media campaign. On May 9, 2013, the Dominique Ansel Bakery's Facebook page leaked what may be New York's first gastronomic birth announcement: "Something beautiful is being unveiled tomorrow (Friday, May 10). Half croissant, half donut... all the crispy sugary goodness of the donut with the flaky layers of a croissant. Wait for it...." Reaction was overwhelming and swift. On May 15, the independent Cronut.org, "a home for cronutophiles," was launched. On May 19, Ansel appeared on *Fox & Friends*, where a Twitter hashtag, #cronutfever, ran on the bottom ribbon. Soon, a secondary market developed, with scalpers lining up to buy the pastries for resale at a premium reportedly of up to $100 per pastry. The bakery continues to feed the frenzy by allowing a limited number of online orders for pickup two weeks hence.

Success has spawned imitators, with recipes for copycat cronuts appearing as early as June 2013. By August 1, Thrillist Maps, available through Google, tracked places to get cronut facsimiles in locales as far-flung as Barcelona, Spain, and Seoul, South Korea. Ansel used some of the notoriety of the Cronut to support local hunger relief organizations, as well as other charities. In August 2013, Ansel sold T-shirts emblazoned with, "Crolanthropy—making the world better one Cronut™ at a time." Proceeds from Cronut T-shirt sales benefited the Food Bank of New York directly, and purchasers of the T-shirts could return in September to buy four, instead of two, Cronuts. The most successful fundraiser to date has been an auction to benefit City Harvest, in October 2013, when a dozen Cronuts were sold for $14,000. Ansel was named the James Beard Foundation's Outstanding Pastry Chef in 2014.

See also BAKERIES and DOUGHNUTS.

"Cronut™ 101." Dominique Ansel Bakery. http://dominiqueansel.com/cronut-101/.
Gopnik, Adam. "Bakeoff: What's Happening to Our Pastry?" *New Yorker*, November 3, 2014.

Cathy K. Kaufman

Cuban

Affluent Cubans, mostly landowning families growing sugar cane, arrived in New York City in the mid-nineteenth century, attracted by its flourishing sugar refining factories. Cubans were the largest Hispanic minority in New York when Cuba's Ten Year War began in 1868 and again after 1885 when war against Spain was rekindled by the Cuban insurgency.

Cuban immigrants enjoyed Cuban food in their home kitchens or the dining rooms of boarding houses like that run by Carmen Millares de Mantilla on 51 West Twenty-Ninth Street. Cuban cuisine has a Mediterranean foundation, featuring an important core of legumes (mostly beans) served with rice, proteins seasoned with pungent marinades (*adobos*) of garlic and citrus juice, and simple tomato and sweet pepper–based cooking sauces (*sofritos*) underpinning most stews and braises. Anyone with memories of Cuban food could have duplicated Cuban recipes in nineteenth-century New York. Caribbean food imports, from bananas to guava paste, were not uncommon in the city, the most important trading port of the United States.

Throughout the nineteenth century, New York maintained active trade with Cuba to supply the sugar refining factories that dotted the East River with the necessary raw material, cakes of raw brown sugar. New waves of Cuban immigrants came to New York after independence was won from Spain in 1898, reaching a peak after the Castro revolution in 1959. The Upper West Side, particularly the area around Amsterdam Avenue, Columbus Avenue, and Broadway, attracted many Cuban immigrants in the late 1950s and 1960s before the area underwent gentrification.

Small storefront restaurants in unfashionable locations served Cuban food. Among them were Cuban-Chinese restaurants run by Chinese immigrants coming from Cuba, a diverse lot. Some had originally come from the southern provinces of China and had lived and worked in Cuba after having left China at different points in time from the end of the nineteenth century through the first half of the twentieth century. Others were born in Cuba, often the offspring of Chinese men and Cuban women of mixed race. They had all fled the island in the aftermath of the Castro revolution and had settled mostly in New York City in the 1960s, where they opened inexpensive but highly popular restaurants modeled after the iconic Cuban-Chinese *fonda* (inexpensive, popular restaurants). These establishments did not serve a hybrid Cuban-Chinese cuisine but rather Cuban and Cantonese foods usually brought to diners on the same blue plate.

Cubans who could afford to dine out for a special occasion would choose a Spanish restaurant or premier restaurant deemed "cosmopolitan." This well-entrenched dining paradigm shifted when a Cuban immigrant named Víctor del Corral opened Victor's Café, a tiny Cuban restaurant, at 240 Columbus Avenue in 1963. Lines of customers attracted by Victor's generous portions and delicious black bean soup formed every night at the door, even when the area was derelict and even dangerous at night. Local hippies would buy Victor's sangria with tropical fruits to drink at Central Park, as if it were jug wine. An unprecedented good review by *New York Times* food critic Raymond Sokolov, who awarded three stars to the restaurant, conferred it an iconic status that attracted throngs of native New Yorkers; even stars like John Lennon, Yoko Ono, Robert Redford, Dustin Hoffman, Al Pacino, Liza Minnelli, and ABC newscaster Bill Evans became Victor's customers.

Such notoriety also impressed New York and New Jersey Cubans, who began to come to Victor's for special occasions and even political events. As the restaurant prospered, del Corral felt an urge to leave his mark, and he would say to anyone who cared to listen that his goal was "to be the first to put Cuban cuisine on the culinary map of New York."

Víctor del Corral put Cuban cuisine on the map, but he also created the blueprint for Latin American restaurants in one of the most demanding food cities in the world, a model widely copied by other Cuban entrepreneurs and successive waves of Latin American restaurateurs throughout the United States. Most importantly, the success of Victor's Café demonstrated that true Cuban cuisine had lasting crossover appeal in the United States and that a solid family-owned restaurant espousing traditional cooking with a contemporary flair could outlive generations and scores of trendier restaurants.

Although many Cuban immigrants have left New York for the suburbs and Miami, today the city has more than twenty Cuban restaurants, ranging from luncheonettes and neighborhood cafés to upscale dining rooms.

See also VICTOR'S CAFÉ.

Pérez, Lisandro. "Cubans in the United States." *Annals of the American Academy of Political Social Science* 487 (1986): 1265–1370.

Presilla, Maricel E. *Celebrating Cuban Cuisine: In Commemoration of Victor's Café 52 25th Anniversary.* New York: Victor's Café 52, 1987.

Presilla, Maricel E. "Cuban American Food." In *The Oxford Encyclopedia of Food and Drink in America*, edited by Andrew Smith, Vol. 1, pp. 357–359. New York: Oxford University Press, 2004.

Siu, Lok. "In Search of Chino Latinos in Diaspora: The Cuban Chinese in New York City." In *Cuba: Idea of a Nation Displaced*, edited by Andrea O'Reilly Herrera, pp. 123–131. Albany: State University of New York Press, 2007.

Siu, Lok. "Chino Latino Restaurants: Converging Communities, Identities, and Cultures." In Special Issue: "Afro-Asia." *Afro-Hispanic Review* 27, no. 1 (Spring 2008): 161–172.

Witchelot, Alex. "Sweet and Savory Memories, Caramelized in Exile." *New York Times*, October 30, 2014.

Maricel E. Presilla

Cuisine

Sphere, a Betty Crocker magazine based in Chicago, begat *Cuisine*. Forum Communications, its owner in 1979, brought *Cuisine* to New York and installed

Patricia Brown as its first editor. She blazed a trail of unique food content for contemporary tastes. In 1984, Carey Winfrey, a former reporter at *Time* magazine and the *New York Times*, took on the mantle as editor, further enhancing the magazine's cutting-edge content.

At a time before the cult of celebrity chefs, food television, and Yelp reviews, *Cuisine* set about to report on America's burgeoning food scene. Subtitled "A Feast for the Senses," each issue covered topics from food trends to election politics to firehouse cooks, as well as usual themes of the time: seasonal food, chefs, wine, and food travel. The magazine began commissioning writers and photographers who usually did not cover food, including Brendan Gill, Daniel Zwerdling, Anthony Burgess, Calvin Trillin, Owen Edwards, and Leslie Bennetts, as well as food writers Christian Millau, Joan Nathan, Karen Hess, Paula Wolfert, Nancy Jenkins, and Lynne Rossetto Kasper. Photographers included John Dugdale, Robert Mapplethorpe, Alen Macweeney, Robert Freson, Brian Hagiwara, and Michael Geiger.

Features such as Critiquing the Critics, Yuppie Pizza, Whither the Great American Food Fad?, and Coffee: Roast Your Own got readers to look at the familiar from a new angle. *Cuisine* commissioned articles and interviewed not only chefs but historians, business people, and critics. Authors were encouraged to go behind the scenes and deconstruct the topic. Wine was covered by Hugh Johnson and books by Richard Sax. A monthly column, Food People, profiled Malcolm Forbes, David Liederman, and Nora Ephron, whose novel *Heartburn* had just come out. Another column, Choice Cuts, excerpted literature from Dickens, Thoreau, Twain, and more.

The Test Kitchen, headed by cookbook author Marie Simmons, created au courant yet approachable food, from weeknight Dinner at Eight to full-on entertaining features. The masthead included design director Mary Shanahan and poet April Bernard.

Cuisine's final owner, CBS Magazines, sold the magazine to Condé Nast, which discontinued its publication after the December 1984 issue. Subscribers were offered issues of *Gourmet* magazine instead. Christopher Kimball, editor of what was then called *The Cook's Magazine*, wrote, in that December issue (Vol. 13, no. 12, p. 160), "*Cuisine* challenged everyone in the food publishing world to be more creative, to look at food in new ways, and to explore better and more versatile food writing."

Bernard, April. *Romanticism: Poems*. New York: Norton, 2009.
Cornfield, Betty, and Owen Edwards. *Quintessence: The Quality of Having "It."* New York: Black Dog and Leventhal, 2001.
Cuisine. Vol. 13, no. 12 (December 2014).
Simmons, Marie. *The Good Egg*. New York: Houghton Mifflin, 2006.

Susan Sarao Westmoreland

Culinary Historians of New York

Culinary Historians of New York is an organization founded in 1985, open to like-minded scholars or enthusiasts who are serious about the group's purpose "to encourage the exchange of ideas and the sharing of information about food and its history" and "to stimulate and share knowledge of the ways food has affected humans (and humans, food) since earliest times," according to its website. At the time of the group's founding, the discipline of culinary history was still relatively new. While food history had gained some limited respect as an academic pursuit, culinary history was considered a folkloristic approach and thus less rigorous. It was (and is) pursued largely by independent scholars who believed in the interdependencies of practical and theoretical knowledge, mainly that one can neither study food without knowing how it is prepared nor study a cuisine without knowing the origins of the foods.

The first organization of culinary historians was formed in Boston in 1980, to share and exchange ideas, to form networks with others, and to provide a forum for presenting current research on food and culinary history. In 1985, with Schlesinger Library, it cosponsored the first American conference on culinary history at Radcliffe College, which attracted more than 180 people. Among the presenters and attendees were many New Yorkers including Karen Hess, Laura Shapiro, Reynaldo Alejandro, Jacqueline Newman, and Anne Pascarelli. These same people expressed an interest in forming a culinary historian group in New York.

"We had more and better people in New York City than anywhere else to set up a strong organization," said Jackie Newman, a professor at Queens College of the City University of New York and scholar of Chinese cuisine. So in 1985, Newman and Alice Ross, an authority of colonial-era cooking and a professor at Queens College, spearheaded two organizational meetings attended by those New Yorkers at the conference and a couple dozen more, including Anne Mendelson, Cara De Silva, Alison Ryley, Marilyn Einhorn, Jeanne Lesem, and Nach Waxman.

A core group formed and met at the Greenwich Village apartment of Larry Maxwell and Marilyn Einhorn, a rare-book dealer; drew up bylaws; elected a board and its first president, Dan T. Richards; and gained official nonprofit status as Culinary Historians of New York. The group held its first program on November 23, 1985, with a presentation by Anne Pascarelli, the culinary librarian at the New York Academy of Medicine, and Reynaldo Alejandro, culinary librarian at the New York Public Library, on available resources for culinary history. Within a few years similar culinary historian groups were formed across the country.

The roster of speakers at Culinary Historians of New York programs over the years reads like a veritable who's who in the food world, many of whom are or were members of the group, including Sandra Oliver, Barbara Wheaton, Karen Hess, Andrew F. Smith, Anne Mendelson, Cathy Kaufman, Laura Shapiro, Gary Allen, Marion Nestle, Michael Krondl, Darra Goldstein, Mark Kurlansky, Nawal Nasrallah, Ken Albala, Elizabeth Andoh, Jan Longone, Rachel Laudan, and William Woys Weaver.

The group continues to host monthly programs on a wide variety of topics from New York City markets, Civil War food, and ramen to cannibalism, Tudor kitchens, and beer. Today Culinary Historians of New York has over 250 members. It publishes an annual scholarly journal, *NY FoodStory*, and awards annual scholarships to promote research in the field of culinary history. The prestigious Amelia award for lifetime achievement has been awarded to Karen Hess, Barbara K. Wheaton, Jacqueline Newman, Betty Fussell, Jan Longone, Andrew F. Smith, and Nach Waxman.

Culinary Historians of New York website: http://www
.culinaryhistoriansny.org.
Klavans, Nancy. "Conference Reviews." *The Digest: A Newsletter for the Interdisciplinary Study of Food* 6, no. 1 (Fall 1985): 8–9, 22–23.

Linda Pelaccio

Culinary Schools

See COOKING SCHOOLS.

Culintro

Culintro, "a community for restaurant professionals," is a professional organization based in New York City, with a location in San Francisco as well, that supports the culinary industry. The organization was founded in 2008 by Stephanie Berghoff and Alina Munoz. Berghoff has a background in professional meeting planning and restaurant public relations, and Munoz came from *Gourmet* magazine. The pair saw a need and opportunity to create community, networking, and professional development opportunities for the restaurant industry, including cooks, chefs, servers, managers, bartenders, and other front-of-house professionals, as well as vendors and supporters, such as public relations people, restaurant architects and designers, and industry media. As stated in its mission, Culintro "fosters an active community of restaurant industry leaders in order to deliver the connections and opportunities that matter."

With over thirty-five thousand members nationally, the organization's activities include (1) professional development events such as panel discussions, networking, and social events; (2) an internship or *stage* (from the French *stagier*) program, which pairs culinary students with leading chefs for work–learn opportunities; (3) a national job board for employers and job seekers; and (4) a blog covering topics such as hospitality industry trends and how-to advice.

The organization is a limited liability corporation with five staffers (including Berghoff) and boards functioning primarily in an advisory capacity in New York, San Francisco, and Chicago. Culintro membership is free at the time of this writing. Revenue is raised via sponsorships from food industry suppliers, admission fees to events, application fees for the *stage* program, and fees to post a job vacancy. Future plans include expansion to additional cities and additional events and programming throughout the year.

Culintro: A Community for Restaurant Professionals website: http://culintro.com.
McCready, Louise. "The Future of Food Journalism." HuffingtonPost.com, February 10, 2010. http://www
.huffingtonpost.com/louise-mccready/the-future-of-food-journa_b_456759.html.

Jonathan Deutsch

Cullen, Michael J.

Michael J. Cullen (1884–1936), the son of Irish immigrants, began his career as a clerk at the A&P grocery store in Newark, New Jersey. He moved up in the A&P hierarchy and became the company's regional superintendent, then left A&P and worked for other grocery store chains, including the Kroger Grocery and Baking Company in the Midwest. In 1930, Cullen decided to strike out on his own: he leased space in an abandoned garage at 171st Street and Jamaica Avenue in Queens, New York, and opened a large grocery store that he named "King Kullen."

Cullen filled his spacious store with a wider range of items—more than one thousand basic food products—than was sold in most groceries. By increasing sales volume, he was able to cut costs, attracting even more customers. King Kullen offered a modern shopping experience: self-service, cash-and-carry, one-stop shopping. The low prices attracted customers willing to drive from a distance, so Cullen offered free parking adjacent to the store. He also launched a massive advertising campaign, with newspaper and radio ads that asked, "King Kullen, the world's greatest price wreckers. How does he do it?"

When Cullen's first store proved an undeniable success, he quickly opened more. By 1932 he owned eight King Kullen stores, with sales of $6 million; traditional grocery stores generated only $25,000 to $50,000 per year. By 1936 fifteen King Kullen stores served Long Island and the Bronx. Following Cullen's model, other entrepreneurs opened even larger stores, which soon came to be called "supermarkets."

Ironically, one reason that supermarkets were successful was the Depression, which hit America just as Cullen opened his first supermarket. Price became the all-important factor in where consumers chose to shop, and supermarkets offered much lower prices than small grocery stores. For the sake of saving money, people were willing to forego the pleasant atmosphere and personal attention of a small grocery for the vast, chilly aisles of a supermarket. Beginning in the early 1930s, many grocery chains closed their smaller stores and opened supermarkets. By 1935 about three hundred supermarkets were in operation across the United States; by 1940 this had jumped to 6,175.

Cullen planned to expand his chain throughout the country, but he died in 1936, just six years after opening his first store. The company he founded remains one of the few supermarket chains to remain in family hands. Cullen was the first to demonstrate that the supermarket model was financially feasible, and the Smithsonian Institution recognizes King Kullen as America's first supermarket.

See also A&P and KING KULLEN.

Humphrey, Kim. *Shelf Life: Supermarkets and the Changing Culture of Consumption*. Cambridge, U.K.: Cambridge University Press, 1998.

Seth, Andrew, and Geoffrey Randall. *The Grocers: The Rise and Rise of the Supermarket Chains*. 2d ed. Dover, N.H.: Kogan Page, 2001.

Zimmerman, M. M. *The Super Market: A Revolution in Distribution*. New York: McGraw-Hill, 1955.

Andrew F. Smith

Cupcakes

Cupcakes, that is, single-serving cakes about the size of a teacup, have been part of the American home baker's repertoire since at least the antebellum era. For much of the second half of the twentieth century they were a fixture at children's birthday parties; however, the broad popularity of these chemically leavened morsels in twenty-first-century America is of much more recent vintage.

The term "cupcake" did not originate with the shape of the cakes but rather the way the ingredients were measured: in cups. Thus, for example, Eliza Leslie's 1827 recipe for "New York Cupcake" (note the singular in the title) specifies four cups flour; four of sugar; another of butter, milk, and wine; plus some saleratus (a precursor to baking soda) to make the batter rise. The mixture is then baked in "some small tins." Occasionally, cupcake recipes instruct the cook to bake the result in actual cups, presumably when a kitchen lacked appropriate-sized pans. Eventually, cupcakes came to be baked in joined muffin tins, but this may not have occurred until the early years of the twentieth century.

Nineteenth-century cupcakes were also not typically iced as they are today, nor were they especially associated with children. It was only in the decades prior to World War II that cupcakes (whether large or individual) were increasingly iced and the small sort of cupcake began to feature more often as a children's treat.

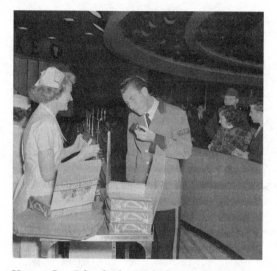

Hostess Cup Cakes display inside the Wonder Bakery building at the 1939 New York World's Fair. Hostess was an early mass-producer of cupcakes, made to appeal to women who did not have the time to make cupcakes for their guests. WURTS BROS./MUSEUM OF THE CITY OF NEW YORK

Starting in 1919, commercial bakeries began making these small cakes. One of the earliest was Indianapolis-based Taggart Bakery with its chocolate cupcakes. In 1925, Taggart was acquired by New York–based Continental Baking Company. The cakes were initially marketed to busy homemakers, as their brand name "Hostess" indicates. The sales approach changed following 1945 as American food companies increasingly began marketing directly to children. In 1954, for example, Madison Avenue came up with sixty-second Hostess cupcake cartoons to "intrigue junior televiewers," as *Television Magazine* put it. Eventually, Hostess Cupcakes were effectively rebranded as a children's treat with their own animated TV spokesperson, Captain Cupcake (joined by Twinkie the Kid).

By the 1960s, these sorts of cakes (whether bought, made from a cake mix, or even occasionally made from scratch) were a fixture at birthday parties. New York–based publishers and women's magazines promoted this idea with recipes and instructions on decorating the cakes to appeal to kids. Arithmetic textbooks used cupcakes as instructional tools. "How many cupcakes can Sue buy for $20 if two cupcakes cost 1 nickel?" asked *Learning to Use Arithmetic* in 1962. (Hostess cupcakes were sold for a nickel with two to a package.)

Cupcakes effectively remained in the peewee ghetto until the turn of the millennium, when a New York–based television show rocketed these homey confections to international fame and fortune. In a 2000 episode of HBO's *Sex and the City*, the show's protagonist, Carrie Bradshaw, sat on a bench in front of Magnolia Bakery eating one of the shop's cupcakes. The Bleecker Street bakery had opened four years previously, specializing in sweet, southern-style baking, including cupcakes among its other offerings. For reasons that are not entirely clear but likely include the contemporary fad for childhood comfort foods (mac and cheese, miniature hamburgers [aka sliders], and s'mores) as well as the advent of the millennial generation, cupcakes became a huge hit, not only in the United States but internationally. It helped that *Sex and the City* was one of the most widely distributed television shows of all time, eventually being syndicated in more than forty-eight countries. See MAGNOLIA BAKERY and *SEX AND THE CITY*.

To give some sense of the explosive growth in popularity of the cakes, consider that prior to 2000 a single cookbook devoted to cupcakes was published, and this a volume of children's recipes. In 2013, as the cupcake frenzy reached its apotheosis, some 250 books with the word "cupcake" in the title appeared; of these about seventy were cookbooks. In 2010, the Food Network jumped on the bandwagon, producing *Cupcake Wars*, a television reality show. Magnolia Bakery was mobbed to such a degree that the owners could not keep up with the demand. In 2010, On Location Tours, which bused tourists around locations made famous by the HBO series, had to take Magnolia off its tour.

Numerous local and chain bakeries have sought to profit from the cupcake phenomenon. The most ambitious was Crumbs bakery, which opened its first branch on the Upper East Side in 2003. Eventually, the company expanded to become the country's largest cupcake chain, with seventy-nine locations in eight states. By 2014, however, it was on the verge of bankruptcy, saved at the last minute by a New York investor. As of 2015, the company had contracted to some twenty-five locations, mostly in New York City. It had plenty of competition. Baked by Melissa, a New York company specializing in miniature cupcakes, boasted twelve locations. Cupcakes of every description could be found in general bakeries, specialist cupcake bakeries, supermarkets, coffee shops, street carts, and food trucks. And, as of 2013, after a brief hiatus when Hostess cakes disappeared off grocery shelves because of financial restructuring, New Yorkers and all Americans could purchase Hostess Cupcakes once more. The brand was rescued by Apollo Management, a New York–based private equity firm.

Leaf, Alexandra. "Cupcakes." In *The Oxford Companion to Sugar and Sweets*, edited by Darra Goldstein, pp. 199–200. New York: Oxford University Press, 2015.
Ward Baking Company website: http://www
.wardbakingcompany.com.

Michael Krondl

Curry Hill

South Asian immigration to New York City began in the 1960s and resulted in two distinct communities known as Little India: one in Jackson Heights in Queens and another in Manhattan in Murray Hill. Curry Hill is the neighborhood in Manhattan that is largely a restaurant and shopping district. The area that today is commonly known as Little India is located in Jackson Heights in Queens at Seventy-Third and Seventy-Fourth Streets between Roosevelt and Thirty-Seventh Avenue.

Located on Lexington Avenue and Twenty-Eighth Street in Manhattan, Curry Hill is populated with Pakistani, Indian, and Bangladeshi restaurants, shops, grocers, and cafes. Many folks refer to Jackson Heights in Queens as Little India, but Curry Hill in Manhattan is a Little India of its own. Kalustyan's (established in 1944) was one of the first ethnic grocery stores to sell Indian spices in addition to Middle Eastern groceries in Manhattan. Curry in a Hurry was one of the first Indian restaurants in Manhattan (established in 1975). Haandi is a landmark Pakistani restaurant in Curry Hill, often populated by Indian and Pakistani college students and South Asian cab drivers, as well as locals. Curry Hill in Manhattan is also the home to excellent vegetarian fare and fusion Chinese and Indian food.

See also KALUSTYAN'S and LITTLE INDIA.

Asia Society. *Asia in New York City: A Cultural Travel Guide*. New York: Balliett & Fitzgerald; Emeryville, Calif.: Avalon Travel, 2000.
Foner, Nancy. *From Ellis Island to JFK: New York's Two Great Waves of Immigration*. New Haven, Conn.: Yale University Press; New York: Russell Sage Foundation, 2002.
Khandelwal, Madhulika S. *Becoming American, Being Indian: An Immigrant Community in New York City*. The Anthropology of Contemporary Issues. Ithaca, N.Y.: Cornell University Press, 2002.

Farha Ternikar

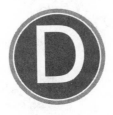

D'Agostino

D'Agostino is one of New York City's major supermarket chains. It was founded by Pasquale (1906–1960) and Nicholas (1910–1996) D'Agostino, brothers born in Bugnara, Italy. Pasquale immigrated to America in 1920 and Nicholas came over four years later. During the 1920s, the brothers helped their father operate a fruit and vegetable pushcart.

Pasquale, after having worked as a butcher's assistant, became a partner in Frank Tucciarone's grocery store at Eighty-Third Street and Lexington Avenue. In 1932, Pasquale and Nicholas bought the store from Tucciarone. Nicholas married his former boss's daughter, Josephine. The D'Agostinos enlarged the store in 1935 and began to offer a wider array of foods, including fruit, vegetables, dairy products, and baked goods; later they added a meat counter. The store did well despite the Depression, and in 1939 the D'Agostinos opened a larger outlet that they named the Yorkville Food Shoppe. They opened two additional stores in the next few years. Despite wartime restrictions, the chain thrived during World War II. In 1943 the *New Yorker* magazine profiled Pasquale, who was hailed as an immigrant who went from "rags to riches"—or, more accurately, from pushcart to supermarket.

The D'Agostinos' target customers were the wealthy "carriage trade" on the Upper East Side. The stores became known for their high-quality meats, purchased daily at Washington Market. After World War II, the D'Agostino stores added freezers and began selling frozen foods. The brothers also converted their outlets from small groceries into supermarkets to compete with the larger chains, such as A&P, Kroger, and Grand Union, that were rapidly opening stores across the city. They changed the name of the company to D'Agostino Brothers in 1950 and began stocking high-end products such as foie gras, canned lobster, crabmeat, and imported products. Advertising focused on the store's "spotless cleanliness," and the brothers were meticulous about in-store and window displays.

When Pasquale died in 1960, there were eight D'Agostino stores. Under Nicholas's management, D'Agostino continued to thrive. In 1986, reinforcing their reputation for personal service, the company introduced "Teledag," which allowed customers to place phone orders, choosing from two thousand foods for home delivery. The following year, the company began accepting credit cards. In 1991 D'Agostino began selling some organic foods. By 1996, the company, still "family-owned and operated," had twenty-six stores.

One reason for the success of the chain was a series of memorable slogans. D'Agostino pioneered the use of image-based advertising and branding; radio and print ads featured tag lines such as "Please don't kiss the butcher," "Please, Mr. D'Agostino, Move Closer to Me!" "Love that D'Agostino!" "If there's no D'Agostino near you—take a taxi!" "If there's no D'Agostino near you—move!" and "Only in New York." Advertising also associated the supermarket visually with New York landmarks, such as the Statue of Liberty and the United Nations building. The store's sturdy, reusable white plastic "D'Ag Bags" served as walking billboards for the chain. In 2014 the privately owned company operated thirteen supermarkets in New York City and one in Westchester.

See also GROCERY STORES; ITALIAN; and SUPER-
MARKETS.

Greenhouse, Steven. "Nicholas D'Agostino Sr., 86, Founder
of Grocery Chain." *New York Times,* June 25, 1996, p. B9.
Murphy, Mark. "If Trouble Can Be Avoid." *New Yorker,*
May 1943, p. 25.
Schmitz, Paul. "D'Agostino Supermarkets, from Pushcart
to Product: Family and Ethnicity as Cultural
Currency." PhD diss, Boston University, 2006.

Andrew F. Smith

Dairy Stores

Dairy stores are part of ethnic New York, strongly
identified with both Jewish and Italian immigrants.
As the name implies, dairy stores traditionally have
specialized in fresh dairy products, although the
role they have played in Jewish and Italian foodways
differs. While there are still a few Italian dairy stores
remaining, Jewish dairy products, by contrast, were
(and still are) often sold in appetizing stores such as
Russ & Daughters, as permitted by the kosher dietary laws. But a few were stand-alone dairy stores.
Among the most famous was a relative latecomer,
Ben's Cheese Planet, founded in 1960 by Ben Gorodinsky at 181 East Houston Street. Famous for its
cream cheese, Gorodinsky sold the shop in 1971 to
Jonah Friedman, who ran the retail store through
2000 and continued to manufacture the cream cheese
in the back for wholesale until 2007, when rising
rents forced relocation to Spring Valley, New York.
Ben's cream cheese is still considered the gold standard for a schmear on a bagel and is sold in New
York City at high-end cheese shops such as Murray's.

Italian immigrants to New York City in the late
nineteenth and early twentieth centuries came largely
from Campania, Puglia, Basilicata, and Sicily. The
southern Italians, especially the Neapolitans, were
famous for their mozzarella and ricotta, fresh cheeses
made daily that added protein and fat to a lean native
cuisine based on legumes, vegetables, and grains. At
a time when residents shopped daily, family-run
latterie—shops specializing in these fresh cheeses,
milk, and butter—proliferated in Little Italy. The
oldest extant is Alleva, established in 1892 by Pina
Alleva and located at the northeast corner of Mulberry and Grand Streets. It is currently run by the
father-and-son team of Robert Alleva Sr. and Jr. The
store now sells imported meats, aged cheeses, olives,
and other Italian products in addition to the homemade mozzarella that still follows Pina's original
recipe.

Down the block, at the northwest corner of Mott
and Grand Streets, stands DiPalo's, founded in
1912 by Savino DiPalo; the store is now run by his
great-grandchildren, Lou, Sal, and Marie. Through
a plate-glass window located behind the counter,
customers can watch the mozzarella curd being cut
and the cheese stretched and twisted into shape;
through the thin plastic wrapping, one can feel the
gentle warmth of the balls stacked on the counter.
Reflecting the frugality of the family's native Basilicata, the homemade burrata started as a way to use
up leftovers from the mozzarella making: the *strac-
ciatella*, bits of stretched cheese curd, would be
stuffed into the following day's new batch. The *strac-
ciatella* is now more luxurious, mixed with expensive
cream for the velvety rich cheese.

Most of these Old World–style retail stores have
folded in recent years, victims of gentrification,
changing neighborhood demographics, a preference for one-stop shopping, and great-grandchildren
no longer interested in maintaining the family vo-
cation. Latticini Barese, in Carroll Gardens, closed
in 2002. Joe's Dairy, a small storefront on Sullivan
Street with a cult-like following, closed in 2013; it
moved its manufactory to New Jersey and now sells
to restaurants and wholesale.

See also APPETIZING STORES; CHEESEMONGERS; ITAL-
IAN; JEWISH; LITTLE ITALY; and RUSS & DAUGHTERS.

DiPalo, Lou, and Rachel Wharton. *Di Palo's Guide to the
Essential Foods of Italy.* New York: Random House,
2014.
Trillin, Calvin. "Mozzarella Story: A Cheese Ritual." *New
Yorker,* December 2, 2013.
Wharton, Rachel. "The History—and Mystery—of the
City's Best Cream Cheese." *Edible Manhattan,* March
6, 2012.

Cathy K. Kaufman

Dean & DeLuca

Dean & DeLuca is a chain of high-end, luxury gourmet
stores that started out as a small shop in New York
City. Friends Giorgio DeLuca, a history teacher-
turned-cheese shop owner; Joel Dean, once a business manager at Simon & Schuster; and Jack Ceglic,
Dean's friend (they were in a relationship), had

dreamed of opening a store to celebrate food, cooking, and eating. Their first shop opened in a cast-iron building at the corner of Prince Street and Greene Street in Manhattan's SoHo. As customers enjoyed previously hard-to-find products like balsamic vinegar, sun-dried tomatoes, ripe cheese, extra-virgin olive oil, and dried mushrooms, the store was a great success.

In the 1980s, as the store began to outgrow its 2,600 square feet, the owners began looking for a larger space. In 1986 they discovered that a manufacturing company and an army/navy store were planning to vacate 10,000 square feet nearby on the corner of Prince Street and Broadway. Partner Jack Ceglic designed the new store to look like an open market. On October 6, 1988, the store reopened to much success. The new store was simple, stark, and white with an airy, industrial feel to it, matching the minimalist art galleries populating the area at the time. There was now room for a wide variety of displays: meat, seafood, cheese, vegetables, oils, and spices—all the ingredients a customer would need to make a fine meal without having to shop at other stores.

Dean & DeLuca also began selling high-quality housewares, including knives, simple white dinnerware, and high-end copper pots and pans. A cafe in the front of the store served high-end coffee drinks and homemade pastries, which customers enjoyed while shopping or at stools overlooking Broadway and Prince Street. Over the years it became a popular epicurean destination for both locals and visitors.

Following the opening of the flagship store, Dean & DeLuca opened smaller stores in Rockefeller Center and in the Paramount Hotel. Over the years, Dean & DeLuca cafes and stores opened in such cities as Washington, D.C.; Helena, California; and Charlotte, North Carolina. In 2003, Dean & DeLuca began licensing stores internationally; the first was in Tokyo. Additional Dean & DeLuca stores in Japan, Dubai, South Korea, Singapore, Qatar, Thailand, and Turkey soon followed.

The Dean & DeLuca brand celebrates high-quality prepared food and the best ingredients, tools, and kitchen items from around the world. Visitors to the retail stores can find different cuts of meats, poultry, fish, freshly made breads, fresh cheeses, a case of desserts, artisanal chocolate, and seasonal fruits and vegetables. There are also many Dean & DeLuca–branded items, from spice collections to teas, as well as ingredients from Portugal, Italy, France, England, and elsewhere around the globe. Some of the stores also have cafes serving coffee, tea, and espresso drinks as well as croissants, cupcakes, and other sweets. In 2014, Dean & DeLuca's located its headquarters in Wichita, Kansas.

See also BALDUCCI'S and ZABAR'S.

Dean & DeLuca website: http://www.deandeluca.com.
"Dean & DeLuca, Inc. History." Funding Universe. http://www.fundinguniverse.com/company-histories/dean-deluca-inc-history.
Hall, Trish. "A Bigger Bite at Dean & DeLuca." *New York Times*, November 9, 1988.
"The Holy Trinity." The SoHo Memory Project, May 21, 2011. http://sohomemory.com/tag/dean-and-deluca.

Tracey Ceurvels

Decker Farm

See STATEN ISLAND.

Deep-Fried Twinkies

Deep-fried Twinkies, a treat now widely seen on the fair food circuit, are widely credited to an English expat in Park Slope, Brooklyn. Christopher Sell, a native of Rugby, England, is the proprietor of Brooklyn fish-and-chips restaurant ChipShop and concocted the delicacy in 2001, when the restaurant first opened. In addition to fried fish, menu offerings included fried candy bars such as Mars and Snickers Bars, both longtime treats in Scotland.

To pass the time one evening, Sell and his coworkers began tossing random junk food items into the shop's industrial deep fryer and found that the Twinkie worked well as a fried treat. The result, which devotees compare to a beignet or a soufflé, is crispy outside and has a soft, pudding-like interior. The deep-fried Twinkie has become a regular on the fair food circuit, joining other fried snacks such as funnel cake and curly fries.

Hostess Brands, the original maker of Twinkies, declared bankruptcy in 2012, making the cream-filled snack cakes challenging to obtain (deep-fried or otherwise) for a while. Interstate Bakeries, the parent company of Hostess prior to the bankruptcy, had been active in promoting the concept of fried Twinkies to vendors at state and county fairs, helping to popularize the treat. After two investment firms purchased the confections company in 2013, Twinkies returned to shelves in the New York area, allowing junk food aficionados to breathe a sigh of relief.

The Park Slope location of ChipShop, where the deep-fried Twinkie originated, closed its doors on December 24, 2014. However, a Brooklyn Heights location on Atlantic Avenue remains open.

Clark, Melissa. "Fry That Twinkie, but Hold the Chips." *New York Times*, May 15, 2002.

Kara Newman

De Gouy, Louis P.

Louis P. De Gouy (1869–1947), a Frenchman by birth, was a New York chef, restaurateur, and cookbook author who also served as *Gourmet* magazine's "Gourmet Chef." De Gouy trained under his father and cooked for the Austrian royal family and with Auguste Escoffier, the famed French chef. During the World War I, De Gouy served as cook for the Fifth Army Corps of the American Expeditionary Force in France and subsequently became an American citizen. He supervised the kitchens of several royal families in Europe and cooked in French, English, Spanish, and American hotels and restaurants, including the Hôtel de Paris; The Carlton in London; the Royal Casino in San Sebastian, Spain; and the Waldorf Astoria in New York City. He was also the chef aboard J. P. Morgan's yacht on the financier's voyage around the world. In 1931, De Gouy opened the Institute of Modern and Practical Cooking in New York City and became a consultant to *Hotel Management* and *Restaurant Management* magazines. In 1940 he joined the staff of the soon-to-debut *Gourmet* magazine as its "Gourmet Chef," a position he held until his death in 1947.

De Gouy's first publication was *The Cookery Book* (1936), one in a series of twenty-five-cent paperbacks put out by the Leisure League of America; his second work, *The Derrydale Cook Book of Fish and Game* (1937), was written for the Derrydale Press, a prestigious publisher of sporting books. In 1939 he published *The Chef's Cook Book of Profitable Recipes*, a manual for "hotels, restaurants, clubs, soda fountains, hospitals, schools, homes."

In 1947 De Gouy collected his recipes and his columns from *Gourmet* magazine into a 1,256-page tome, *The Gold Cook Book* (1947), with more than 2,400 recipes. Oscar Tschirky, former maître d'hôtel of the Waldorf Astoria (and De Gouy's friend for forty years), wrote the introduction. De Gouy died the week the cookbook was published. Two manuscripts he had completed before his death, *The Soup Book* and *The Salad Book*, were both published in 1949.

De Gouy's widow later repackaged his recipes into single-subject collections including books on oysters, breads, hamburgers, cocktails, pies, and ice cream desserts. De Gouy is credited with twenty-one cookbooks, although most of the titles were published posthumously.

See also GOURMET and TSCHIRKY, OSCAR.

De Gouy, Louis P. *The Derrydale Cook Book of Fish and Game*. New York: Derrydale, 1937.
De Gouy, Louis P. *The Gold Cook Book*. New York: Greenberg, 1947.

Andrew F. Smith

DeGroff, Dale

Considered the founding father of modern bartending, Dale DeGroff is credited with reviving and reinventing the profession of mixology and pioneering a culinary approach to recreating the great classic cocktails. Born September 21, 1948, Rhode Island native DeGroff initially moved to New York City in 1969, intending to become an actor. He found himself drawn to saloons and jazz clubs even then, he recalls.

DeGroff began his bartending career in Manhattan in 1975. His training was by no means formal and came at a time when cocktail culture in the United States was not yet widely respected. He worked as a bartender at parties at the Gracie Mansion and at the Hotel Bel-Air in Los Angeles before connecting with well-known restaurateur Joseph Baum in 1985.

Back in New York City, DeGroff was behind the bar at Aurora Restaurant first and later at the Rainbow Room, where Baum steered him toward old cocktail books, such as Jerry Thomas's late-1800s classic *The Bon Vivant's Companion*, for inspiration to reconstruct and tinker with cocktail methods.

DeGroff surely delivered, becoming well known for his cocktail creations at the Rainbow Room, where he presided as chief mixologist for over a decade. He was arguably the first post-Prohibition bartender to emphasize fresh juices and other ingredients for making cocktails and without doubt sowed the seeds of what would become the new millennium's cocktail renaissance.

DeGroff also is widely credited with reinventing the bartending profession and influencing the next generation of mixologists. In particular, he is noted for mentoring Audrey Saunders, who went on to found the Pegu Club and other ventures and subsequently influenced the following generation of bartenders herself.

DeGroff is the founding president of the Museum of the American Cocktail in New Orleans. It is the first museum dedicated to the history of and education about mixology.

See also BAUM, JOE; MIXOLOGY; RAINBOW ROOM; SAUNDERS, AUDREY; and THOMAS, JERRY.

DeGroff, Dale. *The Craft of the Cocktail*. New York: Clarkson Potter, 2002.

Kara Newman

De Gustibus

See COOKING SCHOOLS and LATE TWENTIETH CENTURY.

Delis, German

Six million Germans arrived in America from 1820 to World War I; they were the largest immigrant group in the United States in the middle part of the nineteenth century as a result of agricultural failures and political conditions that drove many central Europeans to emigrate. Germans brought with them a predilection for the foods of their homeland and were particularly enamored of *Delikatessen*, a word for exotic foods that stems from the Latin word *delicatus* (fine, refined, desirable, alluring, voluptuous) and that had also come in Germany to refer to the actual stores in which these foods were sold. (The popular belief that the English word "delicatessen" comes from the German word *essen* [to eat] is incorrect.) As German imperial power grew, the *Delikatessen* in Berlin, Dresden, and Cologne were also known as *Colonialwaren* (purveyors of goods from the colonies). They retailed fancy foods to a rising

bourgeoisie that sought to flatter itself on its newfound purchasing power, social status, and cosmopolitanism.

Dallmayr, a *Delikatessen* store in Munich (which still exists to this day) opened in the seventeenth century; it was called *Königlich Bayerischer Hoflieferant* (Royal Bavarian Purveyor to the Court) because it made daily deliveries to Luitpold, the prince regent of Bavaria. Dallmayr also introduced the German public to bananas, mangoes, and plums, which it brought back from both China and the Canary Islands. The window displays of the *Delikatessen* were so elaborate that the nineteenth-century composer Edvard Grieg compared them to a symphony of symmetry, light, and color; the central element was typically the head of a wild boar. The *Delikatessen* were especially famed for their *wurst* (sausages) since these had been a staple of German cuisine for centuries; each of the dozens of different districts of Germany had developed its own particular type, from *Blutwurst* (pig's blood sausage) to *Weisswurst* (Bavarian white sausage, customarily made from veal).

The first mention of the word "delicatessen" in the *New York Times* appears in 1875, in the context of an amusing court case involving a German delicatessen owner, Caesar Wall, who sued his business partner, August Rath, after Wall's daughter broke up her engagement to Rath and Rath withdrew his funds from the business. But it was H. W. Borchardt, who had opened an iconic food store in his native Berlin in 1853 and then relocated to Grand Street on New York's Lower East Side in 1868, who became the first well-known German delicatessen owner in the United States. Borchardt sold a tempting variety of cooked meats, hard cheeses, fancy canned foods, imported teas, olive oil, and other high-end groceries. Over the next few decades, Borchardt was joined by other German immigrants who opened similar takeout stores but with prices that enabled even the poor to buy small quantities of food for pennies.

By the turn of the twentieth century, the popularity of German delicatessen foods grew rapidly among non-Germans as well, to the extent that by 1895, according to the *New York Tribune*, there were six hundred delicatessens in the city (90 percent of which were located on the Lower East Side), with all but a dozen carrying German names. As a result, according to the *New York Tribune*, Americans of all backgrounds sampled *Kartoffelsalat* (potato salad), *Pumpernickel* (brown bread), and *Lebkuchen* (spice cookies), while *Kalteraufschnitt* (sliced cold cuts) had become "a joy to the housekeeper and a refuge in time of unexpected guests." These delicatessens also sold basic grocery items like milk, bread, and eggs. Black-mirrored signs advertised cold cuts (often Boar's Head or Dietz and Watson) along with light-up signs to advertise beer (typically Rheingold or Schlitz).

During the 1920s, critic H. L. Mencken observed the significant effect of the German migration on American culture, as shown by the nationwide adoption of many German words, including "delicatessen," "hamburger," "frankfurter," and "pretzel." However, the German delicatessen was by this time already beginning to be superseded by the Jewish delicatessen; Jews (many of whom were German, including the Berlin-born Isaac Gellis, who established a prominent sausage factory on the Lower East Side in 1873) had developed their own type of pickled meat and sausage store, at first serving exclusively kosher provisions. See DELIS, JEWISH. The German delicatessen also declined with the overall backlash against German foods that occurred during both world wars; during World War I, in particular, a number of German foods were renamed so that sauerkraut was called "liberty cabbage" and hamburgers were dubbed "liberty steaks."

A few German delicatessens still exist in New York; the best known is Schaller & Weber, opened in 1927 in the Yorkville section of Manhattan, to which many Germans had relocated from *Kleindeutschland* in the early part of the twentieth century. In addition to German sausages, cheeses, breads, and jellies, it sells delicacies like spaetzle (dumplings), liver patés, and the German candies *Gummibärchen* (gummy bears) and marzipan (almond paste).

See also GERMAN and SCHALLER & WEBER.

"A Delicatessen Pioneer." *New York Tribune*, August 2, 1903.
Grimes, William. *Appetite City: A Culinary History of New York*. New York: North Point, 2010.
"Love, Sausages, and Law." *New York Times*, March 27, 1875.
Mencken, H. L. *The American Language: An Inquiry into the Development of English in the United States*. New York: Knopf, 1921. See p. 103, note 36.
Schwartz, Arthur. *New York City Food: An Opinionated History and More Than 100 Legendary Recipes*. New York: Stewart, Tabori & Chang, 2008.

Ted Merwin

Delis, Jewish

The Jewish delicatessen, or deli, is among the most iconic of informal dining establishments in New York City's history. Jewish delicatessens serve a wide variety of foods from Eastern and Central European Jewish cuisines, but they are primarily known for their cured meat sandwiches, smoked fishes, and accompaniments such as pickles, coleslaw, knishes, chopped liver paste, and flavored seltzers. With their unapologetically robust foods and atmosphere, Jewish delis have come to symbolize New York City.

The Jewish deli originates with the mid-nineteenth century German delicatessen stores in New York, which often sold specialty and prepared foods, as well as cured meats and occasionally sandwiches ("delicatessen" is roughly translated as a store for edible delicacies). See DELIS, GERMAN. By the late nineteen and early twentieth centuries, Eastern European Jewish delicatessens had made their appearance, particularly on the Lower East Side. Katz's Delicatessen may have been the first to open in 1888, and it is still the oldest operating deli in New York City. See KATZ'S DELICATESSEN.

Early Jewish delicatessens served unpretentious and reasonably priced smoked or cured meat or fish (often in sandwich form), soups, and other modest foods from regions across Eastern and Central Europe. For example, alongside Romanian pastrami or German salami they served Ukrainian borscht or Polish gefilte fish. Such intermingling of foods under one roof could only have occurred within the context of New World immigration. Perhaps because they offered this amalgam of Jewish immigrant tastes, delicatessens soon became popular gathering spots for many Jews, be they garment workers between shifts or young families looking for a satisfying yet affordable meal.

Some Jewish delicatessens served only kosher meat, but many were kosher style, meaning that they served meat not certified as kosher but did not serve dairy (to avoid mixing with meat) or any pork and shellfish products. With Jewish acculturation to the mainstream, however, the concept of "kosher-style" delicatessens broadened to include smoked meat sandwiches with slices of cheese or luscious New York–style cheesecakes for dessert—if not the occasional ham sandwich. In other words, Jewish delicatessens served the comfort foods of the Old Country along with foods American Jews discovered in the New World.

The heyday of Jewish delicatessens—when they became institutions frequented not just by Jews but by all New Yorkers and tourists—extended from the 1920s through midcentury, with institutions such as Lindy's, Reuben's, the Stage Deli, and the still-operating Carnegie Deli and Katz's Delicatessen. Jews and non-Jews alike flocked to Jewish delicatessens for the food and the scene: the bickering if loving waiters, the din of the boisterous room, and the characters who populated the scene. For example, notorious gangster and alleged fixer of the 1919 World Series Arnold Rothstein preferred a table at Lindy's as his regular "office." See LINDY'S.

Unlike earlier Jewish delicatessens, which were located in Lower Manhattan, several of the delis of the early midcentury operated in Midtown, near Broadway's theaters, and catered to stars such as Eddie Cantor and Fannie Brice, as well as other actors and comedians of the entertainment industry—many of whom were Jewish. Al Jolson is said to have closed his shows at the Winter Garden Theatre by asking his audiences to join him for sandwiches at the nearby Lindy's. Indeed, it was the sandwiches that brought throngs to Lindy's. According to one profile of the deli these included "simple sandwiches" like corned beef, or creamed cheese with lox, and such combinations as "lake sturgeon and Nova Scotia salmon; Wiltshire ham and Swiss cheese; ox-tongue, Swiss cheese, tomatoes, and Indian relish; Fiddler's creek smoked turkey and chicken liver; breast of turkey with pastrami and chicken fat."

The sandwiches and the scene at Jewish delicatessens attracted New Yorkers of every walk of life and visitors to the city as well. In 1961 Craig Claiborne lovingly described Katz's Delicatessen in the *New York Times*: "Known as Katz's Delicatessen, it is a wonderfully aromatic institution that reeks with the robust odors of garlic-flavored salami, pickles, mustard and freshly made sauerkraut....At 10 in the morning or at midnight the customers, from taxi drivers to Madison Avenue executives, appease their hunger with any lavish assortment of sandwiches."

During the immediate postwar period, migration and suburbanization spread Jewish delicatessens across the country. However, as the baby boomers came of age, growing health concerns and new food trends led many Jewish delis to close. Nevertheless, New York City continued to be associated with Jewish delicatessens, even as they began to decline

in numbers. Those that remained into the late twentieth and early twenty-first centuries—Katz's, the Carnegie Deli, the Stage Deli, the Second Avenue Deli, and a few others—became hallmarks of Jewish culture for all New Yorkers. Nearly every New York City mayor in recent history has been photographed in Jewish delicatessens enjoying a pastrami sandwich or other classic deli fare.

Perhaps the most famous New York City Jewish delicatessen moment is Meg Ryan's "I'll have what she's having" scene with Billy Crystal in Katz's Delicatessen during Rob Reiner's 1989 film *When Harry Met Sally*. While not everyone may derive quite as much (feigned) pleasure as Sally does from deli, Jewish delicatessens remain an unparalleled part of the fabric of New York City restaurant culture to this day.

See also CORNED BEEF SANDWICH; JEWISH; KNISH; LOX; PASTRAMI; and SMOKED FISH.

Berger, Meyer. "Sturgeon Saga of the Main Stem." *New York Times*, May 22, 1949.
Claiborne, Craig. "Food News: Meal Is Any Time at Delicatessen." *New York Times*, April 25, 1961.
Sax, David. *Save the Deli: In Search of the Perfect Pastrami, Crusty Rye, and the Heart of the Jewish Delicatessen.* Boston: Houghton Mifflin Harcourt, 2009.

Lara Rabinovitch

Delmonico Brothers

Giovanni Del-Monico (1788–1842) and his brother Pietro Antonio (1783–1860) were born in the Swiss canton of Ticino, on the Italian border. Pietro became a pastry chef and confectioner in Berne. Giovanni took a very different tack, becoming a sailor. By 1818 he owned and commanded a schooner engaged in trade, mainly between the United States and the Caribbean. In about 1824 he sold the ship and settled permanently in Manhattan. He anglicized his name to John and opened a wine shop. At the time, most Americans did not drink wine, so his customers were mostly French and other European immigrants or foreign visitors. To maximize profits, he imported casks of wine from Spain and France and did the bottling himself. By 1826 he was ready to try his hand at something new; he sold the shop and sailed off to visit his family in Switzerland.

While in Switzerland, John Delmonico convinced his younger brother to come to New York and be his partner in opening a cafe. Pietro brought his family to New York and changed his first name to Peter, and in 1827 the brothers opened a small cafe and pastry shop at 23 William Street. They had accumulated considerable capital, and both were experienced businessmen. As the enterprise grew, other members of the family emigrated to take a hand in it, notably nineteen-year-old Lorenzo Delmonico (1812–1881), a son of Peter and John's elder brother, who arrived in 1831 and began working at the restaurant.

To supply their restaurant with fresh vegetables and other provisions, in 1835 the brothers bought a farm in the eastern part of the city of Brooklyn. When John died in 1842, the business was in debt and the farm was sold to raise money. Sixty-one-year-old Peter Delmonico assigned control of the firm to Lorenzo, and under his guidance the restaurant paid its debts and flourished for the next eighty years. In 1848, Peter sold his share of the restaurant to Lorenzo and retired. Peter Delmonico died in 1860. John and Peter Delmonico were buried in the family vault at the old St. Patrick's Church, now the Basilica of St. Patrick's Old Cathedral, at the corner of Mott and Prince Streets in Manhattan.

See also DELMONICO'S.

Thomas, Lately. *Delmonico's: A Century of Splendor*. Boston: Houghton Mifflin, 1967.

Andrew F. Smith

Delmonico's

Delmonico's was one of New York's premier restaurants from 1837 until 1923. It was launched by Swiss immigrant brothers John and Peter Delmonico, who opened a modest cafe and pastry shop at 27 William Street in downtown Manhattan in December 1827. At its six tables, patrons could enjoy European-style pastries, ices, bonbons, cakes, and coffee. In March 1830, the cafe was expanded into a dining establishment listed in the city directory as "Delmonico & Brother, Restaurant Français." It was New York's— and one of America's—first stand-alone restaurant.

After the original restaurant burned down in the Great Fire of 1835, the Delmonicos secured a triangular piece of property at the corner of what is today William and Beaver Streets, across the street from the original. There, in 1837, they opened a larger restaurant, offering salads and other novel French dishes. The eleven-page menu listed a full selection of French dishes (with English translations opposite), such as *potage aux huitres, salade de chicorée, blanquette de veau á la Perigueux*, and *meringues á la crème*, as well as an impressive French wine list. Their clientele consisted of tourists, businessmen, and an increasingly affluent American upper class.

From the beginning, Delmonico's was lauded for the quality of its food and the acumen of its proprietors. Frederick Marryat, an English naval officer, traveler, and novelist who visited Delmonico's in the 1830s, described the "excellent" French food. Half a century later, English visitor and travel writer George Sala celebrated the restaurant. Writing in the 1880s, Sala wondered, "How many tens of thousands of dollars a week Mr. Delmonico is clearing I do not know...but his palatial establishment, as well as scores of these restaurants and cafes, continually overflow with guests." Sala described Delmonico's first floor, with its "immense café, and a public restaurant of equal dimensions, while on the second floor, there are first a magnificent saloon which can be used as a ball room or as a dining hall, and next a series of private rooms for select dinner parties; on the upper floors are a limited number of furnished apartments for gentlemen." (Sala, 1883, p. 90) A visiting Frenchman, Georges Savuvin, upped the ante considerably when he reported in 1893 that the food at Delmonico's was "better and more sumptuous" than that served "in the best restaurant in Paris."

Delmonico's remained one of the city's premier restaurants throughout the nineteenth century, periodically moving north and adding new premises as the city expanded. In 1848, Alessandro Filippini was hired as a cook; over the years he rose to the post of *chef de cuisine*, finally becoming the manager of one of the Delmonico's restaurants. Filippini, who, like his employers, was Swiss, was one of the driving forces promoting the restaurant's culinary renown. When he retired in 1888, he began writing cookbooks; the first, *The Table*, presented simplified versions of dishes he had prepared at the restaurant.

The French-born chef Charles Ranhofer, who had been hired at Delmonico's in 1862 and became Filippini's successor as *chef de cuisine*, flattered his most notable patrons by naming dishes after them. In 1894, Ranhofer produced his masterwork, *The Epicurean*, the most comprehensive French cookbook to have been published in the United States. The book

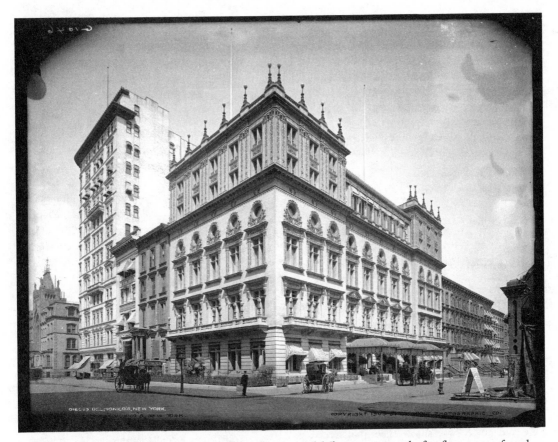

The exterior of Delmonico's, circa 1903. The different floors served different purposes; the first floor was a cafe, and upper floors contained lounges and even apartments for businessmen to socialize and stay in, if needed. LIBRARY OF CONGRESS

described food preparation and service in minute detail and featured menus for every imaginable occasion. Leopold Rimmer, who managed one of Delmonico's dining rooms in its heyday, stated that there was "hardly one hotel in New-York to-day whose chef did not learn his cooking at Delmonico's, every one of them." When *The Epicurean* was published, Rimmer complained that Ranhofer had given "away all the secrets of the house" (Rimmer, 1898).

When Prohibition became law in 1920, French restaurants were hit hard. Fine wines were part of the dining experience, and alcohol accounted for a substantial portion of a restaurant's profits. Restaurants lost customers as America's wealthy decamped for Europe during the summer. In May 1923, after nearly a century of glorious history, Delmonico's closed.

Four books and hundreds of articles have been published about Delmonico's, and Ranhofer's *Epi-* *curean* has rarely been out of print. The Delmonico's name has been subsequently used by many restaurateurs. In 1934 an Italian immigrant, Oscar Tucci, acquired the location of a former Delmonico's at Beaver and William Streets and opened a restaurant named Oscar's OlDelmonico's (later renamed Delmonico's); it survived until 1977. In 1998, the Bice Group opened Delmonico's Restaurant at the same location at the corner of Beaver and Williams Streets. The owners have renovated the restaurant to recreate its nineteenth-century style. Choosing from today's menu, it would be difficult to order a complete dinner for under $80.

See also ANTEBELLUM; DELMONICO BROTHERS; GILDED AGE; MANHATTAN; PROHIBITION; RANHOFER, CHARLES; and RESTAURANTS.

Brown, Henry Collins. *Delmonico's: A Story of Old New York*. New York: Valentine's Manual, 1928.

Choate, Judith, and James Canora. *Dining at Delmonico's: The Story of America's Oldest Restaurant*. New York: Stewart, Tabori & Chang, 2008.

Delmonico's Restaurant Group website: http://www.delmonicosrestaurantgroup.com/restaurant.

Thomas, Lately. *Delmonico's: A Century of Splendor*. Boston: Houghton Mifflin, 1967.

Ranhofer, Charles. *The Epicurean*. New York: Ranhofer, 1894.

Rimmer, Leopold. *A History of Old New York Life and the House of the Delmonicos*. New York: Privately printed, 1898.

Sala, George. *America Revisited: From the Bay of New York to the Gulf of Mexico*. London: Vizetelly, 1883.

Andrew F. Smith

Department Store Restaurants

The first true shopping emporium or "department store" in New York was retailer Alexander Turney Stewart's Marble Palace located at Broadway and Chambers Street, across from City Hall Park. Opened in 1846, the Marble Palace employed the new convention of selling a variety of ready-made retail goods in one location, divided by department or floor. By the second half of the nineteenth century Macy's, B. Altman, and Lord & Taylor stores on the "Ladies Mile" and later Stewart's Iron Palace joined the big-store movement and had outlets spanning Broadway and Sixth Avenues from Ninth to Twenty-Third Streets. See MACY'S.

With their female clientele came a particular need: a place to dine. Few public restaurants admitted ladies eating alone, and the early versions of these emporiums offered makeshift lunch counter–type fare, usually prepared off-site and brought into the store. While local restaurateurs complained about the competition, predicting the failure of department store restaurants because of their substandard fare, eventually these eateries evolved into "tea rooms," with light fare prepared on-site but lacking the same high-end, service-oriented nature of the larger retail experience. See TEAROOMS. By the early twentieth century stores outside of New York City, most notably Marshall Fields of Chicago and Wannamaker's of Philadelphia, created more elegant restaurants on-site, including soda fountains and fashionable grill rooms.

It was not until after the Great Depression that the grand New York City department stores entered into the fray, creating notable and stylish restaurants that were worthy of a trip to the store for their own

sake. These included Lord & Taylor's BirdCage as well as the Soup Bar billed for men and the Milk Bar billed for children. B. Altman boasted a full-sized replica of an antebellum southern mansion façade and garden in its Charleston Garden restaurant.

A latecomer, Bloomingdale's Le Train Bleu, opened in 1979 and was fashioned after a luxury train dining car. It is still in operation today. See RAILROAD DINING.

In the 1970s, New York's economic troubles affected its large-scale retail outlets, and their restaurants began to fade into obsolescence as suburban areas around the city built their own indoor shopping malls, which flourished during the economic rebound of the 1980s and into the 1990s and early 2000s. But a resurgence of elegant, review-worthy department store dining began again in the early 2000s. Notable twenty-first-century department store restaurants included Fred's at Barneys New York, BG at Bergdorf Goodman, Sarabeth's Bakery at Lord & Taylor, Stella 34 at Macy's, Café SFA at Saks Fifth Avenue, as well as restaurants housed in luxury boutiques such as Armani Ristorante at Giorgio Armani, ABC Cocina at ABC Carpet & Home, and the restaurant at Tommy Bahama.

Gold, Jessica. "Rediscovering Retail's Past: B. Altman." *Truth Plus*, May 20, 2011. http://truthplusblog.com/2011/05/20/rediscovering-retails-past-b-altman/.

Leach, William. *Land of Desire: Merchants, Power, and the Rise of a New American Culture*. New York: Vintage, 1993.

"The Charleston Garden, B. Altman & Co., Fifth Avenue, New York, Date Unknown." Restaurant Menus. ScholarsArchive@JWU. Paper 97. 2014. http://scholarsarchive.jwu.edu/restaurant_menus/97.

Whitaker, Jan. *Service and Style, How the American Department Store Fashioned the Middle Class*. New York: St. Martin's, 2006.

Ramin Ganeshram

Depression Food

The Great Depression hit New York City in the early months of 1930, ending eight years of prosperity. A sharp drop in prices coupled with lower profits led many industries to cut their workforces. New Yorkers suddenly found themselves confronted by breadlines and shabbily dressed men begging pennies for coffee. There was no government safety net in 1930 New York. Unemployed workers had to either find new jobs or turn for help to relatives and friends. If these did not come through, they would

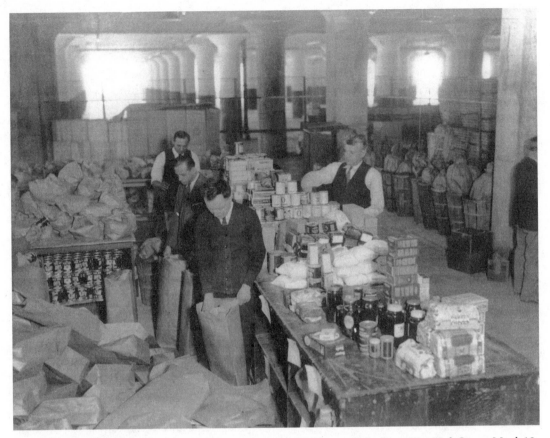

Workmen sort individual 25-pound packages of nonperishable food for needy families in New York City on March 18, 1932. The Emergency Unemployment Relief Committee established the central depot and share-a-meal drive to provide food during the Great Depression. AP IMAGES

often pawn all their possessions and eventually end up on the street, homeless and hungry.

The breadlines that sprang up to serve the newly unemployed offered either servings of bread, fatty stew, and coffee or meal tickets for Lower Manhattan eateries catering largely to down-and-outs. There, poor men could get doughnuts and coffee for a nickel or a hamburger "steak" and a roll for a dime. Women in need tended not to patronize breadlines or these restaurants, instead doubling up with friends or family members and pooling their limited resources. However, charity leaders and civic leaders soon turned against breadlines, which had proliferated even in the city's most visible districts, deciding they were bad for both the city's image and the morale of the unemployed.

In late 1930, New York City banned breadlines, replacing them with a citywide free food distribution program that was deducted out of municipal workers' salaries. Unemployed families would line up once a week to receive their box of food supplies, usually potatoes, carrots, cabbage, turnips, canned tomatoes, beans, rice, macaroni, sugar, coffee, and evaporated milk. For the rest of the decade, official relief programs, variously supervised by the city, state, and federal governments, were a crucial source of food for the poor and unemployed. The relative amounts changed, but nearly all relief distributions included dairy products, inexpensive vegetables (particularly potatoes, cabbage, and canned tomatoes), and beans as a cheap source of protein. Milk was always the centerpiece of the relief diet, either by itself or mixed into recipes such as the near-ubiquitous white sauce. Children in particular were supposed to drink at least a quart of milk every day.

Despite these efforts, some New Yorkers still fell through the cracks. School nurses discovered many children who were sick and listless as a result of in-adequate food at home; hundreds of city dwellers died of malnutrition disorders and outright starvation, particularly in the early years of the crisis.

The Great Depression also changed the habits of many who managed to stay off relief rolls. Workers found their hours and wages cut, while the number of family members they had to support may have increased. In order to survive, many cut back on dining out and ate meat only once or twice a week, and then usually the cheaper cuts. To help them, charity organizations and newspaper food sections began to print pamphlets and articles giving economical recipes and menus that showed how to live on as little as $2.25 worth of food a week. Recipes often relied on milk as well as on meat substitutes such as peas and all kinds of beans. An economical but ample lunch could include macaroni and cheese, shredded cabbage salad, peanut butter sandwiches, applesauce, and milk. However, New Yorkers discovered that these recommended diets were bland, monotonous, and, at their most economical, insufficient. People lost weight so quickly on diets claiming to provide adequate nutrition for less than fifty cents a day that they returned to the traditional foods of poverty—bread, potatoes, fried meat, and coffee—before they wasted away altogether.

Despite the Depression's severity, not all New Yorkers faced economic pressures. A lucky few managed to live, and eat, very well, particularly after the repeal of Prohibition in 1933. As speakeasies closed and people began focusing less on booze and more on food, the restaurant industry rebounded, while the wealthy and cultural elite began to take more interest in the quality and preparation of their food. Dedicated eaters promoted fine dining through groups such as Les Amis d'Escoffier and the Gourmet Society. They enjoyed local and regional specialties such as planked shad, oyster stew, lobster Newberg, Virginia ham, New Orleans gumbo, Lake Superior whitefish, and all kinds of imported foods. The New Year's Day 1939 dinner prepared by the epicure Crosby Gaige included champagne, beluga caviar, chicken consommé, roast Long Island duck, braised celery, Brussels sprouts, and avocado salad, with a ripe brie, coffee, and brandy for dessert. Four months later, the New York World's Fair opened, bringing a wealth of restaurants and some of Europe's greatest chefs to New York. Even as the city was focused on the culinary bounty at the Flushing fair grounds, thousands of New Yorkers remained unemployed and reliant on government food distributions to keep their families from going hungry.

See also BREADLINES and PROHIBITION.

"For Gourmets and Others: Two New Year's Day Menus." *New York Times*, December 25, 1938, p. 25.
Gillett, Lucy H. *Food for Health's Sake: What to Eat.* 2d ed. New York: Funk & Wagnalls, 1937.
Mayor's Official Committee. "Report of the Activities of the Mayor's Committee for the Relief of the Unemployed and Needy of the City of New York, October 31 to June 30, 1931." New York, 1931.

Andrew Coe

De Voe, Thomas Farrington

Thomas Farrington De Voe (1811–1892) was a market butcher, public official, and historian. Apprenticed as a boy to a butcher at Washington Market, he became a leading member of the trade and a prominent spokesperson for city market butchers' interests at a time of rapid, controversial changes in both the meat business and the general market system.

Though De Voe had no formal education, in middle age he developed an interest in the New York City market records owned by the New-York Historical Society. Exploring them while also drawing on his own firsthand market experience, he produced the two best primary sources of knowledge about the nineteenth-century New York City markets and the articles of food they supplied. *The Market Book* (1862) provided chronologies of all the major Manhattan markets since the first New Netherland Dutch settlement. *The Market Assistant* (1867) described the butcher's meats, fish, furred and feathered game, and fruits and vegetables sold at market in different seasons. In addition, De Voe wrote a long paper, published in 1866 as "Abattoirs," summarizing the history of the New York butchering trade and comparing the city's slaughterhouse facilities with Old World counterparts, from a health and sanitation viewpoint.

He eventually gave up his own slaughterhouse and market stall to serve twice as superintendent of markets (1871–1876 and 1881–1884) under reforming mayoral administrations determined to root out rampant bribery and shakedowns from the public markets' stall-licensing and inspection system. During his first term he published a report on the condition of the markets, describing the prevalence of "blackmailing abuse" and proposing improved supervisory measures.

De Voe's sturdy, humorous personality shines through both his published works and his voluminous manuscript materials at the historical society. He is the chief source of information about many areas of the city's food history that otherwise would be complete blanks.

De Voe, Thomas F. The *Market Assistant*. New York: Hurd and Houghton, 1867.

De Voe, Thomas F. *The Market Book, Containing a Historical Account of the Public Markets*. Vol. 1. New York: Printed for the author, 1862.

Mendelson, Anne. "To Market, to Market: A Profile of Thomas F. DeVoe." *NYFoodStory* 1 (2012): 3, 14–15.

Anne Mendelson

Diat, Louis

Louis Diat (1885–1957) was one of New York's most renowned chefs during the first half of the twentieth century. Born in Montmarault, near Vichy, France, Diat learned *la cuisine bourgeois* (home cooking) from his mother, Anne Alajoinine Diat, and his grandmother. At the age of fourteen, he was apprenticed at Maison Calondre, a restaurant in nearby Moulins. Two years later he moved to Paris, where he worked at the Hôtel Bristol and the Hôtel du Rhin. In 1903 Diat became *chef potager* (soup cook) at the Hôtel Ritz. Three years later he transferred to the newly opened Ritz Hotel in London. His next move was to New York, where he became chef of the roof-garden restaurant at the Ritz-Carlton Hotel, which opened in 1910. Diat eventually rose to the position of *chef de cuisine* of the entire hotel. He served in this position until the hotel closed in 1951. During those forty-one years Diat was responsible for hundreds of dinners and banquets attended by the city's notables as well as visiting dignitaries, aristocrats, and royals.

Diat published his first cookbook, *Cooking à la Ritz*, in 1941. It included a recipe for *crème vichyssoise glacée*, a rich, creamy chilled potato and leek soup that Diat claimed to have devised himself, based on a meal he had often enjoyed as a child. He reportedly first served it at the Ritz-Carlton during the summer of 1917, and by 1924 it had become a regular menu item. Others claimed to have invented the soup, but Diat popularized it. Other dishes credited to Diat include many that he named after famous Americans: guinea hen Jefferson, chicken Gloria Swanson, and pears Mary Garden.

Decades before the advent of nouvelle cuisine, with its insistence upon the finest, freshest produce, Diat championed that cause. When he required items that were not typically on the American market at the time, such as baby vegetables, shallots, leeks, and watercress, local farmers were engaged to grow them. Rich cream was shipped daily from Vermont.

Earle MacAusland, publisher of *Gourmet*, commissioned Diat to write for the magazine. When Louis De Gouy, *Gourmet*'s "Gourmet Chef," died in 1947, Diat became the magazine's in-house chef, and the column Menus Classiques appeared under his name. Diat went on to publish three additional books, including the popular *French Cooking for Americans* (1946), which was considered the best French cookbook published in America for the next decade.

After Diat's death in 1957, *New York Times* food editor Jane Nickerson reported in the paper that Diat's articles and cookbooks had been written in collaboration with Helen E. Ridley, a home economics instructor who had also served on the editorial staffs of *McCall's* and *Good Housekeeping* magazines. At the time Ridley began working with Diat, she was the head of the food publicity department at J. Walter Thompson, the Ritz-Carlton Hotel's public relations firm. Her collaboration with Diat, however, was as a freelance writer and not an employee of the advertising agency. Diat supplied the recipes and techniques to Ridley, who translated them into recipes that Americans could follow.

Diat, Louis. *Cooking à la Ritz*. Philadelphia: Lippincott, 1941.

Diat, Louis. *French Cooking for Americans: La cuisine de ma mère*. Philadelphia: Lippincott, 1946.

Andrew F. Smith

Dimsum

Dimsum, especially the Cantonese variety, is one of the most recognizable Chinese food items in New York City. Similar in portion size to *tapas*, dimsum refers to bite-sized food items served in small dishes or bamboo steamers. Among the better-known dimsum items are *har-gauu* (shrimp dumpling), *siu-mai* (shrimp and pork potstickers), and *char-siu bao* (roast pork bun). Over two hundred savory or sweet dimsum with diverse protein, grain, and vegetable ingredients prepared by various cooking methods are regularly served at a wide variety of Chinese restaurants.

Dimsum, literally translated as "a touch of your heart," is frequently eaten during *yumcha* ("drinking tea"). *Yumcha* refers to the routine of people spending time in teahouses to enjoy their favorite Chinese tea and a few dimsum dishes while socializing with others, reading up on the news, or making deals. It began early in the twentieth century in southern China, most notably in Guangzhou, and evolved further in Hong Kong since the 1950s (Lum, 2013). Enjoying Chinese tea and dimsum over *yumcha* is a popular pastime among many Chinese immigrants around the world.

Nowadays, dimsum of all kinds are readily available at a multitude of venues: street vendors, takeout storefronts, neighborhood shops, mass-market or high-end hotel restaurants, haute establishments with an Asian fusion theme, and even the frozen food section of many supermarkets. *Yumcha* remains part of an entrenched subculture in the Chinese immigrant communities in New York City. Nom Wah Tea Parlor is one of the oldest dimsum eateries on Manhattan's Lower East Side, thus making it an easy choice for diners searching for an old-school Chinatown feel. Meanwhile, various other more contemporary Chinese restaurants, such as Golden Unicorn in Chinatown and Asian Jewels in Downtown Flushing, offer a much wider range of dimsum items.

See also CHINESE COMMUNITY.

Lum, Casey M. K. "Understanding Urban Foodways and Communicative Cities: A Taste of Hong Kong's Yumcha Culture as Urban Communication." In *Communicative Cities and Urban Communication in the 21st Century: The Urban Communication Reader III*, edited by Matthew D. Matsaganis, Victoria J. Gallenger, and Susan J. Drucker, pp. 53–76. New York: Peter Lang, 2013.

Casey Man Kong Lum

Diners

Diners originated as horse-drawn wooden lunch wagons in the late nineteenth century. They typically were blue-collar luncheonettes where customers ate their meals standing at a small indoor counter. Over time, these wagons increased in size, and high stools were added so that customers could sit at the counter. Menus were limited to coffee, sandwiches, and a few other items.

Some of New York City's earliest diners were launched by the Women's Auxiliary of the Church Temperance Society in 1893. The Prohibitionist organization opened a late-night lunch wagon that operated from 7:30 p.m. to 4:30 a.m. to draw business away from bars and saloons. The wagon offered tasty "lunches" for ten cents—cheap by New York standards—and the experiment proved a tremendous success: during its first year, sixty-seven thousand ten-cent lunches were served. By 1898 New York City had eight temperance lunch wagons, supplying 230,000 meals annually. The society used the net profits from the wagons to construct free "ice water fountains" to supply clean, fresh water in the city's tenement districts. See TEMPERANCE MOVEMENT.

During the early twentieth century, New York City restricted business hours for street vendors and passed zoning laws to ameliorate the congestion that was gripping the streets. Thereafter diners were transported to fixed locations, where they remained for months or years. Customers at first sat on stools located along a counter; later versions offered booths for customers and waitress service. The diner was basically a small restaurant, not much different from a main-street or highway cafe.

In the early twentieth century Patrick Tierney of New Rochelle, New York, upgraded the wooden wagon to a prefabricated structure that resembled a Pullman dining car, with side panels of enameled metal. (One New York City owner even named his establishment The Pullman Diner.) Its advantage was its modular construction, which made the diner relatively inexpensive to build, buy, and maintain. If a particular site proved unsuccessful, the diner could easily be disassembled and moved to a more promising site. See RAILROAD DINING.

The diners of the 1920s often boasted porcelain enamel interior walls, accented with oak trim, chrome, and glass. Later diners were outfitted with stainless steel exteriors; inside were colorful Formica counters and tabletops, booths upholstered in cushioned leatherette, and fluorescent lighting. An added attraction, beginning in the 1940s, was a tabletop device that allowed diners to make selections from the jukebox by remote control.

When Prohibition took effect in 1920, the free lunch offered by bars disappeared and diners became popular. When Prohibition ended in 1933, diners had established good customer bases and continued to thrive. Most opened early to provide breakfast for people on their way to work; many stayed open late, and some were open twenty-four hours, seven days a week. New Yorkers found all-night diners a good place to sober up after an evening of drinking.

Diner menus depended on the operators and their clientele. Breakfast specials made good use of the grill—various combinations of eggs, bacon, sausage, and hash browns, plus doughnuts, rolls, and coffee—lunch would be soup, cold and hot sandwiches, hamburgers, and hot dogs; and for dinner there were simple entrées like chicken pot pie or meat loaf, with perhaps a daily "blue-plate special"— a set meal, usually meat, potatoes, and a vegetable, served on a single plate, that changed almost daily. For dessert, there was usually pie (often homemade) and ice cream. Diners owned by first- or second-generation immigrants frequently included ethnic fare on their menus.

Just before World War II the owner of one diner construction company estimated that 90 percent of America's diners were within 100 miles of New York City. Early Manhattan diners were located on Manhattan's far west side, near the industrial district, the docks, and Washington Market, the city's huge wholesale food market. As second-generation immigrants moved out of Manhattan into the other boroughs, so did diners. During the 1940s, diner construction picked up in the Bronx and Queens, where two-thirds of all diner construction in the city was located by the 1950s. Few diners existed in Brooklyn and Staten Island. The number of diners in New York City began to decline in the 1960s as fast-food and casual restaurant chains flooded the city.

Greek immigrants revived the industry during the 1970s. Many diners that opened or were renovated during this period were flashier than their forebears with flamboyant touches such as replicas of Greek statuary, fountains, chandeliers, murals, tile work, and lots of mirrors. By the 1990s, it was estimated that two-thirds were Greek-owned. Their multipage menus ranged from the usual pot roast and rice pudding to Greek specialties: stuffed grape leaves, pastitsio, and Greek salad. During the early twenty-first century, many Greek owners retired and sold their diners to new immigrant groups, such as Latinos, Koreans, and Bangladeshis, who serve their own home cooking to a new generation of diner fans. In trendy neighborhoods like Long Island City and Williamsburg, adventurous chefs have turned old diners into cutting-edge restaurants.

The heyday of the stand-alone prefabricated New York City diner has long passed, but many remain scattered throughout the city. There is the Empire Diner in Chelsea, a well-preserved art moderne example from the Fodero Dining Car Company of Bloomfield, New Jersey; the Empire has been home to several upscale restaurants. Others, like the Pearl Diner in the Financial District, have remodeled or covered-over exteriors; but there is no mistaking the original details on the inside. The Airline Diner, near La Guardia Airport, retains its roadside charm but is now a branch of the Jackson Hole hamburger chain. The Jackson Diner in Jackson Heights, Queens, serves Indian food. The Tibbett Diner, in Riverdale, is a newer model but still a classic; the Wythe Diner in Williamsburg, Brooklyn, is now Café de La Esquina, a branch of a Mexican restaurant in SoHo.

See also COFFEE SHOPS; GREEK; and RESTAURANTS.

Baeder, John. *Diners*. New York: Abrams, 1995.
Engle, Michael, and Mario Monti. *Diners of New York*. Mechanicsburg, Pa.: Stackpole, 2008.
Gutman, Richard J. *American Diner, Then and Now*. New York: HarperPerennial, 1993.
Hurley, Andrew. *Diners, Bowling Alleys, and Trailer Parks: Chasing the American Dream in the Postwar Consumer Culture*. New York: Basic Books, 2002.

Andrew F. Smith

Diners Club

Frank X. McNamara, president of a New York finance company, came up with the idea for Diners Club, the world's first independent credit card intended for travel and restaurants. McNamara and two associates launched the service in 1950, initially giving the cards to two hundred friends and acquaintances.

Within months, Diners Club charged an annual $18 per card. Twenty-seven restaurants signed up at the program's onset; each agreed to pay a fee of 7 percent per transaction to Diners Club. The card was first used by McNamara at a restaurant called Major's Cabin Grill, near the Empire State Building; in the credit card industry this transaction is known as "The First Supper." By 1952 more than four hundred restaurants accepted the card. The card's range expanded abroad as restaurants and hotels in Canada, Cuba, and other countries signed up. By 1955 more than twenty thousand people held Diners Club cards, and the following year the company handled $290 million in transactions. In 1959 Diners Club went public, becoming the first credit card company listed on the New York Stock Exchange. By 1960, Diners Club was the largest U.S. card issuer, with 1.1 million members.

The success of Diners Club inspired competitors, including Carte Blanche and a *Gourmet* magazine credit card; but few of these lasted. American Express was the exception. It launched a credit card in 1958, targeted at well-to-do travelers; American Express distributed its cards through its travel offices throughout the United States. The popularity and profits of American Express surpassed those of Diners Club during the early 1960s.

Today, Diners Club cards are mostly held by affluent and well-traveled individuals, but it has been largely eclipsed by its competitors—American Express, Visa, MasterCard, and Discover. Diners Club is currently owned by CitiBank.

Evans, David S., and Richard Schmalensee. *Paying with Plastic: The Digital Revolution in Buying and Borrowing.* 2d ed. Cambridge, Mass.: MIT Press, 2005.

Andrew F. Smith

Dining Car

See RAILROAD DINING.

Distilleries

Distilleries that produced rum, whiskey, gin, and other spirits were an important industry in New York for the city's first three hundred years. William Kieft, the Dutch director-general of the colony, opened his first brandy distillery on Staten Island in 1638, and others soon followed. Rum was distilled in New York by the end of the seventeenth century. At least ten distilleries operated in the city by 1753, and two decades later there were seventeen, producing a half-million gallons of rum annually.

Rum and whiskey were the beverages of choice for the city's poor and working-class drinkers—spirits were cheap, and they gave more of a kick for the price than the more expensive beer and wine. By the mid-1820s New York State had 1,129 distilleries and New York City alone had more than sixteen hundred "spirit sellers," who sold whiskey for thirty-eight cents a gallon. Many German and Irish immigrants, who began arriving in the 1830s and 1840s, went into distilling. There was quite a range in the size of distilling operations: at one, the equipment consisted of a washtub and a cistern. Corn and hot water were placed in the tub and left to soak. Then rye was added, and the mixture was heated and cooled. Yeast was added, and the mash was then drained into the cistern to ferment, producing alcohol.

In 1829 Robert M. Hartley, the founder of the New York Temperance Society, investigated the city's distilling industry, focusing on the dairies that many of them operated as an adjunct to the production of spirits. Hartley found that the cows in these dairies were fed on the mash left after distilling liquor and that the so-called swill milk was one of the distillers' main profit sources. He concluded that those profits were so substantial that, if they were eliminated, the city's alcohol industry would collapse. By 1856 two-thirds of all milk sold in the city came from distillery dairies. Hartley had lifted the lid on a major scandal, and newspapers sent reporters to investigate the distilleries. The first article, in *Frank Leslie's Illustrated Newspaper,* "Startling Exposure of Milk Trade of New York and Brooklyn!" reported that the stables surrounding the distilleries were "disgusting, dilapidated and wretchedly filthy." The controversy heated up and turned violent when one of the newspaper's reporters was murdered while developing a story.

Distillers were well connected with the city's politicians, and they brushed off the newspaper exposés. In the 1860s they faced a much greater threat: federal tax agents who rightly concluded that most Brooklyn distilleries neglected to pay excise taxes on the spirits they produced. Agents tried to close down the offending distilleries, but their owners fought back. The "Whiskey War" commenced in 1869. Eventually, fifteen hundred federal troops were called up and sent into Brooklyn's distilling district to destroy the illegal stills and their whiskey stockpiles. It ended two years later with the withdrawal of the troops.

After the Whiskey War, New York distilleries—legal and illegal—revived, and the industry flourished until the United States declared war on Germany on April 6, 1917. Prohibition advocates linked prohibition and patriotism by denouncing distillers as "unpatriotic" for using grain needed for the war effort. In August 1917, Congress passed the Food and Fuel Control Act (Lever Act), which banned the use of foodstuffs in the production of whiskey and gin for the duration of the war as a way to conserve grain for use by the military and to send to America's allies. New York distilleries closed or were converted for other uses.

Most city distilleries did not reopen after the war ended in November 1918, and those that did were finished off by the passage of the national Prohibition amendment, the Eighteenth Amendment, which went into effect in January 1920. All distilleries were shut down, but illegal distilling operations quickly emerged, and their spirits were sold through speakeasies and other illegal outlets.

Prior to Prohibition, spirits were manufactured by commercial distilleries, whose practices were regulated. The alcohol served in speakeasies, however, was made by amateurs; "bathtub gin" was not just a figure of speech. Liquor sometimes had poisonous wood alcohol as its main ingredient. Imported liquor was available; but it commanded extremely high prices, and much of what was sold as imported spirits was actually domestic bootleg liquor poured into fancy bottles with fake labels. There was no way of knowing where a glass of liquor came from or what it was made from. Many New Yorkers experimented with making bathtub gin and other illegal spirits at home: one-gallon stills were sold at neighborhood hardware stores for about six dollars. In a single year, the deaths of 625 New Yorkers were directly attributed to ingesting poisoned alcohol, and another twelve hundred were chalked up to alcohol-related causes. When Prohibition ended in 1933, the city's distilleries did not reopen.

The Kings County Distillery, opened in 2010, was the city's first distillery since Prohibition. Its bourbon and moonshine (corn whiskey) are fermented in wooden vats crafted by the Isseks Brothers, best known as the makers of New York's iconic rooftop water towers. Kings County Distillery is located in the Paymaster Building in the Brooklyn Navy Yard—not far from where the Whiskey War was fought in the 1860s. In 2011, another distillery opened in Brooklyn: New York Distillery, which produces gin and rye. A great many legal spirits producers now exist throughout Brooklyn, Queens, and other boroughs, bringing New York a bit closer to its earlier days when distilleries proliferated across the city.

See also MILK, SWILL; PROHIBITION; and SPIRITS.

Lerner, Michael A. *Dry Manhattan: Prohibition in New York City*. Cambridge, Mass.: Harvard University Press, 2007.
Spoelman, Colin, and David Haskell. *The Kings County Distillery Guide to Urban Moonshining: How to Make and Drink Whiskey*. New York: Abrams, 2013.

Andrew F. Smith

Dominican

Dominican cuisine made it to New York City with the first wave of Dominican exiles from the Rafael Trujillo dictatorship in the 1930 and 1940s, yet it did not become well known locally until the greatest wave of Dominican immigration to the city between 1980 and 2000. These immigrants helped expand and support a complex chain of food-related businesses. According to the 2010 census there are approximately 1 million Dominicans living in the city.

Even though Dominican immigrants and their descendants are dispersed throughout the boroughs, the most recognized "ethnic enclave" is located in Washington Heights, Manhattan (roughly between 135th and 210th Streets). See WASHINGTON HEIGHTS. In this area alone there are more than 250 small family-owned Dominican restaurants, a few fancy high-priced Dominican American fine dining restaurants, and a network of supermarkets, grocery stores (bodegas), and street food vendors. Rice and beans, *bacalao* (cod fish), stewed chicken, pork chops, boiled tubers, and avocados are in menus associated with "Latino" foods (which refers mostly to Hispanic Caribbean cuisine). For business purposes—broadening the audience through a few staples and taming the seasonings—restaurants choose fares that are common to many Latin American immigrants and do not represent the distinctive flavors which each ethnic group has contributed to New York City. There is a trilogy of uniquely Dominican staple contributions to New York City menus: Sweet Holy Beans (dessert), To Die Dreaming (cold beverage), and The Three Strikes (breakfast).

Sweet Holy Beans

Sweet Holy Beans (*habichuelas con dulce*) is a tradional dessert-like holiday meal eaten in the Dominican Republic only during Lent and Easter (in the

Catholic calendar). There are as many recipes as family traditions, yet a basic preparation is common: red beans—any variety—are cooked until soft, adding evaporated milk, chunks of sweet potatoes (*batata*), sugar, coconut milk, cinnamon, nutmeg, a bit of salt, and cooking until creamy (beans are usually removed and pureed once soft). It is usually served in the afternoon, cold and garnished with raisins and small milk cookies, with an engraved cross.

The origin of this ritual meal, as with many Caribbean foods, is uncertain. The earliest mention of it dates to 1786 in the Dominican Republic historical records. The important shift which makes Sweet Holy Beans a New York City ethnic food is the fact that in Washington Heights it is served all year round, on street corners and in restaurants. For local Dominicans it has become a sort of comfort food to ease nostalgia for the homeland, especially during winter; but it is also consumed by local residents and tourists. The fact that this ritual meal (served only during Holy Week in the Dominican Republic) has become a year-round comfort food speaks of the shifts in cultural meanings (ethnic-memory work) that expand the diverse foodscapes of the city. It is this investment with the local calendar that makes *habichuela con dulce* a New York City street food.

The Three Strikes

The Three Strikes (a free translation of *lo tré golpe* in Dominican Spanish) is a type of hefty breakfast (mashed plantains served with fried eggs, salami, and fried cheese) most suitable for workers, peasants, and others with physically demanding jobs and long hours without break. It is, however, enjoyed by many New Yorkers who live or work around Washington Heights.

Even though mashed plantain (*mangú*) is commonly eaten in the Dominican Republic for breakfast, it is usually served with one small amount of protein, sometimes just a bit of oil, onions, tomatoes, or sardines to add taste (if anything at all, as many in the Dominican Republic cannot afford such luxury). What makes this public plate a New York City invention is how it was born in restaurants: it is served with a combination of three proteins; it is affordable, considering the amount of food; and some restaurants serve it most of the day.

From an "ethnic dish"—an ordinary poor people's food in the Dominican Republic—*mangú* has become a sign of ethnic pride and locality, recognized

by federal and private employees and local communities from Chinatown to Inwood. A huge amount of The Three Strikes was cooked and served during the cleaning and excavation of Ground Zero at the World Trade Center site. This gesture came not from Dominican leaders and politicians but from a dispersed network of Dominican cooks and restaurant workers in Lower Manhattan who donated ingredients and their labor and went to the site to serve it. *Mangú* and plantains have become cultural symbols of Dominicans in New York City; in fact, Washington Heights is sometimes referred to as "*Mangú* City" or "*Plátano* City."

To Die Dreaming

To Die Dreaming (*morir soñando*) is a traditional Dominican cold beverage (slightly similar to a milkshake), which is quite well known in New York City. The drink has been adopted as a regular restaurant and street-food drink in the Alto Manhattan (Washington Heights) and at the many other Dominican food establishments scattered throughout the boroughs, including Staten Island.

The beverage, served in a tall clear glass, is considered a daytime snack, sometimes to accompany breakfast or lunch. It is usually made with fresh squeezed orange juice (or bitter oranges), evaporated milk, brown sugar, cinnamon, nutmeg, a thin piece of skin from a lime, Dominican vanilla extract, and chopped ice. The recipe and preparations vary among individuals, families, and regions and depend on one's budget and the availability of the ingredients.

To Die Dreaming in New York City is not a treat or a children's party drink, as it is in the Dominican Republic. Instead, it has become a daily side beverage for breakfast and lunch. *Morí soñando* (deleting the final *r* of the first word in Dominican Spanish) is an acquired taste and a suitable metaphor for a peaceful exit on a hot New York City summer day.

See also CARIBBEAN.

Díaz, Junot. "He'll Take El Alto." *Gourmet*, September 2007. http://www.gourmet.com/magazine/2000s/2007/09/elalto.html.

Gonzalez, Clara. "Morir Soñando (Milk and Orange Juice)." Aunt's Clara's Kitchen. http://www.dominicancooking.com/976-morir-sonando-milk-and-orange-juice.html.

Marte, Lidia. "Migrant Seasonings: Food Practices, Place-Memory and Narratives of Home among

Dominicans in NYC." PhD diss., University of Texas at Austin, 2008.

Rossetto Kasper, Lynne. "Junot Diaz on Pasteles, Pork Stuffed Chicken, and His Special Relationship with Goat." The Splendid Table. http://www.splendidtable.org/story/junot-diaz-on-pasteles-pork-stuffed-chicken-and-his-special-relationship-with-goat.

Taveras, Karina. "Spilling the Beans on a Dominican Treasure." Daily News, March 18, 2008.

Lidia Marte

Domino Sugar Refinery

See SUGAR REFINING.

Doughnuts

Doughnuts in the United States usually take the form of rings made with either a leavened baking powder or yeast dough. Other shapes, whether chubby, jelly-filled disks or twisted crullers, are also generally considered part of the doughnut clan. While most New Yorkers buy their fried dough in chains and dedicated doughnut bakeries, Entenmann's doughnuts are also available in supermarkets; Greenmarket stands sell cider doughnuts; fresh, hot zeppole and their like are a draw at street fairs; and even classy eateries feature doughnuts on their menus. Korean pastry shops display *pon de rings* (made with a rice flour), Chinese bakeries stack them next to egg tarts and pork buns, and just about any Polish food store has a basket of *paszki* (jelly doughnuts) for sale.

The first documented instance of the term "dough nut" in the United States occurs as a cryptic nom de plume at the foot of a 1791 letter to New York's *Daily Advertiser* devoted to a discussion of public officials in Holland who had a habit of taking *Oeley Koechen en Tee*, that is, Dutch doughnuts and tea. The author recommends that New Yorkers take up this salutary, if exotic, habit. These Dutch treats took the form of a round, yeast-leavened fritter sometimes enriched with raisins and apples. Washington Irving, in his satirical *History of New York* (1809), also suggested that these *olykoeks* (as he called them) were rather obscure among the population at large, noting that they were "at present scarce seen in this city, except in genuine Dutch families." Nonetheless, several Dutch American cookbook manuscripts from the early decades of the Republic contain *olykoek* recipes, implying that at least one segment of New York's population had been enjoying these fried dough balls on a regular basis.

The first printed "doughnut" recipe was inserted, along with other American dishes, by New York publisher G. & R. Waite into a popular English cookbook, Susannah Carter's *The Frugal Housewife* (the copyright reads 1803, though the book was released in late 1802). Much like the Dutch American *oliekoeks* and German American *Fastnachkuchen*, these were leavened with yeast and, though the recipe is vague in this regard, likely formed into nut-size pieces prior to frying. Doughnuts were widespread throughout New England at this point; the name and recipe most likely descended from an obscure Hertfordshire specialty, variously referred to as Hertfordshire "nuts" or "dow nuts" in eighteenth-century English sources. By the 1830s New England cooks had begun to use chemical leaveners to aerate the dough, a variant that a decade later led to the ring shape we are familiar with today.

Most European countries have some form of deep-fried pastry, and each wave of immigrants brought

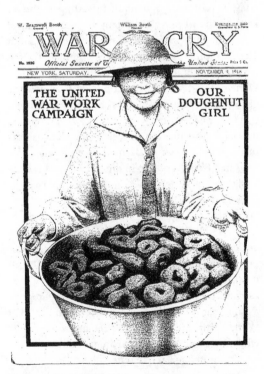

During World War I, the New York–based Salvation Army made and sold doughnuts on the western front to improve morale. This image of a "Doughnut Dolly" appeared on the cover of the Salvation Army's magazine *War Cry* on November 9, 1918.

its own version. Perhaps the most prominent were the Germans and German Jews who brought jelly doughnuts (the name varies according to region) and the Italians with various forms of fried dough including zeppole. See ZEPPOLE.

In the nineteenth century, doughnuts were a largely homemade product long associated with domesticity and rural New England values. During World War I, the New York–based Salvation Army made and sold doughnuts on the western front to improve morale by giving the boys in the trenches a taste of home. This not only polished the army's profile but also boosted the popularity of doughnuts nationwide. During the Depression, the Salvation Army distributed doughnuts and coffee to the down and out. In a little over a month in the winter of 1934 they handed out 2.5 million donuts and 1.5 million cups of coffee.

Several entrepreneurs attempted to tap into the post–World War I doughnut fad, none more successfully than Adolph Levitt, a Jewish immigrant who bought into a New York bakery chain in 1920. Initially, he promoted doughnuts by setting up the fry kettle in the window; eventually, he found a way of automating the process. By the 1930s his Doughnut Corporation of America came to dominate the automatic doughnut machine business nationwide. During World War II, the company provided the gizmos to the Red Cross free of charge, though it sold them the needed doughnut mix. In 1949, it opened up a laboratory on Stone Street where "all five floors of the building [were] devoted to elaborate apparatus that tests every step in the making of this once lowly fried cake," as the *New York Times* reported.

Even more than Levitt's technical ability was his talent at publicity. The Doughnut Corporation of America helped found the National Dunking Association, which, among its other achievements, arranged a great debate at the Hotel Astor in 1941 to determine the origin of the doughnut hole. (They assigned the invention to Captain Hanson Gregory, a claim that has since been disproved.) At the 1939 World's Fair, the corporation set up two exhibits where up to fourteen hundred donut "dunkers" could be accommodated at one time.

Doughnuts came once again into the limelight in 1996 when the Raleigh-based doughnut chain Krispy Kreme opened several branches in Manhattan. The press attention was overwhelming. Writing for the *New York Times*, Roy Blount Jr. described the oily rings as "like fried nectar puffed up with yeast." Others were equally effusive.

Two years earlier Mark Isreal had opened up Doughnut Plant on Grand Street, introducing the city to his version of inventive doughnuts often flavored with fresh fruit and berries he bought at the Union Square Greenmarket. Following Isreal's debut and the Krispy Kreme fad, fine dining restaurants such as Maloney & Porcelli and Craft began to feature doughnuts on their menus. By the early years of the 2000s, a national doughnut revival was in full swing, joined by trendy New York bakeries such Bedford-Stuyvesant's Dough. In 2013, Dominique Ansel fried a circle of croissant dough, filled it with pastry cream, and named it the "cronut." See CRONUT. The pastry became an instant sensation, led to long lines in front of the French chef's Spring Street pastry shop, and was copied within months across the nation and the world.

See also COLONIAL DUTCH.

Blount, Roy, Jr. "Style." *New York Times*, September 8, 1996, p. SM67.
Krondl, Michael. *The Donut: History, Recipes, and Lore from Boston to Berlin*. Chicago: Chicago Review Press, 2014.
"News of Food: Machine Catches Up With Doughnut; It Even Can Imitate a Hand-Made One," *New York Times*, September 26, 1949, p. 28.
Steinberg, Sally Levitt. *The Donut Book*. Pownal, Vt.: Storey, 2004.

Michael Krondl

Downing, Thomas

See ANTEBELLUM PERIOD.

Dr. Brown's Soda

Dr. Brown's is a line of sodas best known for Cel-Ray, a celery soda. Considered a delicatessen staple and New York City classic, the soft drink line originated in New York, where the concentrate for the product still is produced. Dr. Brown's is also known for its black cherry soda and cream soda.

According to the company (and printed on the cans), Dr. Brown's has been around since 1869. As for the brand's namesake, in 1974 Selwyn Cohn, then president of the bottler, told the *Village Voice* that "Dr. Brown" was Dr. Henry E. Brown of New York City, a pharmacist who invented Cel-Ray in

1867—"a druggist who concocted his own tonics and sold them over his soda fountain." See SODA FOUNTAINS.

The sodas were produced by Schoneberger & Noble, a New York–based drink company, which originated the brand. One of its 1910 labels advertised "Dr. Browns [sic] Celery Tonic," made with crushed celery seeds, as a "pure beverage for the nerves" that "strengthens the appetite and aids digestion."

In 1928, Schoneberger & Noble merged with the Carl Schultz and Brownie Corporations (makers of the Brownie chocolate drink) to form the American Beverage Corporation. At this point, production and bottling of Dr. Brown's moved from Water Street in Lower Manhattan to Greenpoint, Brooklyn.

In the 1930s, the brand was advertised in local Jewish newspapers and on the radio. During this same period, Cel-Ray (as well as seltzer) often was referred to as "Jewish Champagne."

In 1953, the U.S. Food and Drug Administration questioned the use of the word "tonic" in the title of the celery tonic beverage, given its lack of proven health benefit; they also took issue with the use of the word "celery" since a minimal amount of the vegetable is used in the soda. In response, the company changed the product's name to Dr. Brown's Cel-Ray Soda, the name still used today.

The sodas enjoyed a wide Jewish following in New York delis in the early twentieth century. But in the early 1980s, as Jewish delis in New York vanished, the company expanded distribution to include delis, gourmet shops, and restaurants in major markets around the country, bringing a formerly "ethnic" drink into the mainstream. See DELIS, JEWISH.

Canada Dry Bottling Company of New York acquired Dr. Brown's in 1982. The concentrate for the sodas still is made in New York and put into cans at Canada Dry's New York facility. The concentrate also is shipped to LA Bottleworks in Montebello, California, where it is packaged in glass bottles.

See also SODA.

Hillinger, Charles. "Drink of the Deli People: Dr. Brown's Cream Soda Making Its Mark Outside of New York." *Los Angeles Times*, July 4, 1986.
Ostrow, Lonnie. "L'Chaim to Dr. Brown, Most Enduring Kosher Soft Drink." *Jewish Star*, August 18, 2014.
Pollak, Michael. "That Old Celery Fizz." *New York Times*, October 14, 2011.
"Scenes." *Village Voice*, July 18, 1974.

Kara Newman

Dufresne, Wylie

Wylie Dufresne is a chef acclaimed worldwide for his inventive, playful, and technically forward cuisine and boundary-pushing flavor pairings. With a small research and development department, he works with new equipment and ingredients, conducting experiments and developing partnerships with experts from scientists to suppliers. Until November 30, 2014, he was the chef–owner of wd-50, which he opened on New York City's Lower East Side in April 2003 with partners Jean-Georges Vongerichten (a three-star Michelin chef with restaurants all over the world) and restaurateur Phil Suarez. Dufresne described the cuisine of his restaurant as modern American. Wd-50 garnered a three-star review from the *New York Times* and one star from the *Michelin Guide*, retained every year since the first New York edition in 2006. Dufresne opened Alder, a more casual version of wd-50, in March 2013.

Dufresne's experimental cooking aims "to understand food better"; he considers it an educational process. Some of his signature dishes include eggs Benedict, which consists of cylinders of egg yolks cooked in a water bath at 70°C and fried hollandaise sauce; shrimp noodles (noodles made from shrimp); and aerated foie gras (foie gras terrine aerated by pressure). Several of his signature dishes at wd-50 included reinventions of traditional dishes, such as fried chicken, pizza, or an everything bagel with lox and cream cheese: the bagel is a frozen, hollowed-out disc; the cream cheese is flattened into a brittle sheet; and the lox is frozen and shaven into minuscule flakes. It tastes like the classic New York breakfast dish but with a presentation that challenges a diner's expectations.

Dufresne was born in 1970 in Providence, Rhode Island, and moved to New York in 1977; his father has been in the restaurant business his whole life. Dufresne began working in restaurants when he was eleven, including at the famed Al Forno's in Providence the summer before college. He earned a bachelor's degree in philosophy in 1992 from Colby College in Maine; this "studying of questions," as he puts it, is training that he uses constantly.

Dufresne says he would have loved to be a professional baseball player and sees many similarities between the mental and physical aspects of both group sports and kitchen work. Instead, he enrolled at the French Culinary Institute in New York, from which he graduated in January 1993. While in culinary school, he worked for Alfred Portale, first at One Fifth Avenue, then at Gotham Bar and Grill. Knee surgery forced a six-month break; his career resumed at Vongerichten's JoJo, where he worked from 1994 to 1997. He helped to open Vongerichten's flagship Jean-Georges, where he became sous chef, and thereafter was chef de cuisine at Vongerichten's Las Vegas property, Prime, until 1999, when he joined his father's latest venture, 71 Clinton Fresh Food, as chef. He remained there until opening wd-50 in 2003, which was one of the first fine dining restaurants to open on the Lower East Side, contributing to a revitalization of the neighborhood that led to the construction of high-priced condominiums, eventually forcing him to close his restaurant to make room for one such building. Dufresne has stated a desire to reopen wd-50 in another location. He is also working on his first cookbook.

Dufresne is often called a chef's chef, a cerebral cook whose complex cuisine walks the line between geeky and fun. He shares his knowledge and teaches in the kitchen, and many of his former cooks and staff members have opened acclaimed restaurants of their own, such as Alex Stupak and Sam Mason, while two of his former pastry chefs have gone on to work at Noma in Copenhagen.

Dufresne has received many awards. While at 71 Clinton Fresh Food he was nominated for the James Beard Foundation's Rising Star Chef of the Year (2000), and in 2001 *Food & Wine* named him one of America's Ten Best Chefs. In 2013 Dufresne won the James Beard Award for Best Chef, New York City, and in June 2014 he received *Food Arts'* Silver Spoon Award, which recognizes a chef or culinary professional's sterling performance and impact on the industry. In April 2014 the international culinary performance organization Gelinaz! organized a surprise dinner for Dufresne at wd-50, for which twenty-eight of the world's best chefs flew to New York at their own expense and cooked for him.

Dufresne is married to food editor Maile Carpenter; they have two children. WD-50.com, the restaurant's website, still includes a menu, as well as photos of some of the dishes.

See also EXPERIMENTAL CUISINE COLLECTIVE.

Begley, Sarah, and Adam Perez. "The Last Days of wd-50." *Time*, October 17, 2014.

"Wylie Dufresne: Chef." http://bigthink.com/experts/wyliedufresne.

Anne E. McBride

Dumpster Diving

Dumpster diving is picking through the trash of an establishment like a supermarket, bakery, specialty food store, or restaurant to find food to eat. In many cases it is a practical response to poverty and food insecurity or simply stems from the idea that something destined for the landfill is "too good to waste." Dumpster diving may also be a manifestation of "freeganism," a sustainable food movement devoted to living off of the food waste of others to both eat in a cost-effective way and draw attention to the inefficiency and unsustainability of the conventional food system.

In a city with the diversity and volume of food—and food waste—as New York City, some dumpster divers report being able to fully live off of the waste of commercial establishments. Some stores are helpful and set aside quality edible waste for dumpster divers, while others actively patrol against it for fear of liability (for example, if a restaurant discards spoiled food and a freegan eats it and becomes ill, is the restaurant responsible?) and potential loss of revenue (could people who take discarded bagels from the trash in the evening be buying them earlier in the day?).

A dumpster-diving (usually by choice) community exists in New York City and beyond where divers share tips via word of mouth, websites, and social media. Important information includes optimal times of day to visit to take advantage of the best products and avoid security guards or hostile managers; types of products typically available; safety and quality concerns with particular foods; and preparation tips, especially for longer-term food preservation. Good information is available online about dumpster-diving opportunities in all five boroughs, with most of the emphasis on Manhattan and northern Brooklyn.

Technically dumpster diving is illegal in New York City as commercial refuse is the property—and responsibility—of the business. Dumpsters are privately owned and are maintained on commercial property. That said, dumpster diving is rarely prosecuted with the exception of occasional trespassing charges. Literature in the dumpster-diving community emphasizes being a good citizen—being polite, re-bagging trash, leaving dumpsters looking neat, and being inconspicuous—so as to maintain good relationships with businesses that could be good food sources.

Most dumpster divers salvage ready-to-eat food such as bagels, fruit, and pastries, although some take fresh vegetables or meat to cook at home. An extreme extension of New York City dumpster diving is the Salvage Supperclub, a pop-up dinner series where guests dine exclusively on salvaged food inside an empty dumpster. A chef-activist, Celia Lam, turns salvaged food into culinary creations that look and taste like a welcome addition to a fine dining menu. Part performance art, part political protest, and part gastronomic experience, the club draws public attention to the vast amounts of food waste in the system and its concomitant environmental impacts.

Freegan.Info: Strategies for Sustainable Living beyond Capitalism. http://freegan.info/freegan-directories/dumpster-directory/manhattan.

Thomas, Emily. "One Man's Trash Is Another Man's 6-Course Dinner." HuffPost Taste, July 15, 2014. http://www.huffingtonpost.com/2014/07/15/salvage-supperclub-dumpster-dining_n_5586457.html.

Jonathan Deutsch

Dutch

See COLONIAL DUTCH.

Dutch-Style New Year's Day Parties

The Dutch custom of visiting family and friends at holidays, such as Easter, Pentecost, or New Year's, was very much a part of social life in the Netherlands and goes back centuries. It was brought to the colony New Netherland when the Dutch settled there in the beginning of the seventeenth century. Jasper Dankaert's diary of 1679–1680 confirms that the custom was not only brought to the New World but continued after the final English takeover of the colony in 1674. He described that on "the second day of Pinxter" he and his companion had various visitors. In the Netherlands holidays are celebrated for two days, a tradition that still prevails.

As we know from diaries and printed sources, the visiting on New Year's Day took on a very elaborate

form, especially in cities such as Albany and New York City, but even in the country it was customary to visit relatives, friends, and neighbors. We have the diaries of gentleman farmer Isaac E. Cotheal of Fishkill, New York, which span the second half of the nineteenth century. Each year he notes how many visitors he received on New Year's. One year it was as many as eight, but in another with particularly bad weather, he noted that he "received no calls."

In cities with houses in much closer proximity, many more visits could be made in a day. The gentlemen would go "calling," while the ladies would stay home to receive. The custom might have had a dual purpose, as a period etiquette book seemed to

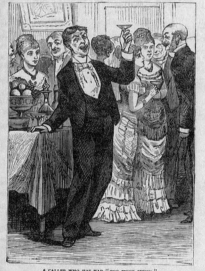

BEWILDERED CALLERS. 327

ably ludicrous. These late visitors leer vaguely at the hostess and her companions, mutter their compliments and good wishes in thick, unsteady voices, gulp down

A CALLER WHO HAS HAD "TOO MUCH PUNCH."

the liquors offered them, and stagger out into the hall, where the servant assists them in making their way out. Sometimes a gentleman who has paid a large number of calls falls helpless at the feet of the hostess, and has

The Dutch custom of visiting friends and relatives on holidays was brought to New Netherland by Dutch settlers at the beginning of the seventeenth century. New Year's Day would be set aside for people to receive visitors, with food and drink served from brunch time until late in the night. Pictured above: a caller who has had too much "punch," from *New York by Sunlight and Gaslight*, by James Dabney McCabe (1882). LIBRARY OF CONGRESS

imply, not only that of extending good wishes to everyone but also of some matchmaking, perhaps. The women would get together a few days later, to discuss "the new faces they have seen and the matrimonial prospects for the year" (Chesterfield, 1860).

Huybertie Pruyn of Albany described a New Year's Day in that city during the period 1885 to 1892. She recalled how the best china and silver were set out on gleaming white tablecloths to serve the "best the household had to offer." Food (and drink) was being served from eleven in the morning until ten at night, and male relatives and friends averaging between two and three hundred in number would come to visit. Tradesmen, messenger boys, postmen, and policemen who rang the bell to wish the household well in the New Year were given a bag with the traditional caraway-flavored New Year's cakes and perhaps a coin or two.

For young males, being old enough to be allowed to come along with their male relatives meant a rite of passage, as is described in a delightful book by Samuel Hopkins called *Grandfather Stories*. He tells about not only the open houses on the first day of the year in Rochester, New York, but also how each house had a reputation for certain foodstuffs. One family might always serve fine pies, another might put out a particularly delicious chicken salad, and yet another would offer not only turkey but also duck and goose.

The most elaborate "New Year's visiting" took place in New York City, where, because of the close proximity of the houses, the gentlemen could strategize and make a very large number of calls in that one day. We have to thank the 1861 diary of John Ward for an insight on how this was done. He described how in that year he and his brother made only a "few calls," visiting thirty-three families. But after returning from the Civil War, he did much better; he and a friend made as many as 107 calls, traveling from Washington Square up to Forty-Seventh Street. Like Hopkins in his book, he also mentions various refreshments—in one case "plum cake"—and one is left to think that these men must have had a very good appetite. He recorded his conversations and mentioned the young ladies he met at the various houses. According to the aforementioned etiquette book, those young ladies could chat "with any one who comes properly introduced" as if they were "intimate friends"—at that time, no doubt, a further enticement for the gentlemen.

As the city became increasingly larger, visits to houses farther spread out took more time. This, combined with the cost and effort of putting on such elaborate gatherings, as well as changing social customs, contributed to the gradual disappearance of New Year's visiting. By the turn of the twentieth century, the custom had vanished.

See also COLONIAL DUTCH and NEW YEAR'S.

Chesterfield, Philip Dormer Stanhope. *Chesterfield's Art of Letter-Writing Simplified … to which is Appended the Complete Rules of Etiquette, and the Usages of Society.* N.p.; 1860.
Rose, Peter G. *Food, Drink and Celebrations of the Hudson Valley Dutch.* Charleston, S.C.: History Press, 2009.

Peter G. Rose

Dylan's Candy Bar

Dylan's Candy Bar, a candy empire founded and made famous in New York City, is the brainchild of Dylan Lauren, daughter of fashion designer Ralph Lauren. The flagship 5,500-square-foot store is located on the Upper East Side, at Sixtieth Street and Third Avenue, cater-cornered to Bloomingdale's. The first two floors carry over seven thousand edible treats, from popular nostalgia items, such as candy cigarettes, candy buttons, and wax bottles, to a huge array of gummy candies, twenty-one exclusive colors of M&Ms, and novelty oversized candy bars. On the top floor is a café, a dessert bar ("dessert pizzas" feature prominently), and a cocktail bar serving such drinks as the "Chocoholic Martini" (two kinds of chocolate-flavored vodka and crème de cacao) and the "Nerdy Mojito" (garnished with purple Nerds).

Dylan's Candy Bar emerged from an events business Lauren started after graduating from Duke University, when she would often use candy in giveaway bags and as decorations for invitations and centerpieces. She was soon convinced that she could sell candy directly by building a lifestyle brand; her father's example here was undoubtedly influential. Lauren's vision was for a "Disneyland and Willy Wonka sort of place," a saccharatopia where customers would be transported to their childhood.

To achieve this vision, Lauren began interviewing candy consultants in 1999 and soon clicked with Jeff Rubin, who had masterminded F. A. O. Schweetz, F. A. O. Schwarz's candy store. Working with designer

Joanne Newbold and architecture firm Allen & Kill-coyne Associates, they built a colorful three-floor emporium that showcased a Pop art design sensibility. Outsized elements inspired by the board game Candy Land included an acrylic staircase embedded with Gummi Bears, a hanging lollipop tree, and candy cane columns.

Dylan's Candy Bar launched in mid-October 2001, just in time for the busy Halloween season; it also happened to be only weeks after the events of September 11. The store was successful from the opening, with as many as ten thousand visitors on Saturdays, and Lauren has speculated that customers saw the store as a space where they could feel "renewed, happy and hopeful" again.

The store has steadily expanded its reach, with locations in Miami, Los Angeles, and East Hampton and plans to expand to Canada, Japan, and London.

A licensing partnership with airport concession operators is also planned. Dylan's ran into controversy in 2013 when workers protesting outside the flagship Manhattan store called for hourly pay equivalent to the $13.99 price of a pound of bulk candy and stable full-time hours. Management and employees compromised on a wage increase to $11 per hour, although most employees remain part-time.

See also CANDY.

Finn, Robin. "Public Lives: Confections of an Enterprising Candy Lover." *New York Times*, November 30, 2001.
Lauren, Dylan. "Sweets Tester in Chief." *New York Times*, June 6, 2009.
Wright, Jennifer Ashley. "The Sweet Life of Dylan Lauren." *Observer*, October 15, 2015.

Max P. Sinsheimer

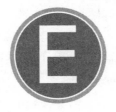

Easter

Easter celebrations in New York City were, early on, observed as seldom as Christmas. Because there was no biblically prescribed date for Easter, neither holiday was observed by Puritan and Evangelical colonists. Catholics and Episcopalians might celebrate, but Easter was not a significant part of the early culture of Manhattan. Starting in the 1850s, as more Catholic immigrants entered the city, newspapers carried accounts of Easter celebrations in Roman Catholic churches; by 1868, the *New York Daily Tribune* reported that, although Easter had passed "almost unnoticed by our Knickerbocker and Puritan ancestors, [it] is yearly more and more observed."

By the mid-1870s, these observations were highly visible and often secular. New York City is famous for originating the Easter parade, which has spawned imitators in other cities. Newspapers began to report on the parade by the late 1870s, noting that it served as a fashionista display for New York's wealthy, who preened in their new clothes along uptown avenues after leaving church services; folklorists trace the wearing of some new article of clothing on Easter to a tradition dating at least to Tudor England, when failure to have one item of new homespun cloth was an omen of bad luck. The parade has morphed into an annual rite where anyone can (and is encouraged to) strut down Fifth Avenue in outrageous garb, with special focus on hats. Irving Berlin's 1933 song "Easter Parade" pays homage to the "bonnet, with all the frills upon it." By the mid-twentieth century, the parade annually attracted an estimated 1 million people to stroll or observe, but the numbers have dwindled dramatically.

In its late nineteenth-century heyday, the parade was an opportunity for public drinking. One critical article in the *New York Herald* bemoaned the Easter intoxication that came not from religious ecstasies but "from a brandy cocktail with a dash of absinthe in it." For those uncomfortable with the culture of the Fifth Avenue parade, smaller parades sometimes took place along racial or ethnic lines. In 1935, the African American community organized its own parade in Harlem. Italian communities brought with them a very different sort of procession, where they follow a figure representing Christ on his march to Golgotha.

Easter foods in New York pay homage to seasonality and Christian traditions as well the promotional savvy of confectioners both large and small. Traditionally, Easter concludes the frugal Lenten season that was an essential part of the Catholic and Eastern Orthodox calendars and welcomes the return of meat and eggs to the table; although relatively few New Yorkers nowadays engage in strict Lenten fasts, meals on Easter Sunday often highlight eggs, which used to become plentiful in the spring. Easter brunch has become a popular pastime, and restaurant menus offer dishes such as eggs Benedict, as well as egg-enriched sweet breads. Spring lamb and cured hams are traditional dinner dishes, again reflecting seasonal rhythms: in times past, Easter coincided with the time when the young animals reached slaughtering age or the salted hams put up the previous winter were finally ready to eat.

The most colorful Easter markets are found in ethnic neighborhoods, especially those with Greek and Russian Orthodox populations, who celebrate

Easter according to the Julian calendar, some days or weeks after the Roman Catholic date. Butcher shops display whole baby lambs or goats, which form the centerpiece of Easter dinner. Elaborately decorated Easter eggs remain a popular tradition: eggshells are gingerly pierced, the contents blown out, and the shells intricately decorated. Greek, Russian, and Ukrainian communities still display these exquisite shells (known as *pysanky* in Ukrainian). The expelled raw egg is baked into *kulich*, a light and sweet bread studded with raisins. A similar bread (with candied citrus substituting for the raisins) is found throughout Italian neighborhoods as the *colomba di Pasqua*, or Easter dove, baked in a special mold. Other bakeries bring out sweet hot cross buns, identified by the thin intersecting lines of icing that evoke the Cross.

Eggs remain at the historical heart of New York's Easter celebrations. Egg trees, of German origin and similar to Christmas trees but decorated with eggs, were the rage in the 1890s: the *New York Times* society pages gushed over a ball hosted by Louis Comfort Tiffany where one of the main entertainments was a dazzling egg tree. Egg trees appeared sporadically in public venues but never gained lasting traction: the Metropolitan Museum of Art displayed an egg tree from the 1940s until sometime in the 1980s, when the tradition petered out. The Easter Bunny, also imported to New York with German immigrants, still delivers colored Easter eggs to children. In years past, hard-cooked eggs were a welcome treat after the Lenten fast, although these eggs nowadays are usually chocolate bonbons wrapped in pastel foils. Children's Easter egg hunts take place in the gardens of many churches after morning services. For older New Yorkers, New York's pastry makers and chocolatiers have created an extravagant array of sophisticated sweets.

See also CHRISTMAS; GREEK; and RUSSIAN.

Barnett, James A. "The Easter Festival: A Study in Cultural Change." *American Sociological Review* 14, no. 1 (1949): 62–70.
"Easter Feast Essentials." NYTimes.com. http://cooking.nytimes.com/topics/easter
Lee, Patty. "New York Candy Makers and Chocolatiers Bring Easter Sweets to the Next Level." *New York Daily News*, March 23, 2013.
Schmidt, Leigh Eric. "The Easter Parade: Piety, Fashion, and Display." *Religion and American Culture: A Journal of Interpretation* 4, no. 2 (1994): 135–164.

Cathy K. Kaufman

Eataly

Eataly is an Old World–style food emporium reimagined for a twenty-first-century international city that never sleeps, and as you might expect, it is exuberantly big (fifty-eight thousand square feet) and almost always bustling with thousands of hungry locals and tourists. Housed on the first floor of the former International Toy Center Building at 200 Fifth Avenue in Manhattan's Flatiron District, Eataly was created by celebrity chefs Mario Batali and Lidia Bastianich, son Joe Bastianich, and Oscar Farinetti, the founder of the original Eataly in Turin, Italy. It offers the most complete selection of Italian regional groceries, spices, pastas, oils, breads, pastries, and takeaway meals in North America, as well as a comprehensive selection of dining opportunities in the form of seven restaurants.

On the rooftop is La Birreria, Eataly's Italian beer garden and brewery offering informal dining under a retractable roof where one can dine on antipasti that includes house-made pickled vegetables, sausages, and house-brewed, imported, and domestic beers. La Piazza is a stand-up food and drinks bar serving salumi (charcuterie), cheeses including mozzarella, and raw bar as well as wines by the glass and bottled beer. At Il Pesce, Chef David Pasternak of Esca proves both his mastery of craft and his appreciation of the pristinely fresh seafood available in New York's famous Fulton Fish Market with his traditional takes on Italian fish cookery. Le Verdure is a seated counter and table area that serves seasonal vegetable dishes. La Pasta and La Pizza share two seated counters where you can dine on artisanal fresh and dried pasta, including tagliatelle, lasagna, and ravioli, while Manzo is a more formal dining experience that features meat, much of it from Italian breeds of livestock raised in the United States. The enigmatically named Pranzo—La Scuola di Eataly (literally "Lunch—The School of Eataly") serves a menu that changes monthly by theme (e.g., truffles) and region and, like all of Eataly, has a mandate to both feed and teach the "gospel" of authentic regional Italian food and culture.

See also BASTIANICH, LIDIA; BATALI, MARIO; and ITALIAN.

Bastianich, Joseph. *Restaurant Man*. New York: Plume, 2012.

Bob Del Grosso

Eater

Eater.com is an all-things-food-focused blog launched in 2005 by Lockhart Steele and Ben Leventhal, two journalists-cum-technology entrepreneurs. Eater began strictly as a New York City–centric gossip website on the restaurant industry, alongside Curbed .com, a New York City–focused real estate chatter blog. In its infancy, Eater had about twenty thousand monthly readers by the end of 2005 as it reported on the comings and goings of New York City's boisterous dining scene. By 2009, the number was about five hundred thousand.

Eater first expanded to Miami, Los Angeles, and San Francisco, and it stayed like that for a few years. In 2009, expansion began in earnest, and now Eater sites include twenty-four cities as well as a national site.

In 2014, the Eater sites collectively drew more than 5 million monthly readers. Eater considers itself the source for people who care about dining and drinking in the nation's most important food cities. In New York, Eater tracks down what restaurants are opening where, what chefs are serving what, and the minutiae of how all those changes go down. Eater has also given credence to the long-form journalism style that many traditional newspapers and magazines have veered away from in recent years, publishing stories on everything from a first-person truffle hunting excursion in Italy to a south-central Wisconsin fish fry guide to a primer on California's reversal on the ban of foie gras. The Eater sites also include punchy, short blurbs on the comings and goings of each city's vibrant restaurant and food scenes. The online-only presence also contributes to a very interactive experience, in which readers are asked their opinions often.

Eater has received accolades from industry professionals to amateurs alike and has become a force in the food world, garnering praise from respected chefs and food critics including David Chang of Momofuku and CNN's Anthony Bourdain. See BOURDAIN, ANTHONY; CHANG, DAVID; and MOMOFUKU RESTAURANT GROUP. Many observers note that as Eater has grown, it has replaced traditional newspaper dining coverage in certain cities as those publications have cut back on reporting.

In 2013, Vox Media bought the Curbed network—Curbed.com, Eater.com, and Racked.com (a style and shopping blog)—reportedly for nearly $30 million; Curbed LLC joined other Vox "verticals," a term used for web-specific content for individual topics or concepts. Since then, Eater has expanded quite quickly, hiring for the first time three restaurant critics, including the former *Village Voice* critic Robert Sietsema, former *Atlanta Magazine* writer Bill Addison, and former *Bloomberg News* restaurant reviewer Ryan Sutton. Eater's reviews are designed to be easily updated and annotated throughout the life of the restaurant.

In July 2014, Eater's editor in chief, Amanda Kludt, was named one of the fifty most powerful women in New York City by the *New York Daily News*, which called her a "national tastemaker." Eater employs about thirty full-time staffers and dozens of part-time and freelance writers. Eater offers several awards, including its Young Guns awards, awarding about twelve to sixteen influential, game-changing chefs, and the Eater Awards, with five categories—Restaurant of the Year, Chef of the Year, Bartender of the Year, So Hot Right Now Restaurant, and Stone Cold Stunner.

Eater website: http://www.voxmedia.com/brands/eater.
Moskin, Julia. "Eater Hires Three Restaurant Critics." *New York Times*, March 13, 2014.
"50 Most Powerful Women in New York." *New York Daily News*, July 3, 2014.
Oppenheimer, Mark. "The Optimist's Blogger." *New York Times Magazine*, March 19, 2010.

Lynne Posner

Ebinger's Blackout Cake

Ebinger's Blackout Cake was a popular chocolate layer cake filled and frosted with a fudgy pudding, coated in crisped chocolate cake crumbs. It was made by Ebinger Baking Company, which was founded in 1898 in Flatbush, Brooklyn, by German immigrants, George and Catherine Ebinger. The Ebingers eventually opened thirty-nine retail outlets in Brooklyn and Queens. Everyone had their favorite item, but blackout cake was prime among them.

Not everyone loved Ebinger's. During World War II it was accused of being anti-Semitic. The company was known for discriminatory hiring practices, excluding not only Jews but also people of color. Most of the retail clerks were of German or Irish descent. In 1962, the Brooklyn Congress of Racial Equality picketed the retail stores. Protesters also conducted a sit-in at the main Ebinger bakery on Bedford and Snyder Avenues so that the delivery trucks could not leave. The protests eventually led to some hiring reforms, but the bakery's popularity was never the same in a city populated by Jews and increasingly people of color.

The bakery never released its recipe for blackout cake. When it closed on August 27, 1972, the recipe died with the bakery. Word of the blackout cake spread from coast to coast as Brooklynites have carried their memories with them.

Today, there are plenty of restaurants and bakeries outside of New York that make a facsimile or what they think is a facsimile. Recipes for blackout cake— or Brooklyn chocolate cake, Brooklyn decadence cake, or chocolate pudding cake—appear in cookbooks and magazines. Many of these recipes are for three-layer cakes frosted with butter cream, which can certainly be delicious; but the original was only two layers and cloaked in a dark chocolate pudding. For home cooks, making a three-layer cake leaves plenty of cake crumbs for the finishing touch.

Schwartz, Arthur. *Arthur Schwartz's New York City Food: An Opinionated History and More Than 100 Legendary Recipes*. New York: Stewart, Tabori & Chang, 2004.

Arthur Schwartz

Edible

The *Edible* magazine franchise focuses on local stories related to food and drink. Publications in the group include *Edible Manhattan & Brooklyn* and *Edible Queens*, as well as *Edible Long Island & East End* and *Edible Hudson Valley*. The franchise also includes community-focused tastings, festivals, and other local events.

Founders Tracey Ryder and Carole Topalian launched the first publication, *Edible Ojai*, in California in 2002 and went on to found Edible Communities (the umbrella organization to most of the magazines; some are independent) in 2005. As of the end of 2014, the franchise included more than eighty titles.

The publications, which span the United States and Canada from *Edible Allegheny* (Pennsylvania) to *Edible Westside* (California), are noted for offering culinary content (and related advertising) tailored to the community they are intended to serve. In many of *Edible's* markets, the print publications are available for free at local restaurants and stores; some are sold at bookstores and other outlets.

Edible Communities, Inc., says (on its website and other materials) that its mission is "to transform the way consumers shop for, cook, eat and relate to local food." Through printed publications, websites and events, the entity "strives to connect consumers with local growers, retailers, chefs and food artisans."

As a whole, the *Edible* franchise is notable for several reasons. First, it focused on publishing hyperlocal food content during a time when most magazines had a national bent. In the first decade of the 2000s, newspaper food sections had the monopoly on local food content, plus the occasional professional-level blog. As newspaper food sections closed and many consolidated, *Edible's* publications thrived. And compared to the limited column inches most newspapers allotted, *Edible's* format encouraged longer-form narrative coverage, leading to awards for many of the deeply researched articles published in its pages.

Another differentiator is *Edible's* business model. Passion (and investment capital) trumped industry experience; local publishers were encouraged to buy into the franchise, even if they did not have previous publishing experience, and *Edible* provided marketing and other support. That model still exists today under the *Edible* umbrella.

Some might also posit that *Edible* was in the right place at the right time, giving ample attention to artisan food producers, farmers, chefs, and bartenders at exactly the moment that New Yorkers (and others) developed a fast-growing interest in the origins of their food, chef and mixology culture, sustainable agriculture, and other food-centric cultures and issues.

Long Island's *Edible East End* started in 2005, the third *Edible* in the nation and the first in the New York area. That was followed by *Edible Brooklyn* in 2006 (the fifth *Edible* publication and the first in New York City), *Edible Manhattan* in 2008 (accompanied by a splashy launch party at South Street Seaport with New Amsterdam market), *Edible Hudson Valley* in 2009, *Edible Queens* in 2010, and *Edible Long Island* in 2012. In 2015, the print versions of *Edible Manhattan* and *Edible Brooklyn* merged into a single publication, *Edible Manhattan & Brooklyn*, although the websites remain separate. Similarly, the two Long Island publications merged to become *Edible Long Island & East End*.

Burros, Marian. "How to Eat (and Read) Close to Home." *New York Times*, August 29, 2007.

"About Us." EdibleCommunities.com. http://www
.ediblecommunities.com/content/index.php?option=
com_content&view=article&id=25&Itemid=200054.

Kara Newman

Egg Creams

An egg cream is a curious New York concoction with
a history as fuzzy as its taste is fizzy. The classic New
York egg cream is an unlikely combination of three
simple ingredients: chocolate syrup, milk, and seltzer,
which are combined to produce a frothy, sweet, carbonated drink. However, the story of the egg cream
is not so simple. The egg cream is a product of Old
New York, an era when candy stores and soda fountains across New York City made flavored sodas using
syrup and seltzer. This was quite different from the
original milkshake (created ca. 1885), which is said
to have been made with sweet cream, a whole egg,
syrup and soda water, shaken together. The egg cream
lay somewhere in between.

Who created the egg cream is a subject for debate,
as is the origin of its name. An egg cream is conspicuously eggless, so many theories have surfaced as
to why "egg" is included in its name. The "egg" may
come from an anglification of *echt*, which is Yiddish
for "good." "Egg cream" may reference the original
milk shake, made with both egg and cream, or it
could be because the foamy head of an egg cream
resembles the effect of egg whites. In the 1880s,
Yiddish theater star Boris Thomaschevsky reportedly came back to New York from Paris, asking for a
drink called "*chocolate et crème*." In the 1890s, Louis
Auster began making a beverage with milk, seltzer,
and chocolate syrup, which he called "egg creams"
and sold by the thousands for five cents at his candy
store on Second Avenue.

Around 1900, Herman Fox founded H. Fox & Co.
(now Fox's U-bet) and created a chocolate syrup
which was used in egg creams everywhere, becoming
synonymous with the new drink. There may have
also been an "Uncle Hymie" who made an egg cream
with syrup, cream, egg, and seltzer in the 1920s but
was defeated by the Great Depression.

There is also debate about its birthplace. Brooklyn has claimed the egg cream as its own, hailing it
as the unofficial drink of Brooklyn since the 1920s.
However, all that can be safely ascertained is that
Brooklynite Herman Fox began his syrup company
in a Brownsville basement. It is actually Manhattan's
Lower East Side which boasts the most egg cream
establishments. Second Avenue, which used to be
known as "Yiddish Broadway" in its 1920s heyday,
claims the drink as its own. Today, it might as well
be known as "Egg Cream Row." Old-school delis and
candy shops that have been around for decades, such
as Gem Spa (which boasts "New York's Best Egg
Cream"), Veselka, B&H Dairy Restaurant, and Paul's
Da Burger Joint, continue the tradition of selling egg
creams. A couple avenues away, one can find them at
Russ & Daughters, Yonah Shimmel Knish Bakery,
and Ray's Candy Store. Other classic egg cream
establishments farther uptown include Lexington
Candy Store, the Second Ave Deli (which migrated
from the East Village to Midtown and the Upper East
Side), and Eisenberg's. There are even whisperings
of a Bronx egg cream, although it is more elusive.

How to Make an Egg Cream

There is still more disagreement about the best way
to make an egg cream. Although advice and rules
have been gleaned over the years, many of the most
famous egg cream makers refuse to give out their
recipes. Beginning this tradition of secrecy, Louis
Auster took his (perhaps original) recipe with him
to his grave, supposedly not letting anyone even
watch him make an egg cream. We know that the
three basic ingredients are syrup, milk, and seltzer;
but the seltzer must be from a tap, and most classic
egg creams use Fox's U-Bet chocolate syrup. While
every candy store or soda fountain once made its
own syrup, and there were dozens of other syrup
manufacturers located in New York City, Fox's U-bet
eventually usurped them all; egg cream purists now
discourage any other syrup.

The ingredients must then be mixed to produce a
frothy head like that of a beer. In order to achieve
this, there is a certain technique for the order of
ingredients, pouring and stirring. Fox's U-Bet syrup
gives out their "Original Brooklyn Egg Cream" recipe,
which reads, "Take a tall, chilled, straight-sided, 8oz
glass. Spoon one inch of U-bet chocolate syrup into
glass. Add 1 inch of whole milk. Tilt the glass and
spray seltzer (from a pressurized cylinder only) off
a spoon, to make a big chocolate head." However,
some add milk, then syrup, then seltzer or even milk,

then seltzer, and the syrup last. This may lead to a different-looking egg cream. While a Brooklyn or Lower East Side egg cream characteristically has a white head, the rarer Bronx egg cream is said to have a brown head because the chocolate syrup and seltzer are mixed first and the milk is added last.

Modern Egg Creams

Today there are some new variations on the classic egg cream. Eleven Madison Park (now closed) created a highbrow version of an egg cream, with a house-made chocolate syrup using Mast Brothers' Madagascar chocolate, mixed with malted milk, vanilla beans, and a splash of olive oil. Ray's Candy Store on Avenue A makes egg creams in many different flavors such as vanilla, chocolate, raspberry, cherry, orange, coconut, tamarind, Sprite, lemon-lime, coffee, and mango. In addition to the classic vanilla and chocolate egg cream, Brooklyn Farmacy (a modern-era soda shop) makes seasonal maple and blueberry egg creams, while Russ & Daughters' new cafe shakes things up by offering a malt egg cream and an egg cream made with "carob buxar molasses," alongside the classic chocolate variety.

See also RUSS & DAUGHTERS and SODA FOUNTAINS.

Bell, Daniel. "The Original Egg Cream—Its Birth, Death and Transfiguration, Or: The Creaming of Uncle Hymie." *New York Magazine*, March 8, 1971.

Fox, Joy. "Sweet Egg-nigma: The Elusive History of an American Classic." *Imbibe Magazine*, June 16, 2011.

Gould, Jillian. "Candy Stores and Egg Creams." In *Jews of Brooklyn*, edited by Ilana Abramovitch and Seán Galvin, pp. 202–205. Hanover, N.H.: University of New England Press, 2002.

Simonson, Robert. "Egg Cream." *Edible Manhattan*, September 1, 2010.

Simonson, Robert. "Iconic Foods: Egg Cream." *Edible Brooklyn*, September 13, 2010.

"The Original Egg Cream." H. Fox & Co., Inc. Recipes. http://www.foxsyrups.com/recipes.php.

Troy, Eric. "What Is an Egg Cream? Did It Ever Contain Eggs?" Culinary Lore, August 31, 2012. http://www .culinarylore.com/sodas%3Awhat-is-an-egg-cream.

Mackensie Griffin

Eggs Benedict

Eggs Benedict is a quintessential brunch dish in America. It consists of an English muffin with a round,

thin slice of ham or Canadian bacon topped by a poached egg, lavished with Hollandaise sauce.

Precisely who originated it is unknown, but the main origin stories point to New York City in the early 1890s. Two restaurants are usually identified as originators: Delmonico's and The Waldorf. See DELMONICO'S and WALDORF, THE. Charles Ranhofer, the famous chef at Delmonico's restaurant, published the first located recipe for "Eggs à la Benedick" in his magnum opus, *The Epicurean* (1894):

> Cut some muffins in halves crosswise, toast them without allowing to brown, then place a round of cooked ham an eighth of an inch thick and of the same diameter as the muffins on each half. Heat in a moderate oven and put a poached egg on each toast. Cover the whole with Hollandaise sauce. (Ranhofer, p. 858)

Ranhofer was known for naming dishes after high-profile customers, but he gives no indication for whom this recipe was named. See RANHOFER, CHARLES.

In December 1942, an article in the *New Yorker* magazine credited Lemuel Benedict, a stockbroker who was a veteran of New York's glamorous Gilded Age restaurant scene. He had dined with Diamond Jim Brady at Delmonico's and with Enrico Caruso, the popular Italian opera singer, in his home. See BRADY, DIAMOND JIM. Lemuel Benedict claimed that forty-eight years earlier (which would have been about 1894), in the throes of a hangover, he had ordered breakfast at the Waldorf restaurant—"some buttered toast, crisp bacon, two poached eggs, and a hooker of hollandaise sauce," with which, continues

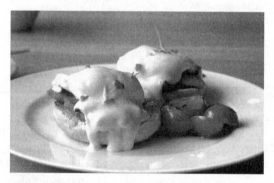

Eggs Benedict, poached eggs lavished with Hollandaise sauce and placed on top of an English muffin with ham or Canadian bacon, likely originated at either Delmonico's or The Waldorf in the 1890s. JON MOUNTJOY

the writer, "he then and there proceeded to put together the dish that has, ever since, borne his name." ("Talk of the Town," p. 14)

Others credit New York's Hoffman Hotel for the invention of eggs Benedict, and the *Oxford English Dictionary* credits Adolphe Meyer, chef at New York's Union Club. To make matters more confusing, the first located printed use of the term "eggs à la Benedict" appeared in the *Overland Monthly* in January 1894 on the lunch menu of the University Club in San Francisco.

What is clear is that recipes for eggs Benedict appeared regularly in American cookbooks and magazines from 1897 on. Eggs Benedict has remained one of the most popular breakfast and brunch choices in American and New York City restaurants ever since.

See also BRUNCH.

Ranhofer, Charles. *The Epicurean*. New York: Ranhofer, 1894.

"Talk of the Town," *The New Yorker* 18 (December 19, 1942): 14.

Tschirky, Oscar. *The Cook Book, by "Oscar" of the Waldorf*. Chicago and New York: Werner, 1896.

Andrew F. Smith

Egyptian

Egyptian food slowly started to take its place among the diverse ethnic cuisines of Gotham in the 1940s, when immigrants began to arrive seeking economic opportunity and, later, political freedom after the several revolutions and wars that have rocked Egypt from the 1950s to the present. Whether from a halal cart in Midtown, a low-capital business for new immigrants, or a white-tablecloth experience complete with belly dancers, New Yorkers can enjoy Egypt's spicy, flavorful sustenance.

When asked where Gothamites go for authentic ingredients and prepared foods, the most frequently mentioned is Kalustyan's in Murray Hill. The shop was originally opened in 1944 and is a mecca for spices, teas, nuts, and condiments from all over the world, including an impressive array of Egyptian ingredients. Upstairs a full-service deli serves pita sandwiches and platters including favorites such as *mujjadara* (a spicy lentil stew); crispy, succulent falafel; *meze*; and an assortment of *torschi* (sour pickles, pickles in brine) that will satisfy the most discerning vegan appetites. Another favorite shop is Sahadi's, now on Atlantic Avenue in Brooklyn; it, too, has a generous inventory of Egyptian ingredients, including hard-to-find *molokheyyah*, a mucilaginous, spinach-like green that is highly popular in Egypt.

If you do not want to cook, then the most authentic neighborhood is Astoria's block-long Little Egypt, on Steinway Street between Twenty-Eighth Avenue and Astoria Boulevard. Jam-packed with restaurants, cafes, bakeries, hookah bars, and street carts, the street is heady with the smell of grilled meats and flavored smoke. Brooklyn Heights's Tutt Café on Hicks Street offers reasonably priced Middle Eastern fare with a touch of fusion. While it has an array of Egyptian delights, it is especially known for its "pit-zas," delicately seasoned pizzas with a pita crust. Another house specialty is *asir limoon*, an Egyptian spin on lemonade: the whole lemon is blended with water, sugar, and mint and served over crushed ice. The result is a soothing, thirst-quenching drink.

Manhattan's Sahara East, on First Avenue between Eleventh and Twelfth streets and prominently advertised as a hookah bar, has resided at this East Village location for over twenty years serving authentic Egyptian food. Although the dining room is small (there is also a tented patio in the back), the restaurant is the closest one will get to an authentic Egyptian dining experience without the white-tablecloth price tag. The menu features the four basic *meze*—hummus, baba ghanouj, falafel, and tabouli—and is known as a unique gathering place to enjoy a flavored *shisha* (tobacco) and some cultural flair.

See also FALAFEL.

Bortot, M. Scott. "New York's Little Egypt District Welcomes Arab Immigrants." iipDigital, November 19, 2010. http://iipdigital.usembassy.gov/st/english/article/2010/11/20101119161919m0.6032221.html#axzz3SDVCfmsr.

Manuel, Shana. "Visiting Egypt and Little Egypt in Astoria, Queens." Culture Weekend, August 11, 2013. http://cultureweekend.com/hookah-hookah-hookah-little-egypt-york.

Riolo, Amy. *Nile Style: Egyptian Cuisine and Culture*. Rev. ed. New York: Hippocrene, 2013.

Schubach, Alanna. "The Five Best Restaurants in Little Egypt." *BQEats* (blog), April 8, 2014. http://blogs.villagevoice.com/forkintheroad/2014/04/best_restaurants_in_little_egypt_nyc.php.

Khaled Younes

Ellis Island Food (1892–1924)

The first national immigration receiving station in the United States was established by an act of Congress in 1892 and located on Ellis Island in New York Harbor. The twenty-seven-acre island, in the upper bay just off the New Jersey coast and north of Statue of Liberty Island, became the entry point for more than 12 million immigrants during its busiest years, 1892 to 1924. Men, women, and children came from over forty countries in Northern, Southern, and Eastern Europe; the Middle East; the Caribbean; Africa; and South America. These were people who had come by way of steamship companies' steerage passage to the harbor. They were put on barges and ferries to be transported to Ellis Island for processing. (First- and second-class passengers did not go through Ellis Island. They were processed aboard steamships and ferried directly to shore.) During this period, more than 70 percent of all immigrants entering the United States came through Ellis Island, making it the most important entry point in the country.

The first meal the majority of immigrants experienced in America came in the form of a boxed lunch sold at concession stands in the ferry and railroad ticketing room. This was the last room they would pass through, after being processed, on their way to the ferries to Lower Manhattan and then railroad lines across America. The boxes sold for fifty cents or one dollar, depending on size, and could contain roast beef, ham, cheese, or bologna sandwiches; a loaf of bread; sardines; sausages; apples; bananas; pies; and cakes. Milk, tea, coffee, and cider were sold separately. Contents and prices were often printed on the boxes in several languages.

Immigrants detained for medical or legal reasons or simply because they had not been processed by the end of the workday were served meals on Ellis Island. By 1901, a wing built next to the main processing hall included a kitchen and bakery, an icehouse, and dining halls to service detainees held for nonmedical reasons, as well as the more than five hundred employees on the island. President Theodore Roosevelt established a commissioner post in 1902 to oversee the daily processing system, which included feeding detainees. The first commissioner began bidding out per-meal food and service contracts. The winning bid also won the boxed lunch concession. Accepted bids averaged eight to ten cents per meal, and detainees' meals were charged back, through the contractor, to the steamship companies.

Contractors used a restaurant model to prepare and serve meals. While the government had amply equipped the kitchens, contractors purchased and transported food, hired cooks and servers, and supervised meal preparation. Contractors were responsible for producing three meals a day, seven days a week. Profits were slim, and the food purchased was the cheapest available. Between 1907 and 1914 close to 1 million meals were served annually. In 1913, the *Washington Post* dubbed Ellis Island the "largest restaurant in the world."

Typical fare varied widely from year to year and from contractor to contractor, and often the food was of poor quality. Meals could include the following: for breakfast, cereals, white bread and butter, apples, bananas, coffee for men, and milk for women and children; for dinner, soups, beef and lamb stews, potatoes, fish, rye bread, coffee for men, and milk for women and children; and for supper, baked beans, rye bread, stewed prunes, tea, and milk for women and children.

Mealtimes were not happy experiences for adult detainees. Groups were brought into the dining halls in rotation, a few hundred at a time. They sat on wooden benches at long tables and were brought individual plates of food. This served the dual purpose of crowd and portion control. Men and women

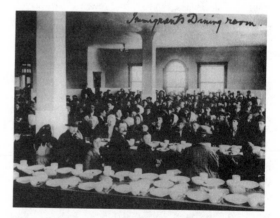

The packed immigrant's dining room at Ellis Island. New immigrants and detainees were served three meals a day in the same room, consisting of bread and cereal or stew depending on the time of the meal. NATIONAL PARK SERVICE FILES, STATUE OF LIBRARY NATIONAL MONUMENT

ate separately, and children ate with the women. Ethnic groups were mixed together, and no translators were on hand to explain unfamiliar food. Many immigrants from the largest ethnic groups, Italians and Eastern European Jews, regarded food such as oatmeal, bananas, or white bread with suspicion.

Women from many civic groups, including the Italian Welfare League, the Catholic Welfare Council, and the Hebrew Immigrant Aid Society, regularly brought milk and cookies to children on processing lines and in detention areas. Aid groups would enlist New York City restaurants to provide detainees with "American" food during holidays—turkey dinners on Thanksgiving, for example. In 1911, the Hebrew Immigrant Aid Society established a kosher kitchen on Ellis Island, and detained Jews were allowed to eat meals separately.

In 1924 Congress established a worldwide embassy visa system for immigration, effectively negating the need for a receiving station. Ellis Island was then turned into a detention center for "alien enemies" and was closed in 1954.

Bernardin, Tom. *The Ellis Island Immigrant Cookbook.* New York: Tom Bernardin, 1991.

Cannato, Vincent J. *American Passage: The History of Ellis Island.* New York: Harper Perennial, 2009.

Diner, Hasia R. *Hungering for America: Italian, Irish, and Jewish Foodways in the Age of Migration.* Cambridge, Mass.: Harvard University Press, 2001.

Moreno, Barry. *Images of Ellis Island.* Charleston, S.C.: Arcadia, 2009.

"Serve 8-Cent Meals: Ellis Island Contractors Run Largest Restaurant in the World." *Washington Post,* October 28, 1913.

Polly Franchini

English Colonial

When the first Europeans arrived in Manhattan and its environs they found native people tied together by matrilineal clans who shared hunting and fishing rights across tribal groups. Largely of the Lenape (Delaware Indian) nation, then broken up into smaller groups that populated different parts of Manhattan Island as well as Staten Island and Long Island, the natives lived by a combined hunter-gatherer and small-scale cultivation proposition. The latter included slash-and-burn methods to grow staples such as native beans, corn (maize), and pumpkins. While the Dutch settlers who claimed the area for the West

India Company in 1614 were the first recipients of the local bounty, which included wild game such as rabbit, deer, bear, buffalo, raccoon, and turkey, pigeons, quail, and other game birds, so too were the English settlers who renamed the colony New York and held sway over the island from 1664 until the end of the American Revolution in 1783.

The seas around English colonial New York teemed with oysters, salmon, cod, halibut, flounder, and other saltwater fish, and colonists adopted the consumption of freshwater fish like perch, carp, and trout. Shad, striped bass, and sturgeon were new to the Europeans as well, but at large the English were less interested than the Dutch in the plentiful local fish, preferring their mainly beef and pork diet. Like their predecessors, however, they consumed a good quantity of the large local oysters, which were generally cooked in the Native American way, over hot coals until they popped open. The first public food sellers in the city were oyster-cart vendors lined up along the old Indian path that later became Pearl Street. Native foods like lobster were considered "garbage" or "throwaway" food by colonists and scorned, although they were abundant and legendary in size. See FISHING and OYSTERS.

Whatever the protein, the English colonists quickly adapted it to their cooking styles and foodways that included boiling, stewing, frying, open-fire roasting, and baking into savory pies. Meats, particularly beef and pork, were cured or dried for the long winter, just as they were in England. They included some dried fish but plenty of beef, ham, and wild game found in the area. Pork in particular was readily available, as accounts of scores of pigs freely roaming the streets of Manhattan attest.

The colonists consumed a prodigious amount of sugar, thanks to availability from other English colonies in the Caribbean, as well as milk, cream, and butter from local dairy cows that were a hybrid of Dutch and New York breeds. Sweet pastries were popular, and recipes for a variety of sweet biscuits (cookies), cakes, fruitcakes, fruit jellies, and both fresh and dried fruit pies abound from this period.

Many English vegetables grew easily in the rich American soil. While corn was first scorned as "pig slop" by the English in America, by the time they settled New York it had become a staple of common fare. Often, corn became the substitute for wheat and barley. Pottages, porridges, and hoecakes—a pancake made from cornmeal—were often eaten at breakfast with ciders and small beers fermented in the home, just as they were in England. Local beans, both fresh and dried, joined sweet peas in the English colonial cooking repertoire, and native berries also came into the English kitchen.

The English also benefited from their predecessors' successful wheat farming, and bread was, as in Europe, a solid part of colonial New Yorkers' diets—particularly among the poor—as were most of the staples common to the British diet of the time. The establishment of robust transatlantic trade over the previous fifty years also meant that the goods from the Far East, India, and the Caribbean, such as tea, spices, and sugar, were easily had for those who could afford them. For the more common colonist, maple syrup and maple sugar were widely available sweeteners. Drinking chocolate imported from the Caribbean was quite popular among wealthy English New Yorkers, and while coffee also came in on the West Indies trade, its popularity as a drink grew after the American Revolution.

As in England, New York City taverns offered places to stay as well as to dine and to share news and discuss politics. While women could not dine in public alone, taverns such as Fraunces Tavern at Broad and Pearl Streets provided a way to broker business and, later, share covert information about the war against England. Tavern fare mimicked home meals in their ingredients and method of preparation. See FRAUNCES TAVERN.

Slaves, another "import," also came from Africa via the Caribbean; and they, too, brought with them native foodways that impacted colonial cuisine, although less so than in the American South where climates similar to much of Africa allowed them to grow native foods and retain their daily and ceremonial foodways. African slaves brought some cooking styles to English New Yorkers, including coal-pot cooking, the hallmark for foods like "pepper pot," a long-simmered stew seasoned with yucca syrup and hot peppers most common in Philadelphia.

Despite the growth of food goods being brought into and out of the city, it was Philadelphia, not New York, that was regarded as the hub of culture and fine comestibles in the American colonies. The largest city (New York was second), Philadelphia also had a more multinational population, which included Germans, Swedes, and other Europeans. However, like Philadelphia, by the beginning of the eighteenth century New York was noted by travelers for its extremely abundant and various food offerings.

See also COLONIAL DUTCH and PRE-COLUMBIAN.

Burrows, Edwin G., and Mike Wallace. *Gotham: A History of New York to 1898*. New York: Oxford University Press, 1999.

DeVoe, Thomas. *The Market Book. Containing a Historical Account of the Public Markets in the Cities of New York, Boston, Philadelphia, and Brooklyn. With a Brief Description of Every Article of Human Food Sold Therein*. New York: Thomas Devoe, 1862.

Ganeshram, Ramin. "Street Food on the Half Shell." *Saveur*, December 9, 2011.

Oliver, Sandra L. *Food in Colonial America*. Westport, Conn.: Greenwood, 2005.

Ramin Ganeshram

Erie Canal

The Erie Canal, the largest public works project in New York State when it opened in 1825, became a major trade and communications route connecting New York City to the Midwest via the Hudson River. The 363-mile long artificial river cut across the top of New York State, connecting the north–south rivers to each other and to the Great Lakes. The canal accelerated the communication, market, industrial, and transportation revolutions of the early nineteenth century and solidified New York City's position as the empire of trade.

The idea for a canal linking the Hudson to the waters west of the Appalachians had been proposed as early as 1768. But it was not until 1808 that the New York State legislature approved a survey for a canal that would connect the Hudson to Lake Erie, opening the lands to settlers and offering a cheaper means of overland transport of goods. Ground was finally broken for the canal in 1817; it took eight years to build. On October 26, 1825, this marvel of engineering opened to great celebration. A procession of canal boats traveled from Buffalo eastward, heralded by cannon booms along the entire route. At the head of the procession was the *Seneca Chief*, which held Governor DeWitt Clinton, the canal's biggest champion, and other dignitaries. From Albany, steamboats towed the canal boats down the Hudson. When they reached New York Harbor nine days later, Clinton ceremoniously poured a container of water from Lake Erie into the Atlantic in a symbolic "wedding of the waters." Balls, processions, speeches, and fireworks occurred in what was the largest public celebration to date in the state.

While a glacially slow form of transportation by today's standards, the Erie Canal offered a far quicker method of carrying goods overland than the antiquated carriages rolling along rudimentary roads. Before the canal opened, overland carriage was so expensive that it trebled the cost of the goods; in fact, it was cheaper to ship goods overseas than it was to carry them a few miles overland in the United States. The Erie Canal lowered the price of carrying heavy goods by 95 percent and sped the time of passage by a similar margin.

Planners predicted the canal would carry 250,000 tons eastward annually. The canal more than delivered on its promise. In its first year, it surpassed that total by more than fifty thousand tons. In 1860, 4,650,000 tons of goods crossed the canal. The canal yielded over $687,000 in tolls its first year. A decade later, that figure had doubled to over $1.375 million and by 1847 had reached well over $3 million. The success of the Erie Canal spurred an era of canal building throughout New York and other states, envious of the commercial success of the Empire State.

The canal brought about changes to agriculture and food marketing across New York State, extending New York City's hinterlands all the way to the Midwest, expanding both the source of agricultural product that came into the city (much of which was redistributed throughout the country and world) and the markets for finished goods that were produced or imported into New York City. Western New York became a central wheat-growing region as the canal made it feasible to get the bulky grain to market at reasonable fares. New York City quickly became the nation's central flour exchange. Farms in eastern New York had produced wheat for decades. But now, their land overused and in competition with farms to the west, these farms turned to dairying and cattle grazing. The Mohawk and Hudson Valleys became major dairy producers and New York, the leading dairy state in the country. Meanwhile, the farms nearest New York City turned from extensive to intensive production, ceding wheat growing, cattle grazing, and dairy production to locales farther afield and concentrating on more perishable goods like berries, lettuces, and other delicate crops.

In New York City, the canal contributed to the development of the Hudson River and the west side docks as the main debarkation point for goods and people. It vastly expanded the food supply coming into Manhattan, contributing to a cheaper, more reliable, and more diverse diet for many New Yorkers. Fresh game from the Midwest, salmon from Lake Ontario, and wheat from Rochester appeared in the markets of Manhattan. It also allowed New York to send perishable goods westward. Contemporaries marveled at the appearance of fresh Long Island oysters in Batavia, over 300 miles away from the sea.

While revolutionary in its impact, the canal's heyday was relatively short. In the 1850s railroads began to replace canals, and by the late nineteenth century the railroads had supplanted the canals as the main source of commercial and industrial transport. Today, the canal is mainly a recreational route. Since 2000 it has been designated by the federal government as a national heritage corridor.

Bernstein, Peter L. *The Wedding of the Waters: The Erie Canal and the Making of a Great Nation*. New York: Norton, 2006.
Klein, Milton. *The Empire State: A History of New York*. Ithaca, N.Y.: Cornell University Press, 2005.
Sheriff, Carol. *The Artificial River: The Erie Canal and the Paradox of Progress, 1817–1862*. New York: Hill & Wang, 1997.

Cindy R. Lobel

Essex House

See RESTAURANTS.

Essex Street Market

The Essex Street Market, one pillar of the urban modernization initiatives of Mayor Fiorello La Guardia, opened in January 1940 as a complex of dreary, rose brick and concrete market buildings stretching along Essex Street from Stanton Street three blocks south to Broome Street, in the heart of Manhattan's Lower East Side. Prior to the market's opening, the Lower East Side reverberated with a boisterous and congested cacophony of street peddlers and pushcart venders, jostling for position in the streets and serving the daily shopping needs of the Italian and Eastern European Jewish immigrants who lived in the neighborhood. If their tenement apartments had a kitchen—a big "if"—it was cramped and often lacked refrigeration. Frequent food shopping was a must, and the market, built at a cost of $525,000, was intended to ease street traffic and improve public safety and food-handling practices. Local store owners welcomed the elimination of the street peddlers, not because they were threatened by the competition (or so they claimed) but because of embarrassment over the "Old World" and backward habits of their poorer landsmen.

The market immediately divided the pushcart venders and peddlers. Those who could afford its $4.25 per week stall rental welcomed the modernized venue, the respite from foul weather, and the psychological step up from "peddler" to "merchant," while the price was too rich for others, driving them out of subsistence businesses and into unemployed poverty. Shop owners soon changed their attitude; although they had expected to benefit from the new ban on peddling, many were stunned when their business did not expand. The reason had more to do with nostalgia than with logistics. Especially among the Jewish merchants, many businesses contracted, as their more affluent customers, who had previously moved to the Upper East Side but sentimentally returned to the old neighborhood for their traditional foods, stopped shopping at the old downtown shops once the colorful pushcarts disappeared and the atmosphere of "coming home" was gone. These well-heeled shoppers, however, still might patronize the old peddlers in the new market; on the occasion of the twenty-fifth anniversary of the opening of the market, one dairy monger reminisced that Saturday night was "mink coat night," the time when former neighborhood denizens came down in their chauffeured cars.

For those living on the Lower East Side, however, the market was a vital community center. Through at least 1960, the New York City Department of Markets gave free cooking classes, many of them in "scientific kosher cookery." But in the 1950s the neighborhood started to change as the Lower East Side became home to Puerto Rican and, decades later, Dominican immigrants. Stalls that had once sold pickles, kosher meats, and bagels gave way to those that sold bacalao, *cabrito*, and plantains. The bustle of the market faded in the 1960s and 1970s as the supermarkets and bodegas sprinkled around the Lower East Side became preferred shopping venues. Private efforts to redevelop the market in the early 1990s stalled, and the New York City Economic Development Council assumed control of the failing market in 1995, pumping $1.5 million into renovations and consolidating the small number of merchants scattered in the cavernous spaces into a single building at 120 Essex Street.

With the increasing gentrification of the Lower East Side and below-market rents offered by the New York City Economic Development Council, the market attracted a new and eclectic mix of merchants. In the twenty-first century, it has been home to an artisanal bread baker, a chocolatier, free-range and heritage butchers, fishmongers, Swedish and Japanese gourmet importers, a socially conscious pastry shop, two cheese shops, and a coffee roaster. It continued catering to the Hispanic clientele, offering Latin American staples such as five-gallon tins of oil and twenty-pound bags of masa, as well as candles decorated with saints and other objects for religious observances.

Although the market has enjoyed a renaissance resulting from the middle-class and luxury residential development in the Lower East Side, it has become a victim of the neighborhood's success. Plans to raze the remaining market building were approved in November 2014, and the lot will form part of the planned Essex Crossing, a six-acre redevelopment zone with commercial and mixed-income housing. The New York City Economic Development Council has promised to relocate the current twenty vendors to a state-of-the-art facility across Delancey Street, at 115 Essex Street. The new space is slated to house thirty-nine stalls and two restaurants.

See also LA GUARDIA, FIORELLO and LOWER EAST SIDE.

Bellafante, Ginia. "A Move for the Essex Street Market." *New York Times*, September 27, 2013.
Essex Street Market website: "History." http://www .essexstreetmarket.com/history.
"Essex Street Market 25 Years Old; 35 Original Tenants Still There." *New York Times*, December 11, 1963.
Wasserman, Suzanne. "The Good Old Days of Poverty: Merchants and the Battle over Pushcart Peddling on the Lower East Side." *Business and Economic History* 27, no. 2 (1998): 330–339.

Cathy K. Kaufman

Exchange Buffet

See RESTAURANTS.

Experimental Cuisine Collective

The Experimental Cuisine Collective is an interdisciplinary assembly of scientists, scholars, chefs, journalists, writers, artists, and intellectually curious food enthusiasts who explore food with academic rigor, using techniques gleaned from the physical sciences, the humanities, and social sciences, as well as the world of the culinary practitioner. Founded in 2007 at New York University by Kent Kirshenbaum (Chemistry Department, College of Arts and Sciences), Amy Bentley (Department of Nutrition, Food Studies, and Public Health at the Steinhardt School of Culture, Education, and Human Development), and chef Will Goldfarb of WillPowder, the group's manifold mission is to use science to understand cooking processes and to create innovative culinary techniques, to educate the public about a healthful and sustainable diet, to understand the cultural context and consequences of new culinary techniques and processes, and to spark interest in the physical sciences through food and cooking curricula addressed to children. The group hosts monthly programs during the academic year, usually (but not always) at New York University, and attracts an international roster of presenters and luminaries, including Hervé This, Harold McGee, Ferran Adrià, and Colman Andrews. The Experimental Cuisine Collective is funded by the National Science Foundation, the New York University Humanities Initiative, and the Steinhardt School.

Membership is open to the public, and notwithstanding the academic and professional credentials of the presenters, the experience is friendly. Meetings begin by attendees briefly introducing themselves and explaining their relationship to food: the "dedicated amateur eaters" are as welcome as the scholars. Most events are free and often include small tastings; a key focus is on the science and food policy that underlie the taste experience, whether it be the responsible harvesting of botanicals to create a sustainable commercial bitters or the creation of steak au poivre by blending various powdered compounds with water and microwaving them to create an edible gel: this 2014 demonstration of "note by note" cookery by Hervé This was not a parlor trick but, as he claimed, a potentially transformative way of eliminating food spoilage and creating new gastronomic pleasures. The demonstration perfectly illustrated the Experimental Cuisine Collective's slogan of "science, society, and food."

Experimental Cuisine Collective website: http://experimentalcuisine.com/about.
Stein, Hannes. "New-New Food: A Foreigner's Perspective." NewsPlink, April 21, 2009. http://www.newsplink.com/2009/04/21/new-new-food.

Cathy K. Kaufman

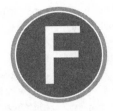

Fabricant, Florence

Florence Fabricant is a nationally renowned American food and wine writer, cookbook author, and *New York Times* columnist. She was born in New York City and grew up in Westchester County, a suburb just north of the city. Her father was an insurance broker, and her mother was a stay-at-home mom who looked after her and her brother.

Fabricant inherited her interest in gastronomy from her parents, both of whom were passionate about entertaining and dining out. They began taking her to restaurants at a young age. She recalls being no more than four years old and going to a Chinese restaurant for Sunday dinners. She was determined to put just the right amount of soy sauce in her egg drop soup—it had to be just so. She also remembers her father taking her to lunch at Chambord, a fancy French restaurant in a storefront on Third Avenue under the El, where she would make him name all of the variously sized bottles of champagne in the window before going in. On Sunday mornings, Fabricant and her father would share toasted bagels with cream cheese and not smoked salmon but anchovies, a food that she adores to this day. These experiences have given her a deep knowledge of New York's food and restaurant scene, going back many decades.

Fabricant obtained a bachelor's degree in French and art from Smith and a master's degree in French from the New York University Graduate School of Arts and Sciences in 1962. After college, she worked at an advertising agency in market research but never really took to it. When her children started school full-time, she found herself trying to figure out what to do. She considered law school, though her husband, a lawyer, discouraged her. Fabricant describes her path to food writing as "falling into it." In 1972, she and her husband were summering in the Hamptons, where they had a house in Wainscott, East Hampton. She was enraged to see people buying iceberg lettuce and prepackaged tomatoes in the middle of summer, when you could go a couple of blocks down the road and buy somebody's fresh tomatoes from a card table on the front lawn. The local weekly newspaper, the *East Hampton Star*, did not have a food column, so she pitched one to the editor. After sending in a sample that met with his approval, she started writing a weekly food column with a recipe, even though she had never before written or cooked professionally.

Within six months of her first column appearing in the *East Hampton Star*, she started getting assignments from the *New York Times*. Fabricant acknowledges that the fact that Craig Claiborne lived in East Hampton and read her articles, as did a number of other *New York Times* staffers, probably helped promote her career. See CLAIBORNE, CRAIG.

Fabricant's first assignments from the *Times* were for the Long Island section. She wrote for that section for many years, contributing recipes, food stories involving people, and reviews of new shops and restaurants. She continued to contribute to that section even after she started writing for what was then the Living section (the Food and Lifestyle section). The first piece she wrote for Living was about how to dip strawberries in chocolate.

Today, she contributes to the weekly Front Burner and Off the Menu columns, is a member of the wine panel, and writes the pairings column for the wine tastings column. She frequently writes features that appear in the Dining section and writes about food and travel for the Sunday Travel section, as well as articles about news in the restaurant industry for the Metro section.

Fabricant continually seeks out the cooks, chefs, entrepreneurs, and restaurateurs who are making a difference in the international food scene. Her influence and credibility with the *Times* can help to put a food business or restaurant on the map.

She is also an accomplished author and has written more than eleven cookbooks; her daughter, Patricia Fabricant, designed five of them. Titles include *The New York Times Seafood Cookbook* (St. Martin's Press, 2003), *The New York Times Dessert Cookbook* (St. Martin's Press, 2006), and *The New York Restaurant Cookbook* (Rizzoli, 2009). Two of her books, *Park Avenue Potluck* (Rizzoli, 2007) and *Park Avenue Potluck Celebrations* (Rizzoli, 2009), were written to raise funds to support The Society of Memorial Sloan-Kettering Cancer Center. Her latest book, *Wine with Food* (Rizzoli, 2014), was written with Eric Asimov, the *Times* wine and food critic, and highlights pairing notes and recipes from their combined experience at the *New York Times*.

She holds L'Ordre National du Mérite from the French government and is a member of Who's Who of Food and Beverage in America. She lives in Manhattan and in East Hampton with her husband, Richard, and together they have two children and two granddaughters.

See also NEW YORK TIMES.

Heritage Radio Network. "Episode 4—Florence Fabricant." *Evolutionaries*. May 22, 2013. http://www.heritageradionetwork.org/episodes/4162-Evolutionaries-Episode-4-Florence-Fabricant.

Layla Khoury-Hanold

Fairway Market

With fifteen stores in the tri-state area and a seemingly endless expansion plan, Fairway Market is no longer the simple family fruit market that Upper West Siders frequented for decades. Fairway's history began in 1933 when Nathan Glickberg owned a series of fruit stands along upper Broadway. In 1954, along with his son Leo, Nathan consolidated them into one storefront on Broadway and Seventy-Fourth Street. At some point along the way, the family named the market "Fairway." While consumer folklore assumes the name refers to fair pricing, the Glickberg family used the name of a toy manufactory that Leo's wife Cynthia's family owned in Pittsburgh. In 1974, the third generation, Howie Glickberg, joined the family venture. Shortly thereafter, amid fractured family tensions from running a business together, Leo stepped away and Howie brought in David Sneddon and Howard Seybert, both Fairway tomato suppliers, as his new partners. It is this trio that forged the first stage of Fairway's significant growth.

In the 1980s, the once overly crowded produce store with aisles barely the width of two shopping carts took over the space next door previously occupied by a D'Agostino supermarket. Glickberg, Sneddon, and Seybert, besides expanding Fairway's real estate, redefined Fairway's mission from a produce-only store to one introducing imported specialty items. In 1980 they hired Steven Jenkins, America's first "master cheesemonger," to develop Fairway's famed cheese portfolio. But even as Fairway branched into specialty food and imported cheese, it did not sell either meat or fish. According to legend, second-generation owner Leo Glickberg had an unspoken agreement with Citarella's original owner. As the two stores were in close proximity, Citarella agreed not to sell any produce and Fairway would refrain from both fish and meat. When Citarella's owner died and a new owner purchased the store in 1983, he negated their oral agreement. Citarella began selling produce, and Fairway immediately retaliated by showcasing meat and fish. The two adjacent businesses were now fierce competitors.

Although Fairway grew in terms of its offerings, it was not until 1995 that it opened the Harlem location, their second store. The three partners purchased an old meat-packing facility and, in lieu of installing refrigeration units, converted the expansive "cold room" into a giant walk-in refrigerator for the dairy, meat, and fish. As a novelty, it hung heavy overcoats outside the room for customers to wear while shopping. With the Harlem store and its adjacent parking lot, Fairway increased its customer base to include consumers from northern suburbs. This new demographic change ushered in the next stage of the company's growth.

In 2006, after Howie's partners retired, he brought in Sterling Investment Partners, and together they set the ambitious goal of two new store openings per year. Although Howie's father Leo and grandfather Nathan were long gone, his son Dan Glickberg, a fourth-generation owner, joined the Fairway team. They opened the Red Hook store in 2007 in a striking 1860s warehouse, which, along with Ikea, revitalized economically depressed Red Hook, Brooklyn. By 2011, Fairway had nine stores open in Manhattan, Brooklyn, Long Island, Westchester, New Jersey, and Rockland County. In April 2013 Fairway Market went public. It is difficult to reconcile the corporate culture that defines Fairway Market today with the family-owned business birthed four generations ago.

See also CHEESEMONGERS; GROCERY STORES; and SUPERMARKETS.

Alexander, Jan. "Fairway Market's Case of Overcooked Ambition." *Institutional Investor*, December 2, 2014. http://www.institutionalinvestor.com/article/3406380/banking-and-capital-markets-corporations/fairway-markets-case-of-overcooked-ambition.html#.VPXPGEKphzQ.
Jenkins, Steve. *The Cheese Primer*. New York: Workman, 1996.
Jenkins, Steven, and Mitchel London. *The Food Life: Inside the World of Food with the Grocer Extraordinaire at Fairway*. New York: Ecco, 2008.
Marx, Patricia. "A Bushel and a Peck: Navigating New York's Food Megastores." *New Yorker*, January 16, 2012.

Jennifer Schiff Berg

Falafel

Falafel originated in the Middle East, but it is ubiquitous in New York City today. It typically consists of deep-fried balls or patties of chickpeas (or fava beans) served with accoutrements such as hummus, vegetables, garlic, spices, tahini, and other sauces. It can be eaten in meze platters or mashed into hollow flatbread, such as pita, and consumed like a sandwich.

Falafel was introduced into New York City's culinary scene by Arab and Jewish immigrants. The first identified print mention of falafel appeared in November 1950, when *Commentary* magazine reviewed Habibi, New York City's "first and only—Israeli night club," located on West Forty-Sixth Street. Its bilingual, Hebrew and English menu listed falafel, defined as "crisp spiced vegetable balls." Falafel was introduced to a broader audience in a column by Craig Claiborne in 1967. Claiborne noted that it was

sold on Atlantic Avenue in Brooklyn. See CLAIBORNE, CRAIG. Falafel was easy to make and eat, cheap, and nutritious. It is vegetarian and vegan and can easily be made kosher and halal—just perfect for multicultural New York. It took off as a street food by the 1980s.

Mamoun's Falafel, a restaurant in Greenwich Village, opened in 1971 and claims to be the first falafel restaurant in the city. Mamoun's has subsequently opened a restaurant in the East Village and in several locations outside of New York City. Today, scores of restaurants, such as Alfanoose in the Financial District, the Kabab Café in Astoria, and Zaytoon's in Brooklyn, specialize in falafel. Added to this are the hundreds of street vendors and food trucks that sell falafel. For the home cook, tens of thousands of recipes can be found in cookbooks, in newspapers and magazines, and on the Internet; and for the less adventurous, falafel mixes are sold in grocery stores.

New Yorkers have put their own distinctive improvisations on falafel. In Flushing, Benjy's Kosher Pizza Dairy restaurant serves falafel pizza, a cheesy slice topped with falafels, tahini, and hot sauce, while Flatiron's upscale Ilili Box adds fiery kimchi to the sandwich.

Bittman, Mark. "Falafel." *New York Times*, February 12, 2008.
Kantor, Jody. "A History of the Mideast in the Humble Chickpea." *New York Times*, July 22, 2002.
Prakash, Alicia. "The 11 Best Falafel Restaurants in NYC." *Thrillist*, November 13, 2014. http://www.thrillist.com/eat/new-york/best-falafel-restaurants-in-nyc.

Cathy K. Kaufman and Andrew F. Smith

Fales Library

The Marion Nestle Food Studies Collection at New York University's Fales Library contains more than fifty-five thousand printed books, making it the largest food studies collection in the United States. The collection began in 2003, with the acquisition of Cecily Brownstone's personal papers and library of approximately seven thousand volumes. Brownstone had been the Associated Press syndicated food writer for thirty-nine years and built her personal research library because there were no libraries for recipe research.

Building a serious collection was essential for students and scholars in New York University's Food Department in the United States, begun by Nestle in

1996. Moreover, a large food studies collection was necessary for the burgeoning field in general. Other major collections of books were donated to the library: *Ladies Home Journal* decided it did not need its cookbook collection, as did the James Beard Foundation. Dalia Carmel has given more than eleven thousand books in memory of her late husband Herbert Goldstein. When Condé Nast closed *Gourmet* magazine in 2009, the collection of more than seven thousand volumes was in danger of being discarded. A generous donation from Rozanne Gold saved the books. Les Dames d'Escoffier of New York City and others have given funds to purchase rare titles lacking from the collection. George Lang, the famous restaurateur, donated his massive collection of more than twenty-six thousand volumes related to food to the library in 2011, making the collection the largest in the country. Other donors continue to give materials, building on the great strength of the collection. Strategic purchases of books, magazines, cook booklets, and ephemera from the nineteenth and twentieth centuries complement the other holdings in the collection, making it a destination for researchers interested in American foodways. In 2013, the collection was named in honor of Marion Nestle, celebrating her career and her vision for building the library.

The Nestle Collection also includes the personal papers of such food luminaries as James Beard, Rose Levy Beranbaum, Cecily Brownstone, Meryle Evans, Betty Fussell, Marion Nestle, and Louis Sherry as well as the archives of Les Dames d'Escoffier, the New York Women's Culinary Alliance, Café Nicholson, Roundtable of Women in Food Service, and many others. Since 2005, food consultant Clark Wolf has helped organize an annual series of panels called Critical Topics in Food that brings together scholars, food writers, historians, and others to discuss timely issues in the food world. Videotapes of these programs are accessible on the web. Taken together, these materials support the research of undergraduate and graduates students, faculty, and other researchers working within disciplines such as food studies, food management, nutrition, performance studies, American studies, and history. These materials are also of use to professionals outside of the university who work as writers, journalists, chefs, or food professionals. The collection is available to researchers by making an appointment at fales.library@nyu.edu.

See also NESTLE, MARION.

Barron, James. "With Latest Donation, N.Y.U. Food Library Joins Big Leagues." *City Room* (blog), April 5, 2011. http://cityroom.blogs.nytimes.com/2011/04/05/with-latest-donation-n-y-u-food-library-joins-big-leagues/?_php=true&_type=blogs&_r=0.
Blotcher, Jay. "Tradition: 101 Cookbooks." *Edible Hudson Valley* (Spring 2013). http://ediblehudsonvalley.com/editorial/spring-2013/tradition-101-cookbooks/.
Taylor, Marvin J., and Clark Wolf, eds. *101 Classic Cookbooks, 501 Classic Recipes*. New York: Rizzoli International with the Fales Library, 2012.
"The Marion Nestle Food Studies Collection." Fales Library Special Collections. http://www.nyu.edu/library/bobst/research/fales/foodcookery.html.

Marvin J. Taylor

Fancy Food Show

The Fancy Food Show was founded in 1955 and is now hosted every summer by the Specialty Food Association at the Jacob K. Javits Convention Center. The Specialty Food Association welcomes tens of thousands of visitors (the 2014 show boasted more than thirty-eight thousand) to the west side of Manhattan to sample hundreds of thousands of products, attend educational programs, and celebrate the best in show with the SoFi awards (Specialty Outstanding Food Innovation, the "Oscars of artisanal food"), begun in 1990.

The Fancy Food Show is remarkable for reasons beyond longevity and volume. The expo is known for launching brands and products that eventually become integral components of that same culinary lexicon. Yerba maté, a South American herb traditionally sipped from a hollowed gourd using a metal straw, with caffeine-like side effects and a vegetal, green tea–like flavor, is one example. Covering the fifty-second Fancy Food Show in 2007 for the *New York Times*, Florence Fabricant remarked on the appearance of maté in commercial bottled beverages. See FABRICANT, FLORENCE. That same year, the Associated Press declared "Tea is the new bottled water, and mate is the new chai." Maté is now nearly ubiquitous, a key ingredient in tea blends, energy drinks, energy bars, even chocolate bars. Ben & Jerry's, Mt. Vikos, La Tourangelle, Honest Tea, and Pop Chips are all brands that launched themselves to national prominence from the halls of the Javits Center. The

Fancy Food Show's increased prominence and educational programming and the SoFi awards reflect a changing culture around food in New York City and the nation.

Fabricant, Florence. "At the Fancy Food Show, Promoting Everyday Luxuries." New York Times, July 12, 2006.
Fabricant, Florence. "Fancy This, Fancy That." New York Times, July 12, 1995.
"History of SoFi: The Industry's Most Coveted Honor." Specialty Food Association. http://www.specialtyfood.com/sofi/history/.

Alexis Zanghi

Farmers' Markets

See GREENMARKETS.

Farm to Table

Farm to table is a cuisine that emerged in the early twenty-first century that emphasizes the importance of local terroir, mer-roir, and regional food culture. A "back to the future" culinary consciousness with a bold, powerful creativeness, the movement celebrates food as lifestyle and entertainment, a peasant versus an aristocratic cuisine, and has coalesced as a potent political force.

In reaction to flavorless, industrial food grown for transport at the expense of taste, farm to table evolved as a way to refer to a "new" type of New York cuisine: food made with locally sourced ingredients, most often from small family farms from upstate to Long Island to the Garden State of New Jersey, using integrated production practices. Because food sources had become ever more remote, there developed community food systems—a practice used interchangeably with "local" or "regional" to foster food security and sustainability, along with food- and agriculture-related businesses including farmers' markets, community and school gardens, and community supported agriculture. See COMMUNITY SUPPORTED AGRICULTURE.

Food aficionados sought control over their food choices, primarily by shortening the distance between producer and consumer and by fostering personal relationships with their food makers and growers—as they increasingly saw great chefs doing. The chefs' renewed dedication to discovering regional dishes, recipes, and the freshest "ingredients-as-inspiration" characterizes farm to table. It is a food-based—food-obsessed—phenomenon that also celebrates the enduring relationships chefs develop with their local farmers, fishermen, foragers, dairy farmers, and artisanal food makers in order to know where their food comes from.

Farm to table developed alongside the idea of a "locavore," the *New Oxford American Dictionary*'s 2007 "Word of the Year," heralding "one who eats foods grown locally whenever possible." The language of locavores soon expanded as a result of its burgeoning popularity: "fin-to-table," "farm-to-fork," and "fin-to-tail" followed as part of a true locavore's vocabulary. By 2013, farm to table emerged as a popular buzzword. But in fact, the effort was ignited decades earlier by some of Gotham's leading chefs.

While it is commonplace now for restaurant menus to list where their food comes from to demonstrate farm-to-table gravitas, Brooklyn's River Café was the first restaurant to name the farm, the varietals, and the region of the ingredients, in 1980. The chef, Larry Forgione, is also credited with coining the term "free range" for the restaurant's commercially produced, naturally raised and fed chickens.

While Forgione worked in Europe, he first noted the reversal of how fresh ingredients were used. "Farmers and makers were producing for restaurants and everyday cooks got to use the same ingredients, whereas in America everybody was producing for the masses, and chefs also had to use what was produced." Forgione returned to New York and started working with farmers and producers.

In addition to Forgione, referred to as the "godfather of American cuisine," a few of Gotham's food rebels resisted corporate ingredients around the mid-1980s, including iconoclastic chefs and the restaurants they owned, primarily The River Café's Michael "Buzzy" O'Keefe; chef Charlie Palmer; Forgione's An American Place; Anna Rosenzweig's Arcadia; Jonathan Waxman, who returned from Alice Waters's Chez Panisse to launch Jams restaurant; Peter Hoffman's Savoy restaurant (now Back Forty), often credited with getting the locavore movement started in New York; and Lutece's chef Eberhard Mueller, who so revered ingredients he traded in his toque, becoming a grower along with his wife, Paulette, at their North Fork Satur Farms.

These chef-owners were at the ramparts of some New York City restaurants, carrying forth Nouvelle Cuisine's simple, casual approach to food prep and cooking. Nouvelle cooking gained popularity after

World War II and continued to the mid-1980s when farm to table took root.

Farm-to-table chef and food leader Peter Hoffman confirmed that nouvelle cuisine opened up things for chefs: "We no longer felt the need to follow the codification of *haute cuisine* and Escoffier." Farm to table embraced the dictum of nouvelle's chic comfort food, continuing to practice the rigors of French technique but without the imports.

Hoffman described how pioneering New York City chefs came to see that the most flavorful berry did not need to be an exotic import but could be grown nearby: "This idea started a shift. We saw great flavors and great taste in local things—not in imported foods and aristocratic cooking. Farm-to-Table was freedom—a celebration of ingredients. A taste of *our* land, *our* waters, *our* place."

Increased food diversity and makers' culinary self-expression led to food as entertainment in restaurants and the media. Without farm to table there would be no Food Network or the plethora of cooking shows and YouTube food channels. By 2010 TV's Food Network was featuring the "grass roots" of food culture: "more diversity in personalities and menus." Food ingredients became the star. New York's PBS featured its own farm-to-table series.

From Farm to Table. WMHT. http://www.wmht.org/topics/home-how-to/food/farmtotable/.

Halweil, Brian. "Talking About? Seeds." *Edible Manhattan*, September 30, 2013.

Lavin, Leeann. *The Hamptons & Long Island Homegrown Cookbook*. Minneapolis: Voyageur, 2012.

Pollan, Michael. "Farmer in Chief." *New York Times*, October 9, 2008.

Salkin, Allen. "Newcomer to Food Television Tries for a Little Grit." *New York Times*, April 20, 2010.

Leeann Lavin

Fast Food

New Yorkers have long had a reputation for being in a hurry (a "New York minute" is the blink of an eye), and lunchtime is no exception. In the early nineteenth century, businessmen in the financial district grabbed a quick meal at places like the Plate House, one of the city's first quick-service lunch establishments. Customers placed their orders, which were relayed to the kitchen by attendants (who shouted them out at top volume), and within seconds the food was delivered. Ten minutes was the usual duration

of the meal, and then the diners were on the run back to the world of commerce.

The Exchange Buffet, which opened in 1885 across the street from the New York Stock Exchange, eliminated the middleman for even faster service: customers lined up to choose food from a buffet and ate it at stand-up counters. Each diner then cleared his dishes, tallied his bill, and told the cashier what he owed. See RESTAURANTS.

In 1889, William and Samuel Child opened a lunchroom on the main floor of the Merchants Hotel in the Financial District. In 1898 they initiated cafeteria-style service there and were the first to provide customers with trays so that they did not have to juggle an armload of dishes. By 1925 there were more than a hundred Childs cafeterias in the city. See CHILDS.

By the 1920s other lunchroom chains began to appear in the city's business and shopping districts. Most chains had only two or three establishments. These shared a name and were advertised as a "system." Some of the larger chains had central commissaries from which the food was distributed to the branch restaurants. One of the most successful of these was W. F. Schrafft's, launched by Frank Shattuck in Boston in 1898.

Another quick-lunch (and breakfast and dinner and in-between) option was Horn & Hardart's automat, which opened its first New York location in 1912. In a completely novel system, customers chose their meal from dishes displayed behind little glass hatches. Dropping one or more nickels into a slot would unlock the hatch so that the food could be removed. Within a few years, Horn & Hardart operated fifteen automats in the city. In September 1922 the company opened a combination automat-cafeteria, which they claimed was the largest restaurant in the city: it had the capacity to feed ten thousand New Yorkers daily. The chain's outlets were supplied from a central commissary, helping to keep costs down. The automats did well during the 1920s, but they really came into their own during the Depression, when many New Yorkers had not much more than two nickels to rub together. In 1933, Horn & Hardart hired Francis Bourdon, a classically trained chef who had worked at top restaurants in Europe and the United States, to run its commissary, a position he held for the next thirty-five years. He brought some prestige to the operation, developed new recipes, and helped ensure food quality and consistency throughout the chain.

After World War II, Horn & Hardart went into decline. Within four decades, most automats closed, many having been converted into Burger King outlets. The last automat in New York closed in April 1991. See AUTOMATS.

Fast-Food Chains

The concept of a chain of identical food outlets with consistent menus and prices came to fruition in the modern fast-food chain. The first one to arrive in New York City was White Castle, which opened several shops in northern Manhattan and the Bronx in 1930. The choices were limited and the service, lightning fast. A small square hamburger on a bun cost a nickel, and soda, coffee, and pie rounded out the menu. The hamburgers were prepared on an assembly-line basis to fill orders as quickly as possible. Outlets were often located near businesses, such as newspaper plants, that operated twenty-four hours a day; and White Castle stands remained open far into the night. White Castle served as a model for the other fast-food chains, such as McDonald's, that moved into the city after World War II. These would later include Burger King, Wendy's, Kentucky Fried Chicken, and Taco Bell, where the food purchased could be eaten on-site or taken out, and the slightly more restaurant-like Chipotle Mexican Grill, Lenny's Sandwich Shops, and Pret-a-Manger.

A few fast-food chains originated in New York. New Yorkers Robert T. Neely and Orville A. Dickinson formed Nedick's Orange Juice Company in 1913, where orange drink, coffee, doughnuts, and hot dogs were sold. Named for the first three syllables of their last names, it later expanded into a chain that sold a wide variety of foods and beverages along with their iconic orange drink. The Nedick's chain folded in the 1980s. See NEDICK'S.

More successful was Nathan Handwerker, a Polish immigrant who opened a hot dog stand in Coney Island in 1916. When the subway arrived at Coney Island in 1920, people from all over the city could visit Coney Island for a nickel, and a hot dog from "Nathan's Famous Frankfurters" (or simply "Nathan's Famous") was a must for beachgoers. Nathan's Famous, Inc., has promoted its operation in a variety of ways. Every summer, on the Fourth of July, Nathan's sponsors a highly publicized hot dog–eating contest on the boardwalk at Coney Island. Contestants down as many hot dogs (and buns) as they can in ten minutes. The 2015 winner ate sixty-two hot dogs. See NATHAN'S FAMOUS.

Foreign Fast Food

New Yorkers have adventurous palates, and the national burger and sandwich chains face stiff competition from Chinese take-out places, pizza joints, Indian buffets and kati roll shops, taco stands, falafel carts, hole-in-the-wall dumpling shops, and an ever-changing variety of food trucks offering meals and snacks from every national and ethnic cuisine (and every possible "fusion" of those).

The Kennedy Fried Chicken chain, with outlets throughout the city, was likely founded by refugees from the Soviet occupation of Afghanistan in 1979, and many of the chain's outlets are run by Afghanis. Filipino immigrants have settled in Flushing, Queens, where a Filipino fast-food chain, Jolly Bee, opened a franchise. Tim Hortons, a Canadian doughnut and coffee chain, operates outlets in New York.

Fast Food Today

New York City's mayors and city council members have passed a number of laws regulating local fast-food outlets, and some of these have affected fast-food operations nationwide. A citywide ban on artificial trans fats (which increase the risk of heart disease and type 2 diabetes) was imposed on all restaurants in 2005. A study published in the *Annals of Internal Medicine* in July 2007 showed that the ban had been effective at reducing the amount of trans fats in the diets of New Yorkers and potentially lowering the incidence of heart disease in the city. Some fast-food chains, including McDonald's, went on to ban trans fat in their products nationwide. See TRANS FAT ELIMINATION.

In 2008, New York City required chain restaurants to post calorie counts in the hope of encouraging New Yorkers to consume fewer calories and less fat. Other cities followed New York's example. In 2010 the federal Affordable Care Act required that all chain restaurants in the United States post calorie counts for their menu offerings. The ruling has made fast-food operators (as well as consumers) more sensitive to the calorie density and fat content of fast-food choices, and some chains have reworked their recipes and introduced new, healthier items. See MENU LABELING.

Today, fast-food chains employ fifty thousand workers in the city. Most are paid minimum wage (in 2015 $7.25 an hour) and work only part-time. Few receive medical insurance, paid sick days, or vacation days. In November 2012 and again in April 2013, workers at McDonald's, Burger King, Wendy's, Taco Bell, and other fast-food chains went on one-day strikes to demand a living wage. This campaign has inspired fast-food workers in other cities to also strike for improved wages. See FAST-FOOD WORKERS STRIKES.

Bromell, Nicolas. "The Automat: Preparing the Way for Fast Food." *New York History* 81, no. 3 (July 2000): 300–312.

Schlosser, Eric. *Fast Food Nation: The Dark Side of the All-American Meal.* New York: Houghton Mifflin, 2001.

Smith, Andrew F. *Hamburger: A Global History.* London: Reaktion, 2008.

Smith, Andrew F. *Fast Food: A Global Perspective.* London: Reaktion, 2016.

Andrew F. Smith

Fast-Food Workers Strikes

With almost 375,000 workers, the restaurant industry is one of the largest and fastest-growing segments of the New York City economy. Fast-food restaurants are an important and rapidly growing segment within the larger New York City restaurant industry. However, despite their size and growth, both the New York City restaurant industry and the fast-food restaurant segment, in particular, include some of the lowest-paying occupations in the entire city. In fact, New York City fast-food workers earn a median wage of $8.86.

New York City fast-food workers began to organize as part of the Restaurant Opportunities Center of New York after 2002. Seeking to change both poverty wages and the lack of mobility to higher-paying jobs in the industry, fast-food workers worked with other members of the Restaurant Opportunities Center and other organizations to successfully raise the minimum wage for all restaurant workers in 2005. They then led the formation of COLORS, a worker-owned restaurant, and inside it the CHOW (COLORS Hospitality for Workers) Institute, which provides training to help low-wage restaurant workers advance to livable-wage fine dining jobs.

In November 2012, New York Communities for Change and the Service Employees International Union organized one hundred New York City fast-food restaurant workers to strike for higher wages and better working conditions. This strike sparked a series of nationwide strikes of fast-food workers—including New York City fast-food workers—in April, May, July, and December 2013. In 2014, fast-food workers across the globe joined these U.S. strikes, including workers in Brazil, Japan, and the United Kingdom. Leading the largest strikes of fast-food workers in American history, these workers' universal rallying cry became a fifteen dollar minimum wage; this has led to several U.S. cities adopting $15 minimum wage proposals, including Seattle and San Francisco. On July 29, 2014, these workers won a tremendous victory when the National Labor Relations Board ruled that McDonald's has liability for the employment conditions in its franchised restaurants, setting a precedent that holds fast-food corporations liable not only for all of the retaliatory firings that occurred against striking fast-food workers but also for the wages and working conditions in the franchised operations.

On July 22, 2015, a state panel appointed by Governor Andrew Cuomo recommended that the minimum wage be raised to $15 per hour for New York City employees of fast-food chain restaurants with at least thirty outlets. The wage increases will take effect gradually over the next three years.

See also FAST FOOD.

Eichelberger, Erika. "Fast-Food Strikes Go Global." *Mother Jones* (May 15, 2014).

Greenhouse, Steven. "With Day of Protests, Fast-Food Workers Seek More Pay." *New York Times*, November 29, 2012.

Greenhouse, Steven. "McDonald's Ruling Could Open Door for Unions." *New York Times*, July 29, 2014.

Resnikoff, Nedd. "New York's Fast Food Workers Strike. Why Now?" msnbc, November 29, 2012. http://www.msnbc.com/the-ed-show/new-yorks-fast-food-workers-strike-why-now.

Saru Jayaraman

Feltman, Charles

Charles Feltman (1841–1910) was a pioneer in the development of Coney Island as New York's, and the nation's, most celebrated amusement park and beach resort. A leading restaurateur, he is erroneously credited with inventing Coney Island's paradigmatic dish, the hot dog.

Born in Germany in 1841, Feltman immigrated to New York at the age of fourteen, eventually settling in Brooklyn. He worked at various jobs for three dollars a week, saved his money, and opened a bakery at Sixth Avenue and Tenth Street in 1866 even before the roads had been cut through the city. His bakery became a success, and always a visionary, he recognized the potential of Coney Island as a weekend resort for city people. He persuaded a railroad company to build a line out to the as yet undeveloped area and there founded his eponymous restaurant. In 1871, his first year on Surf Avenue, thirty-seven thousand customers were served by a staff of fifteen. By 1933 there were 7.4 million and a staff of twelve hundred, with a seating capacity of eight thousand.

Feltman was a brilliant marketer and a pillar of the local Brooklyn business community. He was the first to bring band music to Coney Island and put on shows that he deemed wholesome family entertainment. His fare was the famous Shore Dinners of fresh seafood, including fried clams, served in an upscale atmosphere.

The linkage to hot dog history is the oft-repeated story that Feltman had sold sausages from a cart and was the first to put them in a bun in 1867. There is no credible evidence for this. Though Feltman had a number of sausage grills running for take-out service and in his German-style restaurant, he actually despised hot dog stands and their operators, who he deemed low-class.

Charles Feltman's sons continued the business for many years, but it eventually went bankrupt in 1952, to be replaced by Astroland Park. In 2010 the city tore down the amusement park and the last remnant of Feltman's, its kitchen.

See also HOT DOGS.

"Charles Feltman Dead." *New York Times*, September 21, 1910.
"Charles Feltman Dies in Cassel, Germany." *Brooklyn Daily Eagle*, September 20, 1910.
"Feltman's at Coney Island for More Than Fifty Years." *Brooklyn Daily Eagle*, August 27, 1933.

Bruce Kraig

Filipino

Filipino food entered American consciousness when the American army took the Philippines during the Spanish-American War. Between 1898 and 1946,

the United States ruled the Philippines as an American colony. Many Americans left for Manila from New York on Pacific Mail Lines and Boston Steamship Company ships. In return, Filipino immigrants settled near the ports of the Brooklyn Navy Yard and Red Hook. Some of these settlers had worked as cooks for the American Merchant Marine and the U.S. Navy. They founded New York's first Filipino restaurant in the 1920s, the Manila Karihan Restaurant at 47 Sands Street, Brooklyn. A Works Progress Administration guide from 1939 recorded that the restaurant served Filipino favorites such as *adobong baboy* (pork braised in vinegar), *sinigang isda* (fish in a tamarind broth), *sinigang visaya* (tamarind broth, central Philippine–style), *mixta* (rice and beans), and tropical fruits. But the restaurant's clientele was mostly Filipino.

New Yorkers started frequenting Filipino restaurants after the passage of the Immigration Reform Act of 1965. Large numbers of highly skilled Filipinos entered the city's medical, legal, and financial industries. In 1972, asylum seekers escaping the declaration of martial law by President Ferdinand Marcos brought another wave of Filipinos into the city. This newly educated immigrant class frequented the "Manila Strip," a collection of Filipino-owned stores and eateries on Ninth Avenue between Thirty-Ninth and Fortieth Streets in Manhattan. They settled in affluent tri-state suburbs and established Filipino communities in the Elmhurst, Woodside, and Jackson Heights neighborhoods of Queens. In 1974, cookbook author and restaurateur Nora Villanueva Daza

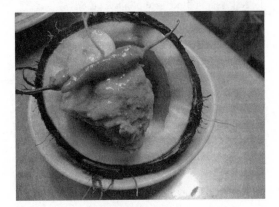

A traditional Filipino meal, beef adobo, made with coconut milk, several different varieties of peppers for seasoning, soy sauce, and sugar for added sweetening. The dish pictured here is served in a coconut shell for a decorative touch. CLARISSA DELOS REYES

opened Maharlika, a restaurant inside the Philippine Consulate General building on Fifth Avenue that paired Filipino music, dancing, and haute cuisine with Western European presentation.

Today's restaurateurs face the challenge of maintaining Filipino culinary heritage while simultaneously appealing to non-Filipinos. It is impossible to define Filipino food as a single set of characteristics because of the culinary range in the Philippine archipelago's seven thousand islands, its diverse population of 90 million people, and the historical influences from four major imperial powers. Contemporary chefs have created their own interpretations of Filipino cuisine by drawing on New York's ingredients and influences. In 1995, Amy Besa and Romy Dorotan opened Cendrillon in SoHo and applied New American Cuisine techniques to traditional dishes. They founded Purple Yam in Brooklyn's Ditmas Park in 2009 and incorporated additional flavors from Korea, Japan, and Southeast Asia. Purple Yam earned the first Michelin Bib Gourmand for a Filipino restaurant in 2013. In 2011, three first-generation Filipino Americans started Maharlika in the East Village. Their dishes are named after important Filipino figures to express pride in serving a cuisine that American imperialists once denigrated. They opened Jeepney, their homage to informal Filipino *turo-turo* street food stalls, in 2012.

In one century, Filipino food in New York has moved from dockside ethnic neighborhoods to the mainstream. This status befits the sixty-seven thousand Filipino Americans who constitute the fourth largest Asian ethnic group in the city.

Alejandro, Reynaldo G., and Eva Maria San Jose-Florentino. *Pinoyork: The Filipino Americans in New York*. New York: Filipino American National Historical Society, Metropolitan New York Chapter, 1998.
Sterne, Michael. "Manila Strip on Ninth Ave. Is Bit of Home for Filipinos." *New York Times*, December 30, 1976.

René Alexander Orquiza Jr.

Fishing

Much of New York City's borders are shoreline: the Hudson and East Rivers, Long Island Sound, the Narrows, and Jamaica Bay spilling into the Atlantic Ocean. Lakes, ponds, and streams are tucked within the city's boundaries. Food from water sources has

a long history in New York City. Native Americans plied the coastlines, hunting the abundant fish, shorebirds, and rabbits. They harvested clams and oysters, heating and drying the meat for immediate and future use. Bounty from the sea also drew a succession of immigrants who became New Yorkers, and to this day, from lifelong New Yorkers to new immigrants, those intent with their fishing poles are common sights along the city's waterways.

Nineteenth-century commerce in local seafood was outstanding, with the oyster in particular. Production, setting, and cultivation of seed in oyster beds was vigorous right off Staten Island shores. Harvests were brought by boat and offloaded on the water side to other boats; "double-deckers" moored in active clusters at "oyster markets" on both the Hudson and the East Rivers. Merchants poised to purchase were welcomed onto the boats dockside. Around the very start of the twentieth century, New York City was known as the oyster capital of the United States; oysters were a ubiquitous street and bar food, and barrels of New York oysters were shipped nationally and internationally. By 1923, however, the industry was shuttered after outbreaks of waterborne typhoid and cholera were traced to local oyster beds.

Marinas for commercial and recreational fishing boats dot all five boroughs. Pursuing "runs" of fish, including cold-water cod, tilefish, hake, halibut, herring, mackerel, bluefish, fluke, flounder, porgys, and other panfish, was a popular seasonal activity through the twentieth century, as was crabbing recreationally for blue claws along marina pilings or commercially for horseshoe crabs used for bait in eel traps. Unfortu-

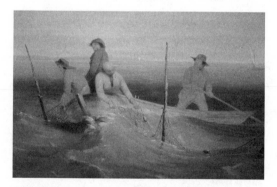

Shad Fishing on the Hudson, an 1846 oil on canvas painting by William Tylee Ranne (1813–1857). Nineteenth-century commerce in local seafood was robust. NEW BRITAIN MUSEUM OF AMERICAN ART

nately, simultaneously, repeated release of industrial chemicals, sewage, and oil spilled from refineries accumulated to negatively affect the health of New York City's waters. People who eat seafood from these waters have access to consumption guidelines issued by the New York State Department of Health. Advocacy for cleaner waters took a definitive step in 1948 with passage of the Federal Water Pollution Control Act; amended in 1972, a toothier Clean Water Act implemented greater pollution control programs. Groups like Riverkeeper, a nonprofit citizen's group that formed initially to advocate for restoration of the health of the Hudson River; students and faculty of the Harbor School on Governors Island; and others work to educate and advocate for cleaner waters. Indeed, the health of New York City's waters has begun to show some improvements through local marine studies.

Whether putting a line into a park lake or surfcasting from a beach, fishing can be very enjoyable, however and wherever it is done in the city. Piers, party boats, bridges, and shorelines still beckon anglers for a nice time on New York waters. If it is not possible to go fishing yourself, Robert Maass conveys the enthusiasm of fishing in New York's vital waters in his 2003 film *Gotham Fish Tales*.

See also OYSTERS.

Hauck-Lawson, Annie. "My Little Town: A Brooklyn Girl's Food Voice." In *Gastropolis: Food and New York City*, edited by Annie Hauck-Lawson and Jonathan Deutsch, pp. 68–92. New York: Columbia University Press, 2009.
Maass, Robert, dir. *Gotham Fish Tales*. DVD. Passion River Productions, 2003.
Mendelson, Anne. "The Lenapes: In Search of Pre-European Foodways in the Greater New York Region." In *Gastropolis: Food and New York City*, edited by Annie Hauck-Lawson and Jonathan Deutsch, pp. 15–33. New York: Columbia University Press, 2009.
"New York City Region Fish Advisories." New York State Department of Health. https://www.health.ny.gov/environmental/outdoors/fish/health_advisories/regional/new_york_city.htm.

Annie Hauck-Lawson

Five Points

Five Points was a Manhattan neighborhood in today's Chinatown that was New York's most notorious slum from its earliest development in the 1820s until the late nineteenth century when much of the neighborhood was razed in an early act of municipal slum clearance. The neighborhood took its name from a five-point intersection formed by three streets: Worth Street, Baxter Street, and Park Street. It expanded out from that intersection to the Bowery on the east, Centre Street on the West, Park Row on the South, and Canal Street on the north. Five Points was an entertainment district, known as much for its bawdy dance halls, saloons, and oyster cellars as it was for its gangs and high crime and mortality rates.

The Bowery especially was a working-class playground, lined with restaurants, oyster cellars, theaters, beer gardens, and dance halls. Oyster cellars lined Canal Street, drawing patrons in by day and night to slurp down the bivalves for which New York was famous in the nineteenth century. Many of the oyster cellars offered all-you-can-eat menus, which became known as the "Canal Street plan." See BEER GARDENS; OYSTER BARS; and OYSTERS.

In 1851, Five Points housed over 250 saloons and groceries, averaging about a dozen per block in the neighborhood. Many of these establishments were "liquor groceries" or groggeries—grocery stores that sold a few food items from barrels but made most of their business by selling beer or liquor by the glass. These "groceries" were not technically saloons, so they could operate on Sundays while saloons could not. Some groceries also had billiard tables, like more formal saloons, and many Five Points groceries attracted prostitutes as well. See GROGGERIES.

Perhaps the most famous of the Five Points groceries in the 1850s was Crown's Grocery. In addition to selling "rum, whisky, brandy, and all sorts of cordials" manufactured on the premises, Crown's stocked hardy produce, preserved meats, spices, pickles, and other provisions. From a counter at the end of the store, Crown's offered "poisoned firewater, doled out at three cents a glass to the loafers and bloated women who frequent the place," explained journalist George Foster in 1850. Crown's frequenters were many—by the end of the decade, the grocery drew as many as one thousand customers a day.

While the women of Five Points could imbibe at the corner groceries, saloons were generally a male bastion, important centers of male working-class sociability in the nineteenth century. Five Points was known for its high number of these "workingman's clubs." They offered respite from the overcrowded tenement apartments of the neighborhood and comradeship for the men who came to have a drink or a free lunch or to gamble on cards, billiards, cockfights, or prize fights. Five Points saloons were associated with their proprietors, often famous for their exploits in politics, firefighting, or boxing. The saloon keepers were among the most respected men in Five Points, offering not just drinks and entertainments to their patrons but also credit, advice, and help finding work. See SALOONS.

After the Civil War, Italian and Chinese newcomers settled in Chinatown, placing their own stamp on the food businesses of the neighborhood, particularly its groceries and restaurants. Groceries became staples of Little Italy and Chinatown, offering provisions but also services such as employment listings, mail pickup, and information from home. Italian cafes lined Mulberry Street, and along Mott Street second-floor restaurants served dumplings, shark fin soup, and chow mein, mainly to Chinese neighbors but in some cases to adventurous native-born New Yorkers who came to Five Points to try the new cuisine. One restaurant in particular, the Port Arthur, distinguished itself by serving a watered-down Chinese cuisine to a white-only clientele. See CHINESE COMMUNITY and ITALIAN.

While the area around Five Points continued to draw new immigrants well into the twentieth century, the intersection itself was razed in 1895 and replaced by Mulberry (now Columbus) Park. This effectively eliminated Five Points from the map of Manhattan.

Anbinder, Tyler. *Five Points: The 19th-Century New York City Neighborhood that Invented Tap Dance, Stole Elections, and Became the World's Most Notorious Slum.* New York: Free Press, 2001.
Foster, George. *New York by Gas-Light and Other Urban Sketches.* Edited by Stuart M. Blumin. Berkeley: University of California Press, 1990.
Sante, Luc. *Low Life: Lures and Snares of Old New York.* New York: Vintage, 1992.

Cindy R. Lobel

Flatbush

See BROOKLYN.

Flay, Bobby

Bobby Flay, a celebrity chef, TV host, cookbook author, and restaurateur, was born Robert William Flay on December 10, 1964, in New York City. He was raised on the Upper East Side of Manhattan.

Flay's interest in food began when, as a kid, he asked for and received an Easy Bake Oven for Christmas. Later he delivered pizza, which was his first job in the food industry. When Flay was seventeen, he dropped out of high school. Meanwhile, his father was the manager of Joe Allen Restaurant in Midtown. One day a busboy was unable to work, so Flay's father told his son to come to the restaurant; he hired him initially as a bus boy, then later as a kitchen helper. The owner, Joe Allen, was so impressed with Flay's cooking that he paid for him to attend the French Culinary Institute. See FRENCH CULINARY INSTITUTE. Flay graduated in 1994, which was the first graduating class.

Upon receiving his culinary degree, Flay went on to work at several restaurants, including Miracle Grill in the East Village and Buds and Jams, which were owned by well-known chef-restaurateur Jonathan Waxman. Under Waxman, Flay developed an interest in bold, vibrant flavors, which soon became his signature style. With restaurateur Jerome Kretchmer, Flay opened his first restaurant, Mesa Grill, in 1991, which was awarded "Best Restaurant" in 1992 by *New York Magazine's* food critic, Gael Greene. Flay soon opened other restaurants, including Spanish-influenced Bolo, which received three stars from the *New York Times* and was noted as New York City's top Spanish restaurant for many years by the Zagat survey until it closed in 2007. As of 2015, Flay owned five restaurants, some of which had several locations: Bar Americain, Bobby Flay Steak, Bobby's Burger Palace, Gato, and Mesa Grill. The original Mesa Grill, located on Fifth Avenue, closed in 2013.

Flay has been the host of thirteen TV shows, most of which appeared on the Food Network, including *Grillin' and Chillin', Hot Off the Grill with Bobby Flay, Bobby Flay's Bold American Food, Bobby Flay's Barbecue Addiction, Brunch at Bobby's,* and *Throwdown with Bobby Flay.* See FOOD NETWORK. He is also a bestselling author of many cookbooks, including *Bobby Flay's Barbecue Addiction, Bobby Flay's Grill It!, Bobby Flay's Mesa Grill Cookbook, Bobby Flay's From My Kitchen to Your Table, Bobby Flay's Boy Gets Grill,* and *Bobby Flay's Burgers, Fries, and Shakes.*

Flay has won many awards. In 1993 he was named Rising Star Chef of the Year by the James Beard Foundation and Outstanding Graduate from the French Culinary Institute. He has been nominated for several Daytime Emmy Awards and won in 2005 for Outstanding Service Show Host for *Boy Meets Grill*. In 2005 Flay was awarded the James Beard Foundation National Television Food Show Award for *Bobby Flay Chef Mentor*. See JAMES BEARD FOUNDATION. He was inducted into the Culinary Hall of Fame in 2007, and in 2009 he won another Daytime Emmy for Best Culinary Program for *Grill It! with Bobby Flay*.

See also TELEVISION.

"Bobby Flay." Biography.com. http://www.biography.com/people/bobby-flay-578278#synopsis.
"Bobby Flay." StarChefs.com. http://www.starchefs.com/chefs/BFlay/html/bio.shtml.

Tracey Ceurvels

Fleischmann, Charles Louis

See BAKERIES; BREAD; and BREADLINES.

Flushing

See CHINESE COMMUNITY and QUEENS.

Food & Wine

Food & Wine magazine was founded in New York City in 1978 by married food writers Ariane and Michael Batterberry along with their business partners, Lindy and Robert Kenyon. Originally titled *The International Review of Food and Wine,* their goal was to offer an alternative to what they perceived as a "stuffy" perspective from other food magazines in circulation and publish articles that would appeal to both male and female readers, rather than cater solely to the "gourmet housewife" set. Early contributors included nontraditional culinary voices such as George Plimpton and Wilfred Sheed.

At first partially owned by *Playboy* magazine magnate Hugh Hefner, it was eventually sold in 1980 with a readership of 250,000 to American Express Publishing. It was sold to Time, Inc. in 2013, and its main offices are still located in Manhattan.

Presented in a convivial, approachable tone, *Food & Wine* features recipes, cooking tips, and articles on restaurants, culinary travel destinations, nutrition, home design, home entertaining, holiday cooking and entertaining, wine pairings, and wine recommendation by price range and wine region. It also features profiles of chefs and other personalities in the culinary and beverage industries.

Food & Wine Classic

Since 1982, the editors of the magazine have held the Food & Wine Classic, an annual event in Wagner Park in Aspen, Colorado. Looked upon as the first major culinary showcase of its kind, the Classic gives journalists and thousands of paying food enthusiasts (more than five thousand ticketed attendees in 2014) a chance to mingle and taste with world famous chefs and sommeliers, who throughout the years have included Julia Child, Jacques Pépin, Jean-Claude Szurdak, Michael Symon, Bobby Flay, Mario Batali, Tyler Florence, Marcus Samuelsson, Hugh Acheson, Emeril Lagasse, Paul Grieco, Mark Oldman, Giada De Laurentiis, Ming Tsai, Eric Ripert, Anthony Bourdain, Tom Colicchio, Danny Meyer, Aldo Sohm, Sissy Biggers, and many more.

Aside from visiting the stalls set up throughout the park for the Grand Tasting, guests are also given the opportunity to attend seminars, panel discussions and participate in charity events.

Dana Cowin

As of 2015 the editor-in-chief is Dana Cowin, former executive editor of *Mademoiselle* and managing editor of *HG* magazine. Since 1995, she has ushered *Food & Wine* from traditional hard copy publication into the digital age and has overseen several prestigious event tie-ins, various books, and multimedia programming. Accompanying the rise of the celebrity chef craze throughout the 1990s and 2000s, she has greatly expanded the readership and influence of the magazine by making it a useful resource suitable for anyone from the master chef to small-town at-home cooks, essentially transforming it into a practical publication that also has a sense of adventure. Said Cowin in 2012, "The idea is to talk about life, but with food at the center."

Top Chef

Top Chef is a James Beard Award–winning reality series co-produced by *Food & Wine* magazine that first aired in 2006 on the Bravo TV network. The show is a cooking competition between sixteen aspiring chefs hoping to win a large cash prize, a feature in the magazine, and a showcase at the Classic in Aspen by competing in timed cookoffs with assorted themes. Each episode includes one "quickfire" and one longer elimination challenge set in different locations, with distinct ingredients and themes.

The series takes place in various American cities, including New York in seasons five and eight. It is hosted by former TV cooking host Padma Lakshmi along with a revolving cast of culinary personalities, including Tom Colicchio, Gail Simmons, Ted Allen, Hugh Acheson, and most recently, former contestant Richard Blais, as well as prestigious guest judges.

The series winners and runners-up ("chef-testants") include several New York–based chefs: Harold Dieterle (Perilla, Kin Shop), Ilan Hall (The Gorbals), Hung Huynh (Catch, The General), Angelo Sosa (Añejo), Stephen Asprinio (Pizza Vinoteca), Jeff McInnis and Janine Booth (Root and Bone), Dale Talde (Talde, Pork Slope, Thistle Hill Tavern), Leah Cohen (Pig & Khao), Ed Cotton (Sotto 13), Andrew D'Ambrosi (Bergen Hill), Manuel Trevino (Horchata), and Ty-Lör Boring (Tipsy Parson). See TELEVISION.

According to its media kit, *Food & Wine* magazine had an average circulation (inclusive of both hard copy and digital) of 941,081 in 2014.

See also BATTERBERRY, MICHAEL AND ARIANE.

Beazley, Aimee White. "The *Food & Wine* Classic Turns 30." *Aspen Peak*, June 11, 2012.
"Delight in the Food & Wine Classic in Aspen, Colorado This June." Travelocity, May 20, 2014. http://www .travelocity.com/inspire/delight-food-wine-classic-aspen-colorado-june.
Food & Wine magazine media kit. http://www.fwmediakit .com/index.html.
Fox, Margalit. "Michael Batterberry, Influential Food Editor, Dies at 78." *New York Times*, July 29, 2010.
Rosenberg, Andrew. "TV Dinners: *Top Chef* Restaurants in NYC." Nycgo.com, October 7, 2014. http://www .nycgo.com/articles/top-chef-restaurants-in-nyc.
Schwartzapfel, Beth. "First Lady of Food." *Brown Alumni Magazine*, September/October 2012. http://www .brownalumnimagazine.com/content/view/3257/40.

Amanda Schuster

Food Arts

An influential trade magazine for chefs, restaurateurs, and the hotel industry, *Food Arts* was founded by New York culinary authorities Michael and Ariane Batterberry in 1988 and acquired the following year by M. Shanken Communications. For twenty-five years, with Michael Batterberry as editor in chief until his death in 2010 and Ariane Batterberry continuing as founding editor and copublisher, *Food Arts* flourished—a celebration of the chef-led American food revolution.

Recalling the genesis of the magazine in its silver anniversary issue, Ariane Batterberry explained that in 1988 "there were restaurant trade publications, but they all focused on fast-food service or feeding at institutions…there was not one magazine for chefs." "Remember," she continued, "there was no Food Network, no James Beard Awards, little to buy from local farmers, and no artisanal anything. There were few tarte Tatins, no molten Valrhona chocolate cakes, and no crème brûlées.…No one had heard the word 'mixologist'" (Batterberry, 2014).

Julie Mautner, *Food Arts*' former Executive Editor recalled in "Farewell to a Renaissance Mensch" (*Food Arts*, December 2010), that "When they conceived *Food Arts*, the Bats [as they were familiarly referred to by their friends] believed that chefs needed information that no one else was providing. And knew that chefs were interested in things far beyond the stove. They saw chefs as artistic, educated, intelligent, business people—and felt they'd embrace a magazine that recognized it." And they did. Eric Ripert, executive chef and co-owner of Manhattan's acclaimed restaurant Le Bernardin, commented, "*Food Arts* became one of the first major magazines to inspire, encourage, and champion so many of us." Anthony Bourdain, author of the popular book *Kitchen Confidential*, wrote that Michael Batterberry "was one of the first people anywhere to treat me as a writer. *Food Arts* was way ahead of its time in that it focused on chefs at a time when everybody else was looking at Bundt cakes or refrigerators" (Mautner, 2010).

"*Food Arts* was born," Ariane Batterberry noted, "just in time to witness, report on, and encourage the explosive expansion of our restaurant world in the U.S." She cited coverage of such transformational events as "the rise of women chefs, and the chef–farmer collaboration; science and technology in the kitchen; artisanal, organic, and heirloom everything; microgreens and microbreweries; baking your own bread; smoking and barbecuing your own meats; creating your own charcuterie. We recorded everything from the advent of sushi to the wood-burning oven" (Batterberry, 2014).

Always relevant, often irreverent, the magazine, with ten issues a year, was a lively read for its fifty-six thousand subscribers, starting with quirky, eye-catching covers. The content included regular features like the Silver Spoon, "awarded for sterling performance" to culinary luminaries from Craig Claiborne to Charlie Trotter; sections devoted to timely topics, recipes, and techniques; and the Mystery Basket challenge for chefs as well as in-depth articles that predicted or analyzed current trends.

"We tried always to be the frontline reporters," Ariane Batterberry recalled. "And new words appeared in our pages: fusion, nuevo Latino, locavore, spa cuisine, kaiseki, forager, predessert—an entire vocabulary that didn't exist 25 years ago" (Batterberrry, 2014).

M. Shanken Communications discontinued publication of *Food Arts* in September 2014. An outpouring of e-mails from culinary professionals expressing their devotion to the magazine included a tribute from Danny Myer, owner of the Union Square Hospitality Group, who wrote, "It's hard to imagine how the fine dining revolution in America could have happened had it not been for *Food Arts*—always looking behind for traditions, ahead for trends—and celebrating the best of the day."

See also BATTERBERRY, MICHAEL AND ARIANE.

Batterberry, Ariane. "Pilot Light: Remembrance of Things Past." *Food Arts* (January–February 2014).
Mautner, Julie. 2010. "Farewell to a Renaissance Mensch." *Food Arts* (December 2010).
"Memories of Michael." *Food Arts* (December 2010).

Meryle Evans

Food Bank

See HUNGER PROGRAMS.

Food Co-ops

During the late 1960s through the 1970s, thousands of food co-ops—alternatives to conventional grocery stores—were established across the United States, many forming in urban centers, including New York City, as well as in college towns. Co-ops focus on healthy and organic foods, often have an anticorporate agenda, and seek to build civic life by addressing problems in the conventional food distribution chain. Food co-ops typically eschew industrial and highly processed foods because of their perceived negative health consequences and are concerned with fair labor practices along the entire chain of food workers, from the field to the check-out counter, and the environmental impact of the food supply chain.

Rooted in the cooperative movement founded in the nineteenth century in Rochdale, England, the co-ops typically follow the seven cooperative principles of (1) voluntary and open membership; (2) democratic member control; (3) member economic participation; (4) autonomy and independence; (5) education, training, and information; (6) cooperation among cooperatives; and (7) concern for community. At their best, food co-ops provide many New Yorkers with healthy food options that are ethically and sustainably sourced, while at the same time giving community members the opportunity to be actively involved in the food system from the local to the global scale. Specifically, members have a voice in the practices and direction of their stores, creating a democratic space for food practice and provisioning enjoyed by tens of thousands of New Yorkers. Co-ops have different labor policies: some pay staff for their labors; others encourage, but do not require, labor; while some require all members to contribute labor to the running of the co-op. Co-ops often face the challenges of working in and serving economically depressed communities; the utopian promise of these ventures as community centers and sources for wholesome, sustainable, and fair food in New York City has had more success than failure.

Established Food Co-ops in New York City

Flatbush Food Co-op is a cooperative grocery established in 1976, and while it has expanded and moved from its original location, it continues to serve Flatbush and the surrounding neighborhoods from its Cortelyou Road location in Brooklyn. Flatbush Food Co-op is open to all, but it encourages membership by offering specific benefits. Staff members are paid for their labor.

Currently, 4th Street Food Co-op is the only cooperative grocery store in Manhattan. It was established in 1995 as a replacement for the Good Food Co-op, which began as a buying club in the 1970s. The co-op is open to the public, but unlike typical food coops, it is run entirely by working members. While the working members serve as unpaid staff, they do receive a discount on co-op goods. Individuals interested in membership, however, may join as working or nonworking members.

Park Slope Food Coop is perhaps among the best-known food co-ops in the world, with current efforts to reproduce a similar cooperative grocery in France under way. It was founded in 1973, beginning like many other coops as a buying club in Brooklyn. Park Slope Food Coop is the largest member-owned and operated cooperative grocery in the United States and aims to provide a meaningful alternative to conventional commercial profit-driven supermarkets. Unlike most cooperative groceries, membership is required in order to shop at Park Slope Food Coop and all members are required to contribute regular working hours to maintain good standing and their shopping privileges.

Newer and Planned Co-ops

Green Hill Food Co-op is located at 18 Putnam Avenue, in close proximity to the Brooklyn communities of Fort Green, Clinton Hill, Bedford Stuyvesant, and Prospect Heights, drawing its name from the closest neighborhoods. Like Park Slope Food Coop, Green Hill Food Co-op is a 100 percent working co-op that requires both membership and regular work hours for shopping.

Bushwick Food Cooperative was formed in 2009. It is a member-owned and -operated co-op with limited hours.

In development are Bay Ridge Food Co-op and Lefferts Community Food Co-op, both of which are located in Brooklyn. Also in development are Queens Harvest Food Coop and St. George Food Co-op located in Staten Island.

Shuttered Co-ops

The South Bronx Food Co-op was located on Third Avenue and East 158th Street in the South Bronx, known to be low-income and underserved by the conventional food system. Much excitement accompanied the formation of the South Bronx Food Co-op in 2007 as it showed promise to bring sorely needed high-quality food to a densely populated area. While the co-op had over 250 members, it was not enough to sustain the store, and local foot traffic was insufficient to keep the store well stocked; it closed in 2010.

The East New York Food Co-op was a Brooklyn-based cooperative grocery in East New York, a low-income community. It opened its doors in 2006, occupying a small, single-room store, and began with twenty members. Membership doubled within a year, but at forty members and with limited stock, the co-op struggled to meet the needs of the community and was shuttered within a couple of years.

Haedicke, Michael A. "Small Food Co-ops in a Whole Foods® World." *Contexts* 13 (2014): 32.
Tirado, Ramona. "East New York Food Coop: First Steps on a Journey of a Thousand Miles." *Linewaiters' Gazette* BB, no. 10 (2007): 1–2.

Christine C. Caruso

Food Deserts

Beginning in the 1960s, grocery stores and supermarkets followed the middle-class migration from the cities to the suburbs, leaving once vibrant urban neighborhoods with scant access to healthy food. Such areas without ready access to healthy, fresh, and affordable food are referred to as "food deserts" and are defined by the U.S. Department of Agriculture as low-income areas in which at least 33 percent of the population lives more than one mile from a supermarket or large grocery store. As of 2009, the U.S. Department of Agriculture determined that 11.5 million Americans live in areas that met these criteria. In food desert communities, where healthy food is unavailable and transportation options are often out of reach or unreliable, residents rely on fast-food restaurants, pharmacies, discount stores, and convenience stores, which typically do not sell fresh foods, to feed themselves and their families. Not surprisingly, studies show that without access to fresh fruits and vegetables, residents have a harder time meeting recommended dietary guidelines for healthy eating. Consequently, residents of underserved food deserts have high rates of obesity, heart disease, and other diet-related diseases.

Historically, New York City has been no exception to this dismal reality of urban food access. According to a 2008 study conducted by the mayor's Food Policy Task Force, nearly three million New Yorkers were living in neighborhoods that have high levels of diet-related disease and large populations with limited opportunities to purchase fresh food. These neighborhoods include Harlem, Washington

Heights, the South Bronx, and numerous others in Brooklyn and Queens.

With obesity rates rising, particularly in children, and the heightened understanding of the relationship between food access and health, solving the problem of food deserts has become a public health priority in New York City and across the nation. Beginning with the creation of the Food Policy Task Force in 2006, the Office of the Mayor and the City Council made access to healthy food and reducing hunger in New York City a priority. To accomplish this goal, the city mobilized a variety of policy and law-making tools to incentivize and promote the development of healthy food retail in underserved neighborhoods. These policy initiatives include the following programs.

The New York City Green Cart Initiative

The New York City Green Cart initiative was designed to address issues of access and proximity to fresh fruits and vegetables by licensing up to one thousand mobile green grocer carts to operate in low-income neighborhoods. As of 2015, there are nearly five hundred Green Carts operating in New York City, with more than ninety of them equipped with Electronic Benefits Transfer machines to accept federal SNAP benefits. See SUPPLEMENTAL NUTRITION ASSISTANCE PROGRAM (SNAP).

The Shop Healthy Initiative

The Shop Healthy Initiative has worked with more than one thousand shops in East and Central Harlem, the South Bronx, and central Brooklyn to increase stocks of fruits, vegetables, and other healthy foods at bodegas, pharmacies, and discount stores that did not historically sell such items.

The FRESH Program

The Food Retail Expansion to Support Health (FRESH) program was created to increase food access in underserved communities by offering zoning and tax incentives to spur the development of full-service supermarkets and grocery stores that devote a certain amount of space to fresh produce, meats, dairy, and other perishables. As of 2015, the program is expected to provide approximately 578,000 square feet of new and renovated food retail space, representing investment of some $80 million.

Community Gardening and Urban Farming Programs

There are numerous programs sponsored by various city agencies that support the creation and maintenance of community gardens and urban farms on vacant municipal lots by providing programs and technical support, tools, supplies, and grants. For example, the city's GreenThumb program is the largest community gardening program in the country, with over six hundred member gardens serving twenty thousand city residents. The New York City Housing Authority's Garden and Greening Program teaches residents how to grow food in more than 740 gardens located on New York City Housing Authority property. See URBAN FARMING.

In addition to city programs, robust participation from a vast network of nonprofit organizations committed to enhancing the availability of healthy food in low-access communities has played a vital role in improving food access throughout the five boroughs. Among them are GrowNYC, which developed and operates over 130 farmers markets throughout the five boroughs, and City Harvest, which works with retailers and residents in low-access communities to increase the quality and variety of available produce and to distribute rescued produce in underserved communities through a fleet of mobile markets. See GROWNYC.

Preliminary studies suggest that residents in underserved food deserts shop at new supermarkets, Green Carts, and other new or improved food retail outlets. However, it remains to be seen whether there will be enough demand to keep these outlets in business and whether these kinds of interventions will be effective at changing people's long-term eating and buying habits.

Citizen's Committee for Children. "Green Cart Implementation: Year One." September 2010. http://www.cccnewyork.org/wp-content/publications/CCCReport.GreenCarts.Sept2010.pdf.
Cummins, Steven, Ellen Flint, and Stephan A. Matthews. "New Neighborhood Grocery Store Increased Awareness of Food Access but Did Not Alter Dietary Habits or Obesity." *Health Affairs* 33, no. 2 (February 2014): 283–291.
Treuhaft, Sarah, and Allison Karpyn. 2010. "The Grocery Gap: Who Has Access to Healthy Food and Why It

Matters." The Food Trust and PolicyLink. http://
thefoodtrust.org/uploads/media_items/grocerygap
.original.pdf.
Ver Ploeg, Michele, Vince Breneman, Tracey Farrigan,
et al. "Access to Affordable and Nutritious Food—
Measuring and Understanding Food Deserts and
Their Consequences: Report to Congress." U.S.
Department of Agriculture, Economic Research
Service, Administrative Publication No. AP-036,
June 2009. http://www.ers.usda.gov/publications/
ap-administrative-publication/ap-036.aspx.

Esther S. Trakinski

Food52

Food52 (www.food52.com) is an online community cookbook, discussion forum, and e-commerce
site. Founded in 2009 by Amanda Hesser and Merrill
Stubbs, the site grew from their work on Hesser's
The Essential New York Times Cookbook (2010), when
Hesser had asked *Times* readers to nominate recipes
from the newspaper's pages for inclusion. Impressed
by the enthusiastic and knowledgeable responses
from these home cooks, Hesser and Stubbs saw an
opportunity to create a new type of interactive
website, where they would curate the culinary knowledge of many passionate amateurs through the technology of the Internet. As Hesser explained in the
Times, they developed "an idea we could package:
in 52 weeks, we'd create the first crowd-sourced
cookbook." Setting up a blogging platform, each
week the pair solicited recipes on a theme and selected finalists from the submissions. The community then voted for winners to be included in the
Food52 cookbook.

Ironically, although it was created in an online
community, the first *Food52 Cookbook* (2011) is a
traditional print work. It has been followed, in print,
by the *Food52 Cookbook: Volume 2* (2012) and *Food52
Genius Recipes* (2015). The latter is based on recipes
from professionals and celebrity chefs, many of which
have been featured on the Food52 website.

Food52 reports roughly 3.8 million unique users
each month, as well as 350,000 registered users. Since
its founding it has raised $9 million from outside
investors, most recently a $6 million stake negoti-
ated in 2014 to help "build its brand" by adding more
video content to the website, extending content
to "home-related" topics, growing beyond its New
York City base, and developing mobile apps that

will help users interact with both the content side of
Food52 and its online store, Provisions.

Launched in 2013, Provisions now accounts for
approximately two-thirds of Food52's revenues, with
the remainder coming from advertising sales. Provisions appeals to well-heeled consumers, with "one-
of-a-kind" items and gadgets with "foodie" snob
appeal, such as ceremonial *matcha* tea sets and basic
versus "upgraded" kombucha home brewing kits. It
is Martha Stewart for a younger demographic.

Although commerce geared to a highly affluent
audience now dominates the Food52 business model,
it maintains its "every cook" appeal through weekly
contests, its extensive online library of recipes (now
totaling approximately 30,000), and its hotline to
answer cooking questions in real time. The sheer
beauty and elegance of the website and the useful-
ness of its culinary information has impressed professional audiences: Food52 received the 2012 James
Beard Award for best publication of the year and the
2013 International Association of Culinary Professionals Award for best website. It shared the latter
accolade with Saveur.com in 2014.

See also HESSER, AMANDA.

Hesser, Amanda. "Recipe Redux: The Community
Cookbook." *New York Times*, October 6, 2010.
Griffith, Erin. "Content, Commerce, and Cooking: How
Food52 is Making Small Community into Big Business."
Fortune, August 7, 2014.
Locke, Michelle. "Web Food Fight: Food52.com vs.
Cook's Illustrated." Salon.com, April 27, 2010. http://
www.salon.com/2010/04/28/us_fea_food_recipe_
showdown.
Perez, Sarah. "Cooking Site and Online Shop Food52
Picks Up $6 Million More." TechCrunch.com,
September 30, 2014. http://techcrunch.com/
2014/09/30/food52-series-a-1.

Cathy K. Kaufman and Tawnya Manion

Food Movement

See LATE TWENTIETH CENTURY.

Food Network

The Food Network is a cable television network that
was launched in New York City on November 23,
1993. It was the first twenty-four-hour television
network to focus solely on food. The Providence

Journal Company, a Rhode Island newspaper and media company, hired Reese Schonfeld, who had cofounded CNN with Ted Turner, to launch the network in late 1991.

Schonfeld felt that rather than build studios in Providence, the network should set up shop in New York. Schonfeld leased existing studios in the city until his wife, Pat O'Gorman, took on the task of seeing to it that a new "studio, control room, editing rooms, and office space" were completed—in less than three months—in an office building. Later the operation moved into the Chelsea Market building.

Since there was no ready pool of "food celebrities" looking for work, new talent had to be located. Donna Hanover, a former TV news anchor (and, at the time, wife of the future New York City mayor Rudy Giuliani), and David Rosengarten, a print journalist, were chosen to be on-air partners for a live food news program. Another live program was *Food Talk* with Robin Leach, a celebrity-focused writer who had hosted a popular television show, *Lifestyles of the Rich and Famous*. Other early programs included *Getting Healthy*, anchored by sports broadcaster Gayle Gardner and Dr. Stephanie Beling, and *Feeding Your Family on $99 a Week*, with chef and cookbook author Michèle Urvater. Chef Emeril Lagasse, formerly of Commander's Palace in New Orleans, hosted other early programs.

In addition to the shows produced in New York, other programs were taped in Nashville, Tennessee, by Reid/Land Productions, a firm with which Schonfeld had previously worked. To fill the broadcasting day, the network licensed the rights to air reruns of a number of existing cooking shows, including those of the ever-popular Julia Child. Also, Schonfeld acquired the rights to the blockbuster Japanese cooking show *Iron Chef*, which introduced American audiences to competitive cooking as a spectator sport. *Iron Chef* was such a hit that it spawned an entire new genre of TV cooking contests. The network's programming eventually settled into a two-tiered approach: instructional cooking shows during the day and nighttime programming that featured entertainment, such as competitions, lighthearted surveys of food history, reality shows, and food-centric travel shows. By 2001 the network was reaching 75 million households, including some of the most affluent TV viewers in America.

Over the years, the Food Network shifted away from instructional television and more toward "lifestyle" shows. While the network found its niche in entertainment—not education—it taught Americans about food in a way that the creators of traditional cooking shows never imagined. It brought glamour to the culinary profession and convinced thousands of Americans that the field is a valid and worthwhile career path. Of course, many young students attending culinary school today dream of becoming tomorrow's television chefs.

Many devoted Food Network viewers are people who have no intention of cooking dinner in their own kitchens, let alone signing up for culinary school. They want to learn more about food so that they can order more wisely in ethnic restaurants or hold their own in culinary conversations with their peers. In this way, the Food Network bestows on viewers a kind of "cultural capital" that allows them to discuss the latest trends, personalities, and events in the food world. With its influence now pervasive throughout America, the Food Network has gone far beyond the realm of public TV daytime cooking shows. It has familiarized viewers with elite food traditions around the world.

In 2008 Scripps Networks Interactive and the Hearst Corporation launched the *Food Network Magazine*. It is published ten times a year and promotes and builds on the chefs and programs on the Food Network. The magazine had 11.5 million readers by 2014.

In 2010 Scripps Networks Interactive, the owner of the Food Network, launched a second cable television channel, the Cooking Channel, which focuses on instructional programs, such as Bobby Flay's *Brunch @ Bobby's*, Emeril Lagasse's *Fresh Food Fast*, and Ben Sargent's *Hook, Line & Dinner*. It has also shown reruns of successful programs that first aired on the Food Network, such as *Chinese Food Made Easy*, *Everyday Exotic*, *Drink Up*, *Indian Food Made Easy*, *Nigella Express*, and *Iron Chef*.

In 2014, the network was being watched in 99 million homes—virtually every American home that had a cable or satellite TV hookup—and its website had 7 million users monthly. While the network's initial audience was primarily female, increasing numbers of men were attracted to the programming. Today, almost half the viewers are male. This can be partly attributed to chefs such as Emeril

Lagasse, Tom Colicchio, and Kaga Takeshi, whose presence on the air made it more culturally acceptable for men to take an interest in cooking. Of the many chefs who have appeared on Food Network programs, one of the most prominent is native New Yorker Bobby Flay, of the Manhattan restaurants Mesa Grill, Bolo, Bar Americain, and Gato. He has appeared as a guest and judge on many shows and was featured on the *Great Chefs* television series. Flay has hosted programs such as *Hot Off the Grill with Bobby Flay*, *Boy Meets Grill*, *BBQ with Bobby Flay*, and *Throwdown with Bobby Flay*. On the Cooking Channel he has hosted *Worst Cooks in America*, *Bobby's Dinner Battle*, and *Beat Bobby Flay*.

Today, the Food Network is a joint venture between Scripps Networks Interactive and the Tribune Cable Ventures, Inc. Its national headquarters is located in Chelsea Market at 75 Ninth Avenue in Manhattan.

See also CHELSEA MARKET; FLAY, BOBBY; and TELEVISION.

Collins, Kathleen. *Watching What We Eat: The Evolution of Television Cooking Shows.* New York: Continuum, 2009.
Salkin, Allen. *From Scratch: Inside the Food Network.* New York: Putnam's, 2013.
Schonfeld, Reese. *Me and Ted against the World: The Unauthorized Story of the Founding of CNN.* New York: HarperCollins, 2001.

Andrew F. Smith

Food Stamps

See SUPPLEMENTAL NUTRITION ASSISTANCE PROGRAM (SNAP).

Food Trucks

Food trucks, like the chuck wagons of the Old West, are vehicles from which food and drink are served. Unlike chuck wagons or today's food carts, however, trucks are motor vehicles that get around on their own horsepower. While food trucks and food carts often serve similar items, trucks are larger—most have room for several people to work inside—much better equipped, and capable of offering a much broader menu.

The current, popular conception of food trucks includes bright, professionally designed graphics; wildly inventive menus; young, marketing-savvy

owners connected to multiple social media accounts; and a hip, white-collar clientele. (Carts can fit this mold, too.) But these self-consciously "gourmet" trucks, for want of a better word, first made headlines not so many years ago. In New York, others have much longer histories: trucks that cater to immigrant communities have been around for decades; trucks that serve sandwiches, soft drinks, and other humble fare to blue-collar workers date from World War II; ice cream trucks, which delight all ages, are known from the 1920s. These genres are not hard and fast, to be sure.

Still older than the ice cream trucks are so-called lunch wagons. Sometimes looked to as forebears of food trucks, these offered modest menus beginning in the late nineteenth century. One, established in 1893 in Union Square by the Women's Auxiliary of the Church Temperance Society, offered "tea, coffee, milk, sandwiches and the like" to night-shift workers. Many such "lunch" wagons, in fact, did business after dark. Typically, they were reconditioned horse-drawn streetcars with indoor seating; although still mobile in theory, often they were stationary in practice. These lunch wagons can be better understood as precursors to diners. See DINERS.

Truly mobile trucks serving ice cream began circulating in New York streets during the first half of the twentieth century. Good Humor, established in Youngstown, Ohio, in the early 1920s and nationally known soon after, sold its wares from gleaming white trucks by men in equally white uniforms. Bungalow Bar, a Queens-based contemporary and local competitor, relied on a homier approach: its trucks are best remembered for their pitched, shingled

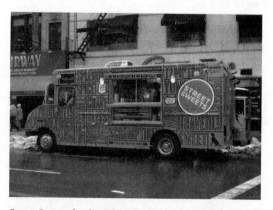

Street Sweets food truck parked outside the Upper West Side Fairway, February 28, 2010. SCOTT BEALE/ LAUGHING SQUID

roofs. By the 1940s, both companies operated hundreds of vehicles, including carts as well as trucks, in the five boroughs.

Today, except for rare promotional appearances, they have vanished from New York streets, giving way to a fleet of prosaic trucks with a jingle of their own and a handful of fancifully decorated gourmet trucks. Most of these latter-day operations are boxy and big; the proprietor can stand inside and dip cones, assemble sundaes, and—especially in the case of the gourmet trucks—prepare custom combinations from ingredients on hand.

The early Good Humor and Bungalow Bar trucks, by contrast, were little more than freezers on wheels, with a seat for the driver in front and cold storage, filled with prepackaged ice cream, in back. Little wonder, then, that a "khaki colored mobile canteen truck" bewildered passersby in Midtown during a 1942 training run. The offer of free food baffled cynical New Yorkers, the *New York Times* reported, but so did the onboard "compact kitchen," staffed by volunteer cooks. However, "several service men, educated to canteens," gladly accepted "plates of cheese sandwiches, slaw salad and mugs of coffee."

Mobile Kitchens on the March

Today's food trucks are descendants of "the catering vehicles that grew popular after World War II" (Engber, 2014). Their acceptance into civilian society surely got a boost from veterans who had patronized mobile canteens in the service. It is quite possible, in fact, that many of the earliest postwar trucks were decommissioned military motor vehicles—just like the first chuck wagon, which was fashioned from a Civil War army-surplus ambulance. (Contemporary accounts are scarce, however, and the lines of descent in any food truck "family tree" are sketchy.)

Workaday vehicles found a niche at facilities like the Brooklyn Navy Yard, but beginning in the 1950s they also settled in beside quiet parks and along busy thoroughfares where quick, inexpensive dining options were wanting. The first such trucks sold hot dogs, sometimes hamburgers; later, their ranks were swelled by Italian American outfits serving massive hot sandwiches laden with sausage. Amenities were few: perhaps a picnic bench, perhaps some homemade onion relish. That is still the case today. Halal trucks, which typically offer chopped, griddled chicken and lamb in addition to pork-free dogs and

burgers, have become common, especially in Manhattan. They are patronized not only by blue-collar workers, many of them new to this country, but also by budget-minded white-collar workers who have been educated to food trucks.

Flavors from Home

According to food critic Jonathan Gold, taco trucks "have been part of civic life…since the 1960s" in car-centric Los Angeles, but their earliest documented U.S. appearance may have been in the residential Riverdale section of the Bronx. In 1966, Craig Claiborne wrote of a shop called Tic-Taco and its truck of the same name, which "travels about the neighborhood purveying the company product." Perhaps owing to what was then exotic fare for most New Yorkers—"the taco is a fried tortilla, and the tortilla is a type of pancake," he explained—Tic-Taco soon vanished without a trace.

By the early 1990s, however, other taco trucks had woven themselves inextricably into the social fabric of Jackson Heights, Queens, and its large Mexican-born population. Despite the familiar-looking contours of the trucks, Jim Leff (1993) wrote in the *New York Press*, "the hanging chorizos and earthy aroma instantly tell you that you'll find no ice cream here." While nearby restaurants catered to "families, groups and courting couples," Leff observed, "when a Mexican worker gets a jones for a slamming dose of Back Home, he'll head to a taco truck." For other demographic groups, the "rotimobile" that sold Trinidadian food for breakfast in the Caribbean heart of Flatbush, Brooklyn, the "mobile soul food kitchen" that supplied fried chicken to West Harlem, and a chimichurri truck serving that Dominican hot sandwich in El Alto, the upper reaches of Manhattan, were similarly alluring.

That chimi truck was the first of many; nowadays they convene after dark along an uptown avenue. In Red Hook, Brooklyn a particularly celebrated group of Latin American trucks parks beside an athletic field on weekends when *futbol* is in season. As for Jackson Heights, today it may be more crowded with trucks, carts, and humbler food stands than when Leff visited in the early 1990s. Most vendors and customers still conduct affairs in Spanish; Ecuadorian fare now rivals Mexican in popularity. Though the trucks themselves are commonly weathered and secondhand, some sport satellite dishes and flat screens that offer entertainment from Latin America—even if the "TV lounge" is no more than a few battered plastic chairs on the sidewalk. Occasionally these trucks appear in Manhattan, seeking out small pockets of their core customers. More often they sit tight on their own turf and, occasionally, play host to traveling food adventurers of all stripes.

The Age of Social Media

Even at the turn of the twenty-first century, published accounts of food trucks were rare. Little changed when newcomers began pulling up to the curb, not in the outer boroughs but in Manhattan's business districts—dessert trucks, a dumpling truck, a pair of pizza trucks. Owners relied mainly on a good parking spot and word of mouth to connect with prospective customers.

A Los Angeles taco truck featuring the Korean-influenced menu of a Seoul-born chef, Roy Choi, is widely credited with kickstarting a frenzy of food truck excitement. In 2008 the Kogi Korean BBQ truck began employing social media, especially Twitter, to build its fan base and to announce its location. In Manhattan, many newer food trucks quickly followed suit—so many that the website Midtown Lunch devised a "Twitter tracker" to aggregate reports of the latest locations and daily specials.

These latest food trucks distinguish themselves in many other ways from the old guard. The proprietors, typically young and English-speaking, often do business from bespoke mobile kitchens. Most trucks, especially the used models, are wrapped in colorful vinyl "skins" that have been professionally printed and branded. Some menus serve traditional fare, albeit from traditions all over the world: Maine lobster rolls, Austrian schnitzel, Moroccan couscous, Taiwanese minced pork on rice. But many trucks describe their dishes as "fusion," "eclectic," or "inventive"—say, southern pulled pork on Belgian waffles, a Korean-Philly "kim-cheesesteak," or Earl Grey tea in ice cream form. Rather than a taste of home, these trucks offer customers what Midtown Lunch calls "an adventure in urban lunching." And while every food truck is a small business, these gourmet trucks are better capitalized than most and often have a formal business plan in tow. Most have aspirations of being not just mobile but upwardly mobile.

Indeed, in 2011 and 2012, at least ten books were published that advised readers on how to fund, start up, market, and run their own food trucks. Television shows such as *The Great Food Truck Race*, whose first cross-country competition concluded in Manhattan, and *Eat Street* celebrated mobile cuisine in New York and farther afield. For its 2011 guide to New York City restaurants, *Zagat* added a new category for food trucks. That spring the recently formed New York City Food Truck Association held its first "rally" on Grand Army Plaza. More than a dozen mobile vendors did business, not on a weekday during working hours but on a Sunday afternoon beside Prospect Park, Brooklyn. Food trucks had become their own reason for being, to be enjoyed for their own sake.

No one, however, enjoys parking on the street in Midtown or the Financial District. Parking and trying to run a successful business, many food truck proprietors discovered, is even more difficult. A November 2011 article in *Crain's New York Business* asserted that the "hip and nascent food truck industry" was "partly a victim of its own success" as a glut of trucks competed with one another (Fickenscher, 2011). And traditional restaurants, reported *Crain's*, were "crying foul—and calling the cops—when the trucks park on their doorsteps, siphoning customers." Tougher city enforcement of parking regulations also made it problematic for trucks to operate in the most heavily trafficked areas. See STREET VENDORS, REGULATION OF. In May 2013, an article in the *New York Times* maintained that, at least in New York, "The Food-Truck Business Stinks" (Davidson, 2013). In this regard, the smaller size of food carts is an advantage: they can squeeze into tighter spaces, and they can legally operate on the sidewalk.

Two truck owners profiled by the *Times* resorted to opening restaurants; one added that he held on to his truck as a "moving billboard" for his stationary venues. Other owners have sought to build a clientele where enforcement is lax or competition, less cutthroat—a practice that also applies to today's trucks that serve immigrant communities, blue-collar workers, and ice cream lovers. This can take time. Since the 1960s, Dominick's Quality Hot Dogs has parked in the same spot in Middle Village, Queens, by the roadside along St. John Cemetery. Dominick's draws a steady stream of customers from near and far, but otherwise it enjoys peace and quiet.

See also STREET VENDORS.

Claiborne, Craig. "From a Taste of a Taco, a New Shop." *New York Times*, November 21, 1966.

Davidson, Adam. "The Food-Truck Business Stinks." *New York Times*, May 7, 2013.

Engber, Daniel. "Who Made That Food Truck?" *New York Times*, May 2, 2014.

Fickenscher, Lisa. "The Rise and Stall of Food Trucks." *Crain's New York Business*, November 27, 2011.

Gold, Jonathan. "How America Became a Food Truck Nation." *Smithsonian Magazine* (March 2012).

Leff, Jim. "Charles Mobile Soul Food Kitchen!!" *Down the Hatch* (November 1994).

Leff, Jim. "Miles of Taco Smiles in Jackson Heights." *New York Press*, October 13–19, 1993, 30.

Shiller, Joyce K. "Meals on Wheels—Night Lunch Wagons in NYC." Norman Rockwell Museum, February 10, 2011. http://www.rockwell-center.org/exploring-illustration/meals-on-wheels-night-lunch-wagons-in-nyc.

Dave Cook

Four Seasons

"There has never been a restaurant better keyed to the tempo of Manhattan than The Four Seasons," declared Craig Claiborne in his October 1959 *New York Times* review of the now-legendary restaurant at 99 East Fifty-Second Street. "Both in décor and menu, it is spectacular, modern, and audacious." When it debuted on July 29, 1959, The Four Seasons set a new standard for American fine dining, with its majestic modern design and innovative, seasonally changing menu that heralded "new American cuisine." In the ensuing decades, The Four Seasons would go on to pioneer such trends as power lunches, spa cuisine, and barrel tasting dinners, staying true to its creators' vision of a restaurant that, like New York City itself, was always evolving.

That vision was the brainchild of Jerome Brody and impresario Joseph Baum of Restaurant Associates. Baum was inspired by the Japanese *shibui* aesthetic espoused by his friend Elizabeth Gordon and haiku poetry, which emphasized the passage of time and the cycle of seasons. "And that's where I came by the idea to use the theme of the four seasons for our restaurant," Baum said, "because everything we wanted to do with it represented change." (Among the names initially proposed for the restaurant was "Season-o-Rama," which one assumes did not make the short list.) Not only would the menu change each season but also "uniforms, trees, graphics, the color of the typewriter ribbons, even the upholstery of the banquettes," as Gael Greene (1970) wrote. To this day, even the color of the match tips is changed every season. Other novelties included fresh herbs grown on the premises and wild mushrooms procured by composer John Cage, an avid mycologist. And classic dishes like crisp duck and Dover sole shared the stage with newly celebrated ingredients like fiddlehead ferns and wild leeks.

Set in the base of the Seagram Building, Mies van der Rohe's modernist skyscraper, the restaurant was designed by architect Philip Johnson and interior designer William Pahlmann, under the visionary guidance of Phyllis Lambert. Her father, Seagram chief Samuel Bronfman, poured millions into the project. In 1989 The Four Seasons was designated an Interior Landmark by the New York City Landmarks Preservation Commission as an exemplar of the International style.

The restaurant, atop a sweeping carpeted staircase, comprises two grand dining rooms with soaring ceilings, French walnut–paneled walls, and undulating metal chain curtains festooning monumental windows. Artwork by such modern masters as Miró, Pollock, and Frankenthaler has graced the walls over the years. A Richard Lippold "sculptured chandelier" composed of thousands of bronze rods is suspended above the bar, a defining feature of the clubby Grill Room. A corridor, adorned until recently with Picasso's massive stage curtain *Le Tricorne*, leads to the serene, sparkling Pool Room, its eponymous centerpiece a bubbling 20-by-20 foot Carrara marble pool. It is anchored at each corner by towering trees—palms in summer, Japanese maple in autumn, birch in winter, cherry blossoms in spring.

A who's who of the New York food and design worlds has shaped The Four Seasons over the years: James Beard and Mimi Sheraton were early menu consultants; Ada Louise Huxtable and her husband Garth designed the tableware. Their Four Seasons snifters and serving bowls are now part of the collection at the Museum of Modern Art. George Lang served as director of The Four Seasons in the late 1960s, a few years before taking over Café des Artistes. Talented chefs have helmed the kitchen, from Albert Stöckli and Seppi Renggli to Pecko Zantilaveevan and Richard Bower. And gifted staff-turned-owners have steered the ship, including Tom Margittai and Paul Kovi from 1973 to 1995 and Alex von Bidder and the suave, madcap Julian Niccolini from 1995 into the twenty-first century—hospitality legends, all.

But much of the aura surrounding The Four Seasons comes from its clientele: sheiks and princes, fashion icons and literary giants, captains of commerce, Hollywood stars, and devoted regulars like the local doyenne who has dined there twice daily for decades and the fellow who comes so often that he is allowed behind the bar to fix his own martinis. In 1979 *Esquire* editor Lee Eisenberg described the Grill Room goings-on in an article titled "America's Most Powerful Lunch," popularizing the term "power lunch" and solidifying The Four Seasons' status as the noontime habitat of the city's movers and shakers.

This is not to say The Four Seasons is all business. An air of celebration, even wackiness, pervades Johnson's celebrated rooms. A first-timer once described her experience at The Four Seasons as "a cross between the waiting room at Bellevue and the first day of Mardi Gras." Ladies have been known to take a dip in the pool after a particularly festive meal, no more clad than the nude nymphs cavorting in the famed Café des Artistes murals across the park.

From day one, servers have spun gossamer turbans of cotton candy at meal's end for the delight of birthday celebrants and anniversary couples. "It was something Joe Baum added to 'unstuffy' the place," recounts Four Seasons maven Regina McMenamin. "To this day, the sight of the cotton candy makes adults scream with laughter!'"

The Four Seasons made "unstuffy" classy. Soon after same-sex marriage was legalized in New York in 2011, the restaurant played host to a star-studded wedding capped by Aretha Franklin singing "I Will Always Love You" to the male newlyweds. For the last few years, the public has been welcomed into the state-of-the-art kitchen for Saturday cooking classes, where everyone from emergency room nurses to small-town mayors forges a camaraderie that spills over to the Bar Room hours after the last sauté pan has been put away.

"We [see] the Four Seasons as the quintessential restaurant of New York," Margittai and Kovi wrote in their Four Seasons cookbook in 1980. Today, countless ducks and Dover soles later, The Four Seasons—with its powerfully modern interior, its balance of restraint and exuberance, its air of magic that continues to enthrall despite lofty prices and a slightly forbidding first impression—remains as vibrant and iconic as New York City itself.

If the Four Seasons' lease is not renewed in 2016 as lamentably looks likely, the storied restaurant will hopefully survive a move to a new space, changing like the seasons, yet remaining essentially the same.

See also BAUM, JOE; BEARD, JAMES; POWER BREAK-FASTS AND POWER LUNCHES; RESTAURANT ASSOCIATES; RESTAURANTS; and SHERATON, MIMI.

Claiborne, Craig. "Dining in Elegant Manner: Four Seasons Termed Spectacular Both in Décor and Menu." *New York Times*, October 2, 1959.
Friedman, B. H. "The Most Expensive Restaurant Ever Built." *Evergreen* no. 10 (1959).
Greene, Gael. "Restaurant Associates: Twilight of the Gods." *New York Magazine*, November 2, 1970.
Margittai, Tom, and Paul Kovi. *The Four Seasons: The Ultimate Book of Food, Wine and Elegant Dining.* Foreword by James Beard. New York: Simon & Schuster, 1980.
Mariani, John, and Alex Von Bidder. *The Four Seasons: A History of America's Premier Restaurant.* New York: Smithmark, 1999.

Meryl Rosofsky

Fourth of July

In a letter to his wife, John Adams wrote, "This *second* day of July, 1776, will be the most memorable epoch in the history of America. I am apt to believe that it will be celebrated by succeeding generations as the great anniversary festival. It ought to be solemnized with pomp and parade, with shows, games, sports, guns, bells, bonfires, and illuminations." Adams did not predicate the exact date, but he was close with other items associated with what is now known and celebrated as Independence Day. Adams's quote is noticeably starved of any reference of the food Americans enjoy consuming on this their nation's birthday.

On that first July 4 in 1776, there were no hamburgers, no hot dogs, and no fireworks sent into the sky. It was not celebrated in New York City until after the British armed forces withdrew from the city at the end of the American War of Independence. From 1784 onward it was celebrated annually in New York City with fireworks, street fairs, parades, entertainment, drinking, food, and patriotic speeches. Later Fourth of July celebrations included military units marching through the streets, large feasts (often prepared by a local tavern keeper) held at community

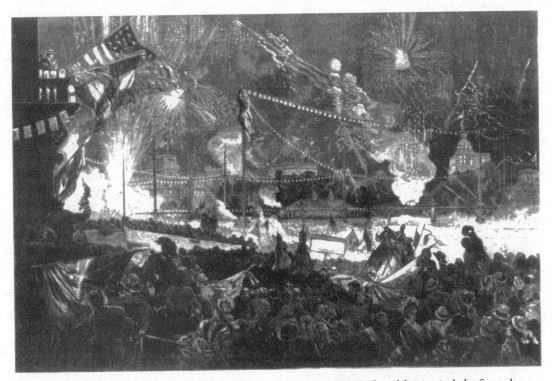

An artist's depiction of the Centennial celebration of Independence Day, 1876. The celebration includes fireworks, decorations, crowds, and food vendors. Originally printed in *Harper's Weekly*, July 22, 1876. LIBRARY OF CONGRESS

centers or Veterans of Foreign Wars halls, and (often raucous) toasts to commemorate and celebrate independence around bonfires that burned late into the night. An official reading of the Declaration of Independence itself was also a popular early tradition (which has since gone away).

Each year the Fourth would ultimately reflect the larger social, economic, and political climate of the country. For instance, the years of the Great Depression would not have been as celebratory as those that came later in the 1950s when America became a superpower. During the 1950s, driving to the beach for a picnic or to a country estate to be with friends or just celebrating in the backyard over a charcoal grill would all become part of America's notable cultural (and consumer) traditions. For New Yorkers, the Fourth has become (as it has for many Americans) a quintessential opportunity to gather with family and friends to unabashedly and unpretentiously embrace our ever-evolving "pursuit of happiness." As is often the case, this happiness is experienced through the palate.

One of the ways Americans have ritualized the Fourth is through the consumption of food. The Fourth of July is a time to gather in backyards over hot grills that cook hot dogs, corn on the cob, and fresh oysters. Meat can be accompanied with cool garden, potato, or fruit salads. Coleslaw is also a refreshing side dish. And if smoked barbecue is your preference, baked macaroni and cheese is also a popular side. Iced tea, cool lemonade, and a variety of sugary, carbonated sodas continue to serve as thirst-quenchers for this popular summer holiday. And, of course, beer and other forms of alcohol are widely consumed (often in copious amounts). In 2015, more than 68 million cases of beer were purchased by Americans over the July 4 weekend.

Some of the earliest foods consumed on the Fourth would have been ice cream and turtle soup. Ice cream purveyors would be out in the summer heat wherever people were gathered, such as along the Coney Island boardwalk and throughout New York's many parks. Today, ice cream is still enjoyed; however, the food most commonly associated with the Fourth is the hamburger, which has become a staple of backyard barbecues.

In 2009, Americans spent $193 million dollars on hamburger patties. The exact date that the first hamburger was served is subject to debate. One version (which food historians seem to agree on) is that what we know as the hamburger was first conceived in Wichita, Kansas, in 1916 by line cook Walter A. Anderson. In the 1930s, White Castle opened locations throughout New York, causing hamburgers to increase in popularity.

Another popular food for the Fourth is the hot dog. When Nathan Handwerker first opened his "Nathan's Famous" in Coney Island back in 1916, he likely never imagined that one day eating the largest number of hot dogs would become such a popular tradition associated with his hot dog stand. In fact, what has become a gluttonous ritual of "competitive eating" may have mortified the "founding fathers," but such events have (since 1972, at least) become another unusual aspect of the American character.

New York City may be best known for hosting the largest Fourth of July fireworks display in the United States. The first advertisement for local fireworks to appear in New York can be found as far back as 1800. But since 1976, Macy's has hosted the show by illuminating the skies over the Hudson and (for some years) the East Rivers with brilliant pyrotechnics that are now visually synonymous with the Fourth.

Adams Family Papers. "Letter from John Adams to Abigail Adams, 3 July 1776, 'Had a Declaration....'" Massachusetts Historical Society.
De Bolla, Peter. *The Fourth of July and the Founding of America*. Profiles in History. London: Profile, 2007.
Heintze, James R. *Fourth of July Celebrations Database*. Washington, D.C.: America University. http://www.american.edu/heintze/fourth.htm.
Smith, Andrew F. *New York City: A Food Biography*. Big City Food Biographies Series. Lanham, Md.: Rowman & Littlefield, 2014.
Travers, Len. *Observing the Fourth: Independence Day and the Rites of Nationalism in the Early Republic*. Amherst: University of Massachusetts Press, 1997.

Nicholas Allanach

Franey, Pierre

Pierre Franey (1921–1996), born in Burgundy, France, was a prominent New York chef and author. At age thirteen Franey became an apprentice in a Paris restaurant, and he worked his way through the traditional culinary hierarchy. By 1938 he was the assistant saucier at Drouant, one of the city's top restaurants. He showed such promise that he was selected to go to New York as *poisson commis* (assistant fish cook) for Le Restaurant du Pavillon de France at the 1939 World's Fair. Franey worked under Henri Soulé, the restaurant's maître d'. By the time the fair closed in October 1940, Europe was at war and France was occupied by German armed forces. See WORLD'S FAIR, 1939–1940.

Rather than return to occupied France, Franey and Soulé remained in the United States. Franey worked briefly in the banquet and room-service kitchen at the Waldorf Astoria. Soulé opened Le Pavillon, a restaurant on New York's fashionable Upper East Side in October 1941, and he hired Franey as a cook. When the United States entered the war in December 1941, Franey enlisted in the U.S. Army and eventually helped liberate France. See WORLD WAR II. Franey returned to New York after the war and rejoined the staff of Le Pavillon. While visiting French restaurants in 1947, he met and subsequently married Betty Chardenet, a French American woman.

Franey moved up the ranks at Le Pavillon, becoming chef de cuisine in 1953. When Le Pavillon hit difficult financial times in 1960, Soulé ordered a staff reduction, but Franey refused to discharge anyone from his *brigade de cuisine*. Newcomer Jacques Pépin, who had been at Le Pavillon for just eight months, joined Franey in protest; and the two walked out, forcing Le Pavillon to close temporarily. Subsequently, both Franey and Pépin went to work for the Howard Johnson's restaurant chain—the money was better and the nine to five working hours were limited.

Franey met Craig Claiborne, the *New York Times* food columnist, in 1959 when Franey worked at La Pavillon. The two became friends, and Claiborne often invited Franey to dine with him when Claiborne was writing restaurant reviews. Claiborne also invited Franey and other top French chefs to cook in his home kitchen. When Claiborne quit the *New York Times* in 1970, he and Franey began publishing a culinary newsletter, but it failed. They also collaborated on many books, including *Classic French Cookery*.

During a 1975 Channel 13 fundraiser, Franey and Claiborne purchased dinner for two at any restaurant of their choice in the world paid for by American Express. They chose Chez Denis in Paris, where they ate a thirty-one-course dinner costing $4,000 (equivalent to $18,000 in 2014). Claiborne's article about the meal in the *New York Times* generated a furor.

When Claiborne returned to the *New York Times* in 1976, he urged the newspaper to hire Franey to write a column, which became The 60-Minute Gourmet. The enduringly successful column was the basis for two cookbooks, published in 1979 and 1981. Franey coauthored five books with Craig Claiborne, including *Classic French Cooking* (1970), a volume in the Time-Life Foods of the World series, and *Craig Claiborne's Gourmet Diet* (1980). Franey cowrote several other cookbooks, including *Pierre Franey's Low-Calorie Gourmet* (1984), *The Seafood Cookbook* (1986), and *Cuisine Rapide* (1989).

Franey also embarked on a career in television, appearing in several popular cooking series. These television appearances gave him great visibility and helped generate a series of engagements as a cooking instructor and lecturer. These, in turn, helped to further his writing career. In all, Franey wrote or coauthored nineteen books; the last one was his autobiography, *A Chef's Tale: A Memoir of Food, France, and America* (1994). Two years after its publication, Franey died of a stroke while giving a cooking demonstration on board the *Queen Elizabeth II*.

See also CLAIBORNE, CRAIG; FRENCH; and LE PAVILLON.

Claiborne, Craig, and Pierre Franey. *Classic French Cooking*. New York: Time-Life, 1970.
Franey, Pierre, Richard Flaste, and Bryan Miller. *A Chef's Tale: A Memoir of Food, France, and America*. New York: Knopf, 1994.
Prial, Frank J. "Pierre Franey, Whose Lifelong Love of Food Led to Career as Chef and Author, Dies at 75." *New York Times*, October 16, 1996.

Andrew F. Smith

Fraunces Tavern

Fraunces Tavern is a landmark restaurant in New York's financial district, noted as the site where General George Washington bid his officers farewell at the end of the Revolutionary War. It has served food and drink on and off since the early 1760s, a time at which taverns were the center of community life.

The current building was built as a private residence in 1719 by Etienne Delancey, son-in-law to New York mayor Stephanus van Cortland. His heirs sold the building to Samuel Fraunces, who converted the structure into a tavern called the Queens Head.

The tavern was a casualty during the Revolutionary War (1775–1783), taking a cannonball through the roof in 1775, but was repaired by the end of the war. British troops occupied the city from 1775 to 1783 and frequented the tavern throughout that period. Samuel Fraunces reportedly passed on information to the American army under George Washington outside the city.

Fraunces sold the tavern in 1785, and it subsequently changed hands many times. After Washington became president in 1789, he hired Fraunces to become his executive steward.

In 1832, 1837, and 1852, the building suffered serious fires. After each fire, the owner rebuilt and added modern additions. By the end of the nineteenth century the building, still located at 54 Pearl Street, bore little resemblance to the original structure. In 1907, the building was restored to its eighteenth-century appearance and opened as a museum and restaurant. In 1965 the building was officially designated a New York City landmark.

Throughout its long history Fraunces Tavern survived as a venerable landmark, if not a renowned restaurant. George S. Chappell, writing about the tavern in 1925, suggests that although ancient, it was still a destination for people who enjoyed a good meal. "The atmosphere of Fraunces is that of a club—quiet, calm, and leisurely—in striking contrast to the bustle of downtown and in perfect accord with what one would hope, but not expect, to find."

Today Fraunces Tavern is a museum and restaurant, and it remains a popular tourist destination. Some consider it the oldest surviving building in Manhattan, although others dispute the claim because of its extensive history of renovations.

See also TAVERNS.

Chappell, George S. *The Restaurants of New York*. New York: Greenberg, 1925.
Fraunces Tavern website: http://frauncestavernmuseum.org.
Sismondo, Christine. *America Walks into a Bar*. New York: Oxford University Press, 2011.
Yeadon, David, and Roz Lewis. *The New York Book of Bars, Pubs, and Taverns*. New York: Hawthorn, 1975.

Peter LaFrance

French

French food culture has been an integral part of the New York City food scene since the early decades of the nineteenth century and remains so to this day.

From the first cafes serving coffee, tea, hot chocolate, and sweets, along with a variety of alcoholic drinks, to the lavish, multicourse tasting menus presented at Manhattan's chicest addresses, the influence of France has been enduring and ubiquitous. Situated along the twisting streets of Lower Manhattan, and especially along Broadway, these earliest cafes and pastry shops offered their clientele a taste of France in a city dominated by Anglo-style taverns, coffee houses, oyster cellars, and chop houses. The majority of these cafes were French-owned, but in the case of Delmonico's, which opened in 1827, its proprietors were two French-speaking brothers from Ticino, Switzerland. See DELMONICO'S.

As the city's small but culturally significant French community developed during the second half of the nineteenth century (comprised of chefs seeking employment opportunities and political exiles fleeing unrest), a French quarter grew up just north of Grand Street and south of Washington Square. There, French was spoken and printed on street signage. One could find boulangeries, butcher shops, general stores, and greasy-spoon-type restaurants (many located in basements), in addition to cafés where absinthe and conversation flowed freely. Even for the poor, a simple meal, including wine, could be had for a modest price. Among those escaping turmoil was Pierre Blot, a chef and cookbook author who opened the city's first French cooking academy in 1865 at 90 Fourth Avenue. Described by the *New York Times* as "a French professor of cooking," Blot offered classes to both servants and ladies. See BLOT, PIERRE.

In the vicinity of Blot's cooking academy, at University Place and Ninth Street, was the upscale Café Martin, opened in 1883 by Jean and Louis Martin. When their cafe relocated to Twenty-Sixth and Madison Avenue in 1904, a location formerly occupied by Delmonico's, the University Place site was taken over by Raymond Orteig, a Café Martin employee, who reopened the hotel/restaurant as The Lafayette. The establishment was known for its *onion soupe des Pyrénées*, loin lamb chops, and *parfait Lafayette au rhum*. A Frenchman and aviation enthusiast, Orteig put up the $25,000 prize in 1919 to stimulate interest in transatlantic flight exploration. It was that purse (equivalent to over $300,000) that inspired Charles Lindbergh to undertake his 33½-hour, nonstop New York–Paris flight in 1927. Orteig

also owned the nearby Café Brevoort, where Mark Twain and Eugene O'Neill were regulars.

The Café Martin flourished in its new uptown home, attracting an affluent clientele. Highly popular among French visitors, the restaurant was considered "the Frenchest French restaurant," with its wine menu featuring over sixty champagnes alone. Beyond its gastronomic significance, Café Martin merits attention for challenging Victorian-era mores with respect to women dining out. While men were permitted to smoke in restaurant dining rooms at the time, women were required to smoke in women-only lounges, often located upstairs from the main dining room. In December 1907, with the new year approaching, the Martin brothers decided that if women wished to smoke at their tables, the staff would not prohibit them from doing so.

Uptown, in the far West Forties and Fifties, where transatlantic ocean liners docked, were a number of restaurants owned and staffed mainly by immigrants from desperately poor, rural Brittany. There, too, one found wholesome food at affordable prices. An important development in the history of French food not only in New York City but in America in general occurred during the summer of 1939 with the opening of Le Restaurant Français at the World's Fair in Flushing, Queens. See WORLD'S FAIR, 1939–1940. There, in the French pavilion, fairgoers (i.e., the public at large) were treated to not only French dining of the highest order but French service of the highest order. A fair brochure explained that the restaurant was conceived to be "an exact copy of a typical Parisian restaurant of the finest class...in an atmosphere identical to that found in the restaurants of the Rue Royale or the Avenue de l'Opéra: same cuisine, same wine, same personnel, same charm."

During the month of June alone, 26,510 fair visitors dined on the likes of *caneton Nantais à l'orange*, *filets de sole Nantua, homard froid Parisienne, fraises Sarah Bernhardt*, and ice cream and pastries to end the meal. The sprawling two-story French pavilion, built at a cost of almost four million 1939 dollars, boasted two areas for dining—the restaurant itself, which featured a spacious terrace with sweeping views of the fairgrounds, and a glass-fronted wine bar, where attendees could choose from an impressive range of French wines

The maître d' of Le Restaurant Français was the imperious and uncompromising Henri Soulé, who had traveled to New York aboard the SS *Normandie* from Le Havre, France, with then eighteen-year-old Pierre Franey. See SOULÉ, HENRI; and FRANEY, PIERRE. Based on the restaurant's tremendous success after two fair seasons, Soulé opened Le Pavillon in Manhattan on October 15, 1941. Located at 5 East Fifty-Fifth Street, opposite the St. Regis Hotel, Soulé's temple of gastronomy became the preferred dining spot of the Kennedys, Rockefellers, and Vanderbilts. Its success spawned other high-profile restaurants such as La Cote Basque (1959), Lutèce (1960), La Caravelle (1961), La Grenouille (1961), Le Périgord (1963), Le Cygne (1969), and Le Cirque (1974), many of which were opened by Pavillon alums. See LE CIRQUE; LE PAVILLON; and LUTÈCE.

At the same time that a French restaurant culture was flourishing in the city, interest in specialty foods from France was on the rise; imported cheeses, the richer and stinkier the better, were especially in demand from the mid-1970s on. This helped launch the artisanal bread movement as a number of New York City bakers jumped on the "baguette bandwagon." In 1975, Les Trois Petits Cochons, the award-winning paté company, burst onto the downtown scene. Located on East Thirteenth Street, the charcuterie/takeout shop served such classics as boeuf bourgignon, coq au vin, blanquette de veau, quiche Lorraine, and crème caramel to Francophile New Yorkers. Culinary icon James Beard was a frequent customer and friend of the owners, Alain Sintourel and Jean-Pierre Paradié. Mimi Sheraton and Craig Claiborne were also enthusiastic fans, whose reviews helped spur the shop's success. See BEARD, JAMES; CLAIBORNE, CRAIG; and SHERATON, MIMI.

The 1970s nouvelle cuisine movement in France also influenced French restaurants in New York City by encouraging chefs to use fresh ingredients, as opposed to canned or frozen, and to eliminate the use of heavy, Escoffier-era sauces. Best known among the nouvelle-style restaurants at the time was Le Plaisir (1979), whose executive chef was the French-trained Japanese Masa Kobayashi. With Francophilia at the table reaching new heights, the French Culinary Institute (recently renamed The International Culinary Center) opened its doors in SoHo in 1984 with an all-star, all French teaching staff. A decade later, Jean-Georges Vongerichten arrived on the scene with Vong, which blended Southeast Asian and French influences. Vong and later his eponymous,

three Michelin–starred Jean-Georges opened in 1997, becoming overnight sensations.

As the twentieth century came to a close, the vast offerings of ethnic restaurants, dietary concerns, and other social factors signaled the demise of many of the city's most venerable French restaurants. In 2004 alone, La Cote Basque, La Caravelle, and Lutèce all closed. Nonetheless, the restaurants, brasseries, and bar à vins at the haute and mid-range levels have continued to draw diners. It would seem that the most persistent presence of French culinary traditions may be the pastry shop, a return to French food's earliest beginnings. Between Payard, Financier, Ladurée, Dominic Ansel (creator of the cronut), Maison Kayser, Millefeuille, and the many other makers of macarons, éclairs, croissants, and pains au chocolates that have sprung up, patisseries remain potent ambassadors of French gastronomy. Most fittingly, forty years after Les Trois Petits Cochons opened on East Thirteenth Street, another French (although Belgian-owned) eatery has taken up residence in its very location, serving croque monsieurs instead of quiche and paté. Plus ça change…

Batterberry, Michael, and Ariane Batterberry. *On the Town in New York: A History of Eating, Drinking, and Entertainments from 1776 to the Present.* New York: Scribner, 1973.

Grimes, William. *Appetite City: A Culinary History of New York.* New York: North Point, 2009.

Schwartz, Arthur. *New York City Food.* New York: Stewart, Tabori & Chang, 2004.

Alexandra Leaf

French Culinary Institute

Dorothy Cann Hamilton founded the French Culinary Institute (FCI) in the SoHo neighborhood of Manhattan, on the corner of Broadway and Grand Street in 1984. It has since grown to become the International Culinary Center (ICC), with locations in California and Italy as well as the original building in Manhattan. "Total immersion," the name of the teaching strategy behind the culinary curriculum, is extremely rigorous. This program places the burgeoning cook in a professional kitchen setting from day one of training. The purpose is to teach the student a comparable amount of basic knowledge (i.e., culinary skills and product knowledge) as you would get from a two-year internship within six or nine months.

The curriculum consists of six hundred hours of intense training. Many of the school's students are fulfilling a lifelong dream and are in the process of changing careers, so the institute offers the option of day classes, which will have the student graduating in six months, or evening and weekend classes, which take nine months to complete.

Hamilton had a desire to travel to Europe even as a young girl growing up in Brooklyn. She convinced her parents to allow her to study at the University of Newcastle upon Tyne in England. Hamilton forged strong bonds with the French women at the university, and because she could not afford to travel home between sessions, ended up spending a lot of time in France, where she was introduced to French cuisine. Upon returning home, her father helped her open the French Culinary Institute using the model she had seen at the schools she had toured in France. She paid the French government to allow her to use its curriculum and invited French chefs to lecture at the institute.

The "French internship" teaching concept has resonated with some of the most prominent culinary icons in the industry. Jacques Pépin, Alain Sailhac, André Soltner, and Jacques Torres have been on the roster of deans at the institute for more than twenty years. See PÉPIN, JACQUES and SOLTNER, ANDRÉ. As the concept has flourished and the curriculum expanded, the dean's list of culinary titans has lengthened.

The institute has grown from two early programs, a classic French culinary arts curriculum and a pastry arts program, to include programs that range from pastry arts, cake design, food media, and Italian and Spanish food studies to farm-to-table practices and intensive sommelier instruction. The Spanish food studies course concludes with a week in Spain, and the farm-to-table program includes field trips and a weeklong program created by FCI graduate Dan Barber and his staff. See BARBER, DAN. The curriculum continues to evolve, and the institute continues to grow, having made a major expansion in 2006.

With the addition of an Italian counterpart to the hugely successful French program, the culinary institution changed its name to the International Culinary Center in 2006. ICC is now an international powerhouse in culinary and wine education. Included in the list of luminaries that makes the institute the global force that it is today are Jose Andres (Dean of Spanish Studies), Emily Luchetti and Cesare Casella (Deans of Italian Studies), and Alan Richman (Dean of Food Journalism and New Media).

The culinary arts curriculum, which for many years comprised four levels, grew to six levels in 2006 with the expansion of the institute's facilities; the other programs differ in their modules. The 12:1 student-teacher ratio ensures close contact between instructor and student. The institute is continually investing in its facilities, which allows students to work with the most up-to-date equipment. ICC places great importance in being an industry leader and staying abreast of industry developments to continually integrate new technologies into the curriculum.

The first four levels of the culinary arts program introduce basic techniques such as knife skills, impart product knowledge, and gradually teach cooking techniques. As the students progressively gain knowledge and confidence, by level 5 they are ready to cook for the Michelin-recommended and Zagat-rated restaurant L'Ecole. This is a full-service restaurant owned and operated by the school. It offers students the opportunity to put their new knowledge to use and cook for actual customers. The students move through every station of the professional kitchen. This is the culmination of the "total immersion" program.

ICC's commitment to the trade is also evidenced by an advanced chef training course. This is a program created for culinary professionals that allows chefs to stay current in a constantly evolving industry.

Graduates of the institute work in nearly every aspect of the food industry, including food styling, print and digital media, catering, management, and of course, restaurants. The institute offers lifetime career services, and with graduates from all over the world, this has created an extensive hiring network. Its distinguished alumni include David Chang of Momofuku fame, Wylie Dufresne of wd 50 and Alder, Dan Barber of Blue Hill, Hooni Kim of Danji, and many others. See CHANG, DAVID and DUFRESNE, WYLIE.

ICC received the International Association of Culinary Professionals (IACP) Culinary School Award of Excellence (an honor bestowed biennially) in

2010, 2012, and 2014. It was also inducted in to the Culinary Hall of Fame in 2013.

See also COOKING SCHOOLS and HAMILTON, DOROTHY CANN.

Dorenburg, Andrew, and Karen Page. *Becoming a Chef*. New York: Van Nostrand Reinhold, 1995.

International Culinary Center website: http://www .internationalculinarycenter.com.

Smith, Andrew F. *The Oxford Companion to American Food and Drink*. New York: Oxford University Press, 2007.

Eirik Osland

FreshDirect

FreshDirect (www.freshdirect.com) was the first major online grocery delivery service to break into the New York City market. It was founded by food broker Joe Fedele and investment banker Jason Ackerman in 1999. Just three years later, they had built a 300,000-square-foot headquarters in Long Island City. Their first delivery to Roosevelt Island went out on July 11, 2002. Today, their company employs over two thousand people and is a familiar name to many New Yorkers, yet their success was far from guaranteed.

A failed national online grocer called WebVan laid some of the groundwork for the genesis of FreshDirect. Started in 1996, WebVan declared bankruptcy in 2001 after receiving over $1.2 billion in funding. Today it is considered one of the biggest flops of the dot-com era. Though the story of WebVan led many to wonder if an online grocery service could become successful, FreshDirect learned from the national chain's mistakes. They started small, delivering to only select locations in the five boroughs. Though the logistics of developing an online delivery system are costly, FreshDirect was founded with only about $60 million. However much their overhead, FreshDirect's success or failure turned on whether enough people would use their service. Though there was a lot of potential for new business in New York City, not enough people were willing to become repeat FreshDirect customers.

For residents of "the city that never sleeps," access to grocery items at all hours is almost a given. Though some New Yorkers live in neighborhoods without access to large or inexpensive grocery stores, many more have options within walking distance. Overall, New York City has more grocery stores per square mile than any other city in the United States. There are bodegas for late-night milk runs and twenty-four-hour pharmacies for toilet paper emergencies. In the midst of this culture, grocery delivery services are both a no-brainer and a particular challenge. When FreshDirect's initial orders suffered from errors like broken eggs, melting ice cream, and late or even missing deliveries, customers were quick to drop the service.

FreshDirect's advertisements offering $50 or even $100 off orders for first-time buyers were a common sight on city subways. Unfortunately, it was not enough to keep customers loyal at full price. FreshDirect churned through new customers, keeping warehouses busy but leaving little room for profit.

At the end of 2007, immigration officials inspected the eligibility of the company's employees to work in the United States. FreshDirect lost over two hundred employees before the winter holiday rush. Their remaining customers complained about sold-out items and poor delivery times. The company had no choice but to restructure with an eye on better customer service. They hired more employees, stopped luring new customers with first-time offers, and started an internal rating system for produce and seafood. All the changes were designed to make repeat customers keep coming back. It was enough to keep the company afloat.

FreshDirect got its first real competition in 2011 with the arrival of Peapod, an Illinois-based online grocer that expanded into New York City. Yet after nearly a decade FreshDirect had so many employees that the city wanted to keep its first e-grocer in New York City. It offered a $127.8 million incentive in the form of tax breaks and cash to allow the company to move its operations to the Bronx, beating out a hefty offer from New Jersey.

While FreshDirect's success in New York City has opened the doors for new companies like Peapod, Good Eggs, and other niche grocery delivery services, its popularity with New York City's residents is far from assured. The subsidized move to the Bronx sparked outrage among neighborhood groups that worried about the delivery trucks increasing air pollution. Controversy aside, at 500,000 square feet, the new facility will allow FreshDirect to more than double its current business. In 2013, it started delivering to Philadelphia, the first foray into a market outside of New York City.

FreshDirect is one of many companies that rely on the Internet for convenience as well as lowered overhead. Rents for a New York City grocery store are significant, and for many food vendors web-based commerce is the only thing that makes financial sense. Though their rocky origins created easy comparisons to WebVan and other early online grocers, they have outlived their predecessors. Over time, FreshDirect learned that the secret to success—especially in a market as large as New York City—is to start slow. Whether other food vendors follow its lead by using e-commerce, a farmers' market booth, or food trucks rather than brick and mortar establishments, their ultimate longevity is a reminder that even in the foodiest city in the United States feeding people is hard work.

Bruder, Jessica. "At FreshDirect, Reinvention after a Crisis." *New York Times,* August 11, 2010.

Fickenscher, Lisa. "Bronx Group Appeals FreshDirect Court Ruling." *Crain's New York Business,* December 5, 2013.

Urbanski, Al. "FreshDirect's Secret to Tantalizing Its Customers." *Direct Marketing News,* April 1, 2013.

Tove K. Danovich

Fulton Fish Market

Fulton Fish Market began its life as Fulton Market, one of the six major public markets that provisioned New Yorkers with fresh food in the nineteenth century. Opened in 1821, Fulton Market replaced the outdated Fly Market, which was the largest east side market during the colonial period. When Fulton Market opened, it was by far the most modern market in the public market system. It was also the most expensive, costing the city over $200,000 for the land, construction, and other expenses.

The original Fulton Market boasted a modern infrastructure and a diversity of stands, including eighty-eight butchers' stalls; thirty-four stands for poultry, fruits, and vegetables; and four sausage stands. It also had stands for hunters selling wild game, dairy farmers vending cheese and butter, and space for cake and coffee shops, hucksters' stands, and tables for "country people" coming from nearby farms to sell their goods. A few months after the market opened,

the Market Committee of the city government offered a few vacant butchers' stalls in the east wing of the market house to "sellers of fish."

In 1838, reflecting on the increased volume of fish in Fulton Market, the city's Market Committee approved the construction of a wholesale fish market, across South Street from the original market house. Fulton had better accommodations for a fish market than Washington Market (which did a large trade in fish and shellfish) because of its direct proximity to the water. See WASHINGTON MARKET. Fishermen could park their fish cars or smacks right against the docks and sell directly to customers from there. By the 1850s, over two hundred smacks lined up daily at the docks of Fulton Market, vending seafood from local waters directly to wholesale customers. Each car could hold about seven thousand pounds of fish. The fish market also received stock from commission dealers who brought fish to New York by steamboat from the waters of New Jersey. In all, the fish market traded close to $1.5 million in the early 1850s. Over the next century, Fulton Fish Market remained the city's central wholesale fish depot. The building itself was rebuilt in the 1840s and again in the 1860s. In 1907, the Tin Building replaced the earlier structure.

In 1924, Fulton Fish Market sold one-quarter of the fish marketed in the United States—384 million pounds. In 1939, under Mayor Fiorello La Guardia, the city opened a second building at Fulton Fish Market: the New Building. The construction of the New Building was part of a general reform of the public market system undertaken by La Guardia and overseen by the newly consolidated Department of Public Markets, Weights, and Measures. La

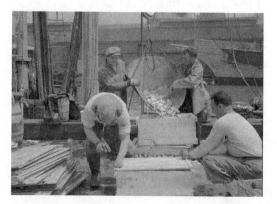

Stevedores packing and icing fish at the Fulton Fish Market, 1943. LIBRARY OF CONGRESS

Guardia's administration created retail market buildings such as the Essex Street and Arthur Avenue Retail Markets in an effort to rid the streets of pushcarts. And they constructed new wholesale market buildings, including the New Building at Fulton Fish Market, in an attempt to modernize the structures and promote a more sanitary environment for wholesale food sales in New York. The New Building thus had refrigerators and freezers, a mechanical conveyor system for getting the fish from the docks into the building's stalls, and fileting areas so that fish could be prepared for sale within the building structure. See LA GUARDIA, FIORELLO.

During its entire history, most of the activity at Fulton Fish Market occurred in the wee hours of the night. Boats pulled up around midnight direct from the sea or carrying the catch that was transported via Long Island Railroad to the Brooklyn waterfront. Vendors unloaded their cargo and wholesale buyers—restaurateurs, fishmongers, and supermarket representatives—came to market between 3:00 a.m. and 9:00 a.m. on Mondays and Thursdays and from 4:00 a.m. to 9:00 a.m. on the other days of the week. The market was closed on weekends. In the 1950s trucks replaced boats as the main conveyance bringing the fish into the market. Unionized workers unloaded the fish onto pallets and hand trucks and distributed it to stalls in the markets, which the shoppers visited.

By the 1950s, only about 6 percent of fish arrived at the Fulton Fish market by boat; the rest came via truck. City officials began to question the logic of keeping the market at South Street Seaport. Bottlenecks caused both traffic and distribution problems on crowded South Street. Some thought the construction of the FDR Drive would relieve this congestion, but in fact it caused other problems, cutting the fish market off from the rest of the neighborhood. Calls to move the Fulton Fish Market to the Bronx began at this time and continued in subsequent decades.

Increasingly, these calls also were related to concerns about corruption in the market. In the 1930s, the market had fallen under the control of organized crime. The Mafia allegedly controlled all aspects of the market, extorting money from suppliers and sponsoring illegal gambling, loan sharking, theft, and murder. Despite decades of trying to rout the Mob from the market, including federal racketeering charges brought by prosecutor Rudolph Giuliani in the 1980s, the market remained under the influence of the Genovese crime family. Finally, while he was mayor, Giuliani closed the market and began steps to move its functions to Hunts Point, in the Bronx, a process that was finally completed in 2005.

By this point, the Fulton Fish Market had become a storied part of the New York City landscape. Tourists and native-born New Yorkers would plan early morning visits to the market, less to buy fish than to interact with characters like "Shopping Bag Annie," who sold cigarettes and other supplies from a shopping cart, and forklift operator "Joe Tuna," whose "meaty biceps jiggle so much," when he rides his cart over the cobblestones, "that the tattoos move like cartoons," according to journalist Dan Barry, writing in the *New York Times* in 2005. The market's move to Hunts Point thus evoked nostalgic laments from many New Yorkers.

Since November 2005, the New Fulton Fish Market Cooperative has operated in Hunts Point. The 400,000-square-foot, refrigerated facility accommodates thirty-seven wholesale seafood businesses doing over $1 billion worth of business per year. Offering one hundred to three hundred varieties of fish a day, it is the second largest seafood wholesale facility in the world, after Tokyo's Tsukiji seafood market. Trucks bring fish from all over the nation and the world to be sold at the market to fish wholesalers, chefs, and retail customers. The market operates from 1:00 a.m. to 7:00 a.m. Monday through Friday. See HUNTS POINT.

Meanwhile, the old Fulton Fish Market buildings have been vacant since the market moved to Hunts Point, and debates have raged over their use. Between 2007 and 2013, the New Amsterdam Market, helmed by urban planner Robert LaValva, held a seasonal open market around the Tin and New Buildings that drew local vendors and manufacturers of food and other artisanal products to sell their goods. The New Amsterdam Public Market Association, Inc., which runs the market, has a political and social mission as well as an economic one: to revive a regional public market system with vendors committed to small-batch, artisanal production and local sourcing. The association hoped that the old Fulton Market buildings would become the permanent home of the New Amsterdam Market. In 2013, their hopes were dashed, however, when the Howard Hughes Corporation gained approval from the city for a proposal to redevelop South Street

232 • Fusion Food

Seaport. The Hughes group's plan includes razing the New Market Building and moving the Tin Building several blocks to the northeast, then renovating and reopening it as a retail food hall. While the New Amsterdam Market still exists and is still seeking a permanent home for its market, it seems that it will not be located at the old Fulton Fish Market. See NEW AMSTERDAM MARKET.

See also PUBLIC MARKETS.

Bagli, Charles V. "Despite Amenities, South Street Seaport Redevelopment Plans Stall over a High-Rise." *New York Times*, February 16, 2015.
Barry, Dan. "A Last Whiff of Fulton's Fish, Bringing a Tear." *New York Times*, July 10, 2005.
DeVoe, Thomas F. *The Market Book: A History of the Public Markets of the City of New York*. New York: Augustus M. Kelly, 1970. First published 1862.
"Fulton Fish Market: New Market Building." Municipal Art Society of New York, 2008. http://www.newamsterdammarket.org/seaportvision/2008_Municipal_Art_Society.pdf.
"History." The New Fulton Fish Market Cooperative at Hunts Point, Inc. "History." http://www.newfultonfishmarket.com/history.html.
Lubasch, Arnold H. "Mafia Runs Fulton Fish Market, U.S. Says in Suit to Take Control." *New York Times*, October 16, 1987.
Tangires, Helen. *Public Markets*. New York: Norton, 2008.

Cindy R. Lobel

Fusion Food

"Fusion food" is a term coined by Chef Norman Van Aken during a speech given in Santa Fe, New Mexico, in 1988. Van Aken borrowed the word "fusion" from jazz music (in which it means jazz mixed with rock or other musical genres); it refers to food composed of ingredients or cooking techniques from two or more distinct ethnic cuisines (for example, Chinese and Mexican). The terms "Pan-Asian," "Asian American," and "New World cuisine" are used synonymously.

The culinary phenomenon of restaurants serving mixed cuisines since around 1988 is fusion in the narrow sense. In the broader sense, it can be said that nearly all of American cuisine is a fusion of various ethnic cuisines. Mixture and cross-sampling of cuisines has been part of the immigrant experience in New York City for centuries. In the nineteenth century, for example, large immigrant populations from Ireland, Italy, Germany, and other European countries settled in New York City, sharing ethnic enclaves and even the same tenement buildings. See IRISH; ITALIAN; and GERMAN. While first-generation immigrants have tended to keep to themselves and preserve cultural markers like cuisine, it is reasonable to assume that there was sharing of cuisines. And second-generation immigrants tended to be curious of cuisines outside their own, literally leaving the home in search of new food experiences.

In nineteenth-century New York City, German and Irish immigrants owned most butcher shops and grocery stores and served as domestics in homes and as cooks in hotels and restaurants. As a result, a considerable number of the city's earlier immigrant population (English, Dutch, etc.) was exposed to new cuisines. Immigrant culinary specialties became staples of New York City–based American cuisine. When did the mixture of cuisines become a fusion, as we understand it from Van Aken? That is hard to say, but it can be stated with certainty that contemporary "American" cuisine is an amalgam, if not a fusion, of many of the cuisines brought here by its immigrant populations.

As for the more recent phenomenon, it started in California. Austrian chef Wolfgang Puck opened his pioneering Asian–French fusion restaurant Chinois on Main in 1983 in Santa Monica. In 1987, chef Nobu Matsuhisa opened his first restaurant, Matsuhisa, in Beverly Hills, offering a combination of Japanese, Peruvian, and European cuisines. Jean-Georges Vongerichten joined the fusion trend in 1985 when he used ingredients like lemongrass and ginger in French preparations in LaFayette in New York City; however, it was not until the opening of Vong in 1993 that he offered a menu that was truly fusion-based, in this case a mixture of Southeast Asian cuisines. See VONGERICHTEN, JEAN-GEORGES. Meanwhile, Van Aken opened his first fusion restaurant, Mira, in Key West, Florida, in 1988.

Vongerichten's Vong may have been the first fusion restaurant to open in New York City, in 1993. Or that designation may go to Chef Nobu's namesake restaurant Nobu, which opened in the Tribeca neighborhood, also in 1993.

By the end of the 1990s, the fusion fad seemed to be on the wane. At the same time that fusion was trickling down into New York City restaurants of all sorts, critics expressed a backlash against the trend. For example, an uncredited review in *New York* magazine listed Le Bernardin as the "Best Fusion

Restaurant of 2001" and credited chef Eric Ripert for his "exhilarating" cooking and "limitless…talent" but also stated unequivocally that "self-consciously crossing borders rarely creates something fresh and delicious." The line between natural fusion and fusion that is imposed on a cuisine unnaturally is drawn by numerous critics, but the distinction is largely subjective.

Not long after that review appeared, a second generation of fusion chefs began to make their presence known in New York City. The difference between them and Puck, Vongerichten, and Van Aken is that these new chefs were by and large of the Asian ethnicity in which their cuisine was based. This second group includes David Chang (with his Momofuku empire of New York restaurants), Danny Bowien (whose New York City Mission Chinese restaurant is equally as popular as the original in San Francisco), Chris Cheung (who was a big part of Nobu's and Vong's success before opening his own restaurant, Tiger Blossom), and Dale Talde (a contestant for two seasons of Bravo's *Top Chef* cooking show and now owner of Talde in Park Slope, Brooklyn), among many others. See CHANG, DAVID.

The newer fusion chefs bring an immigrant experience to their culinary journey. They have grown up eating the Asian cuisines of their forebears, often cooked for them by a grandmother. But unlike earlier generations of New York City immigrants, they were quick to assimilate into American culture and had an openness to cultures other than their own. Their culinary curiosity led them to venture outside the home and try other cuisines, often within their own neighborhoods. Some at a crucial point returned to Asia to immerse themselves in their native cuisine or (as with David Chang) the cuisine of another Asian culture. Their kinship with Latin cuisines, Mexican especially, seems to be centered around an ingredient common to Asian cuisines—namely, hot peppers. And they struggle over whether to call their cuisine "fusion" or other things, not wanting to be considered unhip or passé or feeling that the word does not correctly characterize their restaurants' cuisines.

While fusion is often the vision of a single chef, there are restaurants whose fusion cuisine is the result of shared ethnicities among a couple who own the restaurant. For example, Convivium Osteria on Fifth Avenue in Brooklyn serves Italian–Portuguese dishes, honoring the food of owners Carlo and Michelle Pulixi; and Doma na Rohu in Manhattan's Greenwich Village features cuisine with a German–Czech–Croatian–Austrian mix, recreating owners Michael and Evie Polesny's grandmothers' food.

Whether or not fusion as a trend in New York City is dead, there are nevertheless, according to Yelp, more than three thousand fusion restaurants operating there presently (or 10 percent of the city's restaurants). In addition, at least eighteen food trucks serve fusion foods on the city's streets every day. See FOOD TRUCKS.

Dickerman, Sara. "Fusion Reaction: How America Fell in Love, and Then Out of Love, and Then in Love All Over Again, with Asian-Influenced Cuisine." *Slate*, April 12, 2012. http://www.slate.com/articles/life/food/2012/04/asian_fusion_comeback_american_s_love_hate_relationship_with_asian_inspired_cooking_.html

Esposito, Shaylyn. "Why We Have Norman Van Aken to Thank for the Way We Dine Today." *Smithsonian*, May 29, 2014.

Geiling, Natasha. "Sorry, Wolfgang, Fusion Foods Have Been with Us for Centuries." *Smithsonian*, July 24, 2013.

Hauck-Lawson, Annie, and Jonathan Deutsch, eds. *Gastropolis: Food and New York City*. Arts and Traditions of the Table: Perspectives on Culinary History. New York: Columbia University Press, 2008.

Perry, Charles. "Fusion Food: Birth of a Nation's Cuisine." *Los Angeles Times*, September 16, 1993.

Smith, Andrew F. *New York City: A Food Biography*. Lanham, Md.: Rowman & Littlefield, 2013.

Karl Peterson

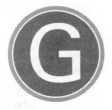

Gage & Tollner

Gage & Tollner first opened in 1879 and remained in continuous operation until it closed in 2004. It was one of New York's most popular dining spots over the years, counting Diamond Jim Brady, Mae West, and Jimmy Durante among its patrons.

When it moved to 372 Fulton Street in Brooklyn in 1892, Gage & Tollner's dining room was the height of Victorian fashion. The walls were covered in wine-colored, flocked velvet. The furnishings and trim were carved from dark oak, cherry, and mahogany. Multi-armed gaslight chandeliers marched down the center of the long, narrow room, their light multiplied by a wall of mirrors on one side and a mirror over a service bar on the other. In fact, gaslight was not romantic. It gave a ghastly glow, which may have been a reason that fashionable women of the day wore heavy makeup when they went out at night.

Gage & Tollner closed in 2004; its site is now a leather goods and jewelry store. But behind the pink fabric that covers the still-flocked walls are all the original decorative details. The gas chandeliers are still there, too—and operable. (Those gaslights were, in fact, ceremoniously lighted every night, until the restaurant closed.)

In 1974, the restaurant building was declared an untouchable landmark by the New York City Landmark Commission. The next year, the interior was declared a landmark, too; at that time it was one of only two restaurant interiors with such protection (The Four Seasons in the landmark Seagram Building was the other). In 1982, Gage & Tollner was also placed on the National Register of Historic Places.

Gage & Tollner has an admirable food legacy. From the beginning, its menu emphasized seafood—Fulton Street led directly to the docks in those days—and fried clam bellies were the most famous item, at least in the twentieth century. Clam bellies are soft-shell clams, also called steamers or Ipswich (Massachusetts) clams, even when they are from Maine. Tossed in flour and fried, the soft bellies remained on the menu through its several owners, until the last owner, Joe De Chirico (who also owns the venerable Marco Polo restaurant in Brooklyn's Carroll Gardens), closed it because Fulton Street was then at its nadir as a shopping street.

The restaurant's glory years could well have been from 1988 to 1992, when African American chef Edna Lewis, whose portrait is now on a U.S. postage stamp, took over the kitchen. She kept seafood at the heart of the menu, adding her own southern American, mainly refined Virginian/African dishes, some of which were already well known from the two cookbooks she had authored. See LEWIS, EDNA.

Schwartz, Arthur. *Arthur Schwartz's New York City Food: An Opinionated History and More than 100 Legendary Recipes.* New York: Stewart, Tabori & Chang, 2004.

Arthur Schwartz

Gay Bars

Gay bars are among the most notable economic and cultural institutions in modern New York City and central to the history of the city's lesbian, gay, bisexual, and transgender communities. The earliest recognizably gay bars evolved in the 1880s and 1890s in the Bowery, a working-class entertainment district whose bars and brothels attracted sailors on shore leave and moral crusaders alike. One of the oldest and most notorious spots, Columbia Hall on Fourteenth Street, featured a beer garden and rooms for rent on the floors above. In the early 1900s, Columbia Hall and other "resorts for perverts" were targeted by moral entrepreneurs like the Society for the Suppression of Vice.

In the midst of both Prohibition and the Great Migration of African Americans from the South in the 1920s, lesbian and gay speakeasies and cabarets proliferated in Harlem, the theater district, and Greenwich Village. As speakeasies spread across New York City, distinctly lesbian and gay subcultures began to take root in the sexually permissive, difficult-to-police atmosphere of the 1920s. Harlem and Greenwich Village were at the epicenter of a lesbian and "pansy" craze, a nightlife fad that saw white, middle- and upper-class customers flock to predominantly working-class and African American establishments in a practice known as "slumming." A highly visible part of New York City's Prohibition culture, lesbians and gay men were depicted in sheet music, Broadway plays, popular novels, and even film. Prohibition brought the establishment of the State Liquor Authority, which included the power to police and shutter lesbian and gay bars, among others. See PROHIBITION. Coupled with the effects of the Great Depression, the 1930s saw a general decline in the visibility and number of lesbian and gay bars. Despite the crackdown on such drinking establishments, Harlem's Ubangi Club opened in 1934 featuring renowned lesbian performer Gladys Bentley. Although World War II saw a swell of lesbian and gay migrants to the city, military police labeled many lesbian and gay clubs off limits, especially in Harlem, where fears of interracial sex and sociability brought even more intense forms of scrutiny.

In the 1950s and 1960s, lesbian and gay bars were essentially an illicit market in New York City. In addition to regulations that banned catering to "homosexuals," New York City passed a 1948 ordinance that banned unescorted women in bars. Police and bureaucrats used these powers to shutter bars and harass lesbian and gay consumers even as lesbians and gay men faced a swell of popular violence. As early as 1952, local gossip columnists linked the city's gay bars to organized crime, especially in Greenwich Village, where gangsters took advantage of the prevailing atmosphere to charge higher prices for cover charges and drinks and blackmail wealthy customers. White, middle- and upper-class gay men sometimes colonized men's bars, like the bars at the Plaza Hotel, The Four Seasons, and the "sweater bars" of the Upper East and West Sides.

See FOUR SEASONS and PLAZA, THE. Simultaneously, the earliest working-class leather bars began to appear in Greenwich Village, often catering to truckers and stevedores in the meatpacking district. Lesbian bars were more tightly concentrated around Washington Square Park and Abingdon Square in the Village, where bars like the Bagatelle, the Sea Colony, and the 181 Club remained popular despite an uptick in raids and street violence in the 1950s and early 1960s.

In 1966, a gay rights organization called the Mattachine Society staged a "sip in" protest at Julius' Bar in Greenwich Village, leading to a reversal in the state ban on lesbian and gay bars. In the late 1960s, the earliest guides to New York City's bars began to appear, the first of which were published by the Mattachine Society's book services. Despite the official end to the ban, lesbian and gay bars continued to face legal scrutiny because of their connection to organized crime and lesbian and gay consumers faced both police and popular harassment. Following a police raid on the Stonewall Inn on Christopher Street on June 28, 1969, riots broke out in Greenwich Village and lasted for three successive nights, marking what many historians describe as the beginning of the gay liberation movement. See STONEWALL INN.

Since the 1970s, lesbian and gay bars have played an increasingly prominent role in the city's nightlife culture. The popularity of disco music in the 1970s made gay male culture highly visible, recognizable, and posh. In the 1980s and 1990s, some gay bars, especially around Times Square, became a battleground over the spread of HIV/AIDS, leading to numerous closures by state and city officials.

In the past two decades, lesbian, gay male, and transgender bars and parties have diversified. Sports bars, leather bars, dance bars, drag, and burlesque have become an important part of lesbian, gay, bisexual, and transgender nightlife culture both in older gay neighborhoods as well as in new ones, like Washington Heights, Astoria in Queens, and Park Slope and Williamsburg in Brooklyn.

See also GREENWICH VILLAGE.

Barnet, Andrea. *All-Night Party: The Women of Bohemian Greenwich Village and Harlem, 1913–1930*. Chapel Hill, N.C.: Algonquin, 2004.

Bérubé, Allan. *Coming Out Under Fire: The History of Gay Men and Women in World War II*. New York: Basic Books, 1990.

Chauncey, George. *Gay New York: Gender, Urban Culture, and the Making of the Gay Male World, 1890–1940*. New York: Basic Books, 1994.

Delaney, Samuel. *Times Square Red, Times Square Blue.* New York: New York University Press, 1999.

Duberman, Martin. *Stonewall.* New York: Plume, 1994.

Heap, Chad. *Slumming: Sexual and Racial Encounters in American Nightlife, 1885–1940.* Chicago: University of Chicago Press, 2010.

Lait, Jack, and Lee Mortimer. *U.S.A. Confidential.* New York: Crown, 1952.

Nestle, Joan. "Bars." Lesbian Herstory Archives. Brooklyn, N.Y.

Christopher Mitchell

German

German food has been, and continues to be, an important part of New York City's culinary landscape. From its earliest days, German immigrants were grocers, bakers, butchers, brewers, and cooks, helping to define the city's collective cuisine. Many foods associated with New York City are German in origin (hot dogs, for example). And several of the most successful food products worldwide were created and originally manufactured in New York City by German Americans (for example, Hellman's mayonnaise). See HELLMANN'S MAYONNAISE and HOT DOGS.

Immigration of German-speaking peoples to New York City took place in three waves. The first significant settlement of Germans in the American colonies took place during the 1670s. A thousand a year arrived in America between 1720 and 1750. Finally, a stream of German-speaking people arrived in the second half of the nineteenth century, fleeing political and religious oppression and famine.

By the time of the American Revolution New Yorkers were already familiar with German delicacies like sauerkraut and pretzels, but it was during the latter half of the nineteenth century that the appeal of German cuisine was felt at all levels of New York society. German Americans dominated bakeries, butcher shops, and groceries, selling pumpernickel, bratwurst, and lager beer. Some worked as domestics and became cooks in restaurants and hotels, cooking sauerbraten and schnitzel and serving bock beer.

The great nineteenth-century swell of German-speaking immigration settled in New York City's Kleindeutschland, the city's first ethnic enclave, found in what is now the East Village, the Lower East Side, eastern Chinatown, and Gramercy. At its height in the 1860s, Kleindeutschland was the third largest community of German-speaking people in the world, eclipsed only by Vienna and Berlin. See KLEINDEUTSCHLAND.

In Kleindeutschland, beer halls were the center of community activity. Unlike taverns, which were exclusively a male domain, beer halls welcomed families to talk and dance and drink beer. In the summer, the activity spilled out into beer gardens. See BEER GARDENS.

The rest of the time, German Americans worked hard. Industrious and ambitious to move up in New York society, today's grocer became tomorrow's beer garden owner and the next day's brewery owner. Within a generation, numerous German Americans gained material success and left Kleindeutschland for newer, more decidedly middle-class ethnic enclaves and neighborhoods. Yorkville, on Manhattan's Upper East Side, was one of these. The impetus for this resettlement to Yorkville was partly upward mobility and partly disaster.

On summer weekends, German American families would travel out of the city into the countryside to have picnics. While on such an excursion in 1904, more than a thousand of Kleindeutschland's residents perished when the *General Slocum* steamship sank in the East River. Rather than remain in the old neighborhood and feel all too keenly the absence of the dead, many joined the trend and started anew in Yorkville. A shift that had started several decades earlier accelerated, such that by 1910 Yorkville had replaced Kleindeutschland as New York City's center of German life and culture. See YORKVILLE.

German American industry found its mark in numerous culinary success stories. Hellman's Blue Ribbon Mayonnaise, Entenmann's baked goods, Gulden's Spicy Brown Mustard—these and many more food products that became household brands in America and around the world were created and manufactured first by German Americans working in New York City. See GULDEN'S MUSTARD.

Some of New York City's most successful restaurants were started by German Americans as well. Lüchow's was opened in 1879 by a former Hanover resident who bought a beer hall after working there for just two years and turned it into an institution that lasted until 1986. See LÜCHOW, AUGUST GUIDO. In Williamsburg, Brooklyn, father and son Carl and Peter Luger opened a series of businesses, including a restaurant, in 1887. When Carl died, the son closed everything except the restaurant, renamed it after himself, and the now famous Peter Luger Steakhouse was born. Luger's survives to this day, on that same spot in Williamsburg.

By the 1950s, many German Americans had left the city. The restaurants that remained in Yorkville's Germantown were no longer the center of a vibrant community and became instead tourist attractions for visitors to the city hoping to catch a glimpse of what used to be. Only one traditional German restaurant is still operating in Yorkville, Heidelberg.

Filling the void, New York City's Steuben Society and its annual Steuben Parade, the largest of its kind in the United States, bring together German Americans to celebrate the achievements of German immigrants and honor their culture. The society hosts many events, and German food and drink are often involved, in the days and weeks leading up to Oktoberfest.

When the annual Oktoberfest celebrations come around every autumn, it may seem as if every bar and tavern in New York City has magically become German. What is traditionally a sixteen-day festival in Germany often goes on for more than a month in New York, although most of the activity is focused on the October weekend that concludes the celebration. Beer gardens in New York City such as Zum Schneider and Hofbräu Bierhaus NYC are among those German restaurants that put on special events for Oktoberfest. However, the festival extends beyond those establishments that serve German food and drink the rest of the year. In some years, more than sixty different establishments in New York City host events. The city's newspapers and magazines publish elaborate guides to getting the most out of Oktoberfest, and residents and tourists alike get their fill of German beer and food.

Beyond Oktoberfest, with the start of the twenty-first century, there is undoubtedly renewed interest in German food in New York City. In addition to Zum Schneider and Hofbräu Bierhaus NYC, restaurants like Lederhosen, Loreley, Der Schwarze Kolner, and Hallo Berlin are serving hefeweizen and currywurst to a new generation, translating German culinary traditions for contemporary New Yorkers. Nevertheless, compared to other ethnic fare offered in the city—for example, Japanese or Thai food—German food remains a very specialized interest.

See also DELIS, GERMAN.

Hooker, Richard J. *Food and Drink in America: A History.* New York: Bobbs-Merrill, 1981.

Nadey, Stanley. *Little Germany: Ethnicity, Religion and Class in New York City, 1845–1890.* Urbana: University of Illinois Press, 1990.

Panchyk, Richard. *German New York City.* Charleston, S.C.: Arcadia, 2008.

Smith, Andrew F. *New York City: A Food Biography.* Lanham, Md.: Rowman & Littlefield, 2013.

Karl Peterson

Gilded Age

The Gilded Age refers to the time period between Reconstruction and the early twentieth century's Progressive Era. Perhaps nowhere did the intense changes that characterize this period in American history come into starker relief than in Gotham, where urbanization, immigration, industrialization and corporate consolidation, debate over political machines, as well as interclass conflict and intraclass solidarity defined the last decades of the nineteenth century. These changes directly influenced New York's foodways as corporate consolidation redefined the food industry, while immigration diversified culinary offerings and class and gender continued to determine access.

If anyone believed that capitalism was stable following the Civil War, the depression of 1873 proved otherwise. Railroad speculation was largely responsible for this first postbellum depression, which left 25 percent of laborers jobless in New York City. The economic elite struggled to find a new way to control the economy, moving from pools to restrain competition to trusts to ultimately corporate holding companies, after the Sherman Antitrust Act rendered trusts illegal in 1890. Like other industries, food companies in Gotham embraced such consolidation. The New York Biscuit Company, a combination of several bakeries, dominated the cracker market. Similarly, the Havemeyer family, which owned massive sugar refineries in Brooklyn, spearheaded the creation of the "Sugar Trust." See NABISCO and HAVEMEYER FAMILY.

Once internally divided between old and new money (an axis that largely pitted merchants against manufacturers), members of the upper crust came to see themselves as part of the same socioeconomic class during this time period. And elite dining establishments were central parts of their highbrow culture. Haute restaurants like Delmonico's defined themselves by their ability to replicate French culinary standards and demanded specific cultural knowledge of patrons, including the ability to read French menus. This helped to ensure that even ordering would be uncomfortable for anyone outside society circles, reinforcing these spaces as exclusive bastions for elite sociability. In 1894, some society women even used Sherry's as a headquarters when they joined the suffrage campaign, partially shielding themselves from ridicule by meeting in this elegant restaurant. See DELMONICO'S; FRENCH; and SHERRY'S.

Corporations required everyone from lawyers to clerks to succeed, fostering the growth of an urban middle class that eventually challenged the elite's culinary hegemony. In the middle of the century, the dining landscape was limited for this developing socioeconomic stratum: men, for instance, might grab a quick lunch at a downtown eating house, eat at a chophouse, or awkwardly ape elite habits at haute restaurants. Pressure for improved dining experiences resulted in a changed restaurant scene by century's end. Clean lunchrooms, table d'hôte restaurants (which provided a multicourse meal at a fixed price), and "coffee and cake saloons" all provided attractive options for middle-class families who did not have the money or cultural knowledge necessary to patronize aristocratic establishments. The ethnic restaurants that immigrants opened provided an additional alternative.

Middle-class New Yorkers could go "slumming" to Chinatown to try chop suey, enjoy lager beer at a German beer garden, or consume a dish of macaroni in an Italian restaurant thanks to the waves of newcomers pouring into the United States in the nineteenth century. A desire for better food and, in some cases, hunger motivated many Italian and Eastern European Jewish immigrants to leave their native countries and join the German and Irish residents who had arrived in the United States decades earlier. Upon arriving in New York, they found work in everything from the construction and garment industries to peddling on street corners. Food provided a comforting taste of the homeland, while also helping to create economic opportunities for immigrant entrepreneurs. Some savvy restaurant proprietors even began to Americanize their food to cater to middle-class palates, resulting in "hybrid" menus that removed ingredients, such as garlic, from meals.

Many immigrants celebrated the quality and quantity of food in their new country compared to what they had known in their homelands, but struggles remained. As Jacob Riis made visible in *How the Other Half Lives* (1890), immigrant life in tenements teemed with difficulties, hunger high among them. The purity of milk presented another danger despite legislation to improve its quality. Fleischmann's Model Vienna Bakery was a notable bright spot for the most des-

perate of New Yorkers: it doled out bread nightly. See BREADLINES and MILK, SWILL.

Like class, gender determined access to food even as more spaces opened for women in the late nineteenth century. A woman attending a restaurant with her family might take comfort in a separate dining room by the Gilded Age, but a male escort remained necessary to ensure her propriety. Society women whose reputation was beyond question were exceptions to this rule with some elite establishments (including Delmonico's) agreeing to serve them lunch. Unaccompanied middle-class females, however, would have had better luck at an ice cream parlor than at Delmonico's. Likewise, they could also dine at department stores' restaurants, such as the one in Macy's, which opened to ensure that women were comfortable when out shopping. See DEPARTMENT STORE RESTAURANTS. While changes in housing (including the popularity of hotels and apartments and the decline in the number of domestic servants) resulted in an increased need to eat outside of the home, etiquette guides continued to celebrate domesticity. Men might not return home for lunch because of growing distances between home and work, and women might be out shopping during the daytime; but dinner increased in importance for individuals concerned about family unity.

New York had the most diverse culinary options and the largest number of restaurants in the nation by century's end. As such, the city served as a culinary bellwether, with newspapers from Boston to Salt Lake City including details about its food scene. Food products also moved in and out of the metropolis from all over the world—oranges and lemons from Italy and Spain, meat from the Midwest (thanks to refrigerated railroad cars), and eggs and milk from Gotham's hinterlands serve as only a few examples. While some expressed concern that New York City was losing its hegemonic place in the United States to Chicago (leading to the consolidation of Manhattan with its surrounding boroughs in 1898), New York's position as the nation's food capital remained secure.

Beckert, Sven. *The Monied Metropolis: New York City and the Consolidation of the American Bourgeoisie, 1850–1896.* Cambridge, U.K.: Cambridge University Press, 2001.

Burrows, Edwin G., and Mike Wallace. *Gotham: A History of New York City to 1898.* Oxford: Oxford University Press, 1999.

Diner, Hasia R. *Hungering for America: Italian, Irish, and Jewish Foodways in the Age of Migration.* Cambridge, Mass.: Harvard University Press, 2001.

Grimes, William. *Appetite City: A Culinary History of New York*. New York: North Point, 2009.

Haley, Andrew P. *Turning the Tables: Restaurants and the Rise of the American Middle Class, 1880–1920*. Chapel Hill: University of North Carolina Press, 2011.

Kessner, Thomas. *Capital City: New York City and the Men Behind America's Rise to Economic Dominance, 1860–1900*. New York: Simon & Schuster, 2003.

Lobel, Cindy R. *Urban Appetites: Food & Culture in Nineteenth-Century New York*. Chicago: University of Chicago Press, 2014.

Lauren C. Santangelo

Gold, Rozanne

Rozanne Gold is a chef, cookbook author, food writer, and restaurant consultant. She cooked for former mayor Robert Wagner and went on to become, at age twenty-three, the first chef to "Hizzoner" Ed Koch at Gracie Mansion, a position she created (in 1977) and used as a platform to showcase New York wines and produce decades before "eat local" became the prevailing mantra. Her menu concept for the Hudson River Club presaged, even catalyzed, the locavore movement, with its focus on Hudson Valley ingredients (including fruit from Fishkill Farms, Manhattan district attorney Robert Morgenthau's historic orchard). In the 1980s and 1990s Gold was consulting chef to two of New York's largest-grossing restaurants, the legendary Rainbow Room, where her "cocktails and little meals" ignited the grazing craze, and Windows on the World, where, as part of the renowned consulting team of Baum + Whiteman, she helped create "The Greatest Bar on Earth" and a global menu featuring spiced veal shank *en papillote* and other showstopping creations. See RAINBOW ROOM and WINDOWS ON THE WORLD.

With her prescient palate, Gold has spotted or sparked food trends—small plates, Mediterranean Rim cuisine, health-conscious cookery—before they happen. But it is the elegant simplicity of her food that is her hallmark and the basis for her "1–2–3" cookbooks featuring three-ingredient recipes. This series inspired The Minimalist column in the *New York Times* and garnered Gold three of her four James Beard Awards. Her 2010 book *Radically Simple* was named by *Cooking Light* one of the best cookbooks of the past twenty-five years.

Gold's gracious, Zen-like demeanor belies the talent and drive that led *Business Week* to deem her a "mover and shaker." But she is equally committed to giving back to her community: in 2011 she rescued *Gourmet's* 3,500-volume cookbook collection and donated it to New York University's Fales Library. See FALES LIBRARY. And in the aftermath of Hurricane Sandy, Gold and her husband Michael Whiteman set up CBE Feeds, a pop-up kitchen that fed 185,000 New Yorkers in need.

Matsumoto, Nancy. "Profile of a Tastemaker: Rozanne Gold." *Edible Manhattan*, May 10, 2011.

Raposo, Jacqueline. "We Chat With: Rozanne Gold, Grande Dame of the New York Food Scene." Serious Eats, October 1, 2012. http://newyork.seriouseats .com/2012/10/rozanne-gold-interview-chef-ed-koch-cookbook-author.html

Meryl Rosofsky

Gomberg Seltzer Works

See SELTZER.

Gordon, Waxy

See BOOTLEGGERS.

Gotham

See IRVING, WASHINGTON and PICNICS.

Gotham Bar and Grill

Gotham Bar and Grill has been a highly regarded downtown destination restaurant since 1985. It had opened a year earlier in a huge, high-ceilinged space on East Twelfth Street formerly occupied by an antique dealer. The inspiration for the restaurant was a Parisian brasserie, and the menu consultant was food writer Barbara Kafka. After the first year, it became clear that a strong vision was needed if Gotham were going to succeed.

On the recommendation of Jonathan Waxman (then of Jams), Alfred Portale interviewed for the position of executive chef and was offered the job; he has held the post since that time. Having trained in French kitchens both in New York City and under Michelin-starred chefs in France, Portale soon married his classical French training with traditional American (and local) foodstuffs like Maine lobster, squab, fresh tuna, and rack of lamb. In so doing, he joined a small but growing number of American chefs with similar sensibilities who helped give rise to "new American cuisine."

Shortly after taking up the reins at Gotham, Portale earned the restaurant three stars from the *New York Times*; it would be the first of many such reviews. (Gotham is New York's only restaurant to receive five three-star ratings.) The review caused a great deal of buzz as such a high rating was customarily reserved for the city's chicest French addresses. In that now famously glowing review, Bryan Miller wrote, "Five months ago, a gifted young chef, Alfred Portale, came aboard from Tucano, where he worked under Jacques Maximin. In a short time Mr. Portale has transformed the Gotham into one of the most exciting 'new' restaurants in town" (Miller, 1985).

The nouvelle cuisine movement, begun in France a decade earlier, helped usher in a new way of thinking not only about French food but about American cooking as well. The ideas of James Beard also helped raise the level and standing of American cooking. See BEARD, JAMES. Regional dishes, too, were embraced for their unique qualities.

With his global pantry sensibilities, Portale was interested in Asian cookery early on and has been credited with creating tuna tartare. His version, made with yellowfin tuna, Japanese cucumber, shiso leaf, miso, and ginger vinaigrette, has been on the menu since the 1980s. The oldest dish on the menu and a perennial favorite is Gotham steak, served with marrow mustard custard, Vidalia onion rings, and a bordelaise sauce. Over the restaurant's thirty-plus-year history, such chefs as Bill Telepan, Wylie Dufresne, Tom Colicchio, David Walzog, and John Schenk worked alongside Portale, turning out as many as three hundred dinners per night.

Grimes, William. *Appetite City: A Culinary History of New York*. New York: North Point, 2009.
Miller, Bryan. "Restaurants." *New York Times*, October 4, 1985.

Alexandra Leaf

Gourmet

Gourmet magazine was launched in January 1941. The magazine's editor, Earle MacAusland, had experience in publishing magazines for a female audience; but he was unable to find corporate backing for his dream magazine, a food journal that addressed elite readers, so he asked for money from his family to start

Gourmet. See MACAUSLAND, EARLE. By the time the first issue came out, Europe was at war, and America would enter later in the same year. MacAusland and his intrepid team of writers and editors, however, assured their audience that the time was perfect for a magazine that celebrated the good things in life.

Gourmet's first editor, Pearl Metzelthin, embodied this spirit. She was born in the United States, raised in Germany and Poland, married to a German diplomat, and stationed in China. She spoke many languages, had studied nutrition, and helped design cooking equipment for airliners in the early days of commercial air travel. Before she became *Gourmet*'s editor, she had capitalized on her globetrotting past by writing *The World Wide Cook Book*, published in 1939.

Metzelthin's influence was clear in the emphasis the magazine placed on travel. *Gourmet* was, from the first, a magazine about eating good food in other countries, giving a new direction to travel journalism and marking a significant departure from traditional recipe sections of women's magazines. Rather than simply providing practical recipes for home use, *Gourmet* provided armchair travel and a fantasy lifestyle to transport readers from the ordinary. The magazine's first food editor, who also provided a recipe column, was a professional chef, Louis de Gouy, who had served as chef to J. P. Morgan on the tycoon's private yacht for a round-the-world trip. See DE GOUY, LOUIS P.

Metzelthin sought out contributors who were known as writers, including Samuel Chamberlain, whose "Burgundy at a Snail's Pace" appeared in the magazine's first issue. Probably her most famous contributor was M. F. K. Fisher. Other writers more famous in their own time, like Stephen Longstreet and Robert Tristram Coffin, wrote about food in the lives of the creative class. That so many of *Gourmet*'s writers were men also set the magazine apart from recipe pages, which typically relied on the idea that women wanted to hear from other women on culinary matters. *Gourmet* addressed readers, both male and female, who were not anxious about what to cook for dinner but were more generally interested in the culinary world around them.

Despite its internationalism and Eurocentrism, however, *Gourmet* simultaneously remained a magazine of New York. Until the 1970s, *Gourmet* only published reviews of restaurants in New York and Europe. The editors also included a column about the city's theater scene, After Dinner, that served to emphasize the magazine's connection to high culture. One reader wrote in 1944 that "The magazine has only one draw back—and that certainly through no fault of yours. Those of us who are—voluntarily or otherwise—exiles from Manhattan suffer acute nostalgia while reading." A year later, another complained about the New York centrism of the magazine: "Your readers are all over the country, and since we very seldom get to New York, but eat every day, I am always much more interested in your articles than I am in your reviews of New York restaurants." To this the editors responded that in fact lots of the magazine's out-of-town readers visited the city at some point and were grateful for the restaurant reviews that could guide them during their sojourn. Other readers, the editors added, seldom or never came to the city but loved the reviews just the same, using them as a kind of armchair travel experience.

Famous food writer Clementine Paddleford contributed a column about new food products she had encountered in New York's gourmet grocery stores. Implicit to this column was the idea that New York was the entrepôt of the gourmet class. See PADDLEFORD, CLEMENTINE. When Samuel Chamberlain published his stories in *Gourmet* about what happened when his family brought their French cook back to the United States with them, he noted that New York was different from all other cities, gastronomically. If the "family had been repatriated to New York City instead of to a little Yankee town, this chapter of our gastronomic adventures would have been very uneventful" (Chamberlain, 1942). Because the chapter was all about fruitlessly searching for French ingredients in local American markets, the story could only have taken place outside New York. In fact, New York could rival Paris: "A well-stocked Lexington Avenue delicatessen would have dazzled us to such an extent that we would have forgotten all about the splendors of the cheese we left behind us." To emphasize how very much the editorial staff identified with a particular version of New York City glamour, they frequently mentioned the magazine's first address—a penthouse suite in the Plaza Hotel.

Having established a style that struck a chord with readers, the magazine remained largely unchanged for its first forty years. *Gourmet* did not jump on food fashion bandwagons, remaining true to its original Francophilia and focus on New York. The magazine was finally jolted into contemporary culture in 1999, when Ruth Reichl was appointed editor. See REICHL,

RUTH. Having spent her adult life in California, writing about the rise of the new American chef, she brought a new sensibility to the magazine. In a daring move that immediately decentralized New York, Reichl contributed a column reviewing restaurants in Minneapolis in the first issue she edited. The magazine lost some of its provincialism under Reichl's leadership, but when the attacks of September 11, 2001, struck the city, Reichl recounted how she and her staff had rallied to help the first responders. Using their kitchens to cook up comfort food classics like lasagna and chili rather than to test the latest fashionable recipe, the editorial staff felt compelled to feed their city.

Chamberlain, Samuel. "Clementine in the Kitchen." *Gourmet* 2, no. 9 (September 1942): 18.
Grauer, Neil A. "*Gourmet's*—and Baltimore's—'Flying Dietitian.'" *Baltimore Sun*, November 23, 1994.
"Louis de Gouy, Chef, Gourmet's Author, 72." *New York Times*, November 15, 1947, p. 17.
Reichl, Ruth. "Letter from the Editor." *Gourmet* 59, no. 9 (September 1999): 24.
Scheer, Bradley T. Letter. *Gourmet* 4, no. 8 (August 1944): 2; Boarts, R. M. Response to letter. *Gourmet* 5, no. 3 (March 1945): 2.
Smith, Andrew F. *Eating History*. New York: Columbia University Press, 2013.

Megan Elias

Gourmet Garage

Gourmet Garage is a small, five-store chain of specialty food markets located in Manhattan. The chain maintains locations in SoHo, Greenwich Village, the East Side, the Upper East Side, and Lincoln Square.

President and chief executive officer Andy Arons began his career in the food business as an importer and wholesaler in 1981. Partnering with two college roommates, he created Flying Food International and rapidly built a business that serviced more than one hundred Manhattan restaurants, such as the famous Four Seasons and Le Cirque. See FOUR SEASONS and LE CIRQUE. Flying Foods' goal was to bring in foods not readily available to New York chefs at the time and to insure immediate shipping to guarantee absolute freshness. Flying Food International was sold to Kraft Foods in 1987, and Arons regrouped with his business partners.

In 1991, Arons opened a mixed wholesale/retail business in SoHo dedicated to supplying New York restaurants with quality fresh ingredients and focused on high-quality produce at reasonable prices. Operating out of a true garage space in Lower Manhattan, the wholesaler would open its doors to the general public once the trucks had left to make restaurant deliveries. Arons realized he had a ready market available for yet another expansion of the wholesale business. Partnering with business food veterans John Gottfried and Edward Visser, Arons formally opened Gourmet Garage as a retailer on Wooster Street in 1992. The SoHo neighborhood in the early 1990s was a strong market for this new brand of retailer. Artists, performers, writers, as well as Wall Street bankers now had a local resource for a wide range of quality specialty products at good prices. The atmosphere of the original store, which has been replicated in each subsequent location, is very much that of a warehouse space. There is a basic, no-frills, relaxed feel to the interior spaces, which includes wooden floors and modest displays that make the produce the focus of consumers' attention.

Following the success of the Wooster Street location, the store moved to a larger space in 1994 and over the next few years began to open additional locations around Manhattan. At the time of this writing, a sixth store is planned for a loft building in the Tribeca East Historic District.

The philosophy of Gourmet Garage is centered in their slogan, "Shop Like a Chef!" which is used in the marketing and advertising materials. The chain has been able to compete successfully in the crowded Manhattan retail food market by focusing on the neighborhood, small-chain feel of the stores and continues to offer a wide range of domestic and international products as well as prepared foods at attractive prices.

See also GROCERY STORES and SUPERMARKETS.

Conover, Kristen. "Gourmet Garage Boasts Truckloads of Bargains." *Christian Science Monitor*, September 22, 1994.
Fabricant, Florence. "Flying Luxury Foods to Tables in U.S." *New York Times*, May 8, 1983.
Gourmet Garage website: http://www.gourmetgarage .com/our_story.
Klenotic, Deborah. "The Neighborhood Gourmet." *UMAS Mag* online (Winter 2005). http://www .umassmag.com/Winter_2005/The_Neighborhood_ Gourmet_848.html.

Carl Raymond

Gramercy Tavern

See MEYER, DANNY.

Grand Central Oyster Bar

James Bond, Agent 007, said "the best meal in New York—oyster stew with cream" was "at the Oyster Bar at Grand Central." Perhaps Bond also loved the Oyster Bar because its roots were British. When the 440-seat Grand Central Terminal Restaurant opened on Saturday, February 1, 1913, it was patterned after the most famous restaurant in the world, the Palm Court at London's Ritz Carlton Hotel. On opening day, 150,000 people came to the terminal. One hundred railroad executives attended the first dinner served at the restaurant, amid potted palms and Persian carpets. The restaurant bore no resemblance to New York's famous nineteenth-century oyster bar dives with sawdust on the floor, and the oysters were no longer from New York's oyster beds.

The early menus, influenced by the Ritz's French chef Auguste Escoffier, were continental. Seafood was minimal. Between the clam fritter appetizer and the cheese finale were meats—venison, prime rib, duck, goose—swimming in French sauces. American exceptions were dessert. Alongside French pastries were strawberry shortcake and blueberry pie.

By 1917, oysters on the half shell (blue points, thirty-five cents for a dozen) and oyster stew were on the menu. The Oyster Bar was a celebrity hangout: Ziegfeld, of the Follies; actors Lillian Russell and Al Jolson; boxer "Gentleman Jim" Corbett. Diamond Jim Brady liked to bet fifty dollars that he could identify Wellfleet oysters blindfolded. Every president since Woodrow Wilson has eaten at the Oyster Bar.

In the 1950s, Americans followed the popular advertising jingle to "see the U.S.A. in your Chevrolet" on 41,000 miles of new freeways created by the Federal-Aid Highway Act. The railroad slid into oblivion. To attract customers, the restaurant went garish: yellow walls, red tablecloths, turquoise columns. Still, in 1973, the sixty-year-old restaurant was shuttered and bankrupt. Like Pennsylvania Station, grimy crime-ridden Grand Central was scheduled for a teardown.

Enter Jacqueline Kennedy Onassis and the Committee to Save Grand Central Station. In 1974, the New York Metropolitan Transit Authority tapped Jerome Brody, former president of Restaurant Associates, who had been involved in resurrecting the Rainbow Room and The Four Seasons, to run the Oyster Bar. He made it a world-class seafood restaurant.

The décor was restored to highlight the herringbone "tile arch system" ceiling of Spanish architect

Rafael Guastavino, who had also designed the main hall at Ellis Island, St. John the Divine Cathedral, and Temple Emanu-El. The menu reflected a new American culinary identity, a cuisine proud of its regional roots. In 1978, the restaurant won wine awards.

The Oyster Bar survived a kitchen fire in 1997 and the death of Brody in 2001. Restaurant ownership passed to the Oyster Bar employees. Executive chef Sandy Ingber, the "Bishop of Bivalves," started at the Oyster Bar in 1990. His menu includes classic and cutting-edge creations: bouillabaisse, fried Ipswich clams, halibut with mango chutney, and Arctic char with wasabi yuzu dressing.

The Oyster Bar has seasonal rituals: shad run in February, soft shell crabs in spring, June "Nieuwe" herring from Holland, fall oyster frenzy. The menu changes daily, depending on what Chef Ingber finds on his 3:00 a.m. foray to the New Fulton Fish Market at Hunts Point in the Bronx. More than thirty varieties of fish and multitudes of clams, crabs, scallops, and lobster are served each day, as well as twenty-five to thirty varieties of oysters, more than 5 million each year. The seafood is served raw, roasted, boiled, broiled, grilled, fried, frittered, steamed, sautéed, stuffed, and stewed. Oyster stew is a menu perennial. Maybe James Bond just loved the Oyster Bar because it is an aphrodisiac paradise.

See also OYSTER BARS; OYSTERS; and RESTAURANTS.

Guastavino website: http://architecture.mit.edu/class/guastavino/news.html.
Ingber, Sandy. *The Grand Central Oyster Bar & Restaurant Cookbook.* With Roy Finamore. New York: Stewart, Tabori & Chang, 2013.

Linda Civitello

Grand Union

See SUPERMARKETS.

Gray's Papaya

See HOT DOGS.

Great Performances

Great Performances, one of the largest privately held catering companies in the United States, plays a major role in New York City's cultural life. The company annually caters over two thousand events around the city and serves as the exclusive caterer for many landmark institutions.

In 1979, photographer Liz Neumark and a flamenco-dancer friend started the company as a waitress service employing women in the arts. Great Performances was conceived as a way to provide female artists with jobs that would allow them the time, money, and freedom to create and perform.

At that time, an all-woman staff serving formal events was a novelty that won them immediate attention. However, Great Performances secured encore engagements because it brought theatrical flair and a highly personalized, energetic level of service to a sleepy, traditional industry. The staff was even willing to pick up an event's food en route to the venue, and this quickly became one of their signature services. By 1982, they were making enough pickups to consider doing the cooking themselves. Without benefit of a business plan—simply as an extension of what Neumark has referred to as the company's "female values"—Great Performances launched an off-premises catering business.

By 1986 Neumark had bought out her partner and set the company's course for future expansion. That same year, Great Performances celebrated a milestone—financially and as a corporate citizen of New York—with its first $1 million event: the Statue of Liberty reopening celebration.

In 1992, the company was named the exclusive in-house caterer at the Wave Hill estate and cultural center in the Bronx. Neumark, recognizing the benefits that exclusive catering contracts offered to enhance revenues, improve profitability, and sustain Great Performances' growth, began to aggressively seek more of these in-house arrangements with iconic New York locations. Today, Great Performances has exclusive or contractual relationships with many institutions, including Jazz at Lincoln Center, Brooklyn Academy of Music, the Plaza Hotel, Asia Society & Museum, El Museo del Barrio, Chelsea Piers, Sotheby's, and Wave Hill.

Great Performances has been an active supporter of many philanthropic activities throughout the years. But it was a personal tragedy for Neumark that caused her to embrace a cause of her own. In 2004 one of Neumark's four children, her six-year-old daughter Sylvia, died suddenly of a brain aneurysm. In 2006, Neumark bought sixty acres in upstate New York and created Katchkie Farm. The purpose was two-fold: to provide Great Performances' city clients with fresh, local food and to serve as the home of The Sylvia Center, an educational nonprofit that introduces children to the pleasures and benefits of eating well through farm visits and cooking workshops.

See also CATERING.

Great Performances website: http://www .greatperformances.com.
Katchkie Farm website: http://katchkiefarm.com.
Stern, Gary M. "Great Performances Indeed—How an Artist Launched One of New York's Premiere [sic] Catering Businesses." The Business Journals. April 22, 2014. http://www.bizjournals.com/bizwomen/ news/profiles-strategies/2014/04/great-performances-indeed-how-an-artist-launched .html.

Doug Duda

Greek

The first wave of Greek immigration to New York City took place between 1890 and 1920. These first immigrants were usually men seeking economic opportunity or persons displaced by the Balkan Wars (1912–1913) and World War I. By the second decade of the twentieth century, these immigrants were settling in Astoria, Queens. Greeks again began to arrive in large numbers after 1945, especially between the 1950s and 1970s, as a result of the economic devastation caused by World War II and the Greek civil war. After 1981, annual U.S. immigration numbers fell to fewer than two thousand. Astoria remains the largest Greek neighborhood in New York City (although its numbers have dwindled as economically successful Greeks have moved to more luxurious suburbs). Astoria remains one of the largest Greek enclaves outside of Greece.

Diners, Restaurants, and Famous Greek Food

Greek immigrants became well-known for opening diners, places where American coffee flows endlessly and breakfast is served all day: the television show *Saturday Night Live* immortalized the fictionalized Olympia diner in John Belushi and Dan Ackroyd's iconic "cheeseburger, cheeseburger" routine. (The diner was actually located in Chicago, but the skit also said much about New Yorker's attitudes toward Greek food.) New York also has many restaurants, tavernas, cafes, bakeries, and food markets focusing on more traditional Greek foods. Virtually all are identified by the distinctive Mediterranean blue and white awning and décor, a motif that continues on the now ubiquitous "anthora" paper coffee cups first popularized in Greek diners and decorated with a Greek key border and line drawing of an amphora or other cultural icon. See COFFEE. While Greek eateries share many similarities with Mediterranean and Near Eastern cuisines, distinctive dishes include mixed mezze appetizers, with tzatziki and *taramosalata*; meat dishes of souvlaki, moussaka, and pastitsio; and many breads and sweets, such as koulouri and baklava. Greek restaurants range from casual hangouts to white-tablecloth ventures. Michael Psilakis is one of the two Greek-origin chefs who won a Michelin star in 2008 with his restaurant Anthos and was named *Bon Appétit's* "Chef of the Year." Psilakis owns the MP Taverna in various locations and Kefi and FishTag in Manhattan.

Greek foods can be found in many of the city's diverse ethnic markets, but the International Grocery at 543 Ninth Avenue, near the Port Authority Bus Terminal, is distinctive in its Greek ownership: the Karamouzis brothers are part of the Greek family that has owned the store for more than thirty years. Nearby is the Poseidon Bakery, and, until recently, there were several Greek butchers whose windows were filled with whole baby lambs and goats for Orthodox Easter.

Ben-Amotz, Allegra. "Michael Psilakis' Guide to Greek Food and Ingredients in New York City." Serious Eats, March 20, 2013. http://newyork.seriouseats .com/2013/03/michael-psilakis-greek-shopping-ingredients-where-to-eat-nyc.html.
Cotsis, Billy. "Astoria...: Little Athens in the Big Apple." Hellenic Travels to the Past, May 9, 2011. https:// herculean.wordpress.com/2011/05/09/atoria-little-athens-in-the-big-apple.
Gill, John Freeman. "Urban History to Go: Black, No Sugar." *New York Times*, June 26, 2006.

Thei Zervaki and Cathy K. Kaufman

Greene, Gael

Gael Greene was *New York* magazine's longtime restaurant critic from 1968 to January 2002. Her reviews described, in vivid detail, her sensual experience with food with tongue-in-cheek innuendo. Throughout her tenure, Greene witnessed the evolution of not only New York food but also America's. Reading her reviews made you her dining companion, and her food descriptions were known for being tantalizing. She would not be at home in *Good Housekeeping*. Her work was powerful, and it sold the five-star experience to the middle class. A few of her notable restaurant reviews for *New York* magazine include "Blue Skies, No Candy" (1976), "Doctor Love" (1982), and "Life of Delicious Excess" (2006). In 1969 she wrote "The Mafia Guide to Dining Out." On her quest, she tested red sauce joints, raided and unraided. She slammed Lombardi's for stingily sauced fettuccini Alfredo and icy veal and extolled Paolucci's broiled sea bass and Italian broccoli. In "Nobody Knows the Truffles I've Seen," she made you fall in love with the pigeon brain and truffle-stuffed chickens of France.

In a summer issue of *New York* magazine, Greene posed with two vanilla ice cream cones covering her breasts to effectively tease her ice cream round-up inside, the hilariously titled "Everything You Always Wanted to Know About Ice Cream But Were Too Fat to Ask." Some of her reviews have enough historical references to make your head spin. She writes with an authority on all things high taste like only a Detroit refugee who escaped to join up with A-listers can.

Greene's sampling of New York food had an obvious high-end bent, but she also dove head first into the culture of "hole-in-the-wall" spots. Still, while some food critics assign prepackaged stereotypes to these lesser-known offerings, Greene was unpretentious when she captured their niches. She was fired after forty years. *New York* magazine told the *New York Times* it was because they did not have the budget to pay food critics. (At the time, Adam Platt was the chief weekly reviewer and wife and husband team Robin Raisfeld and Rob Patronite wrote the Underground Gourmet column and Cheap Eats features.) But she is still not satiated. She ran her independent website called The Insatiable Critic, after the name *New York* magazine gave her. She gave the occupants of New York's eater's paradise a name: foodies. In *The Official Foodie Handbook: Be Modern—Worship Food*, Ann Barr and Paul Levy give Greene credit for coining the term (as does a 1982 *Harpers & Queen* article, "Cuisine Poseur").

Later, in her column Ask Gael, she answered readers' questions about where to take your vegetarian niece or where to find the best modern Chinese. She cofounded City Meals on Wheels, attracting mem-

bers like Nora Ephron, Martha Stewart, and Kathleen Turner as members. She is the self-described "brand name of restaurant journalism." She was criticized, as many food writers of New York regrettably are, for being too cozy with the chefs to reliably pen what consumers crave and deserve. In "I Love Le Cirque, but Can I Be Trusted?" (1977) she wrote, "I send over my serious food-lover friends and stray innocents, who are led to tiny back tables and neglected. They confirm what I already know. Le Cirque can never be a great restaurant."

In her book *Insatiable: Tales From a Life of Delicious Excess*, she chronicled love affairs with famous chefs Jean Troisgros and Gilbert Le Coze and real celebrities like Clint Eastwood and Burt Reynolds. Of her time in a hotel room with Elvis Presley she decided it was "good enough." What always had a purchase on her memory though was the fried egg sandwich that the King asked Gael to order from room service. From 2009 to 2011 Greene was a guest judge on *Top Chef* (seasons 1–3), showcasing her spicy analogies and flair for elegant hats. In her piece "Lessons in Humility and Chutzpah" she taught everyone how to make a reservation like a swell and how to guarantee star treatment you did not deserve ("Pretend you're a secretary and act like you belong with the right purse").

See also CITYMEALS-ON-WHEELS; *NEW YORK* MAGAZINE; and RESTAURANT REVIEWING.

Greene, Gael. "I Love Le Cirque, but Can I Be Trusted?" *New York* magazine, January 31, 1977, pp. 62–67.
Johnston, Josée, and Shyon Baumann. *Foodies: Democracy and Distinction in the Gourmet Foodscape*. New York and London: Routledge, 2010.
Greene, Gael. "Lessons in Humility and Chutzpah." In *American Food Writing: An Anthology with Classic Recipes*, edited by Molly O'Neill, pp. 422–427. Toronto: Penguin Canada, 2007.

Ashley Hoffman

Greenmarkets

In the 1970s the grassroots idea for New York City Greenmarkets blossomed when Barry Benepe, the father of New York's Greenmarkets and one of Gotham's iconic urban city planners, was making a seminal "road trip" through the Hudson Valley with his associate planner, Robert Lewis, where the two were working on architectural development projects. They witnessed decaying family farms despite being blessed with a world-class agricultural cornucopia. Developers were buying up farmland for America's burgeoning suburbia. Envisioning a direct food connection from upstate to New York City, Benepe and Lewis linked the local farmers' plight with the crisis in town, where residents had difficulty finding healthy, locally grown, seasonal ingredients.

Yet, in many ways, it was Mayor Fiorello La Guardia's ban on the city's beloved food pushcarts in 1938—intended as a pivot toward "clean," sanitized indoor markets—that started the inexorable journey that gave rise to today's Greenmarkets. That same year the First Avenue market launched, and Essex Street's indoor market opened in 1940. Soon, supermarkets sprang up. See ESSEX STREET MARKET; LA GUARDIA, FIORELLO; and SUPERMARKETS.

The concept was to transform "dirty" peddlers into clean merchants with an organized business and prices. In other words, the city wanted to "professionalize the peddlers." It was an obsession of La Guardia's—he viewed them all as a sanitary threat, from flower vendors to the Good Humor man.

Karen Seiger, author of *Markets of New York City: A Guide to the Best Artisan, Farmer, Food and Flea Markets*, explains that the endurance of indoor ethnic markets was due in large part to nostalgia for the people who seek out the foods of the old country. But the indoor, "sanitary" markets did not work for farmers who needed to back their trucks right up to their tables to unload and restock. Too much time and labor were needed that would render their already too slim margins nonexistent if they could not deliver their food directly.

In order to get outdoor farmers' markets operational, Benepe and Lewis wrote a proposal for a $7,000 grant. Benepe recalls, "The Foundations we talked to said the city isn't capable of doing this and suggested we find a private non-profit to sponsor financing so we re-wrote it and asked for $35,000 with a plan to run it ourselves and garner a nonprofit sponsor—as part of the existing Council on the Environment of New York City."

First stop: Jack Kaplan, Welch Grape Juice Company owner. The J. M. Kaplan Fund's Ray Rubinow immediately embraced the farmers' market concept, committing funds and talent. In early 1976, with major underwriting from the J. M. Kaplan Fund, a $10,000 investment got plans ramped up for the Greenmarkets.

Benepe first served as a consultant, then appointed Director of the Greenmarket Program for the Council on the Environment, which eventually became GrowNYC. Its board was made up of many city agencies and the mayor—Abe Beame at that time, which made it easier to get city approvals. See GROWNYC. While Benepe worked the city agencies, securing permits and navigating policy politics, Lewis was busy searching for farmers, county by county, to enlist New York and New Jersey growers to participate in their Greenmarket concept. They worked through county cooperative extension agents, who worked directly with farmers; and they worked with New York State's direct marketing bureau, which had connections with farm stands and pick-your-own operations.

In July 1976, the first Greenmarket opened on the Upper East Side at Fifty-Ninth Street and Second Avenue in a vacant lot used by New York police to park their cars. It was the first of its kind in New York City since 1935. Benepe and Lewis unlocked the gates for sixteen farmers and their trucks at 6:00 a.m.; by noon they had sold everything. The two quickly realized guidelines were needed so as not to be seen as a "pass-through" produce market. They needed to establish a "locally grown" benchmark.

According to Benepe, they arbitrarily chose 250 miles because that was roughly where upstate New York's growing region was located from the center of town. Drawing a radius around New York City, "local" extended as far south as Delaware. They also required that growers have 75 percent of their own produce "on-table" with fruits and vegetables grown by the farmer; if selling goods from a nearby grower, that local farm needed to be no more than 25 miles away from his farm. And the locally purchased farmgoods sold could not be found elsewhere in the market, in order to prevent competition with homegrown items. Eventually, the guidelines were expanded to dairy, spirits, and wine.

Two more markets opened that same summer: one at Brooklyn's Flatbush and Atlantic Avenues and another at Union Square. In time, they expanded to fifty-four markets, over 230 participating family farms and fishermen, and more than thirty thousand acres of farmland protected from development. Gotham got its greater share of local produce. Growers and makers proliferated, benefiting from the cross-pollination of culinary concepts and homegrown ingredients.

Benepe and Michael Hurwitz, director of Greenmarket, GrowNYC since 2006, describe the human interaction at Greenmarkets as "wonderful—allowing citizens to engage with farmers, chefs, and each other."

Greenmarkets delivered on the vision to provide fresh, healthy, locally grown food from regional, family farms direct to citizens. According to Hurwitz, demonstrating urban and rural linkages is crucial: "The health of the city is directly linked to that of the rural communities."

See also BENEPE, BARRY.

GrowNYC website: http://www.grownyc.org.

Seiger, Karen E. *Markets of New York City: A Guide to the Best Artisan, Farmer, Food and Flea Markets.* New York: Little Bookroom, 2010.

Wasserman, Suzanne. "The Good Old Days of Poverty: Merchants and the Battle Over Pushcart Peddling on the Lower East Side." *Business and Economic History* 27, no. 2 (1998): 330–339.

Leeann Lavin

Greenwich Village

Greenwich Village is a Lower Manhattan neighborhood that spans northward from Houston Street, running up to Fourteenth Street (Union Square), and from its easternmost boundary of Broadway all the way west to the Hudson River. Its overlapping neighbors include the East Village, NoHo (North of Houston Street), the West Village, the Meatpacking District, and Chelsea.

In the late eighteenth and early nineteenth century, the main source of commerce in the Village (as it is commonly known) was centered in the fresh produce markets and breweries near the Hudson River. At this time, it was a predominantly middle- and upper-class neighborhood, with row houses surrounding a potter's field and public gallows that later became Washington Square Park, and the main buildings of New York University, founded in 1831. In the mid-nineteenth century, waves of European immigrants moved in to work in its factories and warehouses, and the upper classes moved farther north, transforming the neighborhood into the largest Bohemian enclave in the city. Here, a movement of artistic and political individualism, along with the growing student population, gave rise to literary salons, cafés, inexpensive ethnic eateries, saloons, pubs, and art clubs. During Prohibition, its speakeasies, such as Chumley's on Bedford Street, once again attracted uptown New Yorkers. In the 1930s and 1940s, the Village officially established itself as the city's liveliest center for artistic and political expression, known for affordable housing and ethnic food culture.

The Beat Generation

In the 1950s and 1960s, the Village was considered the center of the beat movement and the culture that grew out of it in the coming decades—a place where artists, poets, authors, journalists, playwrights, and musicians frequented its numerous cafés and jazz clubs such as La Lanterna, Café Figaro, Caffé Reggio, Peculiar Pub, Kenny's Castaways, Folk City, the Blue Note, the Village Vanguard, Waverly Inn, Arthur's Tavern, Small's, Café Wha?, and Minetta Tavern. See CAFFÉ REGGIO. Some of the most famous fixtures in this community included Bob Dylan, Jack Kerouac, Allen Ginsberg, William S. Boroughs, Joan Baez, Judy Collins, Ritchie Havens, Diane di Prima, Miles Davis, John Coltrane, Dizzy Gillespie, Nina Simone, Thelonius Monk, Andy Warhol, and Lou Reed.

Stonewall

In 1969, a clash between police and patrons of the Stonewall Inn, a rundown bar owned by the Genovese mafia family that became a haven for the local homosexual community, resulted in successive nights of protests. The Stonewall riots are considered the birth of the gay rights movement and are commemorated each year in June with the Village Gay Pride Parade. Stonewall, as it is now known, is an official landmark. See GAY BARS and STONEWALL INN.

Pizza

Some of the city's best known pizzerias are located within the Village, diverging widely in style from budget-friendly slice joints to upscale eateries and wine bars. Classic Village pizzerias include Joe's Pizza, Bleecker Street Pizza, Arturo's, and John's of Bleecker (known for their brick oven and no-slices policy). With area gentrification neighborhood pizza evolved to Two Boots (an Italian-Cajun hybrid), Mario Batali's Otto, Kesté, and Barbuto, among many others. See BATALI, MARIO. And in some capacity—if not the "original"—there will always be a slice to be had at Ray's. See PIZZA and PIZZERIAS.

Classic Bars and Dining

Village institutions that have survived the times include Portobello, Corner Bistro, Tortilla Flats, Caliente Cab Company, Il Mulino, Bar Pitti, Mamoun's

Falafel, Café Español, Da Silvano, Tea & Sympathy, Elephant and Castle, DoJo West, La Bonbonniere, Knickerbocker, Kettle of Fish, The Duplex, Tartine, Slaughtered Lamb, White Horse Tavern, Cubbyhole, Charlie Mom, Old Homestead, Hogs and Heifers, Cozy Soup and Burger, Cornelia Street Café, and One If By Land, Two If By Sea. See WHITE HORSE TAVERN.

Gentrification

In the 1990s and 2000s rising rents forced a large proportion of the artistic and lower-income demographic out, once again heralding an age of mostly upper-middle-class residents. This gave rise to the prevalence of upscale and chain eateries and bars, the closing of many local favorites, as well as the revamping of area classics such as the Waverly Inn, Riviera Café, and Minetta Tavern. Notable establishments include Danny Meyer's Union Square Café (set to close and relocate in 2015), Babbo, Lupa, Blue Hill, Gotham Bar and Grill, Annisa, Home, Pearl Oyster Bar, Mary's Fish Camp, The Spotted Pig, Corkbuzz Wine Studio, dell'anima, 8th Street Winecellar, Striphouse, and Tertulia, among many others. See GOTHAM BAR AND GRILL and UNION SQUARE CAFE.

James Beard House

The former home on West Twelfth Street of culinary educator and chef James Beard, who died in 1985, is now a center for the James Beard Foundation for culinary excellence. His own kitchen is now used by rising and established chefs to showcase their cuisine for paying foundation members and guests seated throughout the house. See BEARD, JAMES.

Notable Closings

These venerable institutions are gone but never forgotten: Manatus, Dave's Potbelly Stove, Alfama, Lion's Head, Peculiar Pub, Café Figaro, Folk City, Florent, Chez Brigitte, Grange Hall, the Bagel Café, Jimmy Day's, Rose's Turn, the Stoned Crow, Gray's Papaya, Cedar Tavern, Bleecker Luncheonette, Village Gate, Café des Artistes, Peacock Café, Gaslight, Cucina della Fontana, Jack the Ripper, the Bottom Line, and Preacher's.

Both Chumley's bar and Don Hill's nightclub are scheduled to reopen in 2015.

See also NIGHTCLUBS.

Allison, Keith. "The Bar That Launched Pride." The Alcohol Professor (blog), June 30, 2014. http://www.alcoholprofessor.com/blog/2014/06/30/the-bar-that-launched-pride/.

"Greenwich Village." Episode of American Masters, originally aired December 29, 1999. http://www.pbs.org/wnet/americanmasters/episodes/greenwichvillage/about-greenwich-village/620/.

Greenwich Village Society for Historical Preservation. "Village History," October 13, 2006. http://www.gvshp.org/_gvshp/resources/history.htm.

James Beard Foundation website: http://www.jamesbeard.org/about.

Amanda Schuster

Grimaldi's

See PIZZA.

Grimes, William

William Grimes (b. 1950) is a *New York Times* writer and the author or editor of five books, including *Appetite City: A Culinary History of New York*. He was born in Houston, Texas; attended Indiana University; and received a PhD in comparative literature from the University of Chicago (1983). After graduation, he worked for *Esquire* magazine, where he contributed a column on cocktails and wrote articles on food history.

Grimes was hired by the *New York Times* in 1989. After working as an editor at the newspaper's Sunday magazine and as an arts reporter in the culture department, he joined the staff of the Dining section when it was launched in 1997. Two years later, upon Ruth Reichl's departure from the paper, Grimes was appointed restaurant critic. After stepping down from that position in 2004, he wrote book reviews and, from 2008 to 2012, was the newspaper's chief obituary writer. Grimes holds the distinction of having written for almost every section of the paper. He edited *Eating Your Words* (2004), a lighthearted lexicon of food language, and coauthored *The New York Times Guide to New York City Restaurants* (2004). He has written three books, *Straight Up or On the Rocks* (1993, 2002), a history of the American cocktail; *My Fine Feathered Friend* (2002), about a chicken that took up residence in the backyard of Grimes's

Queens home; and *Appetite City: A Culinary History of New York* (2009), which examines the evolution of New York City's restaurants.

In 2011, *Appetite City* was turned into a television series for the public TV channel NYC Life. Hosted by Grimes, the series delineates the history of New York City through its iconic foods, markets, and restaurants. Episodes include "Fine Dining," "Diners," "Street Food," "Green Markets," "Oysters," "Chinatown," "Delis," and "Soul Food." Grimes lives in Astoria, Queens, with his wife, Nancy Grimes, an artist.

See also NEW YORK TIMES and REICHL, RUTH.

Grimes, William. *Straight Up or on the Rocks: The Story of the American Cocktail.* New York: North Point, 2001.
Grimes, William. *Appetite City: A Culinary History of New York.* New York: North Point, 2009.

Andrew F. Smith

Gristedes

Gristedes is a chain of supermarkets in New York City. One of the oldest food retailers in New York, its shifting fortunes and ownership have reflected larger transitions in New York City's food business.

Charles and Diedrich Gristede, brothers who immigrated from Germany, opened Gristedes in 1888. Their original location was on Forty-Second Street and Second Avenue and catered to an upper-class clientele. Gristedes opened another store in Harlem in 1896 and joined the first wave of American chain grocers, including A&P, Kroger, and Grand Union. The business prospered over the next few decades, and by the time Charles Gristede died in 1948, there were more than a hundred Gristedes in Manhattan, the Bronx, Westchester, and Connecticut.

The idea of the chain grocer gained momentum in the 1920s, and the 1930s saw the advent of the nation's first supermarkets. King Kullen, founded in Queens in 1930, is credited by the Smithsonian as the first supermarket. By 1936, there were seventeen King Kullens in the city. The supermarket concept expanded even further in the postwar period so that by the 1960s and 1970s Gristedes had numerous competitors in New York City. Still, Gristedes held its own, generating $60 million in revenue in 1968. That same year, it was sold to the Southland Corporation, which also owned 7-Eleven.

Over the course of the 1970s and 1980s, Gristedes started to struggle against its competition, particularly in light of the expansion of the gourmet food market in the city. While Gristedes had long been a pioneer in varied, high-quality produce, now there were several other reliable sources around the city. Gristedes also showed its age in that many of its stores were smaller than newer supermarkets. Gristedes tried to consolidate its operations by closing most of its stores outside of Manhattan, but that left it less able to weather the increasing cost of delivery and rent as Manhattan's economy surged in the 1980s. In 1986, the company was sold to John Catsimatidis, owner of the Red Apple chain of grocery stores. He closed several stores and overhauled many of the rest in order to make them more competitive with the gourmet food markets, reflecting the trend toward markets with prepared food, hot food, and small dining areas inside the store. Catsimatidis and Red Apple continued buying other stores, including the prominent but troubled Sloan's chain. Between 1991 and 1993, Red Apple bought thirty-three Sloan's stores, continuing to rebrand and consolidate its holdings.

By 1994 Red Apple controlled a significant share of the market, with seventy-five stores and about one-third of Manhattan's customers. This led to complaints that Red Apple had become a monopoly, owning all of the grocery stores in certain neighborhoods and therefore charging high prices. The Federal Trade Commission investigated and ordered Red Apple to divest six supermarkets. By 1997, however, Catsimatidis had divested only one and instead had paid a $600,000 fine.

Gristedes's reputation has been mixed in New York City since the late 1990s. While some residents see it as a staple and a reliable source of groceries, others complain about high prices and small stores. Gristedes is a comparatively small portion of Red Apple's holdings, which also include real estate around the city and petroleum interests in upstate New York. The diverse holdings of Red Apple have insulated the company, and John Catsimatidis, from too much financial damage from Gristedes. As of 2014, Catsimatidis had a net worth of $3 billion, making him one of the wealthiest New Yorkers and putting him in the top 50 percent of the Forbes 400 for 2014. In 2013, Catsimatidis tried to parlay his business expertise into a successful run for mayor, but he was defeated. During the course of that campaign, however, Catsimatidis's detractors often linked their critiques of him with their critiques of his grocery store. A *New York Times* article written that year called Gristedes "the unloved uncle of the New York City grocery scene" and questioned "whether New Yorkers want the proprietor of a maligned grocery chain to run City Hall." Catsimatidis repeatedly distanced himself from Gristedes, explaining that it is a minute part of his business interests and that he has had little involvement with the management of the store over the past ten years.

Gristedes has continued to retool and adjust to the expansion of supermarkets in the city. The growth of supermarkets like Fairway, Trader Joe's, and Whole Foods, each of which operates several large stores with gourmet offerings, has been a blow to Gristedes's share of the market. In addition, all of these grocers now grapple with the lure of online grocery shopping offered by companies like FreshDirect. See FAIRWAY MARKET; TRADER JOE'S; WHOLE FOODS; and FRESHDIRECT.

Although it has often operated at a loss since the year 2000, Gristedes continues to stay afloat. It has begun opening new stores in parts of the city where the rents are lower and the supermarket business is less saturated, like Washington Heights and Hunts Point, in the Bronx. Some Gristedes also include cafes and prepared food sections. Gristedes has also begun offering a limited degree of online shopping.

Gristedes has been a presence in New York City for 127 years. Although the nature of the store has evolved greatly and the company has weathered periods of significant expansion and contraction, it continues to be a familiar entity in the city by reflecting the changing grocery business.

See also GROCERY STORES and SUPERMARKETS.

Grynbaum, Michael M. "A Candidate with a Store Chain around His Neck." New York Times, May 6, 2013.
Ramirez, Anthony. "Gristedes, a Familiar New York Supermarket Brand, Dwindles." New York Times, September 15, 2007.
Schmitt, Eric. "Red Apple Buying Gristedes." New York Times, February 6, 1986.
Smith, Andrew F. New York City: A Food Biography. Lanham, Md.: Rowman and Littlefield, 2013.

Katie Uva

Grocery Stores

Until the mid-nineteenth century, New Yorkers grew, raised, and prepared much of their own food on small farms and in their yards, gardens, and kitchens. What they did not produce themselves, they bought from local farmers at city markets or from street vendors. This pattern began to change during the mid-nineteenth century, when specialty stores emerged.

These stores focused on a particular product, such as imported tea. The Great Atlantic Tea Company (later the Great American Tea Company) was founded by George F. Gilman and George H. Hartford around 1860. It started as a retail tea shop in Manhattan that also sold tea by mail. With the tea trade doing well, Gilman and Hartford expanded their line to include coffee and other luxury products. By 1865 the partners had five small stores in New York City—America's first grocery chain.

The completion of the Transcontinental Railroad, in 1869, made it possible for the company to receive shipments of tea and other specialty goods sent from Asia via San Francisco and then transported east by train. To reflect this new bicoastal operation, Gilman and Hartford changed their firm's name to the Great Atlantic and Pacific Tea Company, subsequently shortened to A&P. Over the next few decades the A&P stores gradually augmented their inventories to include a full range of groceries. The early success of the A&P was condemned by independent grocers, who attacked the company for its predatory pricing and the resulting destruction of small family-owned businesses. But A&P continued to open more stores in the city.

In the late nineteenth century, German, Jewish, Italian, and Irish immigrants flooded into New York City. Many opened grocery stores to serve their fellow immigrants. A notable success among these was a business launched by Irishman James Butler, who arrived in America in 1871. After working in hotels, he and a partner started a grocery store in 1882. They painted the shopfront green and emblazoned their names on it in gold. They kept prices low, and the public thronged the place. Butler bought out his partner the following year and began to open more locations. When Butler died in 1934, there were 365 Butler Grocery Stores in New York and hundreds more outside of the city. As a result of the Depression, the chain collapsed in 1935 and went into bankruptcy; many of its stores were acquired by other chains.

The A&P operation had made it clear that grocery chains were the future of food retailing. The Jones Brothers Tea Company, founded in Scranton, Pennsylvania, expanded its chain to New York and renamed it The Grand Union Tea Company, soon shortened to "Grand Union" in 1928. In 1883 Bernard H. Kroger set up a chain-store operation in Cincinnati and later opened outlets in New York City. Two German immigrants, brothers Charles and Diedrich Gristede, opened their first food store in New York in 1891; Gristede Brothers grew into an upscale chain with locations in New York's wealthier neighborhoods and in Westchester County.

Yet another chain was launched by Michael J. Cullen, the son of Irish immigrants, in 1930. His King Kullen chain stocked more than a thousand basic food products at prices that undercut those at local markets by at least 10 to 15 percent. The Depression was taking its toll as that first store opened, and price became the number-one factor for consumers deciding where to shop. There was also free parking in lots adjacent to the store, drawing in customers in cars. Cullen quickly opened more stores, and by 1936 fifteen King Kullen stores served Queens, the Bronx, and Long Island.

Beginning in the mid-1930s, many grocery chains closed their smaller stores and opened supermarkets. Independent grocers were unable to follow suit, however, and thousands went out of business in New York City during the late 1930s and early 1940s. World War II slowed the growth of supermarkets as wartime restrictions halted the construction of stores, rationing was imposed, and both food products and packaging materials went to the war effort.

In 1945 Italian immigrant Luigi Balducci, who started out selling fruit from a pushcart in Brooklyn, opened a produce store in Greenwich Village—the first in Manhattan to offer high-quality fresh produce, meat, fish, and grocery items all in one place. In the early 1970s the store moved to a much larger space on Sixth Avenue and Ninth Street and added prepared foods, an international array of cheeses, charcuterie, and breads and desserts from top local bakeries: the neighborhood produce stand had evolved into a gathering place for gastronomes. But beginning in the 1980s, conflict within the family caused a rift that eventually led to Balducci's being sold, in 1999, to an out-of-state corporation; the flagship store in the Village closed in 2003.

Nathan Glickberg opened a small fruit and vegetable stand on West Seventy-Fourth Street in Manhattan in 1933. In 1954 he and his son Leo moved the operation around the corner to Broadway, renamed it Fairway Market, and began offering more items. Fairway became a beloved neighborhood grocery store, but in 1974, when Leo Glickberg's son Howard took over, he began transforming it according to his own vision. He eventually expanded it to several storefronts on Broadway but kept the appealing outdoor displays of fresh fruit with hand-lettered signs. Fairway became one of the city's great food-shopping destinations, offering a wide range of prepared foods, imported groceries, cheese, coffee, and olive oil, always at highly competitive prices. In 1995 Fairway opened a second, much larger location on the Harlem waterfront (soon to be developed for recreation as part of the Hudson River Park system); it now has nine stores, including one housed in an old warehouse building in the formerly industrial, newly hip neighborhood of Red Hook, Brooklyn.

One of Fairway's competitors is Citarella, which was started by Mike Citarella as a fish market in Harlem in 1912. In 1941 he moved the store to Columbus Avenue on the Upper West Side. In the 1980s, while still specializing in fresh fish (and famous for its artistic displays of seafood, on ice, in the shop windows), the company expanded its offerings to include specialty meats, prepared foods, pastry, produce, and other gourmet foods. There are now two Citarella outlets uptown, one on Broadway and Seventy-Fifth Street and another on the Upper East Side; a third Citarella's occupies the former Balducci's store in Greenwich Village. Another three branches serve the Hamptons.

Another specialty food shop was launched by Giorgio DeLuca (a former teacher) and Joel Dean (who had worked in publishing) on Prince Street in SoHo in 1977, just as the neighborhood was beginning its transformation from an industrial district to the center of New York's art scene. Nine years later Dean & DeLuca moved to a much larger space on Broadway and Prince Street. Aside from the highest grades of meat, fish, and produce, the store offered prepared foods for takeout; locally made breads, pastries, and chocolates; imported oils, vinegars, and other ingredients and condiments; and its own line of packaged spices. There is a second full-scale Dean & DeLuca store on the Upper East Side as well as three cafés in Midtown. The company has also opened stores and cafes in other American cities and in the Middle and Far East.

More modest neighborhood grocery stores also serve an important function in the city. Corner bodegas, twenty-four-hour convenience stores in Hispanic neighborhoods, sell packaged and prepared food, cold drinks, candy, and household items. Beginning in the 1970s, Korean immigrants began opening small stores that offered a good selection of fresh produce as well as some groceries; like bodegas, these are usually open day and night, 365 days a year. By 1995 there were as many as twenty-five hundred Korean delis in New York City, but by 2005 the number had dropped to about two thousand. In 2011, 70 percent of New York City's small grocery stores were still Korean-owned, but their numbers continue to decline. Rising rents and the upward mobility of the second generation of Korean Americans (their higher education paid for with deli income) are both contributing factors.

During the early 1970s, alternative food distribution systems appeared on the scene, such as food co-ops and community supported agriculture. In 1976, the first Greenmarket was established in Union Square, selling foods grown, raised, and prepared locally (defined as within two hundred miles of the city). Eventually some 120 more Greenmarkets opened around the city, and these, too, reduced sales at city grocery stores. New York–based specialty grocery chains, such as Gourmet Garage, Garden of Eden, and Union Market, have attracted a wide following in the city. National chains Whole Foods and Trader Joe's have had stores in New York City since 2005 and 2006, respectively. Some New Yorkers, though, prefer to dispense with the entire food-shopping experience. For them, since 2002, there has been FreshDirect, an online service that allows customers to place their orders for home delivery from a central warehouse.

See also A&P; CULLEN, MICHAEL J.; D'AGOSTINO; GREENMARKETS; KING KULLEN; and SUPERMARKETS.

Levinson, Marc. *The Great A&P and the Struggle for Small Business in America*. New York: Hill and Wang, 2011.

Smith, Andrew F. *New York City: A Food Biography*. Lanham, Md.: AltaMira, 2014.

Andrew F. Smith

Groggeries

In nineteenth-century New York, groggeries, or grogshops, were synonymous with corner "liquor groceries"—grocery stores in tenement districts where beer and liquor was sold by the glass. By selling food and designating themselves as groceries, these establishments circumvented blue laws, which allowed grocers, but not saloons, to operate on Sundays. In certain neighborhoods, every block had at least one liquor grocery; the notorious Five Points slum had an average of a dozen per block. See FIVE POINTS.

The groggery was a product of the early nineteenth century, a successor to the colonial grocery. During the eighteenth century, groceries sold dried and preserved foodstuffs, coffee, tea, and spices, as well as wines and liquors. The groceries served as adjuncts to the city's public markets, where the vast majority of fresh foods were sold. See PUBLIC MARKETS. But in the early nineteenth century, as the city grew larger and more diverse, some of the groceries expanded their liquor inventory, taking advantage of loopholes in the law that allowed them to essentially operate a saloon without having to adhere to saloon regulations. Meanwhile, as the temperance movement took root in the early nineteenth century, the grocer became vilified as a shady figure who plied his customers with liquor and sold inferior food products simply as a hedge so that he could serve liquor. See TEMPERANCE MOVEMENT. Some groceries, concerned about preserving their reputations, eschewed the sale of liquors and called themselves temperance groceries to distance themselves from the liquor groceries, or groggeries. Other respectable "family groceries" might sell wines and liquors but did not serve it by the glass on the premises as the groggeries did.

Groggeries stocked a motley assortment of food in varying states of freshness. Journalist George Foster catalogued the inventory of one grogshop: "a few maggoty hams and shoulders…some strings of dried onions, a barrel No. 3 mackerel, some pipes and tobacco," and, at the center of the store, large barrels of liquor: gin, whiskey, or schnapps. Often, the liquor sold in groceries was adulterated—the barrels might be filled with straight alcohol colored to look like cognac or brandy. The grocery counter extended into a bar where customers could sit and have a drink (or many). Some grogshops had a curtain separating the grocery counter from the bar, and the back was indistinguishable from a saloon, especially in the evenings. In these back rooms, plenty of drinking took place along with other commercial vices including billiards, gambling contests like cockfights and rat fights, and prostitution. Middle-class reformers and temperance advocates decried the groggeries as centers of vice, dissipation, and disease. But these establishments did serve an important function as the social center of many tenement enclaves.

In the second half of the nineteenth century, the groggeries were replaced by other commercial drinking establishments. Saloons expanded throughout the city, especially in working-class neighborhoods, and took over the drinking functions of groggeries. Illegal saloons nicknamed "blind pigs" or "blind tigers" continued to operate, mainly in the city's slums. But these bars did not purport to carry groceries as the groggeries had. See SALOONS. Meanwhile, the respectable groceries became more of a model to follow for retail food shops throughout the city. This development was linked to changes in food purveying in general in mid-nineteenth-century New York as public markets shifted toward a wholesale function and retail groceries took over retail food provisioning for most New Yorkers. See GROCERY STORES.

Anbinder, Tyler. *Five Points: The 19th-Century New York City Neighborhood that Invented Tap Dance, Stole Elections, and Became the World's Most Notorious Slum.* New York: Free Press, 2001.

Lobel, Cindy. *Urban Appetites: Food and Culture in Nineteenth-Century New York.* Chicago: University of Chicago Press, 2014.

Sante, Luc. *Low Life: Lures and Snares of Old New York.* New York: Vintage, 1992.

Cindy R. Lobel

Growler

See SALOON and SLANG.

GrowNYC

GrowNYC (www.grownyc.org) is a nonprofit organization that collaborates with city government to run farmers' markets, youth education, and community gardens. Formerly known as the Council on the Environment of New York City, GrowNYC was formed in 1970 by an executive order of Mayor John Lindsay. The early years of the decade were an exciting time for the environmental movement, and New York City did not want to be left behind. After celebrating the first Earth Day earlier that year, GrowNYC was started as a think tank for policy decisions. Lindsay hoped to reform crime-ridden, downtrodden New York City into something closer to the European cities he had seen during his travels. However, it was not until after Lindsay left office that GrowNYC became a hands-on organization.

Architect and urban activist Barry Benepe had already succeeded in closing Central Park to traffic on weekends when he heard rumors that local farms were being forced out of business in the area around New York City. See BENEPE, BARRY. Two early 1970s *New York Times* articles by John Hess contrasted the success of a farmers' market in Syracuse, New York, with the difficulties farmers were having selling their goods through the wholesale Hunts Point Market. See HUNTS POINT. Farmers' markets had made their way to the United States but had yet to enter New York City. Benepe found additional support in Bob Lewis, another city planner, and in April 1976 they signed an agreement with GrowNYC. The organization would adopt the Greenmarket program and appoint Benepe as project director. The first market was held in a 200-by-50-foot lot at the corner of Fifty-Ninth Street and Second Avenue in Manhattan. There were seven growers who trucked in their produce from Long Island, New Jersey, and upstate New York. By early afternoon, they had nearly sold out.

Today, the greenmarkets are GrowNYC's best-known project, with fifty-four locations scattered throughout the five boroughs. The success of the program is a major steppingstone for the promotion of the organization's other programs, focused on improving the environment and quality of life for New Yorkers. Though GrowNYC was developed through an executive order, it operates as a 501c(3) nonprofit that often collaborates with the New York City government.

After the Greenmarkets took off, other programs to foster the businesses of local farms as well as the health of New York City's residents emerged. No longer just a think tank, GrowNYC started working to create community and school gardens, recycling outreach, and programs to reach in-need communities.

In 1975, Liz Christy, founder of the first community garden in New York City, created GrowNYC's Open Space Greening Program. This program is responsible for many of the earliest community and school gardens in New York City as well as building rainwater-harvesting systems throughout the city. It continues to serve in-need communities and people of all ages with programs like a food box subscription, which works similarly to community supported agriculture without the season-long commitment. It also hosts three teen-run youth markets that focus on developing small business skills and growing community knowledge of healthy eating. Technical assistance programs help farmers plan for succession planning after retirement or those earlier in their careers to grow their businesses.

After a rebranding effort in 2010 that changed the name from the alienating Council on the Environment of New York City to GrowNYC, the program has grown in the consciousness of New Yorkers. Now there is a name attached to some of the oldest and most beloved food and green space programs.

See also GREENMARKETS.

Benepe, Barry. *Greenmarket: The Rebirth of Farmers Markets in New York City.* New York: Council on the Environment of New York City, 1977.
Hess, John L. "Hunts Point Market, Called 'Grocer's Dream,' Proving Nightmare to Many." *New York Times,* July 31, 1974.

Tove K. Danovich

Gulden's Mustard

Gulden's mustard's post–Civil War beginnings were on Elizabeth Street, near the South Street Seaport—in easy proximity to the requisite mustard seed and vinegar being shipped into the city. It was there, in 1867, that twenty-four-year-old Charles Gulden established the company that would become the country's oldest continuously operating mustard producer and its third largest mustard manufacturer—no mean feat for the son of German immigrants, whose first occupation was as an engraver.

Gulden's mustard began winning awards in 1869, with a "Second Medal & Diploma" from the American Institute of the City of New York for the Encouragement of Science and Invention. The judges were impressed by its fine flavor. They were especially taken with the way Gulden's used American seeds to create a product reminiscent of the flavor and manufacturing process of the Old World mustards of France and Germany. As its popularity grew, more recognition followed, with awards from the World's Columbian Exposition (Chicago, 1893) and the Exposition Universelle (Paris, 1900), among others.

Gulden's was very much a family business; Gulden's father, nephew, and he himself obtained patents for the company—his father for a unique, bulb-shaped mustard bottle and for a precursor to the easy-dispensing modern "squeeze" bottle, which his nephew later improved on, and Gulden himself for a mustard jar cap. Gulden's remained a family business until its sale to American Home Foods in 1962, when it was produced in Saddle Brook, New Jersey. Since 2006, it has been a ConAgra product, made in Milton, Pennsylvania.

The simple ingredients—mustard seed, vinegar, spices, and salt—remain virtually unchanged, although

some color-enhancing turmeric has been added. The exact recipe, however, is still a trade secret. Given New Yorkers' love of franks, corned beef, and pastrami, it is no wonder that the once-hometown and still award-winning Gulden's endures as a mustard-industry mainstay.

See also DELIS, GERMAN and HOT DOGS.

"Charles Gulden." Findagrave. http://www.findagrave.com/cgi-bin/fg.cgi?page=gr&GRid=133453057.
Grace, Roger M. "Gulden's Is Oldest Nationally Sold Prepared Mustard—Not French's." Metropolitan News-Enterprise, December 30, 2004. http:www.metnews.com/articles/2004/reminiscing123004.htm.
O'Reilly, Edward. "Cuttin' the Mustard: Gulden's and the American Institute." *New-York Historical Society Museum & Library* (blog), November 21, 2012. http://blog.nyhistory.org/cuttin-the-mustard-guldens-and-the-american-institute/.

Jane L. Smulyan

Gum

Modern commercial chewing gum got its start through the efforts of Thomas Adams Sr. (1818–1905), a New York City glass wholesaler who was also an inventor and photographer. In about 1857 Adams met the Mexican general Antonio López de Santa Anna, the exiled

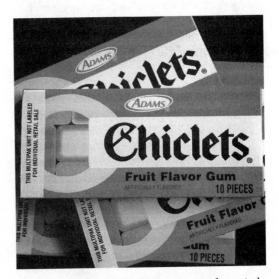

Chiclet's, named for chicle, the gummy sap of a tropical evergreen called sapodilla, were the first widely marketed chewing gum.

former president of Mexico (famous for his conquest of the Alamo), who was then living on Staten Island. Santa Anna needed money to fund his return to power in Mexico. He had become familiar with chicle, the gummy sap of a tropical evergreen called sapodilla, when he visited the Yucatán peninsula; it had been chewed by Mexicans since the ancient Mayan era, and Santa Anna believed that there should be some commercial use for it. But he was thinking of rubber tires, not sweets.

Adams rose to the challenge and imported chicle from the Yucatán. He tried to make rubber from it but found that it would not harden. But the milky-white latex was sweet, and when boiled it turned chewy; so Adams thought it might work as a confection, which he first produced in 1859. At that time Americans chewed spruce gum (made from the sweet resin collected from spruce trees) or a flavored paraffin-based gum called White Mountain.

Thomas Adams and Sons was launched in 1869. Adams patented a gum-making machine that kneaded the chicle and flattened it into long strips. Initially, they were handed out for free by shopkeepers as a means of introducing the product to children. Then the gum—still plain chicle, without added sugar or flavoring—was wrapped in tissue and sold for a penny a stick. Later, sugar was added, and flavors such as licorice (Black Jack) and fruit (Tutti-Frutti) were manufactured. By 1888 Adams was also making candy-coated gumballs, which were dispensed from coin-fed vending machines. To meet increased demand, he built a large factory in Brooklyn.

In 1899 the company formed a monopoly, called the American Chicle Company, with several other gum manufacturers around the country. In 1914, Adams introduced Chiclets, candy-coated tablets of flavored gum. The success of this new product led Adams, in 1919, to construct a five-story, 550,000-square-foot manufacturing facility in Long Island City, Queens. In 1962, the company was acquired by Warner-Lambert Pharmaceutical Company; the Long Island City factory closed in 1981.

Topps Chewing Gum got its start in Brooklyn in 1938, selling penny gum called Change Makers. Topps began marketing Bazooka Bubble Gum after World War II. The pink rectangles of gum, each wrapped in a "Bazooka Joe" comic, quickly became the best-selling gum in America. In 1950, the company introduced thin, flat slabs of bubble gum with a "Hopalong Cassidy" trading card in each package and in 1953 switched over to baseball cards. The company's production plant was moved to Pennsylvania in 1965, but its headquarters remained in New York. In 2007 the company was acquired by Michael Eisner's Tornante Company and Madison Dearborn Partners.

Hendrickson, Robert. *The Great American Chewing Gum Book*. Radnor, Pa.: Chilton, 1976.
Mathews, Jennifer P., and Gillian P. Schultz. *Chicle: The Chewing Gum of the Americas, from the Ancient Maya to William Wrigley*. Tucson: University of Arizona Press, 2009.
Redclift, Michael R. *Chewing Gum: The Fortunes of Taste*. New York: Routledge, 2004.

Andrew F. Smith

Guss' Pickles

See PICKLES.

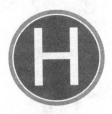

Häagen-Dazs

Häagen-Dazs was the first national brand of super-premium ice cream created in the United States. Its foreign-sounding name was invented to suggest that the product was made in Europe with Old World craftsmanship, a point that was reinforced by putting a map of Denmark on the original containers. Actually, the ice cream maker, Reuben Mattus (1912–1994), was an émigré from Belarus, not Scandinavia, and his wife, Rose, was from Poland. Originally, Häagen-Dazs ice cream was manufactured at the Senator Frozen Products Company in the Bronx.

Mattus came to New York in 1921 with his widowed mother and sister. (His father had been killed in World War I.) The family joined the mother's brother in Brooklyn, where they worked in his Italian lemon ices business. In 1929, Lea Mattus started a new business in the Bronx named Senator Frozen Products. Reuben and his mother expanded their offerings from ices to ice pops, ice cream sandwiches, and chocolate-covered ice cream bars made in their factory on Southern Boulevard. He delivered them to neighborhood stores in a horse-drawn wagon.

For over twenty years, their business was profitable until the early 1950s, when the industry changed to mass-produced ice cream and a price war developed. With his business at risk, Mattus used the problem as an opportunity to create a superior ice cream. It would cost more than other products, but he believed the high quality would justify the price, although he could never convince his mother of the merits.

Mattus developed a recipe using all natural ingredients with a taste and consistency that would distinguish it from ice cream sold in supermarkets. In 1959, he and his wife Rose formed a new company called Häagen-Dazs, reportedly in appreciation of Denmark's treatment of the Jews during World War II. The Häagen-Dazs name was first used October 24, 1960, and the trademark registered on September 4, 1962.

Häagen-Dazs introduced its product with just three flavors—vanilla, chocolate, and coffee—all made with premium ingredients including vanilla beans from Madagascar, Belgian chocolate, and Colombian coffee. Unlike other mass-produced ice creams that use artificial flavoring and nonfat dry milk, Häagen-Dazs uses only real eggs and cream and has a high butterfat content. It is one of the few manufacturers that does not use emulsifiers or stabilizers like carrageenan, xanthan gum, and guar gum. The product is very dense, with little air mixed in during its manufacture.

At first, Häagen-Dazs was sold primarily in small stores in the New York area. Marketing manager Roy Sloane targeted college students, who would then tell their parents about it. It was sold in college towns and promoted on rock stations and at concerts, and he arranged for 7-Eleven stores to carry it. Häagen-Dazs also sold franchises and single stores, with the first store at 120 Montague Street in Brooklyn Heights. A sign on the building reads "World's First Häagen-Dazs Shop Established November 15, 1976." Around that time, the brand took off nationally.

In 1983, Häagen-Dazs was acquired by The Pillsbury Company for more than $70 million. It is sold in over fifty countries.

See also BRONX; ICE CREAM SANDWICH; ICE CREAM SHOPS; and ITALIAN ICES.

Hevesi, Dennis. "Rose Mattus, Co-creator of Häagen-Dazs Ice Cream, Dies." *New York Times*, December 1, 2006.

Mao, Vincent. "Innovate: Reuben Mattus Made New Taste the Name of Häagen-Dazs' Game." *Investors Business Daily*, June 24, 2010.

Nathan, Joan. "Ice Cream's Jewish Innovators." *Tablet Magazine*, August 2, 2012.

Joanne Nicholas

Halal

See ARAB COMMUNITY.

Half Moons

See BLACK AND WHITE COOKIES.

Halva

Halva is a confection of Middle Eastern origin. Since its first recorded appearance in the seventh century, it has migrated throughout Europe and Central Asia as far as India, and in each of these places it has taken different forms and gone by a slightly different name. The most common halva in New York City consists of ground semolina or sesame paste flavored with honey and nuts. It can be found in Indian, Turkish, Middle Eastern, and Jewish food stores, with respective regional varieties. While a ground sesame paste held together with honey or fruit syrup and nuts is most common in Turkish, Jewish, and Middle Eastern varieties, halva in India takes many different forms. The sesame seed–based variety is called *sooji halvah*, while other types are made with beans or carrots. While European halva is generally served as a loaf or bar, Indian halva may take the form of a soft pudding or diamond-shaped cake. Russian-style halva is often coated in, or flavored with, chocolate. Somalian halva, or *xalwa*, served with tea, is made of cornstarch, sugar, and cardamom served in gelatinous cubes, similar to Turkish delight.

Halva is a staple in many diets, usually used as a dessert but in some cases treated as a hearty breakfast food because of its high fat and protein content. Halva is also an important food in several religious settings. In Iran, Azerbaijan, and Albania, Muslims traditionally serve halva on the seventh and fortieth days after a person's death. In the Greek Orthodox religion, halva is a popular dessert during Lent, when

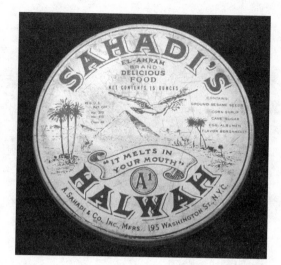

Halva (also spelled *halvah* and *halwah*) is a confection of Middle Eastern origin. The most common halva in New York City consists of ground semolina or sesame paste flavored with honey and nuts. This tin of halva is from Sahadi, a specialty food store that opened on Washington Street in 1898.

many people abstain from animal products. Halva is also a popular Jewish dessert and is considered by Sephardic, but not Ashkenazi, Jews to be kosher for Passover.

The largest American manufacturer of halva, Joyva, is based in Brooklyn. Started by Nathan Radutsky, a Russian immigrant, in 1907, Joyva's original product line consisted solely of halva, although it later expanded to include other desserts and other sesame products. The company is still based in Williamsburg and continues to make its halva by hand. Joyva-brand halva can be found in delis and shops throughout New York and is also shipped to stores around the country.

Clark, Melissa. "For Halvah, Use ½ Cup Nostalgia." *New York Times*, March 24, 2004.

Davidson, Alan, ed. *The Oxford Companion to Food*. Oxford: Oxford University Press, 2014.

Krondl, Michael. *Sweet Invention: A History of Dessert*. Chicago: Chicago Review, 2011.

Katie Uva

Hamburgers

The hamburger—a ground meat patty in a bun—is among New York City's most commonly consumed foods. Precisely when it was first served is unclear.

In the 1890s, some street vendors began selling Hamburg steak—patties of chopped beef. But without plates, knives, and forks, it was a fairly awkward street food. Then someone had the idea of putting the patty in a bun and adding condiments, and the modern burger was born. Cheap and simple, it was a new quick lunch option for working-class New Yorkers.

By the beginning of the Depression, the hamburger was the city's—and the nation's—most popular hot sandwich. It was sold by street vendors, in diners, cafes, restaurants, and drive-in chains. The first hamburger chain to establish operations in New York was White Castle, in 1930. (McDonald's, Burger King, and Wendy's followed decades later. Five Guys, based in Virginia, and the local Five Napkin Burger chain arrived in the twenty-first century.) Lunch spots such as Hamburger Heaven and Bun & Burger made hamburgers their specialty. Upscale burger restaurants, such as BLT Burger, Bareburger, and the Burger Bistro, have recently enthralled New Yorkers. In 2004 restaurant impresario Danny Meyer and his Union Square Hospitality Group opened the Shake Shack—a take on a modern "roadside" hamburger stand—in Madison Square Park. Meyer has since opened outlets in other sections of the city and in other cities around the world. See MEYER, DANNY and SHAKE SHACK.

The hamburger's identity as a cheap, quick meal changed forever when chef Anne Rosenzweig devised a new recipe for the famed 21 Club in 1987. For extra richness and flavor, the chopped meat was formed around a pat of herbed butter, and the burger was served between slices of grilled bread, rather than on a bun. Most shocking, it was priced at $21. Burger connoisseurs pronounced it "the best burger in the world," and it was no doubt also the most expensive at that time.

In 2001, chef Daniel Boulud opened DB Bistro Moderne, a more casual counterpart to his elegant Restaurant Daniel. See BOULUD, DANIEL. The menu featured the "db Hamburger," a ground sirloin patty stuffed with rich, tender, wine-braised short-rib meat as well as foie gras and truffles. At $29 (later up to $35), it quickly became one of the bistro's most popular options and was featured in the *New York Times* and culinary magazines. The gauntlet had been thrown down: who could make a more luxurious burger, and how high could the price climb?

Marc Sherry, owner of the venerable Old Homestead Steakhouse in the meatpacking district, had the answer, at least temporarily: a $41 Kobe beef burger with exotic mushrooms and microgreens on a Parmesan twist roll. Daniel Boulud upped the ante by adding more truffle shavings to his db Burger and upping the price to $50. Then came the Royale Double Truffle Burger for $99 (later $120). This culinary creation, served only during truffle season, won the *Guinness Book of Records* certificate for the most expensive commercial hamburger in the world. But it did not hold the crown for long: in 2008 the Wall Street Burger Shoppe (which closed in 2011) introduced a Kobe beef burger topped with a seared slab of foie gras, truffles, wild mushrooms, and a sprinkling of gold leaf for $175. Hamburgers—both lowdown and high-toned—remain one of the city's favorite foods.

See also FAST FOOD; HAMBURG STEAK; and "21" CLUB.

Ozersky, Josh. *Hamburgers: A Cultural History*. New Haven, Conn.: Yale University Press, 2008.

Smith, Andrew F. *Hamburger: A Global History*. London: Reaktion, 2008.

Tennyson, Jeffrey. *Hamburger Heaven: The Illustrated History of the Hamburger*. New York: Hyperion, 1993.

Andrew F. Smith

Hamburg Steak

A New York physician, James H. Salisbury, had patients with stomach problems: they were unable to digest beefsteak or other meats. He thought they might find it easier to digest beef that had been prepared by scraping it, pressing it into patties about an inch thick, and then broiling them. Condiments, including salt, pepper, butter, Worcestershire sauce, mustard, horseradish, or lemon juice, could be added, if desired. By 1889 recipes for "Salisbury steak" appeared in medical texts as well as in cookbooks. As the preparation originated with medical professionals, it was considered a health food. Salisbury steak became very popular during World War I.

A similar dish, Hamburg (or Hamburger) steak, came to America via German immigrants. The first located record of it is from an establishment owned by Auguste Ermisch, an immigrant from Mecklenburg-Schwerin. His restaurant, at Nassau and John Streets, featured among other dishes "Hamburg steak," which was described by the *New York Times* as "a beefsteak redeemed from its original toughness by being mashed into mincemeat and then formed into a conglomerated mass." Its advantage for commercial food service was that it was an inexpensive dish that could be made by grinding meat scraps that remained after butchering choicer cuts, such as porterhouse or sirloin. Hamburg steak became a nationally popular restaurant dish, especially in places catering to German immigrants, within ten years.

Hamburger and Salisbury steak still appear occasionally on restaurant and diner menus. Unlike hamburger sandwiches, they are served on a plate and eaten with a knife and fork.

See also HAMBURGER and NEW YORK STRIP STEAK.

Smith, Andrew F. *Hamburger: A Global History*. London: Reaktion, 2008.

Andrew F. Smith

Hamilton, Dorothy Cann

Dorothy Cann Hamilton was the founder and chief executive officer of the preeminent French Culinary Institute. See FRENCH CULINARY INSTITUTE. According to Hamilton, as a young girl growing up in Brooklyn she could not distinguish a slice of Brie from a scoop of Camembert. But after spending her college years at Newcastle in England, with the friendship of several French schoolmates and frequent trips to France, she learned that there was life beyond Velveeta.

After college she enlisted in the Peace Corps for three years and then, in 1974, began her career search. "I had a British University liberal arts degree and had taught English at a college in Bangkok. This exotic resume produced scant job offers in a struggling NY economy," Hamilton wrote in her 2009 book *Do What You Love*. "I finally had to resort to the one thing I really didn't want…to go to work for my father's trade school." Her father, John Cann, had started Apex Technical School in Manhattan in 1961, which taught the heavy mechanical trades.

Hamilton started as a receptionist at Apex, and though she saw this job as a last resort, generating the income necessary to pay off her student loans, she found that she enjoyed working with the students and helping to run the school. She was eventually promoted to financial aid director and found time to earn an MBA from New York University. Her interest in the field of vocational education funding led to her becoming an advisor to the U.S. Department of Education on Title IV funding. Through this experience she was elected to the board of directors of the National Association of Trade and Technical Schools.

Birth of a Cooking School

It was during that tenure, in 1980, that Hamilton (along with other educators) was invited to visit the top vocational schools in Europe including a chef training school in Paris. "I was in heaven," she remembers. "When we ate in the school restaurant I found it to be one of the best meals in my life. Why couldn't we have a school like this in the States?" When she returned home she persuaded her father, and Apex started a culinary program, which became the French Culinary Institute in 1984, located in the SoHo district of New York City.

The school was modeled after the highly respected Ferrandi culinary program in Paris, with advice and help from its director, Pierre Remande, and head chef, Pierre Roche. Hamilton encouraged the school's instructor, Antoine Schaeffers, to come to New York City as the first instructor of the French Culinary Institute. One of the first students to enroll was the now famous chef Bobby Flay. See FLAY, BOBBY.

Since its opening, the French Culinary Institute has educated more than twenty-two thousand students, many of whom have gone on to stellar careers—especially in the New York City dining scene—like Bobby Flay, David Chang, Wylie Dufresne, Dan Barber, and Christina Tosi. See CHANG, DAVID and DUFRESNE, WYLIE. Being located in the culinary capital of New York City, according to Hamilton, gives students access to hundreds of great chefs who give class demos and take on students as interns.

In 2006, the International Culinary Center was inaugurated to serve as the home for the school, with programs in Italian and Spanish cuisines as well as pastry, food business, and media. And it recently opened a school in Northern California.

Career Growth

Hamilton's distinguished career in vocational education has earned her accolades and awards from many different organizations. The International Association of Culinary Professionals gave her the Award of Excellence for Vocational Cooking School in 2006 and in 2013 named her Entrepreneur of the

Year. She received the prestigious Ordre National du Mérit from the French government, she was inducted into the Who's Who of Food and Beverage in America by the James Beard Foundation, and she received the coveted Silver Spoon Award from *Food Arts* magazine as a leader in the American restaurant industry.

Hamilton has served as director of the American Institute of Wine & Food and president of the board of trustees of the James Beard Foundation and is a board member of several trade and culinary organizations. See AMERICAN INSTITUTE OF WINE & FOOD and JAMES BEARD FOUNDATION. She conceived the idea for four textbooks for her school, each of which has received awards of recognition.

Hamilton was the creator and host of *Chef's Story*, a twenty-six-part television series of chef interviews which debuted on PBS in 2007, and the author of the companion book *Chef's Story*. She has turned the series into a radio show of the same name for Heritage Radio Network, which introduces listeners to the icons at the forefront of the American revolution of fine dining. See HERITAGE RADIO NETWORK.

In 2009, Hamilton authored a book in which she sums up her own career, titled *Do What You Love: Building a Career in the Culinary Industry*. Hamilton was appointed president of the Friends of the U.S. Pavilion, a nonprofit organization supporting the pavilion for the Milan Expo 2015 World's Fair.

See also COOKING SCHOOLS.

Chef's Story website: http://www.chefsstory.com.
"Dorothy Cann Hamilton & Margo True." *The Main Course*, episode 138. Heritage Radio Network. First aired May 6, 2012. http://hrn.herokuapp.com/episodes/2563-The-Main-Course-Episode-138-Dorothy-Cann-Hamilton-Margo-True.
Hamilton, Dorothy Cann, Lisa Cornelia, and Christopher Papagni. *Do What You Love: Building a Career in the Culinary Industry*. New York: iUniverse, 2009.

Linda Pelaccio

Hamilton, Gabrielle

Gabrielle Hamilton is an American chef and author. She was raised in New Hope, Pennsylvania, by parents who had an appreciation for food. Her father, a set designer and builder, threw lavish, themed parties for hundreds of guests, including an annual lamb roast, while her French mother instilled her love of cooking and eating well in Gabrielle at an early age.

Hamilton's first kitchen job was as a dishwasher at age twelve, but she did not return to the kitchen professionally until after college. She attended Hampshire College in Massachusetts and then moved to New York, where she started a catering business. She sold it in 1995 to escape from cooking.

In 1995, Hamilton left New York City for Ann Arbor, Michigan, to attend the University of Michigan and pursue her dream of becoming a writer, a passion that had been abandoned in favor of making a living. To help make ends meet, she picked up a part-time catering cook job. She quickly befriended the catering company owner, Misty Callies, who became her mentor. Callies showed her that cooking was not only a means to an end but could be a source of pleasure. When Callies opened her own restaurant, Zanzibar, in Ann Arbor, Hamilton joined her but still continued with her master's program. In 1997, she received her MFA in creative writing from the University of Michigan.

After graduation Hamilton returned to New York, where she pursued her dream of being a full-time writer and supported herself with the occasional line cook job. But she found that she missed the structure of a busy schedule, so she returned to cooking full-time. One fateful day she was walking down East First Street and bumped into a man who owned the building where Gabrielle had noticed an empty space. He pointed out the restaurant, which had sat decaying for two years. Though Hamilton had never entertained the thought of having her own restaurant, she found the space charming, and a vision began to take hold.

In 1999, Hamilton opened Prune, a thirty-seat East Village restaurant. She named it Prune after a childhood nickname given to her by her mother. Hamilton has won over legions of fans, cooks, and critics with her own style of rustic American cuisine with European influences. In essence, she cooks the sort of food that she grew up eating, like marrow bones, ratatouille, and liver. She has created a warm and comfortable environment, for both her diners and her staff.

Hamilton was nominated for Best Chef: New York City by the James Beard Foundation in 2009 and 2010 and won the award in 2011. Hamilton's unconventional journey to chef and restaurant owner is chronicled in her critically acclaimed memoir

Blood, Bones and Butter: The Inadvertent Education of a Reluctant Chef, for which she won the James Beard Foundation Award for Writing and Literature in 2012.

Her work has also appeared in the *New Yorker*, the *New York Times*, *GQ*, *Bon Appetit*, *Saveur*, and *Food & Wine* and has been anthologized in *Best Food Writing* every year between 2001 and 2006. She lives in New York City with her two children, Marco and Leone.

Hamilton, Gabrielle. *Blood, Bones & Butter: The Inadvertent Education of a Reluctant Chef*. New York: Random House, 2011.
"Makers Profile: Gabrielle Hamilton." Makers: The Largest Video Collection of Women's Stories. http://www.makers.com/gabrielle-hamilton.
Salkeld, Lauren. "A Q&A with Chef Gabrielle Hamilton." Epicurious. http://www.epicurious.com/articlesguides/chefsexperts/interviews/gabriellehamiltoninterview.

Layla Khoury-Hanold

Hanukah

See CHANUKAH.

Harlem

Harlem is a neighborhood in the north-central section of Manhattan from about 110th to 155th Street. The village of Harlem was established by Dutch settlers in 1658. Early settlers suffered food shortages, but over time their diet improved. Their main foods included salted fish, eels, oysters, butter, oil, vinegar, corn, wheat, and pumpkins. Because of European attitudes to fresh water, virtually everyone drank beer.

Harlem remained rural until after the Civil War, when poor Irish, German, and Jewish immigrants as well as a sizeable middle class moved into the area. In 1917, Harlem held the second largest concentration of Jews (after the Lower East Side) in the United States. Starting in the 1870s, Italian immigrants moved into East Harlem along the East River. They opened ethnic grocery stores, imported Italian ingredients, and launched restaurants. By 1930, the neighborhood was home to some eighty thousand first- and second-generation Italians. Virtually no trace of America's largest "Little Italy" remains except for Rao's Restaurant, Patsy's Pizzeria, and the annual Our Lady of Mount Carmel festival. See ITALIAN; JEWISH; and PIZZERIAS.

Beginning in 1903, the "Great Migration" brought African Americans from the southern states to settle in central Harlem. The migration reached its peak in the 1920s, when tens of thousands of African Americans moved into the area, largely replacing the Jewish population. After World War I, Harlem was a majority African American neighborhood. During the 1920s, the Harlem Renaissance of artists blossomed. See AFRICAN AMERICAN. Puerto Rican and other Hispanic peoples began moving into eastern Harlem after World War II; it was soon called Spanish Harlem.

During Prohibition (1920–1933) Harlem also became known for its culinary scene. Nightclubs such as the Cotton Club featured the greatest African American entertainers and supplied their patrons with beer and other alcoholic beverages. The Cotton Club menu included Chinese dishes, such as "Chinese soup," moo goo gai pan, and egg foo young; other items included baked oysters Cotton Club, filet mignon, broiled live lobster, steak sandwiches, crabmeat cocktails, and scrambled eggs and sausage. See COTTON CLUB.

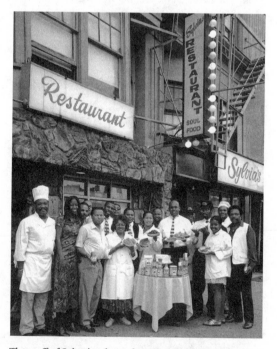

The staff of Sylvia's, a legendary soul-food restaurant in Harlem, presenting some signature dishes and an array of branded sauces and dressings. LIBRARY OF CONGRESS

The Cotton Club was segregated: entertainers were typically African American, as was the staff; but only whites were admitted as customers. Other Harlem clubs were integrated, providing an opportunity for African Americans and whites to socialize. Many African American performers sang songs about food, including the stereotypic foods of pork chops, fried chicken, and watermelon. A new culinary slang emerged in Harlem: restaurants served "yardbird" (chicken) and "strings" (spaghetti).

In the 1960s, some African American culinary traditions were popularized under the rubric of "soul food," such as smothered chicken, ribs, ham hocks, oxtails, chicken livers, hotcakes, cornbread, pigs' feet, chitterlings, collard greens, black-eyed peas, candied yams, sweet potatoes, grits, and rich desserts. The most famous Harlem soul-food restaurateur was Sylvia Woods. She migrated from South Carolina to New York in 1941. She and her husband, Herbert Woods, worked in a Harlem luncheonette consisting of a counter, stools, and a few tables. In 1962, the couple bought the luncheonette and named it "Sylvia's." They served hamburgers, French fries, baked macaroni and cheese, fried chicken, ribs, collard greens, cornbread, and sweet potatoes. Six years later they moved to a larger restaurant on 126th Street. At the time, Harlem was troubled by blight, crime, and drugs. Sylvia's survived and then thrived. It became a major tourist attraction, drawing visitors from all over the world. In the 1990s, Woods launched Sylvia Woods Enterprises, supplying canned soul food and other items to supermarkets. She published two cookbooks: *Sylvia's Soul Food: Recipes from Harlem's World Famous Restaurant* (1992) and Sylvia Woods and Melissa Clark's *Sylvia's Family Soul Food Cookbook* (1999). When she died in 2012 at the age of eighty-six, she was called the "Queen of Soul Food." See SYLVIA'S and WOODS, SYLVIA.

Puerto Rican migration to East Harlem increased during the Depression, eventually displacing the Italian Americans. The Caribbean influx turned to a flood after World War II and reached a peak in 1953 when seventy-five thousand people left Puerto Rico. The mostly rural unskilled immigrants settled predominantly in the northeastern part of Manhattan, which is known as Spanish Harlem or *El Barrio* ("the neighborhood"). Puerto Ricans organized social, cultural, and sports clubs that often sponsored public festivals. The Puerto Rican club Los Jíbaros ("the Puerto Rican peasants") organized festivals that high-lighted the preparation of Puerto Rican specialties. See PUERTO RICAN.

Restaurant fare in Spanish Harlem is diverse. La Fonda Boricua, which opened in 1996, serves "home-cooked" Puerto Rican food; others, such as Café Ollin, serve Mexican food, while still others serve Chinese takeout. In the twenty-first century, Asian and other immigrant groups have begun to move into Spanish Harlem, making it more ethnically—and culinarily—diversified. New upscale restaurants, such as La Condesa with Chilean fare, have emerged.

Despite rich restaurant traditions, grocery and other food stores have languished. In 2007 New York City's Department of Health and Mental Hygiene reported that East and Central Harlem residents had much less access to healthful food in stores than other parts of Manhattan. According to the report, Harlem food stores were half as likely to stock low-fat dairy products and seven times less likely to sell common vegetables. Costco Wholesale opened its first store in East Harlem in 2009. Walmart considered opening several smaller neighborhood food stores to sell fresh produce, but local opposition developed.

In the twenty-first century, Harlem has become more diverse—new groups have moved in, including more well-to-do residents. Gentrification began to dominate Harlem. In 2008, the *New York Times* reported that African Americans made up only 44 percent of "Greater Harlem." Also, health concerns were raised about fried foods served at many Harlem restaurants. Traditional "soul-food" restaurants, such as M&G Diner, Copeland's, Pan Pan, and Louise's Family Restaurant, closed. They were replaced by more upscale diners and restaurants, such as BLVD Bistro, Adel's, Ruth's, Margie's Red Rose Diner, A Taste of Seafood, Miss Maude's Spoonbread Too, and Londel's. Raw Soul, a raw food restaurant, opened in 2004. Two years later, Billie Black's opened—it identifies itself as a "gourmet" soul-food restaurant. The Cecil, "an Afro/Asian/American Brasserie," opened in 2013. Recently, Marcus Samuelsson, an Ethiopian-born, Swedish-raised celebrity chef and restaurateur, opened Red Rooster Harlem in 2010 and Streetbird in 2015. See SAMUELSSON, MARCUS.

Batterberry, Michael, and Ariane Batterberry. *On the Town in New York: The Landmark History of Eating and Entertainments from the American Revolution to the Food Revolution.* New York and London: Routledge, 1999.

Cinotto, Simone. *The Italian American Table: Food, Family, and Community in New York City.* Urbana: University of Illinois Press, 2013.

Gill, Jonathan. *Harlem: The Four Hundred Year History from Dutch Village to Capital of Black America.* New York: Grove, 2011.

Moskin, Julia. "Weaving the Threads of Soul Food." *New York Times,* January 14, 2015.

Andrew F. Smith

Hart-Celler Act

See JACKSON HEIGHTS and POST–WORLD WAR II.

Haute Cuisine

Haute cuisine—French for "high cooking"—refers to the elaborate and refined style of professional cookery that developed in France in the eighteenth and nineteenth centuries. It followed the traditions established by Marie-Antoine Carême (1784–1833) and modernized and codified by Auguste Escoffier (1846–1935). New York City has had two great eras of haute cuisine, when French chefs and French culinary practices dominated upscale restaurants.

The first golden age of haute cuisine began in the 1830s, when hotel restaurants, such as those at the Astor House, the Globe Hotel, the Metropolitan Hotel, and the St. Nicholas Hotel—as well as independent restaurants such as Delmonico's, and private clubs—employed French chefs to oversee their kitchens. When menus were introduced, they were printed in French. These restaurants were frequented by well-to-do New Yorkers as well as travelers and tourists, and they dominated fine dining in New York for the next ninety years. European visitors often commented that these restaurants were comparable to the finest establishments in Paris or London.

Menus at some of these restaurants reached gargantuan proportions, weighing in at a thousand items. After the Civil War, the French chefs of some of New York City's finest restaurants published their recipes in cookbooks. Felix Déliée, who cooked at the New York Club and the Union and Manhattan Club, published *The Franco-American Cookery Book* in 1884. Charles Ranhofer, the chef at Delmonico's, wrote a weighty and comprehensive tome titled *The Epicurean* (1896). Oscar Tschirky, maître d'hôtel at the Waldorf, published *The Cook Book, by "Oscar" of the Waldorf* (1896).

In America French cookery of this kind reached a peak at the beginning of the twentieth century, when fine hotel restaurants run by French or French-trained chefs—at the Waldorf Astoria, the Essex House, and the Ritz-Carlton, among others—were among the nation's premier eating establishments. The lobster palaces of the early twentieth century also featured haute French cuisine.

In New York City, the halcyon days of haute cuisine came to an abrupt end when Prohibition began in January 1920. Expensive French restaurants made much of their profit from the sale of wines, spirits, and liqueurs that preceded, accompanied, and followed the meal. Most featured expensive imported wines as part of the dining experience. Prohibition abruptly made it illegal to serve alcohol, leaving a big hole in restaurant profits, and many, such as the iconic Delmonico's, closed.

While a few hotels, such as the Waldorf Astoria, Hotel Pierre, and the Ritz-Carlton, kept haute cuisine alive in the hands of celebrated chefs such as Louis De Gouy and Louis Diat, their bottom line was badly damaged by the Depression, which began in 1929.

Another exception was The Colony, which survived both Prohibition and the Depression, as well as World War II. Before World War I, The Colony was a somewhat shady bistro with a gambling den upstairs. Gene Cavallero became head waiter in December 1919, and in 1921 he partnered with two other waiters to buy the restaurant. They remodeled the premises in ten days and reopened with a menu of fine French cuisine. The Colony was almost immediately discovered by society matron Anne Vanderbilt (Mrs. W. K. Vanderbilt Jr.), who was followed by other members of New York's fashionable set. By the late 1920s The Colony was so clearly the preferred destination of New York's wealthy that the restaurant closed during the summer months, when well-to-do New Yorkers sailed to France.

Another haute cuisine restaurant, Le Pavillon, was launched in October 1941 by Henri Soulé, who had come to the United States in 1939 to serve as general manager for "Le Restaurant du Pavillon de France" at New York's World Fair, which began in 1939. When the Fair ended in 1940, World War II had begun and France had fallen to the German army. Soulé and members of his staff who remained in New York opened Le Pavillon at Fifth Avenue and Fifty-Fifth Street in October 1941, and it thrived until 1966. In 1958 Soulé opened La Côte Basque, which survived until 2004.

The Colony and Le Pavillon survived the restrictions of World War II–era food rationing and went on to thrive after the war. Their success inspired a host of other restaurants serving a variety of regional French cuisines as well as Escoffier's classics. Pierre Belin and Paul Arepejou, of Le Pavillon's original staff, opened La Poinière in 1954. In 1960 chef Roger Fessaguet left Le Pavillon to become executive chef at La Caravelle, owned by Fred Decré and Robert Meyzen. La Caravelle became the incubator for many of New York's top chefs: Michael Romano worked with Fessaguet until Danny Meyer tapped him to become the chef at Union Square Café; David Ruggerio went on to Le Chantilly, and Cyril Renaud became the chef and owner of Fleur de Sel. Another former Le Pavillon employee, Charles Masson Sr., opened La Grenouille in 1962.

One of New York City's most renowned French restaurants, Lutèce, opened in 1961 with chef (and later owner) André Soltner at the helm. For more than three decades, Lutèce was considered one of the nation's finest restaurants. Le Périgord was opened by Georges Briguet in 1964. Sirio Maccioni, who had come to work at The Colony in 1956, opened the acclaimed Le Cirque with Jean Vergnes in 1974.

Some of the city's most respected French chefs, including André Soltner, Jacques Pépin, Alain Sailhac, and Jacques Torres, facilitated the continuation of French haute cuisine through their mentoring and teaching at the French Culinary Institute (now the International Culinary Center) in New York.

The emphasis on French haute cuisine in New York's fine-dining scene began to fade in 1959, when James Beard was hired to develop seasonal American menus for The Four Seasons, an elegant modern restaurant in the new Seagram Building. Classic French influences receded further in the 1970s, when the lighter, fresher *nouvelle cuisine* emerged in France, and its counterpart, "California cuisine" or "American cuisine," first appeared in the United States. Despite daring forays into exotic cuisines and experiments with molecular gastronomy, many New York chefs and restaurateurs would still credit *la haute cuisine française* as the basis of their contemporary cooking.

See also ASTOR HOUSE; DELMONICO'S; FRENCH; FRENCH CULINARY INSTITUTE; HOTEL RESTAU- RANTS; LA PAVILLON; LOBSTER PALACES; RESTAURANTS; RANHOFER, CHARLES; SOULÉ, HENRI; and TSCHIRKY, OSCAR.

Batterberry, Michael, and Ariane Batterberry. *On the Town in New York: The Landmark History of Eating and Entertainments from the American Revolution to the Food Revolution.* 25th anniv. ed. New York and London: Routledge, 1999.

Grimes, William. *Appetite City: A Culinary History of New York.* New York: North Point, 2009.

Kuh, Patric. *The Last Days of Haute Cuisine: America's Culinary Revolution.* New York: Viking, 2001.

Trubek, Amy B. *Haute Cuisine: How the French Invented the Culinary Profession.* Philadelphia: University of Pennsylvania Press, 2000.

Andrew F. Smith

Havemeyer Family

The Havemeyers were a prominent New York family that made its fortune in sugar refining. Its members were in the sugar business at least since William Havemeyer (ca. 1770–1851) emigrated from Germany in 1799 (by way of an apprenticeship in a London sugar house) and got a job as foreman in the Seaman sugar refinery in Lower Manhattan. When his contract expired in 1807 he set up his own plant along with his younger brother Frederick on Vandam Street in what was then a bustling neighborhood of docks and warehouses on the edge of New York City. At first, the operation consisted of one big room where they did the boiling and refining, but by 1816 the company had expanded operations sufficiently to produce nearly 9 million pounds of sugar annually.

As of 1828, the two brothers' sons, William Frederick (1804–1874) and Frederick Christian (1807–1891), continued in the family trade. In 1842, William F., the senior partner, retired from the business and entered politics. He served three separate one-year terms as mayor in 1845, 1848, and 1873.

In 1856, Frederick Christian's sons Theodore (1839–1897) and Henry Osborne (1847–1907) relocated their operations across the East River to Williamsburg, Brooklyn, where they built a seven-story state-of-the-art factory, the first to be located right on the waterfront. See WILLIAMSBURG. Theodore is better known as one of the founders of the U.S. Open golf tournament than as a sugar baron. It was Henry O. Havemeyer whom the press would crown the "Sugar King." In 1883, Henry bribed and cajoled most of the other sugar refiners in the country to join his American Sugar Refining Company. The trust (reorganized as a corporation in 1891) now controlled 84 percent of the refined sugar market east of the Rocky Mountains. The trust's tentacles reached not only sugar refiners and producers but also coal mines and railroads (sugar mills consumed coal like candy). Even Washington was not immune from the trust's influence. In 1892, it was alleged that the trust had paid off the Treasury secretary and swayed the Senate to pass a tariff favorable to their interests. The trust came under increasing government scrutiny following 1906, though it retained its dominant position well into the twentieth century.

When Henry Havemeyer died in 1907 (of acute indigestion following Thanksgiving dinner, according to the New York Times), his company was still thoroughly intact. His fortune enabled the sugar mogul to acquire a remarkable art collection; following 1929, the family eventually bequeathed almost two thousand works to the Metropolitan Museum.

See also SUGAR REFINING.

Eichner, Alfred S. The Emergence of Oligopoly. Baltimore: Johns Hopkins University Press, 1969.

Frelinghuysen, Alice Cooney. Splendid Legacy: The Havemeyer Collection. New York: Metropolitan Museum of Art, 1993.

"H. O. Havemeyer Dies at L. I. Home." New York Times, December 5, 1907.

Michael Krondl

Hazan, Marcella

Marcella (Polini) Hazan (1924–2013) was born in Cesenatico, Italy, on the Adriatic coast. She grew up in Egypt and moved around northern Italy during the first decades of her life. However, Hazan made her mark as the American "godmother of Italian cooking" while working from her apartment in New York City, where she lived for over thirty-five years.

Marcella and her husband, Victor, also a successful writer, had early ties to New York City. Marcella's father, Giuseppe Polini, worked in New York for five years as head of the men's custom tailor department at B. Altman and Company, whose landmark store was located at the corner of Fifth Avenue and Thirty-Fourth Street. Victor's Jewish parents fled Italy in 1939, settling in New York before returning home fourteen years later.

Marcella and Victor moved to New York in 1955. Victor arrived first, working at David's Fifty-Seventh Street, his father's fur shop. After Marcella arrived in September aboard the S.S. Christofo Colombo, the couple lived in Forest Hills, Queens. Marcella knew nothing about cooking, but, armed with Ada Boni's classic Italian cookbook Il Talismano della Felicita (The Talisman [or Key] to Happiness), she set to learning how to put food on the table. This was more of a challenge than expected because of her lack of English language skills and her shock upon entering the local Grand Union supermarket where she barely recognized the offerings as food (famously labeling the store's freezers as "cemeteries of food"). Marcella tackled the English problem in part by learning baseball terms as she fortuitously became a Brooklyn Dodgers fan during the single season they beat the New York Yankees in the World Series. Her food issues were alleviated when the couple moved to central Manhattan near Victor's work; with access to fresh ingredients she taught herself how to cook while preparing and delivering a full meal for his lunch every day.

Marcella took a job as a biochemist at the Guggenheim Institute for Dental Research at Bellevue Hospital, which she kept until she became pregnant with the couple's only son, Giuliano, now also a cookbook author and chef. In 1962 the couple returned to Italy.

Returning to New York in 1967, Hazan became enamored of Chinese food and enrolled in a cooking class with Grace Zia "Madame" Chu, author of The Pleasures of Chinese Cooking (1962). These classes inspired her, and in 1969 she began offering classes in her apartment at 77 West Fifty-Fifth Street. These classes focused on regional differences in Italian cuisine, rhythms of the Italian meal, and the preparation of unusual ingredients beyond American beef and pork.

An October 1970 Craig Claiborne New York Times article raved about Hazan's food and changed her life. The School of Classic Italian Cooking took off after this publicity. Soon she began contributing to the New York Times, offering classes at a different location (155 East Seventy-Sixth Street) and outside her home (The Forum at Rockefeller Center) and, in 1973, publishing her first book, The Classic Italian Cookbook. Although she expanded her school to Italy, she maintained a New York location until she retired to Longboat Key, Florida, in 1998. Her inability to locate key Italian ingredients in Florida as she had in New York led her to write Marcella Says

(2004). In 2000 she returned to New York for two months each year to teach classes at the French Culinary Institute.

Hazan died on September 29, 2013, but her legacy lives on in New York City. Her life was celebrated in a much circulated *New York Times* tribute by Mark Bittman, the New York location of the International Culinary Center offers a large scholarship in her name in the Italian Culinary Experience program, and New York food importer Gustiamo offers a $250 "Marcella's Favorites Basket" featuring Hazan's staple food products.

See also ITALIAN.

Hazan, Marcella. *The Classic Italian Cook Book.* New York: Harper & Row, 1973.
Hazan, Marcella. *Marcella Says…: Italian Cooking Wisdom from the Legendary Teacher's Master Classes, With 120 of Her Irresistible New Recipes.* New York: HarperCollins, 2004.
Hazan, Marcella. *Amarcord—Marcella Remembers: The Remarkable Life Story of the Woman Who Started Out Teaching Science in a Small Town in Italy, but Ended Up Teaching America How to Cook Italian.* New York: Penguin, 2008.

Arthur Lizie

Hellmann's Mayonnaise

Mayonnaise entered the culinary world during the nineteenth century, but it was difficult to make and spoiled quickly. A self-stable mayonnaise that could be sold in grocery stores was a revolutionary concept. Its invention is credited to German-born Richard Hellmann (1876–1971), who arrived in New York in the autumn of 1903. His first job was with the Francis H. Leggett Co., a wholesale grocer. In 1905 Hellmann and his wife opened Hellmann's Delicatessen at 490 Columbus Avenue, between Eighty-Third and Eighty-Fourth Streets in Manhattan. The couple worked long hours to make the business a success, but with overwork came health problems; in 1911 the Hellmanns sold the delicatessen to Charles Eberhardt and traveled to Europe. While in Paris, Richard Hellmann met a former colleague who managed a wholesale operation that delivered directly to its customers. This was quite unusual. Hellmann took a particular interest in the mayonnaise that was made daily and delivered by hand, the same day, to grocery stores and restaurants.

While in Europe, Richard Hellmann learned via cable that Charles Eberhardt had died, and the Hellmanns returned to New York and resumed running their delicatessen. Inspired by the food distribution system he had observed in Paris, Hellmann decided to wholesale mayonnaise, which had long been a mainstay of his delicatessen. On September 1, 1912, he began selling bottled mayonnaise; on the label were three blue ribbons, indicating "first prize" quality. The glass screwtop bottles could be reused when empty by placing a new rubber gasket under the metal lid. In a brilliant promotional move, Hellmann sold the gaskets for a penny apiece: customers were pleased with the reusable jars, and the trademark on the metal lid was a constant reminder to buy Hellmann's mayonnaise.

Sales soon outstripped Richard Hellmann's ability to whip up mayonnaise in the back of the store. He sold the delicatessen in 1914 and the following year opened a factory at 495/497 Steinway Street in Long Island City. In February 1916, the company was incorporated in New York as Richard Hellmann, Inc. Hellmann then expanded his market beyond New York, opening facilities in other cities, including Chicago and San Francisco. As sales of Hellmann's Blue Ribbon Mayonnaise soared, in 1922 Hellmann began construction on a five-story factory at 34-08 Northern Boulevard Long Island City. When completed, it was "the largest mayonnaise factory in the world." Hellmann's Blue Ribbon Mayonnaise dominated the market in part because of the company's superior advertising. Throughout the early years, Hellmann continued to improve the product, acquire new machinery, and streamline his manufacturing and distribution operations. By 1927 the company owned six hundred trucks that transported cases of mayonnaise from distribution centers to retailers daily. Plants were eventually established in Atlanta and in Tampa Bay, and distribution centers were opened in Dallas and Toronto.

In the mid-1920s the Postum Cereal Company (later to become General Foods) bought up many smaller food companies, including Richard Hellmann, Inc. In January 1932, General Foods folded the Hellmann brand into Best Foods, Inc. On the West Coast, Hellmann's mayonnaise was sold under the "Best Foods" label, while in the East Hellmann's replaced Gold Medal Mayonnaise, another Best Foods brand. The product is the same nationwide and in Canada, where Hellmann's had been sold since the 1920s. In the early 1960s, Best Foods (now CPC International) began to advertise Hellmann's mayonnaise in Europe, and the product was introduced in

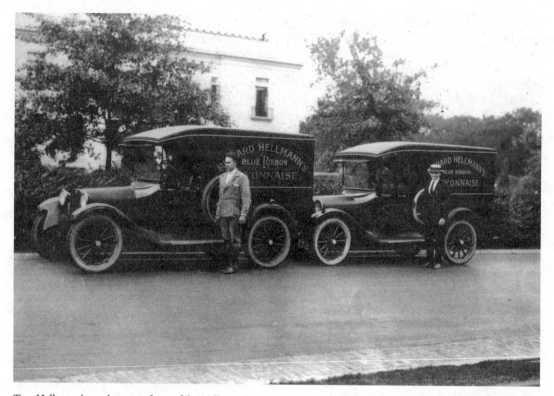

Two Hellmann's employees in front of the Hellmann's mansion, with vehicles advertising Richard Hellmann's Blue Ribbon Mayonnaise. Before selling bottled mayonnaise, German-born Richard Hellman and his wife opened Hellman's Delicatessen at 490 Columbus Avenue, between Eighty-Third and Eighty-Fourth Streets in Manhattan. QUEENS HISTORICAL SOCIETY

Portugal and Spain, as well as in Brazil, Argentina, and Colombia, in the 1970s.

Best Foods was acquired by Unilever Global in 2000. In 2008 Unilever partnered with New York–based celebrity chef Bobby Flay in a promotion called "Build the Perfect Sandwich" and an online show, *Real Food Summer School*, which were designed to clue in consumers to new uses for mayonnaise in sandwiches. Hellmann's-Best Foods dominates the U.S. mayonnaise market, with sales of more than $880 million in 2013.

See also GULDEN'S MUSTARD.

Allen, Gary J., ed. *The Business of Food: Encyclopedia of the Food and Drink Industries.* Westport, Conn.: Greenwood, 2007.
Association for Dressings & Sauces website: http://www.dressings-sauces.org.
Euromonitor. *Sauces, Dressings and Condiments in the US.* London: Euromonitor International, 2013.

Andrew F. Smith

Hell's Kitchen

Hell's Kitchen is a thriving and constantly changing neighborhood on New York City's west side, bordered to the west by the Hudson River, to the east by Eighth Avenue, to the north by Fifty-Ninth Street, and to the south by Thirty-Fourth Street. It is also sometimes referred to as "Clinton," named for former Governor Dewitt Clinton, or simply "Midtown West." Although there are other theories as to how the neighborhood got its name, the *New York Times* is widely credited as describing a notoriously crime-ridden building as "Hell's Kitchen." Other historians cite an unusually high number of customers with food poisoning originating from a neighborhood restaurant. According to this camp, the restaurant and subsequently the neighborhood was nicknamed "Hell's Kitchen." The name has seen an increase in usage in the last few years, and many residents eschew the other two monikers as elitist. Regardless of whether the area is referred to as down-and-dirty

Hell's Kitchen or upscale Clinton, in 2014 costs of apartment rentals rose above the average price of apartments elsewhere in Manhattan.

During the 1600s and 1700s, the early Dutch and English settlers referred to the area as "Bloomingdale," presumably because of the wild flowers that grew in the neighborhood's wide-open green spaces. Later residents included African American laborers who worked on the Croton Aqueduct to bring water from upstate New York to city dwellers. In the 1850s German and Irish immigrants populated the neighborhood, working in the area's slaughterhouses, lumberyards, and rail yards. Many men worked at the Hudson River docks and for the New York Central Railroad, while area women worked as domestic servants for the city's upper class. Quickly constructed tenements emerged to house the never-ending influx of immigrants. As the neighborhood became more crowded, crime became more violent. Street gangs were prevalent, and one particular block became known as "Battle Row."

Hell's Kitchen saw its share of speakeasies and crime during the Prohibition years, and revelers could always find a nightly party and a nightly brawl. After World War II, the neighborhood became even more crowded with returning veterans, and animosity grew between the long-standing Irish residents and the more recently arrived Puerto Rican immigrants. Many theater historians reference this tension as the basis for Leonard Bernstein's and Stephen Sondheim's *West Side Story*.

Today, Hell's Kitchen continues to improve dramatically. Many locals credit the very active and visible gay community for the neighborhood's gentrification as well as the influx of actors, singers, and dancers from the nearby Broadway theater community. Young families who might have moved out to the suburbs to raise their children are staying and making Hell's Kitchen their home. Many local businesses are second and third generation, and a walk up and down Ninth Avenue is like a walk back in time. Esposito's Pork Store has been in business since 1932; International Grocery has been selling spices, rice, grains, beans, and dried pasta for decades; and Poseidon Greek Bakery has been run by the same family for years. Amid the old, new restaurants and sidewalk cafes are opening every day. In addition, trendy coffee shops; clothing stores; wine bars, medical, dental, chiropractic, and plastic surgery offices; and upscale bars; as well as pastry shops, bakeries, ice creameries, cheese shops, and other venues make Hell's Kitchen a welcoming neighborhood.

See also HARLEM; HIGH LINE; LOWER EAST SIDE; and MANHATTAN.

Batterberry, Michael, and Ariane Batterberry. *On the Town in New York: The Landmark History of Eating, Drinking, and Entertainments from the American Revolution to the Food Revolution.* New York and London: Routledge, 1999.

Mike DeSimone and Jeff Jenssen

Heritage Radio Network

Take two shipping containers, a couple of young New York University music techies, and a New York rainmaker who introduced Slow Food to the United States, and what do you have? A radio station that offers cutting-edge programming on food news, farming issues, restaurants, chefs, food producers, policies, history, and just about anything related to food. Located in the back of Roberta's Restaurant in Bushwick, Brooklyn, HeritageRadioNetwork.org, a not-for-profit 501(c)3, is the brainchild of Patrick Martins, an entrepreneur who took his cues from Carlo Petrini, the Italian food activist and founder of the slow food movement.

Martins, a native New Yorker, worked for seven years with slow food, first in Bra, Italy, and then moving back to New York City, where he introduced the movement to New Yorkers. In a phone interview with the author Martins explained his passion for the movement: "The global food chain was broken," echoing Petrini's call, "and it's been a constant struggle to get the world to acknowledge the abuses in agricultural production, policies, sustainability, and to reawaken consumers to both the source of their food and to food's gastronomic value." Petrini was trying to draw attention to the issues with radio programming in Italy, so Martins decided to try it in New York. Up until then, he said, "food media—magazines, TV, radio—was failing to get the word out about the important issues."

He had already formed a mail-order company called Heritage Foods USA, connecting consumers to small farmers of rare and heritage breeds of humanely raised meat, hence the name "Heritage" for the radio project. To get started he enlisted the support of his customers Steve Hearst and Brian Kenny, of Hearst

Ranch, who gave him $5,000 for the shipping containers and believed in what Martins was doing. Hearst continues to be one of the main sponsors of Heritage Radio Network.

Launched in 2009, the station started as something of "a clubhouse for subversive foodies," according to Martins, and has grown into a legitimate media outlet that is a source for both hard news and opinion, particularly appealing to progressives. Heritage Radio Network is an Internet-based radio network active twenty-four hours a day. All programs are archived as podcasts, accessible anytime through its website or other listening sources such as Stitcher and iTunes.

Like National Public Radio, Heritage Radio Network is member-supported and now reaches in excess of 1 million listeners each month in over two hundred countries. At the core are more than thirty weekly shows of original content hosted by a diverse group of food professionals, authors, journalists, historians, and visionaries. Regular programming includes shows such as *Cooking Issues*, *The Main Course*, *A Taste of the Past*, *The Farm Report*, and *Let's Get Real*. The topics are widely varied: food technology, beer, cheese, food history, politics, and cocktails, to name just a few. Shorter, breaking news bites are posted throughout the day to keep listeners current with happenings in the food world.

When asked why an Internet radio network with programming that talks a lot about farming and food supply is based at the back of a pizza restaurant in a formerly working-class neighborhood in Brooklyn, Martins maintains that a New York location allows the station to attract a broad array of pivotal figures in the American food revolution, from Alice Waters to Michael Pollan. Perhaps the location can also be chalked up to the charm of the premises. The rustic studio inside the shipping containers, replete with a wild boar's head mounted on unfinished wood-slat walls, demonstrates the do-it-yourself philosophy of Heritage Radio Network.

See also FOOD NETWORK and RADIO.

"Heritage Radio Network." *Huffington Post* (RSS feed). http://www.huffingtonpost.com/heritage-radio-network.

Heritage Radio Network website: http://www.heritageradionetwork.org.

Linda Pelaccio

Hess, Karen and John L.

New York–born John L. Hess (1917–2005) began working as an editor and reporter at the *New York Times* in 1954. His wife, Nebraska-born Karen Hess (1918–2007), was an excellent cook and a culinary historian.

In 1964 the Hesses moved to Paris, where he wrote and edited copy for a new Paris edition of the *Times*. The Hesses became enthralled with French food and wine, which John Hess wrote about for the newspaper. The couple fell in love with the city's markets, restaurants (witnessing the birth of nouvelle cuisine), and home cooking. Karen Hess spent hours in French kitchens and collected French cookbooks. *Newsweek* referred to Karen as the finest American cook in Paris. When the Hesses returned to New York in 1972, they were horrified at the decline in American food. They began collecting material about American food for what would become *The Taste of America*. Years before others began preaching for local food, the Hesses argued for Americans to revive traditional cooking and seek out farmers and bakers who still produced it.

In a *Times* piece in 1973, John Hess commended the city of Syracuse for permitting farmers to sell their goods on one of the city's streets every Tuesday: "Food lovers should raise a fork today in salute to the Greater Syracuse Chamber of Commerce. Last spring, it got the city to turn a street over to farmers every Tuesday and presto! the village fair was resurrected."

Hess's article was read by New Yorker Barry Benepe, a forty-eight-year-old urban planner, who convinced one of his colleagues, Bob Lewis, that New York City should have a farmers' market as well. With support from the Council on the Environment of New York City, they worked for three years acquiring the necessary permits, locating a site, and convincing farmers to give the new market a try. In July 1976, their efforts bore fruit when the first Greenmarket opened in a vacant lot on Second Avenue and Fifty-Ninth Street. Today, there are fifty-four farmers' markets serving all five boroughs. Benepe and Lewis credited Hess as "the godfather of our inspiration." See BENEPE, BARRY and GREENMARKETS.

John Hess served as the food editor of the *New York Times* for a year and as its restaurant reviewer for nine months in 1974. He despised pretension and loathed the term "gourmet." He believed that Americans would never eat well until they regarded "gourmet" as a dirty word. He was highly critical of most restaurants that he visited; however, he awarded all of Chinatown four stars, proclaiming that the best American food was Chinese food. He attended a home economist's meeting and reported in his column that what was missing was "the taste, the sensuality of good food."

The Hesses were convinced that American food was headed in the wrong direction, and their book *The Taste of America* (1977) was highly critical of contemporary American food culture. The first chapter begins with the question "How shall we tell our fellow Americans that our palates have been ravaged, that our food is awful, and that our most respected authorities on cookery are poseurs?" They took commercial food producers to task and excoriated culinary icons, including Julia Child, James Beard, and Craig Claiborne. When he had an opportunity, Craig Claiborne retaliated: in a review of the American edition of Elizabeth David's *English Bread and Yeast Cookery* (1982), for which Karen Hess had annotated the recipes and written the preface, he savaged the entire production.

Karen Hess went on to publish transcripts and facsimiles of historical American culinary works, accompanied by copious scholarly annotations: Martha Washington's own manuscript cookbook, *Martha Washington's Booke of Cookery and Booke of Sweetmeats* (1981); Mary Randolph's *The Virginia House-Wife* (1984); and *The Carolina Rice Kitchen: The African Connection* (1992). Karen Hess was the first recipient, in 2004, of the Culinary Historians of New York's Amelia Award, honoring lifetime achievement in culinary history, and was a frequent speaker at food history conferences.

John Hess retired from the *New York Times* in 1978 and worked as a freelance writer. In 2003 he published the autobiographical *My Times: A Memoir of Dissent*, in which he again lashed out at Craig Claiborne. Hess started a blog in June 2004 and in one of his last essays criticized Frank Bruni, then the *New York Times* restaurant critic, for giving four stars to an upscale sushi restaurant where dinner could easily cost $500 (excluding drinks, tax, and tip).

See also CULINARY HISTORIANS OF NEW YORK and NEW YORK TIMES.

Asimov, Eric. "Karen Hess, 88, Dies; Culinary Historian Who Challenged Standards." *New York Times*, May 19, 2007.

Daley, Bill. "Karen Hess: Food Historian, Caustic Critic of American Food." *Chicago Tribune*, December 8, 2014.

Hess, John. "A Street for Farmers Benefits a City." *New York Times*, October 15, 1973, p. 58.

Hess, John L. *My Times: A Memoir of Dissent*. New York: Seven Stories, 2003.

Hess, John L., and Karen Hess. *The Taste of America*. New York: Grossman, 1977.

Hess, Karen, ed. *Martha Washington's Booke of Cookery and Booke of Sweetmeats*. New York: Columbia University Press, 1981.

Hess, Karen. *The Carolina Rice Kitchen: The African Connection*. Columbia: University of South Carolina Press, 1992.

Randolph, Mary. *The Virginia House-Wife*. Fasc. ed. Edited by Karen Hess. Columbia: University of South Carolina Press, 1984. First published 1824.

Andrew F. Smith

Hesser, Amanda

Amanda Hesser, a seasoned cookbook writer, former *New York Times* writer and editor, and cofounder of the popular website Food52, is an influential voice in shaping culinary culture in the early twenty-first century. Hesser was born in 1971 in Doylestown, Pennsylvania. She studied economics at Bentley University, a school specializing in business. While enrolled there, Hesser traveled to Europe and discovered a passion for food and culture. After receiving her degree, Hesser decided to study cooking in Europe. Unable to find a traditional culinary program that suited her interests, she arranged a series of apprenticeships with bakers, chefs, and food entrepreneurs and successfully applied for a scholarship from Les Dames d'Escoffier, the philanthropic society of professional women in the gastronomic arts. With financial backing from Les Dames, she set off for Europe.

After several three-month-long baking apprenticeships, Hesser applied to work for Anne Willan at her École de Cuisine La Varenne, at the Chateau du Fey in Villecien, France. The education took two forms: helping to edit Willan's cookbooks while acting as the private cook to Willan's family. Cooking daily with produce grown on the chateau's grounds and talking with M. Milbert, the Old World "peasant gardener," she used her experiences at La Varenne as the basis of her first book: *The Cook and the Gardener:*

A Year of Recipes and Notes from the French Country-side (1999). The book was well received, earning awards for the "Best Book on France by a Non-French Writer" at the Versailles Cookbook Fair and the International Association of Culinary Professionals Literary Food Writing Award.

Following the success of *The Cook and the Gardener*, Hesser was contacted by the *New York Times*: after three rounds of interviews, she was hired as a reporter for the Dining In/Dining Out Wednesday section. She stayed at the *Times* for eleven years, first as a reporter and occasional restaurant reviewer for the daily paper and then as the food editor of the paper's Sunday magazine and its quarterly *T Living*. While at the *Times*, Hesser wrote a series of highly personal articles about her courtship with her husband, Tad Friend, written for the Food Diary feature. Her editor hated it, but Hesser persevered. That kind of intimate "lifestyle" writing would become a staple of contemporary gastronomic essays, especially in the emerging blog medium. As editor of the magazine, she created the Recipe Redux column, which focused on previously published *Times* recipes that had fallen from favor or used little-known techniques that were then tweaked into updated form by professional chefs.

Nonetheless, Hesser's tenure at the *Times* was tainted by minor scandal when she twice ran afoul of the *Times*'s conflict of interest policies. The first involved a favorable review in 2004 of the restaurant Spice Market. Most of the reviews had been disappointing, but Hesser awarded it a staggering, exceptional three stars; the conflict of interest arose (creating embarrassment for the *Times* over the appearance of bias) because its owner, Jean-Georges Vongerichten, had recently written a complimentary blurb for the dust jacket of Hesser's latest book, *Cooking for Mr. Latte*. (The book would win the International Association of Culinary Professionals award for Best Literary Writing that year and Spice Market would continue as a popular, if not critical, success.) Similarly, in 2007, Hesser lauded the latest cookbook by Patricia Wells without disclosing that Wells had previously provided a positive dust jacket blurb for *The Cook and the Gardener*. Hesser left the *Times* in 2008, accepting a buyout that was then being offered to many *Times* employees. While the food world buzzed with rumors that Hesser had been fired, Hesser responded that she was ready for a change. She continued a professional relationship with the *Times*, writing the Recipe Redux column until 2011 and authoring the reinvented *The Essential New York Times Cookbook: Classic Recipes for a New Century* (2010).

The Essential New York Times Cookbook was a monumental undertaking, collecting selected recipes that had been published in the *Times* since the 1850s. Hesser's original idea was to create a culinary history of American cooking as seen through the pages of the *Times*. She soon realized the daunting task she had set for herself and invited *Times* readers to suggest what recipes they thought should be included in the volume. Working with Merrill Stubbs, Hesser sifted through more than six thousand suggestions. Hesser and Stubbs delved into the *Times* archives and tested and selected more than fourteen hundred recipes, yielding an encyclopedic recipe collection of more than 150 years of American food and drink, designed to work in modern kitchens.

Prompted by the enthusiastic responses to her query to the *Times* readership for help in determining content for *The Essential New York Times Cookbook*, Hesser and Stubbs embarked on a new project, Food52, a website that provided a portal for creating a crowd-sourced cookbook in fifty-two weeks, which was published in 2010. Food52 has turned into a thriving online business. Hesser was named one of the fifty most influential women in food by *Gourmet* magazine; she also had a cameo role playing herself in the 2009 film *Julie and Julia*. In 2011, she was identified in *Food and Wine*'s "40 Big Food Thinkers 40 and Under." She lives in Brooklyn Heights with her husband and their twin son and daughter.

See also FOOD52 and NEW YORK TIMES.

"Amanda Hesser." Compass Talent. http://www.compasstalent.com/amanda-hesser.

Hesser, Amanda. "Recipe Redux: The Community Cookbook." *New York Times*, October 6, 2010.

VandeVelde, Christine. "Amanda Hesser." July 2003. http://www.christinevandevelde.com/bookReviews/200307gentry.asp.

Cathy K. Kaufman and Tawnya Manion

High Line

The High Line is an elevated public park, 1.45 miles in length, built along a disused freight-rail trestle on Manhattan's West Side. Conversion to a park began

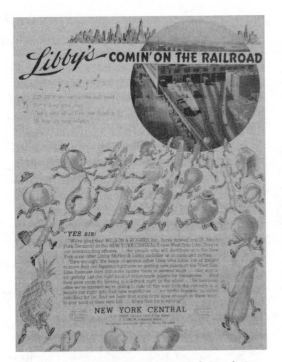

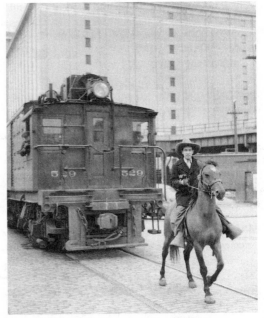

Eleventh Avenue was nicknamed "Death Avenue" because of the high number of pedestrians killed by New York Central's trains, which ran at street level from 1851 to 1929. One of the railroad's early safety measures was to have a flag-wielding horseback rider, called the "West Side Cowboy," precede all trains.

The trains that traveled along the West Side Freight Line tracks were a crucial part of New York City's food distribution network. This 1941 poster, created by New York Central, advertised that Libby's canned foods could now be shipped directly from the cannery to warehouses on the West Side.

with a grassroots community campaign in 1999 and culminated with the opening of the park's first section in 2009. In 2014, the last half-mile of the structure opened to the public.

During its years of operation (1933–1980) the High Line (then known as the "West Side Freight Line") carried freight trains that were a crucial part of New York City's food-distribution network. Nicknamed "the lifeline of New York," the elevated rail brought flour, eggs, cheese, fruit, meat, and poultry into Manhattan, while manufactured goods began their journeys to points west of the High Line. The rail was unique in being the only food freight rail that came directly into Manhattan, though the West Side of Manhattan had long been a center of food markets and distribution.

Beginning in the eighteenth century, farmers from Kings (Brooklyn) and Queens Counties traveled over land or by boat to bring their produce to markets in Manhattan. Before the advent of rail, these farmers' products were sold in local markets only. However, technological advances in the middle of

the nineteenth century changed the scale, scope, and reach of New York's markets.

The advent of steam had a profound effect on New York City's food-distribution network in the mid- to late nineteenth century. First, the focus of the shipping industry shifted from the East River to the Hudson River as steamships required a deeper channel. Second, the railroad arrived. Once the Hudson River waterfront became the locus of the city's shipping industry, it did not take long for rail networks to develop alongside. When the city gave authorization to the New York Central and Hudson River Railway to lay tracks in 1847 along the West Side, the infrastructure was in place for a mighty and long-reaching network to grow.

With both the Washington and Greenwich Markets well established on the West Side, along with the many oyster dealers, who harvested from the brackish Hudson River, the scene was set. Food and grocery warehouses, industrial bakeries, meat-processing plants, refrigerated warehouses, and other related infrastructure were built to support the growing shipping network. The New York Central's trains, which ran along sections of Tenth and Eleventh Avenues at street level, connected with float barges, bringing freight to and from New Jersey and points west.

From 1851 to 1929, the New York Central's trains ran at street level, presenting a traffic-choked and dangerous condition. During the first several decades of operation, 436 New Yorkers were killed by trains despite the railroad's safety measures, which included a flag-wielding horseback rider (the "West Side Cowboy") preceding all trains. Citizen outrage about the carnage ran high, and eventually, the New York Central was required by law to elevate the tracks to save pedestrian lives—hence the birth of the High Line.

The building of the High Line between 1929 and 1934 was part of a larger effort to improve shipping efficiency and decrease food costs in a growing city. Called the "West Side Improvement," the New York Central's project also resulted in the construction of the West Side Highway (now demolished below Fifty-Ninth Street), the St. John's Park Terminal, and the High Line. Along the High Line, warehouses and factories were modified to accommodate the trains and sidings were built directly adjacent to buildings. New York Central promoted the elevated rail as part of an efficient new utopia where trains would load and unload directly into company buildings, decreasing labor costs and increasing the supervision of precious goods. Examples of this infrastructure are still evident today during visits to the High Line.

The area along the High Line, now called the Chelsea Market Passage, was once the space where trains loaded and unloaded at the Nabisco Factory building. Workers unloaded arriving trains laden with sugar, flour, and other raw goods, then loaded departing trains with Oreos, Uneeda Biscuits, and other treats. South of the Fourteenth Street Passage, hooks that once held animal carcasses are still visible on the west side of the park's pathway.

The High Line played an important role in New York City's food distribution through the 1960s, even as interstate trucking supplanted trains as the primary way to distribute food. The last of the neighborhood's meat packers—now serviced entirely by truck—occupies a small building near Washington and Little West Twelfth Streets. Myth has it that in 1980 the last train to travel on the High Line carried three carloads of frozen turkeys.

Today, Friends of the High Line, the nonprofit conservancy that maintains and operates the High Line park, is dedicated to preserving and showcasing

the High Line's food history, while presenting entrepreneurial food vendors to enhance visitors' experience of the High Line. To that end, High Line Food was created in 2011. High Line Food includes a suite of public programs that inspires a connection to community and environment, vendors who serve food with an emphasis on seasonality and sustainability, and a restaurant at the southern terminus of the High Line that opened in 2014. The restaurant's menu favors fish and vegetables, referencing the nineteenth-century produce market that once stood at Gansevoort and Washington Streets, as well as the abundance of seafood that once came from New York City's waterways.

See also MANHATTAN and MEATPACKING DISTRICT.

Buttenwieser, Ann L. *Manhattan Water-Bound: Planning and Developing Manhattan's Waterfront from the Seventeenth Century to the Present.* New York: New York University Press, 1987.
Gray, Christopher. "When a Monster Plied the West Side." *New York Times*, December 22, 2011.
"High Line History." High Line and Friends of the High Line. http://www.thehighline.org/about.
Klein, Aaron E. *The History of the New York Central System.* Greenwich, Conn.: Bison, 1985.
Linder, Marc, and Lawrence Zacharias. 1999. *Of Cabbages and Kings County: Agriculture and the Formation of Modern Brooklyn.* Iowa City: University of Iowa Press.

Timothy C. Ries and Melina Shannon-DiPietro

Hopper, Edward

Edward Hopper (1882–1967), a prominent American realist painter and printmaker, attended the New York Institute of Art while living at 53 East Fifty-Ninth Street. In 1913 he moved to 3 Washington Square, where he lived and worked for the remainder of his life. His wife, Josephine Nivison (1883–1968), was also a painter.

The Hoppers were not food snobs: they often dined at coffee shops, automats, and chop suey joints. Hopper is known to have painted more than eight hundred works, and four of his most famous paintings are set in modest New York City eateries: *New York Restaurant* (1922), *Automat* (1927), *Chop Suey* (1929), and *Nighthawks* (1942).

Many of Hopper's paintings reflect the anonymity, loneliness, and isolation inherent in big-city life. An exception is his *New York Restaurant*, which depicts a charming, bustling restaurant scene. Hopper was trying to depict the crowded glamour of a New York restaurant at lunch time.

Josephine Hopper reported that one of her husband's vices was to drink too much coffee at the automat, where he sat for hours. Horn & Hardart opened its first automat in New York in 1912. These cheap, self-service operations dispensed food through coin-operated windows set into the walls. By the 1920s some automats were open all night—just the thing for "the city that never sleeps" and an appealing subject for a realist painter in the 1920s. Hopper spent a lot of time at the automat on Fifth Avenue and Thirty-First Street. During the day tens of thousands of people streamed through it, but his painting *Automat* shows the place at night, with a lone woman gazing pensively into her coffee cup.

The Hoppers also frequented chop suey houses, inexpensive restaurants that flourished in New York's Chinatown during the early twentieth century. After World War I, Chinese restaurants opened throughout the city as non-Asian New Yorkers discovered the exotic fare. The Hoppers particularly enjoyed eating at The Far East, a chop suey joint one flight up at 8 Columbus Circle. Hopper set his painting *Chop Suey* in this restaurant. In the foreground two women are seated at a table, bathed in sunlight flooding in through the window. The bold lettering of the "Chop Suey" sign can be seen outside this second-floor window.

Nighthawks is arguably Hopper's best-known work. It was painted in the midst of World War II; it may have been based on a local corner coffee shop, on "Greenwich Avenue where two streets meet," as Hopper described it. Nighthawks are predators, and this is a rather desolate image. Unlike the previous three paintings, this view is from the outside, through a window. It is late at night, the street outside is deserted, and the people seated at the counter appear isolated and gloomy. It is a haunting scene that has remained extremely popular.

Hopper's *New York Restaurant* is currently at the Muskegon Museum of Art, *Chop Suey* is at the Seattle Art Museum, *Automat* is at the Des Moines Art Center, and *Nighthawks* is at the Chicago Institute of Art. Reproductions of these images, however, can be found all over New York.

See also AUTOMATS and CHOP SUEY JOINTS.

Barter, Judith A., ed. *Art and Appetite: American Painting, Culture, and Cuisine.* Chicago: Art Institute of Chicago, 2013.
Levin, Gail. *Edward Hopper: An Intimate Biography.* Berkeley: University of California Press, 1998.
Theisen, Gordon. *Staying Up Much Too Late: Edward Hopper's Nighthawks and the Dark Side of the American Psyche.* New York: Dunne, 2006.

Andrew F. Smith

Horn & Hardart

See AUTOMATS.

Hostess

See CUPCAKES.

Hot Dogs

New York City is one of the world's great street food cities. Food carts and, more recently, food trucks abound, especially in Manhattan. Since the late nineteenth century cooked sausages served on buns topped mainly with mustard and chopped onions have been the chief dish served from the several thousand carts that dot the city's streets, parks, and plazas. At the same time, sausage vendors appeared at amusement parks—Coney Island the most famous—and at ballparks. So ubiquitous were the vendors and so celebrated in popular culture in New York that the styles, manner, and name of the sausage sandwiches spread across the nation and are used to the present day.

The sausages are best known as hot dogs. The name "hot dog" is first documented in the mid-1880s in several parts of the country. They appeared in public with German immigrants who arrived in large numbers in the 1850s bringing their sausage food culture with them. Butcher shops in the Lower East Side's "Little Germany" produced varieties of sausages, notably frankfurters and wieners. They were sold to public dining venues such as beer gardens, German restaurants (sausage appetizers were common), and a growing number of street vendors. Wheelbarrows and horse-drawn food carts had been part of the city's food scene for more than a century, and now portable grills for preparing sausages joined the crowd.

When resorts such as Coney Island became popular after the Civil War, sausage vendors flocked to

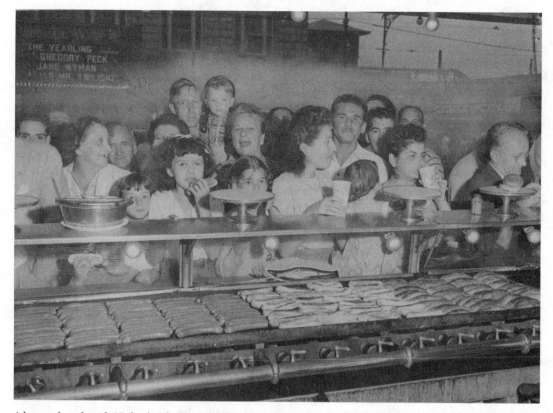

A hungry hoard inside Nathan's, July 17, 1947. The number of hot dogs and buns being prepared at once indicates not only the popularity of the sausage but the ease with which they could be prepared and sold. LIBRARY OF CONGRESS

the areas. By the 1870s small stands were to be found along the beach, to the dismay of conventional restaurant owners who regarded them as unsanitary, fire hazards, and a competitive threat. They flourished, and when a Brooklyn baker created special buns for the vendors' sausages, the hot dog received its classic form. Other popular entertainments, such as baseball and six-day bicycle races, added to hot dog popularity and lore. New York's three big league teams (until 1958) drew large numbers of fans.

The standard and apocryphal story about the name "hot dog" derives from the old Polo Grounds home of the New York Giants. The story goes that on a cold day in April 1901 the New York Giants were playing baseball in their home park, Manhattan's Polo Grounds. Food vendors employed by concessionaire Harry M. Stevens were having a hard time selling their usual peanuts and popcorn to the shivering crowd. Ever the entrepreneur, Stevens hit upon a brilliant idea. He told his men to go out of the park and buy "dachshund" sausages and buns from the butcher and baker across the street. The vendors did, making sandwiches and putting them in their warm vending boxes. They then went into the crowd yelling "Get yer red hots, get yer red hot dogs." "Dogs" came from the dachshund shape of the sausages. In the press box sat the greatest sports cartoonist, T. A. Dorgan, alias TAD. He immediately drew a cartoon of the vendors shouting "hot dogs." When it was printed, supposedly in the *New York Journal*, the word became an instant sensation and spread around the country. Unfortunately, none of this is true as even Harry M. Stevens said in a later interview. But the association of hot dogs with baseball and with Coney Island spread across America: coney is a common hot dog preparation using a meat or spicy sauce.

By the late nineteenth and early twentieth centuries, other ethnic groups arrived in New York and took up the hot dog business. Eastern European Jews made all-beef sausages de rigueur in many dining spots. America's most famous hot dog stand grew out of the Coney Island-Jewish immigrant milieu: Nathan's Famous. Founded in 1916 by Nathan Handwerker, a Jewish immigrant from Poland, the small stand grew by clever marketing and quality products to become an American icon. The family developed a proprietary natural casing all-beef hot dog that is sold in its franchised restaurants and in retail stores throughout the United States. Nathan's uses a flat-griddling cooking technique that is popular in the eastern part of the country.

Greek immigrants have had a major impact on New York hot dog culture. The best-known example is Papaya King. See PAPAYA KING. Originally a fruit juice stand founded on Eighty-Sixth Street and Third Avenue by Constantine Poulos, in 1932 it expanded to hot dogs and fries to accommodate its German–Polish clientele. Poulos's marriage of exotic fruit juice drinks and hot dogs became a New York City specialty and was much imitated. The best known is the celebrated Gray's Papaya (at Broadway and Seventy-Second Street), and at one time there were a host of others such as Papaya Paradise, Papaya Place, Papaya World, Original Papaya, Mike's Papaya or Papaya Jack, Papaya Heaven, and Papaya Circle. Here, too, flat griddled, inexpensive, all-beef hot dogs prevail.

Jews and Greeks, along with Italians, also became manufacturers of sausages. A native of Minsk, Samuel Slotkin founded the Hygrade Provisions Company in 1915 with a small stake and twelve employees. A stickler for natural casing, high-quality frankfurters, he grew the business, buying up other producers and shipping companies to become the standard supplier to the many delicatessens that once graced the city. After his death, the company was moved to Michigan where it was rebranded as Ball Park Franks. Similarly, Gregory Papalexis began in the meat business in 1948, eventually buying up famous hot dog maker Sabrett (founded 1926) and others to form Marathon Enterprises. Like other food industries, hot dog companies underwent consolidation in the latter years of the twentieth century so that most New York hot dogs are made by a handful of companies.

New York's food cart scene has changed to accommodate new cuisines, but the classic New York "dirty water" hot dog cart remains—and often appears in television shows and movies shot in New York. Hot water–bathed, natural casing, usually all-beef hot dogs are set into plain buns, then topped with mustard, chopped onions—often a tomato and onion mixture made by Sabrett—and sometimes sauerkraut. However, the ethnicity of the vendors has changed to mainly South Asian and Middle Eastern.

See also FOOD TRUCKS; GERMAN; and STADIUM FOOD.

Kleiman, Dena. "New York Puts Its Papaya Where Its Hot Dogs Are." *New York Times*, August 21, 1991.
Kraig, Bruce. *Hot Dog: A Global History*. London: Reaktion, 2009.
Kraig, Bruce, and Patty Carroll. *Man Bites Dog: Hot Dog Culture in America*. Lanham, Md.: AltaMira, 2014.
Popok, Barry. "Hot Dog (Polo Grounds Myth & Original Monograph)." BarryPopik.com, July 15, 2004. http://www.barrypopik.com/index.php/new_york_city/entry/hot_dog_polo_grounds_myth_original_monograph/.
The Cries of New-York. New York: S. Wood, 1808.

Bruce Kraig

Hotel Restaurants

During the colonial era, taverns existed in New York where meals were included in guests' lodging fees. Locals might drink at taverns or attend balls in their public rooms, but at this point most New Yorkers took their meals at home.

It was not until the nineteenth century that proper hotels existed in New York. The antebellum period especially saw a luxury hotel building boom in New York. Among the most famous of the early luxury hotels were Astor House (opened in 1836), the St. Nicholas Hotel, and the Fifth Avenue Hotel (both opened in the 1850s). These hotels continued the tavern tradition of the "table d'hôte," where meals were served family style at set times and included in the cost of lodgings. Also like taverns, in addition to serving food to their own guests, hotels hosted banquets for visiting dignitaries and private groups. But the luxury hotels distinguished themselves from taverns by the elaborateness of their restaurants. Hotel dining rooms were lavishly furnished, decorated with marble, velvet, mahogany, and crystal. Hotel meals were events unto themselves. Waiters, dressed in livery, followed a military-style drill, entering the room in formation, lining up behind the tables where guests were seated, and removing covers from dishes, each movement coordinated to the sound of a bell. The menus sometimes consisted of hundreds of items served in a dozen courses. A diner at the St. Nicholas in 1859 could choose from two soups, two kinds of fish, ten boiled dishes, nine roast dishes, six relishes, seventeen entrées, three cold dishes, five varieties of game, thirteen varieties of vegetables, seven kinds of pastry, and seven fruits, with ice cream and coffee. To prepare all these dishes, the hotels had tremendous facilities. The kitchens at the St. Nicholas Hotel could prepare four meals a day for a thousand people. Hotels also offered meal delivery to guests' rooms. See ASTOR HOUSE.

By the mid-nineteenth century, some visitors to New York were chafing against the bundling of meal and lodging costs. In response, more and more hotels switched away from the American plan, where meals were included in the price of board, to the European plan, where guests paid for meals separately from lodging. At this point, some hotels created proper restaurants, serving meals on demand to hotel patrons as well as the general population. For example, in 1857, Astor House announced the opening of an "entirely independent" restaurant, adjoining the hotel, "for merchants doing business in the vicinity." At the same time, a host of freestanding restaurants emerged which hotel guests seeking meals away from their hotels could patronize.

During the Gilded Age, hotel restaurants continued to hold their place at the pinnacle of New York dining. They served as a model of service and décor to restaurants and hotels around the country as well as to individual homeowners. The many hotels around Madison Square featured some of the best dining rooms in late nineteenth-century New York, including the Albermarle, the Gilsey House, the St. James, the Victoria, the Bartholdi, and the Hotel Brunswick, which employed eleven French chefs in its kitchens. See GILDED AGE.

By the early twentieth century, European plan hotels had become the norm. Some hotel restaurants were still renowned—the Rotunda at Astor House, for example, drew locals and tourists alike for a brisk lunch trade, and the Brunswick was still known for its beautiful décor and perfectly cooked steak. But the best restaurants in the city were now found independent of hotels. Through much of the twentieth century, hotel dining was synonymous with mediocre food, a situation that was compounded by the consolidation of New York hotels under national and international chains offering institutional dining services. Hotel restaurants catered mainly to tourists.

This situation has changed, however, as boutique hotels have opened and hotels have made an effort to distinguish themselves by design and amenities. Hotel restaurants have made a comeback, drawing native New Yorkers to their tables. Some of New York's best and most famous chefs are running restaurants in hotels. Hotel restaurant offerings in New York today include April Hoffman's Breslin Bar and John Dory at the Ace Hotel; Danny Meyer's Maialino in the Gramercy Park Hotel; Andrew Tarlow's Reynard in the Wythe Hotel in Williamsburg, Brooklyn; Café Boulud in the Surrey Hotel; The Mark Restaurant by Jean-Georges Vongerichten, Michael White's Ai Fiori at Langham Place; and Daniel Humm and Will Guidara's NoMad. See MEYER, DANNY; BOULUD, DANIEL; and VONGERICHTEN, JEAN-GEORGES.

See also TAVERNS.

Batterberry, Michael, and Ariane Batterberry. *On the Town in New York: The Landmark History of Eating, Drinking and Entertainments from the American Revolution to the Food Revolution.* 2d ed. New York: Routledge, 1998.

Grimes, William. *Appetite City: A Culinary History of New York.* New York: North Point, 2009.

Morabito, Greg. "A Guide to New York City's Best Hotel Restaurants." Eater, June 24, 2013. http://ny.eater.com/maps/a-guide-to-new-york-citys-best-hotel-restaurants.

Sandoval-Strausz, Andrew. *Hotel: An American History.* New Haven, Conn.: Yale University Press, 2007.

Cindy R. Lobel

Hummus

Hummus is a dish made from pureed chickpeas, tahini, lemon juice, garlic, and salt. Served as either an appetizer or a light meal, hummus originated in the lands of the eastern Mediterranean. In Arabic, *hummus* means "chickpea," while the correct name for the dish is *hummus bi tahina*.

In New York, chickpeas were rarely used in cookery until the arrival of immigrants from Spain, Italy, Greece, and other Mediterranean countries at the end of the nineteenth century. Among them were Syrians, most of them Christian from the region that is now Lebanon, who settled on the Lower West Side and on Brooklyn's Atlantic Avenue. See LITTLE SYRIA. They opened grocery stores, including Sahadi's, that sold imported ingredients as well as restaurants featuring lamb, stuffed vegetables, and stews containing chickpeas. In 1943, the food writer Clementine Paddleford visited the Syrian colony and found recipes for a lamb-based dinner that was easy to make under wartime rationing (when beef was hard to find). Among the dishes was one she called "chick pea salad" or "humus bi tahiny," made from chickpeas, "Syrian dressing" (tahini), lemon juice, and garlic.

Until the 1970s, hummus remained a dish that could be found only in Middle Eastern restaurants, particularly on Atlantic Avenue, or on the tables of well-traveled gourmet cooks. Jews in Israel had also fallen in love with dishes such as falafel and hummus that were endemic to their new homeland. New Yorkers who visited Israel fell in love with *chomos* and brought the recipe back to serve as a dip at holiday meals. In the late 1960s and early 1970s, food writers such as Craig Claiborne and James Beard published recipes for hummus that were adopted by home cooks who loved its creamy texture and ease of preparation. As interest in healthy foods grew, hummus was recognized as nutritious, inexpensive, a good source of protein for vegetarians, and not too strongly flavored—even picky children would eat it. Health food stores began to make hummus not just from chickpeas but also from lima beans, black beans, and other legumes and to sell it as a dip or as a sandwich spread.

Following the business model of Israeli hummus companies, in 1986 an Israeli immigrant named Zohar Norman founded Sabra in Queens to manufacture hummus and sell it primarily in the city's kosher markets. A quarter-century later, Sabra is now a joint partnership between Israel's Strauss Group and PepsiCo and dominates the $500-million-a-year hummus industry. Thanks to the company's marketing expertise, hummus has become a popular snack food in millions of American homes. Today, Sabra hummus is sold in more than a dozen flavors, including Classic, Basil Pesto, Chipotle, and Tuscan Garden.

Although industrial hummus is popular in the city and sold in nearly every supermarket, many New Yorkers enjoy the fresh product. Restaurants from around the Mediterranean and the Middle East, including Egyptian, Greek, Persian, Turkish, Palestinian, Syrian, Lebanese, and Yemeni eateries, serve their own versions of *hummus bi tahina*. This includes hummus-centric restaurants such as Hummus Place and Mimi's Hummus opened by Israeli immigrants and featuring three or four varieties of freshly made hummus served with puffy pita bread.

Mishan, Ligya. "Dipping into an Israeli Trend." *New York Times*, March 31, 2009.
Paddleford, Clementine. "Syrian Supper Suggested for Large Parties." *New York Herald Tribune*, June 3, 1943.

Andrew Coe

Hungarian

Hungarian immigrants first came to New York in significant numbers in 1849–1850 following the failed 1848 revolution against Austria. They brought to New York a food tradition that included stews (goulash the most famous), casseroles, cabbage rolls, dumplings, and stuffed peppers and featured such spices as paprika and caraway. Hungarians had a significant impact on New York's restaurant culture in post–Civil War New York. Many of the city's table d'hôte restaurants—prix fixe establishments that served mid-priced meals—served Hungarian food. The best known of these was Hotel Hungaria, on Union Square, which served seventy-five-cent dinners to middle-class families as well as to artists and journalists.

A second wave of Hungarians, dominated by Jewish immigrants, arrived at the turn of the twentieth century. They settled mainly on the Lower East Side, along with many of the other Eastern European Jews who arrived around the same time. See JEWISH and LOWER EAST SIDE. The main Hungarian enclave at this point was in the East Village, east of Avenue A between Houston and Fourteenth Streets, formerly Kleindeutschland or "Little Germany." See KLEIN-DEUTSCHLAND. East Houston Street, lined with Hungarian restaurants and shops, was known as "Goulash Row." One of the most famous of the restaurants was Little Hungary, located at 255–263 East Houston Street. The large establishment housed a cafe, a private room for parties, and a wine cellar. Teddy Roosevelt dined there frequently as police commissioner, and when he returned after his election to the presidency, he made Little Hungary a major tourist destination.

By the 1940s, the Hungarian population center had shifted to Yorkville, on the Upper East Side of Manhattan. See YORKVILLE. That enclave, about 100,000 in the 1940s, grew in the 1950s with the influx of Hungarians fleeing Europe after the revolt against the Soviet Union. Hungarians shared the neighborhood with immigrants from other central European nations including Czechoslovakia and Germany. See GERMAN. Hungarians concentrated around Second Avenue, between Seventy-Ninth and Eighty-Sixth Streets, which became known as "Goulash Avenue." Along the avenue could be found such restaurants as Red Tulip and Mocca and provisions shops like Paprika Weiss (which *New York Times* reporter Joe Berger later referred to as the "Hungarian Zabar's") and Paprika Roth. These stores sold Hungarian specialty goods like red pepper paste, apricot jam, Hungarian sausage, and, of course, paprika. The area was also dotted with Hungarian churches and social clubs like the First Hungarian Literary Society.

By the 1980s, the second generation was moving away from Hungarian Yorkville to other parts of the city. Following the pattern of most ethnic neighborhoods, the businesses lingered for a while; but very few vestiges of Little Hungary remain today. One of the last stalwarts, Hungarian Meat Market and Delicatessen, located on Eighty-Third Street and Second Avenue, closed in 2011 after a fire. A branch store in Fairfield, Connecticut, still thrives, selling Easter ham, szekeley goulash, and stuffed cabbage as well as groceries from Hungary and other central European nations. In Yorkville, Andre's Café, opened in 2005, serves cabbage strudel, *hortobagyi* crepes, wiener schnitzel, and *pasztor tarhonya*, dishes that recall the once-thriving ethnic enclave.

Berger, Joseph. "On the Upper East Side, Memories Fueled by Strudel." *New York Times*, April 7, 2006.
" 'Little Hungary' Restaurant." *Lower East Side History Project* (blog), June 21, 2012. http://evhp.blogspot.com/2012/06/little-hungary-restaurant.html.

Cindy R. Lobel

Hunger Programs

A number of organizations in government programs work within New York City with a mandate to address hunger among its residents and related issues and initiatives. Despite the abundance of available food in New York City as a whole, a marked number of households and neighborhoods have issues with hunger. While a concerted social effort to address hunger in the city began in the early 1980s (after the effects of the city's 1970s fiscal crisis), the percentage of residents experiencing hunger has increased over time. Between 2011 and 2013, over 1.4 million New Yorkers lived in households that did not have sufficient amounts of food. These residents' conditions are largely the result of low income levels and lack of access to healthy or affordable food in certain neighborhoods or, to a lesser extent, particular household or personal issues with finances, psychological health, physical health, and abuse. Most organizations and government programs in New York City have expanded beyond a focus on direct food assistance to also support regional farms and community food projects that produce food for the hungry, perform community outreach and education, conduct research, and develop policy initiatives.

The major hunger-related organizations and government programs working in the city are the Food Bank for New York City, City Harvest, the New York City Coalition against Hunger, the Hunger Action Network of New York State, Hunger Solutions New York, the New York City Human Resource Administration's Emergency Food Assistance Program, and the New York State Department of Health's Hunger Prevention Nutrition Assistance Program. Several of the organizations collaborate on projects as members of the New York City Hunger Free Communities Consortium. There are also many religious and community organizations throughout the city that run neighborhood hunger relief, education, and financial assistance programs (e.g., the Bed-Stuy Campaign against Hunger, the Greenpoint Reformed Church Hunger Program, the Staten Island Hunger Task Force, and The Bowery Mission).

Direct Food Provisioning

The Food Bank for New York City, City Harvest, and numerous religious and community organizations source and provide groceries and meals for those needing temporary or long-term food assistance. The Food Bank for New York City is a non-profit organization formed in 1983, and one of its major activities is emergency food provisioning. It solicits donations of food (both perishable and nonperishable) from the food industry, individuals, and government institutions and purchases discounted food via government programs (such as the Emergency Food Assistance Program, the Hunger Prevention Nutrition Assistance Program, and the

U.S. Department of Agriculture's Food and Nutrition Service's Emergency Food Assistance Program) and supplementally from wholesale distributors. It stores the food at its 90,000-square-foot warehouse at the Hunts Point Cooperative Market in the Bronx and then distributes it to its network of 740 community organizations that run hunger alleviation programs. These programs include food pantries, soup kitchens, senior centers, low-income day-care centers, after-school and summer programs, rehabilitation centers, shelters, and youth services; and the Food Bank for New York City also runs its own combination soup kitchen and food pantry, the Community Kitchen and Food Pantry of West Harlem.

Founded in 1982, the nonprofit City Harvest also distributes food to community organizations (it partners with over five hundred soup kitchens and food pantries throughout the five boroughs), but it sources this food via large-scale food rescue rather than donations or discount programs. City Harvest picks up produce, groceries, and prepared foods that are no longer marketable and would otherwise be thrown away from restaurants, grocers, bakeries, farmers' markets, corporate cafeterias, manufacturers, and farms in the five boroughs. It has a fleet of nineteen refrigerated trucks that travel to these establishments to pick up the rescued food and stores it in a 45,000-square-foot facility in Long Island City (Queens). City Harvest has been expanding the amount of food it rescues since its foundation (exponentially since acquiring the large storage facility in 2011), and in 2015 it projects it will rescue and redirect 50 million pounds of food.

income, and creating economic networks with low-income rural communities.

The Food Bank for New York City partners with the Food Bank Association of New York State, the New York State Department of Agriculture, and Cornell University on an initiative that connects food banks with New York State farmers, and it currently sources some of its produce from a farm in Orange County, New York. City Harvest solicits food donations from twenty regional farms and farmers markets. The New York City Coalition against Hunger (a nonprofit formed in 1983 with the main purpose of coordinating and representing emergency food providers) connects low-income families and individuals in four locations (the Bronx, central Brooklyn, Flatbush, and West Harlem) with community supported agriculture through its Farm Fresh Food Access Program. The program subsidizes community supported agriculture shares based on income, accepts SNAP and WIC (the federal Supplemental Nutrition Assistance Program, formerly known as food stamps, and Women Infants and Children Program), and has flexible share pickup hours. The Hunger Action Network of New York State (a membership organization formed in 1982 that connects local organizations with state-level research, education, and advocacy) runs a low-income community supported agriculture in West Harlem and provides financial, technical, and political support to community food projects in New York City. It assisted in the effort to get the New York State Office of Community Gardens reinstated in 2007 (it was eliminated in 1994, after seven years of operation, because of budget cuts).

Supporting Regional Farms, Urban Farms, and Community Food Projects

In addition to collecting and providing food directly, hunger organizations and programs support other forms of food provisioning for New Yorkers experiencing hunger. Hunger organizations like to procure as much food from regional farms as possible because the food often stays fresher longer (less time from harvest to kitchen) and has a higher nutrient content and diversity (if the farms are biodiverse). They also like to support urban farms, community gardens, and community supported agriculture because low-income urban communities can play an active role in growing their food, supplementing

Community Outreach and Education

Alongside food provisioning, many hunger organizations and programs also emphasize a variety of outreach and education programs for communities and individuals. The New York City Coalition against Hunger, the Food Bank for New York City, Hunger Solutions New York, and the Emergency Food Assistance Program educate low-income communities on their federal food assistance eligibility and assist in enrollment. The New York City Coalition against Hunger has a multilingual Benefits Access Team that works at organizations throughout the city assisting SNAP and WIC applicants with filling out their applications. The Food Bank for New York

City has a Food Stamp Direct Service and Outreach Program through which it identifies in-need populations, conducts one-on-one prescreenings with individuals in those populations, answers applicants' questions, provides electronic application assistance, mediates problems that arise during the application process, and runs SNAP and WIC awareness campaigns in communities. Hunger Solutions New York (a statewide nonprofit started in the early 1980s that focuses on hunger awareness, participation in hunger assistance programs, and antihunger policy) runs a Nutrition Outreach and Education Program, which operates similarly to the New York City Coalition against Hunger's and the Food Bank for New York City's programs. It additionally focuses on increasing participation in the School Breakfast Program and the Summer Food Service Program, federal programs that address the food needs of children in low-income families. The Emergency Food Assistance Program's SNAP Benefits and Nutrition Outreach Program educates the general public about SNAP by disseminating eligibility information and assisting with the SNAP benefit application process throughout the five boroughs of New York City. The SNAP Benefits and Nutrition Outreach Program can be seen at places such as soup kitchens and food pantries, hospitals, senior centers, WIC sites, and public libraries.

In addition to SNAP benefits, these outreach and education programs focus on nutrition and food environments. The Food Bank for New York City and City Harvest both have multipronged nutrition, cooking, and shopping education programs, and workshops. The Food Bank for New York City's CookShop program includes in-school and after-school curricula on food, cooking, and nutrition (CookShop Classroom) which is used in eighteen hundred public schools in low-income areas. It has complementary cooking and food shopping activities for parents and guardians of the students participating in CookShop Classroom (CookShop Families) and nutrition, food systems, and peer education curricula and activities for teenagers (CookShop for Teens/EATWISE). It hosts cooking workshops open to members of particular communities at food pantries through its Community CookShop component. The Food Bank for New York City also runs the Open Market BackPack Program as part of Feeding America's (a nationwide network of food banks) national BackPack Program. Low-income students

choose foods with which to fill up empty backpacks as they learn about the nutritional benefits of the foods, food shopping, and cooking.

City Harvest runs Healthy Neighborhoods, a program that brings together residents, community organizations, after-school programs, and local businesses to change neighborhood food environments. The program runs nutrition education courses for all ages at community organizations; cooking demonstrations at senior centers, supermarkets, corner stores, health clinics, and other community gathering places; food shopping workshops; preschool and after-school nutrition education programs; and retailer and resident communication and action networks. City Harvest also runs Mobile Markets, a program that simultaneously distributes free produce and cooking and health information related to that produce. One hundred and fifty thousand pounds of produce per month are given to low-income communities through this program.

Research and Policy Initiatives

The Food Bank for New York City, City Harvest, the New York City Coalition against Hunger, Hunger Solutions New York, and the Hunger Action Network of New York State all conduct research about the causes of, extent of, and potential ways to reduce hunger and advocate for and help develop policy that addresses hunger. Because the main causes of hunger are poverty and lack of economic opportunity and because hunger causes negative health conditions, these research and policy developments often connect these organizations with organizations and policymakers working in these other related areas.

The Food Bank for New York City conducts research on the extent of food poverty in New York City, demographics of those experiencing food poverty, the degree of access to government nutrition assistance and income support, and the needs of community programs addressing hunger. It communicates the results of this research to community leaders and elected officials, as well as to organizations addressing hunger on a national scale, to influence policy that relates to hunger and poverty at multiple scales.

City Harvest often collaborates on research with other organizations and has produced its own a report on self-sufficiency in New York City (the ability of its residents to afford basic needs like food, shelter, clothing, transportation, and healthcare).

It is connected to public and private sector leaders, philanthropists, and nonprofit organizations (including those not focusing directly on hunger) through research report launches, retail summits, and government meetings to address particular pieces of legislation at the city and state levels.

One of the New York City Coalition against Hunger's main focuses is its research and policy development. It conducts annual hunger surveys that determine the major causes and extents of hunger in New York City that are cited by national publications and used to develop government policies at multiple levels. The New York City Coalition against Hunger has called on the city's mayor and local, state, and federal legislators to commit to its policy initiative, Food Secure NYC 2018, which would eliminate hunger by holistically addressing the interrelated issues of joblessness, labor rights, small business development, and human–environment interaction.

Hunger Solutions New York's research and policy advocacy focus on increasing the availability, eligibility, and enrollment of SNAP and on senior nutrition and child nutrition programs. The Hunger Action Network of New York State collaborates on research with New York City hunger organizations and advocates for universal school breakfasts in New York City, the reduction of food waste, increasing city and state emergency food assistance budgets, healthy food promotion, food democracy, and economic security (i.e., raising the state minimum wage, creating affordable housing, improving the quality of healthcare, creating living-wage jobs, improving child care, improving public assistance benefits, and tax reform).

See also KEY FOOD; CITYMEALS-ON-WHEELS; and SUPPLEMENTAL NUTRITION ASSISTANCE PROGRAM (SNAP).

"Hunger Surveys." New York City Coalition against Hunger. http://nyccah.org/hungersurvey.
Paddock, Barry, and Ginger Otis. "Hunger Crisis: Charities Are Strained as Nearly 1 in 5 New Yorkers Depend on Aid for Food." *New York Daily News*, March 16, 2014.
"Policy Papers." Food Bank for New York City. http://www.foodbanknyc.org/go/policy-and-research/policy-and-research-reports/policy-papers.
"Research and Reports Released in 2014." City Harvest. http://www.cityharvest.org/hunger-in-nyc/research-and-reports.

Alexandra J.M. Sullivan

Hunts Point

The Hunts Point Cooperative Market bills itself as "The Largest Food Distribution Center in the World." It consists of three separate markets: the Hunts Point Terminal Produce Market, the Cooperative Meat Market, and the New Fulton Fish Market. See FULTON FISH MARKET. Each of these entities has its own lease arrangement with New York City. With more than twelve thousand employees, revenues surpass $3 billion, and the customer base is about 23 million. Sitting on 329 acres of gated real estate, the market is situated on a promontory in the South Bronx that juts into, and is surrounded by, the Bronx and East Rivers. See BRONX. The market was built in the 1960s and became a desirable option after construction of highways and warehouses (some refrigerated) with immense loading docks. Huge refrigerated trucks would offload boxed cases of meat and produce (the Fish Market did not arrive until 2005). Trains and planes also contributed to the expansion of these wholesale markets. The Hunts Point Cooperative Market thrived, even as trade on ships declined. Nevertheless, the fortunes of Hunts Point are declining as competition from markets in neighboring states and the creation of vertically integrated food companies (which have their own suppliers and distribution networks) increase. Even Greenmarkets are taking a bite—more like a nibble—out of Hunts Point.

There was a time when Hunts Point (the name and the market) itself did not exist. In 1648, in Manhattan, the first municipal food market was established along the East River, selling "Meat, bacon, butter, cheese, turnips, roots, straw and other products of the farm" (Burrows and Wallace, 2000). Peter Stuyvesant wanted to consolidate market days into one day (Mondays), and markets that existed haphazardly into one location. This effort was only partially successful. Beef was king; butchers were licensed. See BUTCHERS. By 1770, permanent public slaughterhouses had been built. Mulberry Street was called "Slaughterhouse Row." Bakers, oyster sellers, dairymen, and produce and fruit carts followed the butchers, and more extensive markets bloomed. By the early 1800s, there were thirteen public markets competing to feed the rapidly increasing population, which was moving uptown to northern Manhattan and to the Bronx, along with small individually owned markets and butchers. By 1913 New York City's population was 5 million

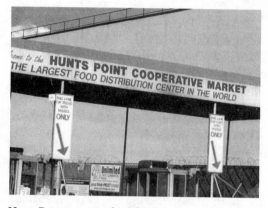

Hunts Point is a major food distribution center that consists of three separate markets: the Hunts Point Terminal Produce Market, the Cooperative Meat Market, and the New Fulton Fish Market.

strong, but the northern population was not well served. Crowded tenements and deregulation of the meat markets propelled people northward, and large wholesale markets, publicly mandated, were needed.

Thomas Hunt, after whom the area of Hunts Point is named, started with 100 acres of fertile agricultural land in 1668. Hunt raised cattle, grew grains, planted orchards, and operated gristmills. The last gristmill is a historic landmark. Farms gave way to development, just as they are still doing today.

The first Bronx Terminal Market was built in 1917 and expanded in 1935; it was intended to provide fresh provisions for the ever increasing population north of 110th Street in Manhattan and in the Bronx. After World War II, urban growth added apartment buildings, schools, and hospitals, as well as immigrant populations to Bronx neighborhoods. By the 1960s, the dilapidated Bronx Terminal Market (near Yankee Stadium), which specialized in Caribbean produce and fruit, was torn down to make way for a mall.

The Hunts Point Produce Market opened on March 21, 1967. Some 122 produce and fruit purveyors moved there from Manhattan, relocating their bins of cabbages, beans, leeks, sage, rosemary, and mint, as well as apples, pears, berries, squash, potatoes, and onions. By 1989, 75 percent of all produce and fruit entering the region was handled there, but by 2012 that had dropped to 22 percent. Of the original 122 purveyors, thirty-eight remain.

After 1960, when slaughtering was banned in New York City, the Hunts Point Cooperative Market (also known as the Hunts Point Meat Market) was established in 1972 (1974 was the official opening) as dealers moved north to take advantage of the area's distribution pathways into and through Manhattan. Boxed beef, shipped from the Midwest and the South, now predominates, although a few purveyors still buy sides of beef delivered on the hook. Master Purveyors specializes in dry-aged beef, which is cut to order for expensive steakhouses, such as Peter Luger. These days, however, a more likely way to see beef carcasses swinging from meat hooks is to rewatch *Rocky*.

Beef (and other meats and poultry) continues to be processed through Hunts Point, although in decreasing amounts. While whole animal (beef) production, including exports, has increased in the United States, per capita consumption of beef in the United States has declined. Beef consumption has decreased from 190 pounds per person in 1999 to less than 150 pounds per person. Goat meat consumption, still a fraction of sales, is increasing rapidly; Muslim, Caribbean, Latin, and non-Muslim Indian populations are the primary consumers.

The Fulton Street Fish Market was one of the last remaining wholesale food markets in Manhattan. It opened in the early 1800s, adjacent to the East River, and continued until the 1970s. After 9/11, the New Fulton Fish Market moved to Hunts Point, where conditions were hygienic and refrigeration was the norm. The official opening was in 2005.

In 1924, the Fulton Street Fish Market sold 25 percent of all seafood sold in the United States. Halibut was king then, but today it is so expensive that only the most upscale restaurants can buy it. Monkfish, once a trash fish, has become trendy. Hake, a fish once reserved for fish sticks, has become popular because it is less expensive, and new customers do not have old habits or preconceptions to overcome. Shellfish is similar; squid and shrimp are ever popular, and the popularity of octopus is on the rise.

A creation of the mid-twentieth century, the Hunts Point Market is adapting to an age that is at once more technology driven and more global and yet nostalgic for the days of an agrarian society. In an effort to keep up, each market at Hunts Point has its own website, with colorful videos and photos, subscriber possibilities, and an ever increasing desire to reconnect with the public, one person at a time. An online presence and a possible TV program for the produce market may help deflect its declining fortunes.

See also CHELSEA MARKET; ESSEX STREET MARKET; MEATPACKING DISTRICT; NEW AMSTERDAM MARKET; PUBLIC MARKETS; and WASHINGTON MARKET.

Burrows, Edwin G., and Mike Wallace. *Gotham: A History of New York City to 1898.* New York: Oxford University Press, 2000.

DiNapoli, Thomas P., and Kenneth B. Bleiwas. "An Economic Snapshot of the Hunts Point Food Distribution Center." Office of the State Comptroller, New York, December 2008. https://www.osc.state.ny.us/reports/economic/huntspoint08.pdf.

Graddy, Kathryn. "The Fulton Fish Market." *Journal of Economic Perspectives* 20, no. 2 (Spring 2006): 207–220.

Krebs, Albin. "Truckload of Onions Opens Hunts Point Market." *New York Times,* March 7, 1967.

Renee Marton

Iceboxes

See ANTEBELLUM PERIOD.

Ice Cream Parlors

See ICE CREAM SHOPS.

Ice Cream Sandwich

Ice cream sandwiches, the simple frozen sweet consisting of a layer of ice cream between two cookies or crackers, were created by an enterprising street peddler in Lower Manhattan at the close of the nineteenth century. In an article in the Sunday, July 13, 1902, edition of the *New-York Daily Tribune* titled "Phases of Ice Cream," a writer reported that the novelty had been invented three years before. The writer said that initially pushcart men had tried to charge two or three cents for the sandwiches, but the neighborhood boys who were the primary customers "would have none of it." They insisted on, and received, a penny sandwich.

Earlier, a columnist in the March 1901 issue of *American Kitchen Magazine*, quoting the *New York Mail and Express*, noted, "As a new fad the ice cream sandwich might have made thousands of dollars for its inventor had the novelty been launched by a well-known caterer. But, strangely enough the ice cream sandwich made its advent in an [*sic*] humbler Bowery pushcart and is sold for a penny." The writer went on to say the ice cream sandwich vendor was the "envy of all other pushcart restaurateurs on the Bowery."

Some newspapers referred to "quarter-inch layers of alleged ice cream" and unsanitary conditions, but the *Tribune* reporter said that although some peddlers made a thinner ice cream with condensed milk rather than rich cream, it was safe to eat. Most press coverage of the ice cream sandwiches emphasized that they were so popular everyone from newsboys and bootblacks to brokers and bankers stood in line together to buy them. The reporters believed such mingling of the classes was extraordinary. To make the sandwiches, the vendors used a tin mold made for the purpose, placing a milk biscuit, Graham wafer, or other cookie in the mold, spreading it with ice cream (flavor not specified), placing another wafer on top, and then, according to the same *Tribune* article, turning it out into "the grimy little paw awaiting it."

The famously ascetic Sylvester Graham, who had died in 1851, would never have approved of his healthful whole-wheat crackers being used for such a self-indulgent treat; but most cookie manufacturers had no such qualms. Peek Frean and others soon advertised wafers suitable for ice cream sandwiches. Fashionable ice cream parlors served dressed-up versions, made with pound cake slices rather than cookies, and served on doily-lined plates with ice cream forks.

Today, supermarket freezers stock an abundance of ice cream sandwiches. Pastry shops sandwich ice cream between pretty pastel macarons rather than pound cake. But ice cream sandwiches are still peddled on New York streets, usually from food trucks rather than pushcarts. The ice cream flavors range from Guinness Stout to pistachio gelato, and the cookies are likely to be salted peanut or chocolate chip, not Graham crackers. One thing has not changed, though: everyone still stands in line together to buy them.

See also CHIPWICH.

American Kitchen Magazine, March 1901, p. xxxiv.
"Phases of Ice Cream." *New-York Daily Tribune,* July 13, 1902. http://chroniclingamerica.loc.gov/lccn/sn83030214/1902-07-13/ed-1/seq-20/#.
Selitzer, Ralph. *The Dairy Industry in America.* New York: Dairy & Ice Cream Field and Books for Industry, 1976.

Jeri Quinzio

Ice Cream Shops

Confectionery shops in Manhattan sold ice cream before the Revolutionary War. An account of eating ice cream in Maryland in 1744 is generally cited as the oldest written record of the frozen treat in the colonies, but colonists probably ate it at an even earlier date. Fancy confectionery shops sold it, and only the wealthy could afford it because of the scarcity of sugar and ice. Ads for ice cream appeared in Manhattan newspapers as early as 1774. In 1777, Italian immigrant Philip Lenzi advertised in the *New York Gazette* that his confectionery shop in Lower Manhattan would begin selling iced creams. Two decades later, Frenchman John Conoit opened what seems to have been New York's first ice cream parlor on Greenwich Street, featuring ice cream, punch, and coffee.

Beginning in the 1790s New Yorkers ate ice cream at pleasure gardens—outdoor venues with pavilions, walking paths, flower beds, and arbors. The entertainment included music, fireworks, and daredevils who soared in hot air balloons. Unlike fancy shops, pleasure gardens attracted the masses by charging moderate prices for ice cream and other treats.

By the mid-nineteenth century, ice cream parlors catered to different social classes. Unless one opted for lavish décor, relatively little capital was needed to operate an ice creamery, making modest ice creameries gateway businesses for new immigrants. Working-class establishments dotted the Bowery, while more elegant parlors served the carriage trade. These public spaces were especially important for ladies who engaged in the new leisure activity of shopping at the department stores found in what is now known as the Ladies' Mile Historic District. Among the most famous ice cream parlors were Taylor's and Thompson's. In addition to the sweets, the parlors served light menus that appealed to women; and they were among the rare places where respectable women could dine without a male escort in the nineteenth century. Courting young couples also retreated to these ice cream parlors in an effort to evade a chaperone's watchful eyes. The upscale parlors were palaces, clad in marble, mirrors, and gold leaf, with blooming plants arrayed to blur sight lines and offer some privacy; red velvet furnishings complemented the interiors. Newspapers cautioned that these parlors were places where single young women might be led astray.

In New York and other big cities, street vendors sold cheap ice cream called "hokey-pokey," hawking it with rhymes such as "Hokey-pokey, sweet and cold; for a penny, new or old." Many hokey-pokey sellers were Italian immigrants, and the treat was especially popular with children. The vendors innovated in ice cream packaging by wrapping hokey-pokey in paper—as either a dab on a square of paper or a slice between two pieces of paper. (The origin of "hokey-pokey" is unknown, but the hawkers may have borrowed it from a popular nonsense song, "Hokey Pokey Whankey Fong.") New Yorkers who could afford more expensive treats patronized ice cream parlors or soda fountains in drugstores, train stations, hotels, and department stores.

Ice cream parlors lost some of their feminine and salacious associations during Prohibition, when closed saloons on Wall Street became ice cream parlors frequented by businessmen before the speakeasies opened at night. Even after Prohibition's repeal, the parlors continued to be popular destinations for children and adults because lack of refrigeration made it almost impossible to keep ice cream at home: although one could crank ice cream at home, it needed to be consumed immediately, before it melted. It was not until after World War II that home freezers became common and ice cream parlors less essential to satisfy sudden cravings.

After World War II, modern street vendors sold frozen treats from refrigerated carts or trucks. Good Humor dominated the truck market until the late 1970s, when the company changed its sales strategy. Since then, independents and a few small companies have owned the truck market.

In the late twentieth century scoop shops replaced the old-fashioned ice cream parlor. The first scoop shops resembled fast-food outlets in design and service. Burton Baskin and Irvine Robbins started the Baskin-Robbins chain in California and franchised shops from coast to coast. Other ice cream brands followed the Baskin-Robbins playbook to build chains.

Many independent scoop shops also opened, often serving distinctive, exotic flavors along with the traditional favorites. New York's ice cream parlors now offer a range of styles based on different ethnic traditions beyond the traditional French, Italian, and American varieties. Spots for Indian kulfi, Lebanese kashta, and Turkish dondurma dot Brooklyn and Queens, while the Chinatown Ice Cream Factory, on Manhattan's Bayard Street, wittily offers such "regular" flavors as durian and pandan, while tempting the adventurous with "exotic" chip mint and vanilla.

Funderburg, Anne Cooper. *Chocolate, Strawberry, and Vanilla: A History of American Ice Cream*. Bowling Green, Ohio: Bowling Green State University Popular Press, 1995.
Grimes, William. *Appetite City: A Culinary History of New York*. New York: North Point, 2009.
Mishan, Ligaya. "A Journey of a Thousand Miles Begins with a Single Scoop." *New York Times*, June 26, 2014.
Schumer, Fran R. "Flavors of Ice Cream Parlors: Nostalgic to New." *New York Times*, August 20, 1986.

J. Anne Funderburg and Cathy K. Kaufman

Indian

See SOUTH ASIAN.

Indo-Caribbean

Immigrants of Indian descent from the Caribbean first arrived in significant numbers in New York at the turn of the twentieth century. Previous Caribbean immigrants were largely of the African diaspora and represented a multicentury movement of people who, at first, largely comprised slaves. In more modern times, these Caribbean New Yorkers found themselves thrown together in a mixed community varying by island and religion and settled for the most part in the Church Avenue and Flatbush Junction areas of Brooklyn.

Overall, voluntary Caribbean immigration to the city reached its height in the 1970s and included newcomers who ethnically identified as East Indian. They hailed mostly from the English-speaking areas of Guyana, Trinidad & Tobago, and, to a lesser extent, Suriname with its Dutch speakers. In 2013 Guyanese and Trinidadian immigrants were among the top ten immigrant groups in the city by population and among the top five in Queens.

Within the borough of Queens, Richmond Hill is home to the largest Indo-Caribbean enclave with a vibrant commerce thoroughfare on Liberty Avenue, heavily dotted with food markets and restaurants, showcasing foods of East Indian immigration, first to the Caribbean and then to New York. A hallmark of this ethnic fare is roti, a soft griddled flat bread that is torn into pieces to eat with curries. New York versions feature curry wrapped in the roti in a "burrito" style, first introduced as a handheld way to eat roti and curry by food trucks selling the fare around the city. This manner of eating has been exported back to the Caribbean, where it has become popular as well.

Indo-Caribbean curries feature beef, chicken, fish, or various vegetables cooked in a version of West Indian curry powder, notable for lacking chili pepper, unlike traditional South Asian varieties. Heat is added with either fresh pepper or pepper sauce while cooking. Pork is relatively uneaten among Indo-Caribbeans because many are either Hindu or Muslim, with religious proscription against the meat.

Purely vegetarian curries and other dishes are common because of the number of Hindus in the population. The variety of fruits and vegetables used in this culinary style is seen in the many Richmond Hill fruit and vegetable stands—as well as those in the older Caribbean neighborhoods in Brooklyn—featuring traditional produce such as *bodi* (long beans), *calabaza* (West Indian pumpkin), *dasheen* (taro), *dasheen* leaves (taro leaves), *eddoes* (a tuber similar to taro), plantain (cooking bananas), *pomme cythere, karaili* (bitter melon), cassava (yucca), and more. The diversity of vegetarian foods is best experienced during the Hindu festivals of Phagwa and Siwali in Richmond Hill.

A mélange of flavors from West Africa, Europe, China, and India, Indo-Caribbean cuisine includes dishes such as fried rice, chow mein, and *pow*, a derivative of *bao* or Chinese steamed buns. Stewed meats that are first browned in sugar and then served with rice dishes speak to the mix of West African and East Indian tradition.

Snack foods that are normally served as street foods in Guyana and Trinidad are particularly popular. Most beloved is Doubles, a hand-held breakfast treat that is eaten all day long among New York Indo-Caribbeans and comprises curried chickpeas sandwiched between ovals of fried yeast-based flatbread.

Baked goods meld traditional European techniques for both sweet and savory. Turnovers can take the form of meat patties as well as sweet fruit–filled pastries. Quick-bread recipes feature tropical ingredients such as coconut, cassava, and calabaza. Guyanese bakers are particular noted for their prowess with flaky pastries such as cheese straws, which feature a butter-based dough that is enriched with cheddar cheese and baked.

Drinks from imported flowers, barks, and herbs are sold both canned and freshly made in restaurants, in snack shops, and sometimes from street vendors, as in the Caribbean. These include sorrel, made from hibiscus flower; ginger beer; peanut punch; mauby, made from carob bark; and sea moss drink, made from carrageen or Irish moss. Alcoholic drinks imported from the Caribbean, such as rum and Carib and Stag beers, remain popular along with nonalcoholic fruit-based sodas such as Solo or Ting.

See also CARIBBEAN.

Bernstein, Nina. "From Asia to the Caribbean to New York, Appetite Intact." *New York Times*, April 20, 2007.
Ganeshram, Ramin. *Sweet Hands Island Cooking from Trinidad & Tobago*, 2d ed. New York: Hippocrene, 2010.
Jaleshgari, Ramin P. "Neighborhood Report: Richmond Hill; An Indo-Caribbean Bazaar, but Some Yearn for the Gap." *New York Times*, September 5, 1999.
New York City Department of City Planning. *The Newest New Yorkers: Characteristics of the City's Foreign-Born Population*. New York: City of New York, 2013.

Ramin Ganeshram

Institute of Culinary Education

The Institute of Culinary Education, known in the industry as "ICE," has been located at 225 Liberty Place in Lower Manhattan since May 2015, and is a 74,000-square-foot center for training and education in all aspects of culinary, hospitality, and related management skills needed for professional success in the competitive world of food and drink. It also is home to diverse avocational offerings, teaching hands-on cooking, baking, and wine and spirits appreciation, offering over seventeen hundred classes to thousands of culinarily curious people each year.

ICE was founded in 1975 by Peter Kump as a small cooking school run out of his New York City apartment. Then known as "Peter Kump's School of Culinary Arts," Kump's mission was to create "recipeless cooks," teaching fundamental techniques to small groups of amateurs with the intention of making them confident and independent in their home kitchens. The techniques-driven curriculum was so successful that, by 1983, the school had expanded to include professional training, opening its Peter Kump's New York Cooking School division, and relocated to a small and rickety brownstone with three teaching kitchens at 307 East Ninety-Second Street. Notwithstanding the space's physical shortcomings, the school flourished, with many of the world's culinary luminaries—Julia Child, Diana Kennedy, Madeleine Kamman, Marcella Hazan, Penelope Casas, and James Beard—teaching classes to rapt students. During the 1980s, the school expanded its offerings to include a professional pastry and baking program under the direction of Nick Malgieri, in addition to its core professional and avocational culinary classes. In 1995, the school opened a second outpost at 50 West Twenty-Third Street, sadly coinciding with the death of Kump. The school was purchased by entrepreneur Rick Smilow, and as more space became available at the modern West Twenty-Third Street facility, the Ninety-Second Street location was closed in 1999.

In 2001, the school expanded its curriculum to include a Culinary Management Division and changed its name to the Institute of Culinary Education to reflect its broader offerings; thereafter programs in advanced pastry studies (2005), hospitality management (2010), and professional development (2012) rounded out its courses of study. ICE also offers a large number of continuing professional development courses, including food media, professional demonstrations, a lecture series called "Meet the Entrepreneurs," business seminars, and study abroad programs. In partnership with the Union Square Hospitality Group, ICE also offers professional wine studies. Along with new programs came expanded space at West Twenty-Third Street: by 2004, the facility had ten teaching kitchens and two lecture halls, working seven days a week throughout the year.

The 2015 move to 225 Liberty Street expanded ICE's facilities to thirteen teaching kitchens and four lecture halls. The school's Culinary Technology Lab features a culturally and technologically diverse array of cooking tools, with traditional stone hearth ovens and rotisseries, a plancha grill, a tandoor oven, and all the specialized implements used in modernist cuisine. A hydroponic herb garden and vegetable farm supply some of the needs of the kitchens, and artisanal production is taught in a chocolate studio that trains students in all of the steps required to process the "bean to the bar." A charcuterie lab includes space for curing and drying specialty products, and there is a kitchen for smoking foods and making stocks.

One of the unique initiatives at ICE has been its collaboration with IBM, utilizing the power of computers to suggest recipes and change the way that chefs approach the creative process. The premise is that, by transforming culinary knowledge into mathematical terms that can be used by a computer, the computer can suggest combinations that might not occur to human chefs—an unexpected culinary synergy. The project produced the 2015 cookbook *Cognitive Cooking with Chef Watson: Recipes for Innovation from IBM and the Institute of Culinary Education*, which marries techniques from traditional and modernist cuisine with provocative flavors.

ICE has international affiliations with the SWISSAM Hospitality Business School in St. Petersburg, Russia; Istanbul's Culinary Institute; and Streets International in Hoi An, Vietnam, a nonprofit culinary and hospitality training center for orphans and young adults. Other philanthropic activities include support for local and international hunger relief organizations and scholarships to study at the Institute of Culinary Education for underserved students.

In 2000, the school was accredited by the American Commission of Career Schools and Colleges and received its "School of Distinction" designation in 2006. In 2003, it was named "Avocational Cooking School of the Year" by the International Association of Culinary Professionals; in 2008, ICE was honored as the IACP "Vocational Cooking School of the Year," and in 2015 was named an IACP "Culinary School of Excellence." Numerous instructors and graduates of the Institute of Culinary Education have also received coveted International Association of Culinary Professionals and James Beard Foundation awards.

See also JAMES BEARD AWARDS; JAMES BEARD FOUNDATION; KUMP, PETER CLARK; and SMILOW, RICK.

"Computational Creativity." IBM Research. https://www.research.ibm.com/cognitive-computing/computational-creativity.shtml#fbid=9OCYHFqs72t.
Institute of Culinary Education website: http://www.ice.edu.
Marcus, Gary. "Cooking with I.B.M.: The Synthetic Gastronomist." *New Yorker*, April 9, 2013.

Cathy K. Kaufman

Inwood

Inwood is the northernmost neighborhood of Manhattan, bordered on three sides by water: the Hudson River to the west, Spuyten Duyvil to the north, and the Harlem River to the east. The southern boundary is generally considered to be Dyckman Street, equivalent to Two Hundredth Street based on the numbered grid; and it stretches just twenty blocks to the north. A triangle of land south of Dyckman Street, bounded by Broadway and Nagel Avenue, which intersects at 193rd Street, is also considered part of Inwood.

A vibrant neighborhood, Inwood is mainly Caribbean and Latin American, with restaurants, groceries, bakeries, and juice bars specializing in Dominican and Mexican food dotting the area. Although Starbucks arrived in Inwood in 2013, many people prefer $1.25 cups of strong *café con leche* available at Dominican eateries all over the neighborhood. A gentrifying stretch along Broadway north of 207th Street has restaurants offering Thai, "new" American, and Italian cuisine as well as coffee bars and more; and a two-block stretch of Dyckman Street west of Broadway is packed with restaurants and wine bars, many Caribbean-themed (including a sushi restaurant with a Dominican touch), that mainly attract young professionals, many with Caribbean and Latin American roots. The wide sidewalk makes it conducive to sidewalk cafes, which are packed on warm days. These restaurants, some playing music, transform the neighborhood on weekends with huge crowds and have been somewhat controversial because of their impact on quality of life. At the western end of Dyckman Street is La Marina, a Latin-flavored restaurant and nightclub overlooking the Hudson River.

Venezuelan food is relatively new to the area. The popular Cachapas y Mas on Dyckman Street began as a food truck in Inwood, took a small retail space, and has since doubled the Dyckman Street space and opened two smaller outposts in Washington Heights. Venezuelan *patacon* sandwiches, using mashed green plantain for the outside of the sandwich, with various fillings, can be found at many Dominican eateries. And the ingredients are similar to Dominican recipes using *tostones* (green plantains), the base for the popular *mofongo*, mashed green plantain, often cooked with garlic sauce and combined with various types of fish, poultry, and meats or eaten with a hearty breakfast as the equivalent of hash browns in a traditional "American" breakfast.

Inwood's history supposedly includes Peter Minuit's "purchase" of Manhattan (for the proverbial $24) on the site that is now Inwood Hill Park, and the neighborhood is home to the Dyckman Farmhouse (now a museum), the oldest existing farmhouse on the island. Perhaps its best-known food legacy is Irish, commemorating the thick presence of Irish families from about the 1930s to the 1980s or so. All that remains is a handful of pubs—Liffy Bar II, Irish Brigade, and Piper's Kilt, the last being the only one that also serves food. One bar, Irish Eyes, closed in 2015. The Broadyke Market is one of the few surviving old-timers and sells Irish soda bread. See IRISH.

The population began shifting from the late 1960s onward with an influx of Dominicans and, in subsequent years, of Mexicans, mostly settling east of Broadway. West of Broadway the population is more mixed, and over a long period in the 1970s and onward, accelerating in the 2000s, there has been an in-migration of non-Hispanics, many from elsewhere in Manhattan, seeking less expensive rents, the beauty of the park, and good transportation. Many are writers, teachers, or artists. One of the newer food attractions is Indian Road Café, on Indian Road (the only "road" in the borough) facing Inwood Hill Park, featuring "new American" cuisine and ample entertainment from local artists.

Since the 1980s, Inwood Hill Park has been home to the annual Shad Festival—Drums along the Hudson: A Native American Festival, which celebrates the park's Native American heritage and coincides with the annual return of spawning shad to the Hudson River. Native American foods are sold at the festival.

See also MANHATTAN.

Drums along the Hudson website: http://drumsalongthehudson.org.
"Goodbye to Glocamorra" (1968). https://www.youtube.com/watch?v=xnG6pLwOflQ.
Uptown Collective website: http://uptowncollective.com.

Myra Alperson

Irish

Irish people have lived in America since the first European settlers arrived in the 1600s. However, the

late 1840s–1850s saw a surge in Irish immigration, when large waves of starving, destitute people fleeing the Great Famine settled in the port cities of Boston, Philadelphia, Baltimore, Buffalo, and New York. By the mid-1850s, the Irish comprised one-quarter of the population of the boroughs of Manhattan and Brooklyn, before eventually spreading out into Queens (particularly the neighborhood of Woodside), the Bronx, and Staten Island.

They settled where the work was hard and the rent was cheap, mainly adjacent to the docks where they landed. In Manhattan the southernmost harbor area known as Five Points—the setting of Martin Scorsese's 2002 movie *Gangs of New York*—and the west Thirties to the Fifties—now known as Hell's Kitchen, Clinton, or Midtown West where the Westies crime gang organized—were the nuclei of Irish food and culture (and consequently an Irish-dominated police force and fire brigade). See FIVE POINTS and HELL'S KITCHEN. Neighborhood pubs emerged and spread throughout the city, and each was often associated

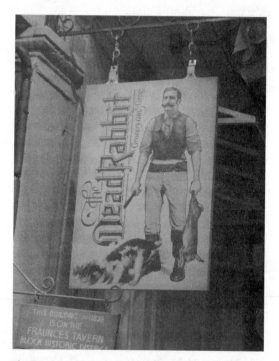

The Dead Rabbit Grocery and Grog, located on Water Street, is an Irish pub that opened in 2013. The name refers to an Irish-American gang that operated in New York City in the 1850s, known for their emblem of a dead rabbit on a spike and their frequent rioting and fighting at the Five Points. JASON BYLAN

with a particular Irish county such as Galway, Cork, or Dublin.

Pubs

Fáilte, the Gaelic word for "welcome," is a common name for pubs where Irish society met to eat home-style food and drink, which evolved into a popular standard of city bar culture, found in almost every neighborhood. Pubs are instantly recognizable by their classic "cottage-style" design. They bear an Irish name, usually that of the owner or previous owner (assuming that person is of Irish descent, which in modern times might well not be); an Irish place; or a Gaelic phrase with Celtic lettering adorning the façade.

Aside from refreshment, pubs also serve as a communal outlet for other key aspects of Irish culture—writing, theater, poetry, and music. Many that exist today hold a weekly Irish session (*seisiún* in Gaelic), when traditional songs are performed on acoustic instruments, often by a house band of musicians, with assorted special guests. In addition, they host writing groups and readings and are places to hear other styles of live music.

Notable Pubs

Some modern-day city pubs are a sort of hybrid between sports bar and classic, or "authentic," pub. However, several of the most famous pubs in the city have withstood the test of time, frequented by some of the most notable New Yorkers throughout history. These include McSorley's Old Ale House at 15 East Seventh Street, which opened in 1854 but only served women beginning in 1970 and installed separate ladies restrooms in 1986; The Old Town Bar at 45 East Eighteenth Street, the setting of several movies including *State of Grace* (1990) and *The Devil's Own* (1997), as well as the opening credits to NBC's *Late Night with David Letterman*; Pete's Tavern at 129 East Eighteenth Street, where O. Henry wrote "The Gift of the Magi"; the White Horse Tavern at 567 Hudson Street, a favorite of Dylan Thomas and allegedly his ghost; P. J. Clarke's at 915 Third Avenue, whose famous patrons include Johnny Mercer, Nat King Cole, Richard Harris, Ernest Borgnine, and Ethel Merman; and Molly's Shebeen at 287 Third Avenue, with both a sawdust floor and a working fireplace. See MCSORLEY'S OLD ALE HOUSE; P. J. CLARKE'S; and WHITE HORSE TAVERN.

In 2013, the Dead Rabbit Grocery and Grog at 30 Water Street (at the former site of the Five Points slum and named for a neighborhood gang) opened as both a pub and a classic cocktail bar, quickly winning many accolades including 2014 Tales of the Cocktail Best American Cocktail Bar and International Bartender of the Year for head bartender Jack McGarry.

Drinks and Food

Pubs contributed several essential culinary and traditional influences on New York City that have endured in various incarnations, crossing both ethnic and class cultures. These once-humble homestyle drinks and dishes are now considered staples in everything from diners and casual bars to cocktail and fine dining establishments.

Stout-Style Beer

Guinness, the dry, dark beer with a creamy foam top, requires taps with both nitrogen and carbon dioxide. It was once a scarcity, served only in certain "destination pubs," such as Eamonn Doran's on Second Avenue, until the late twentieth century, when by popular demand bars were expected to be better equipped to serve it. With the rise of craft beer from the 1990s, Irish stout-style beers are now a common libation of choice.

Irish Whiskey

Thanks to aggressive marketing campaigns that started in the late 1980s, Jameson's, Powers, and Bushmills Irish whiskey are common offerings in every bar and favorite go-tos for "shots." Irish whiskey continues to rise in popularity, with more variety and sippable aged expressions available including single malts.

Irish Coffee

The drink of sweetened strong coffee and Irish whiskey topped with whipped cream continues to be a preferred pick-me-up, with modern-day cocktail bars serving their own spin on the classic. These include frozen versions and fancy syrups as sweeteners.

Fish and Chips

Though some would argue that fried and battered white fish served with fried potatoes (mushy peas optional) and malted vinegar is of English origin, it was the Irish pub that popularized this dish in the city (especially on Friday nights). It now swims its way onto high-end seafood restaurant menus.

Corned Beef

Rock salt–cured beef, though an Irish canning industry technique, was not a popular dish in Ireland because of its prohibitive cost. But it was a common way to preserve rationed meat in the United States during both world wars. In Irish American households it was served with boiled cabbage.

Frank McCourt

Inarguably the greatest Irish immigrant story in New York City history is that of Frank McCourt, author of *Angela's Ashes*, detailing the horrific struggles of his impoverished family in Ireland and Manhattan and his own determination to rise above them. As an academic and author, McCourt was eventually so successful that he became an investor at the upscale pub Angus McInDoe in the theater district before his death in 2009.

Andrews, Evan. "7 Infamous Gangs of New York." History.com, June 4, 2013. http://www.history.com/news/history-lists/7-infamous-gangs-of-new-york.

"Bars and Taverns." Right Here NYC. http://rightherenyc.com/BEEN_HERE_BARS.html.

Jimmy's New York Irish Pub Guide (website). http://www.irishpubguide.com/guide.html.

Olver, Lynn. "FAQs: Irish Food History & Traditions." Food Timeline. http://www.foodtimeline.org/foodireland.html.

Amanda Schuster

Irving, Washington

Washington Irving (1783–1859) was a popular New York writer and editor best known for his satirical *A History of New York* (1809) and the witty yet affectionate prose of the "Rip Van Winkle" and "Legend of Sleepy Hollow" stories collected in *The Sketch Book* (1819). Born in a house on William Street to a Scottish father and English mother, Irving grew up in Lower Manhattan and eventually studied for the bar. In his youth, he was known as a man about town and established a coterie of friends that included scions of old Dutch families. From 1807 to 1808, he and his pals published *Salmagundi*, a satirical journal. A little like today's *Mad Magazine* or *The Onion*, the publication skewered contemporary politics and social mores. The term "Gotham" first appeared in the journal's pages in a mock history of New York. In a similar vein, *A History of New York*, supposedly written by a Dutch New Yorker named Diedrich Knickerbocker, was Irving's first big hit—even though the author's true identity was not known for a year following its 1809 publication.

Irving is best known to food writers for two passages, both in the voice of Diedrich Knickerbocker, the first from *A History of New York* and the other from "The Legend of Sleepy Hollow." The two are largely similar and describe Dutch American tea tables groaning with baked goods and preserved fruit: "There was the dough-nut, the tenderer oly koek, and the crisp and crumbling cruller; sweet-cakes and short-cakes, ginger-cakes and honey-cakes, and the whole family of cakes…" is the way one is described in "The Legend of Sleepy Hollow." Irving had spent part of his youth in the Hudson Valley, so it reasonable to assume that these descriptions are true of Dutch American foodways of his time.

Several of Irving's books proved to be bestsellers and provided a comfortable living, at least for a time. Following 1822, he worked in several European counties as an American diplomat.

See also NOVELS.

Irving, Washington. *The Works of Washington Irving*. New York: Putnam's, 1880.

Jones, Brian Jay. *Washington Irving: The Definitive Biography of America's First Bestselling Author*. New York: Arcade, 2011.

Michael Krondl

Italian

Italian food is ubiquitous in New York City, a major and indispensable part of the unique smorgasbord of flavors, tastes, and imaginaries that is New York City's food. The city's multisensual landscape is unmistakably shaped by a thousand pizza places ranging from joints serving ninety-nine-cent slices to West Village pizzerias where Italian-born and -trained *pizzaioli* bake Neapolitan pizza with personally sourced imported ingredients (buffalo mozzarella, Pachino cherry tomatoes, San Daniele prosciutto, extra virgin olive oil); an over 50,000–square feet megastore of high-quality specialty Italian food in front of the Flatiron Building (Eataly); "family-style" Italian restaurants that serve the ominously large portions of spaghetti and meatballs and fried calamari supposedly eaten at home on Sundays by three-generation Italian families; and endless supermarket and grocery shop shelves of foodstuffs labeled "Italian"—a category that includes "traditional" Gorgonzola cheese made in Wisconsin, rare varieties of capers flown from the island of Pantelleria, and everything in between.

From the late nineteenth century to this day, different waves of Italian migrations, proletarian and middle class, reflecting the significant regional differences of the country, shaped and reshaped Italian food in New York. In fact, today more than ever, New York is an important center for the constant remaking of the Italian food notion.

Between 1890 and the passage of the 1924 Immigration Act, 3 million Italians immigrated to the United States, the vast majority of them through Ellis Island. At the time of the 1930 U.S. census, 1,050,000 first- and second-generation Italian immigrants lived in New York, making up one-seventh of New York's population. Mostly rural people from Italy's south, immigrants to New York congregated in "Little Italies," low-rent tenement districts in Manhattan close to their jobs in construction and the garment industry. Proliferating pushcart markets and food shops contributed dramatically to neighborhood construction. Peddling fruit, vegetables, fish, and bread was the most popular independent occupation for Italian immigrants. They introduced to the city greens like escarole, endive, and broccoli rabe; vegetables like broccoli, zucchini, and fennel; different kinds of clams and seafood; and Italian ice. Food importing operations (some food industries in Italy—notably macaroni, canned tomato products, olive oil, and cheese—thrived almost entirely on the exports to the Italian "colony" in New York) and a domestic food industry dominated by immigrant entrepreneurs catered to a huge ethnic market, while instilling in the immigrants the idea that they could best articulate their identity as Italians in America by consuming Italian foodstuffs and cooking Italian.

Interacting for the first time with Italians from other regions and enjoying the unprecedented opportunities offered by the marketplace, immigrants to New York created a hybrid national cuisine based on the re-creation of what had been the festive food or what they thought the rich people ate in their native towns. Among the hybrid, enriched dishes created as part of this gastronomic and social turnaround were meatballs, veal and chicken Parmesan, lasagna, zeppole, cannoli, and biscotti. Some key seasoning ingredients, like garlic and chili pepper, were used so generously that visiting middle-class Italian travelers often found this new cuisine too greasy, too spicy, and vulgar, like the immigrants that cooked it for them.

Since the 1920s, Italian restaurants formalized and made popular among non-Italian New Yorkers such hybrid Italian cuisine. Restaurants offering menus of spaghetti with tomato sauce, ravioli, minestrone, chicken cacciatore, veal scaloppini, provolone cheese, fruit, and espresso coffee (a technologically advanced version of the beverage, invented in Milan before World War I) and serving wine and grappa in defiance of Prohibition were to be found throughout Manhattan and Brooklyn in the interwar years. Most influential in creating the mystique of Italian food in New York were restaurants in Greenwich Village and the Theater District around Times Square, which catered to an avant-garde customer base of bohemians, artists, and writers. The signature dish of these restaurants, spaghetti with tomato sauce, became arguably the first American ethnic food to break through and be universally known and liked across the boundaries of race and ethnicity. The familiarization of New Yorkers with its culinary complex—dough, tomato sauce, melted cheese, and olive oil—also proved fundamental to pave the way for the success of pizza. See GREENWICH VILLAGE and TIMES SQUARE.

A delicacy local to Naples, pizza made the crossing early in the century with the sizeable Neapolitan contingent of Italian immigrants. It was baked in the basement of bakeries and sold by the slice on the streets of Manhattan's Little Italies, unknown to other New Yorkers until World War II. In the 1950s, a market for pizza was created almost overnight by inventive cooks and entrepreneurs who opened modernized pizza parlors first in the neighborhoods of Brooklyn, the Bronx, and Staten Island, where second-generation Italian Americans had relocated, and then all over the city. The popularization of pizza was helped along by GIs returning from occupied Italy. In the same years, a new smaller wave of southern Italian immigrants reinvigorated Italian food in New York with fresh ingredients and reengaged traditions, by opening food stores, importing businesses, and restaurants in reconstituted Italian communities like Arthur Avenue in the Bronx and Bensonhurst in Brooklyn. See ARTHUR AVENUE; BRONX; BROOKLYN; PIZZA; PIZZERIAS; and STATEN ISLAND.

In the 1970s and 1980s, a tiny group of middle-class northern Italian immigrants in New York City, many of whom had never cooked in Italy, helped reshape Italian food in New York by detaching it from its immigrant origins and relocating it within the "authentic" traditions of Italian regional cooking. Cookbook writers and cooking instructors Giuliano Bugialli, Franco Romagnoli, and especially Marcella Hazan were welcomed by a culture industry eager to let them promote real Italian food among a growing cosmopolitan class of professional New Yorkers who were avid consumers of foreign and ethnic cuisines. Recent immigrant chefs like Pino Luongo (Il Cantinori, Le Madri, Centolire) opened upscale restaurants serving Tuscan and other regional cuisines on the Upper East Side and Greenwich Village. Sometimes called northern Italian cuisine to differentiate it from the down-market red-sauce clichés of early twentieth-century immigrants, this new template for Italian eating popularized dishes like creamy risotto, gnocchi, osso buco, and tiramisu; translated macaroni and spaghetti into "pasta"; and introduced ingredients like pesto, balsamic vinegar, and focaccia to the New York larder. See HAZAN, MARCELLA.

By the late 1990s, two restaurateur-chefs and TV personalities, Lidia Bastianich and Mario Batali, had followed the path opened by Hazan to make Italian food in New York a fully transnational concept. Bastianich, who arrived in New York in the mid-1950s as a refugee from the Italian-Croatian region of Istria, has since opened Buonavia and Villa Secondo in Queens and Felidia, Becco, Esca, and Del Posto in Manhattan and hosted three popular cooking shows on PBS. Batali, an Italian American from Seattle, claims his early work in a traditional *osteria* in Emilia-Romagna as a formative experience in his career, reflected in the restaurants he opened in Manhattan, including the flagship Babbo, the pizzeria Otto Enoteca, Roman-style trattoria Lupa, seafood-focused Esca, and high-end Del Posto (the latter two with Bastianich, with whom Batali also partners on Eataly). Insisting on the importance of "going back" to the source of local ingredients and culinary traditions they can creatively reinterpret, Bastianich and Batali authoritatively promise their customers—many of whom are frequent travelers to Italy themselves—the excitement of consuming a food and a place at the same time. See BASTIANICH, LIDIA; BATALI, MARIO; and EATALY.

Since the turn of the millennium, a new generation of mostly non-Italian younger chefs has further expanded on the same concept of authenticity by embracing Italian regional cooking practices, north and south, such as homemade fresh pasta and *salumi* (cured meats). This group includes Brooklyn restaurants like Al Di La as well as President Barack Obama favorite Missy Robins' A Voce. This last wave of Italian cooking in New York has been significantly inspired by the philosophy of slow food, the movement based in northern Italy that globally promotes the defense and valorization of independent, local, and organic farming; biodiversity; and traditional food cultures and has its American headquarters in Carroll Gardens. See SLOW FOOD.

Finally, the story of Italian food in New York has very recently come full circle with an emerging "red-sauce revival," led by trained young chefs, many of them Italian Americans. Rich Torrisi and his partner Mario Carbone opened Torrisi Italian Specialities on Mulberry Street in the heart of Little Italy, targeting foodies and hipsters with a stylish reworking of old-school dishes. With local, artisanal products, Torrisi showcases "brightly packaged products with names ending in 'o' "—Stella D'oro biscotti, Polly-O ricotta, Progresso bread crumbs. "Nothing from Italy," declares Torrisi in a video on the restaurant's website. "This is American food." Torrisi, and a raft of similar places, offer artful, even playful celebrations of where it all began, at the turn of the twentieth century— the kitchens of poor immigrants entangled between nostalgia and newly found abundance and the shops and humble restaurants of the immigrant entrepreneurs who provided them with the "Italian" food they needed.

See also LITTLE ITALY.

Byock, Lila. "Torrisi Italian Specialties." *New Yorker*, August 2, 2010.

Cinotto, Simone. "Immigrant Tastemakers: Italian Cookbook Writers and the Transnational Formation of Taste in Postindustrial America, 1973–2000." In *Real Italians: Post–World War II Italian Emigration to the United States*, edited by Laura Ruberto and Joseph Sciorra. Urbana: University of Illinois Press, 2015.

Cinotto, Simone. *The Italian American Table: Food, Family, and Community in New York City*. Urbana: University of Illinois Press, 2013.

Hazan, Marcella. *Amarcord: Marcella Remembers*. New York: Gotham, 2009.

Luongo, Pino, and Andrew Friedman. *Dirty Dishes: A Restaurateur's Story of Passion, Pain, and Pasta*. New York: Bloomsbury, 2008.

Simone Cinotto

Italian Ices

Italian ices, also known as water ices, are, despite their name, true New Yorkers. Though similar to Sicilian granita—a simple blend of sugar, water, and juice or flavoring—their smoother texture is closer to sorbet. In Naples, the tradition of making ices dates back to the seventeenth century, and many of those early "gelati" bear a striking resemblance to the Italian ices sold in New York today. Because of their high water content, the New York variant is usually less intense in flavor than a contemporary Italian *sorbetto*, but it is also consequently more refreshing on a muggy summer's day.

Nineteenth-century Italian immigrants brought the ice cream–making tradition to New York, where the ices became a popular treat, typically sold from street carts during summer festivals. To this day, most Italian ice is produced and sold only from March until October. Early versions of New York's Italian ice were mostly available in one or two basic flavors, usually lemon and orange. Today they are produced in at least one hundred flavors including one studded with another iconic New York City treat, Joyva Chocolate Jelly Rings.

From the street carts, ice vendors moved to small shops, often only windows to the sidewalk where long lines still form on hot summer nights. One of the first to do this was Ralph Silvestro, who began selling Italian ice on Staten Island in 1928. Silvestro opened the first retail location of Ralph's Famous Italian Ices there in 1949 and by 2001 had retail locations in all five boroughs (and beyond). In 1944, Nicola Benfaremo began selling lemon and pineapple Italian ices from a stand in Corona, Queens. His son Peter became known as "the Lemon Ice King of Corona," which is now also the unofficial name of the store. The Lemon Ice King of Corona produces over fifty flavors and is known internationally.

Gino Broncanelli began producing Italian ice in Brooklyn in the late 1950s. Gino's Italian Ice is now one of the most iconic wholesale brands in New York City, available almost exclusively in pizzerias. Gino's does not advertise or have a website, and only the familiar white signs with orange boarder and now fading blue letters identify locations. Gino's Italian Ice is still made in its original location in Sunset Park, Brooklyn. On a larger scale, taking Italian ice as far away as China, is Marino's Italian Ice. Marinos Vourderis, a Greek immigrant, introduced Marino's Italian Ices at the World's Fair in 1964. Since then, it has grown to be the largest producer of Italian ice in the world, with all production taking place in their Olympic Ice Cream factory in Richmond Hill, Queens.

Today, neighborhood favorites still thrive. Late-twentieth century newcomers such as Uncle Louie G's and Rita's Italian Ice keep the allure of Italian ice on a hot summer day very much alive on the streets of New York.

See also ITALIAN and STREET VENDORS.

Goldberg, Elyssa. "Frozen in Time." *BKLYNR*, no. 17 (December 5, 2013). http://bklynr.com/frozen-in-time.

Granof, Victoria. *Sweet Sicily: The Story of an Island and Her Pastries*. New York: HarperCollins, 2001.

Mosco, Tom. "A History of Sicilian Cuisine: Sicilian Food II; History." University of Massachusetts Journalism. http://www.umass.edu/journal/sicilyprogram/sicilianfoodhistory.html.

Annette Tomei

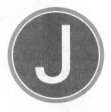

Jack Dempsey's

Heavyweight boxing champ Jack Dempsey, known as "The Manassa Mauler," opened a restaurant at West Fiftieth Street and Eighth Avenue in 1932, across from the old Madison Square Garden where he had some of his greatest triumphs in the ring. In 1938, he opened a second and larger place, Jack Dempsey's Bar, in the Brill Building, 1619 Broadway, which was known as the hub of the music industry—the new Tin Pan Alley. For many years the Broadway eatery was successful, but when Jack Dempsey moved to California it began to fail.

In 1940, entrepreneur Jack Amiel, after having several successful restaurants at the 1939 World's Fair, opened The Turf Restaurant and Bar on the corner of West Forty-Ninth Street and Broadway, also in the Brill Building and right next door to Dempsey's. The Turf was unique for its time, a the-atrical experience for passersby on Broadway. When they looked into the large curved floor-to-ceiling window, they saw a chef cooking on a grill with flames shooting in the air. The Turf became a hangout for the music industry—with its famed "Songwriter's Corner" where sheet music sent from the publishers in the building was pasted on the walls. Frank Sinatra, Ella Fitzgerald, and others were regulars and came in for the renowned cheesecake.

For many years, the two restaurants existed side by side with not much interaction. However, in 1951, Jack Amiel's horse, Count Turf, won the Kentucky Derby, and the restaurant that had been a hangout for showbiz types now attracted sports figures and writers. Amiel himself became a celebrity and was known as the unofficial "mayor of Broadway." The partners next door began to take notice.

Over the years, Amiel had been asked to take over the failing Dempsey's, but now he agreed to do so only if Dempsey moved back to New York. Surprisingly, Dempsey agreed, and that is when Jack Dempsey's Restaurant became a tourist destination and an American institution. The interior became famous, too, with its huge circular bar in the center of the room and photographic murals on the walls of famous boxers on one side and horse racing on the other, including Count Turf winning at Churchill Downs. The highlight was a painting of the 1923 Dempsey vs. Firpo fight, completed by George Wesley Bellows the following year. The restaurant appeared in many films: *Requiem for a Heavyweight* (1962) was shot there, as well as *A Bronx Tale* (1993) and *Somebody Up There Likes Me* (2012). In *The Godfather* (1972), Al Pacino, as Michael Corleone, stands in front of the place waiting to be picked up.

The restaurant was revived when Amiel brought his vast knowledge in running the place, upgraded the menu, and baked his renowned Turf cheesecake on the premises (now known as "Jack Dempsey's cheesecake"). Jack Dempsey sat in the window greeting people, signing autographs, and taking photos with customers. Jack Amiel and Jack Dempsey were business partners for nearly twenty years and were also great friends. In 1973, the Brill family lost their ninety-nine-year lease, and all the commercial leases in the building were null and void. The new landlords, the Downing Corporation (rumored to be England's royal family), doubled and tripled the rents and many tenants were forced out. The restaurant held on as long as it could but finally closed in 1974. The only trace left of those special and exciting times on Broadway is a sign on the corner of West Forty-Ninth Street. It is called "Jack Dempsey Way."

Clark, Alfred E. "Jack Dempsey's Restaurant Is Closing; Original Dempsey's Recalled." *New York Times*, October 6, 1974.

Linda Amiel Burns

Jackson Heights

The foodways of Jackson Heights have always represented the cultures of its resident population, and its restaurants, grocery stores, and butchers all encourage contact among the people of myriad ethnicities who live and shop in the community. Now a neighborhood of nearly 180,000 people, Jackson Heights is located in northwest Queens, bounded to the north by Astoria Boulevard, to the east by Ninety-Fourth Street, to the south by Roosevelt Avenue, and to the west by the Brooklyn-Queens Expressway.

Early Twentieth Century

In 1909, the Queensboro Corporation—led by manager and, later, president Edward A. MacDougall—began purchasing 325 acres of farmland between Woodside and Elmhurst with the express intention of creating a middle-class residential community. The land was developed according to an innovative design model based on single- and two-family houses and apartment buildings built around large communal gardens. In fifteen years, Jackson Heights was the largest planned garden community in the country, replete with golf courses (and nearby Casino Grill), tennis courts (and adjacent tea room), and three commercial districts serviced by rapid transit.

The Queensboro Corporation also offered cooperative ownership of apartments; this, along with restrictive residential and commercial policies, helped shape the early character of the neighborhood, with restaurants and food shops reflecting the culinary interests of the largely middle-class, Caucasian, Protestant residents. In keeping with mainstream American tastes, there was a Schrafft's, a Woolworth's with a luncheon counter, a Horn & Hardart's, several bakeries (including Hanscom's and Shelley's, both branches of New York mini-chains), a Fanny Farmer's, butchers, soda shops, candy stores, and small independent lunch counters. During the wars, common lands were developed as victory gardens, worked by the residents of the community.

Post–World War II

Shifting demographics in the city and the post–World War II housing boom transformed the landscape of the neighborhood. As the Queensboro Corporation developed or sold off much of the common spaces to outside developers, restrictive policies for the newer buildings were relaxed and the population changed. Food also diversified, and new restaurants, butchers, fish stores, groceries, newspaper and candy stores, and delicatessens were added, often owned by previously excluded, second-generation, upwardly mobile Jews and Catholics (particularly Irish and Italians from the nearby working-class neighborhoods of Corona and East Elmhurst) who could now afford to purchase their own homes.

Among the restaurants and stores at the time were Arthur Treacher's, Chock full o'Nuts, and Toddle House (all short-order chain restaurants); Wexler's, Feldman's, and Ellie's (independent appetizing stores); ice cream and candy shops; Wolkes (German), Jahn's (still in operation), and Barracini (Italian); and cuisine-oriented restaurants, such as Dragon Seed ("Exotic Polynesian-Chinese," 1949–1993), The Green Lodge (Turkish-owned American restaurant, closed mid-1960s), Luigi's Italian Restaurant (in operation until 2005), and Cavalier Restaurant (featuring continental cuisine, 1950–2010).

The Hart-Celler Act (1965)

The Immigration and Nationality Act of 1965, also known as the Hart-Cellar Act, marked a radical break from previous national immigration policy that would lead to profound demographic changes in America. By abolishing the quota system based on national origin, the law opened doors to increasing numbers of immigrants from Asia, Africa, the Middle East, and Latin America. The Jackson Heights community would come to reflect this new diversity, aided, in part, by the Fair Housing Act (1968) as well as the public transportation hub of Seventy-Fourth Street–Roosevelt Avenue, which offered access to an affordable city neighborhood—one with open apartment layouts and gardens along with a destination neighborhood for shopping—for these new immigrants. Stores and restaurants catering to and supporting the growing populations of South and East Asians (initially, largely Chinese) appeared, and Jackson Heights began to gain a reputation for international cuisine, most notably Indian.

Though only named "Little India" in 1994 by Mayor David Dinkins, there had been an Indian American population in Jackson Heights for over twenty years. See LITTLE INDIA. In 1973, the commercial district was introduced to Sam and Raj, an electronics and Indian goods store that quickly led to the development of Seventy-Fourth Street between Roosevelt and Thirty-Seventh Avenues as a center for Indian products (food and otherwise), along with several restaurants. Taking over an established diner, the Jackson Diner would serve standard diner fare with sides of *chole*, a spicy chickpea stew, and other southern Indian specialties until the menu became entirely Indian.

As with many ethnic enclaves in New York, there was a large enough customer base to support regional cuisines, including Mumbai, Bengali, or Nepalese–Indian blends, and culinary specialties, such as tandooris (yogurt-marinated baked meats), dosas (thin pancakes made from fermented rice and lentil batter folded around vegetables), chaats (savory snacks), or sweets such as *gulab janum* (syrup-drenched fried dough) and *kheer*, Indian rice pudding. Despite the moniker and the concentration of commercial establishments, such as the Chicago-based grocery and produce chain Patel Brothers, only 6 percent of the current population in Jackson Heights identifies as Indian. Most of the recent immigration from South Asia has been from Bangladesh and Pakistan; altogether they represent 22 percent of the overall Asian population.

More than half (56.5 percent) of the residents of Jackson Heights are of Hispanic origin, and the restaurants, stores, and markets lining Roosevelt Avenue, Northern Boulevard, and parts of Thirty-Seventh Avenue have turned them into the main Latino commercial corridors in the neighborhood. An early establishment was Despaña, which started in 1971 as a chorizo factory and has since grown into an importer of Spanish goods.

A large influx of immigrants arrived in the 1980s from several Central American, Caribbean, and South American countries, mainly Colombia, Ecuador, Peru, and Mexico. The effect on the foodstuffs was immediate: *panaderias* (bakeries), *pelaterias* (ices and ice cream shops), *empanaderias* (specializing in empanadas and other street foods), small restaurants, bars, and bodegas proliferated, each with its own regional flourishes. A particularly diverse market is Los Paisanos, which sells foodstuffs from several countries,

including indigenous fresh, dried, and frozen ingredients that are difficult to find in any other neighborhood. Food trucks have been another local phenomenon, present around the train stations at the three main neighborhood stops as well as at local markets and playgrounds. Several entrepreneurs have gone on to open brick-and-mortar stores.

Current

As of 2012, Jackson Heights had the second highest percentage of internationally born residents in the city; nearly 64 percent were born outside the United States. Besides the nationalities already mentioned, there are pockets of Thais, Filipinos, Koreans, Tibetans, Nepalese, Dominicans, Puerto Ricans, Guyanans, Argentines, and Cubans. Restaurants specializing in these cuisines and more abound. Although there are six supermarkets in the neighborhood, there is also easy access to local produce: Jackson Heights hosts the largest and busiest Greenmarket (urban farmers' market operated by the nonprofit GrowNYC) in Queens, as well as a weekly, seasonal community supported agriculture from eastern Long Island. Chains like McDonald's, Taco Bell, Burger King, and Starbucks are among the other restaurants, wine shops, and cafes dotting the neighborhood. Many, like the patisserie Cannelle, are owned by recent immigrants. Local grocery stores still flourish, providing goods—both specialized and quotidian—and making them accessible to all.

See also ASTORIA and QUEENS.

Jackson Heights Life (blog). http://www.jacksonheightslife.com/community.
Karatzas, Daniel. *Jackson Heights, a Garden in the City: The History of America's First Garden and Cooperative Apartment Community*. New York: Jackson Heights Beautification Group, 1990.
Napoli, Philip. "Jackson Heights: Indians." Seminar 2: The Peopling of New York. Brooklyn College. http://macaulay.cuny.edu/eportfolios/napoli13/indian_nyc.

Lisa DeLange and Alan Houston

Jamaica (Queens)

Founded in 1655, Jamaica is one of New York's oldest neighborhoods. Always a commercial center surrounded by homes inhabited by a range of residents with varied economic statuses, the town was built up around King's Highway—later Jamaica Plank

Road, the original names for Jamaica Avenue—an early American trail predating European settlement that developed into a toll road between Hempstead, Long Island, and Brooklyn's East River ferries. The main thoroughfares are Hillside Avenue, Jamaica Avenue, and Archer Avenue, which are crossed by Merrick Boulevard, Parsons Boulevard, Guy Brewer Boulevard, and Sutphin Boulevard. "Jamaica" is an anglicized version of "Yameca" or "Jameco," the tribe that was in the area and the Algonquin word for "beaver," the quintessential animal of trade and food of colonial America.

Chosen as the county seat in 1683, the town's industries were always a mixture of government (in the form of several courthouses and social services), stores, schools, libraries, and transportation. Developing along with the commuter and transportation aspects of the neighborhood was a mixture of independently owned shops. The nineteenth-century feed and exchange stores, such as Beers Cornell and later J & T Adikes', supported the farmers bringing goods from eastern Long Island to Queens, Brooklyn, and Manhattan. The Long Island Railroad service, which ran through Jamaica starting in 1836 and was electrified in 1886, also made Jamaica a central gathering location in Queens. In May 1895, no less than fifteen liquor licenses were issued to hotels and stores in Jamaica; also that year, Schwarzschild and Sulzberger, one of the largest meat packers and purveyors in the country at the time, opened a branch boasting the capability of shipping anywhere in New York, presumably from their central location. The Elmhurst Cream Company sold milk in glass bottles stamped with "Jamaica."

Photographs from the early twentieth century show many small grocery stores, bakeries, and lunch counters, clearly catering to the more recent German, Jewish, and Italian residents; shoppers; and commuters joining the older Dutch, English, and Irish in the area. Although there were a few national chains sprinkled on the main thoroughfares of Jamaica and Hillside Avenues (notably Woolworth's), smaller, independent lunch counters such as Spooner's, Maple Grove Summer Garden, Dixie Restaurant, Old Corner Restaurant and Grill, The Judge's Chop House, and Happy's Diner, serving popular fare, such as chop suey, oysters, and lunch plates as well as delicatessens (Walter's, Warren's Table Luxuries) and taverns (Beinbrick's Saloon, Hewlett Creed Tavern, Hillside Tavern [still open], Monument Tavern, Archer Restaurant and Bar, Locust Inn, and Caleb Weeks's Giraffe Tavern) abounded. Also along the avenues were single-product grocery stores, like Leo's Market, Fulton Dairy, Mondon Fish Market, Jamaica Market Prime Meats, William Roth's Meat Market, and Lindy's Food Market, as well as a few kosher markets. In 1930, Michael J. Cullen leased a vacant garage and turned it into the country's first supermarket, King Kullen.

With suburban expansion north into Westchester and farther into eastern Long Island, large retailers began to move out into surrounding suburbs where business was more profitable (and there was more area for parking), following the path of many middle-class residents in the latter half of the twentieth century. In the 1980s, there were some important developments: the U.S. Food and Drug Administration established its Northeast Regional Laboratory at York College, training students to become inspectors, and the Greater Jamaica Development Corporation founded a shopping center with Queens-based vendors and a farmers' market (run in conjunction with Down to Earth Markets).

Currently, Jamaica is the largest and most densely populated neighborhood in central Queens, with approximately seventy-seven thousand residents. Jamaica has a long tradition of civil rights advocacy, due in no small part to longtime resident, diplomat, and senator Rufus King (1755–1827) and his son, John. The population has always included large numbers of blacks and some West Indians who attended schools and lived around Rufus Manor from the 1800s. Data from the 1980 census report a 63 percent black population. During the 1990s and early 2000s, the neighborhood began to attract more immigrants from the Caribbean (Guyanese, Trinidadian, Jamaican, Haitian), South and Central America (Ecuadorian, Colombian, Salvadoran, Honduran, Guatemalan), and South Asia (Sri Lankan and Bangladeshi). Shops, bakeries, meat markets, grocery stores, and restaurants clustered along Jamaica and Hillside Avenues are run by, and provide foodstuffs to, people of these various ethnicities. Many are smaller, individual establishments, serving lunch at counters and snacks, in the form of arepas, double-doubles, aloo pies, patties, rotis, kebabs, tamales, *platos tipicos*, *pupusas*, and *fritailles*, still catering to the commercial, civic, banking, and recreational center that is Jamaica.

See also QUEENS.

Copquin, Claudia Gryvatz. *The Neighborhoods of Queens.* New Haven, Conn.: Yale University Press, 2007.

Photographs: Jamaica (New York, NY). The Archives at Queens Library. Jamaica, N.Y.

Smith, Andrew F. *New York City: A Food Biography.* Lanham, Md.: Rowman & Littlefield, 2013.

Lisa DeLange and Alan Houston

Jamaican

Jamaican culture, largely defined by its food, is a rich mixture of ethnic dishes enjoyed at all social levels. Jamaica's complex history resulted in a "melting pot" cuisine, borrowing predominantly from the best of British, Spanish, Chinese, and Indian foods. Whether in Brooklyn, Queens, or the Bronx one can find restaurants serving faithful renditions from the classic Jamaican culinary repertoire.

From a small number of immigrants in the 1920s, New York has become home to the largest Jamaican community in the United States, making up the third largest ethnic group in the city at approximately two hundred thousand persons. Proud of its heritage, these communities demonstrate their cultural identity with dishes reflecting the island's history, beginning with the influence of the Spanish, who occupied and controlled Jamaica from 1509 until the British captured the island in 1655.

This early influence gave Jamaica escoveitch fish—a partly cooked, partly marinated favorite—and the ubiquitous "patty," a pastry-wrapped, hand-held meat pie. These occupiers also imported a variety of domestic animals, with pigs and goats fairing the best. These imports led to jerked pork, curried goat, and mannish water (a celebratory "soup" made mainly with the goat's head and intestines).

The arrival of the British drove the remaining population up into the mountains. Here they partly survived on wild hogs, developing the jerk process of tenderizing, slow cooking, and preservation. Today chicken, fish, seafood, and even tofu are also marinated in this time-honored way. Rubbed in a mixture of scotch bonnet pepper, thyme, scallion, pimento (allspice), and other ingredients, these items are slowly cooked over charcoal and pimento or sweet-wood on "pans" (fifty-five-gallon oil drums cut in half) throughout New York's Jamaican neighborhoods.

The demands of sustaining Jamaica as a huge sugar plantation required feeding a burgeoning population. Foods that were both inexpensive and transportable were required. British sailors and explorers brought breadfruit, mangoes, and coconut plants from the South Pacific, while dried and salted fish, salt beef, and pickled pork parts were imported from America and Britain as part of the rum and sugar trade. These all became part of the culinary lexicon. Additionally, less desirable cuts of locally slaughtered cattle such as the oxtails and offal, passed over by the gentry, were often cooked in one pot, over a charcoal fire. This "one-pot cookery" style still dominates today, with complex dishes such as oxtail and beans, stewed peas (red beans) with pigtail, cow foot soup, or fish tea, often containing "ground provisions" (potatoes, yam, dasheen, etc.) and flour dumplings. With changing times workers from India and China were brought in as indentured servants. They brought their own cooking styles and spices, rounding out the classic Jamaican cookbook.

While this deeply indigenous cuisine, embraced by many chefs throughout New York, is often replicated traditionally in high-street restaurants, it is also being reinterpreted in a contemporary manner, translating the complex flavors of "one-pot dishes" in a more approachable way. Renditions such as oxtail ravioli, butter bean cassoulet, and curried goat shepherd's pie are served at the Rookery in Bushwick. Miss Lilly's, in SoHo, blends salmon with jerk, bok choy, and coconut-flavored mashed sweet potatoes. The Spur Tree Lounge on the Lower East Side draws on the Asian influences with Red Stripe "peppered" shrimp tempura and coconut curried kingfish or Caribbean

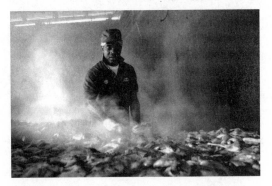

"Jerk" is a Jamaican dish that can consist of chicken (pictured here) or any grilled meat or vegetable marinated in a selection of spices, most commonly including chili, onion, ginger, and allspice, with a sauce made from soy sauce, brown sugar, and sometimes a citrus juice. PUSHCARTFOODS.COM

tapas; each demonstrating both the deep cultural roots and the modern applications that are possible.

While traditional and contemporary abound in a multitude of restaurants peppered throughout the diaspora, Jamaican flavors permeate the home kitchen too. A wide variety of sauces, salsas, jams, and marinades, each capturing the exotic flavors of the island, can be found in supermarkets and gourmet stores throughout the five boroughs, offering an opportunity to "taste Jamaica" at home as well as on the street.

See also RASTAFARI.

Black, Clinton. *History of Jamaica*. London: Harper-Collins, 1988.
Harris, Jessica B. *Sky Juice and Flying Fish*. New York: Simon & Schuster, 1991.
Murrell, N. Samuel. "Jamaican Americans." Countries and Their Cultures. http://www.everyculture.com/multi/Ha-La/Jamaican-Americans.html.
Niederhauser, Andre, and Bill Moore, eds. *A Sample of Modern Caribbean Cuisine*. Coral Gables, Fl.: Caribbean Hotel and Tourism Association, 2013.
Rosseau, Suzanne, and Michelle Rosseau. *Caribbean Potluck*. London: Kyle, 2014.

Bill Moore

James Beard Awards

The James Beard Awards, frequently referred to as the "Oscars of the food world," are prestigious honors bestowed annually to members of the food industry, from chefs and restaurateurs to designers, sommeliers, journalists, and authors. The yearly ceremony furthers the mission of the James Beard Foundation and the passion of James Beard: to recognize and celebrate American cooking. The awards are widely regarded as one of the highest honors in the industry, with a Beard medallion serving as a symbol of excellence. The foundation has created a separate Leadership Awards program with the goal of honoring visionaries working in business, nonprofits, government, and education to create a more healthful, sustainable, and safe food world. With this addition, the James Beard Awards have grown to encompass not only the interpretive potential of fine dining but also the power of American chefs, the culinary industry, and thought leaders to address the pleasures and practicalities of eating and cooking in America.

The awards were established in 1990, combining two of the most prestigious food awards in the country: The Who's Who of Cooking in America (originated by *Cook's* magazine in 1984) and the Food and Beverage Book Awards (originated by R.T. French Co. as the R.T. French Tastemaker Awards in 1966), with the new James Beard Restaurant and Chef Awards. With the foundation becoming more publicly visible in both New York City and the nation at large, the awards were seen as an opportunity to further promote its mission of highlighting the progress of American cuisine by honoring its best and brightest.

The first James Beard Awards took place on May 6, 1991, during the foundation's annual Beard Birthday Fortnight celebration, which was held each year around James Beard's birthday. Sponsored by Seagram's and Champagne Perrier-Jouët, the first ceremony was on the yacht the M.S. *New Yorker*, with one thousand people in attendance and thirty awards handed out. Ruth Reichl, then working for the *Los Angeles Times*, commented that "if the M.S. New Yorker…had sunk, it would have taken American cooking along with it." Among the notable awards, Wolfgang Puck, the first chef to cook dinner at the Beard House (back in 1987), took home Outstanding Chef; New York City's Bouley won Outstanding Restaurant; and James Beard's longtime friend M. F. K. Fisher received the first Lifetime Achievement Award. A reception followed, featuring food from fifteen chefs, a tradition that has continued and expanded as the awards have increased in prominence and scope.

The current structure of the James Beard Awards covers six recognition programs, in addition to the Leadership Awards: Books; Broadcast and New Media; Journalism; Design; Restaurant and Chef; and Special Achievement awards including the Who's Who of Food and Beverage in America, Lifetime Achievement, and Humanitarian of the Year. The Books and Broadcast and New Media Awards are held a few days prior to the main ceremony. Over their history they have evolved to recognize shifts in media and now include honors for video webcasts and online journalism (first awarded in 2000).

The most widely recognized awards are those in the Restaurant and Chef program, which include the categories of Outstanding Restaurateur; Outstanding Chef; Outstanding Restaurant; Rising Star Chef of the Year; Best New Restaurant; Outstanding Pastry Chef; Outstanding Service; Outstanding Wines, Beer, or Spirits Professional; Outstanding Wine Program; Outstanding Bar Program; and Best Regional Chef (for ten defined regions of the United States). Past recipients include some of the most high-profile celebrity chefs and the most popular restaurants across the country, such as Mario Batali, David Chang, Thomas Keller, Alice Waters, The French Laundry, Alinea, and Eleven Madison Park.

The program is overseen by the Restaurant and Chef Awards Committee, one of the six independent committees assigned to each awards program. Each committee includes professionals in the industry who volunteer to serve one- to three-year terms during which they are ineligible for nomination in their program. The Restaurant and Chef Awards Committee also selects each year's recipients of the America's Classics awards, which honor local community restaurant gems, such as John's Roast Pork in Philadelphia, Prince's Hot Shack in Nashville, and Keens Steakhouse in New York City.

The growth of the James Beard Awards in the American cultural consciousness mirrors the rise of food's significance in pop culture. The third annual awards, held in 1994 at the Marriott Marquis in Times Square, aired on the burgeoning Food Network. In 2005, the awards were dedicated to the culinary icon Julia Child, who had died the previous year. The stage was fully decorated in pale green pegboard, ladles, and pots and pans in an homage to her cooking show sets and hosted by Child's friend, CBS anchor Charles Gibson.

In 2007 the awards outgrew its decade-long home at the Marriott Marquis and moved to Lincoln Center, a testament to its large footprint in New York City. Lincoln Center has served as the home base for the awards as they continue to celebrate the ebb and flow of the American culinary scene. In 2011, an increased awareness of the problems within our food system led to new Journalism Award categories encompassing writing on the environment, food politics, policy, and health and nutrition, while in 2012 the Restaurant and Chef Awards, in recognition of the resurgence of bespoke cocktails, gave its first award for Outstanding Bar Program.

The awards have also served as a larger reflection on contemporary American society, reacting to events both local and national. In 2002, the Humanitarian of the Year Award was given to the New York City restaurant community for their efforts to help the city recover in the wake of September 11; in 2006 the same award was presented to a group of twenty New Orleans chefs for their work in the recovery of the city post–Hurricane Katrina. The stage was ornately decorated with a backdrop of city street signs rented from local Louisiana vendors, and the reception included New Orleans chefs cooking local fare alongside an exhibit from the Southern Food and Beverage Museum that explored how the restaurant community worked to support the city after Katrina. And in a time when the gender gap remains a hot-button issue, the 2009 awards ceremony was notable for its theme of Women in Food, which featured an all-female reception showcasing the talents of some of the most prominent female chefs, sommeliers, mixologists, and artisanal producers from across the country.

The annual call for entries begins each October on the James Beard Foundation's website, with up to thirty semifinalists in each of the Restaurant and Chef categories announced the following February. The five nominees in each category are announced in March. In recent years the semifinalist and nominee announcements have taken place in notable food centers across the country, such as Chicago and Las Vegas. The 2015 James Beard Awards will be the first to take place outside of New York City, with the awards celebrating their twenty-fifth anniversary at the Lyric Opera of Chicago.

See also BEARD, JAMES and JAMES BEARD FOUNDATION.

"The James Beard Awards." James Beard Foundation. http://www.jamesbeard.org/awards.
Reichl, Ruth. "Food Oscars:…The Envelope, Please." *Los Angeles Times*, May 16, 1991.
Swanson, Stevenson. "Memories of Julia Child Infuse Culinary Awards." *Chicago Tribune*, May 11, 2005.

Maggie E. Borden

James Beard Foundation

The James Beard Foundation is a nonprofit, membership organization that supports the overall culture of American cuisine. Best known for the annual James Beard Awards and the nearly nightly dinners at the James Beard House in Greenwich Village, the foundation also provides scholarships and hosts an annual food conference and leadership awards ceremony. In recent years, the foundation has added chef boot camps to foster better engagement and dialogue about issues of food systems and culture in the chef community, as well as sponsoring an annual national food festival highlighting the diversity of regional American cooking, all in pursuit of its mission

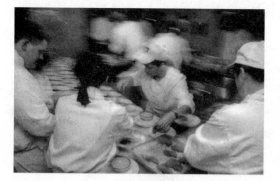

The James Beard Foundation has helped launch the careers of hundreds of young chefs, often showcasing their talents at fundraisers and near-nightly dinners held at the James Beard House in Greenwich Village.
BEARD FOUNDATION

to "celebrate, nurture, and honor America's diverse culinary heritage through programs that educate and inspire."

The establishment of the foundation was a tribute to American cooking icon James Beard (1903–1985). At the International Association of Cooking Professionals conference in March of 1985 (which the late Beard was to have chaired), his close friend Julia Child remarked that action should be taken to continue the legacy of Beard's work and his home, which had served as a meeting place for chefs, fellow cookbook authors, students, and food lovers alike.

Shortly after, Peter Kump, another longtime friend and former student of Beard, embarked on a fundraising campaign to buy the townhouse from the Beard estate, held by Beard's alma mater, Reed College. A coalition of chefs, cooking schools, and fans secured the funds to purchase the house at 167 West Twelfth Street in September 1985, and a certificate of incorporation was then filed for the Culinary Arts Foundation. In July 1986 the organization officially became The James Beard Foundation, with Kump as its first president.

Although Larry Forgione was the first chef to cook at an official gathering in the Beard House (he served hors d'oeuvres at the house's opening), the first fundraising James Beard Foundation dinner took place on January 21, 1987, when the young Wolfgang Puck of Los Angeles's Spago whipped up a menu that included winter greens sautéed with duck livers and grilled salmon with celery cream. Kump was so impressed with the local enthusiasm for the meal that he decided to make dinners at the house a regular

fundraising event, a practice that continues to this day in a format largely unchanged over two decades.

Within a few years, several cornerstones of the foundation began. The James Beard Awards, now considered "the Oscars of food," was announced in 1990, with the first ceremony taking place in May of the following year. Also established in 1991 were the foundation's scholarship program and Chefs & Champagne, a fundraising event held in the Hamptons.

By the mid-1990s the James Beard Foundation was growing in national recognition. A James Beard Award had become a calling card for chefs and cookbook authors, and about one thousand lunches and dinners had been served at the Beard House. Even with the tragic early death of Kump in 1995, the foundation continued to blossom and expand the scope of its membership and programming into the twenty-first century.

The foundation entered a period of substantial instability when a forensic audit in 2004 revealed that Kump's successor as president, Len Pickell, had stolen more than $1 million from the organization. Pickell was eventually arrested and convicted of grand larceny, but his actions brought to light some serious issues with the foundation's finances. In response to these revelations, a number of the awards judges stepped down, and the original board of trustees was forced to resign. Chefs Thomas Keller and Charlie Trotter created an ad hoc advisory board to oversee the transition, led by chair Dorothy Cann Hamilton of the French Culinary Institute (now International Culinary Center). With their help the foundation restructured, forming a new board of trustees, insulating the financing and administration of the awards from the rest of the organization, and hiring Edna K. Morris to serve as interim director. Under the new board of trustees' leadership, the foundation worked to rid itself of the residue of the scandal and reestablish its brand as the "gold standard for American cuisine." Despite the setbacks of the previous year, the 2005 James Beard Awards were a rousing success, paying tribute to the late Julia Child with a replica of her TV kitchen on stage.

The 2005 awards proved to be the turning point for the James Beard Foundation, the fallout from the scandal providing an opportunity to refocus the organization's mission. In 2006, Susan Ungaro, former editor-in-chief of *Family Circle*, was named the foundation's president, and she ushered in a new era dedicated to transforming the foundation into a modern, forward-looking nonprofit. The foundation underwent changes large and small, from the renovation of the Beard House kitchen to bring in restaurant-quality appliances in 2006 to the establishment of the first Taste America national food festival in 2007, in honor of the organization's twentieth anniversary.

Recognizing the growing cultural awareness of food and cooking, the James Beard Foundation has expanded its programming into both the educational and entertainment sectors. The foundation's first Annual Food Conference took place in Washington, DC, in 2010 and focused on issues of sustainability and public health. Now in its fifth year, the Food Conference coincides with the foundation's Leadership Awards, which recognize innovators who are working toward a healthier food system. The foundation also began the Chefs Boot Camp for Policy and Change in 2012, with the goal of providing advocacy and media training for civically and politically minded chefs so that they can be more effective leaders for food-system change. Partnering with the U.S. State Department, the foundation formed the American Chef Corps in September 2012, with the mission of furthering international diplomacy through American culinary initiatives. In 2015, the foundation partnered with the Friends of the USA Pavilion at World Expo Milano to create an interactive exhibition with the theme "American Food 2.0: United to Feed the Planet."

The foundation has also expanded its media presence by adding online newsletters and a blog to its portfolio of calendar and editorial publications, beginning in 2009 with a live blogging of the awards. Yet at its heart the James Beard Foundation remains a member-based organization grounded by its program of dinners at the James Beard House. Membership remains robust, with forty-five hundred members and over two hundred dinners a year. The James Beard House provides a performance space for chefs to showcase their own interpretation of the ever-evolving cuisine championed by the foundation's namesake, the purest display of the foundation's original mission to cultivate and celebrate American cooking. The increasingly international roster of chefs that enter the house's kitchen reflects the James Beard Foundation's enduring position within the food industry. As it enters its third decade, the foundation has extended its reach from its humble roots in Greenwich Village to a global position as the respected custodian of the heritage of American cuisine.

See also BEARD, JAMES and JAMES BEARD AWARDS.

Finn, Robin. "The New Chief Cook and Bottle Washer in Beard's House." *New York Times*, June 2, 2006.
"Foundation History." James Beard Foundation. http://www.jamesbeard.org/about/history.
Hamlin, Suzanne. "Beard House: Promoting Culinary Arts and Itself." *New York Times*, April 24, 1996.
Moskin, Julia. "A New Leader for Beard Foundation." *New York Times*, February 23, 2005.

Maggie E. Borden

Japanese

Prior to the 1950s, New York had a small Japanese population. Much has changed since World War II, notably the influence, acceptance, and popularity of Japanese culture and cuisine. At first, Japanese immigrants would have been more commonly found residing in Southern California, within small fishing communities along the coast. The modest Japanese community in New York before World War II experienced the same adversity as other immigrant groups; moreover, an increasingly volatile geopolitical landscape alongside xenophobic sentiments produced unfavorable conditions for introducing Japanese cuisine to New York.

After Japan's economic recovery from the war, Japanese businessmen began commuting to New York to meet and do business with American corporations. Eventually, these businessmen would immigrate to New York, some even bringing their families to settle for extended, if not permanent, stays. These professionals demanded authentic, high-quality Japanese cuisine. Accordingly, chefs and sushi masters flew in to settle, open restaurants, and feed their hungry compatriots. Japanese nationals continue to immigrate to New York (as of the 2000 census over half of the 37,279 people of Japanese ancestry who live in New York live in New York City), and they crave their home cuisine.

The first Japanese restaurant to open in New York (and, arguably, one of the first in the United States) was Fuji Sushi, which opened in 1954 near Columbus Circle, where it still serves (an admittedly dwindling) clientele of tourists and longtime "old faithful" customers. And the first Japanese restaurant to serve raw sushi to New Yorkers would be Nippon, which opened in 1963. At the time eating sushi would have been considered a unique and adventurous dining experience exclusive to businessmen, celebrities, and

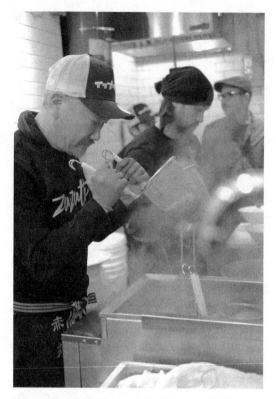

Shigemi Kawahara, known as the "Ramen King," is the founder of Ippudo Ramen, one of the first ramen noodle spots to open in New York. Ramen is a staple of Japanese cuisine and can be prepared with ingredients such as vegetables, meats, eggs, and a flavored stock.
IPPUDO RAMEN

cosmopolitans but not the "average" American diner. Today, Fuji Sushi has opened locations in other cities throughout the Northeast and, like other successful sushi establishments, has expanded its business model to include catering large-scale sushi orders for events and parties.

Japanese food establishments now are quite common inside and outside the city. In fact, Fuji Sushi is likely low on the list of places you should dine to experience high-quality, authentic Japanese cuisine. Despite its current popularity, sushi and Japanese food in general did not initially receive the widespread recognition it deserved. In fact, it is only since the 1970s (thanks to advances in refrigeration techniques) that authentically prepared Japanese cuisine, using raw fish as its main ingredient, was really made available outside of Japan. Of course, even if it were available, it is unlikely New Yorkers would have consumed raw fish until it became acceptable and

fashionable to do so. In 1963, the New York Times food editor Craig Claiborne wrote that sushi and sashimi were "a trifle too 'far out' for many American palettes." Over a half-century later, the American palette has grown to appreciate sushi. There are now sushi establishments throughout the city, which can range from the expensive and exclusive to the affordable and pedestrian.

Sushi is a popular way of experiencing Japanese cuisine. However, there are a variety of other dishes and dining experiences that have grown in popularity throughout New York. As Kat Odell posted on New York Eater, "Japanese food. There's more to it than sushi and ramen. And naturally, New York, with its gastronomic diversity is host to a multitude of Japanese cuisine."

In the Japanese enclave of Astoria, Queens, one can visit a handful of Japanese spots to sample a variety of affordable dishes. For example, the Family Market on Broadway sells bento boxes (with fish, daikon radish, pickled vegetables, rice, seaweed salad) alongside *onigiri* snacks (folded, triangle-shaped rice wedges, wrapped in *nori* seaweed and filled with fish or pickled *ume*) from out of a large cold case to go. The Family Market also sells an assortment of Japanese beers (e.g., Asahi, Kirin, Sapporo), teas, salted snacks, and sweets. The store itself is open late and usually bustling with young Japanese nationals, commuters on their way home from work, and students— all looking for a quick, healthy, and convenient bite to eat. Unlike American fast food, Japanese food is made with fresh ingredients: rice, vegetables, and seafood.

Just up the street, on the same block, is a popular ramen noodle spot called Tamashii. Like traditional ramen noodle bars found throughout Japan, Tamashii has a quick customer turnover rate and seats diners close to maximize space. When you enter Tamashii, the smell of simmering wheat noodles in large pots of chicken, fish, or pork stock welcomes you. Ramen can be served with pork, seasoned boiled eggs, scallions, and bean sprouts. Diners who have yet to experience dining in a noodle bar should know it is customary to slurp (often loudly) when consuming this warm dish.

Like sushi establishments, ramen noodle spots have become increasingly popular throughout the city, some for their affordability and convenience (such as Tamashii), especially with lunchtime crowds and working professionals, others for their reputation, such as old-school players like Ippudo in the East Village, directed by the "the Ramen king," Shigemi Kawahara, who competes with "hipper," American-run joints, like Ivan Ramen. Ippudo is classified as one of the first ramen noodle spots to open in New York. Chef Kawahara opened Ippudo in 2008 in the East Village and continues to explore the possibilities and potential of ramen by working under the banner "keep changing, to remain unchanged."

For diners looking for a more refined and traditional experience, one should "belly up" to the bar at a favorite Japanese spot and request the *omakase*, or chef's choice. In such cases, diners will be subjected to a string of delicate dishes, each designed to enhance and complement the one before. The experience is not just reserved for the palette alone. As Michael Ashkenazi describes in *Food Culture in Japan*, the "presentation of Japanese food is strongly orientated toward the visual. A diner expects the food not only to *taste* good, but also to be visually appealing…at its best, [Japanese food] is an overwhelming sensory aesthetic experience."

Ashkenazi, Michael, and Jeanne Jacob. *Food Culture in Japan*. Westport, Conn.: Greenwood, 2003.
Avey, Tori. "Discover the History of Sushi." *The History Kitchen*, September 5, 2012. http://www.pbs.org/food/the-history-kitchen/history-of-sushi.
Odell, Kat. "The 19 Styles of Japanese Cuisine Found in New York." Eater NY, August 7, 2014. http://ny.eater.com/2014/8/7/6183575/the-19-styles-of-japanese-cuisine-found-in-new-york.
Smith, Andrew F. *American Tuna: The Rise and Fall of an Improbable Food*. Berkeley: University of California Press, 2012.
Smith, Andrew F. *New York City: A Food Biography*. Lanham, Md.: Rowman & Littlefield, 2014.

Nicholas Allanach

Jenkins, Steven

See CHEESEMONGERS and FAIRWAY MARKET.

Jewish

Since the late nineteenth century, Jews in New York have operated a vast array of public eating establishments which have been highly visible on the city's streetscape. Many of these restaurants and other food reflected the regional and national diversity of the Jewish immigrants and their children, millions of whom lived in New York City, the largest Jewish population center in America. Jews from various parts of the German-speaking regions of central Europe, as well as Lithuanian, Ukrainian, and Polish Jews, and those from Romania and the Ottoman Empire opened food stores, bakeries, restaurants, cafes, and taverns, catering to the women and men who came from those places as well as to other Jews. Their customers also eventually included non-Jews, who especially in the middle decades of the twentieth century increasingly patronized such places. To many New Yorkers and tourists, New York food largely meant Jewish food, including bagels and cream cheese, sometimes referred to as "a bagel with a *shmear*," the Yiddish word for "spread," as well as delicatessen food. See BAGELS and CREAM CHEESE. Some of these establishments sold kosher food, which conformed to the complex Jewish dietary laws, while others did not. Even if they sold nonkosher food, they still marked their shops and restaurants with words or symbols that connoted Jewishness and sold items, specifically delicatessen food, associated with European Jewish tastes and culture.

Although public places for the buying and selling of Jewish food did not become highly visible until the latter decades of the nineteenth century with the massive influx of Jews from the lands of Eastern Europe, in the centuries before that, stretching back to the late seventeenth century, Jews found ways to satisfy their need for kosher food and built community around food. Until the beginning of the nineteenth century individuals in the tiny Jewish enclave in New York received kosher food, including *matzah*, the unleavened bread required for Passover, from the city's one synagogue, Shearith Israel. In those early years New York did not always have a *shokhet*, or kosher slaughterer, and Jews had to import kosher meat from Jamaica or from some place in Europe. Some Jews, like Hetty Hays, operated boarding houses for single Jewish men, providing kosher meals. Hays came into conflict with the trustees of the synagogue because of rumors that she served ritually impure (*treif*) food to her boarders. Several other women, mostly widows, ran grocery stores, although no evidence exists that they sold primarily to Jews or that they carried food aimed at the Jewish communities of the city, made up of Sephardic (of Spanish-Portuguese background) immigrants and their descendants as well as an increasing number from

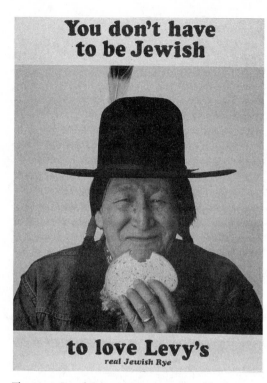

You don't have
to be Jewish

to love Levy's
real Jewish Rye

The iconic Levy's Rye campaign was created by the Doyle Dane Bernbach agency in 1957. People from all different backgrounds were shown in a series of posters enjoying sandwiches on Jewish rye bread, encouraging everyone to eat what had previously been an ethnic food.

northern Europe, Ashkenazim from Poland and the German-speaking states.

With a surge in Jewish immigration after the 1820s, New York's Jewish population grew and diversified. New congregations came into being along with many charitable and other voluntary associations. These institutions relied heavily on dinners and banquets to raise money for their projects. They served food typical of the places they came from, mostly conforming to Jewish dietary law, and invited their members as well as the general public, Jewish and non-Jewish alike, to these food events. These fundraising dinners, some extravagantly catered, may have been the first opportunities for non-Jews in New York to become acquainted with northern European Jewish foods. In this period, until the century's end, countless numbers of Jews, men and women, operated food stores, catering businesses, and taverns. The sources do not indicate if the proprietors of these establishments marked them with Jewish symbols or if they sold food typical of Bavaria, Posen, Bohemia, Lithuania,

and the other places from which so many came. Some stores did sell kosher food as the one synagogue lost its monopoly on the distribution of ritually approved meat and other items governed by Jewish law. The opening of new kosher food venues, however, became a source of community conflict as neither the state nor any organized rabbinic body had the power to prohibit the use of the word "kosher." Observant consumers often found themselves in a quandary as to whose food they could eat.

Like many of the other central Europeans who came to New York in the middle decades of the nineteenth century, a number of Jewish entrepreneurs opened taverns. See TAVERNS. No evidence exists to determine if Jews tended to congregate in those saloons operated by other Jews and if they, likewise, avoided those owned by and frequented by Gentiles. In 1843 a group of young Jewish men, immigrants from Bavaria, gathered at Sinsheimer's, a saloon owned by another Jew. These young men had all been rejected for membership in a Masonic lodge. Sitting at Sinsheimer's they decided to form their own organization, modeled on the Masons. This organization, originally called Bundes Bruder, evolved into B'nai B'rith, the oldest and longest-lasting Jewish organization in the world, one which spread across the nation and the globe. The birth of B'nai B'rith at Sinsheimer's points to Jewish-owned saloons as notable community spaces in the nineteenth century.

The landscape of Jewish food, particularly as consumed in public, transformed and expanded dramatically after the latter part of the nineteenth century and into the twentieth, as the great migration out of Eastern Europe sent millions of Jews to the United States. Most of these immigrants stayed in New York, attracted by the local garment industry, creating there the single largest Jewish city in the world as of 1900. They operated tens of thousands of places to eat in public, as well as butcher shops, bakeries, dairies, fish stores, and other kinds of places where Jews could buy kosher food from their coreligionists to prepare and eat at home.

Jewish food shopping, particularly for meat, fish, and bread, focused on the need to prepare the weekly festive Sabbath meal. While little evidence exists as to what Jewish immigrants ate during the week, the Friday night dinner reigned supreme as the most important, and possibly only, one at which the entire family ate together. That meal typically included a braided challah bread made out of egg dough; gefilte fish with horseradish; chicken soup with noodles, known as *yoikh mit lokshen*; chicken accompanied by kugel, or a pudding made of noodles or potatoes; and a fruit stew, *compot*. Memoirs written by women and men who grew up in New York's Jewish neighborhoods have provided elaborate and sensual detail about these *Shabbos* dinners. Likewise every holiday had its distinctive foods, and Jewish butchers, grocers, fishmongers, and bakers stocked up on the specific items associated with these festivals and holy days.

Jewish immigrants, wherever they came from, had access to foods typical of the places they had left. Romanian Jewish eating establishments like Moskowitz and Lupowitz's on the Lower East Side offered *mamalige*, a starch dish made out of cornmeal, as well as pastrami, dishes made with eggplant, and wine from their many cellars. See PASTRAMI. Isaac Gellis, an immigrant from Germany, introduced kosher sausages and frankfurters in the late 1860s, and hundreds of coffee and cake parlors and dairy restaurants popped up, often operated by Jews from Ukraine. Appetizing shops, owned by Polish Jews, sold smoked and prepared fish dishes and cheeses. See APPETIZING STORES and SMOKED FISH. They tended to sell sweet gefilte fish and herring in sour cream, while shops selling those same items but owned by Jews from Ukraine offered savory gefilte fish and herring in brine. The small community of Jews from parts of Greece, like Janina, who also lived on the Lower East Side, sold their distinctive foods, including olives, eggplant, and a dessert made of sesame called *halavah*. See HALVA.

This kind of ethnic specificity faded in time as Jews living near each other on the Lower East Side and, by the early twentieth century, in Brooklyn neighborhoods like Brownsville and Williamsburg sampled each other's foods and a kind of pan-ethnic New York Jewish cuisine developed, at least in terms of public consumption. Regardless of where Jews may have come from before arriving in New York, they patronized the knish bakery opened by Yonah Schimmel, a Romanian immigrant, on Houston Street in 1890. See YONAH SCHIMMEL KNISH BAKERY. Jacob Harmatz and his brother-in-law, Alex Ratner, opened Ratner's dairy restaurant in 1905, which claimed that it served up to twelve hundred customers a day. These and countless other food spaces, both brick-and-mortar establishments as well as the street vendors who sold hot chickpeas, knishes, bagels, and frank-furters, constituted a crucial element of life on the Jewish street. See KNISH and HOT DOGS. Jewish consumers seemed to have a particular taste for seltzer water, which numerous vendors sold from glass bottles on the streets and delivered in cases of *greptzvasser*, or "belch water," to the tenement dwellers. See SELTZER.

Different Jewish groups tended to congregate in different cafes based on ideology, with socialists, Zionists, and anarchists having their favorite places. The Café Royal on Second Avenue emerged as a particularly favorite spot for actors, playwrights, fans, and others associated with the Yiddish theater which flourished on that street, known as "the Jewish Rialto." New York Jews patronized an array of delicatessens, restaurants, and other places where they could eat out. Although most Jews, until the 1920s, were members of the working class, eating out became such an important part of life that in 1905 Abraham Cahan, the editor of *Forverts*, the most popular Yiddish newspaper, invented the neologism *oysessen*, or "eating out," a word that had not previously existed in the Yiddish lexicon.

Jews in New York also came to be interested in, and tempted by, the foods of other ethnic groups. They gravitated to commercially prepared baked goods and condiments, and American food manufacturers placed daily advertisements translated into Yiddish into the community's newspapers. As early as the 1880s Jewish community leaders, rabbis especially, began to worry about the Jewish interest in Chinese food, which was clearly not kosher. Jewish educational institutions and community centers like the Educational Alliance offered Jewish immigrant women the opportunity to learn how to cook American-style foods. Although these dishes conformed to Jewish dietary laws, as did those included in the Yiddish-language cookbooks published in New York like H. Braun's *The Yiddish Family Cook Book* of 1914, the popularity of the classes revealed an interest in cosmopolitan eating across the boundaries of familiar home foods.

Food in the immigrant neighborhoods became a matter not just of pleasure and culinary adventurousness but also of political conflict. Workers in Jewish bakeries, bagel shops, and butchering establishments all went out on strike, pitting themselves against the Jewish owners who employed them. Jewish housewives, at various times, protested in the street against the high cost of kosher meat, using the tactics of the labor movement against the Jewish butchers, the slaughterers, and even the rabbis who supervised the provision of kosher meat.

Even after the 1920s and the end of the mass Jewish immigration to the United States and the movement of the children of the immigrants into the middle class and into new neighborhoods, the Lower East Side functioned as a mecca for Jewish eating. Jews living uptown and in the other boroughs, as well as Jewish visitors from outside of New York, flocked to the Lower East Side to experience the last vestiges of the immigrant neighborhood. There they frequented Jewish restaurants, like Schmulka Bernstein's on Essex Street, which added kosher Chinese food to its menu in 1959; Katz's (nonkosher) on Houston Street, which had opened in 1917; the Garden Cafeteria, a dairy establishment opened in 1941; and the Second Avenue Deli, opened in 1954. See KATZ'S DELICATESSEN. They also bought kosher wine, rye bread, dried fruit and nuts, and various sweet bakery goods at the remaining shops, often making these shopping expeditions in time for the various Jewish holidays.

By the 1960s and 1970s much of the New York Jewish food culture had transferred to other neighborhoods and to the suburbs as many Jews ceased to eat these foods on a regular basis. Supermarkets like Zabar's and Fairway Market, both owned by Jewish entrepreneurs, sold kosher meat and other Jewish goods, obviating some of the need for kosher meat markets and bakeries. See FAIRWAY MARKET and ZABAR'S. But kosher restaurants and stores continue to function in the twenty-first century. Many of these kosher restaurants, however, began to serve new kinds of foods, particularly Moroccan food and other dishes associated with the Middle East and Israel.

See also DELIS, JEWISH.

Diner, Hasia R. *Hungering for America: Italian, Irish and Jewish Foodways in the Age of Migration.* Cambridge, Mass.: Harvard University Press, 2001.

Grinstein, Hyman B. *The Rise of the Jewish Community of New York, 1654–1860.* Philadelphia: Jewish Publication Society of America, 1947.

Heinze, Andrew. *Adapting to Abundance: Jewish Immigrants, Mass Consumption, and the Search for American Identity.* New York: Columbia University Press, 1990.

Polland, Annie, and Daniel Soyer. *Emerging Metropolis: New York Jews in the Age of Immigration, 1840–1920.* New York: New York University Press, 2013.

Hasia R. Diner

Jones, Judith and Evan

Judith Bailey Jones (b. 1924) and her husband and collaborator Evan Jones (1916–1996) were both influential American culinarians during the late twentieth century. Judith, an editor at Knopf for fifty-seven years, cultivated and published some of America's preeminent cookbook writers. Evan was a journalist and the author of several major culinary works, including a number of cookbooks written jointly with his wife.

Judith Bailey traveled to Europe on a vacation in 1948 and remained in Paris, where she had fallen in love with the food and with Evan Jones, her future husband. They were married in 1951, and the newlyweds returned to the United States, eventually settling in New York, where Judith was hired as an editor at Knopf. The couple cooked together in their spacious home kitchen and often invited friends to join them for dinner. Stanley Kauffmann, a critic with the *New Republic* magazine, once described their East Sixty-Sixth Street apartment as "the best restaurant in New York."

In 1959 Judith Jones was asked to review a manuscript titled *French Home Cooking*, written by three unknowns: two Frenchwomen, Simone Beck and Louisette Bertholle, and an American named Julia Child, the wife of an American diplomat. Jones began testing the recipes and was hugely impressed with their thoroughness and detail. Unlike some other French cookbooks published in the United States, this one was intended for American kitchens, taking into consideration the availability of equipment and ingredients to American readers.

Despite Jones's enthusiasm, Alfred A. Knopf, the publishing company's founder, was not as excited about the manuscript, which had previously been rejected by Houghton Mifflin. Knopf had published French cookbooks written by famous chefs, and he did not think they needed another one on their list. In addition, the voluminous manuscript would be expensive to print. But after extensive internal discussion, Knopf grudgingly agreed to publish it.

It was Judith Jones who came up with a title for the book: *Mastering the Art of French Cooking.* A few months before it was published, she asked Craig Claiborne, the *New York Times* food columnist, to review it. A few days after its publication, in 1961, Claiborne gave it a rave review in the *Times.* Sales were phenomenal, and Julia Child launched a promotional campaign that eventually led to a television contract for *The French Chef* and many subsequent TV series. Judith Jones went on to edit more of Julia Child's cookbooks, plus a posthumous Child autobiography written with her great-nephew, Alex Prud'homme, called *My Life in France* (2006).

Evan Jones's writing appeared in various magazines, and he wrote and edited books on American history; but his culinary breakthrough came in 1975 with the publication of *American Food: The Gastronomic Story*, one of the first attempts to write a history of American food. It contained more than five hundred recipes, selected in collaboration with Judith. Credited with helping to launch an interest in culinary history in the United States, *American Food* went through two additional editions in 1977 and 1990. He followed it with *The World of Cheese* (1976), considered a definitive work at the time, and *The Food Lover's Companion* (1979), a collection of writings about food from sources both predictable (Auguste Escoffier) and surprising (Adolf Hitler).

Judith Jones had many responsibilities at Knopf; one of these was to develop a list of first-rate cookbook writers. This distinguished group eventually included Lidia Bastianich, James Beard, Marion Cunningham, Betty Fussell, Marcella Hazan, Ken Hom, Madhur Jaffrey, Irene Kuo, Edna Lewis, Scott Peacock, Jacques Pépin, Claudia Roden, Nina Simonds, and Anna Thomas, among many others. She also coauthored several cookbooks, including *The L.L. Bean Game and Fish Cookbook* (1981) with Angus Cameron; with her husband she produced *The Book of Bread* (1982), *Knead It, Punch It, Bake It! Make Your Own Bread* (1981), and *The L.L. Bean Book of New England Cookery* (1987).

The Joneses were close friends with James Beard, and Knopf published *Beard on Food* (1974) and *James Beard's Theory & Practice of Good Cooking* (1977). Beard encouraged Judith Jones to choose Marion Cunningham to completely revise *The Fannie Farmer Cookbook* (1979) for its twelfth edition; she also oversaw the thirteenth (1996). Cunningham, with Judith Jones as her editor, published several other cookbooks at Knopf. After James Beard's death, Evan Jones began working on a biography, *Epicurean Delight: The Life and Times of James Beard* (1990).

Knopf published Judith Jones's memoir, *The Tenth Muse: My Life in Food* (2007), and a cookbook about dining alone, *The Pleasures of Cooking for One* (2009). Her most recent cookbook is *Love Me, Feed Me: Sharing with Your Dog the Everyday Good Food You Cook and Enjoy* (2014). Judith Jones is a recipient of the James Beard Foundation's Lifetime Achievement Award.

See also BEARD, JAMES; CHILD, JULIA; and KNOPF.

Jones, Evan. *American Food: The Gastronomic Story.* New York: Vintage, 1975.
Jones, Evan. *Epicurean Delight: The Life and Times of James Beard.* New York: Knopf, 1990.
Jones, Judith. *The Tenth Muse: My Life in Food.* New York: Knopf, 2007.
Jones, Judith. *The Pleasures of Cooking for One.* New York: Knopf, 2009.
Shapiro, Laura. *Julia Child: A Life.* New York: Penguin, 2009.

Andrew F. Smith

Junior's Restaurant

Junior's, a restaurant known for its cheesecakes, has been part of Brooklyn's life in one form or another since 1929. There are now also two Junior's restaurants in Manhattan—one in Times Square, the other in the food court of Grand Central Terminal. But underscoring the restaurant's roots in, and dedication to, its home borough, Alan Rosen, the third-generation owner, announced in 2014, amid an economic and building boom in Brooklyn, that Junior's original two-story building would never give way to yet another high-rise building.

Junior's is a family restaurant, traditionally with Jewish delicatessen undertones and nowadays also soul food overtones, that serves all kinds of people—from bureaucrats, politicians, judges, and lawyers from the nearby civic center to shoppers, African American church ladies on Sunday, and office workers from the booming corporate "backoffice" operations that now surround it. It may not be known for great food, but it does serve a very good hamburger and satisfying fried chicken, and most days the pastrami is juicy, as the brisket always is. Above all else, there is, as you enter, a retail bakery where among the many gaudy goodies is one of New York City's purest pleasures, its cheesecake, the item for which Junior's has become internationally famous.

Junior's cheesecake is a classic New York style: very smooth and thick but not heavy. It is baked on a moist, buttery sponge layer, a Junior's innovation. Other cheesecakes come with a cookie crust or graham cracker crust or some kind of short pastry. At Junior's, it can be had in many flavors—strawberry, pineapple, chocolate swirl—and in several innovative forms—for example, as a filling for chocolate cake layers. But to a traditionalist there is nothing like the unadorned, completely unembellished, pure vanilla and cream cheese flavor of the, hardly plain, "plain" Junior's cheesecake. That one is now sold in New York supermarkets.

Junior's history mirrors the history of Brooklyn since 1929, long before founder Harry Rosen could have had any idea that cheesecake would be his legacy. Harry, Alan's grandfather, started the business with his brother Mike as a sandwich shop called Enduro's, the name of a stainless steel fabricator who supplied restaurants. Harry simply liked the name. Harry saw how Brooklyn was booming; by the end of the decade, the busy downtown corner of Flatbush Avenue Extension and DeKalb Avenue already had the very grand movie palace the Paramount Theater and subway. Along nearby Fulton Street there were genteel department stores, and another movie palace, the Brooklyn Fox, was about to open only two blocks down Flatbush Avenue.

Almost as soon as Enduro's opened, however, the stock market crashed. Somehow, Enduro's survived the Great Depression. But when Prohibition was repealed in 1933, Harry Rosen reconsidered his operation and expanded to adjacent space where he opened a full-scale restaurant with a bar surrounding an elevated bandstand, all in the latest art moderne style.

After World War II, Brooklyn began changing again. Downtown Brooklyn shopping declined. The middle class was leaving for the suburbs. Poor African Americans from the South were moving to New York City for jobs, and many settled in the neighborhoods near downtown Brooklyn—Bedford-Stuyvesant and Fort Greene.

In 1949, Harry decided to downsize and turn the swank Enduro's into a family-style restaurant that he called "Junior's," named for his sons, Walter and Marvin. Junior's Most Fabulous Restaurant Caterers and Bakers opened on election day 1950, with full fountain service and orange vinyl upholstered booths.

The plan was to also have a retail bakery, and to that end Rosen hired Danish-born baker Eigel Peterson. It was not until the late 1950s, however, that Peterson developed Junior's famous cheesecake. And broad fame did not come until the summer of 1973, when Ron Rosenbaum wrote an ecstatic story about it in the *Village Voice*. After that story, *New York* magazine staged a blind tasting of cheesecakes from around the city. In early 1974, the magazine declared Junior's cheesecake the best. Based on that one tasting and one magazine story, Junior's has had a marketing hook for more than forty years. Junior's cheesecake is now sold coast to coast and also sold on television.

See also CHEESECAKE and CREAM CHEESE.

Rosen, Marvin, and Walter Rosen. *Welcome to Junior's: Remembering Brooklyn with Recipes and Memories from Its Favorite Restaurant.* With Beth Allen. New York: Morrow, 1999.

Arthur Schwartz

Kalustyan's

Kalustyan's is a retail store located at 123 Lexington Avenue in the Murray Hill section of Manhattan that specializes in exotic spices, culinary herbs, and specialty foods from around the world. The store, founded in 1944 by K. Kalustyan, a Turkish-Armenian immigrant, originally served the culinary needs of the neighborhood Armenian community. John Bass, a relative of the original owner, sold the business to local Bangladeshi businessman Aziz Osmani and Sayedul Alam in 1988 so that Bass could focus on the large-scale industrial manufacture of spices and seasonings. Since then, the store has gone through several expansions of their retail space to keep up with the public appetite for authentic regional spice blends and international products.

For many years Kalustyan's was one of the few stores in New York City that sold spices and groceries such as lentils, pickles, and chutneys for Indian cookery in New York City. When the Armenian community moved out of Murray Hill and Indian restaurants began to flourish in the area, the neighborhood became colloquially dubbed "Curry Hill." See CURRY HILL. The array of products crammed into the store is dizzying: beyond spices one can find innumerable legumes, rice, salts, sugars, dried fruits and nuts, chutneys, ghee, health products, mushrooms, noodles, olives, pickles, teas, vinegars, and cooking utensils. The spices and spice blends in the store which carry the Kalustyan's label are made to specification at the Kalustyan Corporation's manufacturing facility in New Jersey.

This reputation for quality, consistency, and diversity of product has long caught the attention of food writers; the *New York Times* first mentioned the store in 1958, and Florence Fabricant touted Kalustyan's Indian spice selection in her column in 1978. The store is used as a source for ingredients for America's Test Kitchen, as well as for Food Network stars such as Emeril Lagasse and Bobby Flay. Kalustyan's very popular falafel and Middle Eastern lunch counter is located on the second floor of the retail store, but there have also been forays into fine dining including the short-lived Kalustyan's Cafe which opened in 2004 at nearby 115 Lexington Avenue. Increasingly, the store carries ingredients used in haute cuisine applications, such as volcano rice, Sicilian pistachio oil, Himalayan salt, Australian crystallized ginger, and other gourmet foods. Recent culinary fascinations, such as with molecular gastronomy, cocktail bitters, and microregional spice blends, have also impacted their stock.

See also ARMENIAN.

"Culinary Currents: Kalustyan's Cafe New York." *Nation's Restaurant News*, September 6, 2004.
Fabricant, Florence. "The Spices of India in New York City." *New York Times*, May 10, 1978.
"Food: Rare Delicacies. Third Avenue Grocery Stocks Products Used in Near and Far East Cuisines." *New York Times*, February 3, 1958.

Sherri Machlin

Katz's Delicatessen

Katz's Deli is surely the only eating establishment best known for a fake orgasm. This was not always the case. The Lower East Side institution, founded in 1888, had just celebrated its hundredth anniversary

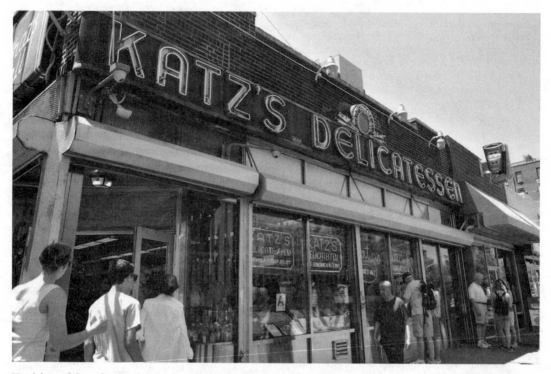

Katz's huge deli sandwiches loaded down with cured meats are no longer the deal they once were, but business remains brisk at this Lower East Side institution.

the year before *When Harry Met Sally* was released (1989). The restaurant was opened as the "Iceland Brothers Deli"; when Willy Katz joined in 1903, it became "Iceland & Katz," then when his cousin Benny joined him in 1910 and bought out the Iceland brothers, "Katz's Delicatessen." Lorna Sass offers an alternate version: the Kostachan brothers founded the deli and Benjamin Eisland and Willy Katz, originally from the same town in Russia, bought it in 1914. Both accounts agree that the next to join, probably in 1917, was Harry Tarowsky, their "landsman."

Back then, wrote Harry Golden in 1962, "Katz's Delicatessen Store...sold a big meal for a dime; a huge club sandwich loaded down with pastrami, corned beef, and salami, all the pickles you wanted, a plate of French fried potatoes, and a bottle of ketchup. Today Katz charges you $1.10 for that deal, and it is still a bargain." At that point, the restaurant was on Ludlow Street. With subway construction in the Forties, it moved to the corner at 205 Houston Street. When a sign maker asked what to put on the new sign, Taroswky said, "Katz's. That's all." And so the sign has read ever since.

During World War II, the deli adopted the slogan "Send a salami to your boy in the Army"; the army was deluged with salamis. The tradition continues today; as of 2014, the deli's site includes an option for "military shipping," and soldiers in Iraq and Afghanistan have continued to receive Katz's salamis.

Katz has long stood out for its scale. In 1953, Walter Winchell claimed that the deli sold over ten thousand sandwiches a day. These sandwiches, described as "prodigious," are served in a space which, by 1989, had expanded from thirty-six seats to 276.

As what had been a Jewish immigrant neighborhood became largely Latino, Katz's remained, with Russ & Daughters and Yonah Schimmel's, an enduring symbol of a former time. See RUSS & DAUGHTERS and YONAH SCHIMMEL KNISH BAKERY. As the same area evolved into one of New York City's hippest neighborhoods, the deli adjusted accordingly. In 1963, it opened from 6:00 a.m. to 1:00 a.m. By 2000, it was already staying open until 3:00 a.m. on weekends, catering to club-goers. As of 2014, Katz's was open all night on weekends. The menu too has evolved. Though never kosher, Katz's would not in earlier times have served meat with cheese; its Reuben sandwich—corned beef, sauerkraut, homemade Russian dressing, and melted Swiss cheese—has long been a bestseller. See REUBEN SANDWICH.

For New Yorkers then, Katz's retains iconic importance as an eatery, an importance it has renewed over the decades. But tourists from around the world now seek out the arrow which shows where Meg Ryan was sitting during her famous scene while, worldwide, many who will never set foot in New York nonetheless know Katz's as the place where Rob Reiner's mother said, "I'll have what she's having."

See also DELIS, JEWISH and LOWER EAST SIDE.

Barron, James. "In 125 Years, Much Has Changed, but the Pastrami Is the Same." *City Room* (blog), *New York Times*, May 14, 2013. http://cityroom.blogs.nytimes.com/2013/05/14/in-125-years-much-has-changed-but-the-pastrami-is-the-same.

Golden, Harry. "Adeline, Cantor." *Pacific Stars and Stripes*, June 20, 1962.

Katz's Delicatessen website: http://katzsdelicatessen.com.

"Huddled Masses? Not on Lower East Side." *Kerrville Daily Times*, March 3, 2000.

"Pastrami from the Lower East Sides." *Kerrville Daily Times*, August 6, 2003.

Sass, Lorna J. "The Great Nosh: Some Landmark New York Delis." *Journal of Gastronomy* 4, no. 1 (1988): 38.

Winchell, Walter. "Theaters in New York Seat Half Los Angeles Population." *Evening Journal*, January 7, 1953.

Jim Chevallier

Key Food

Key Food (full name Key Food Stores Cooperative, Inc.) is a privately held retailers' cooperative of over 160 grocery stores in New York, New Jersey, and Pennsylvania. In 1937, several grocery store owners in Brooklyn formed this cooperative in order to use their purchasing power as a group to get lower prices from their wholesaler distributors (i.e., one of the main purposes of forming a retailers' cooperative). In the time since, the cooperative has steadily expanded in size and scope, while stores in the cooperative have remained independently owned. It now includes specialized markets in addition to the "classic" Key Food—the perishable-focused Key Fresh & Naturals, the organic and gourmet product–focused 55 Fulton Key Food and Urban Market of Williamsburg, the high-variety suburban Key Food Marketplace, the international

product–focused Food World, and the discount-focused Food Dynasty and Food Universe. The cooperative also includes markets with single locations, such as Roslyn Holiday Farms (Roslyn Heights, N.Y.), Locust Valley Market (Locust Valley, N.Y.), Vitelio's Marketplace (Forest Hills, N.Y.), and Milford Farms (Milford, Pa.).

One of Key Food's main organizational and marketing strategies is to tailor each store to its neighborhood demographics. As mentioned, the specialized markets (known as "banners") have general niches into which they fit, but additionally each individual store attempts to fit its neighborhood's desires for particular food products and particular price points. Some stores offer online ordering and, very recently, ordering through the grocery store smartphone application Instacart. Many stores participate in or develop their own community programs as well. Stores have provided a venue for public health organizations to run nutrition workshops (the Community Healthcare Network and a Jamaica store) and cancer charities to hold awareness events (a Zumba flash mob for Relay for Life in a Brooklyn store's parking lot). They have partnered with a local library to fundraise for the library's renovations (the Richmond Hill Library and Lefferts Boulevard store).

In addition to these neighborhood-oriented strategies and activities, the Key Food cooperative employs strategies to unify its stores and its brand. Stores in the cooperative sell the low-cost Key Food–brand products, which include common American food products such as orange juice, apple juice, peanuts, peanut butter, salad dressings, ketchup, maple syrup, waffles, bread, tomato sauce, butter, cooking oil, salt, and French fries. It has a main website for the cooperative to which most searches for individual stores redirect and social media accounts for the cooperative as a whole (some individual stores have their own social media accounts to make announcements only pertaining to their stores). Also, it makes donations to and partners with organizations and businesses on behalf of the cooperative as a whole, such as the Food Bank for New York City, the Bedford-Stuyvesant Campaign against Hunger, Foundation Fighting Blindness, iHeart Radio and Z100's Jingle Ball, and the aforementioned Richmond Hill Library. For its seventy-fifth anniversary in 2012, over sixty stores in the cooperative participated in customer appreciation events that included giveaways, prizes, and entertainment.

Key Food's organizational and marketing strategies have generally been successful; it has been ranked as a top retailer by national distribution company Mr. Checkout (which works with both transnational grocery and convenience store corporations as well as small independently owned stores) and made it onto Crain's 2007 list of the New York area's two hundred largest privately held companies. The Key Food cooperative ranked 66 on the list, with $456.1 million in revenue, and one of its largest member companies, Dan's Supreme Supermarkets, Inc. (which owns several supermarkets under the Key Food banner in New York City and on Long Island), came in at number 160, with $130 million in revenue. There were only two other grocery companies on the list—Inserra Supermarkets, Inc. (dba ShopRite), at number 31 with $1.04 billion and D'Agostino Supermarkets, Inc., at number 135 with $163 million. (To put these rankings in context—Trump Organization was ranked 1, with $10.4 billion in revenue, and Volmar Construction, Inc., was ranked 200, with $65.4 million in revenue.) Key Food has continued to make the list in the years since.

The Key Food cooperative also has had a noticeable involvement in social and economic issues in New York City (along with several other individual grocers and regional supermarket chains). Many Key Food locations in the city report consumers using Supplemental Nutrition Assistance Program (SNAP) benefits at a monthly average of $50,000 or more (according to a report by the Office of Temporary and Disability Assistance of New York State). (SNAP, formerly known as the Food Stamps Program, is a federal program that provides funds for low-income residents to purchase food.) See SUPPLEMENTAL NUTRITION ASSISTANCE PROGRAM (SNAP). Key Food stores have also been built as part of city and state programs addressing food access and security. For example, a Key Food in a "food desert" in Staten Island was funded by a combination of New York Healthy Food & Healthy Communities loans, Food Retail Expansion to Support Health tax incentives, and the owner's own money. These programs supporting both consumers and retailers in these underserved neighborhoods are in contrast to rising rents, city taxes, and interest on the part of national "big box" stores in other neighborhoods. Key Foods and other grocers have closed stores in these neighborhoods (roughly one hundred stores

between 2003 and 2008), which have been replaced by national chains like Walgreens. Unlike other grocers, however, Key Foods has not changed its focus from the city to the suburbs. While it has closed several Manhattan locations in recent years, it has focused on developing new stores in the other boroughs.

There have also been some labor disputes between Key Food's workers and employers. While all stores in the cooperative are unionized, work schedules, working conditions, and compensation are developed at the store level rather than the cooperative level, so labor disputes are handled at this level. In 2009 a Bedford-Stuyvesant Key Food settled a lawsuit by baggers in which the baggers claimed they were not receiving an hourly wage and the stores were employing minors without work permits. In 2011, stock workers at a Brooklyn Key Food filed a suit against their store for wage theft, claiming that they worked between seventy-two and eighty-four hours a week without overtime pay, from 2007 through 2010. These disputes are not unique to Key Food, though; they are similar in nature and number to those at other individual grocers and supermarket chains in New York City.

See also A&P; D'AGOSTINO; GROCERY STORES; and SUPERMARKETS.

Key Food website: http://www.keyfood.com.
"Key Food." Crain's New York Business. http://www.crainsnewyork.com/topics/1379/Key-Food.
"Key Food." DNAinfo. http://www.dnainfo.com/new-york/search?q=key+food&o=r.

Alexandra J. M. Sullivan

Killmeyer's Old Bavarian Inn

See STATEN ISLAND.

Kimchi

Kimchi is widely known as a fermented cabbage dish, but more precisely kimchi refers to a technique used to pickle vegetables to preserve them for longer periods of time. There are more than two hundred types of kimchi, but the most common one is made with napa cabbage, flavored with garlic, ginger, fermented shrimp paste, red pepper powder, and green scallions. For most Koreans, kimchi symbolizes the most basic, affordable side dish that one can have to accompany a bowl of rice, the main staple in the Korean diet. Kimchi has long been thought to be an acquired taste for its strong taste and pungent smell.

In America kimchi products are generally imported directly from Korea or made locally. In New York City, Korean restaurants and supermarkets in Koreatowns in Manhattan and Flushing, Queens, are the main local purveyors of kimchi. In 1980, the Bing Gre Kimchee Pride company was established in Queens and began selling over fifty different types of kimchi. In 2006, the popular restaurant Kum Gang San in Flushing began selling its version, claiming that it contained one hundred times more lactobacilli than other kimchi. These kimchi brands did not reach a broader customer base as they were largely targeting the Korean American community.

In 2008, the trend of fusing kimchi into the American culinary landscape hit New York City by storm when Roy Choi's Los Angeles–based Kogi Taco Truck (think short rib tacos with kimchi slaw and kimchi quesadilla) opened for business. Celebrity chefs in the city began showcasing kimchi in their restaurants: Wylie Dufresne introduced a lobster dish with banana-kimchi sauce at the now-defunct wd-50, Eric Ripert added kimchi jelly on top of a Kumamoto oyster at Le Bernardin, and David Chang made his own kimchi adapted from his grandmother's recipe at Momofuku. As demand for kimchi increased among non-Koreans, second-generation Korean Americans began making small-batch, upscale kimchi for New Yorkers. Brands such as Mama O's of Brooklyn and Mother-in-Law's Kimchi of the Lower East Side emerged with sophisticated and modern marketing strategies. The business-savvy entrepreneurs repackaged kimchi to be more acceptable to a general American audience by selling do-it-yourself kimchi kits and offering fusion recipes such as kimchi chili, kimchi grilled cheese, and kimchi Bloody Mary. In comparison to the first-generation Korean American kimchi purveyors, these products are sold at gourmet groceries such as Zabar's and Murray's Cheese. Kimchi is no longer a foreign, exotic food as more New Yorkers are finding creative ways to incorporate it into their diets and making their own batches at home.

See also KOREAN.

Han, Kyung-koo. "Some Foods Are Good to Think: Kimchi and the Epitomization of National Character." *Korean Social Science Journal* 27, no. 1 (2000): 221–236.
Ku, Robert Ji Song. *Dubious Gastronomy: The Cultural Politics of Eating Asian in the USA.* Honolulu: University of Hawaii Press, 2014.
Yu, Tae-jong, and Young-nan Yu. *Korean Foods.* Seoul: Korea University, 1997.

Chi-Hoon Kim

King Kullen

The King Kullen grocery store on Jamaica Avenue in Queens was America's first supermarket. It was launched by Michael J. Cullen (1884–1936), the son of Irish immigrants. Cullen began as a clerk at an A&P grocery store in Newark, New Jersey. He moved up the A&P hierarchy to become the company's regional superintendent, then left A&P and worked for other grocery store chains, including Kroger Grocery & Baking Co.

Cullen had learned a lot about food retailing, and while employed at Kroger he developed some innovative ideas about how to run a self-service store that would be "monstrous" in size, stocking at least a couple thousand items, all at low prices. It would be a cash-and-carry operation, meaning that no credit would be extended to customers. By increasing sales volume, management could cut prices and stimulate profits. Cullen submitted his proposal to Kroger's president and vice president, but he received no response.

Cullen quit his job and found a partner, Harry Socoloff, vice president of the Sweet Life Food Corporation in Brooklyn. They opened a grocery store, modeled on Cullen's precepts, on August 4, 1930, in a vacant parking garage in Jamaica Estates. Called "King Kullen," the store stocked thousands of food products—about ten times more than other grocery stores—at prices that undercut those at local markets. There was also free curbside parking, drawing in customers with cars, who tended to stock up rather than just buying a few items for immediate use.

Cullen and Socoloff had opened their market almost a year into the Depression, and the tough economic times helped make the new store a success. Price became the biggest factor for consumers in deciding where to shop. The company launched an advertising blitz including newspapers and radio ads that asked, "King Kullen, the world's greatest price wrecker. How does he do it?" King Kullen promised to save shoppers five to ten dollars every week, and customers were willing to travel farther to snag the bargains.

Encouraged by the success of their first location, Cullen and Socoloff quickly opened more stores, and by 1936 fifteen King Kullen stores served Queens, the Bronx, and Long Island. King Kullen undersold small chain and independent grocers by at least 10 to 15 percent, making up the lost profit through high sales volume.

Traditional grocery stores could not compete, and many chains closed their smaller outlets. Thousands of food stores went out of business in New York City during the late 1930s and early 1940s.

King Kullen's success engendered a legion of imitators, and a "space race" commenced. In 1932, the "Big Bear" store in Elizabeth, New Jersey, was set up in an abandoned 50,000-square-foot automobile factory. It attracted two hundred thousand customers and achieved gross sales of ninety thousand dollars every week. Other small retailers, recognizing that their future lay in sales volume, opened similar operations in disused factories and warehouses. Like Michael Cullen, their goal was to generate just a small profit on each item but to make up the difference with a much greater sales volume.

Michael Cullen died in 1936, just six years after opening his first store. King Kullen is one of the few supermarket chains to remain in private hands. Today, the company operates thirty-nine stores on Long Island. Although there were earlier—and larger—grocery stores, Cullen originated and popularized the concept of supermarket chains, and the Smithsonian Institution recognizes King Kullen as America's first supermarket.

See also A&P; GROCERY STORES; QUEENS; and SUPERMARKETS.

Mayo, James M. *The American Grocery Store: The Business Evolution of an Architectural Space.* Westport, Conn.: Greenwood, 1993.
"M. J. Cullen Is Dead; Chain Store Owner." *New York Times,* April 26, 1936.
Seth, Andrew, and Geoffrey Randall. *The Grocers: The Rise and Rise of the Supermarket Chains.* 3d ed. London and Philadelphia: Kogan Page, 2011.
Singer, Lloyd. "Michael J. Cullen: An American Innovator." *Newsday* 1 (May 6, 1990): 21.
Zimmerman, M. M. *The Super Market: A Revolution in Distribution.* New York: McGraw-Hill, 1955.

Andrew F. Smith

King's Arms

See COFFEEHOUSES.

Kings County Distillery

See DISTILLERIES.

Kitchen Arts and Letters

Kitchen Arts and Letters, located at 1435 Lexington Avenue (between Ninety-Third and Ninety-Fourth Streets), is a specialty bookstore that carries a wide variety of titles on food- and drink-related topics from around the world. Most distinctive to its character is the fact that Kitchen Arts and Letter is not a cookbook store. Though it does carry cookbooks, the majority of its titles are curated to provide exposure to the much wider world of food and drink. The store carries books on topics ranging from restaurant economics to food culture and history, from ethnobotany to agriculture.

Nahum (Nach) Waxman opened the store in 1983 after a distinguished eighteen-year career in the book publishing industry. Though the store was small when it first opened (carrying about three hundred to four hundred titles), its commitment to educating food professionals both broadly and deeply attracted the attention of the most important culinary professionals at the time; some of the store's first clients included Julia Child, James Beard, and Laurie Colwin. See CHILD, JULIA and BEARD, JAMES.

Approximately two years after the bookstore opened, a neighboring business moved, allowing Kitchen Arts and Letters to buy out its lease and expand the store. This provided much needed storage and allowed the bookstore to grow to more than twelve thousand titles (plus additional rare and out-of-print items). The majority of its business is still from food professionals; as much as 70 percent of sales can be attributed to chefs, restaurateurs, farmers, writers, and scholars.

The late 1980s marked another important development for Kitchen Arts and Letters: it began importing books from overseas. This included not only English-language books from abroad but foreign-language books as well. These books became an important part of the bookstore's stock over the next decade and now make up more than one-third of sales. The bookstore does not sell many "bestsellers," but instead focuses on less popular books that are of importance to the food community. In some cases, it is the only seller to carry a particular book and may be years ahead of a particular culinary trend.

In 1996, Kitchen Arts and Letters purchased its first computer. Prior to that all business was conducted manually—impressive considering the breadth of collection, depth of knowledge, and commitment to personal interaction. Kitchen Arts and Letters has built a reputation of authority within the culinary community. It is a place to go when you want to have a real conversation about your interests and receive thoughtful recommendations for further reading—indispensable to scholars, chefs, and food enthusiasts alike.

In 2014, Kitchen Arts and Letters opened its first online store in response to the growing number of customers from overseas. Though the virtual store does not list the entire inventory, it is expanding on a regular basis. The true Kitchen Arts and Letter experience, however, remains for those who visit the Upper East Side store, take the time to have a discussion with Nach, and peruse the assortment of unique, rare, and highly specialized books.

See also WAXMAN, NACH.

"About Us." Kitchen Arts and Letters. http://kitchenartsandletters.com/bookstore/about-us.
Barile, Susan Paula. *The Bookworm's Big Apple: A Guide to Manhattan's Booksellers*. New York: Columbia University Press, 1994.
Hughes, Holly. *Frommer's 500 Places for Food and Wine Lovers*. Hoboken, N.J.: Wiley, 2009.

Kristie Collado

Kleindeutschland

Kleindeutschland, or "Little Germany," was Manhattan's main German ethnic neighborhood from the mid- to late nineteenth century. Its borders were Division Street to the south, Fourteenth Street to the north, the East River to the east, and the Bowery to the west.

From the 1830s to the 1880s, hundreds of thousands of German immigrants settled in New York City, fleeing political and economic strife in Germany. By 1860 two hundred thousand Germans called New York home, and most of them lived in Kleindeutschland. Here, German was the lingua franca and German politics were a frequent topic of conversation. The area became a thriving ethnic neighborhood dotted with German clubs (*vereine*), choirs, churches, theaters, schools, and, of course, food businesses. See GERMAN.

By the mid-nineteenth century, German immigrants dominated the bakery and grocery trades of New York and Kleindeutschland housed many of these businesses along Avenues A and B (the German Broadway). German bakeries were located in the cellars of tenement buildings, and in Kleindeutschland every third or fourth cellar might contain a bakery. German bakers produced both the dark brown breads that catered to the palate of fellow German immigrants and the American-style white breads that native-born New Yorkers preferred.

Avenue A, Kleindeutschland's restaurant row, was lined with saloons and eateries that catered mainly to the locals but also with beer gardens that drew New Yorkers from farther afield. The great beer halls were a point of pride in Kleindeutschland, their owners among the neighborhood's economic and cultural elite. See BEER and BEER GARDENS. The *krauthobler* was another familiar sight on the streets of Kleindeutschland in the fall months. Going door to door, the *krauthobler* shredded cabbage (charging a penny a head), which German housewives turned into sauerkraut.

Kleindeutschland reached its height in the 1870s. As the first generation of German immigrants ceded to the second, Germans and German Americans began to spread throughout the city, moving to such neighborhoods as Williamsburg, Brooklyn, and Yorkville, on Manhattan's Upper East Side. See WILLIAMSBURG and YORKVILLE. An influx of new immigrants to New York, from Southern and especially Eastern Europe, began to settle in the area in and around Kleindeutschland, diluting the German presence. Kleindeutschland's demise accelerated after the *General Slocum* disaster, which occurred in June 1904. The fire, on a pleasure cruise carrying thirteen hundred German women and children, quickly overtook the boat, killing over one thousand passengers. The *General Slocum* disaster had a terrible impact on the close-knit German community of Kleindeutschland. Many German New Yorkers, their families decimated, moved to Yorkville or left New York altogether. By the turn of the twentieth century, the area was known as the Jewish Lower East Side. See LOWER EAST SIDE.

Binder, Frederick, and David Reimers. *All the Nations under Heaven*. New York: Columbia University Press, 1996.

Nadel, Stanley. *Little Germany: Ethnicity, Religion, and Class in New York City, 1845–80*. Urbana: University of Illinois Press, 1990.

Ziegelman, Jane. *97 Orchard: An Edible History of Five Immigrant Families in One New York Tenement*. New York: HarperCollins, 2010.

Cindy R. Lobel

Knish

The knish (the "k" is pronounced) is a pillow of dough, stuffed with a filling, most often onion-strewn mashed potatoes. Knishes can be round or square, fried or baked, sweet or savory (the square ones are generally made of potato and fried; the round ones have fillings that include spinach, buckwheat groats [kasha], pastrami, or liver and can also be made in dessert style with fruit fillings combined with farmer's cheese). The pastry's Eastern European roots include a legend from the Polish town of Knyszyn and its first known mention in a Polish-language poem, "The Krakowiec Guild," from 1614. The stuffed dumpling arrived in New York City circa 1900. The influx of Jewish immigrants from the Pale of Settlement made their homes on the Lower East Side of Manhattan, as did the knish. The potato pies were first sold piping hot from pushcarts and then from dedicated eateries, each of which generated a loyal following and heated opinions.

A 1916 *New York Times* headline, "Rivington Street Sees War: Rival Restaurant Men Cut Prices on the Succulent Knish," introduced the battle between Max Green and Morris London, who lured customers with price cuts and tactics such as an oompah band, a cabaret, and a sign advertising the "Ten Knish Commandments," which stipulated the following:

1. All good pure food.
2. Everything strictly fresh.
3. All bread, etc., baked on premises.
4. At any time hot knisches.
5. Strictly union waiters and bakers.

That same year, in a short story, Yiddish writer Sholem Aleichem referenced a newcomer to New York who made a name—and a living—in the dough business:

If you go down to Essex Street, you'll see a sign in the window written in large Yiddish letters—

HOMEMADE KNISHES SOLD HERE—and you'll know that's our in-law....And if you see on the same street, right across the way, another Yiddish sign with the same large letters—HOMEMADE KNISHES SOLD HERE—you'll know it isn't our in-law Yoneh the baker. He now has a competitor, so don't go there.

In the 1940s, knishes still held sway in New York City. In an unpublished Works Progress Administration–funded narrative, folklorist Nathan Ausubel paid homage to Yonah Schimmel's, a knish shop which had occupied a storefront on Houston Street since 1910. Ausubel postulated that the knish "sprang spontaneously from the Jewish people" and credited Schimmel, a Romanian rabbi, as the Americanizer of the food. "Knishes are more than an indigenous food of the Jewish East Side. They are even more than an expression of local culinary patriotism," wrote Ausubel. "Knishes in fact are a passion, an ambrosial ecstasy."

In 1942, knish maker Gussie Schwebel, also of Houston Street, counted Leon Trotsky, Enrico Caruso, and then–New York City police chief Teddy Roosevelt among her clients. She wrote to Eleanor Roosevelt to offer the first lady a taste of knishes (she accepted the offer, but ultimately, a secretary refused the knishes because of the extensive crowds gathered to witness the event). Nonetheless, knishes remained the stuff of politics.

"No New York politician in the last fifty years has been elected to public office without having at least one photograph taken showing him on the Lower East Side with a knish in his face," wrote Milton Glaser and Jerome Snyder in *The Underground Gourmet* in 1966. Izzy Finkelstein, a career waiter at Schimmel's, remembered seeing Eleanor Roosevelt in the shop, purchasing some knishes in conjunction with her husband's campaign.

The pastry pie gained popularity along the Brooklyn boardwalk, from Coney Island to Brighton Beach, as early as the 1920s. Shops like Mrs. Stahl's, Shatzkin's, and Hirsch's formed a knish belt that lasted through the early 1980s and evoked powerful memories and heated opinions over which knish was best. In 2014, knishes were available at Jewish delis and on street carts throughout the five boroughs. Gabila's, the inventor of the Coney Island square knish, migrated to Copiague, Long Island, in 2006, where in autumn 2013 a machinery fire brought about a hiatus in the production, the "Knish Crisis of 2013," which lasted through spring 2014. In Forest

Hills, Queens, Knish Nosh opened its doors in 1952, has sold sweet and savory baked pies on Queens Boulevard since, and opened concession stands in Central Park, including one at Conservatory Water at East Seventy-Fourth Street.

In culture, too, the knish has left an indelible mark. Molly Picon and Fyvush Finkel referenced it on the Yiddish stages of New York City. Manhattan's Second Avenue, home to a high density of Yiddish theaters between Houston and Fourteenth Streets, came to be known as "Knish Alley." The pastry made appearances in the literary works of Henry Roth and Isaac Bashevis Singer, in the sitcoms *Welcome Back, Kotter* and *The Golden Girls*, and in films including *The Night They Raided Minsky's* and Woody Allen's *Whatever Works*.

See also YONAH SCHIMMEL KNISH BAKERY and MRS. STAHL'S KNISHES.

Aleichem, Sholem. "Motl the Cantor's Son: Writings of an Orphan Boy." In *Tevye the Dairyman and Motl the Cantor's Son*, translated by Aliza Shevrin, pp. 319–320. New York: Penguin, 2009.

Ausubel, Nathan. "Hold Up the Sun! Kaleidoscope: The Jews of New York." First draft. Works Progress Administration Historical Records Survey: Federal Writer' Project, Jews of New York, New York Municipal Archives, microfilm no. 176, box 7, folder 243, 21–25.

Glaser, Milton, and Jerome Snyder. "Yonah Schimmel's Knishes Bakery." In *The Underground Gourmet: Where to Find Great Meals in New York for Less than $3.00 and as Little as 50¢*, rev. 2d ed., pp. 239–241. New York: Simon and Schuster, 1970.

Picon, Molly. "Di (Ganze) Velt Is a Te'atr." *Di Groyse Schlagers Fun Kine Un Te'atr*. CD. Tel Aviv: Israel Music, 2005.

"Rivington Street Sees War: Rival Restaurant Men Cut Prices on the Succulent Knish." *New York Times*, January 27, 1916.

Silver, Laura. *Knish: In Search of the Jewish Soul Food*. Waltham, Mass.: Brandeis University Press, 2014.

Laura Silver

Knopf

Publishing giant Alfred A. Knopf, Inc., started as a family affair in 1915 by Alfred A. Knopf, his soon-to-be-wife Blanche Knopf (née Wolf), and his father Samuel Knopf. Alfred's career began in 1912 as a clerk at Doubleday. He soon left to become an editorial assistant for Michael Kennerly, who ran the New York branch of the British publisher John Lane. Seeing a dearth of attention to European authors, especially Russian, by the existing American publishers, the quick-thinking Alfred founded his eponymous publishing house to bring these authors, especially fiction writers, to the American public. The house grew rapidly, moving in 1922 to one of New York City's first skyscrapers, the Hecksher Building on Fifth Avenue and Fifty-Seventh Street, and Knopf soon became a prestige publishing house for authors in the social sciences as well. Among the influential authors in the Knopf stable were Simone de Beauvoir, Sigmund Freud, Joseph Conrad, E. M. Forster, Franz Kafka, D. H. Lawrence, Theodore Dreiser, Langston Hughes, John Updike, Arthur Schlesinger Jr., Toni Morrison, and Samuel Eliot Morison.

By mid-century, Knopf was broadening its range of works including publishing some cookbooks, and was also undergoing generational transition: Alfred retired as president of Knopf in 1957, naming Blanche as his successor. She was one of the first female presidents of a major publishing house in the United States, a position she held until her death in 1966. Critical to Knopf's success in culinary publishing was Judith Jones, who was offered a junior editorial position by Blanche in 1957. See JONES, JUDITH AND EVAN. When the unwieldy manuscript that would eventually become *Mastering the Art of French Cookery*, by Julia Child, Simone Beck, and Louisette Bertholle, crossed Jones's desk, she saw potential where other prominent publishers had passed, considering the work too demanding and exotic for the American audience. Jones, a Francophile, argued passionately for the work, which was published in 1961 to unexpected and overwhelming popularity. Having Blanche as the head of Knopf and Jones as an editor serendipitously paved the way for *Mastering the Art* and may have changed the nature of cookbook publishing, showing that more ambitious works could find an audience.

Mastering the Art catapulted Jones and Knopf to the forefront of culinary publishing, with Jones acting as editor over the next fifty years for many of the most influential culinary books while weathering several mergers, spin-offs, and reorganizations. In 1960, while *Mastering the Art* was in process, Knopf was acquired by Random House to form the Knopf Publishing Group, although the editorial departments of the two houses remained distinct. In 1998, the

Knopf Publishing Group was acquired by the German conglomerate Bertelsmann AG, which owned several other large publishing houses. The economics did not work, and a massive reorganization took place in 2009, with Knopf acquiring Doubleday. Culinary works are now published by several imprints under the umbrella of the Knopf Doubleday Publishing Group.

Knopf's impressive culinary library (including its various imprints) holds many other works by and about Julia Child, including her collaborations with Jacques Pépin in *Cooking at Home*, Noël Riley Fitch's biography, *Appetite for Life*, and Child's autobiography, cowritten with Alex Prud'homme, *My Life in France*. See CHILD, JULIA and PÉPIN, JACQUES. While Knopf has published works by celebrity chefs, such as Lidia Bastianich, Edna Lewis, Nancy Silverton, Marcella Hazan, Joël Robuchon, David Burke, Suzanne Goin, and Susan Spicer, many of its publications are gastronomic writings and memoirs, such as Waverly Root's *The Food of France* and *The Food of Italy*, Adam Gopnik's *The Table Comes First*, Laurie Colwin's *Home Cooking: A Writer in the Kitchen*, Jeffrey Steingarten's *It Must Have Been Something I Ate*, Raymond Sokolov's *Steal the Menu*, Bill Buford's *Heat*, Robb Walsh's *Are You Really Going to Eat That: Reflections of a Culinary Thrill Seeker*, and Peter Mayle's *French Lessons*. Knopf has published a one hundredth anniversary edition of the classic *Fannie Farmer Cookbook* as well as an edition (under the Vintage imprint) of Jean Anthelme Brillat-Savarin's nineteenth-century classic *The Physiology of Taste*, translated by M. F. K. Fisher, with an introduction by Bill Buford.

Knopf has also explored international and ethnic cuisines. Within its library are works by Claudia Roden (*The New Book of Middle Eastern Foods*; *Arabesque: A Taste of Morocco, Turkey and Lebanon*; and *The Book of Jewish Food*); Madhur Jaffrey (three cookbooks on Indian food plus a memoir, *Climbing the Mango Trees*); Penelope Casas (*The Food and Wine of Spain* and *Tapas*); many works by Joan Nathan, one of America's doyennes of Jewish cookery; and Russ Federman, of Russ & Daughter fame. Under its Anchor imprint, culinary works include the Foxfire Americana Library, devoted to preserving Appalachian culture, with volumes on moonshining, baking, pickling and preserving, and meats and small game. Appropriate to her role in establishing Knopf as a preeminent culinary publisher, Judith Jones's work is represented in her autobiography *The Tenth Muse: My Life in Food*, as well as her cookbooks *The Pleasures of Cooking for One*, and *Love Me, Feed Me*.

Clements, Amy Root. *The Art of Prestige: The Formative Years at Knopf, 1915–1929*. Amherst and Boston: University of Massachusetts Press, 2014.
Flamm, Matthew. "Shakeups Hit Random House, Other Publishers." *Crain's New York Business*, December 3, 2008.
Knopf Doubleday Publishing Group website: http://knopfdoubleday.com.

Cathy K. Kaufman

Korean

Korean food has grown increasingly popular in New York since the early 1960s after the United States increased the quota of North and South Koreans allowed to enter the country. Chefs have been embracing Korean ingredients and preparation styles to influence their own cuisines. Traditional Korean cuisine is vegetable-based and centered on spicy and fermented food shared in a familial environment.

In February 2013, *Forbes* magazine named Korean flavors as one of the top ten food trends of 2013 in the United States. *Gochujang* (fermented red pepper paste), *doenjang* (soybean paste), Korean-style barbecue, and kimchi were all highlighted as new and exciting ingredients. However, these tastes and flavors have been around for centuries and are just finally being appreciated by the mass food society. Although Korean cuisine is over five thousand years old, American chefs are experimenting with its ingredients and techniques to create a contemporary approach.

One of the most appealing aspects of Korean cuisine is its bright colorful presentation, with each color in a dish having symbolic importance. For instance, the ingredients in the classic *bibimbap* represent many elements of the natural world: the white component (egg whites and rice) represents the sky, the black components (mushrooms, burdock root) represent the ground, the yellow ingredients (egg yolks) represent the moon, the red ingredients (chili powder, radish, *gochujang*) symbolize the sun, and the green ingredients (watercress, spinach, squash) represent the earth. What appears as a simple dish is reflective of many aspects of Korean traditional culture and spirituality.

The influence of Buddhism on Korean culture is seen in a strong vegetarian emphasis in the cuisine. Generally, vegetable-based side dishes called *namul* are served alongside each meal, whether it is based on barbecue or *sondubu* (soft tofu stew). In a culture that limits beef intake, these simple vegetarian dishes provide a filling meal. In Korean culture, temple cuisine highlights the concept of food as medicine. It is lightly seasoned because of the belief that ingredients such as garlic, green onion, and chives arouse the senses and easily anger individuals. The restaurant Hangwai and the BCD Tofu House are both excellent interpretations of this cuisine in their presentation as well as the overall experience.

This vegetarian-friendly society was disrupted during the Koryo dynasty when the Mongols invaded Korea and introduced many meat dishes, as well as soups, butchery, stocks, braising, barbecue, and *mandu* (dumplings). The Mongols also introduced *soju*, a popular and cheap liquor that can be drunk straight or mixed with beer or other beverages. The introduction of soup to the Korean dining culture also brought along the spoon as a necessary dining instrument. Soup is generally eaten at the end of the meal, to aid in digestion. Boiling soups are eaten in all types of weather, but many traditional Koreans find hot soups and stews to have an internal cooling effect in the hot summer months.

Dining with the family and etiquette are central to the Korean dining experience. Food is shared by everyone at the table. The typical Korean eats with family or friends, and dining alone is not fully accepted in the culture. The meal does not begin until the oldest member of the table begins eating. Younger members of a table generally turn away from their elders when drinking alcohol as a sign of deference. Table manners are specific to Korean culture. When dining in a restaurant, the host presents a toast; diners never fill their own glasses but do fill companions' glasses. The oldest person at the table pays for the meal unless he is a guest. These rules are becoming more relaxed in modern Korean society.

In addition to its unique flavors, Korean cuisine has become popular for its healthy components. Korean food has a high fiber content, many nutritious ingredients, a high soy bean content, and high unsaturated fat and incorporates fermented foods that aid in digestion. Kimchi is perhaps the best-known Korean ingredient, although fermentation and preservation are underlying themes of many Korean foods. Traditional kimchi is white and was transformed into the spicy condiment known by many through trade with the Spanish, who introduced a pepper powder as a cheaper preservative than salt. See KIMCHI.

With the rapid ascent of David Chang, a Korean American chef, and his Momofuku empire, Korean food has exploded on the New York City restaurant scene. Chang's restaurants serve versions of many of the traditional dishes of Korea but use ingredients that are local to New York. See CHANG, DAVID and MOMOFUKU RESTAURANT GROUP. Other chefs, such as Hooni Kin of Danjo and Ben Pollinger of Oceana, are incorporating Korean ingredients and techniques into a modern dining format. What was once a cuisine relegated to certain neighborhoods of New York has now spread to many top restaurants in the city. New York Kom Tang was an excellent venue for Korean barbecue in Koreatown that has sadly closed; it used the traditional method of charcoal for cooking the meats tableside. Miss Korea BBQ is another Koreatown highlight, known for its hot pots. For the novice Korean diner, a meal at Kunjip offers all of the facets of Korean dining, from soups to barbecue. And for the home cook looking to assemble a pantry and begin cooking Korean cuisine, H-Mart is the best grocery store chain to obtain all the essentials of Korean cuisine.

See also KOREAN TACO and KOREATOWNS.

Institute of Traditional Korean Food. *The Beauty of Korean Food: With 100 Best Loved Recipes*. Elizabeth, N.J.: Hollym, 2007.
Pettid, Michael J. *Korean Cuisine: An Illustrated History*. London: Reaktion, 2008.

Michael Traud

Korean Taco

The Korean taco was introduced and popularized in San Francisco about 2008 by Chef Roy Choi and was introduced into New York City about 2009. At first glance, the idea of a Korean taco seems odd. However, Koreans have been eating barbecued meats wrapped in lettuce and topped with various sauces based on soybean paste or red pepper paste for the greater majority of the twentieth century. The *galbi* (Korean barbecue meat) in a lettuce wrap has become popular in New York in a similar manner to the way tacos have been consumed in Mexico.

The Korean taco can be constructed of many layers and can include a variety of toppings, including perilla or sesame leaves, various interpretations of kimchi (cabbage, cucumber, daikon, pear, apple), rice, and fresh vegetables (carrots, beans sprouts, daikon). Moreover, the ingredients in the traditional Korean *bibimbap*—seared meat, kimchi or salsa, fresh vegetables—can be assembled in a Korean taco.

The Korean style of cooking meats is very similar to that used in Mexican tacos. Pork, beef, chicken, or fish are cooked at a very high temperature to caramelize the meat, with various marinades. These marinades contain the sauce elements to both flavor the meat as well as tenderize certain cuts using soy sauce and fruit such as kiwi and Asian pears. These meats are marinated prior to cooking in these sauces to fully develop the flavor for the tacos. For instance, *tacos al pastor* in Mexican cuisine features pineapple both in the marinade for the protein and as a final topping. Toppings for Korean tacos correspond to the *namul* food in a traditional Korean meal. Pickled radish, various kimchi preparations, sautéed and seasoned greens, and mushrooms are all toppings used in Korean tacos, versus the traditional lettuce and onion garnish found in its Mexican counterpart.

The acceptance of the Korean taco in New York City has corresponded with the rise of the modern food truck. See FOOD TRUCKS. One of these, the Kimchi Taco Truck, puts a spin on the traditional taco by adding kimchi to refried beans, fresh kimchi slaw instead of fresh cabbage, and alternative kimchi types such as red cabbage, apple, and pear kimchi and pickled daikon and cucumber kimchi. The Korilla BBQ provides a choice of rice including a bacon kimchi fried rice, a kimchi pickle bar that features various kimchi preparations with a variety of ingredients to the degree of heat of that preparation, as well as the option to add a Korean hot or barbecue sauce. These combinations allow for many different taco interpretations.

The Korean taco theme is expanding with the presence of Korean food elements that are being added to traditional burritos. Other Korean influences include red pepper paste in a traditional Italian pork bolognese or incorporating all the elements of a *bibimbap* into the form of an arancini.

See also KOREAN.

Korean Food Foundation. *Great Food, Great Stories from Korea*. Seoul: Korean Food Foundation, 2012.

Vongerichten, Marja. *The Kimchi Chronicles: Korean Cooking for an American Kitchen*. Emmaus, Pa.: Rodale, 2011.

Michael Traud

Koreatowns

New York City has two major Korean ethnic enclaves, one in Queens and the other one in Manhattan, where Koreans have opened restaurants and businesses to serve Koreans and other residents of the city. New York City has the second-largest Korean population outside of Korea with approximately one hundred thousand ethnic Koreans, of whom two-thirds live in Queens. The Korean population in New York City emerged in the first half of the twentieth century, with a handful of Korean students at major educational institutions such as Columbia University and New York University. The first Korean restaurants opened in the 1960s in Manhattan to serve the approximately four hundred–strong Korean community, composed of occupational immigrants in the medical field, entrepreneurs, and students. For instance, in 1960 Korean entrepreneur Hong Sun-sik opened Mi Cin at 130 West Forty-Fifth Street in the Times Square district. The price of simple Korean à la carte menu items ranged from $1.25 to $4.00. The restaurant also served higher-end dishes such as *sinseollo*, a soup of seafood, meat, and vegetables. Three years later came Arirang House, the first upscale Korean restaurant, which received three stars from the *New York Times* in 1974. The Immigration and Nationality Act of 1965, coupled with expansion of Korean business into the U.S. market, led to a steady stream of immigration from Korea. The number of Korean restaurants grew to eighteen to serve the growing Korean community and began adapting to local preferences by introducing lunch specials, serving food in courses, and offering Korean-style beef barbecue. Despite localization, these establishments could not attract enough customers and many went out of business.

In the mid-1970s Koreans began moving into Queens and opened restaurants, karaoke bars, grocery stores, bookstores, banking institutions, and clothing stores to provide daily necessities for the new immigrant community. Koreatown in Queens developed in Flushing, on Union Street between Thirty-Fifth and Forty-First Avenues. Over the years, it has expanded eastward, along the Long Island Railroad in the neighborhoods of Murray Hill, Bayside, Douglaston, and Little Neck. As Korean businesses thrived, Main Street flourished as one of the busiest commercial areas in New York City and remains a vital source of economic and cultural life for the Korean American community today. The successful establishment of Koreatown in Queens paved the way for Korean businesses to expand back into Manhattan.

In the 1980s, Korean businesses began moving into the neighborhood that encompasses the Empire State Building and Herald Square from Thirtieth to Thirty-Fifth Streets between Fifth and Sixth Avenues. In 1995, Thirty-Second Street between Fifth Avenue and Broadway, the heart of Manhattan's Koreatown, was officially named "Korea Way." Korea Way resembles the streets of Seoul, with businesses and restaurants tucked into all levels of the buildings marked by bright neon signs on their façades.

While both Koreatowns offer similar commercial and business services, the one in Flushing is larger in scale and predominantly serves Korean residents. In recent years, Korea Way has become a culinary destination for tourists and locals alike. In addition to restaurants serving staple Korean dishes such as Korean barbecue and *bibimbap* (rice, vegetables, and meat mixed with *gochujang*, a spicy hot pepper sauce), specialty restaurants offer a wide range of Korean cuisine, such as homemade tofu, *seolleongtang* (beef soup), *mandu* (dumplings), Korean fusion Chinese food, and Buddhist temple food. One can enjoy Korean food at more than a dozen restaurants that are open twenty-four hours a day, seven days a week.

See also KIMCHI; KOREAN; KOREAN TACO; and QUEENS.

Baldwin, Deborah. "Exotic Flavor, Beyond Just the Food." *New York Times*, October 17, 2008.
Lee, Kyou-Jin. "Early History of Korean Restaurants in Manhattan, NY: Focused on 1960's to 1970's." *Journal of the Korean Society of Food Culture* 26, no. 6 (2011): 562–573.

Chi-Hoon Kim

Kosher

See JEWISH.

Kossar's

See BIALYS.

Kump, Peter Clark

Peter Clark Kump (1937–1995) is best known as a cooking teacher, the founder of eponymous cooking schools, and, with Julia Child, cofounder of the James Beard Foundation. Born in Los Angeles, California, he studied speech and drama at Stanford University and earned an MFA at Carnegie-Mellon University. His early career was an amalgam of theater and teaching speed-reading. By the early 1970s, he was drawn to the culinary arts, studying with the preeminent cooking teachers of the day: Simone Beck, Diana Kennedy, Marcella Hazan, and James Beard. A gourmand's trip to Europe, where he claimed to dine every day at Michelin-starred restaurants for lunch and dinner, cemented his love of cuisine.

Returning to New York, he taught his first cooking class in 1974: the students were five friends who were instructed in his techniques-driven method. Infamous was "egg day," where every dish explored egg cookery, including French-style scrambled eggs with caviar, poached eggs in a red wine sauce, hard-cooked eggs for salade Niçoise, and whipped eggs for soufflés. Soon the school outgrew Kump's apartment and his ability to conduct all of the classes; instructors, many of whom were graduates of his program, spent several peripatetic years taxiing equipment and ingredients to rented kitchens throughout Manhattan. By 1979, the school was housed in a funky brownstone at 307 West Ninety-Second Street, where it would remain until February 1998, training both passionate amateurs (Peter Kump's School of Culinary Arts) and aspiring professionals (Peter Kump's New York Cooking School) using Kump's pedagogical methods.

Following Beard's death in 1985, Kump was the driving force behind the formation of the James Beard Foundation, organizing a campaign to raise funds to purchase Beard's Greenwich Village townhouse, which remains the foundation's home. Kump was the first president of the foundation, a post he retained until his death, and was the mastermind behind the James Beard Awards, among the food world's most prestigious accolades. The foundation posthumously honored his lifetime achievement in 1996. Kump also served as president of the International Association of

Culinary Professionals and the New York Association of Cooking Teachers; the latter honored his contributions to culinary education in 1994.

Kump devoted most of his energies to teaching and culinary organizations. His only published cookbook was the 1983 Tastemaker Award–winning *Quiche and Pâté*, although he contributed articles to the *New York Times* and national magazines such as *Food & Wine*. His last project was an expansion of his cooking schools to a second location at 50 West Twenty-Third Street. Construction was well under way when liver cancer claimed Kump on June 7, 1995; just days before his death, he sold the school to entrepreneur Rick Smilow, and the Twenty-Third Street location opened two months later. Smilow would rebrand the school as the Institute of Culinary Education in 2001.

See also INSTITUTE OF CULINARY EDUCATION; JAMES BEARD FOUNDATION; and SMILOW, RICK.

Arndt, Alice, ed. *Culinary Biographies*. Houston, Tex.: Yes Press, 2006.
Miller, Bryan. "Peter Kump, Expert Chef and Cooking Teacher, Dies at 57." *New York Times*, June 9, 1995.

Cathy K. Kaufman

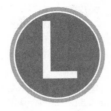

Labor Unions

See RESTAURANT UNIONS.

La Caravelle

La Caravelle restaurant was opened in 1960 by former Pavillon employees Fred Decré, Robert Meyzen, and Roger Fessaguet; the restaurant replaced another French restaurant called Robert's located at 33 West Fifty-Fifth Street. La Caravelle was, in the words of Craig Claiborne, "the finest restaurant in New York on almost every count." (In 1968, Claiborne gave the restaurant four stars in *The New York Times Guide to Dining Out in New York*.)

From the beginning, La Caravelle's menu changed daily, as was customary in Europe; but this was an innovation for American diners at the time. Roger Fessaguet, who arrived in New York City in 1949, was its executive chef. Under his guidance, the kitchen turned out classic French cuisine such as *quenelles de brochet*, roast duck, and a variety of soufflés.

Located in the Shoreham Hotel on West Fifty-Fifth Street, La Caravelle's clientele included the Duke and Duchess of Windsor, Salvador Dalí, Tony Curtis, Marlene Dietrich, David O. Selznick, James Beard, and Janet Leigh. The restaurant's reservation book read like a veritable who's who of theater, fashion, and politics. Among the restaurant's regulars were two generations of Kennedys.

Joseph Kennedy began to frequent La Caravelle with his family after a falling out with Le Pavillon's owner Henri Soulé. Having cooked for the senator at Le Pavillon where he was sous-chef, Fessaguet knew all of Joe Kennedy's favorite dishes. In a bold

move, Fessaguet put on his menu an identical dish that he had cooked at Le Pavillon (*poularde au Champagne*), renaming it *poularde Maison Blanche* in a nod to Joe Kennedy and his newly elected son. The Kennedys were such close and loyal customers of La Caravelle that when John F. Kennedy took office in January 1961, Jacqueline Kennedy asked Robert Meyzen to recommend a French chef for the White House; Meyzen in turn asked Fessaguet.

Despite his insistence, Fessaguet could not convince Jacques Pépin to take the job. (The Howard Johnson's position held greater appeal, and Pierre Franey, who was already working for the company, was lobbying hard.) Consequently, the position went to René Verdon, who was working at the nearby Essex House. Before heading to Washington, Verdon was required to train under Fessaguet for several weeks in preparation for becoming the first family's chef.

At a time when French restaurants were the ne plus ultra of fine dining, La Caravelle was the pinnacle of elegant eating. Enlivening the dining room was a series of murals depicting characteristic scenes of Paris—Les Jardins du Luxembourg, a Bastille Day ball, the church at Saint-Germain des Prés. Of the murals, Mimi Sheraton of the *New York Times* wrote, "The leafy, sun-dappled murals of Parisian park scenes... and the pale, soothing color of walls and draperies reflect a comfortable golden glow of light." The artwork was executed by a student of Raoul Dufy, Jean Pagès, who had also painted murals at La Côte Basque, Le Perigord Park, and other better French addresses in the city.

Upon his retirement in 1984, Fessaguet turned over the restaurant to Rita and André Jammet, who ran La Caravelle to great acclaim until 2004 when the restaurant was closed in part as a result of lease issues. Chefs who helmed the kitchen include Tadashi Ono, Michael Romano, and Cyril Renaud. The same year also saw the closings of Lutèce and La Côte Basque. After the anti-French "freedom fry" backlash that followed in the wake of the World Trade Center attacks, these French restaurants were dealt mortal blows. Mediterranean-diet health consciousness and a growing pan-Latin and pan-Asian dining landscape also siphoned off potential customers.

In its last review of La Caravelle, published some nine months before the restaurant closed, the *New York Times* summed up this venerable address perfectly as it awarded the establishment a final three-star review. "Unlike other Midtown French restaurants which seem like fusty museum pieces, La Caravelle pulses with forward momentum and energy, even while paying respect to the past."

See also LE PAVILLON.

Grimes, William. *Appetite City: A Culinary History of New York.* New York: North Point, 2009.
Kuh, Patric. *The Last Days of Haute Cuisine: America's Culinary Revolution.* New York: Viking, 2001.

Alexandra Leaf

Ladies Who Lunch

The era of the "Ladies Who Lunch," whose heyday was the period between the 1950s and the 1980s, reflects New York's position as the center of fashion, food, and fame. It was a time of beautiful people dining in Gotham's beautiful restaurants.

Some credit *Women's Wear Daily* publisher John Fairchild for inventing the phrase "Ladies Who Lunch." Stephen Sondheim claims to have coined the moniker: the ballad "Ladies Who Lunch" in his 1970 hit play *Company*, sung by Elaine Stritch, was a backhanded salute to the grand dames. *New York* magazine makes its own claim to have introduced the phrase.

Who were these "Ladies Who Lunch" who became such icons? They were, for the most part, upper-class wives of wealthy businessmen, politicians, and royalty—sometimes referred to as "high-society goddesses" or "trophy wives." All were socialites. With feet firmly planted in traditional class and society norms, and a burgeoning women's movement, these women were the foundation of New York's philanthropic efforts. Lunch lubricated their social networking efforts.

There were many popular Ladies Who Lunched—the most photographed included Jacqueline Kennedy Onassis, Lee Radziwill, Slim Keith, Gloria Guinness, Happy Rockefeller, Babe Paley, Pat Buckley, Lynn Wyatt, the Duchess of Windsor, Deeda Blair, Brooke Astor, Gloria Vanderbilt, C. Z. Guest, Nancy Reagan, Betsy Bloomingdale, Nan Kempner, Gloria Vanderbilt, and the Rose Kennedy clan.

Their lunch parade in and out of the restaurants showcased major fashion houses long before the "red carpet." In a time before social media, these women were photographed by the social arbiters of the day: *Women's Wear Daily*, the *New York Post*'s Page Six, and the *New York Times*'s Bill Cunningham, who reported their daily comings and goings from Gotham's glamorous restaurants. The public ate it up, turning to the newspapers for a look at what they were wearing and where they dined.

And many restaurants still had dress codes. Le Pavillon railed against the emerging pantsuit fashion of the day and kept paper skirts for offenders to don. On one memorable occasion Nan Kempner, wearing an Yves St. Laurent pantsuit, refused the paper skirt. She removed her designer pants and wore the thigh-grazing tunic-top as her skirt. See LE PAVILLON.

Escorting the women were equally brilliant and talented men. A quaint custom now, "walkers" was the term used for mainly gay men who accompanied the ladies to lunch. Famous walkers included Jerry Zipkin, Bill Blass, Truman Capote, Billy Baldwin, and Arnold Scaasi.

Lunch protocol gave rise to the importance of where one was seated in the restaurant's dining room. Before celebrity chefs, it was the front of the house that was the face of the restaurant, especially at lunch. The tables closest to the door were held for the prominent clients, where they could be readily seen. The successful maître d' paid attention to the setup of the dining room: who should be seated where. Hosts viewed their dining guests as an "audience in a nonstop show." The maître d' needed to have a finger on the throbbing pulse of Gotham's family fortunes, from old money to the nouveau riche. According to Sirio Maccioni of Le Cirque, Bill Blass was often whispering in his ear, helping to navigate the potential minefield of nouvelle society's indiscretions and successes. See LE CIRQUE and MACCIONI, SIRIO.

Only a few restaurants made it on the Ladies Who Lunch circuit. Yet, their influence transcended their numbers and their time. Most were located in the tony Upper East Side neighborhoods or on streets that hug Central Park in the Fifties and Sixties. See UPPER EAST SIDE. The first restaurant that attracted the ladies was the Colony Club (1903), followed by the Cosmopolitan Club (1909), Le Pavillon (1941), Quo Vadis (1946), Le Côte Basque (1958), La Caravelle (1960), Lutèce (1961), La Grenouille (1962), Lafayette (1965), Orsini's (1968), and Mortimer's (1976). See COLONY CLUB; LA CARAVELLE; and LUTÈCE.

Most of the restaurants served haute French cuisine, and a very few offered French food by way of Italy. Gallic food was acknowledged by food connoisseurs as "important" food. All could trace their pedigree to the French Pavilion at New York's 1939 World's Fair. According to food writer Mimi Sheraton, the chefs remained in the United States to "avoid dangers back home; thus helping shape the postwar dining landscape in New York City." See FRENCH and WORLD'S FAIR (1939–1940).

The richest sauces and dishes were not of interest to the ladies. In the spirit of the Duchess of Windsor, who famously said, "A woman can't be too rich or too thin," the Ladies Who Lunch preferred dainty portions of comfort food with a classic French accent. Favorite menu items included omelets, crabmeat or lobster salad, duck à l'orange, broiled fish, chicken hash, soft-shell crabs, shad roe, and soups. Most of the ladies ordered the same thing every day. Beverages sparked the ambiance. Martinis were popular. Later, the restaurants helped popularize drinking wine with lunch. Others preferred an aperitif or champagne, and in the 1970s and 1980s white wine spritzers flowed. See COCKTAILS and MARTINI.

Borden, Maggie. "Taste Tomorrow: The 1939 New York World's Fair." *The Official James Beard Foundation Blog,* December 3, 2014. http://www.jamesbeard.org/blog/taste-tomorrow-1939-new-york-worlds-fair.
Colacello, Bob. "Here's to the Ladies Who Lunched!" *Vanity Fair,* February 2012.
Haskell, Rob. "Intimate Companions." *W* (November 2012).
Maccioni, Sirio, and Pamela Fiori. *A Table at Le Cirque.* New York: Rizzoli, 2012.
McGrath, Douglas. "An Immoveable Feast." *Vanity Fair* (August 2008).

Leeann Lavin

La Guardia, Fiorello

Fiorello H. La Guardia (1882–1947), the beloved, colorful, and controversial three-term mayor of New York, was a dynamic fighter for honest government and for the underprivileged throughout his career. His Italian immigrant parents were living in Greenwich Village when La Guardia was born. But they soon moved to Arizona, where his father was stationed as a U.S. Army bandmaster. In 1898, La Guardia's father, sickened by tainted meat sold to the army by unscrupulous suppliers, had to leave the service. He died six years later. During La Guardia's public life, he fought against the notorious practices that had led to his father's death and tried to ensure that even the poorest families could eat safely and well. For La Guardia, good food was as critical to public policy as to private pleasure.

In his early twenties, La Guardia moved to New York and studied law. In his practice, he represented immigrants, factory and sweatshop workers, and Lower East Side street peddlers, often free of charge.

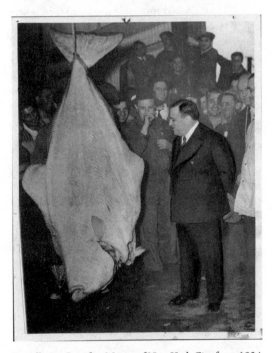

Fiorello La Guardia, Mayor of New York City from 1934 to 1945, was responsible for the opening of Fulton Fish Market's New Building. Here he poses with a 300-pound halibut at the Market in 1939. During his terms, Fiorello strove to make New York food consumption safe and sanitary. *WORLD TELEGRAM & SUN.* PHOTO BY C. M. STIEGLITZ

Elected to Congress from East Harlem in 1916, he supported unemployment insurance and access to affordable food for the disadvantaged.

When he ran for the office of mayor, he campaigned on issues of concern to the poor including housing, jobs, schools, and the high cost of food. He attributed the latter to politically corrupt distribution practices. A progressive Republican, he opposed the entrenched Democratic machine known as Tammany Hall.

As mayor, La Guardia devoted his considerable energies to fighting corruption, expanding social services, and improving living conditions. He cleaned up the streets for the 1939 World's Fair by creating indoor markets for food vendors. Although many vendors opposed the plan because they could not afford to rent space, some of the markets are still thriving.

Shortly before the United States entered World War II, La Guardia, while still mayor, took on the role of national director of the Office of Civilian Defense. He worked to keep food prices down and ensure equitable distribution of foodstuffs during the war. He vehemently warned against profiteering.

La Guardia was responsible for broad food policy issues in New York, nationally, and, later, internationally. However, he was not above offering food rationing advice and cooking tips to housewives during the war. A home cook whose specialty was making spaghetti, La Guardia was said to be the only New York mayor who cooked an election night victory dinner for family and friends himself. On his wartime radio broadcasts, he advised listeners to save fat and pointed out that they should not use the same fat for fish and for meat. He suggested they make bread pudding with stale bread and scolded them for buying too much heavy cream when there was a shortage of milk for children.

After his last term as mayor, concerned about the possibility of famine in postwar Europe, he became director general of the United Nations Relief and Rehabilitation Administration. In that role, he led efforts to feed the millions of displaced persons in Europe with his characteristic passion. La Guardia died of pancreatic cancer in 1947 at home, surrounded by his family.

See also ESSEX STREET MARKET and FULTON FISH MARKET.

Brodsky, Alyn. *The Great Mayor: Fiorello La Guardia and the Making of the City of New York*. New York: St. Martin's, 2003.

Heckscher, August. *When La Guardia Was Mayor: New York's Legendary Years*. With Phyllis Robinson. New York: Norton, 1978.

Jeri Quinzio

Lang, George

George Lang (1924–2011) was a prominent restaurateur and culinary writer. He was born in Székesfehérvár, Hungary, and immigrated to New York in 1946. He worked as a cook and a manager at Chateau Gardens, a wedding banquet facility on the Lower East Side. The owners of Chateau Gardens bought a Greek Orthodox church on East Houston Street, and Lang took charge of its conversion into a second banquet hall—"a muted version of Frankenstein's castle circa 1898," as he later wrote in his memoirs. In 1956, Lang was hired as an assistant banquet manager at the Waldorf Astoria.

This position brought him to the attention of Joe Baum, a manager of Restaurant Associates, who hired Lang in 1960. Lang helped open the Tower Suite in the Time-Life Building and managed several restaurants at the 1964 World's Fair in Flushing, Queens. After the fair closed, he managed The Four Seasons (the crown jewel of Restaurant Associates) for three years. Lang then left to launch his own restaurant-consulting businesses. See BAUM, JOE; FOUR SEASONS; RESTAURANT ASSOCIATES; and WORLD'S FAIR (1964–1965).

Lang is remembered for two great restaurants. In 1975 he took over the restaurant in the Hotel des Artistes. Not far from Lincoln Center, the Café des Artistes was frequented by actors and musicians and, with its atmospheric murals by Howard Chandler Christy, was one of New York's most "romantic" restaurants, according to *New York Times* restaurant critic William Grimes. Plagued by labor problems, Café des Artistes closed in 2009. Lang's second great achievement was the revival of Gundel, one of Budapest's most luxurious and prestigious restaurants, which, in partnership with American billionaire Ronald Lauder, Lang helped restore to its former glory in 1991 and 1992.

Lang wrote four books, including the highly esteemed *Cuisine of Hungary* (1971) and *The Café Des Artistes Cookbook* (1984). His memoir, *Nobody Knows the Truffles I've Seen*, was published in 1998.

See also WALDORF, THE.

Grimes, William. "George Lang, Mastermind Behind Café des Artistes, Dies at 86." *New York Times,* July 6, 2011.

Lang, George. *The Cuisine of Hungary.* New York: Atheneum, 1971.

Lang, George. *Nobody Knows the Truffles I've Seen.* New York: Knopf, 1998.

Andrew F. Smith

Lape, Bob

Bob Lape (b. 1930) is a restaurant critic whose *Dining Diary* radio feature is heard on the CBS flagship in New York. The pioneering newsman got his start covering politicians and murders and brought food news to New York City viewers in the 1970s.

While Lape declared in his high school yearbook that his life goal was to sign a contract with CBS, there was no similarly grand plan to become the "food guy" at the station. A member of the original Eyewitness News team for WABC, he was a hard-news reporter who spent his days following men like President Eisenhower and Edward Brooke, the country's first black congressman. But fate intervened in the form of a chance assignment. *The Eyewitness Gourmet* was born one afternoon when Lape returned from Brooklyn where he was covering a murder and discovered the assignment editor looking around for a restaurant reviewer. The show became the most popular local TV news feature of the 1970s and early 1980s, helping to set the stage for the Food Network in the 1990s. See FOOD NETWORK.

While he was not a complete food industry novice (his first-ever job was delivering farm fresh eggs door to door), he did have a lot to learn about restaurants and haute cuisine. He recalls a *guéridon* (a trolley used for food service) being rolled out and asking, "What's that?" The question got asked a lot—about the *guéridon* and then about sorrel in the sauce and much else at future shoots. Lape was a fast learner and always one step ahead of his viewers.

Those viewers stretched from busy housewives to hungry longshoremen who were known to shout out "Hey, there's that guy who eats" when they would encounter him covering a story. Well into his over twelve thousand stories about dishes or restaurants his popularity was universal—so universal that his

segments reran on *Good Morning America* and on WCBS radio. In 1986, Lape signed a contract with CBS for the *Dining Diary* radio feature, fulfilling the life goal he set out in his high school yearbook. In addition to his TV and radio work, Lape is known for the restaurant review page he created for *Crain's New York Business,* which ran for twenty-four years, and a similar page in the *New York Law Journal,* which had a sixteen-year run.

See also HERITAGE RADIO NETWORK and TELEVISION.

Dining Diary website: http://newyork.cbslocal.com/audio-on-demand/dining-diary/.

Francine Cohen

Late Twentieth Century

New York City's culinary scene is ever-changing, but during the last quarter of the twentieth century it underwent a truly massive upheaval. Large food manufacturing operations and their corporate headquarters left the city, while new startups were launched. Classic French food fell from favor, while innovative chefs and ethnically diverse restaurants came to the fore. Even as the well-heeled enjoyed an embarrassment of indulgent dining options, the number of New Yorkers going hungry increased, and food pantries, soup kitchens, and other programs proliferated to aid those who were food-insecure. A new movement stressing local, organic, and traditionally made foods found its footing; food co-ops and the citywide network of Greenmarkets were created. New culinary schools, professional organizations, and academic programs supported the ever-growing interest in food and cooking. Professional journalism continued to flower, and New York became a major publisher of academic works about food culture.

The exodus of large food and beverage manufacturing operations began in the 1950s, when General Foods and Nabisco left the city. PepsiCo moved its corporate headquarters from Manhattan to Purchase, New York, in 1970, and the company closed its bottling plant in Long Island City, Queens, in 1999 (although its iconic neon sign remains). The Jacob Ruppert Brewing Company, founded in Yorkville in the 1860s, survived until 1965. In 1969 Schlitz closed its Brooklyn plant, and F & M Schaefer, the city's last large brewery, closed in 1976. The Domino Sugar refinery in Williamsburg, the city's last such facility, closed in 2004.

As large corporations left the city and closed their factories, new food and beverage businesses started up. Unadulterated Food Products, Inc., formed in Brooklyn in 1972, sold "natural" fruit juices—including apple—in wide-mouthed glass bottles. In 1988 the company introduced its first flavored iced tea under the name "Snapple." In 1984 the Manhattan Brewing Company opened in an old SoHo industrial building, serving its own beer on tap. When the brewery began wholesaling its products to other establishments, the beer was transported by a horse-drawn wagon. The Manhattan Brewing Company folded in 1995, not long after its brewmaster, Garrett Oliver, left to help start the Brooklyn Brewing Company, which opened in 1996 and is now the city's largest brewery.

Restaurants

As city life grew more casual and the New York palate became more adventurous, haute cuisine restaurants, such as The Colony and Le Pavillon, declined in importance and many closed. This was also true of the once-novel theme restaurants of the 1950s and 1960s. A new generation of chefs and restaurateurs, including Drew Nieporent, Daniel Boulud, Danny Meyer, Jean-Georges Vongerichten, and Keith McNally, developed new restaurant concepts and innovative new menus. Nieporent and his Myriad Restaurant Group operated the groundbreaking Tribeca restaurant Montrachet as well as Tribeca Grill and Nobu New York City. Daniel Boulud, who had been executive chef at Le Cirque, brought classic French cuisine up to date at his restaurant Daniel; five years later he opened the more casual Café Boulud and as of 2015 has a total of eight restaurants in the city. Danny Meyer created the Union Square Hospitality Group, including the Union Square Café and the Gramercy Tavern. Alsatian-born Jean-Georges Vongerichten, who had traveled and trained in Asia, opened his first New York City restaurant, JoJo, on the Upper East Side in 1991. Jean-Georges, on Central Park West, followed in 1997; there Vongerichten introduced the Asian–French fusion cuisine that has become his hallmark. Restaurateur Keith McNally established the long-lived downtown eateries Odeon, Café Luxembourg, Lucky Strike, and Balthazar.

Pastis, which opened in 1999, was one of the earliest arrivals in the not-yet-chic meatpacking district.

Early quick-service chains, such as Childs cafeterias and Horn & Hardart automats, faded once the twentieth century passed its midpoint, while national fast-food chains, such as McDonald's, Wendy's, Taco Bell, KFC, Dunkin' Donuts, Pizza Hut, and Burger King, flooded into the city. Kosher (or "kosher-style") delicatessens specializing in cured meats, pickled fish, and other Old World specialties declined, although a few iconic delis, such as Katz's, the Second Avenue Deli, Carnegie Deli, and Stage Deli, hung on.

Late-century immigrants—Italians, Greeks, Puerto Ricans, West Indians, Chinese, and, especially, Koreans—found that ownership of a small neighborhood grocery store (in New York parlance, a "deli") proved an excellent entry point into the city's economy. Some deli owners include their native favorites; for instance, delis owned by Korean Americans frequently sell kimchi as well as packaged Asian grocery items, while West Indian proprietors offer savory turnovers called "patties." The huge influx of new immigrants following the loosening of racist immigration laws in 1965 led to an unprecedented diversity in the foods and dishes available to all New Yorkers.

Hunger Programs

Simultaneous with the increase in diversity of the city's restaurants was a rise in the demand for, and provision of, hunger programs. School lunch programs for low-income students expanded during the final decades of the twentieth century. The New York City Coalition Against Hunger was formed in 1983 by nonprofit soup kitchens and food pantries to coordinate the activities of emergency food providers. By 2000, the coalition represented more than one thousand hunger-relief groups working in the city. Programs were available for an estimated twenty-three thousand homeless as well as the elderly who are unable to purchase or prepare their own meals. By the end of the century, an estimated one million city residents were food-insecure.

The Food Movement

During the early 1970s, alternative food distribution systems emerged, such as food co-ops and community supported agriculture programs. In 1976, the first New York City farmers' market was set up in an empty lot at Fifty-Ninth Street and Second Avenue. That group of twelve local farmers selling their own produce grew into a network of New York City Greenmarkets, which offer products grown, raised, or prepared within 200 miles of the city. It is not just home cooks who enjoy the abundant fruits and vegetables, meats, dairy products, baked goods, preserves, and even wines that Greenmarkets make available; many of the city's chefs are avid market shoppers, and their menus reflect the bounty they find there. Toward the end of the twentieth century specialty grocery store chains, such as Citarella, Dean & DeLuca, Fairway Market, Gourmet Garage, and Garden of Eden, began to lure customers away from the city's traditional supermarkets.

Professional culinary organizations were started in New York. Les Dames d'Escoffier was established in 1973 by Carol Brock, who was then Sunday food editor at the *New York Daily News*. Membership is by invitation only. An organization of professional women in the food and wine industry, the New York Women's Culinary Alliance was launched in 1981 by chefs Sara Moulton and Maria Reuge. The Culinary Historians of New York was founded in 1985 to stimulate and share knowledge about food history. Slow Food USA was launched in Brooklyn in 2000.

When James Beard died in 1985, cooking-school owner Peter Kump raised funds to buy Beard's Greenwich Village townhouse. With support from other important culinary figures, including Julia Child and Jacques Pépin, Kump helped launch the James Beard Foundation, headquartered in Beard's townhouse on West Twelfth Street. Since 1990, the James Beard Foundation has given awards for excellence to chefs, journalists, and other culinary professionals.

Culinary Schools and Academic Programs

Culinary schools have operated in New York since the nineteenth century, but they proliferated in the late twentieth century. Peter Kump founded the New York Cooking School in 1975; after Kump's death, the school was sold, tremendously expanded, and renamed the Institute for Culinary Education. The Natural Gourmet Cooking School, which focuses on "health-supportive" cooking, was started by Annemarie Colbin in 1977. De Gustibus Cooking School, founded in 1980 by Arlene Feltman Sail-

hac, is based at Macy's in Herald Square; it offers mostly demonstration classes rather than hands-on training. The French Culinary Institute in SoHo, founded by Dorothy Cann Hamilton in 1984, was later renamed the International Culinary Center, having added other world cuisines to its curriculum.

In addition to culinary schools, city universities developed academic food studies programs. New York University opened its Department of Nutrition, Food Studies, and Public Health in the 1990s; the department now offers undergraduate, master's, and doctoral programs in food studies, culture, and food systems. The New School started an undergraduate food studies department in 2007, and other local colleges and universities began offering academic courses on various aspects of food. University presses, such as Columbia University Press and Oxford University Press, began publishing scholarly and reference works about food.

New York's newspapers increased their coverage of culinary matters during the late twentieth century. In 1997 the *New York Times* launched a Dining section that included recipes, restaurant critiques, and wine reviews as well as feature articles on food trends and controversies. The period also saw the debuts of several New York–based food magazines, including *Food & Wine* (1978), *Food Arts* (1988), and *Saveur* (1994). Other magazines, such as the *New Yorker*, *New York* magazine, and *Time Out New York* regularly published reviews and articles about the city's culinary scene.

By the time the twentieth century ended, New York's always-fluid culinary scene had acquired striking new diversity. It was well prepared to face the challenges that emerged in the twenty-first century.

See also BROCK, CAROL; DELIS, GERMAN; DELIS, JEWISH; *EDIBLE*; GRIMES, WILLIAM; HUNGER PROGRAMS; LE PAVILLON; NEW SCHOOL; *NEW YORKER*; *NEW YORK TIMES*; NEW YORK UNIVERSITY; *SAVEUR*; SCHOOL FOOD; SLOW FOOD; and SODA.

Batterberry, Michael, and Ariane Batterberry. *On the Town in New York: The Landmark History of Eating, Drinking, and Entertainments from the American Revolution to the Food Revolution*. New York and London: Routledge, 1999.

Grimes, William. *Appetite City: A Culinary History of New York*. New York: North Point, 2009.

Hauck-Lawson, Annie, and Jon Deutsch, eds. *Gastropolis: Food & New York City*. New York: Columbia University Press, 2008.

Kuh, Patric. *The Last Days of Haute Cuisine: America's Culinary Revolution*. New York: Viking, 2001.

Smith, Andrew F. *New York City: A Food Biography*. Lanham, Md.: AltaMira, 2014.

Andrew F. Smith

Lebanese

See SYRIAN AND LEBANESE.

Le Cirque

In March 1974, Italian-born maitre d'hôtel Sirio Maccioni opened Le Cirque in the Mayfair Hotel, making it the first privately owned hotel restaurant in New York City. He had spent more than a decade building a clientele list of Manhattan hobnobbers while working at Delmonico's and The Colony restaurants. See DELMONICO'S.

Maccioni's talent for lavishing Le Cirque customers with attention along with his insight in selecting French technique-based chefs to execute a cutting-edge menu are the main reasons for Le Cirque's success. Beyond attracting the movers and shakers of the world like Rudolph Giuliani, Martha Stewart, and Donald Trump, Le Cirque is best known to the general public for bringing crème brûlée and pasta primavera to prominence in New York City. These dishes inspired a culinary revolution of sorts as they were replicated across the country. Daniel Boulud, who was executive chef from 1986 to 1992, noted in *Sirio: The Story of My Life and Le Cirque* that the tableside pasta primavera was an example of Maccioni's genius: an Italian dish prepared in a French way. See BOULUD, DANIEL. The crème brûlée was inspired by a dinner in Spain where Maccioni was served *crema catalana*, a popular regional dessert that tops a custard with caramelized sugar. Geoffrey Zakarian dubbed the restaurant a "culinary fantasy land," where exotic ingredients (for those days) abounded—wild game, foie gras, roast baby lamb, and suckling pig.

In 1986, the *New York Times* characterized the energy of the dining room under Boulud as "high-voltage." In 1987 under Boulud Le Cirque earned a four-star review from the newspaper, later winning the James Beard Outstanding Restaurant Award in 1995. In addition to Boulud, the chefs whose careers have been launched at Le Cirque include David Bouley, Andrew Carmellini, Michael Lomonaco, Marc Murphy, Alain Sailhac, Bill Telepan, Jacques Torres, and Geoffrey Zakarian.

In 1997, the restaurant moved from the Mayfair to the New York Palace under the name of Le Cirque 2000, where it remained until 2004. In 2006, HBO released *Le Cirque: A Table in Heaven*, a documentary chronicling Le Cirque 2000 from its opening in that location through the restaurant's reopening in 2006 in its current location at One Beacon Court in Midtown East.

Maccioni's three sons have followed in his footsteps in the restaurant industry, spreading the Le Cirque brand worldwide. The family has launched three Las Vegas restaurants, along with restaurants in the Dominican Republic and India.

See also MACCIONI, SIRIO.

Lynn, Andrea. "2014 James Beard Foundation Lifetime Achievement Award Recipient Sirio Maccioni." *The Official James Beard Foundation Blog*, May 5, 2014. http://www.jamesbeard.org/blog/2014-james-beard-foundation-lifetime-achievement-award-recipient-sirio-maccioni.
Maccioni, Sirio, and Peter J. Elliot. *Sirio: The Story of My Life and Le Cirque*. Hoboken, N.J.: Wiley, 2004.

Andrea Lynn

Lemcke, Gesine

See COOKING SCHOOLS.

Lemon Ice King of Corona

See ITALIAN ICES and QUEENS.

Lenape

See PRE-COLUMBIAN.

Lender, Harry

See BAGELS.

Le Pavillon

Le Pavillon was a New York restaurant that relaunched American interest in haute cuisine after World War II. It started as the restaurant for the French government's pavilion at the New York World's Fair held in Flushing, Queens, in 1939.

Charles Drouant, owner of the Café de Paris and several other restaurants in France, was selected by the French government to run "Le Restaurant du Pavillon de France." It was staffed by workers from Parisian restaurants. Marius Isnard of the Hôtel de Paris in Monte Carlo was selected as chef de cuisine, with the dining room under the supervision of the thirty-six-year-old Henri Soulé. Born in Saubrigues, in southwestern France, in 1903, Soulé began his restaurant career as a busboy at the Hotel Continental in Bayonne and then a waiter at Hotel Mirabeau, where he became captain. After stints at London's Trocadero Restaurant and elsewhere, in 1933 he became the manager and chief of staff at the Café de Paris. The restaurant at the World's Fair received glowing reviews and was frequented by many well-heeled American patrons who appreciated the authentic French cuisine. The *New York Times* called the food served at Le Pavillon's restaurant "an epicure's delight."

By the time the fair closed on October 27, 1940, war had begun in Europe; a defeated France was divided, part under German occupation and the rest controlled by the collaborationist Vichy government. Many employees of the French pavilion's restaurant decided not to return to their home country at that time. Charles Drouant thought he would try opening a French restaurant in New York City. He sought investors, one of whom was reputed to be Joseph P. Kennedy. When Drouant decided to return to France, Henri Soulé took over the project.

Soulé found a promising location on New York's fashionable Upper East Side, and, hoping to trade on the popularity of the restaurant at the fair, he named the restaurant Le Pavillon. Soulé was the owner and manager, and many of his former colleagues joined him, including Pierre Franey, who had been the *poisson commis* (assistant fish cook).

Soulé invited the rich, famous, and powerful to the restaurant's opening on October 15, 1941. Le Pavillon was an unqualified success from the beginning, even as the United States entered the war less than two months later. Franey enlisted in the U.S. Army and helped liberate France. He returned to rejoin the staff at Le Pavillon and moved steadily up the ranks, becoming executive chef in the early 1950s.

New York's wealthiest and most prominent citizens—Astors, Cabots, Kennedys, Rockefellers, and Vanderbilts—were regulars at Le Pavillon. The autocratic Soulé made a virtue of snobbery. Under the guise of protecting the sensibilities of his refined customers, he refused entrance to anyone who did

not meet his standards. Soulé is also thought to have coined the term "Siberia," referring to the tables closest to the kitchen (the least desirable in most restaurants).

In 1955 Harry Cohn, the president of Columbia Pictures, bought the building that housed Le Pavillon. Soulé considered him a loudmouthed vulgarian, and when he dined at Le Pavillon Soulé consistently seated him at a less than prominent table. Cohn charged anti-Semitism. After Cohn tripled the rent, Le Pavillon moved to 111 East Fifty-Seventh Street in 1957. When Cohn died, Soulé rented the old space again, at a much lower price, and opened La Côte Basque, a slightly more casual and affordable alternative to Le Pavillon. Harry Cohn was gone, but rumors of Soulé's anti-Semitism lingered.

Craig Claiborne became the food editor of the *New York Times* in 1957, and he often dined at Le Pavillon. He considered it to be America's finest restaurant—and one of the best in the world.

In 1960, the nation's economy slumped, and the restaurant needed to downsize. Soulé announced that overtime pay would be canceled. Chef Pierre Franey and other workers, including newcomer Jacques Pépin, a rising star who had been at Le Pavillon for just eight months, joined Franey and walked out, forcing Le Pavillon to close temporarily. Neither Franey nor Pépin ever returned to Le Pavillon; the restaurant opened several days later with replacement chefs.

Claiborne wrote an article about the imbroglio. Howard Johnson, owner of the national restaurant chain and a Pavillon habitué, read the article and hired both Franey and Pépin. Although prestige may have been lacking, the money was better and the working hours were less onerous. Chef Roger Fessaguet, who had worked at Le Pavillon since 1948, also left in 1960 to become executive chef at La Caravelle, owned by Fred Decré and Robert Meyzen, both of whom had worked as maître d' at Le Pavillon.

Another untoward event of 1960 occurred when Joseph Kennedy, the father of then senator (and presidential hopeful) John F. Kennedy, was dining at Le Pavillon. A photographer came in and started snapping pictures of Kennedy, who asked the photographer to leave. Soulé announced that he alone would determine who stayed in the restaurant, adding that even though the Democratic convention had not yet been held, the Kennedys were acting as if their son had already been elected president. Joseph Kennedy never returned to Le Pavillon.

When Henri Soulé died, in 1966, Craig Claiborne eulogized him as the "Michelangelo, the Mozart and Leonardo of the French restaurant in America." Le Pavillon survived Soulé's death but closed five years later. It had been one of the most influential restaurants since Delmonico's. See DELMONICO'S.

Though it was replaced by other fashionable French restaurants, adherence to Escoffier's precepts was no longer de rigueur; chefs forged new paths, taking inspiration from other cuisines and creating novel variations on the classics. Soulé's greatest achievement, according to Claiborne, was his nurturing of chefs, restaurateurs, and other individuals who were influential on America's fine dining scene.

See also FRENCH; HAUTE CUISINE; QUEENS; and WORLD'S FAIR (1939–1940).

Batterberry, Michael, and Ariane Batterberry. *On the Town in New York: The Landmark History of Eating, Drinking, and Entertainments from the American Revolution to the Food Revolution.* New York and London: Routledge, 1999.

Grimes, William. *Appetite City: A Culinary History of New York.* New York: North Point, 2009.

Kamp, David. *The United States of Arugula: How We Became a Gourmet Nation.* New York: Broadway, 2006.

Kuh, Patric. *The Last Days of Haute Cuisine: America's Culinary Revolution.* New York: Viking, 2001.

Wechsberg, Joseph. *Dining at the Pavillon.* Boston: Little, Brown, 1962.

Andrew F. Smith

Les Dames d'Escoffier

Les Dames d'Escoffier International is a prestigious professional organization of women achievers in the wine, food, and hospitality industries. Formed in 1973 in response to the all-male fine-dining association Les Amis d'Escoffier Society, the autonomous "Ladies Chapter of New York" (LDNY) was the first such organization in the world, intended to provide women with education, mentoring, and networking opportunities within the culinary and hospitality field. The name references the legendary French chef Auguste Escoffier.

Food journalist Carol Brock, then Sunday food editor at the *New York Daily News,* called together Beverly Barbour, Mary Lyons, Elayne Kleeman, Helene Bennett, and Ella Elvin to formulate the mission and vision of Les Dames.

On November 8, 1976, a landmark investiture and gala for LDNY was held at the French embassy on Fifth Avenue. Les Dames welcomed fifty food and wine professionals as new members, including such luminaries as Marcella Hazan, Paula Wolfert, and Barbara Kafka. Unlike any other culinary industry organization, its members were New York women from across all areas of the food, wine, and hospitality fields. Halston designed the serviettes for the event (the Escoffier group always dined with a napkin tucked under the chin); Tiffany designed the silver napkin rings.

At its first black-tie Regency Hotel dinner, Les Dames New York honored Julia Child as a Grand Dame. Writer M. F. K. Fisher was honored as a Grand Dame at a subsequent reception and supper held in the New York Public Library.

In 1978, women chefs prepared a groundbreaking dinner at the Waldorf Astoria Hotel. (Dame) Leslie Revson, the first woman chef at the Waldorf, headed an all women chef team of fifteen. They prepared an investiture dinner there for 135 people.

Perhaps the New York chapter's most successful and ambitious project was "A Salute to Women in Gastronomy." This one-week extravaganza, held January 16–23, 1994, was announced in a double-page spread ad in the *New York Times.* The event netted more than $100,000 for scholarships and philanthropic causes and resulted in a citation from the City of New York signed by Mayor Rudolph Giuliani. New York members conducted four events each day, including professional seminars, wine and food tastings, book signings, magazine features, and even food-filled documentary forums. In attendance were notables Pierre and Michel Escoffier, Auguste Escoffier's grandson and great-grandson, respectively. The highlight of the week was a benefit at the Rainbow Room attended by Julia Child.

Les Dames New York (a nonprofit 501(c)(3) organization) was the first chapter of what would become an international organization. Within ten years of establishing the New York chapter, chapters were opened in Washington, D.C., Chicago, Dallas, and Philadelphia, and the organization became Les Dames d'Escoffier International (LDEI) as stated in the original constitution. A London chapter was added in 2010. As of 2015, LDEI includes 1,900 members in thirty chapters throughout the United States, Canada, and the United Kingdom.

LDEI now presents the M. F. K. Fisher Award for distinguished journalism and the Grand Dame Award for an outstanding Dame member or nonmember in the food, wine, and hospitality fields. Both awards are presented biennially. In addition, Legacy Awards are presented each year at the LDEI conference, an award that offers the opportunity for recipients to gain hands-on experience and expand their professional expertise.

Two LDEI initiatives bridge various food-producing organizations with food consumers. The Green Tables Initiative, launched in 2005, furthers the connections among urban and rural farms and gardens and school, restaurant, and kitchen tables in LDEI chapter communities. The Global Culinary Initiative embraces global communities through culinary connections that provide educational programming, training programs, and cultural exchange.

Fabricant, Florence. "Food Notes." *New York Times*, January 12, 1994.
Les Dames d'Escoffier International website: http://www.ldei.org.
Les Dames d'Escoffier New York Archives. Fales Library and Special Collections, Elmer Holmes Bobst Library, New York University, 1973–.
Reardon, Joan. *Poet of the Appetites: The Lives and Loves of M. F. K. Fisher.* New York: North Point, 2004.
Rosene, Marcella, and Pat Mozersky, eds. *Cooking with Les Dames d'Escoffier: At Home with the Women Who Shape the Way We Eat and Drink.* Seattle: Sasquatch, 2008.

Carol Brock

Lewis, Edna

Edna Lewis (1916–2006) was born in Freeville, Virginia, an African American community founded by freed slaves after the Civil War. Her family grew much of its own food, and she learned to cook from her mother. Orphaned by the age of seventeen or eighteen and facing the challenges of the Depression, she moved to New York City in the 1930s and lived with an aunt and uncle in Harlem. See HARLEM. She found work as a seamstress, sewing gowns for wealthy women, including Dorcas Avedon, wife of photographer Richard Avedon, while creating African-inspired dresses for herself that eventually became her signature style. She married Steven Kingston, a retired seaman cook and activist (the date is unclear). They were members of the Communist Party, at the time the only integrated organization actively promoting civil rights and racial equality during a period when Jim Crow laws and segregation were rampant.

Lewis was moving in a circle of young, multiracial, artistic friends, among them fashion photographer Karl Bissinger and antiques dealer John Nicholson. She would cook for them occasionally, and, although she had never cooked professionally, in 1948 they asked her to become a partner and the chef at their soon-to-open restaurant, Café Nicholson, on East Fifty-Eighth Street. See CAFÉ NICHOLSON. Lewis's cooking was traditional French, self-taught from classic cookbooks but heavily inflected with her southern family recipes and appreciation of the South's fresh ingredients. The thirty-seat eatery was packed each night, catering to a prominent, bohemian clientele. Marlon Brando, Marlene Dietrich, Rita Hayworth, Greta Garbo, Howard Hughes, Salvador Dalí, Eleanor Roosevelt, Dean Martin, and Jerry Lewis all dined at Café Nicholson and southerners Truman Capote, William Faulkner, and Tennessee Williams were regulars. In a 1951 *New York Herald Tribune* restaurant review, Clementine Paddleford lauded Lewis's "filet mignon… with the most heavenly Béarnaise sauce one could imagine.…Roast chicken…cooked with fresh herbs… it comes brown as autumn chestnuts … cheese soufflé—each bite like springtime on the tongue." See PADDLEFORD, CLEMENTINE.

Her husband Steven became increasingly discontented with Café Nicholson's "bourgeois" nature, protesting that they were "catering to capitalists." At his insistence, five years after opening, Lewis left Café Nicholson. They moved briefly to New Jersey, unsuccessfully farming pheasants, but soon returned to New York City. Lewis became a private caterer and, in 1967, opened a short-lived southern restaurant on Harlem's Seventh Avenue near 125th Street. It was a time when the moniker "soul food" had come to signify any and all food cooked by blacks, particularly in cities outside the South. Lewis disliked the term and often distinguished her cooking from this urban version that relied heavily on canned goods, processed foods, and shortcuts. While Lewis's dishes were not what was considered typically southern, they demonstrated her elegant yet uncomplicated southern-style cookery and choice of ingredients (she remained a proponent of the traditional uses of butter, sugar, lard, and pork) with a knowledge of how to maximize food's inherent flavors starting with what she would later refer to as "nonhybridized," fresh, seasonal produce and meats. In later years, disappointed by what she noticed as a marked decline in the taste of commercially available foods, she spoke out against an overuse of chemicals, additives, preservatives, hormones, and antibiotics in the modern food system. Lewis's philosophy is widely considered a precursor to Alice Waters's California cookery.

In the 1970s, Lewis worked as an educator in the African Hall at the American Museum of Natural History on Central Park West, a caterer, and cooking teacher. See AMERICAN MUSEUM OF NATURAL HISTORY. She started writing her first book, *The Edna Lewis Cookbook* (1972), while bored and recovering from a broken leg. After its publication, she was introduced to publishing icon Judith Jones at Knopf, who encouraged Lewis to find her unique voice when writing down her recipes, memories, and stories of home. See JONES, JUDITH AND EVAN and KNOPF. She traveled throughout the South to broaden her southern regional repertoire, and this memoir of sorts became Lewis's second and bestselling book, *The Taste of Country Cooking* (1976), completed just as her husband died; it is considered one of a handful of essential texts on southern food to this day. The book was highly praised by luminaries M. F. K. Fisher, James Beard, and Craig Claiborne. Lewis would go on to write two more books, *In Pursuit of Flavor* with Mary Goodby (1988) and *The Gift of Southern Cooking* with Scott Peacock (2003).

Already in her early seventies, Lewis took the helm at restaurateur Peter Aschkenasy's short-lived Uncle Sam's (formerly the U.S. Steakhouse in Rockefeller Center) and, in 1989, became head chef at his newly acquired landmark chophouse, Gage & Tollner, on Fulton Street in Brooklyn. See GAGE & TOLLNER. Gage & Tollner had been in continuous operation since 1879 and was a New York institution. There, Lewis added southern notes of pan-fried quail, corn pudding, and her legendary she-crab soup to resuscitate its more-than-one-hundred-year-old menu, garnering publicity and drawing eager crowds. She retired from Gage & Tollner in the mid-1990s and, in 1999, moved to Decatur, Georgia, to live (platonically) with Peacock, whom she had met in 1990 while he was cooking at the governor's mansion in Georgia. They were the "odd couple" of southern cooking: Peacock was a young, gay, white chef

and Lewis was the widowed, elegant grande dame fifty years his senior. Peacock cared for Lewis until her death at their home on February 13, 2006. She is buried in a family plot in Unionville, Virginia.

In her lifetime, Lewis was featured in *Food & Wine, House & Garden, House Beautiful, Essence, Redbook,* the *New York Times, New York Magazine, Ladies' Home Journal, New York Woman,* and *Connoisseur,* among others. *Gourmet* called her the "Dean of Southern Cooks." She was awarded an honorary PhD in culinary arts from Johnson & Wales University in Norfolk, Virginia, in 1996, as well as being the first recipient of the James Beard Foundation's Living Legend Award in 1999. The international Association of Culinary Professionals gave her its Lifetime Achievement Award, and she was honored by Les Dames d'Escoffier and the Women Chefs and Restaurateurs. She was a major impetus behind the founding of the Southern Foodways Alliance and received its first Craig Claiborne Lifetime Achievement Award in 1999. She is one of five culinary legends in the U.S. Postal Service celebrity chef limited edition "Forever" stamp series.

Asimov, Eric, and Kim Severson. "Edna Lewis, 89, Dies; Wrote Cookbooks that Revived Refined Southern Cuisine." *New York Times,* February 14, 2006.
Levy, Paul. "Edna Lewis." *The Independent,* February 22, 2006.
Twitty, Michael. "Edna Lewis." In *Icons of American Cooking,* edited by Victor W. Geraci and Elizabeth S. Demers, pp. 155–168. Santa Barbara, Calif.: Greenwood, 2011.

Tonya Hopkins

Liebling, A. J.

Abbott Joseph Liebling (1904–1963) was a journalist, sports writer, war correspondent, *New Yorker* columnist, and author of the classic *Between Meals: An Appetite for Paris.* A native New Yorker, Liebling grew up in a well-off, bourgeois family. His father was a successful furrier, but Liebling wanted no part of the family business. When he was twenty-two, his father gave him a modest stipend to spend on a year in Paris. Ostensibly, Liebling attended the Sorbonne, but mostly he studied Paris, its people, and its cuisine.

When he returned to New York, Liebling wrote for newspapers and then for the *New Yorker.* He loved the louche life and wrote affectionately about

Broadway's con men and hustlers. His biographer, Raymond Sokolov, said Liebling was the "most important boxing writer in a century" and credited him with inventing modern press criticism in his Wayward Press columns in the *New Yorker*.

His memoir, *Between Meals: An Appetite for Paris*, looked back fondly on his early years and subsequent experiences in Paris. Liebling explained that because he was unhampered by "the crippling handicap of affluence" during his Paris year, he experimented with inexpensive foods and wines and came to appreciate the robust taste of foods such as conger eel stewed in wine, braised beef heart, smoked tripe sausage, and "dark, winy stews of domestic rabbit and old turkey." The wealthy, he wrote, would never know a *pot-au-feu*, "the foundation glory of French cooking." Liebling never lost his taste for the earthy foods and wines of his younger days.

A man of proudly gargantuan appetites, Liebling ate well but not wisely, even when it was clear that surfeit was destroying his health. He became obese and suffered from gout as well as kidney and heart problems, yet he continued to eat and drink excessively and scoff at the abstemious. In *Between Meals*, he wrote of Marcel Proust and the delicate madeleine that inspired *Remembrance of Things Past*: "In the light of what Proust wrote with so mild a stimulus, it is the world's loss that he did not have a heartier appetite."

To say that Liebling had a hearty appetite would be the height of understatement. In France, even in his later years, two dozen snails or oysters and a bottle of champagne for two was a typical start to a meal that might also include sausages, potato gratin, fowl cooked in cream, and more. In New York, according to Sokolov's biography *Wayward Reporter: The Life of A. J. Liebling*, younger journalists would watch in awe as Liebling lunched on martinis, piles of oysters, double portions of lobster *fra diavolo*, and *osso buco*.

Despite his gluttony, Liebling had high standards, and when a dish did not meet them, he was scathing. In *Between Meals*, he described poorly cooked lamb as "tired Alpine billy goat...seared in machine oil." Haricots verts resembled "decomposed whiskers from a theatrical-costume beard," and a mediocre couscous was "cream of wheat with hot sauce." Liebling was fifty-nine when he died of pneumonia and complications in New York, a few months after returning from a trip to his beloved Paris.

Liebling, A. J. *Between Meals: An Appetite for Paris*. New York: North Point, 1986.
Sokolov, Raymond. *Wayward Reporter: The Life of A. J. Liebling*. New York: Harper & Row, 1980.

Jeri Quinzio

Life Savers

Clarence Crane (1875–1931), a Cleveland confectioner, created a novel candy, which he named "Life Savers" for its resemblance to a life preserver. In 1913 New Yorkers Edward J. Noble and J. Roy Allen paid Crane $2,900 for the rights to produce a ring-shaped, mint-flavored hard candy and manufactured them in New York.

Crane packed Life Savers in cardboard tubes; but with nothing between the candy and the cardboard, glue from the seam seeped into the mints, and grocers rejected them. After establishing the Mint Products Company of New York, Edward Noble began packaging stacks of "Pep-O-Mint Life Savers" in foil wrappers and charging a nickel a pack. The marketing angle was to sell them in bars, from a display right next to the cash register. Someone who had been drinking and wanted to hide the evidence might buy a roll of mint candies as breath fresheners. In 1915, the United Cigar Store chain placed racks of Life Savers in their many stores, and the candies were also sold in grocery stores, pharmacies, restaurants, and newsstands.

Life Savers were packed by hand in New York until 1919, when machinery was acquired to expand production. Noble built a plant north of the city, in Port Chester. In 1925 Noble bought out Allen for $3.3 million and changed the name of the firm to the Edward J. Noble Company.

In 1919 Pep-O-Mint, the original Life Saver flavor, was joined by Wint-O-Green, Vi-O-Let, Choc-O-Let, and three others. Fruit-flavored candies debuted in 1921, but they were solid disks rather than rings. By 1929, the technology had been developed to produce fruit-flavored Life Savers with holes, and in 1935 the pineapple, lime, orange, cherry, and lemon flavors were combined in one package—the Five-Flavor Roll. In 1956, Life Savers Candies merged with Beech-Nut, makers of gum and baby food. Life Savers Candies was later acquired by the Wm. Wrigley Jr. Company.

See also CANDY.

Broekel, Ray. *The Great American Candy Bar Book.* Boston: Houghton Mifflin, 1982.

Richardson, Tim. *Sweets: A History of Candy.* New York: Bloomsbury, 2002.

Andrew F. Smith

Lindy's

Lindy's, the delis established by Leo Lindemann in 1921 and 1929 on Broadway near Fiftieth and Fifty-First Streets, enjoy near-mythic status today, not only for their moderately priced food and vibrant atmosphere but especially for memories of the New York–style cheesecake. The originals closed in 1957 and 1969, but since 1979 two more Manhattan eateries have been operating under the Lindy's brand, one on Seventh Avenue at Fifty-Third Street and the other on Seventh Avenues at Thirty-Second Street. They are owned by the Manhattan-based Riese Organization, a major Northeast restaurant and real estate management company. Although Riese acquired a trademark for the name, the New York–centric flavor of the originals is gone, and they play mostly to the deep-pocketed tourist trade. These are "Lindy's" in name only, especially where that cheesecake is concerned.

What put that classic in a class by itself? This can probably be attributed to its particular balance of main ingredients (cream cheese, sugar, eggs, and cream) and to the refreshing addition of grated orange and lemon rind. Then there was that famous cookie-dough crust.

It is perhaps the crust that cheesecake aficionados with long memories remember best. In 1977, writing for the *New York Times*, Craig Claiborne published the "secret" recipe for Lindy's cheesecake that he had acquired from Guy Pascal, then the pastry chef at La Côte Basque restaurant. Pascal, in turn, had figured it out deductively. The former Lindy's employee he'd hired for his struggling Las Vegas pastry shop—and whose cheesecake sales turned around—would not divulge the recipe. By accounting for the number of cakes sold, keeping strict track of ingredients, and watching him out of the corner of his eye, Pascal was able to put together a recipe that rivaled his employee's.

Once Claiborne published it, however, scores of readers wrote in to report that the filling may have accurately recaptured the Lindy's confection but the recipe's light graham-cracker crust was simply

wrong and claimed that it was instead a thin cookie-dough crust. They also made it clear that the "secret" recipe had long been made public by Clementine Paddleford, who, with Lindemann's blessing, got the recipe directly from Paul Landry, Lindy's in-house baker. See PADDLEFORD, CLEMENTINE. Not surprisingly, this recipe conforms to the one typed on Lindy's letterhead business stationery now in the possession of Karen Golumbeck, granddaughter of Joseph Kramer, Lindemann's original partner.

Molly O'Neill's recipe for Junior's cheesecake published in her *New York Cookbook* (1992) hews very closely to the Pascal/Claiborne recipe, though it contains far less sugar than that version. Adding to the intrigue: though Lindemann is credited for making cheesecake famous, he may have acquired his recipe early on from the pastry chef of fellow delicatessen owner Arnold Reuben.

Today, Lindy's cheesecake is baked off-premises and sits on a thin slice of sponge cake. No cookie dough here. A single slice weighs in at nearly eight ounces and costs an almost prohibitive ten dollars. The whisper of citrus wistfully hints at the memory of Lindy's cheesecakes past.

See also CHEESECAKE; CREAM CHEESE; and JUNIOR'S.

Berger, Myron. "The Passing Parade at Lindy's." *New York Times*, August 4, 1957.

Freedman, Dan. "'Lost' Recipe for Legendary Cheesecake Found." *Times Union*, June 13, 2012.

Marks, Gil. *Encyclopedia of Jewish Food.* Hoboken: Wiley, 2010.

Paddleford, Clementine. *How America Eats.* New York: Scribner, 1960.

Jane L. Smulyan

Little India

Indian immigrants have come to the United States in two waves since the 1900s. The first wave consisted of approximately sixty-eight hundred Punjabi Sikhs who immigrated to rural California between 1899 and 1920 to work as manual laborers on farms and on the railroad. The second wave of South Asian immigration is part of the post-1965 or "new" immigration that followed President Lyndon Johnson's repeal of immigration quotas which limited immigration from Eastern and Southern Europe, Latin America, Africa, the Middle East, and Asia and has increased the racial, ethnic, and religious diversity of the United States. The majority of post-1965 South Asian immigrants settled in metropolitan cities such as Chicago and New York. The "new" South Asian immigration can itself be divided into two waves. The first South Asian "new" immigrants were part of the "brain drain"—educated professionals who immigrated to the United States for educational and economic reasons. Many of these immigrants were scientists, physicians, and engineers who, because of their education and technical skills, quickly found jobs and became successful. The second group began to come in 1980, largely through family reunification programs or in search of better educational and employment opportunities, higher standards of living, and political and religious freedoms. Despite these class differences, because of their proficiency in English and the preference for educated immigrants since 1965, South Asians in general have maintained high levels of educational attainment and income relative to other minority groups as part of the "model minority."

Indian immigration to New York City began in the 1960s. The area that is commonly known as Little India today is located in the borough of Queens at Seventy-Third and Seventy-Fourth Streets between Roosevelt and Thirty-Seventh Avenues, in Jackson Heights. Since the 1980s, Jackson Heights has included Indian restaurants, sari shops, and South Asian grocers. In addition to Indian, there are Pakistani, Bangladeshi, and Afghani restaurants. By 1990, Queens had become home to more than fifty-five thousand Indian immigrants. Many non–South Asians do not know the difference between Bangladeshi, Indian, and Pakistani cuisine; and therefore, most of the restaurants are known as "Banglo-Indo-Pak." Since 9/11, there has also been a particular stigma against Pakistani restaurants, which often choose to call themselves Indian as well. There are several historical food institutions in Jackson Heights. Jackson Diner, which opened in 1980, continues to be a popular Indian establishment, catering primarily to non-Indians. The Indian restaurants continue to attract tourists and those seeking vegetarian fare such as *palak paneer*, *chat*, and *chole*. Many of the Pakistani and Bangladeshi restaurants that are known for their tandoori chicken and *seekh kebobs* are owned and run by Muslim South Asian families and serve halal meat.

Since 2000, Indian immigrants and food writers both have been concerned that there continues to be a watering down of "authentic" Indian restaurants in Jackson Heights. However, you can still easily find your share of curries, samosas, dosas, and biryani in Queens. Today "Little India" often refers to two neighborhoods: Jackson Heights in Queens and Murray Hill, aka Curry Hill, on Manhattan's East Side.

See also QUEENS and SOUTH ASIAN.

Lessinger, Johanna. *From the Ganges to the Hudson: Indian Immigrants in New York.* Philadelphia: University of Pennsylvania Press, 1995.

Farha Ternikar

Little Italy

Little Italy was Manhattan's primarily Italian neighborhood from the 1880s until the 1920s. At its height it covered the area bounded by Houston Street to the north, the Bowery to the east, Canal Street to the south, and Broadway to the west.

Most contemporary narratives about Little Italy focus on how the neighborhood went supposedly recently from the oldest and largest Italian immigrant settlement in New York City to a three-block strip on Mulberry Street between Broome and Canal Streets lined with restaurants catering to tourists in search of the flavors of old-time Italian immigrant life and cuisine. In reality, an early "Italian flight" from the area was already under way in the 1920s, and ethnic, if not yet culinary, tourism has been a significant force in defining the neighborhood since the turn of the twentieth century.

The area that became known as Little Italy was primarily Irish in the early to mid-nineteenth century. During the 1880s, new immigrants from Italy displaced the Irish: the area was almost completely Italian when Jacob Riis immortalized it as the worst slum in America—if not in the world—in his famous book *How the Other Half Lives: Studies among the Tenements of New York*, first published in 1890. Thousands of immigrants, overwhelmingly from rural sections of southern Italy, congregated in the area because of the availability of cheap tenement apartments and its proximity to the construction sites and garment factories where most of them toiled. The neighborhood, then referred to as "Mulberry Bend," "Mulberry District," or the "Fourteenth Ward," was not the only Italian settlement in

New York; other major ones existed in Greenwich Village and—the largest of them—East Harlem. In fact, Riis coined the phrase "Little Italy" for the latter, and until World War I, when New Yorkers talked about "Little Italy" they meant Italian Harlem, not its counterpart six miles to the south. See GREENWICH VILLAGE and HARLEM.

At the turn of the century, Italian immigrants striving for a new sense of home turned what would have otherwise been an anonymous tenement district into their place in America. They did so through different cultural tools, from vibrant religious processions to food. The cuisine they invented in the diaspora, best defined by the culinary triangle of tomato sauce, olive oil, and garlic, literally filled the air of Mulberry, Elizabeth, and Mott Streets, becoming attached to their identity as a family-oriented, community-centered, sentimental, and emotional people. The pushcarts that lined the streets of the neighborhood not only provided immigrants with their favorite vegetables, fruits, bread, cheese, and fish—much of which were unfamiliar to other New Yorkers and unavailable in other parts of the city—but also defined Little Italy in the eyes of adventurous visitors as a moderately dangerous, yet exotic and appealing destination. "What strikes one first is the beauty and the variety of the vegetables and fruits sold there in what is supposed to be one of the poorest quarters," reported a writer. "Peaches with blooms on, and the softest and the most luscious plums, the cleanest salads, the most unusual vegetable leaves and roots. You are in Little Italy, Elizabeth Street, with deep cellar stores and cellar restaurants, and the odor of fried fish and oil; the cries of the venders in that open-mouthed Latin of the southern Italians are hurled at you." Magazine and newspaper articles suggested to readers that, especially because of the food, a visit to the area was an experience as close as possible to actually traveling to Naples. See STREET VENDORS.

However, the Spartan eating places of the area did not attract many visitors until the 1920s. With the end of mass immigration, these establishments had stopped catering to single immigrant men, and the restaurants in nearby Greenwich Village had popularized the Italian fare of pasta dishes, thick vegetable soups, and meats simmered in spicy tomato sauce among an early cohort of non-Italian customers—artists, students, and white-collar workers. Accordingly, it was in the 1920s that Little Italy finally got its name. This renaming was part of a reconfiguration of the city's cultural geography that firmly identified Harlem in white New Yorkers' minds with African American culture—obliterating its Italian component—and consolidated the adjacent immigrant neighborhoods of the Jewish ghetto, Chinatown, and Little Italy into a single Lower East Side visiting package for an expanding ethnic tourism interested in experiencing cultural difference at the table as well. Ironically, the name came to identify an area that had just begun to de-Italianize as the most successful among immigrant renters were fulfilling their dream of becoming homeowners in the outer boroughs. See RESTAURANTS.

In the 1930s and early 1940s, the local restaurant scene further expanded to include fancy and upscale Italian eateries alongside the simpler places that had appealed to Bohemian eaters. Researchers with the Works Progress Administration's Federal Writers' Project found Moneta's, at 32 Mulberry Street, to be "an effective stage for the rendezvous of brilliant judges, lawyers, writers, celebrities and beautiful women." Throughout the postwar era, as more and more Italian American residents left, restaurants remained the central institution defining the identity and economy of the area. Bypassed by the urban change that transformed New York in the 1950s and 1960s and still dominated by three- or four-story tenement houses, Mulberry Street's Little Italy continued to be imagined as a vibrant immigrant community regardless of contrary evidence, its restaurants commanding media attention also because of the occasional Mafia shooting on their premises, which somehow perpetuated the association with both danger and pleasure that had presided over the "invention" of Little Italy earlier in the century. In the 1970s, movies like *The Godfather*, *Mean Streets*, and other lesser classic Mob movies were shot on location, featuring neighborhood landmarks such as Ferrara Pastry Shop and Luna Restaurant and globally disseminating the image of Little Italy as the quintessential place for consumption of Italian American life and food. See MOVIES.

It was first a heavy influx of new post-1965 Chinese immigrants who moved from Chinatown into its abandoned tenements, and later real estate investment overflowing from gentrifying SoHo and East Village into the neighborhood, that completed the conversion of Little Italy into a miniature ethnic theme park. By the early 1990s, the Feast of San Gennaro, first held in 1926, had grown from a one-day religious celebration attended by immigrants only to a weekly affair attracting thousands of international tourists with the lure of street stands offering sausage and pepper sandwiches, fried calamari, and *zeppole* (deep-fried dough and sugar puffs). In a further twist of irony, the successful theming of a much reduced, deprived of any significant Italian population, and totally safe Little Italy was accomplished amid the flourishing of community associations aimed at "preserving the character of Little Italy and stemming the exodus of its residents." Tellingly, only a couple of grocery stores selling Italian cheeses, cold cuts, and olive oils (Alleva and DiPalo's) survive on Mulberry Street, surrounded by some thirty-eight Italian restaurants. See CHINESE COMMUNITY and SAN GENNARO, FEAST OF.

Characteristically, Little Italy restaurants still largely serve old-time classics of Italian American cuisine with very little concessions to the regional Italian cuisine that in the last two decades has become dominant in Italian restaurants of other parts of Manhattan. They seem much more interested in appearing authentic to the image of the New York Italian food celebrated in Francis Ford Coppola's and Martin Scorsese's movies than to what Italians in Italy eat: dishes like chicken Scarpariello (chicken casserole with sausage and peppers), fettuccine Alfredo (noodles tossed with Parmesan cheese and butter), and lobster Fra Diavolo (lobster in spicy tomato sauce topped over spaghetti) feature prominently and invariably on their menus. The last addition to the Little Italy restaurant scene is in fact a creative, playful, high-quality reelaboration of the same "red-sauce" cuisine that came to represent so strongly the identity of the neighborhood, notwithstanding the demographic change it has experienced for a very long time. The young Italian American chefs at Torrisi Italian Specialties, at 250 Mulberry Street, offer revisited versions of Italian American classics, skillfully prepared with local and artisanal prime ingredients but respectfully celebrating the long tradition of cooks and restaurateurs that made Little Italy and its food famous worldwide.

See also ITALIAN.

Bercovici, Konrad. *Around the World in New York*. New York: Century, 1924.

Cinotto, Simone. *The Italian American Table: Food, Family, and Community in New York City*. Urbana: University of Illinois Press, 2013.

Gabaccia, Donna. "Inventing Little Italy." *Journal of the Gilded Age and Progressive Era* 6, no. 1 (January 2007): 7–41.

Kosta, Ervin. "The Immigrant Enclave as Theme Park: Culture, Capital, and Urban Change in New York's Little Italies." In *Making Italian America: Consumer Culture and the Production of Ethnic Identities*, edited by Simone Cinotto, pp. 225–243. New York: Fordham University Press, 2014.

Sifton, Sam. "Torrisi Italian Specialties." *New York Times*, June 8, 2010.

"Tony Moneta," "Foreign Restaurants," 1940. Works Progress Administration, Federal Writers' Project, *Feeding the City*, reel 144, Municipal Archives of the City of New York.

Simone Cinotto

Little Odessa

Little Odessa is the nickname for a part of Brighton Beach, a sunny seaside town in south Brooklyn that is heavily populated with Russians and Ukrainians. Historically, Brighton Beach did not always have a deep Eastern European connection. The area was made up of farms owned by the descendants of English colonizers until 1868, when affluent businessman William A. Engeman bought several hundred oceanfront acres with designs on reproducing the sophistication of Brighton, England.

Initially, the area flourished. The year 1878 saw the arrival of the Brighton Beach Bathing Pavilion and Ocean Pier, and the racing track was opened a year later, which brought a flurry of activity to the neighborhood. The track was shut down in 1908 with the advent of the Hart-Agnew law, an anti-gambling bill. Its closing led to people losing interest in the area, triggering an exodus. As a result, the Eastern European Jews living in cramped tenements on the Lower East Side and in Brownsville moved to the area. The neighborhood soon was taken over—the music hall became a Yiddish theater, and Russian Jewish food was widely available. There were even knish eating competitions.

In the 1930s and 1940s Jewish immigrants came to Brighton Beach to escape the Nazis, and Little Odessa became a hub of culinary entrepreneurship. Arguably the most famous example of this was Mrs. Stahl's, a no-frills knishery started by a Galician (modern-day Ukraine) émigré who was actually named Feige Goldenberg. See KNISH and MRS. STAHL'S KNISHES.

The 1965 Hart-Celler Act dramatically shifted immigration law, opening doors to Eastern Europeans and heralding the arrival of more Russian Jews to New York City; but the aging population and growing crime rate led to Little Odessa's decline in the late 1960s and 1970s. It was around this time that the term "Little Odessa by the Sea" came about.

The arrival of immigrants after the fall of the Soviet Union, this time not necessarily Jewish, revived the neighborhood. Initially, there was tension between the waves of immigrants, with the previous settlers calling the new arrivals *kolbasnaya immigraciya* ("sausage immigration"), but the two communities soon learned to live together. The neighborhood by this point was very much established; it was even celebrated in the 1994 thriller movie *Little Odessa*.

Today Russian and Ukrainian culture still holds strong. Shops line the boulevard with stalls out front selling Russian fare. Offerings include *pirozhki*, baked or fried buns with sweet or savory filling; sweet pastries; and Russian candies galore. Russian supermarkets stock *vareniki*, blini, caviar, smoked fish, pickles, as well as self-serve cooked food and other Russian staples. Shops selling vodka are plentiful, as perhaps expected. It does not stop at food: Russian fashion, furniture, books, and music are also well represented in the area.

The boardwalk along the beach is the glittering jewel in the neighborhood's crown. Glitzy restaurants pepper the boardwalk offering Russian and Ukrainian cuisine, with lashings of vodka, of course. With ample outdoor seating, they are an excellent venue for people watching; the older Ukrainian and Russian generation can often be seen basking in the sun.

The restaurant scene in Brighton Beach accurately reflects the ethnicities that populate the area. You can eat at Soviet-style *stolovayas* or more upscale Ukrainian and Russian restaurants, and there are options for delicious Uighur and Uzbek cuisine. Gentrification has slowly crept in, with more mainstream eateries and cafes cropping up; but the area, with its signs in Russian and its faded seaside glamor, is still undeniably Russian.

See also BRIGHTON BEACH; RUSSIAN; and UKRAINIAN.

"Brighton Beach." Brooklyn Public Library. http://www
.bklynlibrary.org/ourbrooklyn/brightonbeach.
Fertitta, Naomi, and Paul Aresu. *New York: The Big City and Its Little Neighborhoods*. New York: Universe, 2009.
Idov, Michael. "The Everything Guide to Brighton Beach: Inside the Land of Pelmeni, Matryoshkas, Tracksuits, and of Course, Vodka." *New York Magazine*, April 13, 2009.
Silver, Laura. *Knish: In Search of the Jewish Soul Food*. Waltham, Mass.: Brandeis University Press, 2014.

Asia Lindsay

Little Syria

Little Syria is the affectionate name given to the area of Lower Manhattan that stretched alongside Washington Street, from Battery Place north to Liberty Street. Between the 1880s and the 1940s, this area was home to the nation's first Arab American community and was a thriving commercial district.

Arab-owned groceries and restaurants in Little Syria were the first to import and serve traditional Arab and Middle Eastern food products. In addition to hummus and falafel, New Yorkers could sample distinctive products like *halwa* (halva, a sweet sesame paste), pistachios, *arak* (liquor distilled from grapes), and Turkish coffee (coffee ground with cardamom). See HUMMUS; FALAFEL; and HALVA. An October 2, 1892, *New York Daily Tribune* article remarked that the restaurants on Washington Street served "coffee of the consistency of mud, but delightful to the taste" and that "the proverbial hospitality of the Arab suffers no loss at the hands of his Syrian representative."

It is difficult to overestimate the impact that Little Syria had, and continues to have, on the national Arab American community. Not only did Little Syria's textile factories and warehouses supply merchants and peddlers across the country, but its Arabic press, including the nation's first Arabic-language newspaper, *Kawkab America* (1892), had international distribution. The presses on Washington Street also published the first works of famed poet Kahlil Gibran. The grocery stores shipped their products to Arab immigrants throughout the country. And the success of the Arab-owned restaurants in Lower Manhattan, with names like The Sheik, Mecca, Near East, and the Arabian Inn, spurred the development of Arab and Middle East restaurants in numerous cities.

The population of Little Syria began to decline in the 1930s. By 1946, lower Washington Street had been almost completely abandoned by order of the City of New York, to make room for the construction of the Brooklyn–Battery Tunnel. Later the neighborhood's northern area became part of the site of the World Trade Center. The only remnants of the community in Lower Manhattan are the former St. George's Melkite Church at 103 Washington Street, which became a designated New York City landmark through the efforts of citizen activists, and two buildings adjacent to the church once used as a community center and a tenement building.

See also ARAB COMMUNITY; EGYPTIAN; and SYRIAN AND LEBANESE.

Benson, Kathleen, and Philip M. Kayal, eds. *A Community of Many Worlds: Arab Americans in New York City.* New York: Museum of the City of New York; Syracuse, N.Y.: Syracuse University Press, 2002.
Felton, Ralph. "A Sociological Study of the Syrians in Greater New York." Master's thesis, Columbia University, 1912.
"Little Syria, NY: An Immigrant Community's Life and Legacy." Arab American National Museum. http://www.arabamericanmuseum.org/little.syria.ny.exhibit.

Matthew Jaber Stiffler

Lobster Newberg

Lobster Newberg leads the pantheon of classic New York dishes. For about one hundred years, from its creation at Delmonico's in the mid-1870s until the coming of nouvelle cuisine in the 1970s, you could find a form of Newberg on many New York menus. See DELMONICO'S. It might have been spelled "Newburg" or "Newburgh," and instead of lobster, the seafood could have been shrimp, crab, a seafood mixture, or a lobster, seafood, or fish cake. The really essential element was an egg yolk–thickened sauce flavored with either Madeira or sherry. It started as an elegant restaurant dish but ended up in cookbooks for home cooks, sometimes with a béchamel-based sauce, eventually with a sauce made with a can of creamy soup.

This is Charles Ranhofer's version, exactly as written in his monumental work *The Epicurean*, published in 1894; he also called the dish "lobster Delmonico":

Cook six lobsters each weighing about two pounds in boiling salted water for twenty-five minutes. Twelve pounds of live lobster when cooked yields from two to two and a half pounds of meat with three to four ounces of coral. When cold detach the bodies from the tails and cut the latter into slices, put them into a sautoir, each piece lying flat, and add hot clarified butter; season with salt and fry lightly on both sides without coloring; moisten to their height with good raw cream; reduce quickly to half; and then add two or three spoonfuls of Madeira wine; boil the liquid once more only, then remove and thicken with a thickening of egg yolks and raw cream. Cook without boiling, incorporating a little cayenne and butter; then arrange the pieces in a vegetable dish and pour the sauce over.

The story of lobster Newberg is possibly even more delicious than the dish itself. It starts on an evening in 1876 when Ben Wenberg, a wealthy sea captain who plied the fruit trade between New York and Cuba and a regular at Delmonico's on Fourteenth Street and later at Twenty-Sixth Street, came in for dinner and told Charles Delmonico about a new way he had learned to cook lobster. He, the captain, would show Delmonico's staff how to do it. He ordered from the kitchen a freshly boiled lobster, sweet cream, clarified sweet butter, cognac, and sherry. He provided, from a silver snuffbox, a secret ingredient.

The procedure must have been pretty much the way Ranhofer outlines it. Naturally, as soon as the great chef tasted the dish, he pronounced positively that the secret ingredient was cayenne pepper. The dish was added to the menu as lobster à la Wenberg, and it was a hit.

Wenberg later had an argument with Charles Delmonico, and the restaurateur decided to remove the dish from his menu. Patrons, however, continued to demand it. Delmonico put it back on the menu as lobster Delmonico, but it was not selling with that name. So Delmonico changed the name again—to Newberg, simply reversing the *W* and the *N* in Wenberg's name. Lobster Newberg remains a favorite on New York menus.

See also RANHOFER, CHARLES.

Thomas, Lately. *Delmonico's: A Century of Splendor.* Boston: Houghton Mifflin, 1967.
Ranhofer, Charles. *The Epicurean.* New York: Dover, 1971. First published 1894.

Arthur Schwartz

Lobster Palaces

Lobster palaces were expensive, opulently decorated after-theater restaurants that opened in New

York in the late nineteenth century, thrived until 1912, and finally died with the advent of Prohibition in 1920. They rejected the formal menus and manners of the city's finer restaurants, such as Delmonico's, opting instead for a more relaxed dining experience with live entertainment—orchestras, dancing, chorus lines, and floor shows. Lobster palaces served a variety of dishes, from haute cuisine to exotic foreign fare, but a late-night meal of whole lobsters, accompanied by champagne and fine wines, was their signature offering. Their liquor licenses permitted them to serve alcohol throughout the night, and habitués would sometimes stay until dawn. The far-reaching reputation of New York's lobster palaces drew an international clientele who thrilled at mingling with actors, musicians, singers, and other celebrities, courtesans, showgirls, visiting royalty, self-made men (mainly bachelors), wealthy playboys, and their assorted admirers. Even New York's social elite occasionally dropped in, just to glimpse the spectacle.

Louis Sherry, one of the creators of the lobster palace concept, started as an owner of a catering business in 1881. When it proved a success, he opened a restaurant at the corner of Fifth Avenue and Thirty-Seventh Street. The restaurant's décor and the creations of its French chefs soon attracted New York's social elite as well as those who loved good food. Sherry employed sixteen chefs, with an additional two hundred kitchen staff. When this proved too small, in 1898, he commissioned the architect Sanford White to construct a four-story lobster palace and hotel complete with a ballroom opposite Delmonico's restaurant at Forty-Fourth Street and Broadway.

Another lobster palace inventor was Thomas Shanley, an Irish immigrant, who opened a small restaurant at the corner of Sixth Avenue and West Twenty-Third Street, then the heart of the theater district, in 1891. Actors from the nearby theaters became regulars, and the business grew. The theater district moved north to Longacre (later Times) Square, and Shanley opened two additional restaurants on Broadway. In 1910 Shanley opened a new restaurant on Broadway between Forty-Second and Forty-Third Streets. Shanley offered "light entertainment" in addition to the food and liquor. The place was lavishly decorated, and the food was excellent; but these were of secondary importance to patrons who came mainly for the entertainment: Shanley's featured a full orchestra and was the first restaurant in the city to have one. Thomas Shanley is credited with launching New York's first lobster palace. A 1900 menu from Shanley's features "LIVE LOBSTER, Broiled, Large" at the top of the first page, with deviled lobster, lobster fricassee, and lobster Newberg as alternatives, as well as every imaginable type of fish and shellfish, steaks, chops, Hamburg steak, frankfurter sausages, omelets, and French Champagne by the "pint" or "quart."

The Café Martin was another acclaimed lobster palace. French immigrants Jean-Baptiste and Louis Martin owned a small hotel with a restaurant on the corner of Ninth Street and University Place in Manhattan that was a favorite dining spot for French visitors. In 1899 Delmonico's vacated its premises on Madison Square, at Twenty-Sixth Street near Fifth Avenue, and moved uptown. The Martins leased the building and opened a lobster palace, lavishly decorated in the art nouveau style and featuring novel "banquettes," which offered diners privacy. Café Martin opened to great fanfare in February 1920 and quickly became a favored meeting place for New York's upper crust. Diamond Jim Brady was a regular, and when the popular British actress Lily Langtry visited the city, she held court at Café Martin. But New York's theater scene was again moving uptown, so in 1912 Louis Martin acquired the failing Café de l'Opera, on Broadway between Forty-First and Forty-Second Streets. There he created one of the largest and most extravagant lobster palaces ever. It was shuttered less than two years later—the heyday of the lobster palace was over as the fashionable set moved on to other entertainments.

Chicago restaurateur George Rector opened a lobster palace on Broadway between Forty-Third and Forty-Fourth Streets after spending $200,000 on improvements and décor. Its entrance was a Greco-Roman façade complete with electrical lighting and the city's very first revolving door. Rector hired staff away from Delmonico's to run the kitchen. Rector's grand opening in 1899 was attended by New York's swankiest citizens, many of whom made frequent return visits during the following decade. Rector declared that he and his staff had but a single motto: "The guest is right, right or wrong."

Other popular lobster palaces included Bustanoby's (with its famous Pré-Catalan Room), Café des Beaux Arts, Churchill's, Faust's, Healy's Golden Glades, Maxim's, John Murray's Roman Gardens,

Reisenweber's Café (with its famous Paradise Room and Four Hundred Club), The Pekin, and The Tokio. They were typically located on or near Longacre Square, the new heart of the city's theater district. Around them developed a "lobster palace society" of fashionable, rather racy New Yorkers, largely the nouveau riche.

Like many other restaurants, lobster palaces made most of their profits on liquor. When Prohibition began, in January 1920, the lobster palaces shut down. Less glitzy cabarets and nightclubs emerged in 1913 and "cafe society" replaced "lobster palace society" in the 1920s and 1930s.

See also GILDED AGE; HAUTE CUISINE; RECTOR, CHARLES AND GEORGE; RESTAURANTS; and TIMES SQUARE.

Batterberry, Michael, and Ariane Batterberry. *On the Town in New York: The Landmark History of Eating, Drinking, and Entertainments from the American Revolution to the Food Revolution.* New York and London: Routledge, 1999.
Erenberg, Lewis A. *Steppin' Out: New York Nightlife and the Transformation of American Culture, 1890–1930.* Chicago: University of Chicago Press, 1984.
Grimes, William. *Appetite City: A Culinary History of New York.* New York: North Point, 2009.
Street, Julian. *Welcome to Our City.* New York: John Lane, 1913.

Andrew F. Smith

Local 338

See BAGELS.

Loft's Candy Stores

Loft's was a famous chain of New York candy shops that thrived from 1895 until its demise almost a century later in 1990. William Loft (ca. 1828–1919) and his wife, who came from London to New York City in the 1850s, crafted handmade chocolates in their kitchen. In 1860 they opened a small shop on Canal Street that also manufactured candy for out-of-town sales. In 1895, their son, George W. Loft (1865–1943), struck out on his own. With only $550, he opened his first store in 1895 and quickly expanded the business, opening other retail outlets in New York. The shops sold low-cost assortments and advertised that they only made a "penny-a-pound

profit" on their candies. Their low-cost candy undersold their competitors, and the company made its profits on sales volume. In 1915, George Loft reported that New Yorkers bought 100,000 pounds of his company's candy every day.

In 1919 the firm built a manufacturing facility on Fortieth Street in Long Island City, Queens. The renamed Loft, Inc. was one of America's first retail candy store chains. By the 1920s, it was the largest retail candy company in America, with seventy-five outlets. Loft's sponsored local radio programs, and with this effective publicity the business grew. It was estimated to be worth $13 million in 1929, when stockholders took control and ousted the Loft family.

After a protracted corporate battle, Charles Guth (1876–1948), president of Mavis Candies, became president of Loft, Inc. in April 1930. Under Guth's leadership, Loft, Inc. acquired two other candy retailers, the Happiness and Mirror chains. The combined operation owned 175 candy shops, soda fountains, and tearooms. Loft's had been using Coca-Cola syrup in its soda fountains, but when that company turned down Guth's request for a larger discount, he bought bankrupt National Pepsi-Cola Company and became president of both companies. He put Loft chemists to work on reformulating Pepsi-Cola syrup, and he used Loft staff to restart the Pepsi-Cola Company in July 1931. Pepsi sales took off. By 1935, Pepsi generated a $2 million profit and was the second-largest soft drink company in America. Guth left Loft in 1935 to work full-time on Pepsi, where he was president and general manager.

The Loft Candy Company was all but bankrupt by the mid-1930s, when Phoenix Securities Corporation, which specialized in revamping failing corporations, took charge of it. Walter Mack, head of Phoenix, decided that the company should produce five-cent candies rather than "fancy" chocolates. He also decided to sue Guth, claiming that Guth had used Loft employees, resources, and facilities to restart Pepsi and that the successful Pepsi-Cola Company should really belong to Loft, Inc. After a protracted court case, Mack won and Loft and Pepsi were reunited.

Loft candy stores were subsequently spun off and acquired by Philadelphia businessman Albert M. Greenfield (1887–1967), who owned the City Stores Corporation. Greenfield expanded Loft's operations outside the New York area, and by 1957 the company operated three hundred stores on the Eastern Seaboard and the Midwest. At its height Lofts had more than twenty-one hundred employees and sold more than 350 different products, including boxed chocolate assortments, gift baskets, and candy bars, the most famous being their butter crunch bar and their Parlay—"heavenly honey nougat dipped with creamy caramel, rolled in crisp chopped pecans, covered with Loft's rich milk chocolate." It also offered holiday treats, such as chocolate Easter bunnies; and it was one of the first companies to offer kosher chocolates wrapped in silver and gold foil to simulate Chanukah "gelt" (coins).

Loft candy stores and the Barricini chocolate company (founded in 1931) merged in 1970. By the mid-1970s there were 287 Barricini-Loft stores, which sold their own brand of chocolates, imported chocolates, nuts, hard candy, and ice cream. Over the next decade, the firm faltered, and many of the retail outlets were closed. By 1990 all stores had closed, and Loft's candies were only a sweet memory.

See also CANDY; CHANUKAH; CHOCOLATE, CRAFT; EASTER; and PEPSI-COLA.

Loft, George. "How New York's 'Penny-a-Pound-Profit' Candy Man Got His Start." *Candy and Ice Cream* 26 (April 1915): 10.
Smith, Andrew F. *New York City: A Food Biography*. Lanham, Md.: Rowman & Littlefield, 2014.

Andrew F. Smith

Lombardi's

Lombardi's is a pizzeria located at 32 Spring Street on the border of Manhattan's Little Italy. Opened in 1905, Lombardi's is widely considered the first pizzeria in the United States.

Lombardi's can trace its history back to 1897, when Neopolitan immigrant Genarro Lombardi opened an Italian grocery and provisions shop at 53½ Spring Street. Lombardi's shop was in the center of the thriving neighborhood of Little Italy, home at its height to over ten thousand Italian immigrants. See LITTLE ITALY and ITALIAN. Neopolitan immigrants brought with them a tradition of pizza making. In Little Italy, they borrowed or rented bakers' ovens to cook breads and pizzas, which they ate at home. Naples pies were made from thin crusts topped with buffalo mozzarella cheese, tomatoes, and simple ingredients like sausage or vegetables, cooked at high temperatures in wood-fired ovens. Eventually, some

Neopolitan immigrants were able to open bakeries where they sold pizza as well. Lombardi was among this group. In 1905, Lombardi successfully applied for a license to operate the city's first pizzeria.

While carrying over the Neopolitan traditions, New York's pizzaiolas made accommodations to the new environment, substituting cow's milk mozzarella for buffalo mozzarella and using coal instead of the more expensive wood to fire the ovens. New York pizzas were also larger than the Neopolitan originals, a nod to the new country with its notable abundance. Lombardi sold whole (20-inch) pies for a nickel, wrapping them in brown paper. He also sold partial pies and slices. Lombardi trained some of the best-known pizza makers in New York, many of whom went on to create their own, long-running pizzerias, including John's of Greenwich Village, Totonno's of Coney Island, and Patsy's Pizzeria in East Harlem.

The original Lombardi's remained open for almost eighty years, passing from Gennaro Lombardi to his son John and then his grandson Gennaro (Jerry). In 1984, the restaurant, suffering financially and physically (its oven cracked as a result of vibrations from the Lexington Avenue subway line), closed. Ten years later, Lombardi, along with partner Joan Volpe and family friend John Brescio, revived the restaurant, opening in a defunct bakery down the street from the original location but reinstalling the door of the original coal oven in the new space.

The public face of the new Lombardi's was its thirty-two-year-old manager, a self-styled pizza expert named Andrew Bellucci. Bellucci was thought by many to be the restaurant's owner, a misconception he did little to dispel. Bellucci publicized the history of Lombardi's and its excellent pizzas and, at a time when New York pizza had lost some of its luster, promised to lead a revival of the old, thin-crust, coal-fired Neopolitan style of pizza. The ubiquitous Bellucci appeared on local and national food and news programs to celebrate the history of pizza in New York, and Lombardi's in particular. Bellucci also invited chefs from around the country to visit Lombardi's and study pizza making. So it was a shock to many in the New York food world and beyond when Bellucci was arrested in 1996 for embezzling hundreds of thousands of dollars from a New York law firm where he had worked in the late 1980s. Bellucci served a thirteen-month prison term after pleading guilty for the crime. Lombardi's continued to serve

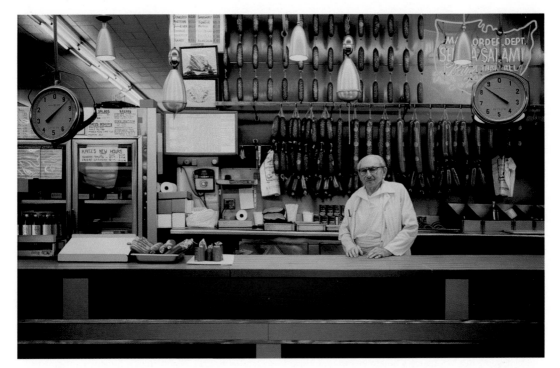

Katz's Delicatessen (1993), an oil painting by artist Max Ferguson. Katz's is famous for its long links of salami displayed behind the counter, heaping pastrami and corned beef sandwiches, and, of course, the orgasm Meg Ryan faked here in *When Harry Met Sally* (1989). © MAX FERGUSON/PRIVATE COLLECTION/BRIDGEMAN IMAGES

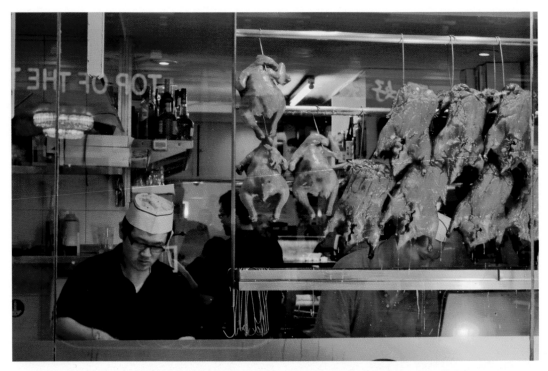

Ducks crisping in a Manhattan Chinatown restaurant window, October 8, 2011. Manhattan's Chinatown is home to the densest population of Chinese people in the Western hemisphere, but there are actually numerous other Chinatowns throughout New York City. Flushing, a Korean–Indian–Chinese enclave close to the last station of the number 7 subway line in northern Queens, has suddenly expanded into the city's biggest, most affluent Chinatown.
GARRY KNIGHT

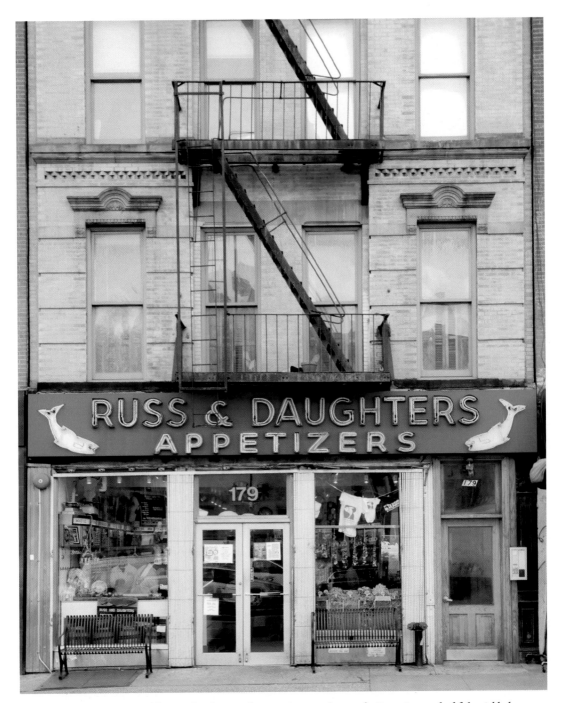

The storefront of Russ & Daughters, a family-owned appetizing store known for its caviar, smoked fish, pickled herring, and other traditionally Jewish offerings. In 2014 it celebrated its one hundredth year in business. PHOTO BY MICHAEL HARLAN TURKELL / COURTESY OF RUSS & DAUGHTERS

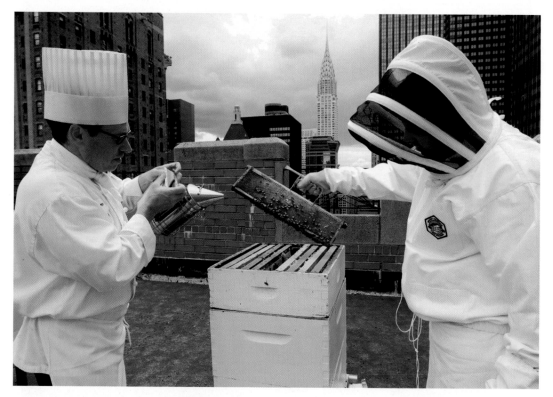

Sous chef Josh Bierman (left) and culinary director David Garcelon inspect honeybees from hives on the twentieth-floor roof of the Waldorf-Astoria Hotel, June 2012. The hotel harvests its own honey and helps pollinate plants in the skyscraper-heavy heart of the city, joining a mini-beekeeping boom that has taken over hotel rooftops from Paris to Times Square. AP PHOTO/KATHY WILLENS

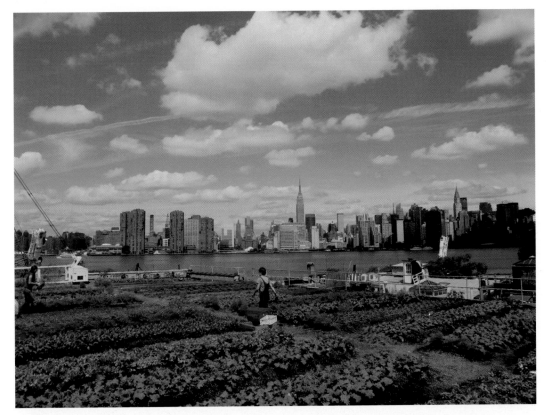

Eagle Street Rooftop Farm is a 6,000-square-foot organic vegetable farm located atop a warehouse rooftop in Greenpoint, Brooklyn. Community organizations such as Eagle Street are using rooftop gardens to educate schoolchildren and underserved communities about fresh produce and urban farming. © EAGLE STREET ROOFTOP GARDEN. PHOTO BY ANNIE NOVAK

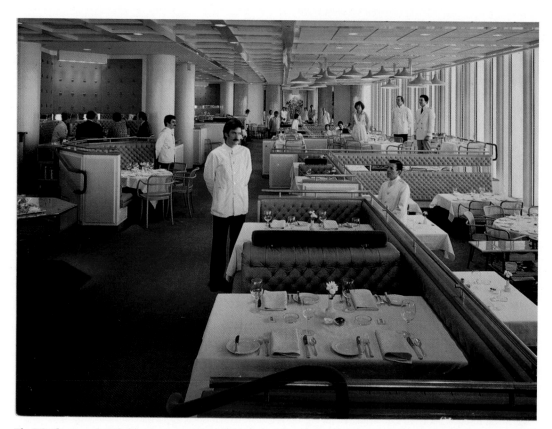

The Windows on the World restaurant in the World Trade Center before September 11, 2001. The restaurant was well known for its unique menu and for allowing diners to view the city below as they ate. MICHAEL WHITEMAN

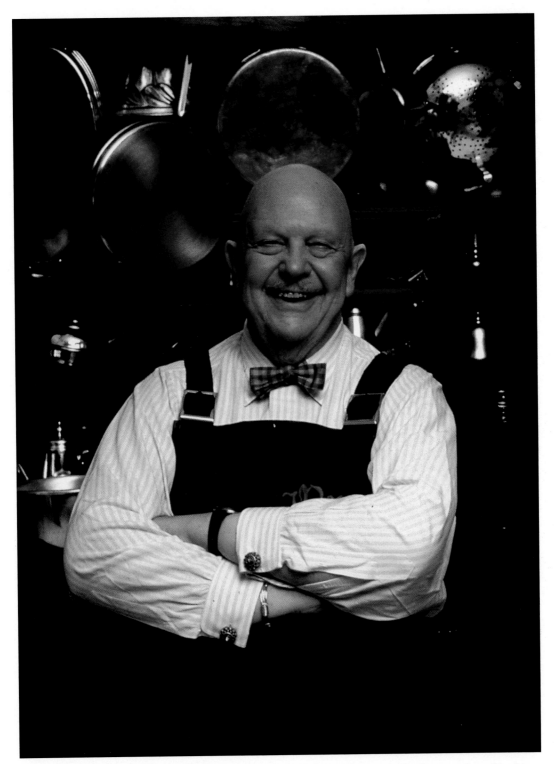

James Beard, an iconic American cook. After his death in 1985, a foundation was created in his name that utilizes his estate for food-related fundraisers and distributes awards named after him for culinary accomplishments. PHOTO BY DAN WYNN. COURTESY OF THE JAMES BEARD FOUNDATION

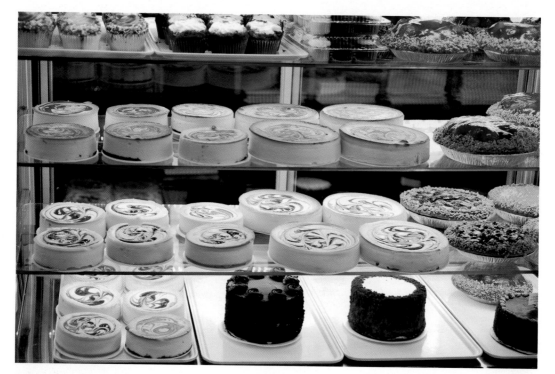

Junior's, a Brooklyn restaurant established in 1950, became famous for its distinctive cheesecake. It was lighter and less sweet than Lindy's cheesecake, with a thin layer of sponge cake as a base and vanilla flavoring. Today, Junior's sells cheesecakes in myriad flavors and sizes.

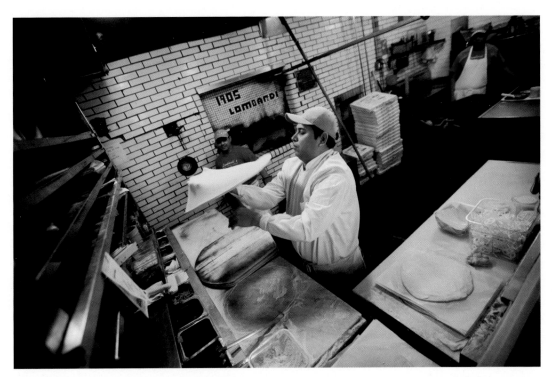

Workers prepare pizzas in the kitchen at Lombardi's Pizza in the East Village, January 2014. Opened in 1905, Lombardi's is widely considered the first pizzeria in the United States. JOHN MINCHILLO/AP PHOTO

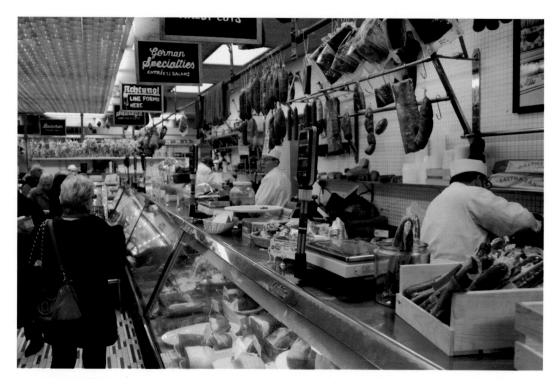

The German deli and butcher shop Schaller & Weber is a reminder of Yorkville's history as a gathering point for German immigrants. SCHALLER & WEBER

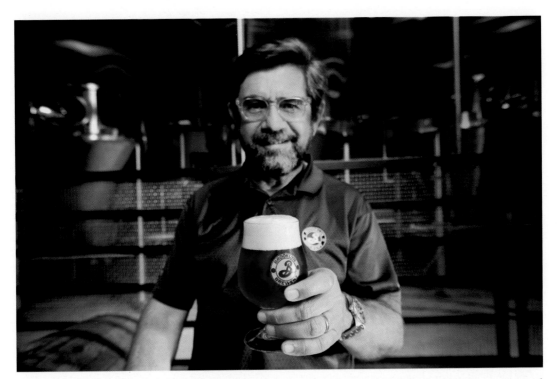

Steve Hindy, founder and president of Brooklyn Brewery, with a glass of his own lager. The Brooklyn Brewery is one of the largest exporters of craft beer. BRETT CASPER

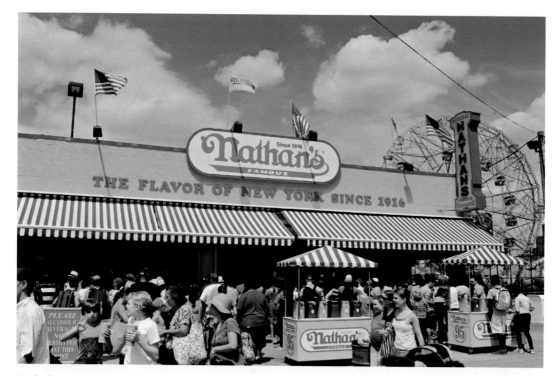

By the late 1930s Nathan's Famous was an established Coney Island institution, serving fifty-four thousand hot dogs on Memorial Days alone. The original landmark restaurant covers a whole city block and still attracts hundreds of thousands of diners and much media attention during its hot-dog-eating contest. WENDY BERRY

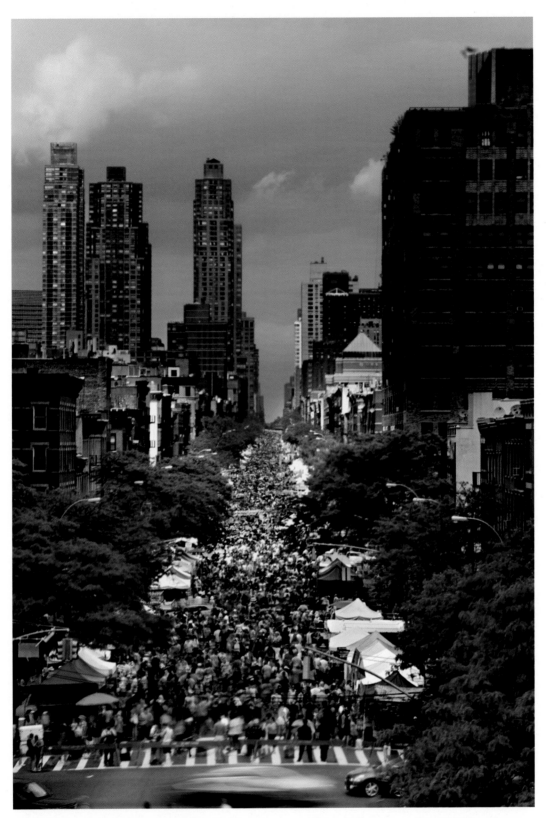

This aerial view of the Ninth Avenue Food Festival showcases its popularity. Each year more than 200,000 people are drawn to the Hell's Kitchen area of midtown to "eat the world in 20 blocks," as food writer Molly O'Neill once quipped.
COURTESY NINTH AVENUE ASSOCIATION

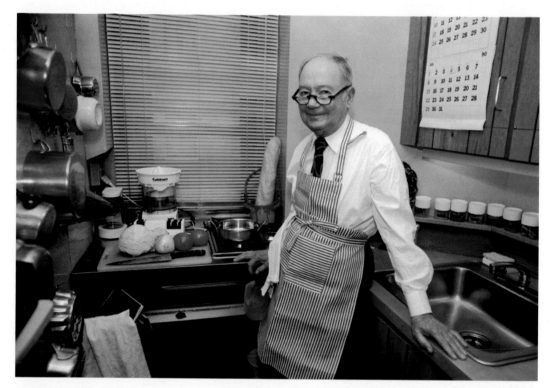

Craig Claiborne poses in his kitchen in New York City, May 1990. Claiborne was the food critic and editor for the *New York Times* from 1959 to 1987. AP PHOTO/RICHARD DREW

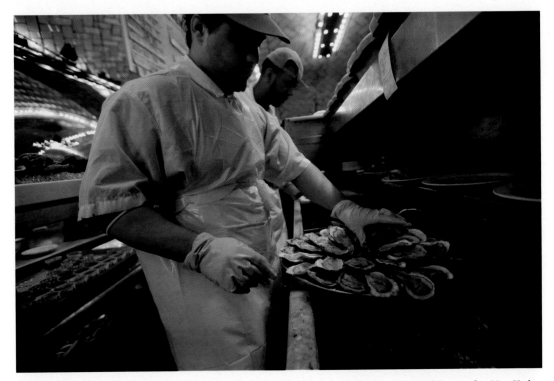

An employee of the Oyster Bar lays out a plate of freshly shucked oysters inside Grand Central Terminal in New York, January 9, 2013. Located on the lower level of the terminal, the Oyster Bar first opened its doors in 1913. AP PHOTO/ KATHY WILLENS

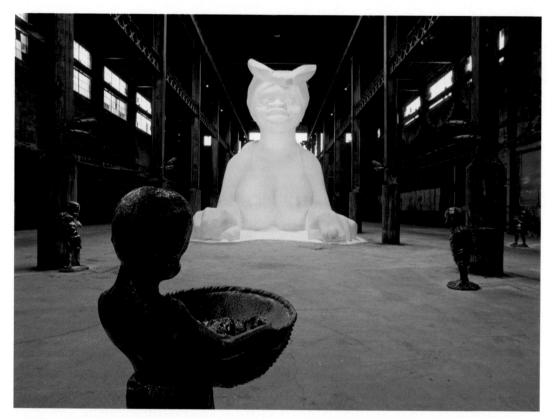

A Subtlety, or the Marvelous Sugar Baby was a 75-foot-long sphinx-like sculpture made from sugar and carved polystyrene in the abandoned Domino Sugar Refining plant in 2014. Constructed by artist Kara Walker, the nude "mammy" figure evoked antebellum stereotypes of black women in a setting freighted with meaning. ARTWORK © KARA WALKER. PHOTO BY JASON WYCHE. COURTESY OF SIKKEMA JENKINS & CO., NEW YORK

delicious pizza without him at the helm. Indeed, Lombardi's has expanded since 1994 from its small, narrow space that accommodated thirty seats to include the space upstairs and next door so that it now takes up the entire corner of Mott and Spring Streets.

Today, Lombardi's is an institution on Spring Street, drawing locals and tourists to taste the pizzas, cooked in the coal-fired oven at temperatures of eight hundred to nine hundred degrees. The restaurant still vies for the title of best pizza in New York City. And it holds on to its title as the first pizzeria in New York and the United States, though because of its ten-year hiatus, it ceded its title as oldest New York pizzeria to its spawn Totonno's.

See also PIZZA and PIZZERIAS.

Boyles, Tom. "Who Is the Father of American Pizza?" *PMQ Pizza Magazine* (November–December 2003).

Doherty, Caitlin. "Lombardi's Pizza Restaurant, New York City." InterestingAmerica.com, January 12, 2011. http://www.interestingamerica.com/2011-01-12_Lombardi_Pizza_NYC_by_C_Doherty.html.

Levine, Ed. *Pizza: A Slice of Heaven: The Ultimate Pizza Guide and Companion.* New York: Universe, 2005.

Mariani, John. *How Italian Food Conquered the World.* New York: Palgrave Macmillan, 2011.

Cindy R. Lobel

Loubat, Alphonse

See WINE and WINE-MAKING.

Lower East Side

The Lower East Side is a neighborhood in Manhattan that runs from Houston Street to Canal Street, from the Bowery to the East River. Historically, the Lower East Side stretched up to Fourteenth Street, but the section of the neighborhood that covers Alphabet City has become known, since the 1960s, as the East Village. Famous for its immigrant past, the neighborhood has more recently undergone gentrification. Young hipsters, professionals, and families are attracted to the upscale apartments and businesses of the area. Today's Lower East Side has a lively food scene with some notable restaurants and food shops that reflect both its past and its present.

Farmland during the colonial period and middle-class residential area in the early nineteenth century, the Lower East Side saw construction of blocks of tenement buildings during the great wave of immigration to New York that began in the 1830s. During the mid-nineteenth century, much of the area that is today's Lower East Side was the German immigrant neighborhood Kleindeutschland. German restaurants, bakeries, groceries, saloons, and beer gardens proliferated. See KLEINDEUTSCHLAND.

In the late nineteenth century, with the great wave of Jewish immigration to the United States and New York in particular (80 percent of the Jews who immigrated through Ellis Island settled in New York City, most on the Lower East Side), the neighborhood—especially east of the Bowery—became associated specifically with Jews. Hundreds of thousands of Jews poured into the district, its population 550,000 at its height—one of the most densely populated neighborhoods in the world. Streets were crowded with people, including peddlers pushing carts and selling all manner of goods. Hester Street was a major shopping street, nicknamed in Yiddish the *chazzer mark*, or "pig market," even though pork was about the only thing these Jewish shops and carts did not offer. Surrounding streets like Orchard, Essex, and Grand also were lined with shops and blocked with pushcarts selling dry goods as well as live poultry, kosher meats, produce, herring and other fresh and preserved fish, baked goods, and pickles. The area around Essex Street became known as the pickle district; eighty businesses brined, packed, and sold pickles to local residents and markets around the country. See JEWISH and PICKLES.

Other Jewish food businesses on the Lower East Side included matzah factories, kosher wineries, and bakeries. See MATZAH and BAKERIES. Russian and Romanian restaurants lined the streets along with Jewish cafes and teashops that drew such radicals and intellectuals as Emma Goldman and Alexander Berkman. Jewish delicatessens also opened, a kosher adaptation of the German Gentile shops that had sold cured meats, frankfurters, and prepared foods to New Yorkers since the 1850s. Appetizing stores—the dairy counterpart to the deli (kosher laws forbid mixing meat and dairy in the same meal)—sold smoked fish, cream cheese, blintzes, and other dairy and parve (neither meat nor dairy) delicacies. While the Lower East Side once housed dozens of these

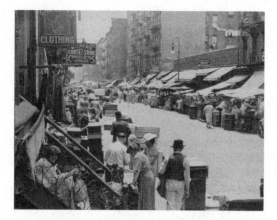

Looking south on Orchard Street from East Houston in the Lower East Side, 1939, with vendors crowding the streets. RARE BOOK AND MANUSCRIPT LIBRARY, COLUMBIA UNIVERSITY, COMMUNITY SERVICE SOCIETY COLLECTION

establishments, today only two remain—Katz's Deli (kosher style but not kosher) and Russ & Daughters Appetizing Store. Many of Russ & Daughters' employees are second- and third-generation Lower East Siders, not Jews but Latinos, demonstrating the fusions that the constantly changing neighborhood has engendered. Other rare holdouts from the old Jewish east side include Economy Candy on Rivington Street, Kossar's Bialys on Grand Street, Yonah Schimmel Knish Bakery on Houston, and Sammy's Roumanian Steak House on Orchard Street. Streit's Matzoh, the only extant matzah business in the neighborhood, is slated to move to New Jersey in 2015, its building purchased by a real estate developer with development plans for the site. See KATZ'S DELICATESSEN; RUSS & DAUGHTERS; and YONAH SCHIMMEL KNISH BAKERY.

With dwindling Eastern European immigration and outmigration of Jews from the Lower East Side to the suburbs, the Jewish population of the neighborhood began to decline significantly from the 1930s forward. In the mid-twentieth century, the ethnic character of the area shifted toward a Latino population, particularly Puerto Rican, and part of the neighborhood (especially around Alphabet City) became known as the Spanglish "Loisaida." Jewish shops and restaurants were replaced by bodegas and Puerto Rican eateries serving tostones, *maduro*, *pernil*, and other Caribbean specialties. See PUERTO RICAN.

Since the 1960s, the boundaries of Chinatown have spread over the Bowery and into the Lower East Side. The area south of Seward Park in particular is home to many immigrants from the province of Fujian. Dumpling shops, Chinese bakeries, dimsum parlors, and Asian groceries line Division Street and the nearby blocks of Canal Street and East Broadway. See CHINESE COMMUNITY.

While parts of the Lower East Side were blighted during the 1970s, the neighborhood started to gentrify beginning in the 1990s as the gentrification of the East Village began to cross Houston Street. Bars and clubs opened on Ludlow Street and surrounding blocks, and the neighborhood became known for its nightlife. Meanwhile, a restaurant renaissance began as chefs like Wylie Dufresne took advantage of the relatively inexpensive real estate in the area. At the turn of the twenty-first century, once-dicey Clinton Street became a restaurant row, featuring establishments like 71 Clinton Fresh Food, wd-50, and Clinton Street Baking Company. Other notable restaurants and bars have opened in the last several years, including gastropub Freeman's, Stanton Social, Schiller's Liquor Bar, Dirty French, and Cherche Midi. Rents have increased so quickly and real estate development has progressed so rapidly on the Lower East Side that even some of the vanguard restaurants like wd-50 have been forced to move on; Dufresne's Clinton Street restaurant closed its doors in late 2014. See DUFRESNE, WYLIE.

Despite the changes to the Lower East side, reminders of the neighborhood's immigrant past and present still exist, such as Prosperity Dumpling and Congee Village. The old Essex Street retail market, established by Mayor Fiorello LaGuardia to try to force pushcart vendors indoors (and thereby to regulate them), reflects the old and new Lower East Side. Produce stands selling plantains and cassava abut Saxelby Cheesemongers and Heritage Meat Shop. See ESSEX STREET MARKET and PUBLIC MARKETS. Also combining the old and new Lower East Side is Russ & Daughters Café, which opened in 2014 and serves bagels and lox and *kasha varnishkas* as well as caviar flights and curated cocktails to today's Lower East Siders, some of them the great- and great-great-grandchildren of the neighborhood's original residents.

See also DELIS, JEWISH.

Asimov, Eric. "And to Think I Ate It on Clinton Street." *New York Times*, April 10, 2002.
Beck, Peter. "Tasting a Neighborhood: A Food History of Manhattan's Lower East Side." https://sophiecoeprize

.files.wordpress.com/2014/07/beck-sophiecoe2014-tastinganeighborhood1.pdf.

Diner, Hasia. *Hungering for America: Italian and Jewish Foodways in the Age of Migration*. Cambridge, Mass.: Harvard University Press, 2003.

Federman, Marc Russ. "The Soul of a Store." In *Gastropolis: Food and New York City*, edited by Annie Hauck-Lawson and Jonathan Deutsch, pp. 195–208. New York: Columbia University Press, 2010.

Polland, Annie, and Daniel Soyer. *Emerging Metropolis: New York Jews in the Age of Immigration, 1840–1920*. New York: New York University Press, 2013.

Ziegelman, Jane. *97 Orchard: An Edible History of Five Immigrant Families in One New York Tenement*. New York: Harper, 2010.

Cindy R. Lobel

Lox

Lox, a Yiddish word, originated from the German word for salmon, *lachs*. Long before its arrival in Gotham in the early twentieth century, lox's roots can be traced to Native Americans, who used the fish in dried and smoked form as sustenance and currency, as well as Scandinavians, who were known to preserve salmon in saltwater brine.

While there are an array of terms bandied about colloquially (and interchangeably) for cured salmon, lox technically only consists of the fish's belly, which is the most delectable, rich, fatty part of the salmon and features the widest grains of fat and slightly less saltiness. There's no smoke, heat, or drying whatsoever involved in lox proper; it's simply subjected to a salt brine for three to six months and then rinsed lightly. Oft-confused treatments of the lusciously pink fish include hot-smoked salmon, which cooks the fish to a smokier, drier, meatier texture; gravlax, a method of brine curing; and Nova salmon or lox, which is gently cured before being cold-smoked. To cloud things further, in the early 1900s most salmon in New York came from Nova Scotia (or Quebec's Gaspé Penninsula).

In the early twentieth century, salmon in the United States was wild-caught, usually out West, and packed in salt to preserve the fish for the long train journey to New York. Much of this fish then traveled even further, to Europe, while a portion ended up in smokehouses in Brooklyn, to be smoked with a mix of wood chips and charcoal and then sold in appetizing shops, particularly on the Lower East Side. By the 1940s, the invention of refrigeration rendered traditional salt-cured fish passé, ushering in the popularity of smoked salmon.

The advent of the bagel–lox–cream cheese trifecta dates back to the 1930s on the Lower East Side, according to Mark Russ Federman of the lineage: "At one time, every appetizing-store owner in the neighborhood claimed to be the originator of this creation.... Before the lox, cream cheese, and bagel troika came into being, smoked fish was traditionally eaten with butter schmeared on thick slabs of dark pumpernickel or rye bread." His family's business was established in 1914. See BAGELS; CREAM CHEESE; and RUSS & DAUGHTERS.

Contrary to popular belief, the neighborhood's Eastern European Jewish population didn't come to the United States with a long-abiding affinity for salmon, in any form, "...but they did bring with them a taste for salt-preserved fish like herring." And the prices were right for the rosy-hued fish: "Because huge quantities of salmon were available, the prices were very cheap—pennies for a quarter of a pound. Lox quickly caught on among residents of the Lower East Side, and they took the taste for it with them when they moved out of the neighborhood" (Federman, 2013). For context, in the 1920s and 1930s, lox fetched approximately 35 cents per pound, while smoked sturgeon was priced at $4 per pound.

A few miles north, Russian immigrant Barney Greengrass set up shop, initially in 1908 at 113th Street and St. Nicholas Avenue in Harlem, before moving a bit farther south in 1929 to the current location on Amsterdam Avenue between Eighty-Sixth and Eighty-Seventh Streets. In 1938, Greengrass was dubbed the Sturgeon King by New York senator James J. Frawley. Currently, it's a third-generation family spot, run by Gary Greengrass. See BARNEY GREENGRASS.

"By the 1950s, 'bagels and lox' had become an insult—a disparaging term used by Jewish immigrants to describe their counterparts who had become too American. Bagels and lox had no analog in the old country. It was food as collage—pickled Italian flower buds [capers] and Scandinavian-style fish heaped over English-style cheese," Heather Smith wrote in the now-defunct food magazine *Meatpaper* in 2012.

While the distinction between actual lox and its slew of smokier cousins remains blurry, discrepancies in sales are pretty clear. As of 2003, Russ & Daughters' salmon sales consisted of a fairly paltry 15 to 20 percent coming from lox, while the Coney Island shop Banner Smoked Fish reels in just 5 percent of smoked salmon sales from lox. Acme Smoked Fish, the largest smoked-fish house in the continental United States (located in Williamsburg, Brooklyn), sells far more smoked salmon than actual lox—25,000 to 30,000 pounds per week of smoked salmon versus 1,000 pounds per week of lox.

In 2014, Russ & Daughters opened a full-service café a few blocks from the hallowed original store. Next up: a café and retail outpost in the Jewish Museum that will be the family's only kosher eatery.

See also APPETIZING STORES and SMOKED FISH.

Altman, Alex. "Where Lox Unlocks the Past." *Time,* June 19, 2008. http://content.time.com/time/world/article/0,8599,1816662,00.html.

Clark, Melissa. "Smoked Salmon Any Way You Slice It." *Diner's Journal* (blog), *New York Times,* April 13, 2011. http://dinersjournal.blogs.nytimes.com/2011/04/13/smoked-salmon-anyway-you-slice-it.

Federman, Mark Russ. *Russ & Daughters: Reflections and Recipes from the House That Herring Built.* New York: Schocken, 2013.

"The Raw Truth about Lox." *Jewish Daily Forward,* July 11, 2003. http://forward.com/articles/7669/the-raw-truth-about-lox.

Smith, Heather. "A Fish and Bread Journey: The Natural and Social History of Bagels and Lox." *Meatpaper,* July 15, 2012. http://meatpaper.com/wordpress/2012/07/a-fish-and-bread-journey-the-natural-and-social-history-of-bagels-and-lox.

Alexandra Ilyashov

Lucas, Dione

British-born Dione Lucas (1909–1971) was the first woman in America to host a TV cooking show and perhaps the best-known spokesperson for French cuisine in America in the 1950s. She promoted cooking as a high art with little to do with housewifery.

Lucas claimed to be among the first women to graduate from the prestigious Cordon Bleu Cooking School in Paris. Along with fellow student Rosemary Hume, she established the Cordon Bleu Cooking School and Restaurant in London. In 1942 Lucas moved to America, opening a Cordon Bleu Cooking School and Restaurant in New York City. In 1947 she was the first woman to host a television cooking show, *To the Queen's Taste* (1947–1949, CBS), and she continued to host prime-time cooking shows including *The Dione Lucas Cooking Show* (1953–1956, WPIX), with only minor interruptions for the next decade.

She operated several restaurants in New York, wrote and co-wrote many cookbooks (including *The Cordon Bleu Cook Book* [1947], *The Dione Lucas Book of French Cooking* [1947], and *The Gourmet Cooking School Cookbook* [1964]), published recipes and articles in popular magazines, gave cooking demonstrations, and ran cooking classes across America. An indication of her status in New York, her image featured in a cartoon by Peter Arno, on a 1949 front cover of the *New Yorker* magazine. Lucas is pictured on a television screen above men drinking in a New York bar.

In the mid-1950s she toured Australian capital cities. She held cooking demonstrations in major department stores, receiving great publicity because of her celebrity status in America.

Lucas's potential to market products to postwar American women was recognized, and her work and her image were very quickly commercialized. With one hundred thousand viewers, she had one of the largest and most loyal TV audiences of any daytime cooking show. *The Dione Lucas Cooking Show*, sponsored by Caloric gas appliances, gained her a reputation as the nation's leading saleswoman of gas appliances.

Lucas had a mixed reputation. Duska Howarth, her New York publicist and friend, wrote that Dione was endlessly generous, well meaning, and talented in what she did and that she worked hard all the time and must have been exhausted; however, she had a tendency to cover up embarrassing situations with elaborate fibbing. Robert Clark, writing in *The Solace of Food*, noted that although she was the most visible figure on the New York food scene of the early 1950s, she was "a strange bird and…she maintained an entourage of fanatical hangers-on."

Her impact on American (and Australian) food culture has been largely overlooked in favor of those who followed her. The late Craig Claiborne (1970) described her as "the high priestess of high cookery" and summed up her influence: "Dione Lucas pioneered French cooking in this country…when the average American couldn't distinguish a crepe Suzette from a flapjack or a scrambled egg from an omelette."

See also TELEVISION.

Claiborne, Craig. "Tools of Her Trade in Dione Lucas's Shop." *New York Times*, March 5, 1970.

Clark, Robert. *The Solace of Food: A Life of James Beard.* South Royalton, Vt.: Steerforth, 1996.

Howarth, Jessmin, and Dushka Howarth. *"It's Up to Ourselves": A Mother, a Daughter and Gurdjieff; A Shared Memoir and Family Photo Album.* New York: Gurdjieff Heritage Society, 1998.

Schinto, Jeanne. "Remembering Dione Lucas." *Gastronomica* (Winter 2011): 34–46.

Jillian Adams

Lüchow, August Guido

August Guido Lüchow (1857–1923), an émigré from Hanover, Germany, was one of New York City's foremost German American restaurateurs. Arriving in New York in 1879, he soon found work in a little *biergarten* owned by Oscar von Mehlbach on East Fourteenth Street, just off Union Square. Three years later, with a loan from William Steinway, the city's preeminent piano manufacturer, Lüchow bought the place and began turning it into a full-fledged restaurant serving fare like pig knuckles, venison, *sauerbraten*, roast goose, *huhn im topf* (chicken in a pot), and *wienerschnitzel*. Lüchow's would eventually expand to fill several storefronts, with a Gentlemen's Grill, Café, Garden (the original outdoor beer garden, enclosed and topped with a skylight), Hunt Room, and Nibelungen Room. What had been the stables housing the beer wagons and draft horses later became The New Room.

The wood-paneled walls were hung with European paintings as well as stag heads and other hunting trophies; the Nibelungen Room featured murals representing scenes from Wagner's operas. Hundreds of beer steins lined the walls throughout. A string quartet played during meals. At holiday time the restaurant displayed the city's tallest indoor Christmas tree, which was lighted with great fanfare at dinner every night of the season.

In the 1880s Union Square was a center of both high and low culture, lined with concert halls, theaters, and music halls. William Steinway's piano showroom and concert venue, Steinway Hall, was nearby. He often dined and held banquets at Lüchow's, as did other members of New York's musical elite, including the composers Antonin Dvorak and Richard Strauss and the tenor Enrico Caruso. The future U.S. president Theodore Roosevelt often visited Lüchow's, and the hearty German fare and free-flowing lager

also drew a wide range of musicians, actors, artists, and writers, including H. L. Mencken and O. Henry. Andrew Carnegie, J. P. Morgan, and Diamond Jim Brady entertained their friends with lavish dinners at Lüchow's.

World War I brought the closure of many of the city's venerable German restaurants. See WORLD WAR I. Lüchow's survived through this period (but removed the umlaut from its name as a concession to anti-German sentiment) and, more remarkably, hung on through Prohibition. After August Lüchow's death, in 1923, his nephew-in-law, Peter Eckstein, took over, and the restaurant went into a decline. A new owner, Jan Mitchell, who bought Lüchow's in 1950, restored some of its former glory by reinstating seasonal events such as the bock beer festival and kept the city's last prominent German restaurant going until 1967, when he sold it to Riese Brothers, a national restaurant management firm. By this time Fourteenth Street had turned seedy and dangerous, and Lüchow's décor and cuisine had lost their luster. In 1982 the restaurant again changed hands: Peter Aschkenasy, the principal of Restaurant Associates, moved the restaurant to the plaza of an office building on Broadway between Fiftieth and Fifty-First Streets, but it closed for good four years later. The original building, having fallen into severe disrepair, was razed in 1995.

Mitchell, Leonard Jan. *Lüchow's German Cookbook: The Story and the Favorite Dishes of America's Most Famous German Restaurant.* Garden City, N.Y.: Doubleday, 1952.

Patrick, Ted, and Silas Spitzer. *Great Restaurants of America.* Philadelphia: Lippincott, 1960.

Bonnie Slotnick and Andrew F. Smith

Lucky Peach

Lucky Peach is a print quarterly and mobile app, and in the realm of food magazines it has positioned itself as the smart, cool kid in the room, the Vassar to *Bon Appétit* and *Saveur*'s Harvard and Yale. Founded in 2011 by David Chang of Momofuku with Peter Meehan (coauthor of Chang's *Momofuku* cookbook) and Zero Point Zero Production, *Lucky Peach* has come a long way since its inaugural, ramen-themed issue.

Since that first issue, *Lucky Peach* has featured contributions from rising stars and established figures from Manhattan and beyond, including René

Redzepi (chef of Noma, DK), Momofuku Milk Bar's own Christina Tosi, then–*Village Voice* columnist Robert Seitsema, Mario Batali, Michael Pollan, and even Ted Nugent (as part of *Lucky Peach*'s apocalypse issue). Its coverage is just as eclectic as its contributors. Past issues have focused on topics from "All You Can Eat" to "Before and After the Apocalypse." In 2014, *Lucky Peach* won five James Beard Awards for its food coverage, including an especially meditative essay on canning and preserves by *New York Times Magazine* writer John Jeremiah Sullivan.

Few publications rival *Lucky Peach* for creative presentation. Instead of glossy photography, readers of *Lucky Peach* are greeted with intricate illustrations and custom fonts. Instead of instructional how-tos, LuckyPeachTV (a YouTube channel) features behind-the-scenes office hijinks and a psychedelic cartoon series about four friends of indeterminate species in search of the perfect meal. It is the food magazine for readers who prefer vinyl.

Initially published as part of the ever-expanding McSweeney's Publishing, *Lucky Peach* split off on its own in 2013. The results have been unbridled success. Still helmed by Chris Ying as editor-in-chief, Meehan and Chang remain on the masthead, alongside Manhattan luminaries like Mark Ibold (as its "SE Pennsylvania Correspondent") and Anthony Bourdain (as "Film Critic Emeritus").

See also CHANG, DAVID and MOMOFUKU RESTAURANT GROUP.

Beaujon, Andrew. "Lucky Peach Gets Five James Beard Awards." Poynter, May 6, 2014. http://www.poynter .org/latest-news/mediawire/250738/lucky-peach-gets-five-james-beard-awards/.
Dixler, Hillary. "Lucky Peach Goes Solo, Splits from McSweeney's." Eater NY, September 3, 2013. http:// www.eater.com/2013/9/3/6377949/lucky-peach-goes-solo-splits-from-mcsweeneys.
LuckyPeachTV. YouTube. https://www.youtube.com/ user/LuckyPeachTV.

Alexis Zanghi

Luger, Carl and Peter

See PETER LUGER'S.

Lunch

In the colonial period and early republic, lunch (then called "dinner") was a family meal, which in many households included apprentices and slaves. Men, women, and children ate together in the early afternoon, making this the main meal of the day and only taking something small for supper before going to bed. Occasional formal luncheons marked important occasions, such as the farewell luncheon George Washington gave for his troops at Sam Fraunces's tavern at the end of the Revolution. See FRAUNCES TAVERN.

Beginning early in the nineteenth century, merchants and businessmen began to move farther uptown away from the hustle, bustle, and dirt of the business districts. Unable to return home for lunch, they began to eat together in the taverns and private clubs and eventually freestanding restaurants that emerged to serve this new market.

Workingmen, too, were bound to new timetables. Where once apprentices and masters dined together over their workbenches, now workers were rung in and out of the factory by bells that allowed them one hour for lunch. They had to find their lunch where they could and eat it on street curbs or standing up. Saloons welcomed this new midday clientele with "free lunch" that was typically small and salty. The new kinds of business that were part of the market revolution required a clerical class, who in turn required lunch. Some dashed "home" to boarding houses, while others patronized chop houses or ordered food to be delivered from taverns to their desks. See SALOONS and TAVERNS.

Looking back from the end of the nineteenth century, one New Yorker recalled that the many downtown eating places that served businessmen and clerks alike did not offer much to entice the palate. Most served greasy fare on crude china with weak tea or coffee and not a bottle of wine in sight. An enterprising French Canadian, however, introduced table d'hôte meals and French cooking to the city shortly after the Civil War. Journalist Edgar Fawcett (1854) recalled "my amazement at dining for the first time" in this establishment, owned by Dennis Donovan, where the proprietor offered "a good French breakfast and luncheon at fifty cents."

Women of the employer class typically ate a light, cold lunch at home and saved the larger, hot meal of the day for after 5:00 p.m. when their husbands came home. With the development of department stores and cultural institutions that catered to the middle class, these same women left home to enjoy the city; and like (but not with) their husbands,

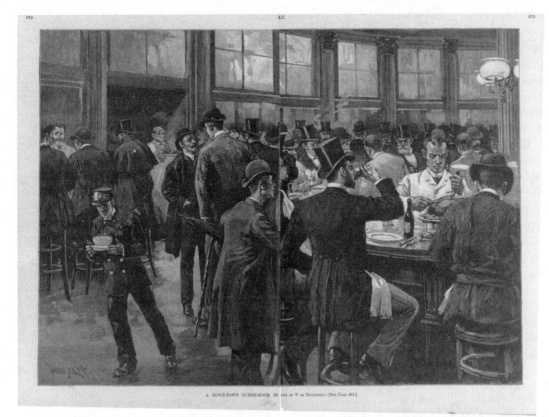

A downtown lunchroom in New York, drawn by T. de Thulstrup (1848–1930), a Swedish-born illustrator whose work featured in *Harper's Weekly* for three decades. Lunchrooms were frequented by both businessmen and blue-collar workers in the mid-day. LIBRARY OF CONGRESS

they also needed to lunch downtown, around the shopping district of "Ladies' Mile." Some hotel restaurants served "ladies," while others did not, so department stores themselves quickly stepped in to solve the problem of hungry shoppers with on-site tearooms, lavishly decorated and serving sandwiches and sweets. For working-class women, street carts or food brought from home remained the only options. See DEPARTMENT STORE RESTAURANTS; HOTEL RESTAURANTS; and STREET VENDORS.

By the end of the nineteenth century, lunch pioneers William and Samuel Child saw a niche for sanitary and modern lunch restaurants. They opened their first restaurants in the Wall Street neighborhood in the 1890s, catering to the business crowd, and eventually operated nine restaurants around New York City. The Childs amazed the public with their first self-serve cafeteria in 1898 at 130 Broadway. That model was soon picked up by Schrafft's and Horn & Hardart (of automat fame), two multi-

city restaurant chains. See CHILDS; SCHRAFFT's; and AUTOMATS.

When the clerical workforce had expanded significantly to include young women, these first members of the pink-collar class provided business for restaurant chains and drugstore lunch counters. F. W. Woolworth opened its first lunchroom in New York in 1910 in its Fourteenth Street store after trying out a limited menu in a Philadelphia shop. Because Woolworth had a reputation for value but also for modern efficiency, it provided a respectable spot for lunchers on a budget. This same combination helped lunch counters survive the Depression.

With the decline of the five and dime in the postwar period, the traditional drugstore lunch counter became a rarity, while establishments that New Yorkers term "coffee shops" and others call "diners" or "greasy spoons" survived and prospered. A postwar boom in immigration from Greece to the metropolitan area helped to expand Greek domination of the coffee shop. New Yorkers of all ethnic backgrounds and classes became as familiar with spinach pie as they were with grilled cheese sandwiches. Coffee shop lunch menus typically included a few Greek American classics as well as the mainstays of Anglo-American food—omelets and cheeseburgers served "deluxe"—with lettuce and tomato. See COFFEE SHOPS; DINERS; and GREEK.

Rising wages for the lower middle class made the coffee shop a place that was both ubiquitous and egalitarian. A further democratization of "fine" dining and concurrent growth of the fast-food industry displaced the coffee shop by the end of the twentieth century. While the elite lunched powerfully at The Four Seasons in the 1990s, office workers munched pizza slices from Sbarro. The British lunch chain Pret A Manger entered the American market in New York in 2001, miraculously converting a city accustomed to mile-high deli sandwiches to slim, triangular packages of lunch. Competing with the new chains and old delis, food trucks rolled into the midday scene toward the end of the new century's first decade. Boosted by the widespread adoption of Twitter, food trucks attracted followers who sought out their favorites wherever they happened to be in the city. See FOUR SEASONS and FOOD TRUCKS.

The most notable innovation in New York lunch since 2010 has been the transformation of the previously reviled food court into a space attractive to determined urbanites. The many small food stations of Chelsea Market, the food court of the renovated Grand Central Station's lower level, and the covered market atmosphere of Eataly have proved to be popular lunch venues. Following the success of Brooklyn's Smorgasburg and The Flea, open-air food courts now tempt office workers in midtown Manhattan. See CHELSEA MARKET; EATALY; and SMORGASBURG.

See also POWER BREAKFASTS AND POWER LUNCHES.

Batterberry, Michael, and Ariane Batterberry. *On the Town in New York: The Landmark History of Eating, Drinking, and Entertainments from the American Revolution to the Food Revolution.* London and New York: Routledge, 1998.
Fawcett, Edgar. "Old Restaurants of New York." *Lippincott's Monthly Magazine,* no. 54 (July–December 1854): 709–711.
Ferling, John. *Jefferson and Hamilton: The Rivalry That Forged a Nation.* London: Bloomsbury, 2013.
Lewine, Edward. "The Kaffenion Connection: How the Greek Diner Evolved." *New York Times,* April 14, 1996.
Lobel, Cindy. *Urban Appetites.* Chicago: University of Chicago Press, 2014.
Pitrone, Jean Maddern. *F. W. Woolworth and the American Five and Dime: A Social History.* Jefferson, N.C.: MacFarland, 2003.
Rose, Peter G. "Dutch Food in Life and Art." *Culinary Historians of New York Newsletter* 16, no. 1 (Fall 2002): 1–4.

Megan Elias

Lunchrooms

See RESTAURANTS; SCHRAFFT'S; and TEAROOMS.

Lutèce

From the moment it opened its doors in 1961 at 249 East Fiftieth Street, luxe French restaurant Lutèce was notable for its chef, André Soltner, who presided over the kitchen for thirty-four years. He was one of the first chefs in America to emphasize the freshest possible ingredients and was considered America's first superstar chef.

The 1950s and 1960s witnessed the rise of French cuisine in America, including New York. Lutèce was among those old-guard French restaurants that offered elegance and luxurious meals. André Surmain and then twenty-nine-year-old André Soltner opened Lutèce with a vision of the restaurant as a luxurious monument to rarefied cuisine, naming it for Lutetia, the mellifluous Gallic appellation for Paris. Together they ran the restaurant until 1973, when Surmain returned to Europe.

Soltner was the heart of Lutèce and was often spotted greeting customers at the front, including many of New York's well-heeled and celebrity diners. But his genius lay in the kitchen. Reared in Alsace, France, with its fertile terroir, he combined the freshest possible ingredients with traditional French techniques.

Soltner specialized in traditional, even rustic fare with accents of his native Alsace. Signature dishes included pastry with salmon mousse, puffy Alsatian onion tart, and sautéed foie gras prepared with dark chocolate sauce and bitter orange marmalade. Compared to other grand, often-intimidating

French restaurants, Lutèce was lauded for its warm and unpretentious atmosphere. The Soltners lived above the restaurant, and some praised its *maman et papa* charm.

Ark Restaurants purchased Lutèce in 1994. This led to the legendary dining shrine's closure in 2004, concluding a more than forty-year run.

See also FRENCH and SOLTNER, ANDRÉ.

Daria, Irene. *Lutèce: A Day in the Life of America's Greatest Restaurant*. New York: Random House, 1993.

Sheraton, Mimi. "America's Best French Restaurant." *Time*, March 10, 1986.

Soltner, André. *The Lutèce Cookbook*. With Seymour Britchky. New York: Knopf, 1995.

Sokolov, Raymond. *New York Times*, January 14, 1972.

Michele Kidwell-Gilbert

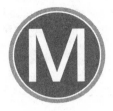

MacAusland, Earle

Earle R. MacAusland (1891–1980) was the founder and publisher of *Gourmet*, subtitled *The Magazine of Good Living*. *Gourmet* was the first glossy, color food and travel magazine published in the United States, and by building a sophisticated, food-savvy readership, it paved the way for the many American food magazines on the market today.

MacAusland was born in Taunton, Massachusetts, and moved to New York when he was in his thirties to go into publishing. He sold advertising for publishers of women's magazines and was quite successful, but when he tried to launch a magazine of his own in the early years of the Depression, the effort left him bankrupt. Still, MacAusland never gave up the dream of publishing his own magazine.

In the late 1930s MacAusland began to rough out a plan for a magazine focused on food and drink. His father and brother agreed to underwrite the printing of the first issue, which was released in January 1941. Its intended audience was the well-heeled sophisticate who had enjoyed fine food and wine while touring Europe. MacAusland promoted the magazine to members of gastronomic organizations, such as the Wine & Food Society.

MacAusland himself had no professional expertise in food and cooking, so he hired a small group of eminent culinarians to edit and write the magazine. Pearl Metzelthin, author of *The World Wide Cook Book* (1939), was appointed the magazine's editor. Louis De Gouy, a French chef and cookbook author with considerable experience in restaurants in the United States and Europe, was hired as the magazine's "gourmet chef," a position he held until

his death in 1947. A third collaborator was Samuel Chamberlain, a writer, artist, and photographer whose articles and illustrations—often describing beloved places in France—enlivened the magazine's pages for many years. Chamberlain eventually became *Gourmet*'s associate editor. Clementine Paddleford, a food journalist who wrote a column for the *New York Herald Tribune*, later joined the team, writing the column Food Flashes, about the latest culinary trends and products. Illustrator Henry Stahlhut created the cover art for the first issue and continued to illustrate *Gourmet* covers until around 1960.

MacAusland distributed copies of the inaugural issue to potential corporate advertisers; he also sent sample copies to the rich and famous. He signed up a number of advertisers, but more important, he found two financial backers: Ralph Reinhold of Reinhold Publishing (later Van Nostrand Reinhold) and Gladys Guggenheim Straus, a granddaughter of the Swiss-born philanthropist Meyer Guggenheim. Straus was dubbed cofounder and made vice president of *Gourmet*, but she also worked as assistant editor. Despite this support, MacAusland still had to spend his days selling advertising while also putting in long nights editing the magazine.

The United States entered World War II in December 1941. *Gourmet* gamely kept going for the duration, despite rationing and transportation restrictions that made many food products hard to come by. Years later, MacAusland wrote that the war had actually helped *Gourmet* find its footing. For those lucky enough to have dined at the finest restaurants in France before the war—and those who hoped to do so in the future—*Gourmet* offered a vicarious sampling of haute cuisine while enabling its readers to try the dishes at home (if they could find the ingredients). Culinary historian Anne Mendelson (2001) has written, "Hardship (and later the war) fostered a taste for images of a happier past and perhaps a happier future." Shortly after the war, MacAusland moved *Gourmet's* offices into a penthouse at the Plaza Hotel, where they remained for twenty years. See WORLD WAR II.

As the years went on, MacAusland courted the finest of food writers, such as Jane Grigson, Joseph Wechsberg, Elizabeth David, and chef Louis Diat, author of *Cooking à la Ritz* (1941). (Diat became the magazine's in-house chef when Louis De Gouy died.) MacAusland also published writers from other genres, such as science fiction master Ray Bradbury and even F. Scott Fitzgerald (whose article appeared posthumously). MacAusland hired the New York City caterer and cookbook author James Beard, who had just published *Hors d'Oeuvre and Canapés* (1940), as associate editor. Beard became the magazine's restaurant critic in 1949. He left in 1950 after feuding with MacAusland over a gaffe—Beard had reprinted one of his *Gourmet* columns almost verbatim in an advertising booklet. The two eventually buried the hatchet, and Beard returned to the magazine in 1969. M. F. K. Fisher, whose *Serve It Forth* appeared in 1937, also wrote for *Gourmet*, but after her translation of Brillat-Savarin's *Physiology of Taste* was published in 1949, MacAusland believed that she was too sophisticated for *Gourmet*.

Gourmet celebrated its tenth anniversary, in 1951, by bringing out *The Gourmet Cookbook*; Earle MacAusland is credited as author. Food critic Charlotte Turgeon praised the book, as well as the magazine, in her *New York Times* review: "Never compromising with short cuts or substitutes, *Gourmet Magazine* has weathered war and rationing without lowering its standards and is celebrating its first successful decade with the publication of a splendid volume." *The Gourmet Cookbook* was the first of many cookbooks published by the magazine under MacAusland's leadership.

MacAusland was interested in "good living" as expressed though fine dining, fashion, entertaining, and travel. Being a "gourmet," the magazine repeatedly affirmed, was not dependent on a person's wealth, class, or social status. Rather, a gourmet was one who prepared meals with love and care and shared them with congenial company—something

anyone could do. Of course, *Gourmet* also served as a "dream book" for armchair travelers whose trips to Burgundy, Istanbul, or Bangkok began and ended within the covers of a magazine.

Earle MacAusland died in 1980. *Gourmet* was sold to Condé Nast, publishers of *Vogue*, in 1983, and the print edition of *Gourmet* folded in 2009.

See also BEARD, JAMES; DE GOUY, LOUIS P.; DIAT, LOUIS; *GOURMET*; PADDLEFORD, CLEMENTINE; and WECHSBERG, JOSEPH.

Kamp, David. *The United States of Arugula: How We Became a Gourmet Nation.* New York: Broadway, 2006.
Kuh, Patric. *The Last Days of Haute Cuisine: America's Culinary Revolution.* New York: Viking, 2001.
Leibenstein, Margaret. "Earle MacAusland." In *Culinary Biographies*, edited by Alice Arndt. Houston, Tex.: Yes, 2006.
Mendelson, Anne. "60 Years of Gourmet." *Gourmet* 61 (September 2001): 71, 110–111, 133, 153, 203, 219.
Shapiro, Laura. *Something from the Oven: Reinventing Dinner in 1950s America.* New York: Penguin, 2004.

Andrew F. Smith

Maccioni, Sirio

Sirio Maccioni (b. 1932) was born in Tuscany and began his path toward restaurant destiny while still a teenager by working as a busboy to support his family after his father's death. Later, Maccioni enrolled in restaurant and hotel training programs in Paris and Hamburg, followed by European apprenticeships at hotel restaurants at the Plaza Athénée in Paris and the Hotel Atlantic in Hamburg. A position on the high seas brought him to New York City, where he worked as a waiter at the Wall Street eatery Delmonico's. See DELMONICO'S. Later, he moved to the renowned Colony restaurant as maître d'hôtel. While there, he spent thirteen years bulking up his Rolodex with the city's most prominent people until he was ready to launch his own restaurant. In March 1974, Maccioni opened Le Cirque, in the Mayfair Hotel, making it the first privately owned hotel restaurant in New York City. See LE CIRQUE.

Maccioni is widely credited as the main reason for Le Cirque's decades of success. His database of high-powered clientele, his gift at schmoozing and giving attention to customers, as well as his insight into choosing chefs and adding menu dishes contributed to the restaurant's longevity and appeal. The restaurant was one of the first to bring exotic ingredients (at the time), like foie gras or suckling pig, to a restaurant setting. It was also Maccioni who selected a virtually unknown Daniel Boulud, making him the executive chef from 1986 to 1992. See BOULUD, DANIEL. The restaurant subsequently netted a four-star review from the *New York Times* under the chef's tenure. Maccioni was also credited with bringing crème brûlée to the United States and the actual invention of pasta primavera; both became iconic Le Cirque staples, introducing them to American palates and restaurant menus across the country. According to Michael Lomonaco, a former Le Cirque line cook, Le Cirque was the most important restaurant in the United States in the mid-1980s and among the top five in the world, all the result of Maccioni's guidance.

In 1997, the restaurant moved from the Mayfair to the New York Palace Hotel under the name Le Cirque 2000, where it remained until 2004. In 2007, HBO released *Le Cirque: A Table in Heaven*, a documentary chronicling the closing of Le Cirque 2000 through the restaurant's reopening in 2006 in its current location in Midtown East. Maccioni documented his life story and culinary journey in the autobiography, *Sirio: The Story of My Life and Le Cirque* (2004), cowritten by Peter Elliot, along with *A Table at Le Cirque* (2012), cowritten with Pamela Fiori.

There have been numerous awards along the way, including the James Beard Restaurant of the Year in 1995; the Impresario dell'Anno (Entrepreneur of the Year) award at Affreschi Toscani, a festival in Tuscany; and 2002 Father of the Year by the National Father's Day Committee. The New York Landmarks Conservancy designated the distinguished Maccioni as one of its living landmarks, and he was distinguished with a James Beard Foundation Lifetime Achievement Award in 2014. His three sons, Mario, Marco, and Mauro, have followed their father's footsteps into the Le Cirque restaurant business.

Lynn, Andrea. "2014 James Beard Foundation Lifetime Achievement Award Recipient Sirio Maccioni." *The Official James Beard Foundation Blog*, May 5, 2014. http://www.jamesbeard.org/blog/2014-james-beard-foundation-lifetime-achievement-award-recipient-sirio-maccioni.

Maccioni, Sirio, and Peter J. Elliot. *Sirio: The Story of My Life and Le Cirque*. Hoboken, N.J.: Wiley, 2004.

Rossi, Andrew, dir. *Le Cirque: A Table in Heaven*, 2007. DVD. New York: First Run Features, 2011.

Andrea Lynn

Macfadden, Bernarr

Bernarr Macfadden (1868–1955) was an early health-food guru who promoted salads and other raw produce, as well as weekly fasts. He was born Bernard Adolphus McFadden in Mill Spring, Missouri. He suffered health problems as a child, but his stamina, strength, and vigor improved when he began an extensive bodybuilding program as a young man, engaging in weightlifting and wrestling while also coaching and teaching. He changed his name to Bernarr Macfadden, which he believed sounded much stronger than his original name.

With only fifty dollars in his pocket, Macfadden moved to New York City in 1893. He developed a physical training program for clients and, in his off-hours, wrote articles on physical culture. Macfadden toured England for two years, promoting his theories, and then began a lecture tour of the United States. In 1899, having failed to find a magazine or newspaper willing to publish his articles, he founded *Physical Culture*, America's first "muscle magazine," which was a vehicle for his philosophies and advice on health, exercise, fasting, and nutrition. The success of *Physical Culture* permitted Macfadden to launch a publishing empire that cranked out newspapers and magazines. He also wrote more than a hundred books.

The winter of 1902 was a bitterly cold one, and many New Yorkers were out of work. Macfadden opened a cafeteria for the unemployed in City Hall Park that charged a penny per course. When it closed in the spring, it had actually turned a profit.

When the Depression hit in 1929, Macfadden established a $5 million foundation to help launch a chain of "penny cafeterias" to feed the city's destitute. He opened the first in December 1931 and five more subsequently. The cafes served a vegetarian menu of "cracked wheat, Scotch oatmeal, lima bean soup, green pea soup, soaked prunes, seeded raisins, whole wheat bread, butter, raisin coffee and cereal coffee." (Macfadden did not approve of "real" coffee—it was available but at an extra charge.) Each dish cost one cent. Macfadden said he charged for the food so that the unemployed would not feel that they were accepting charity. His penny restaurants served fifteen hundred to three thousand customers per day, with turnover encouraged by the lack of physical comforts: there were no tables or chairs, just counters where customers ate standing up. At the depth of the Depression, the penny cafeterias served an estimated eleven thousand New Yorkers a day. They operated through 1941.

Macfadden believed that the majority of Americans ate too much, and he advocated eating only two meals a day. He also decried the American habit of eating many different types of food at the same meal; he believed that this was "a crime against any stomach and that disease is an almost inevitable result." The health regimen that Macfadden developed included specialized diets and fasts. He fasted every Monday, and when he was ill, he frequently abstained from food for several days at a time. He recommended drinking a dozen or more glasses of water every day but eschewed alcohol, ice water, coffee, and tea. Whole milk, Macfadden felt, was the greatest of all foods; he developed milk-only diets for specific therapeutic applications.

While Macfadden was not a vegetarian, he advocated eating meat sparingly and rarely touched it himself, although he did consume milk and eggs. He opposed the use of seasonings and condiments such as salt, pepper, vinegar, and spices, which he believed were "undoubtedly harmful and provocative of disease" (Macfadden, 1920, p. 101). He prescribed a diet rich in fruits, vegetables, and whole grains and warned against white flour and sweets. He particularly encouraged the consumption of raw beets, carrots, cabbage, corn, tomatoes, turnips, citrus, figs, raisins, legumes, nuts, and eggs. Macfadden promulgated his dietary principles in many articles and books, including *Strength from Eating: How and What to Eat and Drink to Develop the Highest Degree of Health and Strength* (1901) and *Eating for Health and Strength* (1921). Like C. W. Post and the Kellogg brothers—fellow health-food advocates who made their fortunes in breakfast cereal—Macfadden created and sold his own ready-to-eat mixture of wheat, oats, and nuts under the name "Strengthfude." Macfadden even opened his own sanitarium in Battle Creek in 1907, but neither the cereal nor the institution did very well, and he relocated the latter to Chicago within a few years.

See also DEPRESSION FOOD and RESTAURANTS.

Adams, Mark. *Mr. America: How Muscular Millionaire Bernarr Macfadden Transformed the Nation through Sex, Salad, and the Ultimate Starvation Diet.* New York: Harper, 2009.

Macfadden, Bernarr. *Eating for Health and Strength.* New York: Physical Culture, 1921.

Macfadden, Bernarr. *Strength from Eating: How and What to Eat and Drink to Develop the Highest Degree of Health and Strength.* New York: Physical Culture, 1901.

Macfadden, Bernarr, *Macfadden's Encyclopedia of Physical Culture.* Rev. ed. New York: Physical Culture, 1920.

Andrew F. Smith

Macy's

The largest department store company in the world, Macy's was started in 1858 by Rowland Hussey Macy as a "fancy dry goods" store on Sixth Avenue and Fourteenth Street. Its original merchandise included ribbons, laces, artificial flowers, handkerchiefs, hosiery, and gloves. When Macy's opened, Ladies' Mile was still a distance downtown on lower Broadway, but by the 1870s, with the growth of the city and construction of the elevated train lines, Manhattan's shopping district shifted uptown, and Macy's was at the center of the new Ladies' Mile. By that point, Macy had expanded his merchandise line significantly, in search of increased revenue. Macy's new stock included rugs, furniture, decorative items, bicycles, gardening sets, and beach equipment along with a new "picnic department," offering crackers, jams, preserved meats, and other provisions. Macy's also introduced a year-round candy department; prior to that point, they had sold confections only around Christmastime.

In 1878, Macy's opened a ladies' lunchroom on the second floor to serve the needs of its patrons who wanted a bite to eat while out shopping. While Parisian department stores innovated the in-house restaurant, Macy's introduced the custom to the United States. Several other department stores quickly followed suit. In its early years, the restaurant served cold food, prepared off premises, alongside hot drinks like tea, coffee, and hot chocolate. An 1892 guidebook wrote that Macy's and other department store restaurants did a large business but catered mainly to the tourist trade. The guide derided them as "not first-class in cooking or in service."

In 1888 brothers Isidor and Nathan Straus became partners in Macy's, and in 1893 they gained majority control of the firm. Under their supervision, the store expanded into one of the world's largest department stores. During the 1890s, the store's inventory grew to include ready-made clothing, shoes, jewelry, instruments, photography supplies, optical goods, saddlery, infants' haberdashery, and fire-arms. In 1893 the Straus brothers established a grocery department that featured a complete line of staple and fancy goods such as fine wines, chocolates, coffees and teas (Macy's was the first store to sell tea bags), assorted cheeses, smoked meats, and tropical fruits and vegetables, even out of season.

In 1902 Macy's moved uptown to its current flagship location at Herald Square. The store boasted sixty-five departments, including a restaurant on the eighth floor touted as the world's largest—it seated twenty-five hundred people—as well as a separate Japanese tearoom on the fifth floor. Macy's restaurant served one million people in 1908. By 1914, Macy's expanded grocery department included 265 kinds of wine, claret, and champagne; "dietetic" foods such as yogurt, granola, and wheat bran; an assortment of liquors; and its own brand of premixed cocktails. Macy's also was the first large retail store to sell kosher foods.

In the next few decades, Macy's grew to take up the entire block of Thirty-Fourth Street between Broadway and Seventh Avenue, touting itself as "the world's largest store," with over one million square feet of retail space. In 1922 Macy's went public and began a period of expansion, opening branch stores and buying up competitors such as Bamberger's, Lasalle & Koch, and Davison-Paxton.

In the 1940s Macy's expanded to the West Coast, taking over the San Francisco department store O'Connor Moffatt and Company and renaming it Macy's in 1947. The San Francisco Union Square store became the West Coast flagship. There, Macy's introduced the flower show. The annual tradition is still held in San Francisco's Macy's as well as in New York, Chicago, Minneapolis, Philadelphia, and Washington, DC. The Union Square (San Francisco) store also is where "The Cellar" was born when, in 1971, the firm decided to convert the bargain basement of the store into its housewares department. In 1976 the Herald Square store followed suit. Today, The Cellar offers a huge collection of housewares as well as packaged foods and a large, cafeteria-style restaurant.

In 1994 Macy's was acquired by the Federated Department Store Conglomerate (eventually changing its name to Macy's, Inc.), which became the largest department store company in the world. In subsequent years Macy's, Inc. took over many of its competitors, rebranding them as Macy's, including I. Magnin, A&S, Jordan Marsh, and Stern's. In 2005,

Macy's took over the May Department Store Group, which included such names as Strawbridge & Clothier, Filene's, and Marshall Fields. Today, Macy's operates over eight hundred stores around the country.

The Herald Square store remains Macy's flagship. It houses ten restaurants, including four Starbucks, an Au Bon Pain, a McDonald's, Cucina and Co., the Cellar Bar and Grill, the Herald Square Café, and Stella 34. A noteworthy feature of the Herald Square store is De Gustibus Cooking School, located on the eighth floor. Founded in 1980 by Arlene Feltman Sailhac, De Gustibus offers cooking classes and demonstrations by renowned chefs from New York City and beyond. Virtually every American chef of note has appeared at De Gustibus including Julia Child, James Beard, Rick Bayless, Wolfgang Puck, and Michael White. These chefs offer demonstrations in cooking techniques followed by a tasting for customers who pay one hundred dollars per class. Today DeGustibus is owned and run by Salvatore Rizzo.

Macy's also operates a few branch stores in the outer boroughs. The Macy's Thanksgiving Day Parade, ushering in the Christmas shopping season since its founding in 1924, has become a national Thanksgiving Day ritual.

See also DEPARTMENT STORE RESTAURANTS.

Howard, Ralph M. *History of Macy's of New York 1858–1919*. Cambridge, Mass.: Harvard University Press, 1943.
Leach, William. *Land of Desire: Merchants, Power, and the Rise of a New American Culture*. New York: Vintage, 1994.

Cindy R. Lobel

Madden, Owney

See BOOTLEGGERS.

Mad Men

Mad Men was a television series that aired on the AMC network from 2007 to 2015. Set in New York during the years 1960 through 1970, it was based on the golden years of the advertising industry and the drinking, decadence, and debauchery of the era's greatest creative minds in advertising. From its first year on air until its last in the spring of 2015, *Mad Men* was the recipient of multiple accolades including several Emmy and Golden Globe Awards.

Rocketing to cult status by the end of its first season, viewers teetered between loving and loathing Don Draper, Roger Sterling, Pete Campbell, and the agency's compelling females Peggy Olson and Joan Harris.

Among the real-life New York locales depicted in the show, the fictionalized agency on Madison Avenue was stumbling distance from two infamous, martini-saturated lunch haunts: The Oyster Bar and Keens Steakhouse. See OYSTER BARS. After-work indulgences could be found by way of stripteases at the Slipper Room, bubbly conversation with a bunny at the New York Playboy Club, celebrating with a mistress at Sardi's, or among the drawn knives at Benihana. See SARDI'S. There were hops-fueled jukebox cha-chas at P. J. Clarke's, steak tartares at The Four Seasons, liquid dinners at The Oak Room Bar, and chicken Kiev at the now-defunct Jimmy's La Grange. See P. J. CLARKE'S; FOUR SEASONS; and PLAZA, THE. Marriage proposals were anticipated over steak at the Minetta Tavern, and New York City swans could be wooed at Barbetta before being returned to the sophisticated sanctuary of The Barbizon.

Beyond being safe havens for affairs or makeshift offices, New York City hotels such as The Pierre and the Hotel Elysée were places to toast new accounts or lament the lost ones. At the Waldorf, Don famously exclaims his enthusiasm for the hotel's in-room dining, "best kitchen in the world—got a salad named after it." See WALDORF, THE and WALDORF SALAD. Just outside of the city, the neon orange A-frame of a Howard Johnson's dining room served as a modular cornucopia of milkshakes, fried clams, saltwater taffy, and perfumy orange sherbet for Don and his wife.

Whether the characters were partaking in "liquid consultation" during office hours, entertaining in their Westchester homes, or staggering back to them, the cocktails in the show were featured almost as predominantly as the cast. This contributed to the cocktail renaissance of mid-century classics such as the Old-Fashioned, Manhattan, vodka gimlet, whiskey sour, Gibson, white Russian, Tom Collins, mint julep, and Bloody Mary. See OLD-FASHIONED COCKTAIL; MANHATTAN COCKTAIL; and BLOODY MARY.

As the calendar crept closer to the close of the 1960s, director Matthew Weiner's indefatigable commitment to historical authenticity inevitably meant an evolution of the venues, menus, and cocktails to reflect the times. Where once the Old Fashioned was a Don Draper standby, viewers watched him take a tiki turn by way of the Blue Hawaii at the close of season 4. Where once there were dining dens that evoked the formality of the 21 Club, by the end of season 5 faux Polynesian crab Rangoon and mai tais are served under a thatched ceiling resembling Trader Vic's, giving a culinary whisper to the geography of Hawaii and California throughout season 6 and the first half of season 7.

See also TELEVISION.

Della Femina, Jerry. *From Those Wonderful Folks Who Gave You Pearl Harbor: Front-Line Dispatches from the Advertising War.* New York: Simon & Schuster, 1970.
Swanson, Abbie Fentress. "Mad Men Mapped: A Guide to NYC Locales Frequented by Our Favorite Characters." WNYC, June 4, 2012. http://www.wnyc.org/story/204140-map-new-york-city-mad-men.

Georgette L. Moger

Magnolia Bakery

Magnolia Bakery was opened by partners Allysa Torey and Jennifer Appel on the corner of Bleecker and Eleventh Streets in the West Village in 1996. At the time, Bleecker Street was just beginning its transformation from a neighborhood shopping street to an enclave of high-end designer boutiques. Fitted out like an old-fashioned small-town bakery, Magnolia served classic American desserts such as red velvet cake, banana pudding, and an icebox cake made with Nabisco Famous Chocolate Wafer cookies. But its biggest crowd-pleaser was a vanilla cupcake lavished with a topknot of supersweet confectioner's sugar frosting. In 1999 Torey and Appel published *The Magnolia Bakery Cookbook: Old-Fashioned Recipes from New York's Sweetest Bakery.* Before the book was published, Appel had left and opened the competing Buttercup Bake Shop on East Fifty-First Street.

In a 2000 episode of the hit HBO television series *Sex and the City,* Carrie (played by Sarah Jessica Parker) and Miranda (played by Cynthia Nixon) sat on a bench outside the Magnolia Bakery, eating cupcakes as they discussed their love lives. The scene put Magnolia on the national and eventually international radar, and tourists lined up to buy cupcakes at the small storefront. The bakery became a key stop on *Sex and the City* bus tours. Eventually the demand was so great that the tour companies had to buy cupcakes elsewhere (from Billy's Bakery in Chelsea) and serve them on the buses—Magnolia was too small to handle the volume.

Magnolia was also mentioned in other television programs, such as *Saturday Night Live*, and in films, such as *The Devil Wears Prada*. On some days the bakery sells two thousand cupcakes, with sales of more than $40,000 a week from cupcakes alone. The *Sex and the City* episode is also credited with launching the "cupcake craze" that swept America and the world during the following years.

Entrepreneur Steve Abrams purchased the bakery in 2006. He opened additional branches in New York—in the tourist hubs of Rockefeller Center and Grand Central Station—and established locations in Chicago, Los Angeles, Dubai, and Tokyo. Abrams plans to add three more stores each year, with each location producing its baked goods in-house. He has expanded the product line, which has grown to sixty items.

In 2004 Allysa Torey published *More from Magnolia: Recipes from the World-Famous Bakery and Allysa Torey's Home Kitchen*. Torey's book *At Home with Magnolia*, which includes savory as well as sweet recipes, was published in 2006. The recipes from the first two Magnolia books were combined in *The Complete Magnolia Bakery Cookbook*, which came out in 2009.

See also CUPCAKES; SEX AND THE CITY; and TELEVISION.

Appel, Jennifer, and Allysa Torey. *The Magnolia Bakery Cookbook: Old-Fashioned Recipes from New York's Sweetest Bakery.* New York: Simon & Schuster, 1999.
Bushnell, Candace, and Darren Star. "No Ifs, Ands, or Butts." *Sex and the City*, season 3, episode 5, directed by Nicole Holofcener, aired July 9, 2000.

Andrew F. Smith

Mallomars

During the early twentieth century, American cookie manufacturers began to experiment with marshmallow, a delicate, pillowy confection then made from gelatin (or gum arabic), sugar, and cornstarch. In the early 1900s the National Biscuit Company (later Nabisco), with its baking plant on Ninth Avenue and Fifteenth Street in Manhattan, introduced the "Marshmallow Crème" cookie, a disk of vanilla shortbread topped with marshmallow and enrobed in dark chocolate. These were distributed in wholesale boxes (to be weighed out by the grocer) and did not sell particularly well. The National Biscuit Company's bakers went back to work on the product, and on August 13, 1913, the cookie, now with a graham-cracker base, was relaunched as the "Mallomar." The new product was sold in retail packages—eleven Mallomars to the ten-cent package (some grocers offered two packages for fifteen cents). As the pure chocolate covering melted in the heat, Mallomars were sold only during cooler weather, from late September to April.

Mallomars were distributed nationally, but sales were best along the East Coast and in the South. Labeled as "Chocolate Mallomars Cakes" from the 1940s on, Nabisco promoted them with advertising campaigns in *Life* and other national magazines. "Kids are mad for Mallomars!" was the slogan in the 1960s. Despite the advertising, national sales of Mallomars dwindled as the price of chocolate rose in the 1960s. By the 1980s, Mallomars had lost its "leadership status" and was considered a "ghost brand" by Nabisco, yet the company has continued to make them. Today, 70 percent are sold in the metropolitan New York area; most of the rest are sold in Florida, where many New Yorkers have relocated.

Mallomars are similar to other chocolate-and-marshmallow biscuits and confections enjoyed in Europe, and the three main ingredients are the same as those used in "s'mores," traditional campfire treats. Mallomars are also similar to Whippets, which have been made in Montreal since 1927. Because of the cooler Canadian climate and different formula for the chocolate, Whippets are sold all year round.

Despite the fact that hard chocolate coatings can be made to withstand warm temperatures, Nabisco has continued to manufacture and distribute Mallomars only during the cooler months. Some aficionados stockpile the cookies in the refrigerator or freezer for later consumption, but others prefer to keep them as a seasonal specialty, considering the Mallomar's return in the fall as cause for celebration.

Nabisco closed its Manhattan factory in 1959 but continued to make Mallomars in its Philadelphia plant. When that was closed, production was shifted to Canada, where all Mallomars are made today.

See also NABISCO.

Cahn, William. *Out of the Cracker Barrel: From Animal Crackers to Zu Zu's.* New York: Simon & Schuster, 1969.

Andrew F. Smith

Manhattan

Manhattan, a small island (about 23 square miles) surrounded by the Hudson estuary, has one of the world's most eclectic and vibrant foodscapes—twenty-four thousand restaurants; thousands of delis, bodegas, grocery stores, gourmet shops, food trucks, and street vendors; and nineteen weekly Greenmarkets operate in Manhattan. Newspapers and magazines published in Manhattan have greatly contributed not only to the island's food culture but to the whole country's sense of what people should eat. In this, their influence was second only to that of the media mavens of Madison Avenue.

It all started with the Lenape Indians who settled on the island in prehistoric times. They found a cornucopia of native edibles to gather, hunt, fish, and cultivate. These included thousands of species of fish (notably herring, salmon, mackerel, halibut, trout, pike, and eels), sea mammals (seals, porpoises, and whales), fowl (ducks, geese, swans, and turkeys), shellfish (crabs, lobster, oysters, mussels, and scallops), and mammals (deer, bears, rabbits, foxes, and beavers). They also gathered tempting tree fruits, berries, nuts, seeds, flowers, barks, and roots and cultivated several food plants, the most important being maize, squash, and beans.

The Dutch acquired the island from the Lenape in 1626. At its southern tip they established a small village, New Amsterdam, which was the administrative center for the colony of New Netherland. When the British occupied the island in 1664 they renamed the village "New York"; over time it expanded northward on the island and became a bustling city. It was not until 1898 that Manhattan joined the other four boroughs (Brooklyn, Queens, Staten Island, and the Bronx) to create "greater New York." Manhattan is the smallest borough in terms of land area and the most densely populated. As of 2014, it was home to 1.6 million residents.

The harbor surrounding Manhattan was well protected, providing a safe haven for deepwater ships. Edible commodities and other goods—grains, raw sugar, molasses, spices, wines, and agricultural

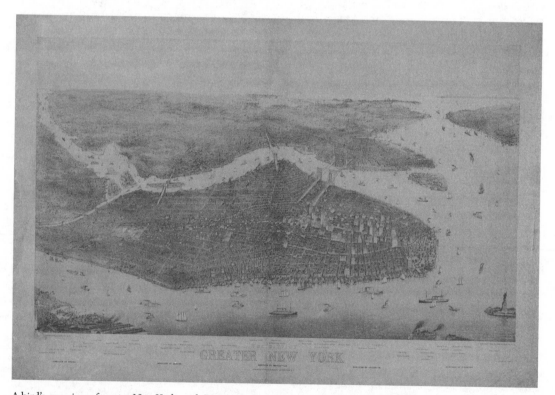

A bird's-eye view of greater New York, with Battery Park at the tip of Manhattan on the right, and showing the Bronx, Queens, Brooklyn, and Richmond, with the Hudson River in the foreground. Steamboats are carrying supplies and passengers to the harbors, alongside sailboats and fishing vessels. LIBRARY OF CONGRESS

products—landed at and departed from Manhattan's docks. The island became the sugar-refining center for America, a position it held until the mid-nineteenth century. The Hudson was the only river on the East Coast that was navigable for any distance. The importance of the city's location was greatly enhanced by the 1825 completion of the Erie Canal, connecting the Hudson with the Great Lakes. Wheat that grew abundantly in upstate New York and the Midwest could be shipped down the canal to Manhattan, where it was milled into flour. Bread, biscuits, and flour became major export items, and in the nineteenth century Manhattan was one of the world's largest milling, baking, and exporting centers. Imported molasses was made into rum, which was shipped throughout America. Domestic grain was converted into whiskey in Manhattan's distilleries, which dotted the island until the mid-nineteenth century. Barley and hops were used for making beer, and breweries operated in Manhattan until the 1960s.

Immigrant Foods and Beverages

Modern Manhattanites—and the millions who visit the city each year—can thank the masses of immigrants who have settled on the island for the incredible diversity of its culinary offerings. The Dutch allowed a mixed population of other Europeans, Jews, and Africans to settle on the island. Successive immigrant groups have brought their own culinary offerings to be folded into the city's simmering stewpot. German immigrants introduced lager beer, as well as the traditional foods that would evolve into the American hamburger and hot dog. Southern Italians brought pizza and pasta. German and Eastern European Jews contributed bagels, lox, and the pastrami, corned beef, and sour dill pickles of delicatessen culture. Following the Civil War, former slaves came north to New York, where they ruled and ran the kitchens of popular Manhattan restaurants. French chefs arrived to cook in upscale restaurants, introducing New Yorkers to haute cuisine. Chinese restaurateurs, adapting their native cuisine, served up chop suey, an "exotic" dish that was acceptable to Western palates. West Indian shopkeepers offered savory filled turnovers called "patties." Latino immigrants—first Puerto Ricans, followed by other Latin Americans, including a mighty wave of Mexicans—offered *chicharron, alcapurrias, mofongo, sancocho,* burritos, and tacos. Japanese chefs intro-

duced sushi to Manhattan in the 1960s. Korean immigrants lured locals with the manifold flavors of kimchi. An estimated 160 languages are spoken in Manhattan, and there are at least that many cuisines represented in Manhattan restaurants.

Restaurants

Taverns, including the colonial-era Fraunces Tavern on Pearl Street, were common drinking and eating establishments from Manhattan's earliest days. By the mid-nineteenth century, restaurants and cafes also flourished in the city, as did oyster houses and other inexpensive options. Manhattan offered an estimated five or six thousand restaurants and eating houses, ranging from the elegant and exclusive Delmonico's to dockside bars where workingmen could cadge a free lunch to accompany their tot of rum or mug of beer.

Delmonico's was created by Swiss immigrants John and Peter Delmonico, who in 1827 opened a little cafe on William Street. In March 1830, they expanded the cafe into a more upscale establishment that was listed in the city directory as "Delmonico & Brother, Restaurant Français." Manhattanites developed a taste for sophisticated French food, and increasing numbers of French chefs arrived to cook in Manhattan.

"Quick food" was an important selling point for Manhattan's restaurant trade beginning in the 1830s. Faster and more efficient ways of feeding workers began to emerge in the city. One example was the Exchange Buffet, which opened in 1885 across the street from the New York Stock Exchange. In later years, many other quick-service chains, such as the Horn & Hardart automats, were launched in the city. National fast-food chains, such as White Castle, appeared in Manhattan beginning in the 1930s.

Although Prohibition exacted a heavy toll on Manhattan's finer restaurants, the haute cuisine scene resurfaced after World War II. Le Pavillon, an offshoot of the French Pavilion at the 1939 World's Fair, held in Queens, reintroduced Manhattanites to elevated French cuisine. Lutèce opened in 1961, with Chef André Soltner at the helm, and for more than three decades it was considered one of the country's top restaurants. Le Périgord was opened by Georges Briguet in 1964; Sirio Maccioni started up Le Cirque, with Jean Vergnes as chef, in 1974.

New types of eateries arrived on the scene during the 1950s. Restaurant Associates was the leader in creating dramatic specialty and theme restaurants, such as the Hawaiian Room at the Lexington Hotel (Polynesian, complete with hula dancers), La Fonda Del Sol (South American), Zum-Zum (German sausage), Quo Vadis (French and Italian), the Forum of the Twelve Caesars (a riff on an imagined ancient Rome), the Hudson River Club, Tavern on the Green (in Central Park), The Four Seasons, and Windows on the World (atop the towering World Trade Center).

Markets

Public markets were set up in Manhattan beginning in the late seventeenth century. By 1867 there were eleven of them; the largest and most important were the Washington and Fulton Markets. During the mid-nineteenth century, as prosperous New Yorkers moved northward, central markets declined in importance. Grocery store chains, such as A&P, D'Agostino's, and Gristede's, and "gourmet shops" like Balducci's, Citarella, Dean & DeLuca, and Fairway, came to the fore during the twentieth century. The national chain Whole Foods opened its first New York City store in Manhattan's Chelsea neighborhood in 2005.

Culinary Schools and Organizations

In the nineteenth century, Manhattan's wealthier residents, as well as its restaurateurs, required skilled cooks. Immigrant "hired girls" did not have the knowledge to satisfy the palates of sophisticated diners. Juliet Corson opened the New York Cooking School in 1876 to train professional cooks, and others followed her example. During the twentieth century, Manhattan offered middle- and upper-class women the opportunity to improve their own culinary skills. After World War II, Dione Lucas, an English emigrée, opened the Cordon Bleu Cooking School at her Manhattan restaurant. Caterer and cookbook author James Beard began teaching classes in the kitchen of his Greenwich Village townhouse. By 1975 Manhattan had forty-five cooking schools or groups offering classes.

The late twentieth century saw an increased demand for career-oriented culinary schools. Peter Kump's New York Cooking School, founded in 1975, expanded into a professional school that was renamed The Institute for Culinary Education in 2001. The Natural Gourmet Cooking School, started by Annemarie Colbin in 1977, teaches future chefs the concepts of healthy cooking. The French Culinary Institute in SoHo, founded by Dorothy Cann Hamilton in 1984, later expanded its curriculum and was renamed The International Culinary Center.

Some of Manhattan's colleges and universities have developed academic programs in food studies. New York University introduced its Department of Nutrition, Food Studies, and Public Health in the 1990s. It offers undergraduate, master's, and doctoral programs in food studies, culture, and food systems. The New School has an undergraduate food studies department, and other city universities offer numerous academic courses on various aspects of food.

Several important culinary organizations originated in Manhattan. Les Dames d'Escoffier, which offers membership by invitation to women in the food, beverage, and hospitality industries, was founded in 1973 by Carol Brock, then Sunday food editor at the *New York Daily News*. It originated as a female counterpart to the men's organization Les Amis d'Escoffier. In 1981 the chefs Sara Moulton and Maria Reuge started an educational organization for female food and wine professionals, the New York Women's Culinary Alliance. The Culinary Historians of New York was founded in 1985 to stimulate and share knowledge about food history.

For the past sixty years, New York's culinary scene has been stimulated by newspaper columnists and magazine writers at the *New York Times*, the *New Yorker*, *Gourmet*, *New York* magazine, *Food & Wine*, *Bon Appétit*, and *Saveur*, all of which have their editorial offices in Manhattan. Manhattan is also the nation's center for cookbook publishing—and many of those books popularize recipes from some of Manhattan's best restaurants. Many national food and beverage advertising and marketing campaigns originate in the city's cluster of media companies.

Not every resident is able to enjoy the borough's rich culinary offerings: tens of thousands of people living in Manhattan are food-insecure, and it is a cruel irony that an estimated 41 percent of the restaurant workers in Manhattan fall into that category. In 1982 a group of volunteers started the nation's first "food rescue" to collect surplus food from restaurants, caterers, bakeries, and grocery stores and distribute it to the hungry. Today, City Harvest salvages about 50 million pounds of food a year—wholesome, nutritious produce, prepared food, and grocery items that otherwise would go to waste. The New York

City Coalition Against Hunger was formed in 1983 by soup kitchens and food pantries to coordinate the activities of emergency food providers. The coalition represents more than eleven hundred groups devoting themselves to hunger relief. Nutritious meals and groceries are supplied to the homeless as well as to the elderly and homebound who are unable to purchase or prepare their own meals.

See also BROCK, CAROL; CHINESE COMMUNITY; CULINARY HISTORIANS OF NEW YORK; DELI'S, GERMAN; DELI'S, JEWISH; DELMONICO'S; *FOOD & WINE*; GERMAN; *GOURMET*; GROCERY STORES; ITALIAN; JAMES BEARD FOUNDATION; JEWISH; KATZ'S DELICATESSEN; LES DAMES D'ESCOFFIER; NEW SCHOOL; *NEW YORKER*; *NEW YORK TIMES*; NEW YORK UNIVERSITY; NEW YORK WOMEN'S CULINARY ALLIANCE; RESTAURANT ASSOCIATES; RESTAURANTS; and *SAVEUR*.

Batterberry, Michael, and Ariane Batterberry. *On the Town in New York: The Landmark History of Eating, Drinking, and Entertainments from the American Revolution to the Food Revolution.* New York and London: Routledge, 1999.

Grimes, William. *Appetite City: A Culinary History of New York.* New York: North Point, 2009.

Hauck-Lawson, Annie, and Jon Deutsch, eds. *Gastropolis: Food & New York City.* New York: Columbia University Press, 2008.

Ray, Krishnendu. "Exotic Restaurants and Expatriate Home Cooking: Indian Food in Manhattan." In *The Globalization of Food*, edited by David Inglis and Debra Gimlin, pp. 213–226. Oxford and New York: Berg, 2009.

Smith, Andrew F. *New York City: A Food Biography.* Lanham, Md.: Rowman & Littlefield, 2014.

Andrew F. Smith

Manhattan Brewing Company

See LATE TWENTIETH CENTURY and MICROBREWERIES AND BREWPUBS.

Manhattan Clam Chowder

Manhattan clam chowder is a clam-based stew made with a tomato broth. French, Nova Scotian, or British fishermen may have introduced chowders (from the French *chaudière*, a "kettle") into New England, and they had become important dishes in America by 1732. Early American seafood chowders were made with fish, clams, or other seafood; potatoes (and crumbled crackers for thickening); and flavorings such as lemon, cider, ketchup, or curry. Regional differences emerged within New England. Nantucket Islanders did not add crackers or potatoes. Chowder makers in Massachusetts and Maine enriched the soup with heated milk or cream. Tomatoes were sometimes added in Rhode Island, Connecticut, and elsewhere.

The first located recipe titled "Manhattan Clam Chowder" was published by Virginia Elliot and Robert Jones in *Soups and Sauces* (1934). This recipe substituted tomatoes for milk. The name "Manhattan clam chowder" caught on, but it had no real association with New York City. Ann Roe Robbins, in her *100 Summer and Winter Soups* (1943), wrote of tasting Manhattan clam chowder at the Greyhound Inn, on the shore road to Atlantic City. Robbins, a New York City cooking teacher, recalled this as one of the best meals of her life. Subsequently, most American soup cookbooks offered two recipes—one with tomatoes and one without.

The debate as to whether real clam chowder should contain tomatoes was touched off by Representative Cleveland Sleeper, who introduced a bill in the Maine legislature in the late 1930s to "make it an illegal as well as a culinary offense to introduce tomatoes to clam chowder." Eleanor Early picked up Sleeper's sentiments, remarking in her *New England Sampler* (1940) that there was "a terrible pink mixture (with tomatoes in it, and herbs) called Manhattan Clam Chowder, that is only a vegetable soup, and not to be confused with New England Clam Chowder, nor spoken of in the same breath." She wrote that tomatoes and clams had "no more affinity than ice cream and horse radish." She believed that it was a "sacrilege to wed bivalves and bay leaves, and only a degraded cook would do such a thing." Early equated Manhattan clam chowder with a "thin minestrone, or dish water, and fit only for foreigners" (pp. 349–350). She proclaimed that traditional Boston clam chowder was rich, creamy, and devoid of tomatoes.

Within a few years of the outbreak of the "chowder wars," Chef Louis P. De Gouy, author of *The Soup Book* (1949), prefaced his chapter on chowder with this observation: "Clam chowder is one of those subjects, like politics and religion, that can never be discussed lightly. Bring it up even incidentally, and all the innumerable factions of the clambake regions raise their heads and begin to yammer." His six clam chowder recipes may have added to the consternation: the recipe for New England clam chowder called for potatoes, celery, carrots, leeks, and, surprisingly, "3 peeled large tomatoes." His two "Manhattan-manner" chowders originated, he wrote, in "Gloucester, Swampscott, Nahant, Cohasset, Scituate, all around the Cape and up and down Narragansett Bay from Point to Providence." He continued, "They make all the varieties up there, no matter what you call them." One of these recipes was made with tomatoes; the other was not.

Whatever its real origin or ingredients, Manhattan clam chowder still has its critics. Culinary impresario James Beard once referred to it as a horrendous soup, "which resembles a vegetable soup that accidently had some clams dumped into it." Despite such disparagement, Manhattan clam chowder still appears in cookbooks and on restaurant menus. Today, almost by consensus, it is made with tomatoes and contains neither potatoes nor milk.

See also BEARD, JAMES and DE GOUY, LOUIS P.

De Gouy, Louis P. *The Soup Book*. New York: Greenberg, 1949.

Early, Eleanor. *A New England Sampler*. Boston: Waverly House, 1940.

Elliott, Virginia, and Robert Howard Jones. *Soups and Sauces*. New York: Harcourt, Brace, 1934.

Robbins, Roe. *100 Summer and Winter Soups*. New York: Thomas Y. Crowell, 1943.

Smith, Andrew F. *Souper Tomatoes: The Story of America's Favorite Food*. New Brunswick, N.J.: Rutgers University Press, 2000.

Andrew F. Smith

Manhattan Cocktail

Who first thought to blend rye whiskey, Italian (dry) vermouth, and cocktail bitters into the drink we now call the Manhattan cocktail? No one really knows, although the combination is so obvious that several bartenders might have thought of it at approximately the same time, so it is possible that the drink does not have a single, clear origin story. The Manhattan first appears in print in the early 1880s, a few years before its close cousin, the martini. See MARTINI. This era marked the ascendance of vermouth as a cocktail ingredient. Prior to this, cocktails were simpler beverages—generally spirit, water, a sweetening agent, and a dash of either bitters or a liqueur. The spirit—usually whiskey, brandy, or gin—took the fore, with the other ingredients accenting the flavor of the base ingredient. The drinks were generally boozy and bracing, and indeed, in many cases, they were consumed in taverns by men on their way to work in the morning. See TAVERNS.

Cocktails as a class of beverage arose in the late eighteenth century. The first printed definition of the word appeared in 1806, in a newspaper in Hudson, New York. The paper defined a cocktail as "a stimulating liquor, composed of spirits of any kind, sugar, water and bitters." Early newspaper accounts of cocktails indicate they were exactly that simple. Through the course of the nineteenth century, the cocktail accrued additional ingredients as bartenders began to experiment with products new to the United States. Bartenders found that liqueurs such as Benedictine, maraschino, and chartreuse added depth of flavor and complexity to mixed drinks, but the ingredient that most changed the cocktail was vermouth.

Writing in his *Martini, Straight Up*, Lowell Edmunds traces the introduction of vermouth into the United States as happening no later than 1851. In that year, the French company Noilly Prat & Cie sent a shipment of one hundred cases of French (or dry) vermouth to the Port of New Orleans. Edmunds states that the Italian firm Martini and Rossi claims to have exported its Italian (sweet) vermouth to the United States in 1834, but he could find no evidence to support this claim. Vermouth took a while to catch on, but by 1900 Noilly Prat was exporting twenty-five thousand cases a year to the United States, and by 1910 that number had tripled to seventy-five thousand cases.

The rise of vermouth-accented cocktails marked a dramatic change in American drinking habits. Prior to about the 1870s, cocktails were boozy and spirit-forward, knocked back quickly in the morning by workers en route to the job. Economic growth in the last decades of the nineteenth century, however, led to a rise in after-work tippling, when drinkers could sit and sip their cocktails slowly. A couple of strongly boozy drinks, though, are usually enough to make an average drinker sleepy, so wine-based vermouth provided a way to lighten the profile of a cocktail, smoothing its rough edges and making it possible to enjoy multiple drinks without getting besotted. Vermouth also lent an air of European urbanity to the affair. Though vermouth appeared in other cocktails before the Manhattan came along, it was the Manhattan that cemented its reputation as a cocktail ingredient.

The earliest cocktail manuals, those published in the 1860s, do not include many vermouth-accented cocktails. By the 1880s, though, vermouth was a common cocktail ingredient. In 1882, in fact, a newspaper in Olean, New York, published the first known mention of the Manhattan cocktail, describing it as "a mixture of whiskey, vermouth and bitters." The earliest recipe for the Manhattan appeared in the 1884 book *The Modern Bartender's Guide*, by O. H. Byron, and through the remaining years of the nineteenth century, the drink became increasingly common in cocktail manuals.

Early recipes call for equal parts whiskey and sweet vermouth, with a dash of bitters and sometimes a dash of sugar syrup, maraschino liqueur, or curaçao. Some writers specifically call for rye whiskey, though others simply say whiskey without specification and at least two pre-Prohibition recipes call for bourbon. In the northeastern United States at that time, rye was still the most common whiskey poured, a fact that would not change until Prohibition, so rye was probably the base of the first Manhattan.

The drink gets progressively more boozy in later manuals, and by 1900 the recipe had generally settled into the form we know now: two parts whiskey, one part vermouth, bitters. The garnish varied between a twist of lemon peel and a preserved cherry, depending on the source.

But what are its origins? According to one story, the Manhattan was invented in 1874 at the Manhattan Club for a banquet hosted by Jeanette "Jennie" Jerome (also known as Lady Randolph Churchill) to celebrate the election of Samuel Tilden as New York's governor. This story, however, has a serious problem. Tilden was elected governor on November 3, 1874, and took office January 1, 1875. At this time, Jennie Jerome was in England, with her husband Lord Randolph, for the birth and christening of their son, Winston, the future prime minister of the United Kingdom. It is still possible that the drink was invented at, and named for, the Manhattan Club, but Jennie Jerome's participation is unlikely.

Another prevailing theory also has scant evidence. In the early twentieth century, Henry Collins Brown (founder of the Museum of the City of New York) edited an annual historical volume called *Valentine's Manual of Old New York*. His 1923 issue contains an essay by William F. Mulhall, a former bartender at the Hoffman House, which stood at Madison Square Park until its demolition in 1915. Mulhall recalls the diners and rogues who sat at his bar and recounts tales of the drinking habits of nineteenth-century New Yorkers. Mulhall writes, "The Manhattan cocktail was invented by a man named Black, who kept a place ten doors below Houston Street on Broadway in the [1860s]—probably the most famous mixed drink in the world in its time." The cocktail historian David Wondrich attempted to locate this bar for his 2007 book *Imbibe!*, about the early history of the American cocktail. He found city records from the 1870s that indicated a William Black operated a saloon, though it was on Bowery, not Broadway, and it was above Houston, not below. Mulhall's account is possible but, lacking further evidence, just speculation.

Historians generally accept the theory that the Manhattan was invented in, well, Manhattan; the first newspaper accounts of the drink place it at Manhattan bars. The Manhattan cocktail rose quickly in popularity, though, spreading across the United States and to Europe. The Manhattan quickly became one of the most popular cocktails around. Soon, however, would come along a vermouth-enhanced drink that would eclipse even the Manhattan: the martini.

See also MIXOLOGY.

Brown, Henry Collins, ed. *Valentine's Manual of Old New York*. New York: Valentine's Manual, 1923.
Byron, O. H. *The Modern Bartenders' Guide*. New York: Excelsior, 1884.
Edmunds, Lowell. *Martini, Straight Up: The Classic American Cocktail*. Baltimore: Johns Hopkins University Press, 1981.
Wondrich, David. *Imbibe! From Absinthe Cocktail to Whiskey Smash, a Salute in Stories and Drinks to "Professor" Jerry Thomas, Pioneer of the American Bar*. New York: Perigee/Penguin, 2007.

Michael Dietsch

Manhattan Special

Manhattan Special is a coffee-flavored soda that has been produced in New York City since 1895. The full name of the product is Manhattan Special Espresso Coffee Soda. The product is named not after the island of Manhattan but for Manhattan Avenue in the Williamsburg section of Brooklyn, where the soda still is made in the same factory.

Manhattan Special was created in 1895 by Italian immigrants Michael Garavuso and Teresa Cimino. Cimino's great-grandchildren, siblings Aurora Passaro and Louis Passaro, currently run the company.

Boldly flavored and supersweet, the soda is made with roasted and ground coffee beans and cane sugar. A diet version made with NutraSweet also is available, as is a decaffeinated version. The company also makes sodas in cherry, orange, sarsaparilla, lemon-lime, and vanilla cream flavors.

Aurora Passaro has said that she does not believe the soda was inspired by any particular Italian coffee drink but may have been "an American answer to an Italian craving." Italian immigrants rejected American-style coffee and frequently drank espresso with sugar. In summertime, that espresso often was cooled but not diluted with ice. Created during a time when drugstore soda fountains added flavored syrups to fizzy water, Teresa Cimino brewed heavily roasted espresso, sweetened it with cane sugar to make a syrup, and added carbonated water. According to the Passaros, the recipe is little changed today.

A departure from the company's otherwise sweet history: Manhattan Special also made headlines in 1983 when Albert Passaro, father to Aurora and Louis and then president of Manhattan Special, was found shot dead in his basement in Woodhaven, Queens, after an apparent robbery. The brother and sister team subsequently took over the soda business at a young age.

Manhattan Special is a cult favorite among Italian Americans in particular and New Yorkers in general. Despite America's fast-growing taste for iced and sweetened coffee drinks fostered by the growth of Starbucks and other coffee chains, Manhattan Special remains a regional taste.

See also SODA.

Bowen, Dana. "Brooklyn Brew." *Saveur*, no. 113 (July 2008).

Wharton, Rachel. "Eating Along the G Line." *New York Daily News*, June 8, 2014.

Wilson, Michael. "A Modern Comeback for a Taste of Brooklyn." *New York Times*, July 7, 2008.

Kara Newman

Martini

The martini is perhaps the quintessential American cocktail, a bracingly cold mixture of gin (or vodka) and dry vermouth, served with an olive or a lemon twist. Fans of the drink are full of opinions on whether to shake or stir the drink, how much vermouth to use, and whether gin or vodka makes for the best martini.

Just as fans disagree on its proper composition, students are equally divided on the origins of the drink and its name. Neither historian nor etymologist has been able to uncover how the drink arose. One story suggests that the martini derives from the martinez. Because both drinks feature gin and vermouth, that idea seems plausible on the surface.

As for the origins of the word "martini," the stories vary. One tale says it was named for the Martini & Rossi brand of vermouth, which began exporting to the United States in 1868. Another story claims its name derives from a brand of rifle, the Martini-Henry, which the British army used in the late 1800s. Though neither story has any concrete evidence in its favor, the Martini & Rossi story seems more plausible on its surface than does the Martini-Henry story.

The "dryness" of the martini has evolved over time. If we acknowledge the martinez as forebear to the modern martini, we should note its ingredients. The first martinez recipe was recorded in the 1884 book *The Modern Bartender's Guide*, by O. H. Bryan. It calls for equal parts Old Tom gin and sweet (Italian) vermouth, plus bitters and orange curaçao—in other words, quite unlike the modern martini.

That is not to say that the martini was always as dry as it is today. The first known martini recipe was printed in Harry Johnson's *New and Improved Bartender's Manual*, in 1888. Johnson's martini is quite similar to Bryan's martinez, giving some credence to the thought that the martini was initially a misnamed martinez. Johnson calls for Old Tom gin, sweet vermouth, simple syrup, and curaçao.

Old Tom was sweeter and milder than the London dry style of gin that dominates the gin market today. London dry arose in the late 1800s after the development of the column still made it possible to distill a neutral tasting spirit. A nineteenth-century Old Tom gin would have tasted more like grain and less like botanicals, whereas London dry gins developed to taste clean and neutral, less like whiskey, and with the botanicals front and center.

Liquor importers started bringing London dry gin into the United States near the end of the nineteenth century, and the drier style became increasingly popular among bartenders. So around the turn of the century, fewer recipes for either the martinez or the martini call for Old Tom and more call for either

Plymouth (a gin style similar to London dry but a little softer) or London dry.

At around the same time, the martini landed in New York. By 1887, the Hoffman House was already serving the drink, as the *Evening World* reported on October 11 in an article called "Fine Fancies in Drinks." The paper reports that "the whiskey, Holland gin, Tom gin, hickory, Manhattan, Turf Club, vermouth, absinthe, Martini, and bourbon cocktails are served at all times."

The drink was already ensconced in Republican politics by 1892, when the New York *Sun* ran a front-page piece on April 28 by an unnamed reporter, covering the Republican convention that year in Albany, where downstate politicians "drove the bartenders frantic with calls for metropolitan Martini cocktails and hayseed mixtures of gin and tansy." It was not just the Republicans. Tammany Hall Democrats, the *Sun* observed the following year, headed south on early trains to Washington, DC, "reinforcing their enthusiasm early in the day with Manhattan and Martini cocktails."

On June 3, 1894, on page 10, the *Brooklyn Daily Eagle* inventoried "A Variety of 'Bracers,'" or morning cocktails, from "Brooklyn's best-known hostelries." These were the drinks that "individuals with a propensity for getting all the good things of this life" would consume en route to work. Whiskey with seltzer was the most popular tipple, followed by Manhattans, old-fashioneds, and martinis.

The July 12, 1895, issue of the *Brooklyn Daily Eagle* recounts the dangers of getting too absorbed in one's cocktail, in a page 12 story called "Bittel Is Still at Liberty." The story concerns a convicted counterfeiter, John Bittel, who escaped his captors at the Cosmopolitan Hotel, which still stands today, at Chambers Street and West Broadway. While the federal marshals who guarded him took a martini break in the hotel's cafe, Bittel slipped away from them, down the elevator, and out the front door of the hotel.

On page 10 of the magazine supplement for the June 29, 1902, issue of the *New York Times*, a columnist going only by the name "Bobbie" documents a drink served at the Calumet Club, at Twenty-Ninth Street and Fifth Avenue. The hall cocktail, Bobbie reported, was "a great improvement on the popular Martini." A September 2, 1906 column on page 2 of the magazine section of the *Times* goes behind the scenes of an unnamed Times Square restaurant, depicting waiters calling out orders for such cocktails as martinis, horse's

necks, Manhattans, gin rickeys, and Tom Collinses. On July 15 of the same year, in a piece on page 2 of the magazine section, the *Times* detailed what was passing for fine dining in Manhattan that year: "There is no cocktail more delicate than a Martini, made of very dry gin and two kinds of vermouth, the French and the Italian."

The martini story gains another Gotham influence from the bartender Martini di Arma di Taggia, who worked at the Knickerbocker Hotel. In either 1911 or 1912 (the year varies according to who is telling the story), Martini di Arma di Taggia created the drink for a famous Knickerbocker customer, John D. Rockefeller. Clearly, this story is false. However, Martini, the bartender, was responsible for a major innovation in martini, the cocktail. He was the first person to marry gin and dry French vermouth alone (without the sweet Italian).

This evolution in the martini is responsible for the term "dry martini." Today, tipplers assume that a dry martini is one with very little vermouth, or even no vermouth at all, but that is historically inaccurate. When the term "dry martini" first appeared in cocktail manuals, the writers meant to say, "Here's how you make a martini with London dry gin and dry vermouth." The word "dry" was there to indicate that this was not a "sweet martini," made with sweet gin and sweet vermouth.

See also THREE-MARTINI LUNCH.

"Behind the Scenes in a 'Smart' New York Restaurant." *New York Times Magazine Supplement,* July 15, 1906.
"Bittle Is Still at Liberty." *Brooklyn Daily Eagle,* July 12, 1895.
["Bobbie"]. "With the Clubmen." *New York Times Magazine Supplement,* June 29, 1902.
"Covers for Two: A Gastronomic Study." *New York Times Magazine Supplement,* September 2, 1906.
Edmunds, Lowell. *Martini, Straight Up: The Classic American Cocktail.* Baltimore: Johns Hopkins University Press, 1981.
Grimes, William. *Straight Up or On the Rocks: A Cultural History of American Drink.* New York: Simon & Schuster, 1993.
"New York Republicans. The Circus Begins in Albany with Willis as the Clown." *The Sun* (New York), April 28, 1892.
Regan, Gary. *Joy of Mixology.* New York: Clarkson Potter, 2003.
"A Variety of 'Bracers'. Calculated to Make Hats Fit in the Morning." *Brooklyn Daily Eagle,* June 3, 1894.
Wondrich, David. *Imbibe! From Absinthe Cocktail to Whiskey Smash, a Salute in Stories and Drinks to*

"Professor" Jerry Thomas, Pioneer of the American Bar. New York: Perigee/Penguin, 2007.

Michael Dietsch

Mason, John L.

John Landis Mason (1832–1902) was a tinsmith who invented a screw-on lid for a glass preserving jar, which came to be called the "Mason jar." The Mason jar revolutionized home fruit and vegetable preservation.

Born in Vineland, New Jersey, Mason grew up in Philadelphia. He began experimenting with metal lids for glass preserving jars as an improvement on existing methods of sealing the jars, which included corks, flat metal tops sealed with wax, or flat glass tops held on with wire bails or other types of clamps. None of these methods were completely satisfactory because air frequently leaked into the jars, causing the food to spoil.

John Mason found the solution: a glass jar with a tightfitting screw-on top made of zinc. On November 30, 1858, Mason patented the self-sealing zinc lid and glass jar. He later added a rubber gasket, or "ring," under the lid to exclude air more perfectly. The screw-on lid greatly simplified the canning process and made the jars genuinely reusable (only the rings needed to be replaced). In 1859 Mason formed a partnership with T. W. Frazier, Henry Mitchell, and B. W. Payne, and they set up a factory at 257 Canal Street in New York City to produce the jar lids. They contracted out to various glassblowers, who followed Mason's pattern for the threaded design at the mouth of the jar.

As the jars were fairly inexpensive to make, they could be sold cheaply, and their popularity soared. By 1860 Mason jars were being shipped throughout the United States. When Mason's patent on the design ran out, in 1879, many other companies began mass-producing similar jars, even using Mason's name on their products. He continued to apply for patents for new inventions, but none were successful. He moved into a New York City tenement apartment, where he died, a charity case, in 1902.

Glass Container Manufacturers Institute. *Mason Jar Centennial, 1858–1958.* New York: Glass Container Manufacturers Institute, 1958.

Leybourne, Douglas M. *Collector's Guide to Old Fruit Jars.* North Muskegon, Mich.: Altarfire, 2000.

Toulouse, Julian H. *Fruit Jars: A Collectors Manual.* Camden, N.J.: Thomas Nielson/Everybodys, 1969.

Andrew F. Smith

Mast Brothers Chocolate

See CHOCOLATE, CRAFT.

Matzah

Matzah, the Hebrew word for the unleavened bread most commonly available during the Jewish holiday of Passover, is certainly not a food unique to New York, but it has left an indelible, if small, mark on the landscape of the city. Matzah is ancient in origin. Made of just flour and water and, when strictly kosher, baked for no more than eighteen minutes, it is one of the most distinctive foods of the Jewish people, who are prohibited from eating leavened bread during Passover. This flat, large, cracker-like bread likely first appeared in New York City with the first handful of Portuguese Jewish immigrants in the seventeenth century. These Jews, like hundreds of generations before them, ate the plain unleavened bread, also known as "the bread of affliction," during Passover to commemorate the quick fleeing from harsh Egyptian rulers, as described in the biblical book of Exodus.

However, it was not until the German Jewish influx in the mid-nineteenth century that matzah began to be produced in significant quantities in the United States. In New York City, synagogues were largely responsible for the baking of matzah during this period; the unleavened bread was as much a religious symbol as a substitute for bread during the eight-day Passover holiday. The ultraorthodox Jewish community, particularly in Brooklyn, continues to bake traditional matzah in a similar fashion by hand in wood-burning ovens.

By the end of the first decade of the twentieth century the Cincinnati-based German Jewish immigrant Behr Manischewitz popularized commercial matzah—eventually in its now popular square, rather than traditional round, shape. The Manischewitz family's continued operations in the Midwest dominated commercial matzah manufacturing for the growing number of Eastern European immigrant Jews on the East Coast at the same time, centered primarily in New York City. Then in 1932 the company opened a new factory in Jersey City. Manischewitz's main competitor in the growing commercial matzah industry was (and still is) Streit's, a family-run business that began operating on the Lower East Side in 1916 and continued for nearly one hundred years on Rivington Street. It is possible to see fresh matzah roll off conveyer belts at Streit's year round as a small market exists for

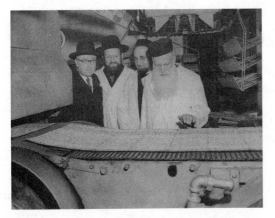

Streit's, a family-owned and -operated matzah bakery, began operating on the Lower East Side in 1916 and continues to this day on Rivington Street. It is still possible to see fresh matzah roll off conveyer belts at Streit's year round, just as in this undated photo. COURTESY STREIT'S MATZOS

matzah (and matzah meal) in the months beyond Passover for Jewish foods such as the dumpling-like matzah balls usually served in chicken soup.

However, the spring holiday of Passover remains the most common time to see matzah in New York—in restaurants, delicatessens, and even in bodegas. Matzah is so distinctive that New York artist Larry Rivers created a vast triptych covering four thousand years of Jewish history against the tan backdrop of a slab of matzah called *The History of Matzah (The Story of the Jewish People)* (1982–1985). In New York matzah has become a staple of deli menus and has come to symbolize not only a biblical holiday but also, more generally, the culinary culture of the Jewish people.

See also JEWISH and PASSOVER.

Sarna, Jonathan D. "How Matzah Became Square: Manischewitz and the Development of Machine-Made Matzah in the United States." In *Chosen Capital: The Jewish Encounter with American Capitalism*, edited by Rebecca Kobrin, pp. 272–288. New Brunswick, N.J.: Rutgers University Press, 2012.

Lara Rabinovitch

Maxwell's Plum

Maxwell's Plum was noted as a flamboyant restaurant and singles bar, located at First Avenue and Sixty-Fourth Street in Manhattan. "More than any place of its kind," summed up the *New York Times* upon its closing, Maxwell's Plum "symbolized two social revolutions of the 1960's—sex and food."

Maxwell's Plum opened in April 1966 under the ownership of Warner LeRoy, son of famed Hollywood film producer Mervyn LeRoy (who produced *The Wizard of Oz*) and later known for his similarly showy restaurants Tavern on the Green and the Russian Tea Room. See TAVERN ON THE GREEN and RUSSIAN TEA ROOM. Maxwell's was famed immediately for its scale, serving more than twelve hundred customers a day; its celebrity clientele (regulars included Richard Rodgers, Cary Grant, Bill Blass, Barbra Streisand, and Warren Beatty); and theatrical art nouveau décor. The *Times* described its "kaleidoscopic stained-glass ceilings and walls, Tiffany lamps galore, a menagerie of ceramic animals, etched glass and cascades of crystal." Along with the original location of Thank God It's Friday (TGI Friday's) on the next block, First Avenue became known as a playground for the "swinging singles" set of the 1960s and 1970s.

Regarding the food, the wide-ranging menu featured everything from hamburgers and chili con carne to Iranian caviar and stuffed squab. In the early 1970s, Maxwell's Plum received four stars, the *Times*'s highest rating, from food critic Craig Claiborne. However, the rating eventually slipped to two stars and then one star as the menu switched rapidly from traditional American to trendy California cuisine, then to continental, Pacific Northwestern, and French.

Chefs through the revolving door included many names well recognized today, such as California chefs Mark Peel and Nancy Silverton, both recruited in 1985 from Spago in Los Angeles; Seattle's Kathy Casey, who lasted only three weeks in 1987; and Geoffrey Zakarian, an alumnus of Le Cirque and the 21 Club.

Maxwell's Plum closed in July 1988. LeRoy died in 2001. In 2013, Jennifer Oz LeRoy, Warner LeRoy's daughter, announced plans to open a Maxwell's Plum in downtown Manhattan; as of the summer of 2015, that restaurant had not yet opened.

Miller, Bryan. "Maxwell's Plum, a 60's Symbol, Closes." *New York Times*, July 11, 1988.
Horne, Sarah. "Jennifer LeRoy Plots Comeback with Maxwell's Plum Revival." *New York Post*, June 25, 2013.

Kara Newman

McNally, Keith

See LATE TWENTIETH CENTURY.

McSorley's Old Ale House

McSorley's Old Ale House, located at 15 East Seventh Street in Manhattan, is New York City's oldest continually operating Irish bar and an icon of old New York. The saloon was founded by John McSorley, an immigrant from County Tyrone, who claimed to have opened it in 1854, although city tax records suggest that it opened a few years later. McSorley's offered the Irish working-class men who lived around the Bowery, as well as a diverse clientele of labor organizers like Samuel Gompers, businessmen, and financiers, a taste of the old country's neighborhood ale houses. It still maintains this atmosphere, perhaps because of the ethnic heritage of each of McSorley's subsequent owners, all of whom were either Irish immigrants or Irish Americans, including its current (as of 2015) owner, Matthew Maher, who immigrated to New York in the 1960s after being promised a job at the bar. All vow to continue the enterprise as John left it on his death in 1910.

There have been few concessions to modernity. McSorley's sawdust-strewn floors, rickety chairs, and gloomy dark walls covered in memorabilia seem frozen in time: a yellowed newspaper clipping announces the assassination of President Lincoln. McSorley's has been proudly, quirkily independent of many modern city regulations. Until recently, cats openly roamed, and generations of barkeeps refused to touch its vintage gaslight chandelier hanging over the bar, festooned with ancient turkey wishbones and enshrouded in capes of dust accumulated over the decades. In 2011, Maher reluctantly acceded to Board of Health requests to clean the fixture. He performed this act of housekeeping sacramentally: according to tradition, the wishbones are hung by soldiers heading off to war, to be reclaimed upon their safe return. The ones still hanging are memorials to the fallen, ranging from World War I doughboys to Iraq and Afghanistan service personnel.

The drinks menu at McSorley's has not changed since John's day, offering only ale, "light" or "dark." Nowadays served in twin half-pint glass mugs and brewed under a proprietary license to Pabst, in John's day the ale was brewed nearby at the Fidelio Brewery on First Avenue and served in pewter mugs, which

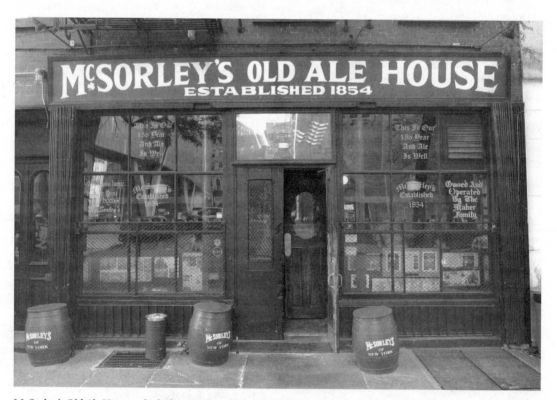

McSorley's Old Ale House, which claims to have been established in 1854 in Manhattan's East Village but may actually have opened a few years later, is nevertheless New York City's oldest pub. LEONARD J. DEFRANCISCI

became a much-pilfered souvenir upon John's death. His son Bill inherited the bar and navigated it successfully throughout Prohibition, when the ale was brewed in the basement by a retired brewer, Barney Kelly, and cut with nonalcoholic beer to reduce its alcohol level but not its popularity. Bill made no effort to mask the saloon's activities in the 1920s, when the bar remained a haunt of police officials and Tammany Hall politicians who turned a willfully blind eye to the violation of the Volstead Act. A mug (by then made of earthenware) cost fifteen cents or two for a quarter. This Prohibition pricing scheme may be the origin of the contemporary practice of serving two small mugs per order. The food menu is nearly as perfunctory: the signature dish is a ploughman's lunch of sharp cheese, raw onions, soda crackers, and mustard, mimicking the free lunch that was served in John's day to encourage drinking.

By the early twentieth century, McSorley's clientele included many notable artists. The Ashcan School painter John Sloan was a regular, portraying the bar's interior five times from 1912 to 1930; E. E. Cummings wrote a poem about the bar; and folk musician Woody Guthrie was an habitué. Who you would not find among the patrons, however, were women. The motto, attributed to John, of "Good Ale, Raw Onions, and No Ladies" aptly summarized the saloon's strictly enforced policy: women were not admitted until 1970 and only begrudgingly, after a lawsuit brought by the National Organization of Women was summarily decided in the women's favor. It would be another sixteen years before a ladies' restroom was added.

See also PROHIBITION and SALOONS.

Barry, Dan. "Dust Is Gone Above the Bar, But a Legend Still Dangles." *New York Times*, April 6, 2011.
Dennison, Mariea Caudill. "John Sloan's Visual Commentary on Male Bonding, Prohibition, and the Working Class." *American Studies* 47, no. 2 (2006): 23–38.
Mitchell, Joseph. "The Old House at Home." *New Yorker*, April 13, 1940.

Cathy K. Kaufman

Meatpacking District

New York's Meatpacking District, centered on Gansevoort Street along the Hudson River on Manhattan's Lower West Side, has transitioned from economic powerhouse to archetypal "seedy" New York neighborhood to an upscale enclave for New York

trendsetters. It is so named because until the 1970s it was home to hundreds of meatpacking businesses. Only a handful of meat packers remain, replaced by boutiques, high-end hotels, expensive restaurants, and high-rises. Above the neighborhood sits High Line Park, where an elevated train once ran. The Whitney Museum, designed by the architect Renzo Piano, is at the corner of Washington Street and Gansevoort Street.

People initially moved into the Meatpacking District in the 1820s. Beginning in the 1840s, townhouses and tenements were constructed in the area. When the Lower West Side railroad was completed in 1869, businesses moved into the neighborhood. An open-air farmers' market, later named Gansevoort Market, opened in 1879. It initially focused on sales of produce, but after the development of reliable refrigeration in the 1890s, two-thirds of the market was eventually taken up by meatpackers. In 1884, the West Washington Market, mainly a meat and poultry market, was constructed around West Street and Tenth Avenue.

The construction of two piers along the Hudson River attracted major wholesalers into the area. By 1900, 250 slaughterhouses and packing plants filled the district, and after 1906, the Manhattan Refrigerating Company supplied underground refrigeration, which added greatly to meatpacking abilities. In 1926 the *New York Times* said that the far west side of Fourteenth Street was one of the most important markets in the world. By the 1940s, it had become the largest meat and poultry receiving market in the world, bringing economic stability to the neighborhood.

By the 1960s, however, the neighborhood began to decline. A decline in local butcher shops and the rise of supermarkets changed the distribution and consumption of meat and dairy products. The development of frozen foods and containerization technology were factors in the move from local meat distribution to national shipping patterns. The High Line railroad was closed in 1980.

While meatpacking continued to be the major economic activity in the neighborhood through the 1970s and 1980s, a new alternative nighttime economy emerged. The neighborhood became known for illicit activities including prostitution, drug dealing, and sex clubs.

By the turn of the millennium, however, the neighborhood was again trending upward. The Meatpacking District is one of many neighborhoods in New York that has changed drastically, following in the

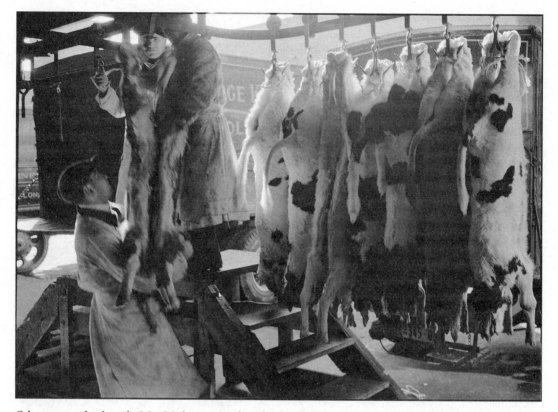

Calves on meat hooks at the West Washington Market. The slaughterhouses, meat markets, and packing plants that once contributed vital economic activity to New York City have largely closed, and the Meatpacking District has gentrified.
SOL LIBSOHN (1914–2001) / FEDERAL ART PROJECT / MUSEUM OF THE CITY OF NEW YORK

footsteps of gritty-to-gentrified neighborhoods such as Times Square and Williamsburg, Brooklyn. With the formation of Friends of the High Line in 1999, the Meatpacking District started to gentrify. In the early 2000s, the development of the High Line Park attracted high-end businesses catering to young professionals, including high-fashion boutiques, corporate retail, and upscale restaurants and nightclubs. In 2004, *New York* magazine named the Meatpacking District "New York's most fashionable neighborhood." High Line Park opened in 2009 and has attracted many visitors to the neighborhood. In 2001 there were still twenty-five to thirty meatpacking businesses left in the neighborhood. By 2015, there were approximately five left, all located in the Gansevoort Market Co-op, which is a block of buildings that the city owns and rents to these companies at subsidized rates.

In 2007, the Greenwich Village Society for Historic Preservation announced that the New York State Parks commissioner approved adding the Meatpacking District neighborhood to the New York State and National Registers of Historic Places. In 2014, the Greenwich Village Society for Historic Preservation claimed victory against two developers who wanted to build tall buildings in the Meatpacking District. According to the Greenwich Village Society for Historic Preservation, this is an important victory in their efforts to preserve the scale and character of the Meatpacking District.

See also BUTCHERS; HIGH LINE; and MANHATTAN.

"Meatpacking District Approved for Listing on State & National Registers of Historic Places." Greenwich Village Society for Historic Preservation. April 11, 2007. http://www.gvshp.org/_gvshp/preservation/gansevoort/gansevoort-04-11-07.htm.
Shockley, Jay. *Gansevoort Market Historic District Designation Report*. New York: New York City Landmarks Preservation Commission, 2003.
Wasserman, Suzanne R., dir. *Meat Hooked!* DVD. New York: Phizmonger Pictures, 2012.

Suzanne Wasserman

Menu Labeling

Late in 2006, aiming to reduce the prevalence of obesity and its consequences—notably heart disease and type 2 diabetes—New York City Mayor Michael Bloomberg's Department of Health and Mental Hygiene proposed something new: to require fast-food chain restaurants—those with more than ten outlets nationally and that already provided nutrition information to customers—to display the calorie content of their food items on menu boards. City health officials knew that most people do not understand calories well, do not know how many calories they are eating, and typically underestimate them, especially from large portions. Calorie labeling, they predicted, would encourage choices of lower-calorie options, especially if accompanied by explanations that most people require about two thousand calories a day to maintain current body weight. The city also predicted that menu postings would encourage fast-food companies to reduce the number of calories in the items they serve. It estimated that calorie labeling could lower the number of obese New Yorkers by 150,000 over the next five years and prevent more than thirty thousand cases of diabetes.

The proposal gained nearly universal support from a wide range of health and nutrition advocacy groups and health associations. Indeed, the only obesity expert who publicly opposed the measure was later found to have been paid by the New York State Restaurant Association (NYSRA) to do so.

The NYSRA filed Freedom of Information Law requests and lawsuits to delay or block implementation. It complained that the proposal was impractical, expensive, punitive, and unconstitutional on the grounds that it was preempted by the Nutrition Labeling and Education Act of 1990 and First Amendment rights. It sued the city. In September 2007 a federal judge ruled in favor of the NYSRA, but his ruling gave the city an opening to try again. He suggested that calorie labeling would be possible if the rules applied to all chain restaurants, regardless of whether they voluntarily provided nutrition information.

The city went back to the drawing boards and in January 2008 rewrote the proposal to comply with this decision. This time it required calorie labeling of all chain restaurants with fifteen or more outlets nationwide, a stipulation that encompassed about 10 percent of the city's twenty-three thousand restaurants. The NYSRA again took the city to court. The National Restaurant Association issued a statement of nonsupport. Restaurants, it said, should be free to decide how to provide nutrition data to their customers.

But in April 2008 the judge ruled that calorie labeling is in the public interest and does not violate the First Amendment. He said it seemed reasonable to expect some consumers to use the information to select lower-calorie meals and that such choices would help reduce obesity. The New York State Restaurant Association again appealed, but the judge allowed the law to go into effect while this appeal was in progress.

In June 2008 the appeal was denied, and the regulation went into effect. The Health Department kicked it off with a campaign: "Read 'em before you eat 'em" and "2,000 calories a day is all most adults should eat."

While the city measure was under litigation, leaders in other places were developing their own initiatives. Although some states passed laws forbidding calorie postings, many cities in other states passed or were considering local ordinances. Some fast-food chains had voluntarily started their own labeling programs. These postings differed in so many particulars that the National Restaurant Association appealed to Congress to pass preemptive national legislation.

Thus, buried in the 2010 Affordable Care Act is a provision mandating national calorie labeling in chain restaurants with twenty outlets nationwide. When the Supreme Court affirmed the act as constitutional two years later, it also made menu labeling constitutional. The U.S. Food and Drug Administration issued the final regulations in November 2014.

Is calorie labeling effective? The city's preregulation baseline data indicated that only 4 percent of customers looked at calorie labeling when it was hidden in brochures, posters, and tray liners. Although the percentage at Subway restaurants was higher, only one-third of the customers who reported looking at the information chose lower-calorie options. Later studies showed little effect of calorie labeling on overall choices, although the subsets of individuals who actually pay attention to the labels do report that calorie postings influence their purchases. An additional benefit is that the regulation induces the chains to reduce the calories in some of their items.

New York City led the way in getting calories posted on menu boards. In this and other public health initiatives aimed at reducing obesity-related chronic disease, this experience demonstrates the value of initiating innovative food regulations at the local level and inspires other communities to develop their own regulations. See RESTAURANT LETTER GRADING and SODA "BAN."

See also BLOOMBERG, MICHAEL.

Farley, Thomas A., Anna Caffarelli, Mary T. Bassett, et al. "New York City's Fight over Calorie Labeling." *Health Affairs* 28, no. 6 (2009): w1098–w1109.

Kiszko, Kamila M., Olivia D. Martinez, Courtney Abrams, et al. "The Influence of Calorie Labeling on Food Orders and Consumption: A Review of the Literature." *Journal of Community Health* 39, no. 6 (2014): 1248–1269.

Ludwig, David S., and Kelly D. Brownell. "Public Health Action Amid Scientific Uncertainty: The Case of Restaurant Calorie Labeling Regulations." *Journal of the American Medical Association* 302, no. 4 (July 22, 2009): 434–435.

Marion Nestle

Menus

A restaurant menu describes the dishes available for order at a restaurant. The menu usually suggests a sequence of courses (appetizers, entrées, desserts) and may recommend or promote specialties or suggestions, but the patron has a considerable amount of choice. The menu as a type of document emerged in the late eighteenth century at the same time that the restaurant first supplemented other, long-standing ways of dining away from home. The key element of novelty in both restaurants and their menus was choice. Food offerings at inns and taverns were restricted, and meals were usually served at set times. Food shops offered a range of selections but only to take home. The restaurant patron can decide to dine at a time of choice, pick his or her table companions, and make a selection from a menu, what was usually referred to in nineteenth-century restaurants as a "bill of fare."

Paris was the innovator in dining styles, and it took about seventy years in the case of the United States and even longer for Britain for the restaurant model to be adopted. The first real restaurant in New York (and in the United States) is usually thought to be Delmonico's in Lower Manhattan, which was established first as a pastry shop by two brothers from Ticino (Italian Switzerland) and then expended during the 1830s into a French restaurant. The oldest surviving New York menu (in the Museum of the City of New York) is from 1838, an eleven-page list of dishes offered by Delmonico's including many kinds of meat and fowl with truffles and an impressive wine list.

Before the Civil War, most of the fancy restaurants in New York and elsewhere were in hotels. Grand hotels such as the Astor House and Metropolitan in New York opened at the end of the 1830s and in the 1840s. They often provided a separate restaurant for women (a "Ladies' Ordinary," as it was called) where women could dine alone or in all-female groups. The oldest menu in the extensive collection in the New York Public Library (from 1843) is from the ladies' restaurant at the elegant Astor House Hotel on Lower Broadway. Comparison with an even older menu (1841) from the main restaurant at the same hotel, in the collection of Henry Voigt, shows that as yet no distinction was made between male and female tastes. The gentlemen were offered seventeen entrées, all rendered in French, including mutton cutlets, duck with olives, macaroni "à l'Italienne," and fried marinated calf's head. The women were presented with twelve "side dishes" (the same thing as entrées) listed in English, among them mutton cutlets, duck with olives, macaroni, and calf's head (here served with brain sauce). The rest of the ladies' menu is similarly hearty: sautéed kidneys with *fines herbes*, stewed mutton with turnips, breaded veal cutlets with tomato sauce. Even before the Civil War, however, restaurants catering to women shopping or later working at clerical or retail jobs offered ice cream and other desserts and later light fare such as salads and sandwiches. In the 1850s Taylor's, a so-called ice cream saloon, attracted ladies shopping at the great Stewart's Dry Goods store nearby on lower Broadway.

Restaurant menus, especially at hotels, were not organized according to individual à la carte offerings. Hotel guests could adopt what was known as the American plan, by which the meals were included in an overall lodging price and outside guests simply paid a sum (ranging from one to three dollars before the Civil War) that entitled them to whatever they wished, much as might be the case today on a cruise ship or at a grand brunch, except not self-service. The diner informed the waiter which of the dishes on offer he or she desired, but as there were routinely as many as eight courses, the meals consumed by even the most abstemious diners seem large to us. By the 1870s, menus more frequently listed prices for items separately. The Grand Hotel at Broadway and Thirty-First Street in 1879 had an extravagant menu of over ten courses, each item having its own price: oysters and clams, soup (five offered), fish (four), entrées that were roasted (four) or boiled (mutton in caper sauce), game

❖ MENU ❖

Chaud
Consommé
Bouchées à la régence
Croquettes de chapons
Huîtres, béchamel aux truffes
Terrapène à la Maryland
Canards à tête rouge
Thé & Café

Froid
Saumon à la parisienne
Filets de boeuf à la Lucullus
Galantines de poulet à la Victoria
Langues de boeuf à l'écarlate
Aspic de foies-gras, historié
Pâté de bécasses, Pithivier
Cailles piquées, grouse
Mayonnaise de volaille
Salade de homard
Sandwiches
Rillettes
Canapés

Entremets de douceur
Gelée aux cerises   Oublies à la crême
Gateau noisette   Pain d'abricots
Mottoes   Pièces montées   Bonbons
Glaces de fantaisies
Tutti-frutti   Biscuit glacé
Dessert   Petits fours   Fruits

Vins
Moët Impérial Brut   Pommery sec
Pontet Canet   Apollinaris

Le 20 Décembre, 1888
DELMONICOS

Delmonico's dinner menu. Delmonico's is thought to be the first real restaurant in the United States, with the oldest surviving menu dating to 1838, featuring many kinds of meat and fowl with truffles and an impressive wine list. This menu is from 1888. RARE BOOKS DIVISION, THE NEW YORK PUBLIC LIBRARY. ASTOR, LENOX, AND TILDEN FOUNDATIONS

(squab or reedbirds), pastry, ices and jellies, and fruits. The most expensive dish was *filet de boeuf grillé à la Béarnaise* at $1.10.

Up to this point the menus were plain and forthright in appearance. They might be decorated with vignettes, and hotel menus often showed a representation of the grand building's façade. With the advance of color engraving, menus by the 1890s were carefully and beautifully designed. The swank Café Martin near Madison Square in 1903 featured an art nouveau color female figure of chaste but Beardsleyesque inspiration. The fancy and louche Mouquin's has a menu lamenting the advent of Prohibition (June 19, 1919) titled "Farewell Dinner to Personal Liberty" with an exotically dressed young woman sitting forlornly in a green martini glass.

The period from 1920 to 1970 may not have been the golden age of American gastronomy, but it was an era of magnificent and extravagant menu design. Oversize menus with vivid colors represented romantic scenes, far-off locations, female beauty, art deco design, and symbols of progress and mechanization. The fanciest restaurant in New York, Le Pavillon (established in 1941), offered large, cumbersome menus but with illustration limited to a tableau of a cooking pot, knife, glasses, and wine bottle.

The menu at Le Pavillon was in French with no English translation. The leading restaurants were French and to varying degrees accommodated those not familiar with French gastronomy with some English translation. Menus from establishments with generic American or "continental" cuisine might include French touches to convey sophistication. The Rainbow Room at the newly completed Rockefeller Center in 1934 featured soups called "Essence of Tomate Xavier" and "Green Turtle aux Vieux Madère."

This era also saw the advent of menus that not only described dishes but extolled them. Toffenetti's on Times Square pioneered this practice. A menu from the 1950s describes the meat sauce for "Spaghetti à la Toffenetti" as "made from a traditional recipe of old, discovered by Mrs. Toffenetti in the archives among the ruins of the castle of Bonpensier in Bologna." Dishes with less elaborate description are nevertheless "juicy," "hot," "tender," "fresh," or "luscious." Even high-end restaurants such as The Forum of the Twelve Caesars in the early 1960s used fervid if not completely serious descriptions to heighten interest: "Fiddler Crab A LA NERO—Flaming, of course."

Contemporary menus are less exuberant and tend to divide between earnest descriptions of local sourcing—so that we learn where and under what careful nurturing every chicken or raspberry was born—or austerely plain. Craft on Nineteenth Street combines these elements so that while the dishes are severely pruned of all description (merely the name of the principle ingredient under categories such as "roasted" or "shellfish"), there is a listing of farms and purveyors. The menu remains more than merely informative, but there are several ways of trying to present the meal as enticing.

"Bottolph Collection of Menus." New York Public Library Digital Collections. http://digitalcollections.nypl.org/collections/buttolph-collection-of-menus.

Grimes, William. *Appetite City: A Culinary History of New York*. New York: North Point, 2009.

Heiman, Jim, ed. *Menu Design in America: A Visual History of Graphic Styles and Design 1850–1985*. Cologne, Germany: Taschen, 2011.

Lobel, Cindy R. *Urban Appetites: Food and Culture in Nineteenth-Century New York*. Chicago: University of Chicago Press, 2014.

Voigt, Henry. *The American Menu* (blog). http://www.theamericanmenu.com.

Paul Freedman

Merchant's Coffee House

See COFFEEHOUSES.

Mexican

Mexican food in New York City is a relatively recent phenomenon. In 1980 there were fewer than seven thousand Mexicans in the city (largely from the state of Puebla); by 2013 there were almost two hundred thousand. As a result, early representation of the cuisine was limited to a few high-end Manhattan establishments serving an Americanized interpretation, such as the celebrated Zarela (now closed), and local outer-borough spots serving the immigrant population fast-food staples including *atole*, churros, tacos, and tamales. The immigration explosion and the growing popularity nationwide for the ancient corn, bean, and chili-based Mexican cuisine has blurred the lines between high and low in recent years, creating a spectrum of restaurants, bodegas, taco stands, and food trucks that promote an ongoing quest for authenticity.

By the early 2010s Mexican enclaves had been established in Sunset Park in Brooklyn, Jackson Heights and Corona in Queens, and "Little Mexico" on the Upper East Side of Harlem. In these areas shoppers could find locally produced masa (corn dough), freshly made tortillas, dried yet still pliable chilis, and imported mole pastes. The large population of immigrants also encouraged a rise in local Mexican-style cheese production.

Outside the Mexican neighborhoods, celebrity chefs (Mexican and not) have opened a wide range of establishments focusing on Mexican cuisine, ranging from swanky clubs and bars serving elevated versions of Mexican classics to casual eateries that attempt to bring south of the border specialties to a mid-level market. There is perhaps no better marker of the influence of Mexican cuisine in today's New York than the appearance of women selling steaming tamales out of coolers on street corners as well as the prevalence of dishes such as chilaquiles, *pozole*, and huevos rancheros on the brunch menus of the city's best-known spots. Whether it is by lining up at Chelsea Market for the newest and most sought-after tacos or traipsing to Queens for the torta of the moment, New Yorkers' interest in Mexican food is thriving, as is their love for the incredible history and flavor that comes from our neighbor to the south.

Arellano, Gustavo. *Taco USA: How Mexican Food Conquered America*. New York: Scribner, 2012.

New York City Department of City Planning. *The Newest New Yorkers*. New York: Department of City Planning, 2013.

Alexandra Olsen

Meyer, Danny

In 1985, with little restaurant experience, St. Louis–born Danny Meyer launched what became one of New York City's most revered and informal restaurants, Union Square Cafe, in a then-seedy neighborhood that he helped revitalize. Boasting fine wines and an eclectic menu that experts advised against, Union Square Cafe helped lead the way in such trends as flavored mashed potatoes, different specials every night of the week, and people eating at the bar. It also banned smoking before there were legal bans. Meyer went on to become chief executive officer of one of the world's most dynamic restaurant organizations, Union Square Hospitality Group, which

includes nearly a dozen New York dining establishments that have garnered an unprecedented twenty-five James Beard awards. The *New York Times* has called Danny Meyer "the greatest restaurateur that New York has ever seen."

Born March 14, 1958, as a middle child in St. Louis, Meyer was raised in a Europhilic family. His parents exposed him early on to Europe, where he experienced the gracious hospitality in family-run inns and the hug that came with the food that he says made it taste better. He fell in love with all kinds of food as a seven-year-old, eating everything from French ratatouille and wild strawberries with crème fraiche to later winning a cooking competition in summer camp for his native St. Louis barbecue.

Meyer graduated from Trinity College in Hartford, Connecticut, with a degree in political science. He worked as a political field director in Chicago for John Anderson's 1980 independent presidential campaign, toying briefly with the idea of going into politics himself one day.

Meyer ultimately chose to live in New York and got a job as a sales representative for a security company, traveling the country. His affability won him clients and brought him large commissions, and he became the company's top salesperson. But Meyer yearned to pursue his love of food, and in 1983, with the encouragement of his family, he chucked his lucrative career to take a low-paying job as an assistant manager at Pesca, an Italian seafood restaurant in Lower Manhattan. He soaked up what he could for eight months, then returned to Europe as a cook's apprentice in Italy and Bordeaux, plucking dead birds, learning about wine, and impressing the staff with his *côtes de porc*—his grandmother's version of St. Louis spareribs.

While Meyer had toyed with the idea of being a chef, he decided his real forte would be as a "restaurant generalist," running his own place. He returned to New York to really start cooking. After scouting more than a hundred prospective sites, he used his savings to lease and remodel an old, stale-smelling vegetarian restaurant in the emerging Union Square neighborhood, with its nearby Greenmarket. (Supported by the restaurant, the Greenmarket would grow to be the largest in the city.) Experts told Meyer that the eclectic menu he developed with a novice chef was doomed. Meyer stuck to his instincts and opened Union Square Cafe on October 20, 1985. He got rave reviews with such dishes as confit of duck with garlic mashed potatoes, his grandmother's mashed turnips with fried shallots as a side dish, and filet mignon of tuna marinated with soy, ginger, and lemon.

In 1998, with the opening of the restaurants Tabla and Eleven Madison Park, Meyer founded the Union Square Hospitality Group. Meyer helped set the American restaurant table on a course of enlightened hospitality, putting his employees first and the customers second. Meyer has said that employees who are excited to work spread their enthusiasm to customers. He also believes that to be successful, you must first meet the needs of employees, then guests, followed by the community, suppliers, and finally investors—in that order. Now more than twenty-five years later, Union Square Hospitality Group grosses in excess of $50 million a year and has more than twenty-two hundred employees. Along with its catering company, Union Square Hospitality Group has also begun foreign licensing. The culture of hospitality has extended beyond the restaurant and food service industries: in 2010 Union Square Hospitality Group launched Hospitality Quotient, a learning and consulting business designed to foster success and customer loyalty by adapting a "company culture of hospitality," regardless of the industry.

Meyer says he prides himself on hiring nice people who are smarter than he is. And he has produced several books, including the award-winning *Union Square Cafe Cookbook* (1994), with his chef-partner Michael Romano, and an acclaimed memoir-cum-business manual on hospitality, *Setting the Table* (2006).

Even more important than his delicious dishes, Meyer also dished out a bounty of hospitality. Remembering his solo dining excursion in restaurants internationally where he would be rebuffed by hosts, Meyer welcomed the solo diner with extra courtesy and respect. Publishers and advertising executives began coming in for lunch, and Meyer would often introduce them to each other. He kept records of birthdays, customers' favorite dishes, favorite waiters, and favorite tables. His goal was to build a community of regulars and have them make his restaurant their clubhouse. They did—and the restaurant began winning James Beard Awards, for outstanding restaurant, outstanding service, and more.

After ten years of success with Union Square Cafe, Meyer felt it was time to grow. In 1995 he opened Gramercy Tavern, which won acclaim for its down-home luxury dining. Other Meyer eateries followed, including Blue Smoke, with real pit barbecue; Shake Shack, offering burgers, hot dogs, and frozen custard; and The Modern, his deluxe eatery at the Museum of Modern Art. Meyer says he makes every restaurant different, and each reflects his diverse culinary and cultural passions.

See also GREENMARKETS and UNION SQUARE CAFE.

Bounds, Gwendolyn. "Hospitality for Everyone." *Wall Street Journal*, October 3, 2006, p. A17.
Meyer, Danny. *Setting the Table*. New York: HarperCollins, 2006.
Schlosser, Julie. "Keeping Tabs on a Food Empire." *Fortune* (July 24, 2006): 42.
Union Square Hospitality Group website: http://www.ushgnyc.com.
Wilsey, Sean. "A Movable Feast: Danny Meyer on a Roll." *New York Times Magazine*, August 4, 2011.

Scott Warner

Microbreweries and Brewpubs

Microbreweries, sometimes called craft breweries, are small independent breweries that focus on producing quality beer, consumed mainly off-premises. There is some disagreement about how small a brewery must be to qualify as a microbrewery, but the Brewers Association defines the category as having annual production of fewer than fifteen thousand U.S. beer barrels. A related term, "brewpub," is a pub or restaurant that brews beer, with a significant portion of sales of brewed beer occurring on-site (the Brewers Association defines it as at least 25 percent). What is now known as the craft brewing movement began in 1976 with a single brewery in California, called New Albion Brewing Company. It took almost ten years for the movement to reach New York City.

In 1984 the first brewpub opened in New York City. The Manhattan Brewing Co. (Broome/Watts Street) featured a brewery on the third floor of a converted Consolidated Edison electric substation with a large eating area on the second floor. It lasted almost seven years in one incarnation or another, from 1984 to 1991, when it fell victim to a combination of high overhead costs, the raised drinking age in New York, and the residual effects of the Black Monday stock market crash in 1987. Garrett Oliver, the brewmaster of the Manhattan Brewing Co., went on to become the brewmaster of Brooklyn Brewery in 1994. See BROOKLYN BREWERY.

Zip City/The Tap Room (3 West Eighteenth Street) was a brewpub that opened in 1991 at the same location that once housed the Women's Christian Temperance Union. The establishment went through two incarnations. As Zip City it lasted from 1991 until 1997, when the owner dramatically emptied 3,100 gallons of unsold beer into the sewer. As The Tap Room under the ownership of the brewhouse supplier, it lasted only a few more years.

One of the most impressive of the first New York City brewpubs was the Commonwealth Brewing Company New York (10 Rockefeller Plaza), located on ideal real estate. This rather grand brewpub had a brewery and bar on the ground floor and a split-level upstairs dining area. A sister establishment to Commonwealth Brewing Company Boston, it lasted from July 1996 to May 2001.

On the Upper West Side, the West Side Brewery (Seventy-Sixth Street and Amsterdam Avenue) opened in 1993 brewing a house brew, but when it closed seven years later it was no longer brewing any beer. A. J. Gordon's Brewing Company, also on the Upper West Side (212 West Seventy-Ninth Street), opened in 1996 and closed two years later.

The East Side featured The Carnegie Hill Brewing Company (1600 Third Avenue), lasting from July 12, 1995, until March 2002. Another East Side brewpub, The Typhoon Brewery (22 East Fifty-Fourth Street), gained more of a reputation for its food than its beer. Yorkville Brewery (1359 First Avenue) was a short-lived establishment that lasted two years, from 1996 to 1998.

In the midst of Times Square, sitting above a major subway station, the Times Square Brewery and Restaurant (160 West Forty-Second Street) was one of the longest-lasting members of the first brewpubs established in New York City. It opened its doors in 1996 and lasted until 2013.

When the Chelsea Brewing Company (Pier 59, Chelsea Piers) opened in 1996 its position on the pier looking west over the Hudson made it a destination for the view as well as the beer. One of the longest-running microbrewery businesses, it closed in June 2014.

The Heartland Brewery (35 Union Square West), still in operation as of the writing of this entry, opened its doors at its original location on Union Square West in April 1995. Since then, Heartland has grown into a five-restaurant chain.

Not all of the brewpubs and microbreweries have been in Manhattan. If you paid a visit to the slowly gentrifying Park Slope neighborhood of Brooklyn in the mid-1990s, you could find the Park Slope Brewing Company at Van Dyke and Dewight Streets. The beer developed a reputation, and the belt-driven ceiling fan system made the visit worthwhile. The brewery lasted from 1994 until 1997.

Microbreweries in New York City today have an advantage over their predecessors in that there is a cadre of brewers who have experience and are at least familiar with business planning. They are also spread out over all five boroughs of the city: Manhattan, the Bronx (including Bronx Brewery and Gun Hill Brewing Co.), Queens (Finback Brewery, Big Alice Brewing Co. and Transmitter Brewing in Long Island City, SingleCut Beersmiths, and Rockaway Brewing Company), Brooklyn (Sixpoint Brewery and Brooklyn Brewery), and Staten Island (The Flagship Brewing Company, opened in 2014, returning craft brewing to Staten Island after the Old World Brewery closed in 2003).

See also BEER and BREWERIES.

Bryson, Lew. *New York Breweries*. Mechanicsburg, Pa.: Stackpole, 2003.
Hindy, Steve, and Tom Potter. *Beer School*. Hoboken, N.J.: Wiley, 2005.
Oliver, Garrett, ed. *The Oxford Companion to Beer*. New York: Oxford University Press, 2012.

Peter LaFrance

Middle Eastern

See ARAB COMMUNITY.

Milk, Raw

Although most milk available in the New York City area is now pasteurized—treated with heat to kill pathogens—"raw" (nonpasteurized) milk is available in limited quantities, though it is a product surrounded by intense public-health debates. All animal milk sold in New York City was raw until about 1890, when heat treatment of milk to kill pathogens was still semi-experimental. In 1893 the philanthropist Nathan Straus and the pediatrician Abraham Jacobi organized a program for pasteurizing and bottling cows' milk at small neighborhood facilities and distributing it to families at nominal cost. Simultaneously, the Newark, New Jersey, pediatrician Henry L. Coit developed a program for producing and bottling unpasteurized milk on dairy farms where trained microbiologists certified that it met exacting sanitary standards. In 1910 New York began requiring that milk sold in the city be pasteurized, with the exception of "certified raw milk" approved by Coit's "medical milk commissions."

Soon thereafter, discoveries about milk's nutrient content helped boost an already flourishing dairy industry in New York State and nearby New Jersey and Connecticut. Meanwhile, a raw foods cult popularized by pseudoauthorities like the New York "physical culturist" Bernarr Macfadden fostered some demand for unpasteurized milk, despite the difficulty and expense of distributing it in pristine condition. Though nearly all milk reaching city consumers after about 1920 was pasteurized, certified raw milk retained a small fan club.

Local raw milk producers disappeared as the economic advantages of pasteurized milk from organized dairy farm co-ops and large commercial processing plants progressively routed any competition. Public-health authorities, meanwhile, increasingly urged a high-handed zero-tolerance policy toward retail sale of raw milk under any circumstances. This approach eventually succeeded but not without controversy.

For many years city consumers could buy raw milk from the famous Walker-Gordon dairy of Plainsboro, New Jersey, known for the richness of milk from its herd of Jersey cows. After it shut down in 1971, the smaller Gates Homestead Farms of Chittenango, New York, tried to fill the same market, supplying milk in black cardboard cartons to health-food stores. No other retail outlets continued to carry raw milk. At least officially, it could be bought only with a doctor's prescription.

Gates went bankrupt in 1982, ending legal raw milk sales in the city. The State Departments of Health and of Agriculture and Markets have since prohibited retail sale of raw milk except on the producing farm. However, a new and growing clientele seeking raw milk for near-miraculous healthful properties (never conclusively demonstrated through any rigorous medical study) has begun challenging the ban.

By declining to debate any suggestion that raw milk sales might be safely permitted under some conditions, state health authorities have helped create a semiclandestine business. In 2004 a *New Yorker* Talk of the Town article described an illegal delivery by an out-of-state farmer to a "private raw milk coven."

Since 2007 the Farm-to-Consumer Legal Defense Fund, an arm of the Weston A. Price Foundation, has promoted a legal stratagem called "cow shares," in which participants receive raw milk as official part owners of a herd or farm. Any change in this situation hinges on the unlikely event of a liberalized bill being adopted by the state legislature. Meanwhile, an undetermined number of New Yorkers embrace cow share arrangements on freedom-of-choice grounds.

See also MILK, SWILL.

Meckel, Richard A. *Save the Babies: American Public Health Reform and the Prevention of Infant Mortality, 1850–1929.* Baltimore: Johns Hopkins University Press, 1990.
Mendelson, Anne. " 'In Bacteria Land': The Battle over Raw Milk." *Gastronomica: The Journal of Food and Culture* 11, no. 1 (Spring 2011): 35–43.
Selitzer, Ralph. *The Dairy Industry in America.* New York: Dairy Field/Books for Industry, 1976.

Anne Mendelson

Milk, Swill

"Swill" milk (milk produced by cows fed the spent mash produced by industrial-scale breweries and distilleries) sickened and killed an alarming number of cows and people in the early- to mid-1800s, becoming a subject for sensational journalism and, ultimately, a catalyst for improved milk safety measures. For several generations in early Dutch New Netherland and English New York, cows pastured and stabled near every settlement supplied household wants for milk, butter, and cheese. But around 1800, medical authorities began placing an unprecedented stress on fresh, unsoured, drinkable cows' milk as the foundation of children's health. This emphasis produced a huge demand for the most perishable form of milk, making it especially profitable for suppliers just as farmland for producing it was being pushed farther and farther away from the growing urban population.

The changed supply-and-demand equation created two divergent branches of the embryonic milk industry. In the long run, the more important would be formed by farmers in nearby parts of the Hudson Valley and Connecticut, who switched their focus from butter and cheese to fluid milk when railway lines were built to connect the countryside with the burgeoning urban market. But city entrepreneurs had previously gotten an advantage by exploiting wastes from New York's many industrial-scale breweries and distilleries.

Eagerly discovering gold in these otherwise useless byproducts, beer or liquor producers and a greedy new class of milk producers invented mutually helpful arrangements for building sheds next to brewers' or distillers' operations, crowding every possible cow into them and dumping the hot slops into the hapless animals' feeding troughs. This diet actually increased their milk output, enabling "swill" dairymen to sell milk to city dwellers for a pittance while turning a comfortable profit. The cows, however, sickened and died at an alarming rate while producing bluish, creamless, unnaturally watery milk.

The swill milk business grew rapidly from the late 1820s. By the late 1830s the temperance reformer Robert M. Hartley had become concerned about its terrible cost in human and bovine mortality. He denounced the industry in a sweeping inquiry published in 1842 and supported by many leading physicians. Unfortunately, public health was only starting to be recognized as a civic responsibility. Such health officials as existed had no authority to conduct serious investigations or shut down overcrowded, foul-smelling facilities where sick cows lapped up alcoholic swill guaranteed to poison ruminant digestive systems.

Various advocates and newspapers intermittently revived the issue. They were aided by the accelerating shift of large-scale brewing and distilling operations from East Coast cities to the Midwest, along with the appearance of new regional rail links between country dairy farms and city distributors via a "milk train." Equally important was a dawning era of aggressive competition between illustrated periodicals made possible by faster printing presses, colorful eyewitness reporting, and new image-printing technology. In the spring of 1858, Frank Leslie, publisher of a major weekly journal, enlisted a crew of reporters and sketch artists for a team project, "Our Exposure of the Swill Milk Trade." The *Frank Leslie's Illustrated Newspaper* account still stands as one of the most powerful exposés in the history of American journalism.

Trying to rough up illustrators and reporters, the milk handlers unwittingly helped the paper to burnish its crusading image in a series of circumstantial accounts, accompanied by sensational engravings, which began on May 1. Perhaps the crowning horror was a front-page depiction of a semiputrified carcass being dissected "for examination of the intestines" in the presence of "the health wardens, Frank Leslie and his corps."

The city Common Council—deservedly nicknamed the "Forty Thieves"—hastily produced a whitewashing "investigation" of the swill dairies. Leslie's and other newspapers, however, kept up pressure until a new mayor, Daniel F. Tiemann, requested a real investigation from the New York Academy of Medicine. Its damning report, published in 1860 after much stalling by the milk dealers' stooges at City Hall, finally led to an official—though laxly enforced—ban on swill dairies and impure milk in 1862.

Vestiges of the swill milk industry hung on in New York for nearly twenty years longer. But after the late 1850s milk from grass-fed cows, shipped by rail from dairy farms in Orange and Westchester Counties, began to dominate the market. Though usually safer than swill milk, it had its own truth-in-advertising problems. The middlemen who distributed the milk for retail sale frequently diluted it with large amounts of sometimes germ-laden water, adding thickeners and colorants to disguise the swindle, or mixed true grass-fed and swill milk.

The situation, however, was improving. After about 1880, facilities for chilling milk and filling it into glass bottles under careful sanitary supervision began replacing haphazard street sales from bulk containers. Meanwhile, the infant science of bacteriology succeeded in identifying the most dangerous milk pathogens by microscopic analysis just as civic health authorities trained in this new discipline were being granted real policing powers. These developments delivered the coup de grace to swill milk by the early 1880s. After the next decade, debates over milk safety would shift to the pros and cons of an entirely new measure, pasteurization.

See also MILK, RAW.

Duffy, John. *A History of Public Health in New York City, 1625–1866.* Vol. 1. New York: Russell Sage Foundation, 1968.
Selitzer, Ralph. *The Dairy Industry in America.* New York: Dairy Field/Books for Industry, 1976.

Anne Mendelson

Mitchell, Joseph

Joseph Mitchell (1908–1996) was born in the farming community of Fairmont, North Carolina, and moved to New York when he was twenty-one. He began his long career at the *New Yorker* shortly thereafter.

Mitchell wrote about the people and places he encountered on his legendary long walks through the city. His stories captured New York's characters as well as its tastes, sounds, and smells, from kippered herring breakfasts at the Fulton Fish Market to calypso picnics in Harlem. In a story titled "All You Can Hold for Five Bucks" he wrote about the grand, greasy dinners called "beefsteaks" that were run by political groups and labor unions. He called them "a form of gluttony as stylized and regional as the riverbank fish fry, the hot-rock clambake, or the Texas barbecue." In "Old Mr. Flood," Mitchell chronicled the "seafoodetarian" who at ninety-three believed that if he lived solely on seafood he would reach his goal of 115. Richard Severo, who wrote the *New York Times* obituary of Mitchell, called him "the poet of the waterfront... of the clammers on Long Island and the oystermen on Staten Island."

For years, Mitchell was one of the *New Yorker*'s prized writers. Then, after 1964, silence. He worked in his office but produced nothing. When asked, he said the piece he was working on was not quite ready. In 1992, much of his work was collected in *Up in the Old Hotel and Other Stories*, for which he wrote a brief introduction.

Mitchell died in 1996. Subsequently, portions of a memoir he was writing came to light and were published in the *New Yorker*. As it did in his earlier works, food resonates throughout the excerpts, from stories about gathering wild persimmons for his mother's pudding as a boy to his recollections of the aromas of spice warehouses on the Lower West Side of Manhattan.

See also NEW YORKER.

Mitchell, Joseph. "Days in the Branch." *New Yorker*, December 1, 2014.
Mitchell, Joseph. *Up in the Old Hotel and Other Stories*. New York: Pantheon, 1992.
Severo, Richard. "Joseph Mitchell, Chronicler of the Unsung and the Unconventional, Dies at 87." *New York Times*, May 25, 1996.

Jeri Quinzio

Mixology

Mixology is the art of preparing mixed drinks. The term came into use as early as the mid-1800s and tended—as is the case today—to refer to the preparation of cocktails in higher-end establishments rather than neighborhood bars or pubs.

Although Americans have enjoyed combining other ingredients with their alcoholic beverages since the earliest colonial days, recipes for cocktails first began to appear in print in the early nineteenth century. The first definition appeared in 1806, when the editor of a New York magazine, *The Balance*, defined the cocktail as "a stimulating liquor, composed of spirits of any kind, sugar, water, and bitters."

By the late eighteenth century, bars were featured in luxury hotels. By the 1800s, many of these hotels housed the more opulent barrooms. As bars became popular, a new profession emerged: the bartender, who served up increasingly more complicated drinks. New York's Metropolitan Hotel, which opened in 1852, was among those with a prominent bar. Jerry Thomas, regarded by many as the first "mixologist," became principal bartender at the hotel in 1858. Over the next eighteen years, Thomas would become America's most famous bartender, embodying bravado and showmanship. He was also the first American to publish a cocktail book. See THOMAS, JERRY.

The golden age of mixology came to an end with the enactment of Prohibition. During the Prohibition years (1920–1933) in New York City, bar culture evolved into drinking in illicit speakeasies. An estimated 100,000 illegal bars popped up all over the city during this period. See PROHIBITION and SPEAKEASIES.

The Dry Era, which lasted from 1919 until the Twenty-First Amendment to the U.S. Constitution repealed the Eighteenth Amendment in 1933, completely transformed bar culture and mixology in the United States and, of course, New York City. Drinking publicly was illegal and expensive, but consumption of alcohol remained an essential part of the nightlife experience, something that undoubtedly increased the allure, excitement, and certainly the danger of the scene.

Because production of alcoholic beverages was illegal and obtaining high-quality spirits was difficult and expensive, demand regularly exceeded availability. This inevitably led to shortages and changed the role of the mixologist from someone who crafted cocktails from high-quality liquors, spirits, and other fresh ingredients to someone who concocted palatable drinks—usually sweet and colorful—with inferior products for establishments that made a sizeable profit from the sale of alcoholic beverages. During this period, a number of bartenders left the United States to practice their craft elsewhere.

After the passage of the Twenty-First Amendment, bartenders continued to offer the sugary-sweet, colorful drinks that had gained popularity and whose flavor profiles generally lacked the balance and complexity of the more classic cocktails. This trend has continued since, with concoctions such as Sex On the Beach and the notoriously strong and sweet New York (Long Island) drink the Long Island Iced Tea being more infamous examples.

However, in the late 1990s and early 2000s, mixology made a return to New York City, creating a second golden age for cocktails. Mixologists such as Dale DeGroff, Audrey Sanders, Gaz Regan, and other newcomers such as Harlem's Karl Franz Williams have worked to reestablish and maintain the quality and creativity of mixology. Newer establishments like Death and Company and Pegu Club have joined classic outposts like Bemelmans Bar and 21 Club in continuing the mixology traditions of New York City.

See also DEGROFF, DALE and SAUNDERS, AUDREY.

Curtis, Wayne. "Old Fashioned." *The Atlantic*, January 1, 2009. http://www.theatlantic.com/magazine/archive/2009/01/old-fashioned/307205.
"Experience the Cocktails and Chronicles of Harlem's Revival." https://www.sidetour.com/experiences/experience-the-cocktails-and-chronicles-of-harlem-s-revival.
Mixology101 website: http://www.mixology101.com.
Regan, Gary. *The Joy of Mixology: The Consummate Guide to the Bartender's Craft*. New York: Clarkson Potter, 2003.
Regan, Gary. "Masters of Mixology: Ada Coleman." Liquor.com, August 22, 2012. http://liquor.com/articles/masters-of-mixology-ada-coleman/.
Smith, Andrew F. *Drinking History: Fifteen Turning Points in the Making of American Beverages*. New York: Columbia University Press, 2013.
Wondrich, David. *Imbibe! From Absinthe Cocktail to Whiskey Smash, a Salute in Stories and Drinks to "Professor" Jerry Thomas, Pioneer of the American Bar*. New York: Perigree, 2007.

Rachel Monet Finn

Modernist Cuisine

Modernist cuisine has become one of the preferred terms of reference for what was once called "molecular gastronomy." It refers to using science, and often technology, to better understand cooking so as to be able to push the boundaries of what was previously known and possible in the kitchen. Chemist Hervé This and physicist Nicholas Kurti began using the label "molecular gastronomy" in 1988 in France to describe their work (initially as "molecular and physical gastronomy," until Kurti's death in 1998). In March 2011, *Modernist Cuisine: The Art and Science of Cooking*, by Nathan Myhrvold with Chris Young and Maxime Bilet, was hailed as the most important book to be published since Auguste Escoffier's *Le Guide Culinaire*. Myhrvold, the former chief technology officer of Microsoft, initially set out to write a cookbook of sous-vide techniques, but the project soon ballooned to include techniques and dishes developed in his cooking laboratory in Seattle and by top experimental chefs around the world. Many of the techniques and practices explored in the book are improvements on traditional cooking methods that can benefit home cooks just as much as professional cooks. What it, and practitioners of experimental cooking in general, most importantly teaches is the value of questioning the established method of doing things. Why do we make stocks or blanch vegetables a certain way, for example? Thinking of it as a frame of mind, as proponents of the movement are likely to explain in presentations, demonstrations, or articles, can make it more accessible since that does not necessarily require highly technological equipment or hard-to-find ingredients.

One of the key moments in the early days of molecular gastronomy took place in 1992 in Erice, Sicily, at a workshop that brought together scientists and chefs, organized by Kurti, This, and author Harold McGee, whose seminal book *On Food and Cooking* already served as bible to chefs interested in better understanding why foods behaved a certain way when cooking or baking them. One of the lasting contributions to gastronomy made by these meetings is in helping these two different professional groups to realize what they could learn about their own work by collaborating with the other.

In New York, Wylie Dufresne was probably the earliest, and most prominent, practitioner of modernist cuisine and adopter of its intellectual approach, first at Clinton Fresh Foods and then at wd-50. He worked closely with McGee and with scientist and artist David Arnold, among others, to research scientific questions and principles that allowed him to develop flavor combinations, textures, and overall dishes never seen before, such as an everything bagel with lox and cream cheese—but the bagel is a frozen, hollowed out disc, the cream cheese is flattened into a brittle sheet, and the lox is frozen and shaven into minuscule flakes. The dish tastes like the classic New York breakfast, but Dufresne reinvented it, challenging notions of what is iconic.

Dufresne's kitchen became a training ground for a generation of chefs, notably pastry chefs, who then set out to push their own boundaries. Sam Mason went on to open Tailor, Rosio Sanchez and later Malcolm Livingston became the pastry chef at noma in Copenhagen, and Alex Stupak opened the restaurant mini-empire Empellon, focusing on Mexican cuisine.

In the early 2000s, the movement was especially noticeable in New York's pastry kitchens. Acclaimed chefs including Johnny Iuzzini and Michael Laiskonis, executive pastry chefs of the three Michelin–starred Jean Georges and Le Bernardin, respectively, and Will Goldfarb at Room4Dessert and with his product company WillPowder, collaborated with food scientists, chemists, and other experts to push the boundaries of what they could do with eggs or with ice cream, to name but a couple of examples. Iuzzini, who went on to become a consultant and TV personality, was known for four-course dessert tastings. Laiskonis left Le Bernardin and became the creative director of the Institute of Culinary Education, where his projects have included working with IBM on developing cognitive cooking and pushing the limit of creativity for chefs. Put simply, "Chef Watson" is a computer that generates recipes based on recipes and ingredient pairings, resulting in "computational creativity" that can mine much larger quantities of data than a human brain ever could.

Goldfarb was one of the founders of the Experimental Cuisine Collective, which launched at New York University in 2007 as a collaboration between the chemistry and food studies departments. The organization, which as of 2015 has more than twenty-five hundred members, meets monthly around presenters whose work sits at or near one of the many intersections of science and food. Its audience is as varied as the membership. The university also has offered classes on experimental cuisine and culinary physics. Meanwhile, the Culinary Institute of America's Hyde Park campus began offering a culinary science major in 2013, where courses taught by scientists and chefs explain the scientific principles behind what students otherwise learn in the kitchen, preparing them for careers in restaurants and in the food industry.

Another important figure of modernist cuisine in New York has been Dave Arnold, who was director of technology at the French Culinary Institute (now the International Culinary Center) and the technology contributor at *Food Arts*. In his educational role, Arnold held seminars and worked with students who wanted to learn more about the principles behind modernist cuisine. He also collaborated with chefs as a resource of vast and invaluable knowledge, including with Dufresne. Arnold went on to found the Museum of Food and Drink, whose first mobile exhibit was a puffing gun that cereal companies use to make their products. See MUSEUM OF FOOD AND DRINK.

In recent years, modernist cuisine has made its home in many kitchens. Its technology and ingredients have become part of a chef's tool kit the way a knife or sauté pan are, with results on a plate that do not always betray its adoption.

See also DUFRESNE, WYLIE and EXPERIMENTAL CUISINE COLLECTIVE.

Barham, Peter, Leif H. Skibsted, Wender L. P. Bredie, et al. "Molecular Gastronomy: A New Emerging Scientific Discipline." *Chemical Reviews* 110, no. 4 (2010): 2313–2365.

McGee, Harold. *On Food and Cooking: The Science and Lore of the Kitchen*. Rev. ed. New York: Scribner, 2004. First published 1984.

Myhrvold, Nathan, Chris Young, and Maxime Bilet. *Modernist Cuisine: The Art and Science of Cooking*. Bellevue, Wash.: Cooking Lab, 2011.

This, Hervé. *Molecular Gastronomy: Exploring the Science of Flavor*. New York: Columbia University Press, 2006.

Anne E. McBride

Momofuku Restaurant Group

Momofuku Restaurant Group is the umbrella business group for David Chang–owned restaurants throughout the world. See CHANG, DAVID. The name "Momofuku" has dual purpose: it means "lucky peach" in Japanese and pays homage to the inventor of instant ramen, Momofuku Ando.

Chang's first restaurant, the ramen-themed Momofuku Noodle Bar, opened in August 2004 in the East Village, introducing New Yorkers to Chang's Asian-influenced new American style, as well his signature pork buns. Noted in Peter Meehan's *New York Times* review of the restaurant, Chang translated the lessons he learned working at Tokyo ramen and soba shops and created his own Americanized version of the dish rather than trying to replicate the authentic Japanese version. The French Culinary Institute–trained chef also became known for his seasonally focused menu, a throwback to Tom Colicchio's Craft influence.

Momofuku Ssäm Bar opened in August 2006. This restaurant introduced New Yorkers to dishes that included thinly sliced country hams in the style of prosciutto, whole-rotisserie duck, dry-aged ribeye, and the reservation-only bo ssäm pork shoulder that serves six to ten people. The restaurant earned a two-star *New York Times* review. Momofuku Ko debuted in March 2008. With just twelve seats, it is the smallest of the group's restaurants and, at the time, the most high-end restaurant offering of the group. Serving only a tasting menu, Momofuku Ko received two Michelin stars in 2009 and has held onto them for six straight years. In 2014, both Ssäm Bar and Ko were included on San Pellegrino World's 100 Best Restaurant list.

It was also in 2009 that Chang and the Momofuku Restaurant Group acquired the dessert talent of Christina Tosi, previously at Wylie Dufresne's wd-50, opening up Momofuku Milk Bar inside a space in the expanded Momofuku Ssäm Bar. See DUFRESNE, WYLIE. The pastries under Tosi drew so much buzz that Milk Bar expanded to five New York City locations, all serving crack pie, cereal milk soft serve, and compost cookies. Inspired by the à la carte experience of dimsum, Má Pêche, which translates to "mother peach," opened in Midtown in April 2010 to accommodate the business lunch crowd. Located in the Chambers Hotel, the offerings also include to-go lunches, desserts, and coffee.

Booker and Dax opened in January 2012 as Momofuku Restaurant Group's first bar in the city. The group has recently launched international endeavors like a Momofuku-only building in Toronto, which houses three Momofuku restaurants and a bar, as well as Momofuku Seiōbo in Sydney, Australia. A few years ago, Chang joined forces with McSweeney's publishing and Peter Meehan to launch *Lucky Peach*, a quarterly publication that has received food writing accolades, including five James Beard Awards in 2014. See LUCKY PEACH. Future plans include a line of miso sauces and kitchenware.

Momofuku website: http://www.momofuku.com.
Roberts, Daniel. "David Chang Broke All the Rules." Time.com, September 26, 2013. http://business.time.com/2013/09/26/david-chang-broke-all-the-rules.

Andrea Lynn

Moulton, Sara

Sara Moulton is an American chef, author, and television personality. She was born on February 19, 1952, in New York City. Her love of cooking developed out of her familial relationships. Her paternal grandmother, Ruth Moulton, attended one of the early culinary schools in Boston and gave Sara her first cookbook, *Mud Pies and Other Recipes*. Likewise, her mother, Elizabeth Day, loved to cook, using ingredients like fresh fennel, endive, mushrooms, and shad roe, which were considered exotic in the 1960s. Moulton cooked often as a child, helping her mother prepare for dinner parties and making creative Sunday lunches out of leftovers.

After graduating from The Brearley School, a rigorous private girls' school on Manhattan's Upper East Side, Moulton left New York City for Ann Arbor, Michigan, to attend the University of Michigan. A year after graduation she was still working as a short-order cook. This worried her mother, who wrote to Craig Claiborne and Julia Child to ask what her daughter should do if she wanted to become a chef. See CLAIBORNE, CRAIG and CHILD, JULIA. Child never answered, which was unusual since she was known for responding to all queries, but Claiborne did and said she should go to cooking school, recommending Ecole Hôtelière de Lausanne in Switzerland or the Culinary Institute of America in Hyde Park, New York.

In the fall of 1975, Moulton attended the Culinary Institute of America. She excelled in her studies and graduated second in her class of 452 students. In 1976, after graduation, she was hired as a sous chef at Harvest restaurant in Cambridge, where she had previously completed a three-month externship as a garde manger. Moulton's next job was as a chef manager for a catering company, Caras & Rowe.

While peeling hard-boiled eggs one day, one of Moulton's workers mentioned that she was a volunteer on Julia Child's show. Moulton asked if she thought they needed another volunteer. The next day her worker reported back saying that Child wanted to hire her. Moulton promptly went to the corner pay phone to call Child. "Oh dearie, I've heard all about you!" exclaimed Child. "Do you food style?"

Although Moulton had not had any professional food styling experience, she said yes. She then went to work behind the scenes on *Julia Child and More Company* and the cookbook that went with it. While working on Child's show two days per week, she was hired as a chef at Cybele's (one of Caras & Rowe's restaurants), working five days per week. In 1979, Moulton took a brief leave of absence from the restaurant in order to take advantage of a *stagiaire* opportunity that Child had arranged at Henri IV Restaurant in Chartres, France, working under master chef Maurice Cazalis. Though he barely let her cook on the line, it was an eye-opening experience.

In 1981, Moulton returned to New York City. Child continued to serve as an inspiration but also as a bit of a guardian angel, helping Moulton land another behind-the-scenes job as on-air food editor at *Good Morning America*. She also continued working in restaurants, serving as the chef tournant at La Tulipe, a three-star restaurant. Restaurant cooking was still very much a male-driven profession, and in 1982 Moulton founded the New York Women's Culinary Alliance, a professional organization designed to foster networking and education for women in the culinary fields. It continues to be an invaluable resource and organization for women in the industry. See NEW YORK WOMEN'S CULINARY ALLIANCE.

After seven years working in restaurants, she left the eighty-hour workweek behind and focused instead on recipe testing and development. This allowed her and her husband to start a family. In 1983, Moulton worked as an instructor at Peter Kump's New York Cooking School (now known as the Institute of Culinary Education), which ignited her passion for teaching. See INSTITUTE OF CULINARY EDUCATION.

In 1984 she took a job at *Gourmet*, working in the test kitchen for four years and then as the executive chef in the dining room for twenty-one years. She only quit when the magazine shuttered in 2009. See GOURMET.

While at *Gourmet*, Moulton went on to become a star in her own right as one of the first on-air personalities for Food Network. Between 1996 and 2005, she hosted *Cooking Live* (1996–2002), *Cooking Live Primetime* (1999), and *Sara's Secrets* (2002–2005). Moulton describes *Cooking Live* as her favorite job, not only because she was teaching but also because she learned so much doing it. Over the course of fifteen hundred hour-long episodes, she took callers' questions live, answering five to six questions and cooking five recipes every night.

In 2001 Moulton was named Culinary Institute of America's Chef of the Year, and in 2002 she was inducted into the James Beard Foundation's Who's Who of Food and Beverage in America. Sara is also an accomplished cookbook author, having published *Sara Moulton Cooks at Home* (2002), *Sara's Secrets for Weeknight Meals* (2005), and *Sara Moulton's Everyday Family Dinners* (2010), the latter of which won an International Association of Culinary Professionals Cookbook Award. Since 2008, Moulton has been the host and co-producer of *Sara's Weeknight Meals* on PBS. The show was nominated for a James Beard Award in 2013, while Moulton herself has been nominated three times as Outstanding Personality/Host.

Moulton, Sara. *Sara Moulton Cooks at Home*. New York: Broadway, 2002.
Moulton, Sara. *Sara Moulton's Everyday Family Dinners*. New York: Simon & Schuster, 2010.
Moulton, Sara. *Sara's Secrets for Weeknight Meals*. New York: Broadway, 2005.
Sara Moulton.com (website). http://saramoulton.com.

Layla Khoury-Hanold

Movies

The semiotics of food and film coincide in movies about New York because the city that never sleeps is also the city that never stops eating. Food reveals the cultural and culinary diversity of the city: the rigidity of Gilded Age dining etiquette (*The Age of Innocence*, 1993); anorexic ballerinas (*Black Swan*, 2010); corruption when Al Pacino as real crusader cop Frank Serpico in *Serpico* (1973) refuses food "on the arm," or free; and human flesh as possible future food (*Soylent Green*, 1973).

However, until the 1950s, movies about New York were filmed on Hollywood sets, from upper-class dinner parties in *Dinner at Eight* (1933) and *The Thin Man* (1934) to starving actresses trying to finagle a meal in *Stage Door* (1937) and the 1930s *Golddiggers* series. Depression struggles for food were at the core of *Mr. Deeds Goes to Town* (1936), director Frank Capra's movie about feeding farmers. *Imitation of Life* (1934) is a meal made in heaven when maple syrup saleswoman Claudette Colbert meets African American Aunt Delilah (Louise Beavers), who has a secret pancake recipe. The inspiration was Alice Foote MacDougall, whose business grew from the Little Coffee Shop in Grand Central Station in 1921 to six restaurants worth $2 million six years later.

Communal automat dining was democratic and photogenic. In *Easy Living* (1937), all the food doors open accidentally and the stampede for free food is on. In *That Touch of Mink* (1962), an automat worker reaches through the food door and slaps a surprised patron in the face. *Just This Once* (1952), *Metropolitan* (1990), and *Dark City*, a 1998 neo-noir, have scenes set in automats.

Alcohol figures prominently in New York movies. Middle America's reaction to bootleggers and drunken parties in movies such as *Lights of New York* (1928) and *Platinum Blonde* (1931), made during Prohibition, contributed to the censorship of the Motion Picture Production Code. Joan Crawford's *Dancing Lady* (1933) dances because beer is legal again under the New Deal. Revisionist Prohibition gangster movies like *The Roaring Twenties* (1939), starring James Cagney and Humphrey Bogart, gave way to studies of individual alcoholics in *I'll Cry Tomorrow* (1955), about Broadway star Lillian Roth; *Lost Weekend* (1945), with terrifying animated hallucinations; and alcoholic newspapermen in *Come Fill the Cup* (1951). In *Enchanted* (2007), princess Amy Adams dodges a poisoned appletini, fitting for the Big Apple.

In the 1950s, the French New Wave and Italian neorealism influenced American filmmakers, who realized that nothing trumped the streets of New York for grit and glamour. Both are in *Breakfast at Tiffany's* (1961), as the elegant Holly Golightly (Audrey Hepburn) stands in front of Tiffany's jewelers on Fifth Avenue. With a black elbow-length gloved hand, she pulls a croissant and a cardboard cup of coffee out of a paper bag, illustrating the difference between her dreams and her budget. Less elegant is breakfast at Buddy's in *Elf* (2003): spaghetti topped with chocolate sprinkles, mini-marshmallows, M&M's, Hershey's syrup, maple syrup, and crumbled Pop Tarts.

Spaghetti is a staple in New York movies. Over a plate of spaghetti in *Godfather II* (1974) the young Vito Corleone (Robert De Niro) says that he is going to make his enemy "an offer he can't refuse." Jack Lemmon demonstrates his tennis racket spaghetti straining technique in *The Apartment* (1960). In Disney's animated *Lady and the Tramp* (1955) a shared single strand leads to a kiss. Spaghetti is the last straw in the *Odd Couple* (1968). As fussbudget Felix eats dinner, slob Oscar orders, "Remove that spaghetti from my poker table." Felix retorts, "Ha! It's linguini." Oscar throws the plate against the wall: "Now it's garbage."

Italians are deeply connected to food in movies, as in life. Ernest Borgnine's Academy Award-winner *Marty* (1955) weighs whether to buy the butcher shop where he works (tenderloin, 59 cents). Borgnine trades his meat cleaver for a taxi in *The Catered Affair* (1956), about working-class parents struggling to provide an upper-class wedding dinner for their daughter. Baker Nicholas Cage is *Moonstruck* (1987) over bookkeeper Cher through multiple meals. The wise guys in Martin Scorsese's *Goodfellas* (1990) cook and eat lavishly even in prison. One of the most famous movie lines is in *The Godfather* (1972), after the execution of the Don's treacherous driver, when Clemenza orders, "Leave the gun. Take the cannoli."

In *Do the Right Thing* (1989) Spike Lee serves up a tragic slice about racial tensions between African Americans and Italian Americans. Based on real incidents, the movie takes place in the fictitious Sal's Pizzeria during one pressure-cooker, insufferably hot summer day. In *Jungle Fever* (1991), Lee uses dinner to show that the African American family is in a higher socioeconomic class than the Italian American family.

Servers, plentiful in New York movies, vacillate between despair and dreams. Mia Farrow's abused Depression-era waitress loses herself so deeply in a movie that one of the actors steps off the screen to be with her (*Purple Rose of Cairo*, 1985). *It Could Happen to You* (1994), originally titled "Cop Gives Waitress $2 Million Tip," was based on a true story. In *Jungle Fever*, in a Harlem restaurant that specializes in soul food—barbecue, pinto beans, crab cakes, and blackened catfish—African American waitress Queen Latifah does not want to serve a racially mixed couple. Waitress Michelle Pfeiffer falls for ex-con short-order cook Al Pacino in *Frankie & Johnny* (1991). In *Sea of Love* (1989) detective Pacino goes undercover as a waiter at O'Neal's Balloon across from Lincoln Center. In 1973, a real-life drama played out in O'Neal's when actress Sylvia Miles dumped a plate of food on the head of film critic John Simon.

New York food is also the subject of documentaries. *Farm to Table* (2013) is about the Brooklyn restaurant EGG, which grows produce on its own farm. Filmmaker-turned-guinea pig Morgan Spurlock made himself sick eating fast food in *Supersize Me* (2004). *I Like Killing Flies* (2004) tucks into Shopsin's Diner in Greenwich Village. Three-star chef Paul Liebrandt is the subject of *A Matter of Taste* (2011). *The Best*

Thing I Ever Done (2011) was shot at Di Fara's Brooklyn pizzeria. New York City's Food Film Festival, an annual event since 2011, has shown *Food Porn*. Mickey Rourke feeding a blindfolded Kim Basinger in the theatrical feature *9 1/2 Weeks* (1986) was food porn before the term was coined.

Background food is ubiquitous in New York movies. Street vendors sell hot dogs and pretzels. Chinese is the food of choice for a Mafia meeting to plan an execution in *The Godfather*, it is the first meal shared by the interracial couple in *Jungle Fever*, and Chinese herbs are the catalyst for Mia Farrow's transformation in *Alice* (1990). In *The Terminal* (2004), stranded immigrant Viktor (Tom Hanks) eats JFK Airport's fast food and leftover airline food.

Americans' fascination with food in the twenty-first century moved food to the main course. Chefs Catherine Zeta-Jones and Aaron Eckhardt duel over food and gender in the romantic comedy *No Reservations* (2007). Julie (Amy Adams) blogs and cooks her way through Julia Child's *Mastering the Art of French Cooking* in her tiny apartment kitchen in *Julie & Julia* (2009).

It would not be New York without Jewish food. Much of *Funny Girl* (1968) takes place in the saloon owned by Fanny's mother. In *Crossing Delancey* (1988), Amy Irving thinks she deserves better than her pickle salesman suitor. In *Quiz Show* (1994), Rob Morrow observes that in the upscale restaurant that claimed to invent the quintessential Jewish Reuben sandwich, there were not many Reubens. They would all shudder at WASP *Annie Hall*'s (1977) culinary sin: pastrami on white bread with mayonnaise. "I'll have what she's having," says a hopeful female diner after Meg Ryan's fake orgasm in the real Katz's Deli in *When Harry Met Sally* (1989).

New York has many iconic celebrity restaurants. Woody Allen filmed *Manhattan* (1979) and *Manhattan Murder Mystery* (1993) in Elaine's. It is in the Russian Tea Room that Dustin Hoffman reveals to his agent that he is the female soap star *Tootsie* (1982). Aging comics gather at the Carnegie Deli to reminisce about the comic who achieved immortality through the sandwich named after him, in *Broadway Danny Rose* (1984). In a classic case of life imitating New York City's unique connection to food and film art, the Carnegie Deli has a real sandwich on its menu: the Woody Allen.

See also NOVELS.

Abrams, Nathan. "'I'll Have Whatever She's Having': Jews, Food, and Film." *Reel Food: Essays on Food and Film*, edited by Anne L. Bower, pp. 87–100. New York and London: Routledge, 2004.

Cinotto, Simone. *The Italian American Table: Food, Family, and Community in New York City*. Chicago: University of Illinois Press, 2013.

Diner, Hasia R. *Hungering for America: Italian, Irish, & Jewish Foodways in the Age of Migration*. Cambridge, Mass.: Harvard University Press, 2001.

Reid, Mark A. *Redefining Black Film*. Berkeley: University of California Press, 1993.

Linda Civitello

Mrs. Stahl's Knishes

Mrs. Stahl's Knishes stood at 1001 Brighton Beach Avenue, in Brooklyn, from circa 1935 to 2005, beneath the elevated subway tracks on Coney Island Avenue at Brighton Beach Avenue. See BRIGHTON BEACH. The shop sold a variety of knishes (a handheld stuffed pastry in the Eastern European tradition)—kasha (buckwheat groats), potato, mushroom, apple, and cherry cheese—and was also known for potatoniks (cousins of potato pancakes), a flat, oniony bread called a pletzel, and cherry lime rickeys. Fist-sized hunks of stuffed dough, Mrs. Stahl's knishes were unique for their construction: they appeared round, as many knishes are, but were, in fact, a circular-shaped coil of filling-stuffed dough, turned in on itself, like a snail.

The knish shop's founder, Mrs. Fannie Stahl, was born Feige Goldenberg in Kulikov, Galicia, in 1887 to Bella and Baruch Goldenberg, a ritual slaughterer and a cantor. Mrs. Stahl—she took her married last name from the maiden name of her husband's mother—arrived in New York City on Valentine's Day 1914. She supported her five children as a domestic, a cook in a kosher cafeteria on the Lower East Side, and, at the suggestion of her daughter Dora, by making challah and pastries. Mrs. Stahl began her business sitting on the sands of Brighton Beach with a basketful of knishes (so as not to arouse suspicion from the police). Mrs. Stahl later sold her wares from a stall beneath the boardwalk and, in the mid-1930s, opened up her eponymous shop a block from the ocean. Remembered by one of her employees as "a queen and a delightful person and a very hard worker," Mrs. Stahl was a successful, philanthropy-minded businesswoman and proud supporter of Hadassah, a Jewish women's organization.

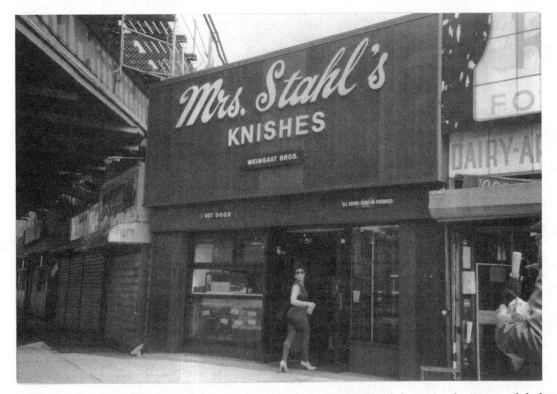

The storefront of Mrs. Stahl's Knishes, which sold not only her uniquely shaped knish, but many other European baked goods. Her recipe was sold after the closing of the store and can now be found in restaurants and bagel shops along the East Coast. LAURA SILVER

After her death in 1961, Mrs. Stahl's daughters and sons-in-law ran the business. Soon thereafter, it was sold to Sam and Morris Weingast. Les Green purchased the business in 1985 and, in 2005, citing changing demographics in the neighborhood, sold Mrs. Stahl's knish recipe to Mike Conte of Conte's Pasta in Vineland, New Jersey. The pasta man made his kitchen kosher, produced Mrs. Stahl's product line, and shipped items to bagel stores in the New York City metropolitan area and beyond—as far north as Great Barrington, Massachusetts, where, in 2015, a local bagel shop continued to identify them with a placard, "Mrs. Stahl's Knishes."

See also KNISH and YONAH SCHIMMEL KNISH BAKERY.

Silver, Laura. "From under the Subway to 'Subway': Mrs. Stahl's Now Made in Jersey." *Brooklyn Papers*, January 21, 2006.
Silver, Laura. *Knish: In Search of the Jewish Soul Food.* Waltham, Mass.: Brandeis University Press, 2014.

Laura Silver

Murray's Cheese

Murray's Cheese, opened in Greenwich Village in 1940, is the city's best-known address for a wide range of specialty cheeses. The shop's current location (and third home) on Bleecker Street is steps from its original site on Cornelia Street. Opened by Murray Greenberg and his brother in what was then a predominantly Italian neighborhood, the shop began as a simple butter and egg purveyor and gradually expanded its offerings to include cheese, pasta, olive oil, salami, and sausages; for bread, there was Zito's bakery just around the corner.

Trading in off-condition items, Murray's was known for its fair prices, and as a result, the store was always busy. At some point in the 1950s, Louis Tudda, a young Italian American from Cornelia Street, began working for Murray, first as a stock boy and later as a counterman. By the 1970s, when Murray was ready to retire, Louis was ready to buy the business, so ownership transferred to him. Working with his brother-in-law Benny, Louis ran the business much as Murray had, continuing to trade in off-condition cheeses. The plate-glass windows of the store were papered with handwritten signs advertising the cheeses on offer and their deeply discounted prices. The majority of Louis's customers were Italians from the neighborhood.

A peculiarity of the store was that the cash register that sat on the counter was never used. At some point, it had stopped working, so customers' purchases were tallied up in pencil on a brown paper bag. One of Murray's customers in the late 1980s was Robert Kaufelt, a former supermarket executive who had recently moved to Cornelia Street. Learning one day that Louis had lost his lease and was closing, Kaufelt suggested relocating to the spot on the corner being vacated by the J Durando Meat company. Louis was not interested, so Kaufelt bought the business, and in May 1991 Murray's moved to its second home at the corner of Bleecker and Cornelia. Louis stayed on in the new location for another year before moving to Italy, and one of his countermen, Frank Meilak, also went to work for Kaufelt; thirty years later, when Murray's was celebrating its seventy-fifth anniversary, Meilak was still with the company.

In its new location, some regulars continued to frequent the store but gone were the off-condition items. Instead, during the mid- to late 1990s, extraordinary cheeses (raw milk, mixed milk, ash-covered) from France, Italy, and Spain began to turn up in the glass-fronted cases, attracting the attention of chefs from some of the city's best restaurants. Faced with a rapidly expanding business and little room in which to grow, Murray's opened a second location in Grand Central's food court in 2000. It was an instant hit but did not alleviate the cramped quarters downtown. So in 2004 Murray's moved once again, this time across the street to 254 Bleecker. After several renovations, the new store (including its subterranean cheese caves) is roughly ten times the size of Murray Greenberg's original shop.

In 2005 a partnership with the Kroger's supermarket chain was begun, and today there are nearly two hundred Murray's Cheese kiosks inside Kroger's markets. Additionally, Murray's has expanded to Long Island City, where it has a large warehouse and newly created cheese caves. So what began as a modest neighborhood shop trading in Italian staples has grown into an important national brand. With its home base still located on Bleecker Street,

Murray's Cheese remains a vital part of Greenwich Village's rich food culture and a reminder of a vanished past.

See also CHEESEMONGERS.

Murray's Cheese website: http://www
.murrayscheese.com/.
Wharton, Rachel. "Murray's Cheese." *Edible Manhattan*, March 6, 2012.
Zarin, C. "The Big Cheese." *New Yorker*, August 23, 2004.

Alexandra Leaf

Museum Food

"A museum is not the first place I look for a good meal. And yet, why not?" wrote *New York Times* restaurant critic William Grimes in 2001. During the last few decades New York City's museums have greatly improved their food service. The older museums typically had utilitarian self-service cafeterias to accommodate school groups and the like quickly and cheaply. Some have also offered smaller, more upscale cafes or dining rooms to members and their guests, like the Metropolitan Museum of Art's Trustees' Dining Room and its Patrons Lounge, which overlook Central Park. In addition to serving good meals, museums have hosted exhibitions related to food and beverages.

Museum Restaurants

As early as 1905 the Metropolitan offered table d'hôte and à la carte meals in a basement dining room, which became a self-service cafeteria in 1922. Repeated renovations failed to make the space very inviting, so in 1953 the museum relocated the restaurant to the Pompeian Court, an atrium gallery of ancient Roman sculpture on the ground floor. Preeminent New York City decorator Dorothy Draper designed the space around a rectangular pool that featured The Fountain of the Muses, a sculpture by Carl Milles. The Fountain Restaurant lasted until 1981, when the water feature was turned into a sunken dining area. In 2003 Restaurant Associates was hired to create new dining options for the museum. Meals are also served in the Petrie Court, and there is a self-serve cafe in the American Wing. Both feature glass walls facing Central Park. Visitors can also visit the Iris and B. Gerald Cantor Roof Garden, with a stunning vista of Central Park accompanied by live chamber music, light fare, and drinks. The Great Hall Balcony Bar, tables set up along three sides of the balcony overlooking the Great Hall, offers cocktails and appetizers, themed to match current exhibitions, on Friday and Saturday evenings. The museum serves its own "Metropolitan martini," an interpretation of the Cosmopolitan cocktail.

In 1993, the Museum of Modern Art (MoMA) opened its Italian-themed restaurant Sette MoMA for fine dining on the museum's seventh floor (*sette* is Italian for "seven"); it later moved to the second floor. On the walls was a rotating selection of food-themed works from the museum's collection. Though the food itself received mixed reviews, museum administrators and restaurateurs took note that upmarket restaurants in museums had merit. When MoMA expanded in 2004, restaurateur Danny Meyer was selected to create new dining establishments in the museum. For the ground floor he created The Modern, a French restaurant with a wall of windows overlooking the museum's sculpture garden, as well as the adjacent, more casual Bar Room, led by Alsatian-born chef Gabriel Kreuther. The Modern received a coveted Michelin star shortly after it opened, and the restaurant would eventually earn three stars from the *New York Times* in 2013. Other MoMA restaurants include Café 2, featuring seasonal Italian fare, and the fifth-floor Terrace 5, a second cafe that overlooks the sculpture garden, with a more limited menu.

Other museums and cultural institutions followed MoMA's lead, opening their own upmarket restaurants. Stephen Starr, the Philadelphia restaurateur, opened Caffè Storico, a high-end Italian restaurant, at the New-York Historical Society Museum and Library in 2011, and Café Serai at the Rubin Museum in Chelsea. Taking its cue from the museum's Tibetan collection, it serves thali plates, chicken tikka masala, handmade momo (Tibetan dumplings), and specialty teas. Another restaurant that reflects the museum's collection is the Neue Galerie's Café Sabarsky, serving Austrian-style meals and desserts.

When The Museum of Arts and Design (formerly the Museum of Contemporary Crafts) relocated to Columbus Circle, it opened the restaurant Robert (named for Robert Isabell, a prominent New York City event planner) on the ninth floor, with a spectacular view of Central Park. Operated by Ark Restaurants, it serves Mediterranean-influenced contemporary American food.

One of the more unusual museum culinary experiences is at MoMA's PS 1 in Long Island City. The contemporary art space boasts a cafeteria run by the French-Canadian chefs Hugue Dufour and Sarah Obraitis. The museum cafeteria, called M. Wells Dinette, offers a constantly changing menu featuring items like foie gras, marrow bones, blood pudding, and goat liver. In 2012, the *New York Times* gave M. Wells Dinette two stars, the only cafeteria to have achieved this distinction.

In 2009 the Solomon R. Guggenheim Museum opened The Wright restaurant, named after the museum's architect, Frank Lloyd Wright. The Wright's sleek design includes a ceiling that echoes the concentric curves of the iconic building itself; in 2010 the restaurant received the award for Outstanding Restaurant Design from the James Beard Foundation.

In 2013 Chef Saul Bolton moved his Michelin-starred restaurant Saul from Boerum Hill to the Brooklyn Museum of Art, the city's second-largest museum. The new Saul, operated in collaboration with Restaurant Associates, is decorated with murals by Paul Kelpe. Its menu features some of Bolton's classic dishes, including a passion fruit baked Alaska.

Until it closed, prior to moving downtown in 2014, the Whitney Museum of American Art presented a striking contrast in its food service. Visitors in search of modern and contemporary art were offered the distinctly homey and old-fashioned selections at a branch of Sarabeth's, a New York City–based chain of small restaurants. At its new location in the Meatpacking District, its patrons can dine at Untitled, a new restaurant from Danny Meyer.

Museum Food Exhibitions

Just as dining has become an important aspect of the New York museum experience, food has taken its place as an important subject for exhibitions. In November 1988, *The Confectioner's Art* opened at the American Craft Museum. The show, curated by food historian Meryle Evans, celebrated artistry in sugar and chocolate from around the world. In 2004 the Museum of Chinese in America, in Chinatown, hosted a major exhibition about Chinese restaurants in America. See MUSEUM OF CHINESE IN AMERICA (MOCA). In 2006 the Cooper Hewitt, Smithsonian Design Museum hosted *Feeding Desire: Design and* the *Tools of the Table 1500–2005*. See COOPER HEWITT, SMITHSONIAN DESIGN MUSEUM. In the autumn of 2010 MoMA presented *Counter Space: Design and the Modern Kitchen*. It explored the evolution of the home kitchen during the twentieth century.

In November 2012 an exhibition called *Lunch Hour NYC* opened in the main building of the New York Public Library. See NEW YORK PUBLIC LIBRARY. The show delineated a century of New York lunches, explaining how the city reinvented that meal. A highlight was a panel of chrome-and-glass food dispensers from the automat. The New-York Historical Society mounted a major exhibition called *Beer Here: Brewing New York's History* in 2012, and in 2013 the Drawing Center in SoHo held the first major exhibition focusing on the visualization and drawing practices of master chef Ferran Adrià, the chef and owner of the now-closed elBulli restaurant, on Spain's Costa Brava. See NEW-YORK HISTORICAL SOCIETY. In late 2012 the American Museum of Natural History opened a long-running exhibit called *Our Global Kitchen: Food, Nature, Culture*, which looked at every aspect of the world's food systems—growing, transporting, cooking, eating, tasting, and celebrating food. See AMERICAN MUSEUM OF NATURAL HISTORY.

See also MUSEUM OF FOOD AND DRINK.

Coffin, Sarah D., and Ellen Lupton. *Feeding Desire: Design and the Tools of the Table, 1500–2005*. New York: Assouline/Cooper-Hewitt, National Design Museum, 2006.
Grimes, William. "Table Hopping; Stick with Cézanne, but the Real Apples Are Also Tasty." *New York Times*, May 2, 2001.

Margaret Fiore and Andrew F. Smith

Museum of Chinese in America (MOCA)

Founded in 1980 to preserve and present the history, heritage, and culture of people of Chinese descent in the United States, the Museum of Chinese in America (MOCA) is a small, nonprofit organization with fifteen staff members and a nineteen-member board of directors. It maintains headquarters at 215 Centre Street and a collections and research center on Mulberry Street.

The museum holds over sixty thousand artifacts, documents, oral histories, photographs, and textiles including the personal effects of five consecutive generations of the Marcela Chin Dear family. Dear's grandfather arrived in Manhattan in the late 1800s, and his descendants began a string of enterprises along Mott Street, including import/export, a general store, a liquor store, and A Bit of the Orient (aka the Rice Bowl), a restaurant proffering *heung ben ball low*, a dessert of fresh pineapple and marshmallow "dipped in the flame of Puerto Rican rum." Other cross-cultural finds in MOCA's collection are a 25-pound Sorico Extra Fancy Texas Patna Rice sack; Fu Man Chews, a 1960s Chinese Checkers board game with gumballs instead of marbles; a suite of imprinted glassine bags; chopstick and fortune cookie wrappers; mustard, teriyaki, and sweet-and-sour sauce packets; and a cardboard takeout box from McDonald's "Chicken McNuggets Shanghai."

Food, the first aspect of Chinese culture experienced by many outsiders, is often a springboard to stereotyping, and MOCA did not explore aspects of Chinese American foodways in depth until 2004, when it opened the traveling exhibition *Have You Eaten Yet?* This analysis of the diasporic Chinese restaurant as a site of cultural exchange updated traditional narratives and drew crowds to Chinatown, helping the ethnic enclave recover from the 9/11 attacks.

The museum's permanent exhibition begins with the story of a 1784 shipload of Appalachian ginger bound for Canton, a millstone used for grinding soybeans in 1850s Idaho, and a porcelain soup plate custom-made in China for New York State Governor Dewitt Clinton. The exhibit further explores Chinese American culture by singling out fifty-two outstanding Chinese American leaders, four of whom were involved in the nineteenth-century food business: a potato pioneer, the developers of the Bing cherry and the Valencia orange, and a trapper who turned Salinas Valley mustard "weed" into a cash crop. Side-by-side displays devoted to chop suey and nightclubs include menus, chopsticks, forks, and La Choy–brand Chinese American food radio advertisements. Also, MOCA hosts public programs on culinary topics, presents "From Coffeehouses to Banquet Halls" walking tours, and sells food-related books and periodicals for children, general audiences, and academics.

Museum of Chinese in America website: http://www
.mocanyc.org.

Sze, Lena. "Chinatown Then and Neoliberal Now: Gentrification Consciousness and the Ethnic-Specific Museum." *Identities: Global Studies in Culture and Power* 17, no. 5 (2010): 510–529.

Harley J. Spiller

Museum of Food and Drink

Although the Museum of Food and Drink (MOFAD) is not yet a physical location one can visit, it is an idea that is well on its way to being realized. Headed by president and founder Dave Arnold—also known as the creator and former director of the Department of Culinary Technology International Culinary Center—and executive director Peter Kim, MOFAD is expected to feature a series of rotating exhibitions that provide an in-depth look at topics related to food history, culture, science, production, and commerce.

Following a successful Kickstarter campaign in June/July 2013, which raised over $100,000, MOFAD went on to launch its first exhibit, called *BOOM!*, a 3,200-pound "puffing gun" that explosively puffs food. The puffing gun has been displayed in parks, schools, and many other locations to teach the science behind every puff and the puffing gun's key role in the larger narrative of breakfast cereal's rise from obscure health food to global, multibillion-dollar industry. This exhibit debuted on August 17, 2013, at New York City's Summer Streets festival. Also, MOFAD has held a series of roundtables featuring experts and advocates to discuss provocative food-related topics such as GMOs and New York City's soda regulation.

A brick-and-mortar home for MOFAD is one of the long-term goals, but according to published interviews with Kim, that permanent home may still be years away. In the meantime, MOFAD is anticipated to develop a series of traveling exhibits and digital initiatives that will be available around the country, if not around the globe.

Museum of Food & Drink website: http://www.mofad.org.

Rudess, Ari. "Details on the Museum of Food and Drink with Dave Arnold and Peter Kim." Serious Eats, July 15, 2013. http://newyork.seriouseats.com/2013/07/we-chat-with-peter-kim-about-the-museum-of-fo.html.

Kara Newman

Museum of the City of New York

The Museum of the City of New York (MCNY) is located on Manhattan's Museum Mile of Upper Fifth Avenue. Founded in 1923 to preserve and present the history of New York and its people, MCNY offers permanent and temporary exhibitions of art and material culture that relate to the history and culture of New York.

The Museum's collection contains over 1.5 million items, encompassing furniture; decorative arts; theater ephemera; prints, including a large collection of Currier and Ives lithographs; and photography, including original works by Jacob Riis and Berenice Abbott. Notably, the museum also has a very large collection of historic toys and was the first institution in the country to establish a curatorial department for toys.

In 2005, the MCNY began a major $93 million phased renovation that included infrastructure updates as well as a completely revamped floor plan. The renovation also reflected a rethinking of the museum's content and how it presents New York's history to the public. The museum did away with such long-standing exhibitions as the old period rooms that showed elite and middle-class New York room interiors from the colonial period through the nineteenth century; the showcases of nineteenth-century toys; and the old seaport exhibit that explored figures from the past like DeWitt Clinton and Henry Hudson. In their place are revolving, interactive exhibits like "Growing and Greening New York: PlaNYC and the Future of the City," "City as Canvas: Graffiti Art from the Martin Wong Collection," and "Making Room: New Models for Housing New Yorkers" as well as longer-term, ongoing exhibits like "Activist New York," "Gilded New York," and "Timescapes," a twenty-two-minute film that surveys the history of New York from the Dutch settlement to the present. Among the food-related exhibits the MCNY has mounted are "A Moveable Feast: Fresh Produce and the NYC Green Cart Program" in 2011, and, in 2012, "From Farm to City: Staten Island 1661–2012," which addressed various aspects of the borough's history including its important oystering and brewing industries in the nineteenth century.

The museum also maintains a lively, interactive website that features online exhibitions such as "Mapping Staten Island," and "America's Mayor:

John V. Lindsay and the Reinvention of New York." An important part of the museum's mission is its educational programs. Through the Frederick A. O. Schwarz Children's Center, the MCNY welcomes tens of thousands of children from the five boroughs for hands-on programs that explore the city and nation's history and urban development in general. It also offers a slate of professional development opportunities for New York City teachers.

Chalsty's Café, located on the second floor of the museum and operated by Great Performances catering company, sells artisanal sandwiches, salads, soups, and other light bites to museum-goers and the general public.

See also MUSEUM FOOD.

Pogrebin, Robin. "Museum of History Unveils Its Future." *New York Times*, August 11, 2008.
Museum of the City of New York website: http://www.mcny.org.

Cindy R. Lobel

Myriad Restaurant Group

See NIEPORENT, DREW.

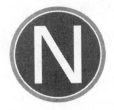

Nabisco

During the mid-1800s, each sizeable American town had one or more cracker bakeries. Crackers and cookies were sold unpackaged directly out of barrels and boxes and without any way to keep them fresh. As they were soon perishable, deliveries had to be made quickly by horse or wagon. Upon arrival the crackers quickly became stale and dried out as the barrel or box was emptied over days, resulting in uneven degrees of freshness experienced by the consumer.

During the Civil War, soldiers and sailors survived on hardtack, a hard, dried cracker that was portable and nourishing but solid almost like wood. After the war, the continued demand for these crackers stimulated the growth of commercial biscuit and cracker production for the general population. At the same time, large parts of the country were moving to an urban economy that led to fundamental changes in eating, working, and home life especially for ready-made food, as there was less time and space to cook and prepare food in cities. Refrigeration and railroads were revolutionizing the transportation of food between cities at an unprecedented speed. To be competitive American bakeries had to learn to be more efficient, improve their ovens and mechanize the process, and be inventive with packaging and distribution. Business people of the time who had studied the baking industry saw that there was a need and opportunity for unification and consolidation.

The New York Biscuit Company

William Moore, a Chicago-based lawyer, formed the New York Biscuit Company in 1890 under the laws of Illinois. It brought together twenty-three bakeries in ten northeastern states. The company prospered from the start, as it was composed of the most celebrated baking firms in the country. Within a year, it had branches in leading cities in the East Coast producing some of the most popular crackers and biscuits. One of those bakeries was the Holmes & Coutts Bakery of New York City, known for its variety of sweet biscuits including the early sugar wafers. It was housed on the east side of Ninth Avenue between Fifteenth and Sixteenth Streets.

The Nabisco Birth

Like the New York Biscuit Company's successful merger in the East, the American Biscuit & Manufacturing Company, founded by Adolphus Green, another Chicago lawyer, brought the same success for the baking firms of the midwestern states.

However, instead of working together, the New York and American companies were soon engaged in an escalating economic battle (and a personal rivalry between Green and Moore). There was also a third western baking combination, the United States Baking Company (with bakeries located in Ohio, Mississippi, and Pennsylvania), that remained neutral in this battle. After years of financial confrontations and price-cutting practices, bakers from all sides wanted to end this biscuit warfare and asked for a consolidation. The result was Nabisco, born on February 3, 1898, in Jersey City, New Jersey.

The National Biscuit Company (abbreviated NABISCO) was established through the merger of American Biscuit & Manufacturing Company, New York Biscuit Company, and the United States

Baking Company. Nabisco, often referred to as N.B.C. (or NBC) was initially located in Chicago, Illinois. The merger of those three trusts brought together 114 bakeries, over 400 ovens, and $6.5 million in cash and supplies in hand to start the business.

Nabisco in New York

Nabisco headquarters moved to New York in 1906 because of the success of its Uneeda brand's biscuits and because of Manhattan's rise as the U.S. financial center. It was located at the Ninth Avenue site of the former Holmes & Coutts Bakery. A new building was erected and was named Uneeda Biscuit Works. This was the official National Biscuit Company's Manhattan bakery until 1958, when it moved into a new modern facility in New Jersey.

The Uneeda Biscuit

The first product that Nabisco introduced was the Uneeda biscuit, which was unique for its patented packaging; it featured a cardboard carton and a waxed inner wrapper. This innovative packaging was called "in-er-seal" and became the landmark of the industry's move from bulk containers and barrels to convenient self-serve packages.

Adolphus Green, the president of the company, aspired to create the best soda cracker and to protect it if possible with some sort of package that would preserve its crispiness. Green thought that the "word cracker had too long been associated with stale and soggy products. The word biscuit used to describe a thin, hard bread that would keep without spoilage for some time and had a more dignified status." After receiving hundreds of name suggestions, he decided on the "Uneeda Biscuit."

Uneeda Biscuit also marked the beginning of the advertising era. In an effort to draw the attention of consumers, Green invented the most imaginative type of advertising. The portrait of a boy dressed in boots, oil hat, and slicker clutching the Uneeda Biscuit box became one of the most widely used advertising motifs in the history of advertising. It was soon reproduced in posters, banners, cards, booklets, and reprints. The Uneeda Biscuit boy helped end the era of anonymous unpackaged foods and introduced that of brands and trademarks in colorful, artistic, and individual packages.

The Oreo Cookie

On March 6, 1912, at Nabisco's Manhattan Bakery, the cookie named Oreo was produced for the first time. The Oreo cookie consisted of two firm chocolate cookies with rich vanilla frosting in the middle and sold for 30 cents per pound.

The Oreo was first registered in 1913 as Oreo Biscuit. By 1921 it had become Oreo Sandwich and by 1948 Oreo Creme Sandwich. It changed to Oreo Chocolate Sandwich Cookie in 1974. Today's design was developed in 1952 and includes the Nabisco logo by William Adelbert Turnier. During the years since its first appearance, the Oreo cookie has been produced in many different flavor varieties and shapes. Recent ones include the Limited Edition Cookie Dough Oreo Flavor Creme and the Marshmallow Crispy Flavor Creme. The company claims that it is the most popular cookie in the world. See OREOS.

Nabisco baked over five hundred varieties of cookies, crackers, bread, cereals, and fruitcake. These include such popular products as Oreos, Triscuits, Barnum's Animal Crackers, Nilla Wafers, and Ritz Crackers. Its most iconic New York brand was Mallomars. See MALLOMARS.

Nabisco was headquartered in New York until the 1950s. Many of its products were manufactured at its bakeries on Ninth Avenue between Fifteenth and Sixteenth Streets—a block where the street sign now reads "Oreo Way." This former Nabisco plant is now home to Chelsea Market. See CHELSEA MARKET.

Nabisco's Corporate History

National Biscuit Company adopted Nabisco as the family name to identify the company and all of its products in 1941, although the actual corporate name did not change until 1971. The company went through a series of mergers and acquisitions and changed names. In 2000, Philip Morris Companies Inc. acquired Nabisco Holdings Corp., Nabisco, Inc., and its subsidiaries. In 2001, Nabisco was acquired and merged into the Kraft Foods business. In October 2012, Kraft Foods split into two new separate companies and the bulk of the Nabisco business went with the global snacks company called Mondelēz International.

See also COOKIES and NEW YEAR'S CAKES.

Cahn, William. *Out of the Cracker Barrel: The Nabisco Story from Animal Crackers to ZuZu's.* New York: Simon & Schuster, 1969.

Eber, Hailey. "The Big O." *New York Post,* February 26, 2012.

Food Timeline website: http://www.foodtimeline .org/foodcookies.html#oreos.

Nabisco website: http://www.mondelezinternational .com/Brands.

Santlofer, Joyce. "'Hard as the Hubs of Hell': Crackers in War." *Food, Culture and Society* 10, no. 2 (2007): 191–209.

Wallace, Emily. "The Story of William A. Turnier, the Man who Designed the Oreo Cookie." Indy Week, August 24, 2011. http://www.indyweek.com/ indyweek/the-story-of-william-a-turnier-the- man-who-designed-the-oreo-cookie/ Content?oid=2640604.

Thei Zervaki

Nathan's Famous

Nathan's Famous Hot Dogs on Brooklyn's Surf Avenue is America's most famous hot dog stand. Begun as a small stand with a single counter in 1916, Nathan's Famous is now a publically traded corporation. It is a brand of franchised fast food stands and retail hot dogs sold in supermarkets nationwide. While the original landmark restaurant covering a whole city block still attracts hundreds of thousands of diners and much media attention during its hot dog eating contest, it is also the home of a national chain that sold 450 million sausages in 2013.

Born in Poland in 1890, Nathan Handwerker was one of millions of Eastern European Jews who immigrated to New York City. Arriving in 1912, he worked in various restaurants on the Lower East Side, including Max Garfunkel's Max's Busy Bee on the Bowery. Always attentive to detail and enthusiastic, young Nathan opened a small Busy Bee unit soon thereafter. By 1915 he had moved to Coney Island where he worked cutting rolls at Feltman's restaurant. See FELTMAN, CHARLES. This grand shore beer garden leased fast food stands just outside the main dining room. The later famous entertainers Eddie Cantor and Jimmy Durante worked at nearby Carey Walsh's saloon and often went to Feltman's stands for hot dogs after work. Friends with Nathan, they urged him to open his own place, where he could be free to sell them hot dogs for a nickel, rather than for the ten cents Feltman and others charged. After saving up three hundred dollars, Handwerker did just that, with a nine-by-sixteen-foot stand at the corner of Schweigert's Alley and Surf Avenue.

The nickel hot dogs worked wonders, but it was the quality of the products and astute marketing that made Nathan's famous. The natural casing hot dogs were made by the new Brooklyn manufacturer, Hygrade Provisions Company (and later by the iconic New Jersey-based company, Sabrett) according to a spice recipe devised by Nathan's wife, Ida. Flat griddled on thick metal sheets, one for cooking, one for warming, the sausages had perfectly browned exteriors and much desired snap when eaten. First-rate crinkle-cut French fries became a featured item. Nathan developed the cutting technique and later machinery as a way to make perfectly cooked fries. The potatoes came from personally selected preferred Maine suppliers and were kept in special temperature-controlled warehouses. With a limited menu and cheap, high-quality items, Nathan's grew over the next two decades with an ever-expanding facility.

Marketing was integral to the restaurant's success. Worried that his cheaper hot dogs might seem unhealthy to potential customers, Nathan dressed some local men in white physician coats and had them eat at the stand. The theory was that if doctors ate there, the food must be wholesome. It worked and business grew. Still, the stand had no name until 1925 when customers urged that a sign be put up. Based on a popular tune of the time, "Nathan, Nathan, why you waitin'?," the eponymous name was put on a large sign, one that would be the brand name ever after: Nathan's Famous. By the late 1930s Nathan's Famous had become an established Coney Island institution. On Memorial Day alone, fifty-four thousand hot dogs were served from the now expanded stand.

Nathan's Famous became a national brand in the 1950s when Nathan's son, Murray took over operations. An advertising agency began serious promotions with fishing contests to highlight the restaurant's seafood additions to the menu. In 1972 hot dog eating contests were begun, events that became national media phenomena by the 2000s. In 1968 Murray turned Nathan's into a public company, eventually developing a number of franchised outlets. After some business vicissitudes, the company was sold to a private equity group and Murray retired having built a major hot dog company.

By 2014 Nathan's operated some three hundred outlets in the United States and overseas and was one of the main retail premium hot dog brands. Its products were made by the John Morrell Food Group, an old Cincinnati company and later a unit of Smithfield Foods headquartered in Illinois. On-going promotions included the Nathan's Famous hot dog eating contest held annually on the Fourth of July, with qualifying events held around the United States. This business model was a far cry from Nathan Handwerker's comment that "you had only one mouth to feed and you could drive only one car and Coney Island is the keystone." But modern Nathan's Famous is a prime example of how small companies can become big players in the national food market.

See also HOT DOGS and STADIUM FOOD.

Abelson, Reed. "Murray Handwerker, 89, Dies; Made Nathan's More Famous." *New York Times*, May 15, 2011.

Handwerker, Murray. *Nathan's Famous Hot Dog Cookbook*. New York: Grosset and Dunlap, 1968.

Bruce Kraig

Nation's Restaurant News

The *Nation's Restaurant News* (NRN) is the major American trade publication covering the foodservice industry. Available today both as a magazine and online (NRN.com), it was founded in New York in 1967. NRN reports on virtually all aspects of the foodservice industry from consumer and market trends, to names in the news, operational issues, national and international business developments, franchising, health and nutrition, current technology, advertising and social media, as well as food, health and beverage ideas—even recipes. Based in New York with reporters in American cities across the country, the publication also addresses current industry challenges such as advertising and marketing. Its opinion section features articles and discussions on diverse subjects, such as the minimum wage issue, scheduling practices and the effect of American elections on the restaurant industry. NRN's website, NRN.com, is the go-to place for job seekers nationally as well as for breaking news in the industry, which is available daily.

The publication also issues e-newsletters, videos, and in-depth reports, such as its Top 200 rankings, and it has a presence on LinkedIn, Facebook, and Twitter. It is currently owned by Penton Media, part of the Penton Restaurant Group, which also owns NRNJobPlate for job seekers and employers all over the country.

Nation's Restaurant News website: http://nrn.com.

Judith Weinraub

Natural Gourmet Institute

The Natural Gourmet Institute for Health and Culinary Arts is a cooking school based on the core belief that food should be delicious, beautiful, and health supportive. NGI began in 1977 as the Natural Gourmet Cookery School in the Upper West Side apartment of the Institute's founder, Annemarie Colbin. Colbin started teaching a small number of students her core nutritional principles: that meals should be whole, fresh, natural, seasonal, local, balanced, in harmony with tradition, and delicious. Borrowing from French, Japanese, and macrobiotic culinary traditions, Colbin's approach toward holistic nutrition was considered quite radical at the time, and sourcing ingredients was often a challenge.

The school soon outgrew Colbin's home kitchen and moved to its current location in the Flatiron District of Manhattan at 48 West Twenty-First Street in 1983. Annemarie Colbin is today Chairman Emeritus of the Natural Gourmet Institute, and has authored numerous articles and books on nutritious cooking such as *Food and Healing* and *The Natural Gourmet*. Public perceptions of the relationship between food and health have changed dramatically since the program's early days, and thus the school has evolved to encompass a Chef's Training Program, a robust roster of Public Classes, and numerous community outreach programs, such as weekly live cooking demonstrations at the Union Square Greenmarket.

Several alumni of NGI have gone on to establish high-end vegetarian restaurants in New York City, such as *Pure Food and Wine* and *Dirt Candy*. While the curricula for both public and professional classes remain heavily plant-based, the school is not exclusively vegetarian or vegan, but rather emphasizes that all food choices should support the health of the individual. The prolific public course offerings are always evolving; current options include *Tempeh*

Temptations, Vegan Umami, and Spices: The Heart and Soul of Indian Cuisine, as well as training in basic knife skills, fermentation, gluten-free baking, and raw food preparations. And for those who just want to sample the offerings of the Natural Gourmet Institute without putting on an apron, the school offers a Friday Night, four-course, BYOB prix fixe dinner. The menu is designed, executed, and served by students in the Chef's Training program and is as much a value to the customer as it is the burgeoning chefs, who use the training as an opportunity to learn menu planning for up to one hundred people at one sitting.

The school also puts its values into practice by relying on green energy (hydropower) to fuel its kitchens, sourcing food from local farms, composting, and utilizing the entirety of plants and vegetables, from root to stalk to frond. The Natural Gourmet Institute's CEO, Anthony Fassio, is also the chair of Slow Food NYC, an organization whose mission is to counteract the negative effects of fast food on society, and which seeks to further build bridges between NGI and vendors that support the biodiversity of plant species.

See also COOKING SCHOOLS.

Colbin, Annemarie. The Natural Gourmet: Delicious Recipes for Healthy, Balanced Eating. New York: Ballantine, 1989.
Colbin, Annemarie. Food and Healing. 10th anniversary ed. New York: Ballantine, 1996.
Marano, Hara Estroff. "Vanity Fare." Psychology Today 1, no. 4 (2008): 55–56.
Natural Gourmet Institute website: http://www .naturalgourmetinstitute.com.

Sherri Machlin

Nedick's

Before the word "ubiquitous" became attached to Starbucks, before the terms "fast food" and "wallet-friendly" were appropriated by McDonald's and Dunkin' Donuts, there was Nedick's, the original ubiquitous fast-food, wallet-friendly enterprise. For nearly seven decades, beginning in 1913, Nedick's was the stop of choice for the on-the-go New Yorker—cash strapped or not.

Nedick's name derives from its founding owners: Robert Neely, a wealthy real estate investor, and Orville A. Dickinson, who ran a small store in the Bartholdi Hotel, at Broadway and Twenty-Third Street in Manhattan. The initial site was a little booth adjacent to Dickinson's hotel store. The partners fashioned their business after Clements, an Atlantic City juice operation, establishing the city's first orange drink stand. Four years later, there were thirteen locations; by 1929, there were 140 stands citywide, with a growing presence in other Mid-Atlantic Seaboard cities—and soon thereafter, Chicago. At its peak in those early days, there were more than 180 leaseholds, and between 1921 and 1927 the company grossed $10 million. That's a lot of ten-cent juice, franks, coffee, and donuts.

The Great Depression took its toll on Nedick's. By 1934, only forty locations remained, and the ten-cent menu had been reduced to a nickel. Rents, however, remained constant—"prohibitive," according to Mr. Neely. Now the sole owner, he watched as title to the assets of Nedick's, Inc., passed to Morris Wertheim, A. M. Rosenthal, and R. T. Johnson, who had purchased them at auction for $48,000. See DEPRESSION FOOD.

Customer loyalty, brand-name recognition, and savvy stewardship prevailed, however. When the new owners eventually partnered with Max Geller of Weiss & Geller, a Manhattan advertising agency, Nedick's turned a financial corner. Their first innovation was to add vitamin B1 to the orange drink and to advertise it that way. This had worked for sales of bread and milk, and it worked for Nedick's.

Then, there were state-of-the-art radio spots that sold listeners on the benefits of fortified orange drink—and the 1944 introduction of mascot-like "Little Nick," who regularly sang its praises on air. There was also the "Ten-Cent Breakfast." Breakfast was offered at a loss, but it incentivized customers to return throughout the day. Between 1941 and 1946, Nedick's business tripled.

Almost from the start, Nedick's non-threatening competitors included Chock Full o' Nuts, some small chain restaurants, and the occasional "wildcat" stand. See CHOCK FULL O'NUTS. But in the 1950s and 1960s, the looming presence of the likes of McDonald's and then Dunkin' Donuts gradually overshadowed Nedick's. By the late 1970s they dominated, and Nedick's frank on a butter-toasted, split-top roll was no longer viable in the competitive fast-food world. In the early 1980s the chain with the lively orange-and-white décor ceased operations.

In 2003, the Riese organization briefly attempted to reestablish the brand. Even with a vastly expanded menu, the Penn Station site failed to create traction with consumers. Riese soon put its acquisition back into retirement. The once-mighty and always-scrappy Nedick's was both the perfect product of the time it came of age and ultimately its victim as well.

Hinckley, David. "It's Good Again Like Nedick's!" *New York Daily News*, January 14, 2003.
"The Man Behind Nedick's." *New Yorker*, February 25, 1928.
"Nedick's: Little Nick Brings Them In." *Broadcasting-Telecasting: The Newsweekly of Radio and Television*, October 18, 1948. http://americanradiohistory .com/Archive-BC/BC-1948/1948-10-18-BC.pdf.
"Nedick's Sells a Loss Leader." *Sponsor: For Buyers of Broadcast Advertising*, January 1947. http://archive .org/stream/sponsor4647spon/sponsor4647spon_ djvu.txt.
"Title to Nedick's Will Pass Today." *New York Times*, April 13, 1934.

Jane L. Smulyan

Nestle, Marion

Scholar, author, and educator Marion Nestle (b. 1936) is the New York University professor who established food studies as a legitimate subject for investigation and scholarship in the United States. Now the Paulette Goddard Professor at NYU's Department of Nutrition, Food Studies and Public Health, and professor of Sociology, Nestle focuses her research on how science and society influence dietary advice and practice. Her popular website and blog, Food Politics, reflects the concerns of food activists, social scientists, historians, and nutritionists in America and beyond.

Born in Brooklyn, Nestle moved with her family to Los Angeles when she was twelve. She earned a bachelor's degree at the University of California, Berkeley, and was elected to Phi Beta Kappa. She continued her academic studies at Berkeley where she completed her doctorate in molecular biology and, later, a master's in public health nutrition. From 1971 to 1976, she taught biology at Brandeis University. From 1976 to 1986, she was a lecturer and associate dean of the University of California School of Medicine, where she taught nutrition to medical students, directed a nutrition education center, and ran a public lecture.

In 1986, Nestle moved to Washington, D.C., where she served as the staff director for nutrition policy and the senior policy advisor in the Department of Health and Human Services in the Office of Disease Prevention and Health Promotion, and managing editor of the 1988 Surgeon General's Report on Nutrition and Health. In 1988 she moved to New York City when she was recruited by NYU to chair its Department of Home Economics and Nutrition. At that time, food studies was not yet considered an academic field, but Nestle had become aware of the increasing interest in the subject, in large part as a result of her travels with the Oldways Preservation & Exchange Trust, a group that brought together academics, food writers, and chefs. When the opportunity arose, Nestle, with the help of food consultant Clark Wolf, initiated undergraduate, master's, and doctoral programs in food studies in 1996.

An article in the *New York Times* describing her goals for the program attracted immediate attention, and fifteen students immediately enrolled for the following semester. Nestle continued to chair the growing department for fifteen years until she stepped down in 2003 to focus on writing and lecturing. A popular speaker and panelist all over the country and the world, she travels extensively. She is also the go-to resource for print, television, and online journalists in need of clear explanations for just about anything related to food studies, in particular how science and society and the food industry influence dietary advice and practice, on the politics of food safety, and on the effects of the food industry marketing on children's diets and health. Among her other concerns are the American food supply, food portion sizes, and the ways in which science and society interact to influence personal food choices.

She is the author of several books, most prominently *Food Politics: How the Food Industry Influences Nutrition and Health* (2002), which put under a microscope the ways in which industrialized food producers and the regulatory agencies and legislative bodies affect American eating habits, and *Safe Food: Bacteria, Biotechnology, and Bioterrorism* (2003), both from the University of California Press. *Food Politics* received many awards: from the Association of American Publishers, the James Beard Foundation, and World Hunger Year. Her other books include the *What to Eat* (2006), *Pet Food Politics: The Chihuahua in the Coal Mine* (2008), *Feed Your Pet Right* (coauthored with Malden Nesheim, 2010), *Why Calories Count: From Science to Politics* (also with Malden Nesheim, 2012), and a book of cartoons, *Eat Drink Vote: An Illustrated Guide to Food Politics* (2013). Her *Soda Politics: Taking on Big Soda (and Winning)*, which is about food advocacy and the soda industry, was published by Oxford University Press in 2015.

Nestle also tweets from @marionnestle and blogs regularly at FoodPolitics.com. From 2008 to 2013, she wrote a monthly Food Matters column for the *San Francisco Chronicle*, and has an ongoing appointment as a Visiting Professor at Cornell University's College of Agriculture, Division of Nutritional Science.

See also FALES LIBRARY and NEW YORK UNIVERSITY.

Food Politics website: http://www.foodpolitics.com.
Marion Nestle oral history. *Voices from the Food Revolution: People Who Changed the Way Americans Eat.* New York University Fales Library and Special Collections, New York, 2009.
Nestle, Marion. *Food Politics: How the Food Industry Influences Nutrition and Health.* Rev. and exp. ed. Berkeley: University of California Press, 2013.

Judith Weinraub

New Amsterdam

See COLONIAL DUTCH and MANHATTAN.

New Amsterdam Market

New Amsterdam Market was a public outdoor market that operated under the Franklin Delano Roosevelt Drive at Fulton Street in front of the original Fulton Fish market from 2007 to 2014. A project of the New Amsterdam Market Association, the nonprofit enterprise was founded in 2005 by former New York City Department of Sanitation and Metropolitan Transit Authority employee Robert LaValva in a nod to New York's long history of practical markets in the oldest part of the city. The purpose of the association was to take over the original Fulton Fish Market site of the Tin Building (built 1904) and New Market (built in 1939) that were abandoned when the markets moved to the Bronx in 2005.

Historically, the highly regulated public market system was the retail source of most fresh food in New York throughout the colonial period and the early nineteenth century. In the second half of the nineteenth century, technological change and a more laissez-faire government led to the decline of the public market system as the primary retail source of New Yorkers' food. Public markets such as Fulton and Washington Market took on a wholesale function. The face-to-face interactions between the producer and consumer of foodstuffs were replaced by more impersonal interactions and food came to New York from much farther afield as its hinterlands spread far away thanks to transportation and technological advances.

Placed in a location central to the shopping and tourist district of Pier 17 at South Street Seaport, the New Amsterdam Market intended to follow the long historical tradition of other indoor markets in New York, such as the still-operating Essex market with the higher-end artisanal food products more akin to London's Borough Market.

When the market was unable to obtain a lease to the buildings from the city's Economic Development Corporation, LaValva instead gained a permit for an open-air market to take place just in front of the building site, in a parking area underneath the elevated FDR Drive, the highway running along Manhattan's east side. The first market was held on December 16, 2007 and featured local fish, meat, cheese, prepared food, and produce purveyors. As it grew, New Amsterdam Market was seasonal, operating on Sundays from April to December and at its height had relationships with over four hundred food purveyors, among them established New York artisanal vendors such as Brooklyn's Acme Smoked Fish, Murray's Cheese, and Russ & Daughters, the Lower East Side store selling Jewish appetizing specialties. These long-standing food sellers joined with farmers and new food artisans from within one hundred miles of the city, such as Long Island wine makers, Hudson Valley cideries, Connecticut beekeepers and fishermen, farmers from New York, Pennsylvania, New Jersey and New England, and many more.

In 2008, General Growth Properties, a spinoff of Texas-based Howard Hughes Corporation, created the permanent Fulton Market Stalls, selling a variety of retail goods and prepared foods. These stalls were located directly across from the New Amsterdam Market and in January 2011, the Howard Hughes

Development Corporation became the city's Economic Development Corporation's partner to develop the South Street Seaport area, of which New Amsterdam Market was a part. The corporation would not lease the Tin and New Market buildings, intending the buildings for other use, setting off a maelstrom around historical preservation and public access to locally produced foods.

On July 14, 2014, founder Robert LaValva publicly announced New Amsterdam Market was permanently closed to the public with the last market having been held on June 21 of that same year. In August 2014, the market's board announced plans to find a new president and reopen the market in its open-air format.

See also ESSEX STREET MARKET; FULTON FISH MARKET; PUBLIC MARKETS; and WASHINGTON MARKET.

Bittman, Mark. "A Food Market for New York." *New York Times*, March 12, 2013.
DeVoe, Thomas. *The Market Book: Containing a Historical Account of the Public Markets in the Cities of New York, Boston, Philadelphia, and Brooklyn. With a Brief Description of Every Article of Human Food Sold Therein.* Thomas Devoe: New York, 1862.
Hanania, Joseph. "Duel at the Old Fulton Fish Market." *New York Times*, January 24, 2014.
Plagianos, Irene. "New Amsterdam Market Plans to Return with New Leadership." DNA Info New York, August 4, 2014. http://www.dnainfo.com/new-york/20140804/south-street-seaport/new-amsterdam-market-plans-return-with-new-leadership.

Ramin Ganeshram

New School

The roots of the New School's Food Studies Program can be traced to the culinary arts courses it offered in partnership with Gary A. Goldberg's cooking school during the 1980s, 1990s, and early 2000s (and the Restaurant School of New York before that), when the university offered thousands of non-credit, continuing education courses to adult students. One-session cooking classes ended with dinner and wine in the cozy kitchen and dining room of the Culinary Arts Program's townhouse on Greenwich Avenue (and later on Twenty-Third Street), while more serious students devoted weeks of study to professional certificates in cooking and baking. In 2007, the New School seized its opportunity as the only university in the United States with curricula in the liberal arts and urban policy, an in-house design school (Parsons School of Design), and a cooking school, to create an innovative, interdisciplinary food studies program.

The program was designed in the New School's tradition of offering socially relevant courses to a broad range of degree seeking and non-credit students, but focused on emerging conversations about food production, environmental sustainability, food science, and gastronomic trends. It launched in 2007 with a mix of credit and non-credit courses on food policy, food writing, and restaurant management; a series of conferences cosponsored with Just Food, Farm Aid, and World Hunger Year; a series of public events, including the inaugural "Culinary Luminaries" panel on Julia Child; and the first of its many collaborations with the local *Edible* magazine empire.

Gary Goldberg and the New School ended their partnership in 2008, but the Food Studies Program continued to grow. The program now offers an AAS, BA, BS, and minor in food studies, collaborative degree programs for culinary professionals with the International Culinary Center, online courses for credit, MOOCs, and the *Inquisitive Eater* blog. In the words of its director, Fabio Parasecoli—professor of food studies and author or editor of numerous books on food and culture—the New School's food studies program is designed to produce "liberal artisans."

The program works closely with key culinary partners in New York City, including the James Beard Foundation, just a block away from the New School's home on Twelfth Street in Greenwich Village; the Restaurant Opportunity Center and its cooperative Colors restaurant, which was founded by former employees of Windows on the World at the World Trade Center; growNYC, which has hosted pop-up food studies classes at the Union Square Greenmarket; and the annual "Edible Institute," among others. Food design programs in collaboration with Parsons and its Paris outpost are in the works.

Cacciola, Jesse. "Brain Food." *Edible Manhattan*, July 21, 2011.
Florence Fabricant. "Food Notes: New School Cooking." *New York Times*, August 19, 1987.

Almaz Zelleke

Newspapers

See *NEW YORK TIMES* and *VILLAGE VOICE*.

New Year

In the early years of the city's existence, New Year's Day was the main secular holiday. Both the Dutch and their successors, the English, exchanged gifts. It was a festive day of visits to the homes of friends, family, and acquaintances, and refreshments were served to all comers. Some revelers celebrated New Year's by "going from House to House with Guns and other Fire Arms, and being often intoxicated with Liquor"—a practice that was recorded as early as 1675. Despite laws enacted to prevent such activities, and a doubling of the city police presence on the holiday, the tradition of celebratory shooting continued until the 1840s.

City residents also upheld the custom of New Year's Day visits into the nineteenth century. New York City was the nation's first capital of the United States after the passage of the Constitution. On January 1, 1790, President and Mrs. George Washington, whose home was on Cherry Street, were visited by Vice President John Adams and other dignitaries. Martha Washington served the guests tea, coffee, and cake.

For many, New Year's Day was simply a day off from work and an occasion for drinking; by evening the streets were frequently littered with the semiconscious forms of those who had overindulged. On New Year's Day in 1837, New York's mayor, Cornelius W. Lawrence, graciously opened his home to the public. Gentlemen came, tendered their greetings, and left; a few drank "a single glass of wine or cherry bounce, and a morsel of pound-cake or New Year's cookies," reported diarist Philip Hone. Then less-refined visitors crowded in the door demanding their share of the refreshments. They devoured the beef and turkey, wiped their greasy fingers on the curtains, drank the mayor's liquor, and discharged "riotous shouts of 'Huzza for our Mayor!'" The police were called in to restore order.

There was drinking in the homes of the wealthy, too, along with sumptuous repasts that featured hot oysters, salads, boned turkey, quail, and hot terrapin. Hostesses offered their visitors rare wines, cognac, bourbon, and sometimes Champagne. An English visitor to New York City in 1870 found that eggnog was "the peculiar beverage of New Year's day," but guests might also be offered apple toddy, milk punch, brandy smash, and mixed drinks, such as the popular Tom and Jerry, a sort of eggnog spiked with rum and brandy and served hot. By the end of the nineteenth century, however, the temperance movement had found some traction among well-to-do New Yorkers. When George Sala, an English writer, made his rounds on New Year's Day in 1880, he was offered coffee, bouillon, and chocolate, but no alcohol. Temperance was not the only reason for the decline in New Year's visits. According to etiquette maven Abby Buchanan Longstreet, writing in 1869, the "generous" hospitality of the past was "too burdensome, . . . with not even standing room in popular households." The most fashionable New Yorkers were now escaping to their country houses for the holidays or celebrating in public.

By the 1890s dining out on New Year's Day offered a welcome alternative to home visits. The traditional menu at the Fifth Avenue Hotel in 1897 included oysters, green turtle soup, terrapin, and, of course, New Year's cake, while the city's Hungarians feasted at the Grand Central Palace in 1899 with specialties like fish soup, veal paprikas, stuffed cabbage, and noodles and cottage cheese.

Over time, the focus of the celebration shifted to New Year's Eve. For entertaining at home there were theme parties with games and supper. A 1904 manual, *Entertainment for All Seasons*, suggested a "turning over a new leaf" décor and a buffet of lobster

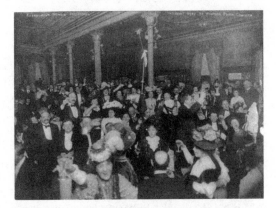

A large crowd celebrating New Year's Eve at Restaurant Martin, December 31, 1906. Around this time it started to become more popular to celebrate New Year's Eve rather than New Year's Day. The tradition of toasting the new year and the old is evident by the number of cocktail glasses in the hands of the revelers. LIBRARY OF CONGRESS

Newberg, Newmarket sandwiches (chopped celery, hard-boiled eggs, capers), Neuchâtel sticks (celery filled with cheese), and snow pudding. But many revelers flocked to hotels and restaurants for more lavish suppers and Champagne toasts. New Year's Eve was becoming a time to let loose publicly, with normal standards of behavior temporarily suspended. In advance of the December 31, 1907, festivities at Martin's Café, a tony lobster palace, it was announced that the normal ban against "respectable" ladies smoking would be suspended for the evening. Newspaper accounts carried the story, reporting that many of the women were awkward, novice smokers. The publicity launched a vigorous debate over behaviors considered acceptable for women in public. Breaking rules was common: by 1921, the *New York Times* reported that despite the onset of Prohibition making selling liquor unlawful, Oscar of the Waldorf expected six hundred to seven hundred merrymakers who would presumably carry their own.

In 1910, the *New York Times* estimated that 100,000 men and women would be out and about, some 3,500 of them at four new restaurants, the Ritz Carleton, Rector's, The Martinique, and Louis Martin's. Taking advantage of New Year's Eve in 1912, a smattering of hotel workers tried to strike. The job action was unsuccessful, but pointed to the importance of public, rather than private, celebrations of New Year's. As high-end restaurant and hotel workers gained union representation in the twentieth century, they negotiated double pay for New Year's work.

Beginning in 1904, street celebrations began to concentrate around Times Square, and in 1907 the first lighted ball was lowered on a flagpole atop One Times Square in a midnight countdown. The Times Square celebration became a national event with the advent of radio, interrupted only for two years during World War II, and a global celebration watched by millions after the arrival of television.

Today, an estimated 750,000 visitors and locals crowd Times Square to watch the ball drop and celebrate the incoming New Year. As watchers can't take packages or bags into the Times Square area due to security issues, many visitors dine before or after the midnight celebration.

For those less inclined to brave the cold weather, many restaurants, clubs, and bars have special prix fix menus and many require advance reservations weeks or months in advance. One of the hallmarks of these restaurant meals is Champagne: more Champagne

is sold on New Year's Eve than on any other night. In anticipation of 2013, one of New York toniest restaurants, Eleven Madison Park, boasted a special rolling cart of Champagne that circulated through its dining room on New Year's Eve, teasing dinners with its offerings that included the coveted Krug Grand Reserve. Others invite guests over to their home or apartment. Still others stay home, enjoy the proceedings on television and sip Champagne at the appointed time.

When the clock strikes midnight, New Yorkers like to welcome in the New Year with a glass (or more) of Champagne and the singing of "Auld Lang Syne."

See also DUTCH-STYLE NEW YEAR'S DAY PARTIES; NEW YEAR, CHINESE; and RESTAURANT UNIONS.

Haley, Andrew P. *Turning the Tables: Restaurants and the Rise of the American Middle Class, 1880–1920.* Chapel Hill: University of North Carolina Press, 2011.

Meryle Evans, Andrew F. Smith, and Cathy K. Kaufman

New Year, Chinese

Chinese New Year, also known as Spring Festival, is the most important festival on the Chinese calendar. Called Nónglì Nián by the Chinese, the centuries-old holiday is celebrated between January 21 and February 19. It originated during the Shang dynasty (1600–1100 B.C.E.).

In New York, the holiday is celebrated with parades through the streets of Chinatown with elaborate floats, marching bands, lions, dragon dancers, magicians, acrobats, and fireworks to ward off evil spirits. Smaller New Year's parades take place in Flushing, Queens, one of the largest and fastest growing Chinese enclaves outside Asia, and in Brooklyn. The holiday ends fifteen days later on *Yuanxiao*, or Lantern Festival.

There are many traditions and beliefs associated with the Chinese New Year, a number of them associated with food. On the eighth day of the lunar month before the holiday, *laba*, a porridge of sweet rice, millet, berries, seeds, and beans, is prepared and eaten. On the twenty-fourth day of the month, the Kitchen God who hangs at the hearth is burned and, accompanied by fireworks, sent aloft for the Jade Emperor in Heaven with sticky rice cakes or a pudding of nuts, candied

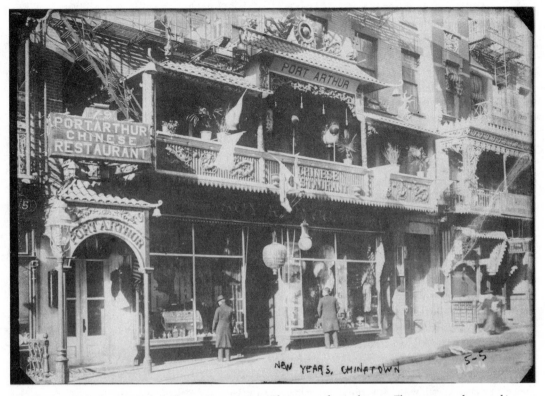

New Year's outside the Port Arthur Chinese Restaurant in Chinatown, date unknown. The streets are decorated in preparation for the celebrations that will occur over the next fifteen days and nights. LIBRARY OF CONGRESS

fruits, sweets, and honey. Most Chinese business owners host a banquet for employees the last week of the old year and give them red envelopes with dollars inside.

Other traditions include decorating homes with symbols of longevity, settling debts, and eating honey to be poison-free for a healthy New Year. Chinese who return to their ancestral homes celebrate the New Year with a Reunion dinner on New Year's Eve. Dishes served at the dinner might include long noodles (to extend their lives), a whole fish (for prosperity), and sweet rice (for a sweet year). In New York, Chinese beliefs and behaviors have been simplified, and are varied but are still of great importance. Traditional foods at the Reunion dinners and throughout the fifteen-day holiday include pork and cabbage dumplings called *jiaozi* and New Year's cakes called *niangao*. Friends and relatives share greetings, gifts, and sweets, and dress in new red or gold clothes to symbolize health and strength. New Year's Day is a feast day. No one takes out garbage lest it cast out family fortunes, and most businesses close the first three to five days of the year.

Guests are welcomed throughout this holiday with tea and sweets from an eight-section round or octagonal "Tray of Togetherness." It symbolizes luck, and is filled with red melon seeds for happiness, kumquats for prosperity, sweet coconut for togetherness, lotus seeds for many children, candied melon for good health, etc. Some modern families have a nine-sectioned-tray—the extra section wishing for wealth.

Families serve a vegetarian stew called *jai*, or *yu-sheng*, a shredded vegetable and raw fish salad. Each vegetable is symbolic of a desired outcome: gingko for silver, black moss for wealth, dried bean curd for happiness, bamboo shoots for good health. Tradition dictates that guests bring oranges or tangerines for prosperity.

Each Chinese year is named for one of twelve animals that visited Buddha. The Year of the Horse started on January 31, 2014, the Year of the Sheep began February 18, 2015, and the Year of the Monkey begins on February 8, 2016. Many Chinese in New York and around the world practice these traditions as touchstones to their past, part faith, part folklore, and part custom. All bring happiness and honor family and friends.

See also CHINESE COMMUNINTY; DUTCH-STYLE NEW YEAR'S DAY PARTIES; and NEW YEAR.

Jenkins, Nancy Harmon. "Tracking Down Oriental Ingredients." *New York Times*, February 5, 1986.

Jackie Newman

New Year's Cakes

Like doughnuts, pretzels, coleslaw, pancakes, waffles, and wafers, cookies were brought to New Netherland by the Dutch in the seventeenth century and became part of America's culinary heritage. And like the Dutch word *koolsla*, or "cabbage salad," which became "coleslaw," the Dutch word *koekjes* was adopted into American English with surprisingly little change. In the manuscript cookbook of Maria Sanders van Rensselaer (1749–1830) we glimpse the gradual Anglicization of the Dutch word *koekjes*, in a recipe titled *Tea cookjes*—buttery, crunchy little morsels baked in a Dutch oven with "fire above and below." See COLONIAL DUTCH.

The story of the American word "cookies" begins with New Year's cakes, which were served at Dutch-style New Year's Day parties in New York some two centuries ago. See DUTCH-STYLE NEW YEAR'S DAY PARTIES. The special treat for New Year's Day celebrations in the Netherlands was *Nieuwjaarskoeken*. Originating in eastern Holland and nearby parts of Germany, *Nieuwjaarskoeken* were paper-thin round wafers baked in special wafer irons that imprinted different images on each side. Some of these images depicted religious stories, such as the Crucifixion or the Resurrection, while others were secular in nature, featuring birds, flowers, and so on. Dutch housewives prepared enormous quantities of these wafers for New Year's Day, because the wafers were not only consumed by family and guests but also distributed to children, who went from house to house singing New Year's songs, collecting their share of the wafers along the way.

In the New World, the character of Dutch New Year's cakes changed greatly over time, as the carved wooden New Year's cake boards held in museums and private collections attest. These boards were used to stamp designs on the American version of Dutch New Year's cakes. The American cakes were not iron-baked wafers but oven-baked "little cakes" made from dough rolled out with a pin.

How did an iron-baked wafer become an oven-baked little cake imprinted with a cake board? It appears that American New Year's cakes were a fusion of the original Dutch *Nieuwjaarskoek*, described above, and a Dutch spice cookie called *speculaas*. A traditional treat for the Dutch holiday of Saint Nicolas Day, celebrated on December 6, *speculaas* is formed by molding dough in fanciful wooden forms, a procedure similar to that used to form American New Year's cakes. Cookies much like *speculaas* are still familiar in this country today, such as the large "Santa Claus cookies" popular at Christmas and the smaller, often cinnamon-scented "windmill cookies."

The American version of New Year's cakes was originally popularized by the New Year's Day parties staged by Dutch-American families in New York City and elsewhere along the Hudson Valley, areas of historic Dutch settlement. As the food historian William Weaver explains in *America Eats*, "By the end of the eighteenth century, when New York City served as the capital of the United States, New Year's cakes were in vogue among upper-class Americans, who imitated the New York custom of open-house visiting on New Year's Day." An early, humorous reference to New Year's cakes occurs in Washington Irving's 1809 *History of New York, by Diedrich Knickerbocker*, which credits a "mighty gingerbread baker" for being "the first that imprinted New Year's cakes with...mysterious hieroglyphics...." Weaver also explains that New Year's cakes were adopted early on by certain Protestant groups outside the New York area, in particular, the Quakers and Congregationalists. These groups were drawn to the cakes because they celebrated a secular holiday rather than Christmas, which these groups still disdained at the time.

American New Year's cakes were likely invented by commercial bakers, who found it much more expedient to roll out dough and stamp it with a cake board than to bake wafers in irons. Many early American families thought of New Year's cakes as store-bought products, and some prominent families, who could expect many New Year's Day callers, bought the cakes in enormous quantities. However, New Year's Cakes were also made at home. Recipes geared to the smaller cake boards typical for home use appear in the manuscript cookbooks of influential Dutch-American families such as the Van Rensselaers, the Van Cortlandts, and the Brooklyn Lefferts, among many others. Many recipes also appear in

American cookbooks published from 1796 to the time of the Civil War and even beyond.

Crucially, some American cookbook recipes are titled "New York cookies" or simply "cookies" in reference to the cakes' Dutch ancestry. This naming brings us to the lasting legacy of New Year's cakes, which was first predicted by certain recipes for the cakes that show up in American cookbooks in the early 1840s. In these recipes eggs have been added (the original American New Year's cakes were eggless), and the typical original seasoning of caraway seeds has been replaced by then-popular American flavors like rose water, grated lemon zest, and nutmeg. Most significant of all, the distinctive stamping with a cake board has disappeared; instead, the dough is just rolled out and cut into rounds. These far-flung adaptations were no longer really New Year's Cakes, of course, and soon enough, the recipes in cookbooks are no longer so titled. Instead, the recipes are called simply "cookies." In modern terms, these "cookies" are sugar cookies of a rather plain sort—the kind of sugar cookies that a housewife could bake cheaply and conveniently, in huge batches, to feed a houseful of hungry children. Over time, many other "little cakes," as Anglo-Americans once referred to the genre, would also come to be known as "cookies."

Commercial New Year's cakes survived well into the twentieth century in areas of historic Dutch settlement. Baker Otto Thiebe of Albany offered his customers a traditional caraway-flavored version until his death in 1965. But the lasting gift of these cakes was the wonderfully evocative word "cookies," one of the many contributions to American culture of the Dutch settlers of the New World.

See also COOKIES.

Barnes, Donna R., and Rose, Peter G. *Matters of Taste: Food and Drink in Seventeenth-Century Dutch Art and Life*. Albany, N.Y.: Albany Institute of History and Art; Syracuse, N.Y.: Syracuse University Press, 2002.

Leslie, Eliza. *Directions for Cookery, in Its Various Branches*. New York: Arno, 1973. Facsimile of the 1848 edition.

Rose, Peter G. *The Sensible Cook: Dutch Foodways in the Old and the New World*. Syracuse, N.Y.: Syracuse University Press, 1989.

Rose, Peter G. *Food, Drink and Celebrations of the Hudson Valley Dutch*. Charleston, S.C.: History Press, 2009.

Webster, Mrs. A. L. *The Improved Housewife*. Facsimile ed. New York: Arno, 1973.

Weaver, William Woys. *America Eats: Forms of Edible Folk Art*. New York: Harper & Row, 1989.

Peter G. Rose and Stephen Schmidt

New York Academy of Medicine

The New York Academy of Medicine was founded in 1847 as an organization to promote learning among health care professionals from a wide range of disciplines and practices. According to its original charter it was organized for "the advancement of the art and science of medicine, the maintenance of a public medical library, and the promotion of public health and medical education." The library has been open to the public since 1878.

Since 1927 the Academy has been housed in a stunning Romanesque revival Palazzo on the Upper East Side of Manhattan at 103rd Street and Fifth Avenue. The building is faced with various shades of gray limestone and sandstone, inscribed with classical medical aphorisms, and the front portal, gleaming doors, and marble entryway are among the lesser known architectural gems of the city. It is also adjacent to Central Park and the Conservatory Garden. Apart from lecture rooms, offices and other spaces, it houses the Drs. Barry and Bobby Coller Reading Room (formerly the Malloch Room), which holds one of the finest history of medicine collections in the world, including more than thirty-two thousand books and manuscripts. Among them is the Ebers Papyrus, one of the most important documents of medical practice from ancient Egypt. The strength of the collection focuses on the fifteenth through eighteenth centuries and is built upon several important donations and acquisitions, principally from the collection of Edward Clarke Streeter, which was made in 1928. The reading room itself is a beautiful, quiet place furnished with massive tables and comfortable leather chairs, and is lined wall to wall with shelves bearing rare books.

Not well known is that the library is also a premier site for research in the history of food, partly through the collection of texts donated by Margaret Barclay Wilson in 1929. Wilson taught physiology and hygiene at Hunter College from 1893 to 1933 and was a fellow of the academy. She was also friends with Andrew Carnegie; they both came from Dunfermline, Scotland. Her collection includes more than five thousand works on nutrition, cookbooks, banqueting guides and carving manuals as well as natural history. In her day, she was known as an expert on nutrition and food chemistry and even had a collection of unusual foods on display in her laboratory, which she would gladly show to visitors. The greatest treasure in the collection is one of only two existing copies (the other in the Vatican Library) of the ancient Roman cookbook

De re coquinaria attributed to Apicius, copied in the ninth century at Fulda. Wilson saw it in the Phillips Library in England, which was gradually being sold off after the death in 1872 of the great bibliomaniac collector Baronet Thomas Phillipps. When the Apicius went up for auction, she purchased it and donated it to the Academy. In 2006, the fifty-seven-leaf manuscript was rebound by Deborah Evetts, with support from the Culinary Trust and with underwriting by Brown-Forman Corporation and Kitchen Aid.

There are few other libraries in the world where one can read virtually every single great classic in Western gastronomy, from the late middle ages to the nineteenth century, in one room. The first printed cookbook, *De honesta voluptate*, by Bartolomeo Sacchi (better known as Platina), is here in several editions in multiple languages. Christoforo di Messisbugo's *Banchetti* of 1549 and Bartolomeo Scappi's monumental *Opera* of 1570 are both in the collection. Marx Rumpolt's *Ein new Kochbuch* of 1581 is also housed here, as well as many English works of the same era. The library has a copy of François Pierre de La Varenne's classic seventeenth-century *Cuisinier François*, as well as Eliza Smith's *The Compleat Housewife, or Accomplished Gentlewomen's Companion* of 1744, and Hannah Glasse's *The Art of Cookery, made Plain and Easy*, in the 1748 edition. Amelia Simmon's *American Cookery, Made Plain and Easy* in the 1748 edition, the first truly American cookbook, is here and is also represented in the third (1804) edition. There is also an extensive collection of nineteenth century menus and culinary ephemera.

Other highlights of the collection include historic editions running the gamut of the history of nutrition and gastronomy in the West. These naturally include the works of Hippocrates and Galen but also the Deipnosophists of Athenaeus, which includes fragments of the first cookbook in the West, the *Hedypatheia* or *Life of Luxury* by Archestratus, written about 330 B.C.E There are editions of the Roman agricultural author Cato the Elder and satirists Juvenal and Petronius, as well as the natural historian Pliny. There are early printed editions of medieval works such as the *Regimen of Salerno* and the *Ortus Sanitatis* or *Garden of Health*, with its famous woodcuts of monstrosities. There are also editions of virtually every single work on nutrition from the five hundred years preceding Wilson's donation. One gets the distinct impression that she opened her copy of Georges Vicaire's massive bibliography of gastronomic texts (also held by the library) and proceeded to purchase every single title. For the researcher in the history of food there are few comparable repositories on earth.

New York Academy of Medicine website: http://www.nyam.org/library/collections-and-resources.

Ken Albala

New York City Coalition Against Hunger

See HUNGER PROGRAMS.

New York City Wine and Food Festival

The New York City Wine and Food Festival (NYCWFF) is an annual four-day fundraising celebration of food, wine, and cocktails under the mantra "Eat. Drink. End Hunger." All net proceeds benefit two hunger relief charities: Share Our Strength's No Kid Hungry campaign and the Food Bank of New York City. What started as a one-night event in 2007 quickly grew into a long weekend of ticketed tastings, dinners, culinary classes, and parties that "bring[s] together the world's greatest chefs, winemakers, spirits producers and personalities to educate palates and entertain attendees in high style."

NYCWFF was launched in 2008 by Lee Brian Schrager as a sister festival to the Food Network South Beach Wine and Food Festival. Both derive cachet with support from *Food & Wine* magazine, the Food Network, and the Cooking Channel. In 2014, the festival had more than one hundred sponsors and vendors from the food, beverage, hospitality, and travel industries and raised more than $1 million for hunger relief from the fifty-five thousand attendees. Personalities from the Food Network and the Cooking Channel, restaurant chefs, cooking teachers, food writers, wine and spirits purveyors, and opinion leaders host or participate in a variety of events, and tickets range from a modest $20 for panel discussions to above $300 for a variety of intimate dinners with celebrity chefs. The signature events are the Grand Tasting Walk-Arounds held on Saturday and Sunday at Pier 94, off Fifty-Fifth Street and the West Side Highway: ticket holders can nosh at hundreds of stations, watch demonstrations, attend book signings, and, for an additional premium, gain access to a special wine and spirits tasting room.

While most of the NYCWFF is geared to titillating the palates of the general public, there are events for members of the trade, making the festival a mecca for the culinary world.

NYCWFF website: http://corporate .nycwineandfoodfestival.com.

Thei Zervaki

New York Cooking School

The New York Cooking School was founded by Juliet Corson in November 1876. Although not New York City's first cooking school (Pierre Blot ran two very short-lived ventures in the 1860s: the Culinary Academy of Design and his confusingly named New York Cooking School), Corson's school became famous for its various curricula, geared to different social classes, especially the economic needs of working-class families.

Corson's New York Cooking School was established in the wake of the severe economic downturn of the panic of 1873. At that time, Corson was the secretary of the Women's Educational and Industrial Society of New York. In 1873, the society opened the Free Training School for Women, teaching sewing, bookkeeping, and other suitable vocations to help women qualify for jobs. Under Corson's initiative, the school added a cooking class in 1874. Although she had no formal background in cookery, Corson studied French and German cookery books and presented lectures while dishes were demonstrated by professional chefs. What made Corson's efforts so successful was her clever emphasis on the delicious economy of European provincial cookery, incorporating such thrifty novelties as tarragon vinegar. When several of her well-heeled colleagues at the society took notice and asked for culinary instruction, Corson opened the New York Cooking School, initially in her home on St. Mark's Place.

As the school became more successful, it moved to East Seventeenth Street, where it eventually offered four curricula: the First and Second Artisan Courses, designed to teach, respectively, the young daughters and then the grown daughters and wives of working-class men; the Plain Cook's Course, geared to young housewives of "moderate circumstances" and to training young women for positions as cooks in middle-class homes; and the Ladies' Course in Middle Class and Artistic Cookery, which incorporated elements of French haute cuisine. Corson's first book, *The Cooking Manual* (1877), attempted an uplifting answer to her rhetorical opening question, "How can we live well, if we are moderately poor?" Its first chapter focused on marketing, and Corson could be seen leading students to New York City's public markets to teach them how to select the best foods for the cheapest prices. Tuition was charged on a sliding scale, and no one was denied instruction because of inability to pay. The higher fees for "artistic cookery" subsidized the other classes and the printing of her 1878 recipe pamphlet, *Fifteen-Cent Dinners for Workingmen's Families*, which was distributed free to families earning "one dollar and fifty cents, or less, per day." The school became a model for cooking education in other cities, and Corson continued to supervise the school until 1883, when her ill health forced the school to close.

See also COOKING SCHOOLS and CORSON, JULIET.

Baumgarthuber, Christine. "Workingman's Bread." *The New Inquiry*, December 10, 2012.
Sapiro, Laura. *Perfection Salad: Women and Cooking at the Turn of the Twentieth Century*. New York: Farrar, Straus and Giroux, 1986.

Cathy K. Kaufman

New Yorker

The *New Yorker* magazine was launched in 1925 by the husband-and-wife team of Harold Ross and Jane Grant, who positioned it as a sophisticated, urban humor magazine. To date there have been only five editors: Ross held the position until his death, in 1951, and was succeeded by William Shawn, Robert Gottlieb, Tina Brown, and David Remnick. The *New Yorker* began publishing serious articles about food and beverages during the 1930s. Alabama-born Cecile Craik, under the pen name Sheila Hibben, originated the "Markets and Menus" column in 1934 and was the magazine's first restaurant critic. She brought acerbic wit and intelligence to her campaign for the preservation of regional American food, observing that it could be the equal of French cuisine if given the attention and respect it deserved. She scorned convenience foods and praised fresh, local ingredients that were affordable even during the Depression.

In accordance with the magazine's sophistication, many *New Yorker* writers wrote about French food.

The journalist and gourmet A. J. Liebling was hired by the magazine in 1935 and began contributing articles—many focusing on French cuisine—the following year. Liebling had made his first trip to Paris while in his twenties. He returned as a war correspondent during the first few months of World War II, and again visited France during the 1950s. His book *Between Meals: An Appetite for Paris* (1962), about the culinary changes he observed over the years, was first serialized in *The New Yorker*. In 1956, Robert Shaplen wrote two articles about Delmonico's, the iconic New York restaurant that had closed in 1923. Mary Frances Kennedy Fisher, who became one of America's preeminent food writers, began her affiliation with *The New Yorker* in 1964. She contributed articles about eating caviar at the Café de la Paix in Paris, about tripe, "secret ingredients," and casseroles, and also reviewed cookbooks.

Joseph Mitchell was hired by *The New Yorker* in 1938. Many of his articles focused on the city's eating and drinking places and the people who inhabited them. His 1939 article, "All You Can Hold for Five Bucks," described the traditional New York City "beefsteak," an all-you-can-eat steak dinner. In 1940, Mitchell wrote about John McSorley, the owner of the venerable McSorley's saloon (founded in 1854) on East Seventh Street. Mitchell collected these stories and published them in *McSorley's Wonderful Saloon* (1943).

Czech-born Joseph Wechsberg wrote about two of the twentieth century's great French chefs: Fernand Point at La Pyramide, in Lyon, and Alexandre Dumaine, at the Hostellerie de la Cote d'Or in Burgundy. Wechsberg published two collections of his *New Yorker* articles: *Blue Trout and Black Truffles: The Peregrinations of an Epicure* (1953), and *Dining at the Pavillon* (1962), the story of New York's premier French restaurant at the time.

In 1963, Calvin Trillin became a *New Yorker* regular. His beat from the sixties through the eighties included his "U.S. Journal" and "American Chronicles" columns, often covering regional American foods. One of his best-known pieces is about the superlative barbecue of Kansas City (Trillin's hometown); he also wrote essays on bagels and Buffalo wings. In a piece for the "Shouts and Murmurs" humor page, "Doing it the Lard Way," Trillin earnestly campaigned to change the national Thanksgiving dish from turkey to spaghetti carbonara.

Anthony Bourdain, the New York chef turned author turned television personality, gave a foretaste of his best-selling *Kitchen Confidential* in a *New Yorker* article titled "Don't Eat Before Reading This"—an insider's look at the seamy underbelly of the restaurant kitchen.

John McPhee began writing for *The New Yorker* in 1965. His meticulously detailed prose lends itself to long, in-depth pieces. For the article "Giving Good Weight," about the early years of New York City's Greenmarkets, McPhee spent time working on a farm upstate and manning a farmer's stand back in the city. His story "Brigade de Cuisine" painted a portrait of a chef who, with his wife, ran an extraordinary little country inn within a hundred miles of New York City (the chef wished to remain anonymous, so his name was changed and the location only vaguely suggested).

Food also turns up in poems published by *The New Yorker*. In 1942, Vladimir Nabokov's first published piece, the poem "A Literary Dinner," savages a fashionable dinner party in rhyming couplets. Sylvia Plath's 1958 poem "Mussel Hunter at Rock Harbor" details her hunt for "free fish-bait: the blue mussels." The magazine published Ogden Nash's "Curl Up and Diet" and "Quick, Hammacher, My Stomacher!" ("Man is a glutton. He will eat too much even though there be nothing to eat too much of but parsnips or mutton.")

Under David Remnick's editorship, beginning in 1998, *The New Yorker* began to publish themed issues, and "The Food Issue" was launched in 2002. Each year this special issue includes brief memoirs, longer-form nonfiction, and fiction with a food angle by writers like David Sedaris, Chimamanda Ngozi Adichie, Adam Gopnik, and Gary Shteyngart. Wayne Thiebaud, renowned for his still-lifes of cakes and pies, has created the covers for most of the special food issues, and food-centric cartoons abound. In 2007, Remnick edited a collection of the best food and beverage articles from *The New Yorker* and published them as *Secret Ingredients: The New Yorker Book of Food and Drink*.

Some of the magazine's food-related cartoons have become iconic, such as Carl Rose's 1928 drawing of a mother telling her daughter, seated at the table: "It's broccoli, dear," only to have the little girl snap back, "I say it's spinach, and I say the hell with it." Rose credited E. B. White with the dialogue. In 1932 James Thurber skewered pretentious wine-speak with the caption to his drawing of a foursome at the dinner table: "It's a naïve domestic Burgundy without any breeding, but I think you'll be amused by its presumption." Also well-known is Al Ross's 1973 rendering of two boys looking up at a McDonald's sign reading, "Over 11 billion served." One boy asks the other: "How many thousands do you figure you've eaten?" Yet another popular cartoon is Robert Weaver's 1989 rendering of a diner waitress clarifying a menu item for a bewildered customer: "It's macaroni. We call it pasta as a marketing ploy."

On its current multiple platforms, even the online blogs occasionally focus on food. In 2014, Sophie Brickman blogged about "The History of the Ramen Noodle," her account of a lecture given by ramen scholar George Solt at a meeting of the Culinary Historians of New York.

See also CULINARY HISTORIANS OF NEW YORK and LIEBLING, A. J.

Remnick, David. *Secret Ingredients: The New Yorker Book of Food and Drink*. New York: Random House, 2007.

Margaret Fiore and Andrew F. Smith

New-York Historical Society

The New-York Historical Society (NYHS) is a history museum and library located on the Upper West Side of Manhattan. The Society, founded in 1804, is the oldest museum in New York City. NYHS offers temporary and permanent exhibitions of art and material culture that relate to the cultural, social, and political history of New York and the nation at large. Among the most popular and well-known temporary exhibits that the Society has hosted since 2003 are Slavery in New York (the museum's largest themed exhibit in two hundred years) and New York Divided: Slavery and the Civil War. In 2012, the NYHS held an exhibit, Beer Here: Brewing New York's History, about the history of brewing in New York.

In addition to the museum, the NYHS maintains a library with over two million manuscript and over four hundred thousand printed items relating to the history of New York and the United States. The archive houses a number of collections useful to historians studying food and drink including the George B. Corsa Hotel Collection; the Bella Landauer Collection, which includes menus, trade cards, and other publicity materials relating to food-related businesses; a menu collection with over ten thousand historical menus from around the United States; and the papers of several colonial merchants and wholesale grocers.

The Society sponsors an active educational program and a prestigious fellowship program that funds scholars doing research in its collections.

A 2011 renovation of the Society's 1908 building included the addition of Caffè Storico, an Italian restaurant run by restaurateur Stephen Starr (who also owns Buddakan and Morimoto as well as a number of restaurants in Philadelphia).

Fabricant, Florence. "Amid New York History, Caffè Storico Speaks Italian." *New York Times*, December 5, 2011.
Gray, Christopher. "Where the Streets Smelled Like Beer." *New York Times*, March 22, 2012.
Raskin, Laura. "New-York Historical Society Gets $65 Million Makeover." *Architectural Record*, June 16, 2011.

Cindy R. Lobel

New York Magazine

New York magazine, an influential city-focused publication, has thrown a spotlight on New York City's restaurant culture for more than four decades.

In general, the publication's focus is broader than just food. As its mission, the magazine says it "covers, analyzes, comments on, and defines the news, culture, entertainment, lifestyle, fashion, and personalities that drive New York City."

New York began life in 1963 as the Sunday magazine supplement of the *New York Herald Tribune* newspaper, where Clay Felker was hired as a consultant. Soon after the *Tribune* went out of business in 1966–1967, Felker and partner Milton Glaser purchased the rights and reincarnated the magazine as a standalone glossy.

On April 8, 1968, Felker published the first issue of *New York* as founding editor, with an elegant cityscape on its cover.

The magazine was influential from its very first issue. It showcased colorful and important voices, such as Tom Wolfe, Gail Sheehy, and Jimmy Breslin, and was considered a cradle of New Journalism. Hollywood found cinematic stories in its pages; articles published in the magazine became the basis for *Urban Cowboy*, *Saturday Night Fever*, and other films. It was also the launching pad for *Ms.* magazine, which began as a "one-shot" sample insert in the December 1971 issue.

In terms of food coverage, Felker was noted for his fascination with power and status—and he decreed that restaurants were as important as business or politics.

Nick Pileggi, writer and early New York contributing editor for *New York,* observed: "Cities were really down when he started all this. We had just come out of the fifties, where the cities were slums.... Clay is out there reviewing restaurants. Little ones, cheap ones. None of the newspapers were doing it. And all of that was critically important to the people who wanted to stay in the city."

The food writer and early New York contributing editor Mimi Sheraton noted that Felker "made service [journalism] fashionable—that was his genius." That included restaurant reviews. From 1968 through 2000, Gael Greene, aka "The Insatiable Critic," was the magazine's chief restaurant critic, though she continued to write as a columnist until 2008. See GREENE, GAEL and SHERATON, MIMI.

In the 2000s, the magazine continued to win acclaim for its food writing, led by restaurant critic Adam Platt, who won a James Beard Award in 2009, and Underground Gourmet critics Rob Patronite and Robin Raisfeld, who expanded New York's coverage to artisan food products, beverages, and Greenmarkets.

Digital food coverage also has been a particular strength, helping to supplement ongoing food news as the magazine reduced its print output, moving to a biweekly format in March 2014. Among *New York's* content-specific websites, Grub Street focuses on food and restaurants.

Bernard, Sarah, and Aaron Latham. "My God, What Trouble You Could Cause!" Clay Felker obituary. *New York,* July 6, 2008.
McLellan, Dennis. "Clay Felker, 1925–2008." *Los Angeles Times,* July 2, 2008.

Kara Newman

New York Public Library

The richness of the New York Public Library's culinary collection is inextricably linked to its mission and its unique position as both a public library and as an independent research library. Unlike most research institutions, the library is not affiliated with a college or university and is therefore not beholden to a singular academic curriculum; the library's collection development policy aims—and has always aimed—to reflect both the traditional works of the academy and the culture of the public it serves. As a result, the library's holdings include popular, less scholastic content rarely found in other research libraries, including a wealth of food-related material.

The NYPL encompasses a branch library system and four research libraries. While special collections of manuscript receipt books, antiquarian cookbooks, and restaurant menus reside in the research collections, the web of branch libraries throughout the Bronx, Manhattan, and Staten Island houses circulating food titles, which include new release and recent backlist cookbooks, food history monographs, and popular interest food periodicals. These materials largely reflect the communities they serve, with an emphasis on regional and ethnic cuisines, local restaurant cookbooks, and New York food interest titles.

Unlike the branches, the four research libraries offer subject-based collections to a community of scholars. Food is a ubiquitous thread weaving its way through the diverse collections, reflected in the holdings of each research center—The New York Public Library for the Performing Arts; the Science, Industry and Business Library; the Schomburg Center for Research in Black Culture; and the Stephen A. Schwarzman Building, for humanities and social sciences scholarship.

One collection of note at the Stephen A. Schwarzman Building is the Helen Hay Whitney Collection, which consists of seventeen culinary manuscripts, and over two hundred printed cookbooks. Whitney, the wife of financier Payne Whitney, was a poet, a race horse breeder, and clearly a woman with a keen eye for culinary riches. Her collection of mostly English-language manuscripts, housed in the Manuscripts and Archives Division, spans from the fifteenth to the nineteenth century and includes rarities such as a fifteenth-century compilation of recipes that closely resembles those found in *Forme of Cury,* a fourteenth-century manuscript housed at the British Museum. The Rare Book Division and the General Research Division are responsible for the printed cookbook titles bestowed to the library by Whitney. The cookbooks range in date from the fifteenth to the twentieth century, with the earliest being a first edition English translation of Girolamo Ruscelli's *The Secretes of the Reverende Maister Alexis of Piemont,* from 1558. The majority of the remaining titles were published in the seventeenth and eighteenth centuries and represent works intended for everyday use in the kitchen.

The Miss Frank E. Buttolph Menu Collection, another culinary resource unique to the library, is housed entirely within the Rare Book Division. While the collection has grown in recent decades and now includes thousands of additional menus from other named donors, it was Buttolph who was responsible for the birth of the collection and for the bulk of its holdings. According to all accounts, she started collecting menus for NYPL at the turn of the twentieth century. By the time she left in the 1920s, she had amassed approximately twenty-five thousand menus from restaurants, hotels, and ocean liners around the world. They include the menus from the inauguration of the Statue of Liberty in 1886, bills of fare from the Fifth Avenue Hotel, and menus from President McKinley's funeral train procession. The collection now totals nearly forty-five thousand menus and extends to the present day. In 2011, the Library launched *What's on the Menu?*, a crowd-sourced digitized menu transcription platform. As of this writing, over seventeen thousand menus have been digitized for inclusion in *What's on the Menu?* and over one million dishes, or items, have been transcribed, enabling researchers to source specific food and drink names such as turtle soup or Diet Coke.

With dozens of languages represented across thousands of titles, the periodicals collection is one of the great strengths of the library. While scholarly journals, such as *Gastronomica*, are represented in the holdings, much of the culinary research value stems from popular culture, women's history, shelter, and industry-specific titles. Trade journals document the changing landscape of the food industry, from hospitality to supermarkets to liquor and home kitchens. Journals and zines focusing on women's history, agriculture, home brewing, and baking spread across the collection and mirror a popular culture in a way that few other research libraries can.

And lest we forget the printed cookbook, the veritable bread and butter of the culinary history world. While they are increasingly making their way into the collections of major university libraries as valuable texts in women's history, material culture, and printing history, the NYPL has been collecting cookbooks since its founding in 1911. All four research libraries, regardless of subject focus, have cookbooks: dance nutrition at the Performing Arts Library, African American cuisine at Schomburg Center, home economics at the Science, Industry, and Business Library, and scores of antiquarian and recently released cookbooks at the Schwarzman Building. All these continue to make the NYPL one of the finest research institutions for food research and culinary history—as well as simply helping you decide what to make for dinner.

See also COOKBOOKS and MENUS.

Ryley, Alison. "Mrs. Whitney's Cabinet Enlarged and Opened: Some Resources in Culinary History at the New York Public Library." *Biblion* 2, no. 1 (Fall 1993): 19.
Stark, Lewis. *The Whitney Cookery Collection*. New York: The New York Public Library, 1946.

Rebecca Federman

New York Strip Steak

New York Strip Steak, also called New York Steak, New York Strip, New York Sirloin, Delmonico Steak, or Kansas City Steak (particularly in the Midwest), is properly a strip loin steak, usually boneless, cut from the *Longissimus dorsi* muscle or short loin primal, along the back mid-section of the steer, between the ribs to the front and sirloin to the rear, and above the flank. The short loin is not a particularly well exercised muscle, given its position on the steer, giving it good tenderness and marbling. While not as prestigious or high-demand a cut as tenderloin or rib steak, the short loin is popular for its ease and flexibility in butchery, good value, attractive presentation, and tenderness. In butchery terms and for restaurant purchasing purposes, the cut is called "Loin, Strip Loin Steak, Boneless."

There is no definitive story of how the short loin became associated with New York more than other cuts, or came to carry the name New York Strip. One prevailing theory is that the designation was primarily a marketing strategy that developed in the early twentieth century when meat began being sold in small sub-primal cuts to restaurants rather than as entire sides or quarters. Anything "New York" had some cachet, so the cut was so labeled to distinguish strip loin steaks from sirloins, top loins, and other similarly named cuts. There is another, possibly apocryphal scenario that, like much New York City food lore, traces its origins to Delmonico's Restaurant. See DELMONICO'S. That story is that one long-standing signature item on the Delmonico's menu was a short loin steak called a "Delmonico steak." As the Delmonico steak gained traction beyond New York City, it took on the name of its home. To this day, New York Strips are also called Delmonico Steaks, though, confusingly, Delmonico cuts can also refer to rib steaks or sirloin steaks.

Because they are well-marbled and have minimal tough connective tissue, New York Strips are tender enough to cook quickly using direct heat with methods

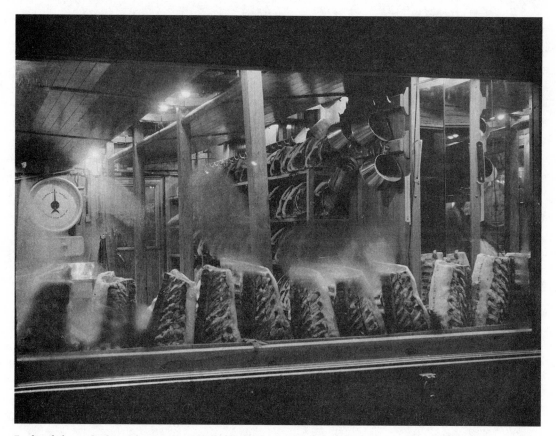

Racks of ribs on display in the meat locker of a steak house, circa 1950. The New York Strip cut is located between the ribs of the cow and its rear, above the flank. MUSEUM OF THE CITY OF NEW YORK

such as sautéing, grilling, or broiling. They appear on the menus of most New York steakhouses today as well as casual dining (chain restaurants), and restaurants nationally. New York Strip Steaks are also available in the meat case of most supermarkets and butcher shops, within and beyond New York City.

Herbst, Sharon Tyler. *The Deluxe Food Lover's Companion*. Hauppauge, N.Y.: Barron's, 2009.

North American Meat Processors Association. *The Meat Buyer's Guide: Beef, Lamb, Veal, Pork and Poultry.* Reston, Va.: North American Meat Processors Association, 2007.

Jonathan Deutsch

New York Times

No news source has influenced what New Yorkers eat more than the *New York Times*. For more than seventy years it has hired professionals to write about food. The newspaper began publishing a "Housekeep-er's Column" in 1875; its unnamed editor published readers' recipes and answered their questions, as well as offered the editor's own recipes. In 1942, the *Times* hired Jane Nickerson as the paper's first food editor. Nickerson's emphasis on food news, rather than just recipes and cooking tips, laid the foundation for the newspaper's coverage of culinary trends during the following decades.

When Nickerson retired, in 1957, the *Times* hired the Mississippi-born Craig Claiborne as its food critic and writer. Claiborne was well qualified for the job, having been trained at L'École Hôtelière in Lausanne, Switzerland. He was among the first restaurant critics to dine out incognito, and the first newspaper writer to rate restaurants using a star system. Claiborne continued to write for the *New York Times* on and off for the next thirty-five years.

Claiborne was the first of many talented food writers to join the *New York Times* staff. Raymond Walter Apple Jr., known as Johnny, came to the *Times* in 1963. Apple served as a correspondent, bureau chief, and later associate editor, reporting on domestic politics, foreign affairs, and, beginning in the 1970s, food. He traveled far and wide, usually with his wife, Betsy (invariably mentioned by name in his stories), discovering obscure local specialties and reveling in world-class restaurants on five continents. Some topics were oysters, mutton, clotted cream, cheesesteaks, mangosteens, and Scotch whisky. In the autumn of 2002, he covered a sweet potato festival in Louisiana and herring fishing in Sweden—while also reporting on the U.S. midterm elections.

Native New Yorker Florence Fabricant became interested in food when she spent her junior year of college in France. She began writing a column called "In Season," for Long Island's *East Hampton Star* in 1972, and very quickly became a celebrity, earning praise from Craig Claiborne. By December of that year she was writing for the *New York Times*, where she has remained a columnist and reporter ever since. Her weekly column "Front Burner" covers the latest in food products, kitchen equipment, classes, and events, and Fabricant's "Off the Menu" postings keep New Yorkers apprised of restaurant openings, closing, and moves.

Growing interest in wine led the *New York Times* to appoint a weekly wine columnist, Frank Prial, in 1972. Eric Asimov, who had been writing the "$25 and Under" restaurant reviews for the paper, took over as Chief Wine Critic in 2004 after Prial's retirement. Since 2011, the *New York Times Magazine* has featured a wide-ranging beverage column called "Drink," by Rosie Schaap.

As culinary journalism, and especially restaurant criticism, became a mainstay of local and national newspapers, attempts were made to put some distance between journalists and the food companies, restaurants, and advertisers they wrote about. Some publications forbade their critics and writers to go on press trips or to accept free meals or merchandise. Newspapers had been publishing restaurant reviews for years, but the professional standards for critics were set by Brooklyn-born Mimi Sheraton, who served as restaurant critic of the *New York Times* from 1975 through 1983. Sheraton, who was the paper's first full-time restaurant critic, initiated the trick of dining out in disguise to avoid preferential treatment from restaurant staff. Her predecessors were Raymond Sokolov, John Hess, and John Canaday, and her successors include Marion Burros, Bryan Miller, Ruth Reichl (who went on to become the editor of *Gourmet* magazine), William Grimes, Frank Bruni, Sam Sifton, and Pete Wells.

Marian Fox Burros joined the *New York Times* as a food reporter in 1981. Aside from her one-year stint as restaurant critic, she has covered the more serious and scientific side of food—additives, caffeine, mercury in tuna, diets, dietary supplements, artificial sweeteners, pesticides, cholesterol—while also reporting about food items new to the market and compiling an annual roundup of mail-order holiday food gifts.

Molly O'Neill, who had written for the *Boston Globe* and *New York Newsday*, began a ten-year stint as a reporter for the *New York Times* in 1989 and subsequently became the weekly food columnist for the paper's Sunday magazine. In 1995 she was the first food writer nominated for a Pulitzer Prize.

In September 1997, the *Times* revamped its "Living" pages into a "Dining In, Dining Out" section that appeared on Wednesdays. The new section included recipes, restaurant reviews (which previously had been published on Fridays), reports on new food products, calendars of culinary events, and articles of local interest as well as broader coverage of food issues and happenings around the United States and the world.

Amanda Hesser began working as a reporter for the *New York Times* in 1997; she wrote restaurant reviews and also edited the Sunday magazine. Hesser was the editor of *The Essential New York Times Cookbook* (2010), taking on the task of testing recipes from the newspaper's entire 150-year history.

Several influential columns geared to efficient but delicious cooking were launched by the newspaper. The "60-Minute Gourmet" ran from 1976 through 1993 under chef Pierre Franey's byline. Franey's farewell column noted that in 1976, "the notion of preparing an entire home-cooked meal in less than an hour was formidable." The column led to several popular *60 Minute Gourmet Cookbooks*. Mark Bittman's practical column "The Minimalist" ran in the *Times* from 1997 through 2011. His aim was to help readers "create exciting dishes with the smallest number of ingredients and the least fuss." The column grew into a blockbuster book, *How to Cook Everything* (1998), with several sequels. Bittman continues to write for both the Wednesday food section and the Sunday *Magazine*, often addressing issues of healthful eating and food sustainability.

Kim Severson wrote about food for the *San Francisco Chronicle* for six years before arriving at the *New York Times* in 2004. She often writes about regional American food and has covered everything from Girl Scout cookies and Jamaican beef patties to the fate of New Orleans restaurants after Hurricane Katrina.

Severson has won four James Beard Awards for journalism.

Julia Moskin, who began reporting on food news and trends for the *Times* in 2004, frequently writes the section's main feature story. Melissa Clark, who worked as a professional cook before deciding to become a writer, has since 2007 penned the paper's weekly column "A Good Appetite," which offers new twists on classics for readers who cook family dinners.

In 2014 the *Times* renamed the Dining section "Food" and launched a comprehensive companion website called "Cooking" that offers a database of more than sixteen thousand recipes.

See also CLAIBORNE, CRAIG; FRANEY, PIERRE; GRIMES, WILLIAM; HESSER, AMANDA; JAMES BEARD AWARDS; NICKERSON, JANE; O'NEILL, MOLLY; RESTAURANTS; RESTAURANT REVIEWING; SHERATON, MIMI; and SOKOLOV, RAYMOND.

Johnston, Josée, and Shyon Baumann. *Foodies: Democracy and Distinction in the Gourmet Foodscape.* New York: Routledge, 2010.
Smith, Andrew F. *Eating History: Thirty Turning Points in the Making of American Cuisine.* New York: Columbia University Press, 2009.

Andrew F. Smith

New York University

The New York University food studies program, begun in 1996, is the largest stand-alone academic food studies program in the United States. Employing interdisciplinary approaches from the humanities and the social sciences, NYU food studies examines food as a bio-cultural system focused on the urban environment. Its curriculum prepares students to analyze the current American food systems, global connections, and local alternatives. Located within NYU's Steinhardt School of Culture, Education and Human Development, the NYU Food Studies program is emblematic of the Steinhardt School's mission of focusing teaching and research at the intersection of theoretical and applied approaches to knowledge. Further, its administrative location, housed in a department alongside nutrition and public health programs, has afforded the program a privileged optic into food in the modern biomedical system, allowing students to examine the connections among expertise and everyday experience, illness, wellness, and the politics of health and food professions. The program also offers experiential travel learning courses in global, domestic, and local venues.

More specifically, the NYU food studies curriculum has emphasized the ways individuals, communities, and societies relate to and represent food within a spatial, cultural, and historical context. It examines the political, economic, and geographic framework of food production, while attending to the study of consumption, including gastronomy, and media portrayals of chefs and cuisines, along with attention to problems that follow consumption, such as the re-making of bodies, accumulation of waste, and burdens of externalizing costs. The role food plays in urban culture, flows of people, commodities, produce, and media products, is the prime locus of the program's investigations.

NYU food studies offers degrees at the undergraduate, master's, and doctoral levels. The master's program, consisting of approximately 120 students, is the largest of the three. The master's program includes forty credits of core, specialization, elective, and research courses. Students select one of two areas of concentration: Food Culture, which explores food consumption from a humanities or social science perspective, or Food Systems, which focuses on issues of sustainable food production from a perspective of political economy, though there is much crossover between the two. Students complete the master's degree program with a capstone project that ranges from a traditional thesis-type research paper to more applied or creative projects. Applied projects have included book proposals, computer applications, websites, food or beverage production or marketing projects, restaurant or market concepts, screenplays, and long-form journalism.

NYU food studies students combine academics with hands-on experience in the form of internships and classes in its teaching kitchen and the NYU Urban Farm Lab. Alumni find employment in food production companies, nonprofit food organizations, publishers, public relations and marketing firms, magazines, food distributors, food producers, restaurants, and educational institutions. The master's and undergraduate programs include a strong applied/practical component, while also emphasizing the development of critical thinking and research skills.

Program Origins and Development

While food had always been well-represented topic in the disciplines of anthropology and folklore, in the

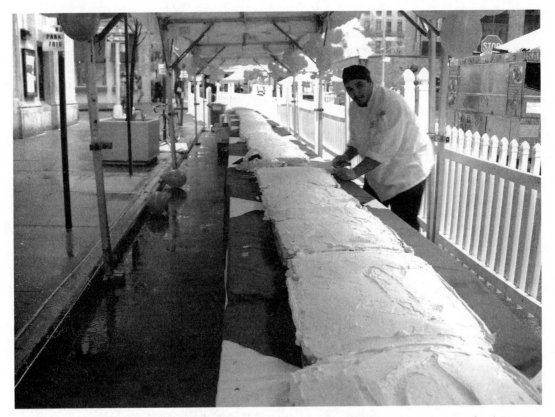

Among the many food-related events at New York University is the annual Strawberry Festival, a street fair that includes carnival games, live music, and New York City's longest strawberry shortcake. Here a pastry chef frosts cakes in preparation for the 2007 festival. JEFFREY BARY

late twentieth century it became ripe for broader academic inquiry. The rise of social history as well as the emergence of such fields as women's studies, ethnic studies, material culture, and other programs that gave voice to the academic study of the everyday and the less powerful, created venues of discourse for food as a primary subject matter. Previously regarded as a quotidian topic more suitable for amateurs, academic interest in the interdisciplinary study of food grew in the late 1980s and 1990s. NYU food studies arose as part of the burgeoning academic interest in the cultural and social study of food in the late twentieth century. Practitioners in this field, originating in anthropology, folklore, and the Annales school, regarded the study of food as key to understanding cultures and societies, and individuals' lives within them. Eating, after all, is much more than ingesting nutrients for biological survival: food plays a significant role in social relationships, is a highly symbolic element in religious rites, aids in developing and maintaining cultural distinctions, and assumes enormous significance in shaping individual identities. Food also helps to designate class, ethnicity, and gender.

Contributing to the continued growth of the NYU food studies program was the emerging food movement in the late twentieth century that arose as an attempt to counter the worst aspects of the industrialization of food. Those involved sought to demonstrate the connection between good food and sustainable agricultural practices and to create better-tasting, higher quality food for restaurants and consumption at home. Scholarly and political attention to food matters deepened as the field of food studies emerged, and as popular books by Eric Schlosser (*Fast Food Nation*) and Marion Nestle (*Food Politics* and *Safe Food*) exposed to an interested public the questionable practices of the food industry and the government's willingness to accommodate corporate demands.

In addition to its origins in interdisciplinary study in the humanities and social sciences, NYU food studies bears a unique imprint from its evolution from a home economics department at NYU, established in the 1920s as part of the School of Pedagogy. As women's opportunities expanded after the feminist movement of the 1960s and 1970s, home economics departments were falling out of favor and out of necessity began transforming themselves into programs more relevant to contemporary needs and attitudes.

By 1987, the NYU home economics department had evolved into a nutrition, food management, and hospitality program and hired Marion Nestle, as department chair in 1988. Nestle earned a PhD in molecular biology and an MPH in public health nutrition from University of California, Berkeley. Nestle, who had previously held positions at Brandeis University and the UCSF School of Medicine, arrived at NYU after serving as senior nutrition policy advisor in the Department of Health and Human Services and editor of *The Surgeon General's Report on Nutrition and Health* from 1986–1988. Nestle recognized a potential, untapped synergy with New York City's abundance of distinctive food traditions and practices, restaurant culture, and food-related media and publishing mecca. She believed that there would be people in the culinary industry, for example, who would seek retraining in other aspects of the food industry (publishing, cookbook writing, nonprofits, public relations), and along with food industry professional Clark Wolf, worked to establish a program that took an academic approach to food as opposed to an applied culinary approach. This program, eventually attained the name "food studies," was approved by NYU administrators and hired food historian Amy Bentley as the first tenure-track faculty member. Classes began in the fall 1996 semester. Jennifer Berg (MA 1996 and PhD 2006) helped shape the original curriculum, and serves as clinical associate professor and director for the Graduate Program in Food Studies.

NYU Food Studies in the Twenty-First Century

NYU food studies continues to grow and develop in the early twenty-first century, and is viewed as a leader by many other food studies programs that have been created in the United States and globally. In addition to Nestle, Bentley, and Berg, current faculty include Krishnendu Ray (sociology), Carolyn Dimitri (economics), and Gustavo Setrini (political science). As a result of the continuing national conversation in issues of agricultural sustainability, global food systems, and health and nutritional disparities among populations, the program expanded its food system offerings. In 2012, after several years of planning, the department broke ground on an urban garden on campus, called the NYU Urban Farm Lab.

Still maintaining food culture/food systems areas of emphasis, NYU food studies has implemented curriculum cohesion with an eye to the following three foci: Planning, Policy, and Advocacy (urban planning, economics, nutrition, business, sociology, social sciences, and allied programs); Business and Social Entrepreneurship (business, economics, nutrition, marketing, consulting, public relations); and Media and Cultural Analysis (journalism, communication, and the humanities). These three areas cross a production/consumption divide.

See also FALES LIBRARY and NESTLE, MARION.

Nestle, Marion. *Food Politics: How the Food Industry Influences Nutrition and Health.* San Francisco: University of California Press, 2003.
Schlosser, Eric. *Fast Food Nation: The Dark Side of an All-American Meal.* New York: Houghton and Mifflin, 2001.

Amy Bentley and Shayne Leslie Figueroa

New York Women's Culinary Alliance

The New York Women's Culinary Alliance is a professional organization whose mission is to foster networking, education, and cooperation for women in the culinary and beverage fields in the New York metro area.

In the early 1980s, New York City restaurant kitchens were dominated by men (still true to some degree today). The NYWCA was founded in 1981 by American chef, cookbook author, and TV personality Sara Moulton as an "old girls' club," a tongue-in-cheek nod to the "old boys' club" environment of the restaurant world. This was a period when women began changing careers, breaking out of typical gender-based roles like teacher, nurse, or housewife. As more women turned to the labor market, the food industry provided opportunities for women to create new careers.

At Moulton's side was charter member Maria Reuge, a food editor at *Gourmet* magazine and wife of Chef Guy Reuge, with whom Sara cooked at La Tulipe restaurant. Seventy-five women showed up to the first meeting, held at Reuge's restaurant. Other charter members included: Miriam Rubin, the first female chef at The Four Seasons; Georgia Chan Downard, who produced Sara Moulton's Food Network show *Cooking Live!*; Peggy Collins of Sarabeth's Bakery; Sandy Gluck, then a chef at Café New Amsterdam; cookbook author Jean Anderson; and food editor Michele Scicolone, who worked in the test kitchen at *Ladies Home Journal* at that time.

The Alliance quickly became a multifaceted organization representing all food professions, including magazine editors, recipe testers, cookbook authors, food journalists, food stylists, public relations professionals, and chefs. It served as a one-stop shop for members who wanted to network with and learn from their Alliance sisters. All members were required to work full-time in the food or beverage industry, live in the tri-state area, and maintain active member status through volunteering, hosting programs, or attending events.

Today the NYWCA continues the organization's original mission, providing members with continuing education opportunities, and sponsoring ongoing food and wine tastings, workshops, field trips, and business-related seminars. It places a strong emphasis on the preservation and sharing of culinary information through member-generated programs. The NYWCA plays an active role in supporting the food community in New York City through outreach programs, volunteer opportunities, and fund-raising for women's health and nutrition.

See also MOULTON, SARA.

NYWCA website: http://www.nywca.org/culinary-alliance/history.

Layla Khoury-Hanold

Niblo's Garden

Niblo's Garden, a restaurant and entertainment complex occupying a full block at the northeast corner of Broadway and Prince Street (today's SoHo neighborhood), was reputedly, during the 1830s, the finest eatery in New York. Founded by William Niblo, an Irish immigrant with a flair for the dramatic, it was the most elegant of his several gastronomic ventures: in 1814, he had opened the Bank Coffee House on Pine and William Streets and, in 1822, a boarding house on Fourth Street in Greenwich Village. When Niblo purchased the block in the mid-1820s, it held only an open-air venue used as a circus and two brick houses. Originally named Sans Souci, an allusion to the summer palace of Prussia's Frederick the Great, Niblo created a pleasure garden, described in the popular press as "a romantic retreat," by landscaping the block with shrubbery, intimate tables, and gravel paths and distributing caged songbirds throughout.

Shortly after purchasing the property, the nearby Bowery Theater was destroyed by fire. Niblo seized the opportunity, erecting a formal theater that seated thirty-two hundred and a hotel and eatery that opened on May 18, 1829; the entire enterprise was renamed Niblo's Garden. It attracted a fashionable crowd, as much for the entertainment as for the cuisine. In 1832, an English visitor, Thomas Hamilton, described his very pleasant dinner as including "oyster soup, shad, venison, partridges, grouse, wild-ducks of different varieties, and several other dishes less notable.... The wines were excellent." Hamilton did, however, critique the service as chaotic and the presentation as inelegant.

Niblo's soon lost its élan as the preeminent dining spot with the rise of Delmonico's, but it continued to play a pivotal role as a leading theater, home to Broadway musicals and the Philharmonic Society. Niblo himself retired in 1858, and the theater was closed in 1895.

See also COFFEEHOUSES.

Batterberry, Michael, and Ariane Batterberry. *On the Town in New York: The Landmark History of Eating, Drinking, and Entertainments from the American Revolution to the Food Revolution.* New York: Routledge, 1999.
Feldman, Benjamin. *East in Eden: William Niblo and His Pleasure Garden of Yore.* New York: Wanderer, 2014.

Cathy K. Kaufman

Nickerson, Jane

Jane Nickerson was the first food editor at the *New York Times*. She has been largely overlooked due to the prominence of her successor, Craig Claiborne. *New York Times* food journalist Molly O'Neill wrote that Nickerson was one of the first food journalists to apply ethics to her craft and noted that there was news in a vast majority of Nickerson's coverage of food.

Nickerson was born on May 19, 1916, in New York City to Eunice Fogg Nickerson and Ralph Brown Nickerson; she grew up in West Medford, Massachusetts. She recalled helping to cook large family meals in summers while in Cape Cod.

Nickerson graduated from the all-female Radcliffe College in 1938 and the following year began her journalism career as an editorial assistant for the *Ladies Home Journal*. She moved on to the *Saturday Evening Post* before being hired by the *New York Times* in 1942. During her time at the *Times*, she penned the column "News of Food" and covered features about food. She guided her readers through the rationing of World War II and the changing food technologies of the time. She reviewed cookbooks and interviewed both home cooks and restaurant chefs.

Nickerson reviewed restaurants and often took along with her the Associated Press food editor, Cecily Brownstone, renowned chef James Beard, and her future husband, Alexander Steinberg, as dinner companions.

The *New York Times* started its own radio program for women that focused on fashion and food in 1948 with Nickerson serving as an on-air contributor to the show.

Nickerson married Steinberg in 1950, and by 1957 she was a mother and ready to leave the *Times* and join her husband in Florida where they planned to continue having more children.

After a few years off to raise her four children, Nickerson became the food editor at *The Ledger* in Lakeland, Florida, in 1973. It was a *New York Times*-owned newspaper at the time. Nickerson ultimately spent from 1973 until 1988 as the food editor at *The Ledger*.

She died in 2000 at the age of 83.

See also NEW YORK TIMES; CLAIBORNE, CRAIG; and O'NEILL, MOLLY.

O'Neill, Molly. "Food Porn." *Columbia Journalism Review* 42, no. 3 (September/October 2003): 38–45.

Mendelson, Anne. "Review of Craig Claiborne's Revised New York Times Cookbook." *Journal of Gastronomy* 6, no. 1 (1990): 78–95.

Voss, Kimberly Wilmot. "Dining Out: New York City Culinary Conversation of James Beard, Jane Nickerson, and Cecily Brownstone." *NYFoodStory: Journal of the Culinary Historians of New York*, 2014.

Kimberly Wilmot Voss

Nidetch, Jean

Jean Nidetch (1923–2015) was an overweight housewife living in Queens when her struggle with her own size led to the founding of Weight Watchers and turned her into a successful businesswoman.

Born in Brooklyn on October 12, 1923, Jean Slutsky did not seem destined for wealth or renown. Her father drove a taxi, her mother was a manicurist. Without enough money to accept the partial scholarship she had received from Long Island University, Jean began a business administration course at City College. After her father died in 1942, she left school and went to work at a series of jobs in New York, including one at a company that published tip sheets for horse players, and another at the Internal Revenue Service.

In 1947, she married Mortimer Nidetch, and followed him to jobs in Tulsa, Warren, Pennsylvania, and New York, where she worked at various low-skilled jobs. In her autobiography, *The Story of Weight Watchers*, she described herself at this point as an overweight woman married to an overweight husband, surrounded by overweight friends.

Nidetch's friends, however, were instrumental to the development of what became Weight Watchers, the now international company that offers support, assistance, and products to people trying to lose weight. In 1962, desperate about her increasing size, she went to the New York City Department of Health Obesity Clinic, where, weighing in at 240 pounds, she was given a strict diet typical of the time. Struggling with sticking to it and occasionally succumbing to a passion for chocolate-covered marshmallow cookies, she turned to six of her friends, and invited them to share the diet and meet once a week to talk and compare notes. The model for Weight Watchers was born, and the organization was officially founded on May 15, 1963. Eventually, she lost seventy-two pounds, her husband seventy, and her mother fifty-seven.

As other friends joined the group's weekly meetings, Nidetch developed a reward system that celebrated their successes. One of the people participating in the program was a businessman named Al Lippert, who encouraged her to turn the program into a business. With his financial savvy and backing, she did. Aspiring dieters pay the company to become a member of Weight Watchers either at in-person meetings or online. The meetings follow Jean Nidetch's model, where dieters can discuss their struggles and successes with the group.

By 1968, Weight Watchers operated franchises across the United States. In 1978, it was sold to the H.J. Heinz Company, which owned it until 1999. Weight Watchers International became a publicly traded company in 2001.

Jean Nidetch died April 29, 2015, at age ninety-one.

See also WEIGHT WATCHERS.

McFadden, Robert D. "Jean Nidetch, 91, Dies; Eyeing Her Girth, She Helped Start Weight Watchers." *New York Times*, April 29, 2015.
Nidetch, Jean. *The Story of Weight Watchers*. New York: New American Library, 1979.
Nidetch, Jean. *The Jean Nidetch Story: an Autobiography*. New York: Weight Watchers Publishing Group, 2009.
Weight Watchers website: http://www.weightwatchers.com.

Judith Weinraub

Nieporent, Drew

Drew Nieporent has been a particularly prolific and successful restaurateur in New York over the last twenty-five years. As the founder of the Myriad Restaurant Group, he has opened restaurants all over the United States and internationally, including such esteemed NYC establishments as Tribeca Grill, Nobu New York City, Nobu Fifty Seven, Nobu Next Door, Bâtard, and Crush Wine & Spirits. He has won numerous awards, among them James Beard Outstanding Restaurateur and Humanitarian of the Year.

Nieporent received a degree in hotel management from Cornell University in Ithaca, New York, in 1977. His first job was as a waiter on a luxury cruise ship line. His first management post was at New York City's Maxwell Plum, owned by Warner Le Roy, who then hired him as restaurant director at Tavern on the Green. See MAXWELL'S PLUM. He further honed his skills at prestigious French restaurants, such as Le Périgord, La Grenouille, and Plaza Athénée's Le Regence.

Nieporent's first restaurant was Montrachet, which he opened with chef David Bouley in 1985, and which was an early step in the gentrification of the Tribeca neighborhood. Montrachet earned three stars from the *New York Times* and kept that rating for twenty-one years. In 2008, the restaurant reopened as Corton, maintaining its three *New York Times* stars and receiving an unprecedented two Michelin stars with chef-partner Paul Liebrandt at the helm. Today, his latest concept, in the same location, is Bâtard, which recently received three stars from the *New York Times*.

In 1990 came Tribeca Grill, which continues to be one of New York's landmark restaurants. It was opened with partner Robert De Niro, and an all-star roster of investors including Bill Murray, Sean Penn, and Mikhail Baryshnikov.

In 1994, again with partner De Niro, now joined by sushi master Nobu Matsuhisa, Nieporent launched Nobu New York City. Nobu NYC, Next Door Nobu, and Nobu Fifty Seven have all earned the coveted three-star rating from the *New York Times*. In 1995, The James Beard Foundation voted Nobu as Best New Restaurant, a major coup for a fledgling restaurant. Today, the Nobu empire spans thirty restaurants in six continents.

Nieporent was one of the few American restaurateurs to go bicoastal. In 1994, in collaboration with De Niro, Robin Williams, and Francis Ford Coppola, he opened Rubicon in San Francisco.

Nieporent is on the Board of Madison Square Garden's Garden of Dreams Foundation, Citymeals-on-Wheels, Downtown Magazine NYC, and DIFFA, an Honorary Chair of the City Harvest Food Council, and Culinary Director of the Jackson Hole Wine Auction. He has co-chaired Share Our Strength's Taste of the Nation event in New York City since 1997.

Myriad Restaurant Group website: http://www.myriadrestaurantgroup.com/our_team_dn.php.
Smith, Andrew F. *New York City: A Food Biography*. Lanham, Md.: Rowman & Littlefield, 2014.
Wells, Pete. "Expressing Himself with Joy." *New York Times*, August 26, 2014.

Eirik Osland

Nightclubs

Nightclubs, places of public accommodation where patrons can enjoy drinks, staged entertainments, and often food and dancing, originated in New York City in the early years of the twentieth century. Various writers have claimed that their antecedents are found in the raucous minstrel shows, concert saloons, dance halls, rathskellers, and even rent parties that drew in different audiences in nineteenth-century and early twentieth-century New York. While these venues traditionally married some forms of entertainment with drink, the glamorous nightclubs are the offspring of the lobster palaces of Gilded Age New York. The lobster palaces, grandiose restaurants described as "magnificently gorgeous at any cost," were located in and around the Times Square theater district offering postshow suppers. Patrons went to see and be seen; they were luxury for those not part of "Mrs. Astor's 400" and, with their all-night liquor licenses, had more than a whiff of the louche. Showgirls from the nearby theaters would sashay in to drink champagne, making lobster palaces famous for their "hot birds and cold bottles." If the lobster palaces challenged the Victorian morality of the late nineteenth century, the nightclubs of the first decades of the twentieth century destroyed it.

Reisenweber's, a lobster palace at Fifty-Eighth Street and Eighth Avenue, is credited with creating the first true nightclub in or around 1901, when it introduced a floor show of chorus girls. Within a few weeks, every lobster palace with a dance floor was offering shows, with dinner and drinks soon relegated to an important but supporting role. The press called these new entertainments "cabarets," after the bohemian Parisian nightspots. Headliners such as W. C. Fields, Sophie Tucker, and Florenz Ziegfeld's Follies regaled New Yorkers in the 1910s and 1920s.

Nightclubs were expensive to run, with their often elaborate sets, high wages to top talent (who earned more in a week than the average American earned in a year), and large staffs to cosset patrons. High operating costs meant high prices for drinks, and nightclubs invented a novel revenue source: the cover charge. Not surprisingly, nightclubs drew the attention of antiliquor crusaders as venues of debauchery, especially as the "dance craze" swept New York in the years leading up to World War I. The Charleston, foxtrot, and tango, danced to the music of black and Latin American artists, replaced the waltz and suggested sexual freedom. The racial and socioeconomic overtones of these dances and musical forms, as well as the fact that, in the 1910s and 1920s, black and white patrons mixed with relative freedom at the Midtown nightclubs, were thought by some to threaten white culture and added perceived urgency to the dry movement. When Prohibition took effect in January 1920, the wherewithal of nightclubs was shattered, at least temporarily.

Although New York City was notoriously lax in enforcing Prohibition, raids did take place, and the loss of liquor revenues killed many of the original, flashier clubs. New clubs sprang up by the mid-1920s. While Midtown continued with the early model, albeit less flamboyantly, Greenwich Village became home to clubs catering to college students, while in Harlem the Cotton Club opened in 1923. Home to such jazz greats as Duke Ellington, Cab Calloway, Count Basie, and Louis Armstrong, the Cotton Club symbolized the social, racial, and political issues of the times, sharply dividing the black community. Some leaders felt that abiding by Prohibition would show to white America that the black community was responsible, moral, and equal to white society, while others saw the nightclubs, with their illegal liquor trade, as a much needed economic opportunity. The Cotton Club's whites-only patron policy for much of its early years did little to ease tensions, especially as it was soon owned by white gangster Owney Madden, diverting money from the Harlem community.

Nightclubs emerged from the shadows after Prohibition, and a new aesthetic took hold, when the epitome of urban glamour was a night at The Rainbow Room, The Stork Club, or El Morocco. The exploits of well-heeled New Yorkers and celebrities at these playgrounds were covered by gossip columnists in local and national publications, fueling New York–style nightclubs throughout the country. The still-extant Latin-themed Copacabana in midtown Manhattan became a household name, memorialized in the 1978 Barry Manilow song. Stalwarts such as the Cotton Club, however, could not navigate changing musical tastes, and the original closed in 1940 as bebop and scat—jazz meant to be listened to, rather than danced to—became the rage. In Greenwich Village, clubs such as the Village Vanguard opened in 1935; it is still operating and was a stage for such greats as Thelonius Monk and Miles Davis. More traditional spots, such as Café Carlyle, longtime home to Bobby Short, still command a premium in price and New York glamour, although the equally famous Oak Room at the Algonquin closed in 2012, a victim of economics in the intimate cabaret setting. One can still experience an updated version of the old lobster palaces, complete with extravagant floor shows worthy of Las Vegas, by heading out to the Russian nightclubs in Brighton Beach, where bottles of vodka are deposited on tables and groaning buffets tax the appetite, including lobster salads on the high-end menus of restaurants Tatiana and Romanoff.

See also LOBSTER PALACES and PROHIBITION.

Erenberg, Lewis A. *Steppin' Out: New York Nightlife and the Transformation of American Culture, 1890–1930.* Westport, Conn.: Greenwood, 1984.

Lerner, Michael. *Dry Manhattan: Prohibition in New York City*. Cambridge, Mass.: Harvard University Press, 2007.

Mackay, Ellin. "Why We Go to Cabarets." *New Yorker*, November 28, 1925.

Perletti, Burton W. *Nightclub City: Politics and Amusement in Manhattan*. Philadelphia: University of Pennsylvania Press, 2007.

Cathy K. Kaufman

Ninth Avenue Food Festival

The biggest, oldest food fair in New York City, the Ninth Avenue International Food Festival, has been drawing food lovers to Hell's Kitchen since 1973. The two-day event takes place every year on the weekend after Mother's Day and spreads over about twenty blocks of the midtown portion of the avenue, drawing more than two hundred thousand people.

In 1973, the Ninth Avenue Association was formed to spotlight the neighborhood, which has a turbulent history. See HELL'S KITCHEN. The association launched the food fair the same year to raise money for charities in the community. Besides food and art booths, there are representatives from wellness groups and community organizations.

The avenue's traditional plethora of cheap ethnic eateries has evolved to include trendy new spots, and so has the festival. The fair now offers everything from classic Italian sausage and peppers to egg creams and elk burgers, with music and dance performances like ballroom dancing or tango on the Fifty-Fifth Street stage.

Haute cuisine it may not be, but you can, as food author Molly O'Neill has said, "eat the world in 20 blocks." There's takoyaki, octopus balls doused with teriyaki sauce and dusted with flakes of seaweed and bonito; Portuguese "meatballs," made with beef and blood sausage; and flaky strudels and rich pies, such as the Greek cheese pie filled with cream cheese, feta, and mint. Corn dogs, crêpes, and even Frito Pies (Texas chili with cheese and chips served in a corn chip bag) are easily found. There are oysters on the half shell;

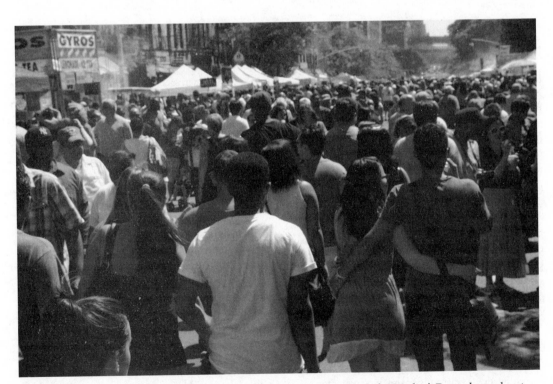

The two-day Ninth Avenue Food Festival takes place every year on the weekend after Mother's Day and spreads out over about twenty blocks of the midtown (Hell's Kitchen) portion of the avenue. COURTESY NINTH AVENUE ASSOCIATION

potato pierogies; grilled turkey legs or ears of corn; a seafood salad of squid, sea legs, and baby salad shrimp; and fried dough in all configurations. In recent years the fair has assumed a greater international profile, with booths featuring the foods of Argentina, Brazil, China, Colombia, Cuba, the Dominican Republic, Ethiopia, France, South Korea, and many more countries, as well as regional North American fare, including the foods of Cajun country and the South.

Some detractors claim the fair is not what it used to be, that it is just a bigger version of any other street fair, with too many sock sellers and not enough booths from the eclectic collection of ethnic eateries that line the avenue. But whether you see it as merely a bigger street fair or a fitting reflection of the wonderfully diverse population of New York City, the Ninth Avenue International Food Festival is an opportunity to taste the world in one city neighborhood.

See also STREET FAIRS.

Molly, O'Neill. *The New York Cookbook*. New York: Workman, 1992.
Ninth Avenue Food Festival website: http://www.ninthavenuefoodfestival.com.

Jennifer Brizzi

No-Cal Soda

In 1904, Russian immigrant Hyman Kirsch founded Kirsch Beverages, a soft drink business in a 14-by-30-foot store in Williamsburg, Brooklyn. It sold ginger ale and grape, celery, black cherry, and other fruit-flavored sodas. At first, he produced twenty-five cases by hand per day and distributed them by horse and buggy. The company slowly expanded during the following years and it relocated to College Point, Queens, where by 1976, it produced 6,000 cases per hour.

In addition to running the soda company, Kirsch founded and served as vice-president of the Jewish Sanitarium for Chronic Diseases (later renamed the Kingsbrook Jewish Medical Center) in Brooklyn. Many of its patients suffered from diabetes, and could not drink sugary soda drinks. Hyman, his son Morris and the company's chemist, Dr. Samuel Epstein, sought an artificial sweetener that did not have a metallic off-flavor, thinking that it would be a boon to diabetics. They came up with calcium cyclamate. Kirsch Beverages introduced the first sugar-free soft drink, No-Cal ginger ale, in March 1953; it was bot-

tled in College Point, Queens. Additional flavors soon came along, including cola, root beer, black cherry, and chocolate. But when the big national soda companies introduced their own diet colas in the 1960s, the modest New York enterprise lost most of its market. In 1970 the U.S. Food and Drug Administration banned cyclamates as carcinogens and No-Cal shifted to other sugar-free sweeteners.

Hyman Kirsch died, age ninety-nine, in 1976. The family sold the business in July 1980, and No-Cal brand disappeared from the market. "No-Cal Soda Pop" was relaunched in January 2005 by INOV8 Beverage Company in Rye, New York, with "retro" packaging and flavors including vanilla cream, cherry lime, clementine, and chocolate. Sales were not great and the brand fizzled out. However, the idea of no-calorie soda remains one of New York's and America's favorite beverage concepts.

See also SODA.

"Hyman Kirsch, 99, Made Diet Sodas; Originator of No-Cal Dies Brooklyn Philanthropist." *New York Times*, May 13, 1976.

Andrew F. Smith

Novels

Despite the title of *The Bostonians* (1886), Henry James sets key food scenes in New York City. That choice makes sense in historical context: the city was becoming known as one of the best food towns anywhere. As Alessandro Filippini noted in 1891: "There is no place in the civilized world where the market for the supply of food is so well provided as in New York, both as to variety and excellence, and even as to luxuries."

James's novel shows the city's high-end dining choices through the choices of two characters pursuing a beautiful woman. One, hoping to show off, takes her to the city's most "celebrated restaurant," Delmonico's, where he "preside[s], in the brilliant public room of the establishment, where French waiters flitted about on deep carpets and parties at neighbouring tables excited curiosity and conjecture." See DELMONICO'S. Her other suitor also plans a dinner, far less showy, at "a very quiet, luxurious French restaurant, near the top of the Fifth Avenue." His "plan" is that "she should sit opposite him at a little table, [while] they waited till something extremely good, and a little vague, chosen out of a French carte, was brought them." See FRENCH.

Like James, novelists have long been fascinated by the choices available in New York—choices ranging from the most elegant dining in the country to the diverse ethnic fare of an immigrant-shaped city to the depressing grub of the city's countless poor. Whether an elegant dish like Delmonico's "saddle of lamb *à la Colbert*" of Caleb Carr's *The Alienist* (1994) or street food like the "frostbitten" yam of Ralph Ellison's *Invisible Man* (1952), such choices characterize novels' inhabitants and enrich their settings.

James Fenimore Cooper may have been the first novelist to draw on the city's immense financial and cultural capital. *Home as Found* (1838) depicts a wealthy family just returned from Europe. Describing a dinner party in great detail, Cooper emphasizes that the meal comes to table in an early version of service *à la Russe*, the predecessor of the modern course structure that was only then coming into fashion in France and not common in America until the end of the century.

New York was well known for wealth and culture, but life in the city was marked by extraordinary extremes. Movement across class lines fascinates novelists and readers alike, and few have captured those extremes better than Edith Wharton. In *House of Mirth* (1905), Lily Bart learns her father is bankrupt while nibbling "*chaufroix* and cold salmon"—leftovers from fancy dinners being the Bart's only gesture toward economy. The rest of the novel chronicles Lily's increasingly desperate attempts to maintain social status, only to recognize that canvasback ducks and fresh asparagus are themselves a kind of prison.

As far as Lily falls, though, there are deeper depths in the crowded tenements explored by Jacob Riis in *How the Other Half Lives* (1890). Riis's nonfictional work, which was terrifically influential on how novelists and others thought about urban poverty, offers little commentary on tenement food except to say he found it "disgusting." See TENEMENT MUSEUM. In *Maggie: A Girl of the Streets* (1893), however, Stephen Crane conjures up the overstuffed tenements: "a dark region" filled with "[a] thousand odors of cooking food"—odors, not smells—where a good dinner consists merely of "grease-enveloped" potatoes. When Maggie first leaves this neighborhood to go to "deh show," she finds a much different world with "[a] battalion of waiters" serving beer and "Little boys, in the costumes of French chefs, . . . vending fancy cakes."

Such movement between social—and culinary—extremes shapes many New York novels. Tom Wolfe's *Bonfire of the Vanities* (1987), for example, pairs the meteoric fall of one of Wall Street's "Masters of the Universe" with desperate hopes of upward mobility in the city's teeming lower and middle classes. Scenes of the rich dining on "vegetable pâté" transformed into "a painting in sauce" alternate with depictions of district attorneys eating deli sandwiches—one "held half a roast-beef hero up in the air like a baton"—because they are too "terrified to go out into the heart of the Bronx and have lunch at a restaurant!" See BRONX. Food becomes central to the novel's view of a fractured city where the divide between the haves and the have-nots is a cliff.

In Wolfe's novel, simple fare becomes a false claim of authenticity by the wealthy, but elsewhere it takes on other meanings. In *The Amazing Adventures of Kavalier and Clay* (2000), for example, Michael Chabon evokes Brooklyn's creative class subsisting on "the thrice-picked-over demi-carcass of a by now quite hoary chicken." See BROOKLYN. Chabon's characters are hardly alone in seeing food as mere sustenance while worrying about other things. In J. D. Salinger's *The Catcher in the Rye* (1951), Holden Caulfield notes the "Swiss cheese sandwich and a malted milk" he invariably orders. To others, though, Manhattan's drugstores and diners can be sites of real longing. In *You Can't Go Home Again* (1940), Thomas Wolfe reveals George's dream of being one of New York's truckers, secure in communal routines amidst "the male smells of boiling coffee, frying eggs and onions, and sizzling hamburgers." See DINERS.

Just as often, though, novelists use food to convey their characters' intense longings for home, for their own pasts. In Saul Bellow's *Herzog* (1964), the main character's memories of his mother intertwine with her love of fish. Herzog finds himself "loitering near the fish store, arrested by the odor" and the sight of the fish "packed together, backs arched as if they were swimming in the crushed, smoking ice, bloody bronze, slimy black-green, gray-gold." Similarly, in *Home to Harlem* (1928), Claude McKay's Jake may dream of "brown gals," but the first thing he does on returning to the city from Europe during World War I is to find "a Maryland fried chicken feed—a big one with candied sweet potatoes." See HARLEM.

But, as Henry James knew, food choices in New York are also self-defining. In Chang-Rae Lee's *Native Speaker* (1995), Henry Park may be nostalgic for the Korean American food of his youth—Flushing's restaurants full of "plates of grilled short ribs and heated crocks of spicy intestine stew"—but he feels most American when he orders too much Chinese food like anyone else. See CHINESE; KOREAN; and QUEENS. And Don DeLillo's *Cosmopolis* (2003) follows the choices of one of the richest men in the world, whose sense of himself depends precisely on being able to have what he wants when he wants it, whether "a plate of pancakes and sausages" in a nondescript coffee shop or "yebeg wat in berber sauce" from a just-closed Ethiopian dive. Brillat-Savarin may have claimed "Tell me what you eat, and I shall tell you what you are," but he could never have imagined a city with so many choices.

See also MOVIES.

Golemba, Henry. " 'Distant Dinners' in Crane's *Maggie*: Representing 'the Other Half.' " *Essays in Literature* 21, no. 2 (Fall 1994): 235–250.

McWilliams, Mark. *Food and the Novel in Nineteenth-Century America*. Lanham, Md.: AltaMira, 2012.

Xu, Wenying. "Sexuality, Colonialism, and Ethnicity in Monique Truong's *The Book of Salt* and Mei Ng's *Eating Chinese Food Naked*." *Eating Identities: Reading Food in Asian American Literature*. Honolulu: University of Hawaii Press, 2007.

Mark McWilliams

NYC Food Film Festival

The NYC Food Film Festival is a competitive film festival that is also billed as a multi-sensory series of events, where audience members partake of the exact foods they see on the screen. It takes place in October each year, and is the flagship production of the Food Film Festival, a larger entity that runs similar festivals in Chicago and Charleston and curates smaller events around the country.

The Food Film Festival was created and launched in 2006 by George Motz, a documentary film maker and Travel Channel host who continues to serve as the festival director. In addition to screenings of the original films in competition, festival events include parties and receptions featuring themes related to the films. Recent events have included a barbeque party, a low country seafood bash, a Peruvian feast, the Edible Adventures series, which highlights particularly unique foods, and the popular Food Porn Party, celebrating the most beautifully photographed food.

Each year's festival screens approximately thirty films, which include world as well as New York City premieres. The submission requirements are fairly loose, with the main stipulation being that the film is about food ("a one-hour film with a two-minute food scene should not be considered to be a 'food film' "), and that the term "food porn" not be taken literally—sexually explicit films are excluded. Films submitted to the festival are judged in seven categories: Best Feature Film, Best Short Film, Best Super-Short Film, Best Food Porn Film, the Audience Critic's Award, the Made in New York Award, and the Food Filmmaker of the Year Award. The judging panel is made up of members of the food and film communities and recent panels have included the Travel Channel's Andrew Zimmern, chef Brad Farmerie, and NBC's Cat Greenleaf.

Recent films that have been screened in the festival include Patricia Perez's *Finding Gaston*, Charles Grantham's *Balls*, Robert Cole and Dennis Rainaldi's *Hog on Hog*, and George Motz's *Head On: Shrimping in the Low Country*.

The film festival has been supported by In The Raw, Warsteiner, Jarlsberg, Bloomberg, and Stumptown Coffee Roasters, among other partners. All events during the festival benefit nonprofit organizations such as the Food Bank of New York, The Billion Oyster Project, and GrowFood Carolina.

See also MOVIES.

NYC Food Film Festival website: http://thefoodfestival .com.

Carl Raymond

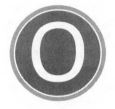

Old-Fashioned Cocktail

One of the oldest and most enduring of classic cocktails, the Old-Fashioned adheres to the original definition of the cocktail as a simple mixture of spirit, sugar, bitters, and water. Its origins lie in the Whiskey Cocktail, which was typically served "up"—that is, not on the rocks—and enjoyed as a morning eye-opener during the first half of the nineteenth century. In 1881, the *Brooklyn Eagle* reported that the drink was a "bracer up" much favored by "the Brooklyn boys."

By the end of the century, bartenders began altering the drink with dashes of various elixirs newly arrived from Europe, such as curaçao and maraschino liqueur. Disgruntled conservative tipplers, disliking these innovations, reacted by asking for an "Old-Fashioned Whiskey Cocktail." Thus the drink won the name by which we know it today. Under its new title, the cocktail was prepared and served in its eponymous glass—a heavy-based rocks glass. The water and bitters were muddled with lump sugar, and the drink was served over ice with a twist.

A drink of nationwide popularity, the Old-Fashioned belongs to all cities and no city. Likewise, no one person can be identified as the creator of what is basically the original cocktail formula. Nonetheless, claims of parentage were noisily made from time to time. "Colonel" Jim Gray, for thirty years the head bartender at the famous Fifth Avenue Hotel on Madison Square, declared in a 1908 *New York Sun* article to have invented the Old-Fashioned in 1881. He didn't, but he most certainly served a great many of them.

Prohibition did not extinguish New Yorkers' thirst for the drink. Following Repeal, the *New York Times* reported, "The most popular drinks in the Times Square and Grand Central districts as well as the hotels along Park Avenue seem to be the Scotch-and-soda and the 'old-fashioned' cocktail." Among those ordering it were women, who, empowered by the democratic attitudes of the speakeasy, now felt free to drink in public. In the post-Prohibition era, the drink was usually served with fruit, and remained popular in that form through the 1960s, when traditional cocktails were eclipsed at bars and clubs by vodka and fruity and fruit concoctions. See PROHIBITION.

With the turn of the twenty-first century and the advent of the classic cocktail renaissance, the Old-Fashioned returned to form, prepared by newly earnest bartenders as it had been in the late-nineteenth-century, as an elemental whiskey drink adorned with only traces of sugar, bitters and an orange or lemon twist. Served at sophisticated Manhattan cocktail dens such as Pegu Club, Death & Co., and PDT, it was newly adopted by young urban drinkers. At many of the trendiest cocktail bars, it became the most frequently ordered drink.

Simonson, Robert. *The Old-Fashioned: The Story of the World's First Classic Cocktail*. Berkeley, Calif.: Ten Speed, 2014.
Wondrich, David. *Imbibe!* New York: Pedigree Trade, 2007.

Robert Simonson

O'Neill, Molly

Cookbook author and food writer Molly O'Neill (b. 1952) has usually been ahead of the curve. She is the founder of One Big Table, an innovative, mostly online community of food writers, bloggers, and thinkers based in Berne, New York, that serves as a useful resource for both current and aspiring food writers. In 2011, One Big Table gave birth to Cook 'n' Scribble, a home for virtual food writing workshops and podcasted lecture series as well as in-person food writer retreats and mentoring opportunities. Its online interactive courses and its retreats focus on subjects like food writing, food memoirs, food history, and blogging about food. The stated goal is to keep food writing lively, literate, and smart.

Molly O'Neill is the oldest of five children, and the only girl. She grew up in Columbus, Ohio, and in 1975 graduated from Denison University. She later studied at La Varenne in Paris. She has been a chef, a restaurant critic, a reporter, a columnist for the *New York Times Sunday Magazine*, and a reporter for that newspaper. She is the author of several books, among them the award-winning *New York Cookbook* (1992); *A Well Seasoned Appetite* (1995); *The Pleasure of Your Company* (1997); *Mostly True: A Memoir of Family, Food and Baseball* (2006)—one of her brothers, Paul O'Neill, is a retired major league baseball player who won five World Series while playing for the Cincinnati Reds and the New York Yankees; *American Food Writing: An Anthology with Classic Recipes* (2007); and *One Big Table* (2010). O'Neill, who traveled 100,000 miles assembling recipes from home cooks across the United States for this last title, has said that the ten-year project was impelled by her desire to investigate reports that Americans had stopped cooking at home. They hadn't.

In 2014, O'Neill launched a series of what she calls Little BIG Books: small collections of recipes reflecting a specific American region or cultural group. Each book contains twelve recipes selected by O'Neill, as well as a profile of the author.

O'Neill, Molly. *Mostly True: A Memoir of Family, Food and Baseball*. New York: Scribner, 2006.
O'Neill, Molly. *One Big Table*. New York: Simon & Schuster, 2010.
One Big Table website: http://onebigtable.com.

Judith Weinraub

Oreos

Oreos are sandwich cookies consisting of two cocoa-flavored disks filled with a vegetable oil-based sugar frosting. The treat was developed by New York-based National Biscuit Company (Nabisco); the patent was filed on March 6, 1912. See NABISCO. It has been suggested that the company came up with the product to compete with an almost identical confection, Hydrox Biscuit Bonbons, produced since 1908 by the Kansas City-based Loose-Wiles Biscuit Company under the brand name Sunshine Specialties. (For a time, Loose-Wiles boasted of having the biggest bakery in the world at its Long Island City location.) No matter the inspiration, Nabisco's version was vastly more successful, selling 450 billion cookies in the century since its inception, making it the best-selling packaged cookie of the twentieth century. Today, the brand is owned by Mondelez International.

Prior to World War II, Oreos were primarily marketed to the modern woman. A 1919 ad for the cookie features a fashionable young woman speaking into a telephone, "I must have Oreo Sandwich for Dessert." A 1927 *Good Housekeeping* ad suggests that they are great to have on hand if you've kept too busy with bridge games to have made dessert. A silver platter of the cookies is displayed next to a stack of fine china. However, by the 1950s Nabisco shifted its sights to a more gullible demographic and began aiming the ads squarely at children and their mothers. A 1954 *Good Housekeeping* ad explains, "Let them have another, Mother, they're pure NABISCO cookies....Kids just love 'em." A contemporary ad features a freckle-faced girl with her tongue stuck out. The copy encourages the kids to "Open up an Oreo Creme Sandwich and take a lick." In the following decades, the industrial confections became a favorite with several generations, undoubtedly because the sandwich cookies were fun to eat.

The cookie was originally sold in two versions, the familiar cocoa colored one and another made with vanilla wafers. The vanilla version was discontinued in the 1920s but revived later in the century. The cookie's stamped design was reformulated several times before the current embossed pattern of stylized flowers was settled on in 1952. Today, Oreos are available in over a hundred variations, in multiple sizes, with fillings flavored with vanilla, chocolate, caramel, mint, berry and lemon, cocoa, some chocolate dipped, and others turned into wafers or cones. The cookies are often mixed into ice cream and used as the basis for other recipes. Restaurants and high-end pastry shops often make Oreo-like confections substituting buttercream and fine chocolate for the original's inexpensive ingredients.

Whereas the gastronomic charm of Nabisco's invention is somewhat dubious, its role as comfort food for generations and consequently its prominent place in American culture is incontrovertible. Beginning in the late 1960s, Oreo came to be used as a pejorative term for African Americans who were seen to be acting too "white." In 1971, Lionel, a black character in the Queens-based sitcom *All in the Family,* explains the term to the show's notoriously bigoted Archie Bunker: "He's what we call an Oreo cookie.... Black on the outside and white on the inside." In a rather different take on the confection, architecture critic Paul Goldberger dubbed the cookie "the stuff of legend" in a 1986 *New York Times* article marking the confection's seventy-fifth anniversary. In his view, "It stands as the archetype of its kind, a reminder that cookies are designed as consciously as buildings, and sometimes better."

In the late 1990s, Nabisco and its ad agency, FCB, thought it would be useful to analyze the cookie's appeal through a series of focus groups. Both adults and children considered the cookies almost magical. Eating the cookies rekindled childhood memories, evoked feelings of nostalgia and made the responders relive "the good things" of childhood. The study was proof, once again, of the powerful magic practiced by the wizards of Madison Avenue on the American palate.

See also COOKIES.

Boland, Ed, Jr. "F.Y.I.: 450 Billion Oreos to Go." *New York Times.* July 28, 2002.

Oreo official website: http://www.oreo.com.

Winston, William, and Larry Percy. *Marketing Research That Pays Off: Case Histories of Marketing Research Leading to Success in the Marketplace.* Hoboken, N.J.: Taylor and Francis, 2014.

Michael Krondl

Organic Food

Typically idealized by consumers as a food grown entirely without the use of additives, such as pesticides, herbicides, and chemical fertilizers, organic food receiving federal certification must adhere to a strict list of allowed and prohibited substances throughout its production and processing, restricting the use of synthetic substances. Organic food has been the fastest growing segment in the food industry since the 1990s. In an interesting twist, in a city known for cuisine, the development of retail markets for organic food in New York City lagged behind the rest of the nation. As in the rest of the nation prior to the late 1990s, organic food was available in New York food cooperatives and health food stores. Although precise information is not readily available, three food cooperatives existed at this time, located in Manhattan or Brooklyn: The Flatbush Food Co-op, the Park Slope Food Co-op, and the Fourth St. Co-op (formerly Good Food Co-op). See FOOD CO-OPS. A handful of health food stores, such as the Westerly Market and Food for Health, were purveyors of organic food.

Yet, during the 1990s, in the United States, organic food marketing began shifting from health food stores to conventional supermarkets. The timing of this coincided with the 2002 rollout of the National Organic Program, promulgated by the U.S. Department of Agriculture, which by the authority of the Organic Foods Production Act of 1990 established the first regulatory and uniform certification system for organic foods in the United States. Part of the impetus for creating a national certification system was to facilitate commerce of organic foods, and to assure the consumer of the integrity of organic food. Over this same time period, the quintessential organic foods retailer, Whole Foods Market, was on a buying spree, purchasing independent natural products stores around the country, such as Bread and Circus, Fresh Fields, and Bread of Life. By the time Whole Foods finished purchasing regional natural product chains, the store had created a successful business and had gained a reputation for being the premier retailer of organic food. Yet despite its large presence in the United States, it was not until 2001 that Whole Foods Market opened in New York City, a date much later than other similar metropolitan regions, such as Boston and Washington, D.C.

In 2015, the main ways for New York City residents to procure organic food are shopping at farmers markets, supermarkets (including the eight Whole Foods Markets), the local bodegas, or through one of the many direct-from-farmer arrangements. The most well-known direct-from-farmer scheme is community supported agriculture (CSA), in which a consumer pays a fee, upfront, to the farmer, for the promise of a share of the harvest over the course of the season. In 2015, approximately one hundred such CSA arrangements existed. Other new, creative business models have emerged, attempting to exploit the current vogue of supporting the local economy while eating organically. One such example is Good Eggs, which acts as an intermediary between consumers and farmers and "foodmakers," taking orders from consumers and then delivering the promised food, in approximately two days.

Despite consumer demand for organically produced food, not all of the food sold through these market channels is certified organic. While few expect all food sold by a supermarket to be organic, or to be local, consumer expectations regarding food purchased directly from farmers are much higher. Furthermore, the relationship between organically produced and locally produced is subject to interpretation. For example, research shows that consumers substitute between organic and local when buying food. From the supply side, few farmers offer organic food at the farmers markets in New York City. More specifically, of the seventy-two farm stands registered for a Saturday at Union Square, the largest farmers market in New York City, only five had official organic certification. Similarly, not all of the CSAs are operated by certified organic farmers. In any case, it may be that consumers desiring the attribute of organic more than local may choose to shop at a supermarket, while those preferring local food may choose to frequent a farmers market or a CSA. Those demanding both organic and local can use a business like Good Eggs, which allows the consumer to specify desired attributes, including local and organic, or can seek out the few organic vendors at the farmers markets.

The sale of organic food raises questions about access and equality in New York City. Residents of Manhattan have access to organic food, while those residing in the other boroughs are more limited in their ability to buy organic food easily. Whole Foods, for example, has stores in Manhattan and one in Brooklyn, but has no presence in other boroughs. Year-round farmers markets are more likely to be located in Manhattan than in the other four boroughs. Social justice advocates have expanded the availability of CSAs in areas outside of Manhattan, but as previously mentioned, CSAs do not necessarily sell organic food. And even within Manhattan, there is unequal access to organic food, with the more affluent consumers having more opportunity.

This inequity may be what led Good Eggs to restrict its business to Brooklyn; by bringing organic, fresh, and local into a locality with little supply of organic food, they appear to have a stronghold on the market for organic food.

See also COMMUNITY SUPPORTED AGRICULTURE; GREENMARKETS; SUPERMARKETS; and WHOLE FOODS.

Dimitri, Carolyn, and C. Greene. *Recent Growth Patterns in U.S. Organic Foods Market.* Agricultural Information Bulletin 777. Washington, D.C.: U.S. Department of Agriculture, Economic Research Service, 2002. http://www.ers.usda.gov/media/249063/aib777_1_.pdf.

Dimitri, Carolyn, J. Geoghegan, and S. Rogus. "Two-Stage Determinants of the Organic Food Retailing Landscape: The Case of Manhattan, NY." *Journal of Food Products Marketing* (forthcoming).

Good Eggs website: https://www.goodeggs.com/about.

Meas, Thong, Wuyang Hu, Marvin T. Batte, Timothy A. Woods, and Stan Ernst. "Substitutes or Complements? Consumer Preference for Local and Organic Food Attributes." *American Journal of Agricultural Economics* 97, no. 4 (2015): 1044–1071.

"Union Square Greenmarket Saturday." GrowNYC. http://www.grownyc.org/greenmarket/manhattan-union-square-sa.

"Whole Foods Market History." Whole Foods. http://www.wholefoodsmarket.com/company-info/whole-foods-market-history.

Jared Michael Guy Fernandez
and Carolyn Dimitri

Oxford University Press

Oxford University Press is the world's largest university press, publishing some six thousand books a year, with offices in more than fifty countries. Its origins date to 1478, when, as a natural outgrowth of the University of Oxford's theological interests, the university began working with printers to publish bibles, prayer books, and works of Christian scholarship. Publishing activity remained sporadic for a century, until Elizabeth I granted the university permission to set up its own printing press in 1586. The press's reputation grew considerably with the publication of several major reference works, chief among them the *Oxford English Dictionary*, the first fascicle of which was published in 1884. The press, looking to expand its operations, opened the New York office in 1896, originally to distribute the Authorized King James Bible. By the 1920s the New York

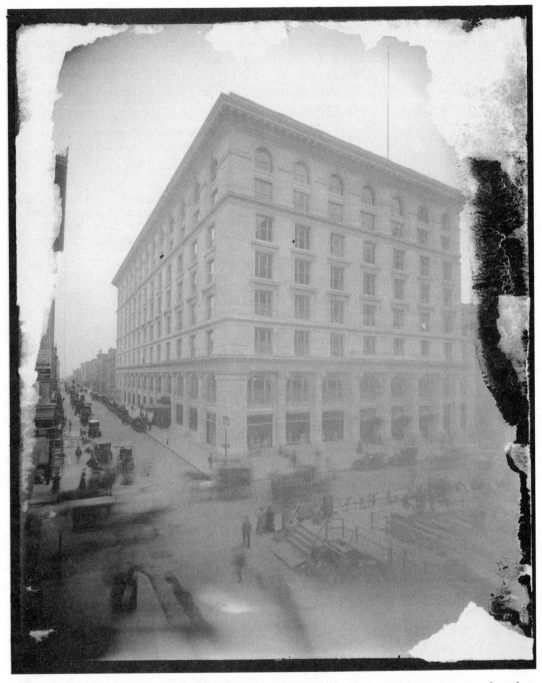

Oxford University Press USA is housed in what was formerly the B. Altman & Company department store, shown here sometime between 1900 and 1910. LIBRARY OF CONGRESS

office was publishing books of its own, and in the 1990s the office moved to its present location at 198 Madison Avenue, which at one time was the B. Altman building. See DEPARTMENT STORE RESTAURANTS.

Food was not a focus for the press until the late twentieth century, when the Oxford office published two modern classics. *The Oxford Companion to Wine*, first published in 1994 and now in its third edition, was edited by the British wine critic Jancis Robinson.

The *Companion* won every major wine book award and had a significant impact on consumer understanding of wines and wine culture. *The Oxford Companion to Food*, first published in 1999 and now in its fourth edition, was originally edited by British diplomat and food historian Alan Davidson. After Davidson's passing in 2003, the former restaurateur and food writer Tom Jaine assumed editorial oversight. It covers the history of foodstuffs worldwide, with a particular emphasis on European and British cooking.

The New York office took the successful companion format and ran with it, publishing, in relatively short order, *The Oxford Encyclopedia of Food and Drink in America* (edited by Andrew F. Smith, first edition 2004, second edition 2012) and its one-volume successor, *The Oxford Companion to American Food and Drink* (also edited by Andrew F. Smith, 2007), *The Oxford Companion to Italian Food* (by Gillian Riley, 2007), *The Oxford Companion to Beer* (edited by Garrett Oliver, 2011), and *The Oxford Companion to Sugar and Sweets* (edited by Darra Goldstein, 2015). The strength of these works is that they gather dozens, and sometimes hundreds, of authors, meaning that entries are generally written by recognized topic experts. (*The Oxford Companion to Italian Food* is an outlier in that it was authored, rather than edited, by Gillian Riley.) Shorter-format food dictionaries published by Oxford University Press include *Eating Your Words: 2000 Words to Tease Your Taste Buds* (William Grimes, 2004) and *The Diner's Dictionary: Word Origins of Food and Drink* (John Ayto, 2012).

Beyond reference and lexical books, Oxford University Press publishes a wide range of monographs, handbooks, and academic works on issues relating to food and drink. Those with a focus on the politics of food include *Feast: Why Humans Share Food* (Martin Jones, 2007), *Food Politics: What Everyone Needs to Know* (Robert Paarlberg, 2013), and *Soda Politics: Taking on Big Soda (and Winning)* (Marion Nestle, 2015). Food histories include *Chop Suey: A Cultural History of Chinese Food in the United States* (Andrew Coe, 2009) and *Planet Taco: A Global History of Mexican Food* (Jeffrey Pilcher, 2012). Food science and technology books include *Beer: Tap Into the Art and Science of Brewing* (Charles Bamforth, 2009), *The Science of Cheese* (Michael Tunick, 2013), and *Your Brain on Food: How Chemicals Control Your Thoughts and Feelings* (Gary Wenk, 2014).

Oxford University Press remains a department of the University of Oxford, transferring 30 percent of its annual surplus to the university's coffers. Delegates appointed from the academic staff of the university must review and approve book proposals, including those originating from the New York office.

Asimov, Eric. "Settling in, Glass in Hand, to Read of Wine." *New York Times*, December 6, 2006.
Fabricant, Florence. "The Oxford Companion to Food: 6 Pounds, with Light Touches." *New York Times*, November 24, 1999.
Gadd, Ian, Simon Eliot, and W. Roger Louis, eds. *The History of Oxford University Press*. Oxford: Oxford University Press, 2014.
Oxford University Press website: http://global.oup.com.

Carl Raymond

Oyster Bars

Historically, oysters have been among New York's most popular and cherished foods, enjoyed by the poor, the rich, and everyone in between. From colonial times, street vendors sold freshly shucked oysters, and they could also be had, doused with ketchup, for a penny apiece at huts and shanties along the East River. The city's first oyster cellar was established in 1763 in the basement of an old building on Broad Street. Longshoremen, stevedores, and sailors kept such modest restaurants busy serving up big bowls of oyster soup for five cents. Oysters were also sold from "floating-houses," which kept oysters alive for several days by placing them in baskets in the cellar and attic of the oyster-boat.

The golden age of oyster cellars occurred in the nineteenth century when oyster saloons dotted the city. Mainly constructed in cellars, the saloons typically identified themselves with a bright red balloon, which was illuminated with a candle in the evening. The greatest concentration of oyster places was found along Canal Street, and many operated on what was called the "Canal Street Plan"—twelve cents bought you as many oysters as you could eat. But rumor had it that if a customer ordered too many, the server would start handing over spoiled ones.

By 1835, an estimated five thousand New Yorkers were engaged in retailing oysters. Oyster shuckers, many of them African Americans, quickly opened oysters for waiting customers. A good shucker could open 3,500 oysters a day, but the average was about 2,500.

One of the city's iconic oyster establishments belonged to Thomas Downing, an African American who was born free in Virginia, then a slave state. He arrived in New York in 1819 and worked as a painter before opening an oyster house on Broad Street, near the U.S. Custom House. In the center of the city's business district, it became a favorite meeting place for the city's political and economic elite. About 1862, Downing moved the business into the Merchants' Exchange at Fifty-Five Wall Street. When Downing retired, his son took over the business, but it closed about 1871.

Charles Dickens ate at Downing's when he visited New York in 1842. He wrote that he considered such places "pleasant retreats" with "wonderful cookery of oysters, pretty nigh as large as cheese plates." Another British visitor reported that there was hardly a square in the city without several oyster saloons. They were aboveground and underground, in shanties and "palaces."

Another iconic New York City oyster bar was Dorlon's, in the Fulton Fish Market. It was founded in 1847 by Alfred P. Dorlon, who worked at his father's stall wholesaling oysters. Dorlon and his brother opened an oyster stall of their own and placed a few tables with stools out front, where people could sit and eat. Over the next ten years, Dorlon's expanded to become one of New York's most fashionable oyster bars, even though it was described in the late 1860s as plainly furnished, without tablecloths or carpets. Dorlon's claimed that they had never served a bad oyster. Fashionable New Yorkers en route to or from the opera or a society soirée would stop at Dorlon's, but common folk also frequented the place. Everyone—rich or poor—had to stand in line waiting to be served. The business survived until 1888, by which time the Fulton Fish Market had become very seedy and was no longer a dining destination. See FULTON FISH MARKET.

By 1874, more than 850 oyster establishments dotted Manhattan alone. Oyster "palaces," illuminated by gaslight and furnished with chandeliers, carpets, mirrors, paintings, and other artistic enhancements, catered to the upper class. Tables could be closed off with curtains, providing customers with a discreet place to conduct business.

The Scottish poet and journalist Charles Mackay, who visited New York in 1859, noted that oysters were served at breakfast, dinner, and supper. They were prepared in a hundred different styles: pickled, stewed, baked, roasted, fried, and scalloped, and made into soups, patties, and puddings. They were served with or without condiments. Another visitor, George Makepeace Towle, noted that oysters were served in every imaginable way: "escolloped, steamed, stewed, roasted, 'on the half shell,' eaten raw with pepper and salt, devilled, baked in crumbs, cooked in *pâtés*, put in delicious sauces on fish and boiled mutton." Still, most New Yorkers preferred their oysters freshly shucked and raw.

Not surprisingly, the oyster beds in New York Harbor were over-harvested, and many of them were closed in the late nineteenth century. Other oyster beds became contaminated, since raw sewage was still being dumped into the city's waters. When a typhus outbreak in the 1890s was attributed to tainted oysters, still more beds were closed by health officials. By 1916, most oyster beds in New York Bay had been closed or destroyed by pollution. Oysters were brought in from Long Island and elsewhere, but they were no longer a cheap food and a simple pleasure for the masses.

Most oyster bars closed in the early twentieth century. The exception was the Grand Central Oyster Bar, which opened in 1913 on the lower level of the newly completed Grand Central Station. See GRAND CENTRAL OYSTER BAR. It continues to flourish, bringing in oysters from Long Island, New Jersey, Connecticut, Massachusetts, Washington State, Canada, Mexico, and New Zealand. In addition to raw oysters on the half-shell, its signature dishes include oyster pan roast and oyster stew.

See also OYSTERS.

Foley, Joseph, and Joan Foley. *The Grand Central Oyster Bar and Restaurant Seafood Cookbook*. New York: Crown, 1977.

Hewitt, John H. "Mr. Downing and His Oyster House: The Life and Good Works of an African-American Entrepreneur." *New York History* (July 1993): 229–252.

Kurlansky, Mark. *The Big Oyster: History on the Half Shell*. New York: Random House, 2006.

Mensch, Barbara. *South Street*. New York: Columbia University Press, 2007.

Reardon, Joan. *Oysters: A Culinary Celebration*. Rev. ed. New York: Lyons, 2000.

Andrew F. Smith

Oysters

Oysters are plentiful, trendy, and sought out all over New York City. Oyster appreciation in New York goes back to the Lenape, the nomadic native people who inhabited the area more than 6,500 years ago and lived by hunting, fishing and foraging. Lacking metal tools to open their oysters, they wrapped them in seaweed and heated them over hot embers until they gaped open. See PRE-COLUMBIAN.

By 1524, when white settlers arrived from Europe, there were still 15,000 Lenape in what would become New York City; the land was filled with hundreds of mounds of buried oyster shells—called middens—which gives us an idea how many of the bivalves the Lenape devoured. Middens continued to be discovered throughout the twentieth century—from a few yards across to several acres wide—especially when roads were being built or railroad tie laid for the Metro North Hudson line, or, most recently, in 1988, below some Metro North railroad tracks dug up for repairs.

Oysters thrived in New York then, in the mild brackish water off its shores spiked with the fresh, nourishing water mixing in from the Hudson River, and they grew big. Unlike most other creatures they continue to grow during their ten to fifteen year lifespan, reaching 8 to 12 inches across if not harvested.

Oystermania

British colonial rule replaced that of the Dutch West India Company in 1664 and the area economy evolved from being hunting-based to depending on fishing and agriculture. Within a century, New York was the leading city in prostitution, alcohol consumption, and oyster eating, and boatloads and streetcars full of the shellfish fed the oyster-hungry population.

The first cannery in the city commenced operation in 1819, packaging oysters (and cod) for storage. The Erie Canal that was completed in 1825 made way for barges to ship oysters to the Midwest and beyond, although this job was taken over by the railways not long afterward. Later, oysters were packed in salt in barrels for shipping. See ERIE CANAL.

By the 1820s most of the city oyster beds were running low on oysters, and by the 1830s cultivation began at City Island in the Bronx with the creation of artificial reefs made from shells and oyster seed; tiny young oysters were planted to enrich the supply, brought in from Maryland and Virginia. The oyster business thrived, and Prince's Bay on Staten Island was the center of the industry, stimulating the shipbuilding business as well. At one point, Tottenville on Staten Island had six to eight shipyards. In 1837, the restaurant of the Astor House Hotel on Broadway between Vesey and Barclay Streets offered "boiled cod & oysters" and "oyster pie." See ASTOR HOUSE. Oyster cellars proliferated, elegant and low-brow both, with the same patrons sometimes frequenting both kinds on different days. By 1874, there were 850 oyster houses in the city, mostly for men only, serving the mollusks raw and sprinkled with vinegar and pepper, lemon in the fancier places.

Oyster wholesalers and retailers who couldn't afford storefronts gussied up the ends of their double-decker barges to make faux two-story buildings and lashed them side by side to the docks on the Hudson or East River. They installed fancy windows, doors, and balconies, and painted them pink, yellow, or green, creating rows of gently bobbing oyster shops.

By 1880, the average American ate 660 oysters a year and over the next forty years New York area beds produced 700 million a year. Oyster stands were as ubiquitous throughout the city as hot dog stands are today, selling oysters for a penny each, or stew for a dime. In 1882 at Coney Island, a dime got you a frankfurter on a bun or a plate of oysters.

Although every formal dinner started with oysters, most families, rich or poor, could afford two oyster dinners per week. Juliet Corson's 1885 *New Family Cookbook* had a recipe for raw oysters on the half shell with a dusting of cayenne and a squeeze of lemon juice, to be served with salt, brown bread, and butter. But Americans were starting to look beyond the raw oyster for ways to consume their beloved mollusk. They would stuff them, fry them, or make soup out of them. They made pan roasts, oyster bisque, oyster Newberg, smothered oysters, oyster omelets, oysters over steak, oyster stuffing for poultry, and oyster loaves: French rolls stuffed with oysters stewed in white wine.

Oyster Scarcity

Typhoid and cholera outbreaks were blamed on oysters, and as the twentieth century began there was too much sewage from the city's growing population for the oyster lairs to stay clean. Twenty to fifty gallons of seawater move through an oyster's gills

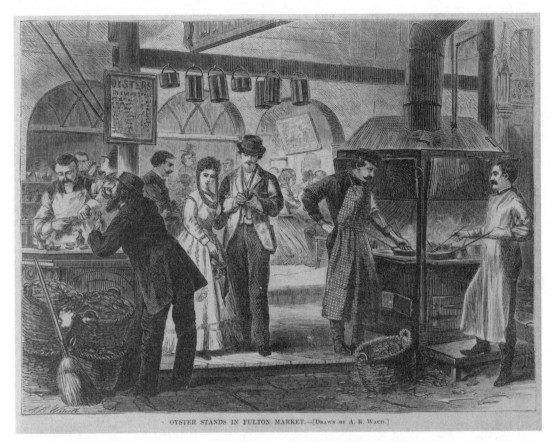

OYSTER STANDS IN FULTON MARKET.—[DRAWN BY A. R. WAUD.]

Oyster stands in Fulton Market, drawn by A. R. Waud (1828–1891). Oysters drawn from the Hudson River were both popular and cheap during the nineteenth century—as the sign says, "Oysters in every style" were available at any given time. LIBRARY OF CONGRESS

each day, and the water was increasingly tainted. The shellfish beds of Jamaica Bay produced a quarter to a third of the city's oysters, and in 1915 and again in 1921 they were shut down because of contamination. In 1927, oystering ended for good in New York City, and, although seven years later the U.S. Supreme Court ordered the city to stop dumping garbage in the water and put it in landfills instead, it was too late for the oyster.

Nevertheless, the oyster craze continued. Commodore Cornelius Vanderbilt opened the Grand Central Oyster Bar in 1913 and the seafood landmark Lundy's opened in 1934 in Brooklyn, seating 2,200 to 2,800 people with a long shellfish bar open to the street for eating oysters without going inside. See GRAND CENTRAL OYSTER BAR. Although today there are still oysters in the harbor, between rocks at the seawall at the Battery and the pier off TriBeCa,

they were planted there to build up reefs and filter organic waste. They're powerless against heavy metals and PCBs, though, and are surely not for eating. Nor are the ones from proposed oyster reefs cultivated to diffuse the force of waves from superstorms like Sandy.

But New York oyster lovers don't have to look far for their oysters, and seem to be willing to pay high prices for quality and variety. There are dozens of kinds to choose from—from fairly local to far-flung—and they are easy to find around town. Dozens of city bars and restaurants lure customers with happy hour oyster specials, often a dollar per oyster, usually a Blue Point from Long Island Sound or another eastern one. Grand Central Oyster Bar offers more than thirty varieties at a time, in rotation, from the United States, Canada, and Mexico, including several from nearby waters, to please the locavore.

Although oyster varieties vary in size, flavor, salinity, and texture, there are three main types, the saltier *Crassostrea virginica* being the eastern one. Although summer oysters can be softer and flabbier due to spawning, modern refrigeration means they're good year round, especially now that many are farmed. And there are still wild ones out there, worth seeking for their bold flavor.

See also OYSTER BARS.

Coomes, Steve. "Oyster Craze: Oyster Farms and Harvesters Are Struggling to Feed a Growing Restaurant Demand for the Shellfish." *Seafood Business Magazine*, June 2014.
Egan, Hannah Palmer. "Demystifying New York's Favorite Mollusk, The Oyster." *Village Voice*, June 26, 2013.
Kurlansky, Mark. *The Big Oyster: History on the Half Shell*. New York: Ballantine, 2006.
Riffee, Mark. "Tribes of New York." *New York Times*, March 30, 2011.
Root, Waverley, and Richard DeRochemont. *Eating in America: A History*. Toronto: HarperCollins, 1976.

Jennifer Brizzi

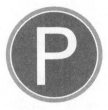

P. J. Clarke's

P. J. Clarke's, at Third Avenue and Fifty-Fifth Street, is one of New York City's most famous saloons. It is one of the few nineteenth-century saloons to have survived. The building, constructed as a four-story apartment house in 1869, was reportedly converted into a saloon in 1884 by Michael J. Jennings, an Irish immigrant with close ties to Tammany Hall, the Irish-dominated political organization that controlled New York City from the late nineteenth century until the Depression. Jennings was also heavily involved in the liquor business. He hired Patrick J. Clarke, an Irish immigrant who arrived in 1903, as a bartender. Jennings likely lent Clarke the money to buy the saloon in 1911. With the advent of Prohibition in 1921, Clarke's continued to operate as a speakeasy.

When Prohibition ended, Clarke's resumed its function as a neighborhood bar, frequented by many writers, such as Charles R. Jackson, who lived less than a block away. During the mid-1930s, Jackson went on a drunken spree for several days at Clarke's. During the 1940s, he turned that experience into a novel, titled *The Lost Weekend* (1944). The following year the movie producer Billy Wilder picked up the film rights to the book. Wilder created a replica of the interior of Clarke's for the film set. The movie, released in 1945, made the saloon famous, and it was visited by celebrities like Nat King Cole, Frank Sinatra, Johnny Mercer, and Woody Allen. It has been frequently cited in books, articles, movies, and plays.

The building was sold to John and Dan Lavezzo in 1941, although P. J. Clarke continued to run the bar until his death in 1948. When the Lavezzo family took over the saloon in 1949, they changed the name from Clarke's to P. J. Clarke's in his honor. The watering hole morphed into a popular restaurant, serving hamburgers and other simple fare.

In 1967, the Third Avenue saloon was slated for demolition to make way for an office tower. The outcry from celebrities, locals, and preservationists managed to save most of the structure, but the two upper floors were removed, and a skyscraper was erected around the little old brick building. Today, the Clarke Group owns P. J. Clarke's. In 2010 it hired chef Larry Forgione, a pioneer in New American Cuisine, to update the menu, which now includes a raw bar, steak, seafood, and classic American dishes made with local ingredients. There are now several outposts of P. J. Clarke's—near Lincoln Center and in the Financial District, and also in Woodbury, New York; Washington, D.C.; and São Paolo, Brazil.

See also IRISH; SALOONS; and SPEAKEASIES.

Clarke, Helen Marie. *Over P. J. Clarke's Bar: Tales from New York City's Famous Saloon*. New York: Skyhorse, 2012.

Andrew F. Smith

Paddleford, Clementine

Clementine Paddleford (1898–1967) was one of the most influential American newspaper food columnists and editors ever. During her thirty-plus years at the *New York Herald Tribune* she shaped the future of food writing by invigorating it with narrative stories from the people (usually women) *behind* the recipes. Previously newspaper food stories usually just included recipes. But she is one of the least known food reporters in the modern era, in part because she had throat cancer and spoke out of a voice box, and thus could not talk about food effectively.

Born on September 27, 1898, on a Stockdale, Kansas, farm, Clementine Haskin Paddleford's view of food was shaped in her mother's kitchen, where the farm-fresh fare was rooted in local tradition. Growing up, the bookish Paddleford was more interested in writing letters and telling stories than in milking cows. By the time she was fifteen, she was writing news stories for the Manhattan, Kansas, *Daily Chronicle*. After graduating from Kansas State University with a degree in journalism in 1921, the aspiring reporter promptly moved to New York City. By 1924 she had a job as women's editor with *Farm & Fireside*, a prototypical "home arts" magazine. In 1931, a chronic hoarseness developed in Paddleford's throat that was diagnosed as throat cancer. The thirty-one-year-old writer opted for a radical surgery in which her larynx and vocal cords were removed. She spoke out of a voice box for the rest of her life, yet continued to write and was undeterred in conducting interviews.

During the Great Depression, the intrepid journalist persuaded editors at the *New York Herald Tribune* to give her a small food column, most of which chronicled prices at the city's produce markets. Within six months the *Tribune's* readers were clamoring for more and Paddleford was offered a permanent staff position. During World War II, the *Herald Tribune* columnist wrote many stories on how to work around the shortages in the kitchen caused by rationing and the loss of many imported foods. In 1948 Paddleford started her position as roving editor for *This Week* magazine, a Sunday supplement in more than thirty-four major newspapers— including the *Herald Tribune*—with approximately 12 million readers. Her assignment was a weekly series devoted to "How America Eats." During the first twelve years of the column, Paddleford traveled more than eight hundred thousand miles by train, plane, automobile, mule, and on foot. She ate every dish at the table as she found it, and then again when the recipes were tested in *This Week's* kitchen.

By the1950s, Paddleford had amassed more than three thousand cookbooks and countless filing cabinets crammed full of notes. Her usual routine was to show up at the *Herald Tribune* offices at 5:30 a.m. The 1950s were the meaty years of the "How America Eats" series; Paddleford learned to pilot a Piper Cub plane to speed up her research. In 1953 the columnist's international travels took her to England, where she reported on the coronation of Queen Elizabeth II. The *New York Herald Tribune* dubbed her "Hop-a-long Paddleford," and on December 28, 1953, *Time* magazine referred to her as the "best known food editor in the United States." Due to her voice condition, she was not able to give speeches and didn't embrace television; thus, there is no footage of her.

The early 1960s found Paddleford continuing to log air miles across the continent. During that time she published her most important work, *How America Eats* (Charles Scribner's Sons, 1960), the culmination of more than two thousand interviews with home cooks across the country. In it, she wrote smartly and sassily about everything from a mess hall for lumberjacks in the Pacific Northwest, to chili parlors in Texas, to a dinner of imported Italian truffles at the Four Seasons restaurant in Manhattan. By the early 1960s, Paddleford was at the height of her popularity. She was even featured in a cartoon in a 1964 issue of the *New Yorker*: it depicted a man and a woman sitting in lawn chairs while their faithful dog brings them the newspaper; the caption reads, "I am pretty fed up with teeth marks on Clementine Paddleford." She was given the New York Newspaper Women's Club Award at least seven times.

The final chapter of Paddleford's life coincides with the death of the *New York Herald Tribune*. In 1967, the *New York Times* bought the *Herald Tribune*. That same year Paddleford died from multiple cancers. Her legacy was nearly forgotten, but modern food writers have rediscovered her in recent years and find her prose holds up remarkably well.

Alexander, Kelly, and Cynthia Harris. *Hometown Appetites: The Story of Clementine Paddleford, the Forgotten Food Writer Who Chronicled How America Ate*. New York: Gotham, 2008.

Kelly Alexander

Paintings

Paintings depicting New Yorkers dining offer insight into how life was experienced in earlier New York. Although helpful for showing restaurant interiors and the dynamics of social interaction during meals, in general emphasis is not placed on literal illustration of the pleasures of the table.

At first glance, Thomas Cole's *The Pic-Nic* (1846) seems like a romantic juxtaposition of transcendental nature with people enjoying a picnic inserted into the pastoral vista. However, the reality behind this nostalgic reverie is quite different. With companion Cornelius Ver Bryck recently deceased, Cole transforms his friend into Orpheus. The terrain correspondingly evokes Brooklyn's Green-Wood Cemetery, where Cornelius was interred. Cole's fascination with food can be inferred from his numerous journal entries about meals as well as his preparing a picnic for critics attending a National Academy of Design spring annual. In the painting, it is difficult to ascertain what was transported in the cooler as only scraps remain, while the steaming kettle makes it apparent tea was enjoyed.

The Ashcan School shared a profound fascination with the life around them whether beautiful or unseemly. Also known as The Eight, the members were Arthur B. Davies, William Glackens, Robert

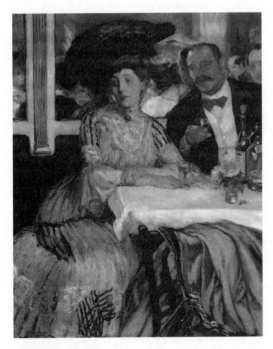

The Ashcan school, a progressive American artistic movement around the turn of the twentieth century, frequently depicted scenes of New York City restaurants. William Glackens's *Chez Mouquin* (1905) renders the renowned uptown restaurant where the Ashcan coterie and their wives often dined, enjoying its French atmosphere and gaiety as reflected in mirrors. ART INSTITUTE OF CHICAGO

Henri, Ernest Lawson, George Luks, Maurice Prendergast, Everett Shinn, and John French Sloan. The most progressive American group of their time, they emphasized genre scenes of urban life, humble subjects, popular cultural haunts, the dynamism of New York City. Notably, many paintings by The Eight depict restaurant settings.

For example, William Glackens's *Chez Mouquin* (1905) renders the renowned uptown restaurant where the Ashcan coterie and their wives often celebrated, enjoying its French atmosphere and gaiety as reflected in mirrors. Reminiscent of their Parisian student days, it functioned as headquarters when in 1908 The Eight devised their famous rebellion against the National Academy of Design. Elegant in blue but with evident boredom as she awaits her husband's return, Jeanne Louise Mouquin sits with James Moore, owner of the rival Cafe Francis. Meanwhile, George Luks suggestively refers to Glackens's *Chez Mouquin* in his *The Cafe Francis* (1906). In his work, Luks portrays an older, potent James Moore with one of his lady friends. Moore owned the Cafe Francis, which he advertised as "New York's Most Popular Resort of the New Bohemia." Glackens and Luks both focus upon a couple within a vital restaurant setting and, along with fellow artists and writers, patronized each establishment.

Petitpas, a small Lower West Side French restaurant-cum-boardinghouse, was another gathering spot for the creative intelligentsia. It was also famous as the residence of philosopher-painter John Butler Yeats, father of the poet William Butler Yeats. John Sloan's *Yeats at Petitpas'* (1910) depicts the famed haunt, a favorite with members of The Eight, George Bellows, and their spouses. In this composition, Yeats is surrounded by reigning intellectuals, Sloan's wife standing next to Celestine Petitpas, and Sloan himself. George Bellows's *Artists' Evening (at Petitpas') (Mason 19)* (1916), likewise demonstrates insight into its unique, genteel ambience.

Associated with The Eight but not a member of it, Guy Pène Du Bois painted *Mr. and Mrs. Chester Dale Dining Out* (1924), the subjects of which seem not to have ordered any food. Seated at a table in the fashionable Fifth Avenue Hotel Brevoort with a waiter hovering, Chester Dale peers at his wife while she avoids his gaze, with both exhibiting stiff body posture and claw-like hands. On a surface level, this affirms personal isolation and lack of a true intimacy prefiguring the ultimate unraveling of their marriage.

But there may be another interpretation possible as Chester Dale and his painter wife, Maud, were major patrons of Pène Du Bois and collected splendid art.

For these artists, Chinese establishments represented the exotic. John Sloan's *Chinese Restaurant* (1909) depicts an event that the artist witnessed while visiting a Chinese restaurant in his neighborhood. The scene before him unfolds with an immediacy as a girl wearing a festive red chapeau appears to pay more attention to a cat than to her date. Capturing the details of the restaurant, Sloan emphasized vertical lines in a somber interior excepting that shock of red in the hat. Belonging to a later generation and known to dress in Chinese garb, Max Weber describes his *(Memory of a) Chinese Restaurant* (1915) in analytic cubist forms. Commemorating numerous visits to "China-Town" and glorious repasts savored, his canvas pulsates as visual, tactile, auditory, gustatory happening, transforming itself into sensual experience.

A number of works reflect the reality of single, newly employed women and their public roles. In the early decades of the twentieth century, restaurants and bars remained a male preserve, with solitary women assumed to be prostitutes. Formerly they might not have been encouraged to enter restaurants unaccompanied by male escorts, but now dining on their own or with other women, they encountered respectful treatment. Prints by Isabel Bishop depicted working-class women enjoying ice cream and soda during their lunch break. In *New York Restaurant* (1922), Edward Hopper explores psychic tensions between a couple, with the woman wearing a bright red hat reminiscent of Sloan's *Chinese Restaurant*. She appears distant and oblivious of her companion. The addition of the female waitress within this elegant setting signifies the emerging modern world. Reginald Marsh's *Girls (Red Buttons)* (1936) features two fashionably-attired young women standing together in Childs Cafeteria with an outdoor scene visible through the glass window offering a perfect example of Marsh's interest in a slice of daily life and its harsh reality. The somewhat anxious postures of the two women seem to suggest that they are awaiting the arrival of their dates. Isaac Soyer treats an unpretentious *Cafeteria* (1930) with a note in the window reading "ladies invited." This is analogous to the recent social innovation in which dining establishments advertised "tables for ladies" in order to welcome mobile female customers.

Other significant scenes of individuals at dining tables involve those unable to afford the costs associated with eating out easily. Henry Kallem, a member of the Twenty-Eighth Street Group of Modernists, executed within a geometric framework *Municipal Lodging House* for the Works Progress Administration. Established in 1908 by New York City, this residence daily provided 2,500 homeless men free meals during the Great Depression. Jacob Lawrence's *Bread, Fish, Fruit* (1985) was created as focal point for his traveling *Migration of the Negro* series. One of the foremost exponents of social realism, his narratives portray the struggles of blacks, especially those like himself who grew up during the Harlem Renaissance. Jack Levine, with a George Grosz tableau, satirically criticizes America. His *The Reluctant Ploughshare (Soldier's Return)* (1946) depicts a soldier's homecoming and discovering others more concerned with their food than his arrival.

America's succeeding generation of artists relished personal expressive freedom. An early Jackson Pollock, *The Tea Cup* (1946), portrays people seated around the table enjoying tea, whereas his wife Lee Krasner's *Mosaic Table* (1947) focuses upon Little Images. The Abstract Expressionists enjoyed disputing the meaning of aesthetics and visual integrity while smoking a cigarette or drinking a five-cent cup of coffee in the Waldorf Cafeteria. As time progressed, they originated The Club's interactive programs and met at bars such as the Cedar Bar, where conversations flowed. Paul Georges's *Kaldis at the Cedar Street Bar* isolates the painter whereas Red Grooms's *Cedar Bar* (1985) integrates intriguing personages in this their unofficial Metropolitan hangout.

Gerdts, William H. *Art Across America: Two Centuries of Regional Painting, 1710–1920.* 3 vols. New York: Abbeville, 1990.

Zurier, Rebecca, Robert W. Snyder, and Virginia M. Mecklenburg. *Metropolitan Lives: The Ashcan Artists and Their New York.* Washington, D.C.: National Museum of American Art; New York: Norton, 1995.

Michele Kidwell-Gilbert

Papaya King

Though admittedly a strange pairing, papaya and hot dogs have been a staple of New York's fast food scene since 1932. That is when Gus Poulos, a Greek immigrant who had arrived at Ellis Island in 1923 at the age of sixteen, opened Hawaiian Tropical Drinks on the corner of Eighty-Sixth Street and Third Avenue in Manhattan.

According to legend, Poulos discovered papaya while on vacation in Miami (some accounts say it was Cuba). He converted his deli into a juice stand, but New Yorkers were not interested until Poulos hired women in hula skirts to give out free samples on the sidewalk.

Because the juice stand was in a heavily German part of town, Poulos introduced a frankfurter to the menu in 1939. (His German American wife, Birdie, might have also had something to do with it.) The hickory-smoked hot dogs are made of beef seasoned with garlic, oregano, and an enigmatic blend of "South American spices." The natural casings are imported from Germany and provide a real snap when biting into the dog.

The stand's popularity grew, and Poulos opened more outlets, including ones in Philadelphia and Miami. One of the regular customers—supposedly a Brooklyn Dodger—began referring to Hawaiian Tropical Drinks Company as "Papaya King." Poulos officially changed the name in the early 1960s.

By then, the restaurant had become a tourist attraction. The Beatles were rumored to have eaten the dogs, which the store claims are "tastier than filet mignon," before their 1964 *Ed Sullivan Show* appearance. The success of Papaya King led to a slew of imitators: Papaya Prince, Papaya World, and Papaya Plus, among many others. Poulos and his heirs have sued some of the knock-offs over the years, including one called Papaya Kingdom.

Poulos died in 1988 and his son and nephew took over the business. In 2010 caterer Wayne Rosenbaum and a group of investors bought Papaya King. In 2013, a location was opened on St. Mark's Place, and the next year in June 2014, the first Papaya King truck hit the streets.

Broder, Mitch. *Discovering Vintage New York: A Guide to the City's Timeless Shops, Bars, Delis & More.* Guilford, Conn.: Globe Pequot, 2013.

Kleiman, Dena. "New York Puts Its Papaya Where Its Hot Dogs Are." *New York Times.* August 21, 1991.

Papaya King website: http://www.papayaking.com/index.php/about.

Reed Tucker

Park Slope

Park Slope is a Brooklyn neighborhood bordered by Prospect Park, Windsor Terrace, Prospect Heights, and Gowanus. It was part of land inhabited by the Gowanus Indians, who were adept hunters, gatherers, and growers. European settlers later farmed here. After the Civil War, when transportation to Manhattan improved, this previously sparsely populated area was mapped into grids. Tracts of land were bought by developers who then built stately brownstones and townhouses in rows identified by similarities of decorative motifs. Houses of worship and schools of similar stature laced the community to serve it.

Park Slope has two main commercial strips: Seventh and Fifth Avenues. In the twentieth century, food stores all along these avenues included delicatessens, luncheonettes, soda parlors, candy stores, fishmongers, butcher shops, produce stores, bakeries, and grocery stores. On Seventh Avenue between Carroll and Fourth Streets alone, Al's Candy Store, Irv's Stationery (with candy, too), Pergola Meat Market, Herzog's Delicatessen, Finnegan Brothers groceries, Lehigh Fruits and Vegetables, Ebinger's bakery, Pino's pizzeria (with marble window counter), and Steve's greasy spoon met the food needs of the community. Bars and grills—Mooney's, Caulfield's, Stack 'O Barley, Snooky's, McFeeley's, the Eagle, and the Coach Inn—dotted corners and side streets. The Montauk Club and the Fordes family's Michel's Restaurant were among Park Slope's more exclusive places to dine. Many of these Park Slope small businesses were family owned and were conducive to frequent, even daily, marketing or stops. This encouraged a rapport with merchants who came to know well the needs and preferences of their customers.

Park Slopers experienced neighborhood challenges. In 1960, a midair collision in a snowstorm brought one plane crashing down onto the corner of Sterling Place and Seventh Avenue near the Ward mansion. The completion of the Verrazano-Narrows Bridge in 1964 intensified urban flight to the suburbs. However, in the 1970s, young families attracted to substantial brownstones at low prices bought and renovated them. The Park Slope Civic Council promoted beautifully restored homes on Spring House Tours, and when the term "Brownstone Brooklyn" was coined, it was readily applied here. The Park Slope Food Coop was founded on Union Street in 1973 and in line with the "back to the land" movement of that time period (albeit urban-style), founding members bagged bulk natural foods. Now with around fifteen thousand owner-members, all of whom perform two and three-quarter hours of work monthly, the PSFC has grown to be the nation's largest and a model for the cooperative food movement. See FOOD CO-OPS.

Park Slope's vibrancy continues to this day. Premier housing and good schools are proximal to the Brooklyn Museum of Art and the Brooklyn Public libraries, both at Grand Army Plaza and on Sixth Avenue and Eighth Street. Outdoors, Greenmarkets, farmers markets, craft markets, and the popular P.S. 321 flea market pop up on specific places and days of the week. Real estate is at a premium, and the brick-and-mortar service stores of the twentieth century have transitioned or largely been replaced by upscale specialty shops. Two corners of Ninth Street serve as examples. In the second half of the twentieth century, the Park Town Coffee Shop offered breakfast, lunch, milkshakes, newspapers, and candy at Ninth Street and Eighth Avenue. Nicknamed Benny's, its corner was a popular teenage meeting spot. In a similar spirit, albeit with a revised menu, Dizzy's "fine diner" offers hearty fare on the spot now.

One block east, across from the park entrance at Ninth Street and Prospect Park West, "LEWNES—SODA FOUNTAIN—LUNCHEONETTE" was spelled out in stained glass transom windows in a one-story building. In 1980, when the city was rife with crime, Charles Musemeci opened the bright and welcoming Raintree's restaurant on the site, still tipping a hat to the history of the soda parlor and neighborhood gentility. In its early years, when it was a challenge to persuade Manhattanites to visit Brooklyn, Musemeci generously opened Raintree's doors to civic groups for their fundraising and motivational events. Raintree's closed in 1999. The century-old building has been razed and replaced by a condominium boasting floor-through corner apartments with park views.

Street pizza eaten out of hand while standing on the sidewalk transitioned to sit-down pies, some eaten with fork and knife, as illustrated by the arrival of Two Boots in 1989. Notable numbers of Szechuan, and then Hunan, -style restaurants opened in the late 1970s and 1980s, enriching Park Slope with a wider range of flavors from around the globe. The Purity is one coffee shop that has spanned the turn of the century, and Prospect Hall has changed from a Polish National Home to the Grand Prospect Hall for banquets and events. And though McFeeley's closed on Union Street, the family's popular Sante Fe Grill continues.

Locavore and specialty foods are served at Al di La, Talde, Stone Park Café, Franny's, Thistle Hill, Apple-

wood, Rosewater, Flatbush Farm, Bierkraft, and Fleisher's, among many others, including an artisanal candy store. Food trucks rally along main avenues and by Grand Army Plaza these days. Vibrant avenues and comparatively quieter residential streets are full of Park Slope's food businesses and their customers.

See also BROOKLYN.

New York City Landmarks Preservation Commission. *Park Slope Historic District Designation and Historic District Designation Report*. New York: Landmarks Preservation Commission, 1973. http://www.nyc.gov/html/lpc/downloads/pdf/reports/0709.pdf.

Hauck-Lawson, Annie. "My Little Town: A Brooklyn Girl's *Food Voice*." In *Gastropolis: Food and New York City*, edited by Annie Hauck-Lawson and Jonathan Deutsch, pp. 68–89. New York: Columbia University Press 2009.

Annie Hauck-Lawson

Passover

Passover (*Pesach* in Hebrew) commemorates the Jewish exodus from Egypt. The holiday begins on the fifteenth day of the Hebrew month of Nissan, which generally falls in late March or April on the Gregorian calendar. *Pesach* refers to the Pascal lamb, offered as a sacrifice on the eve of the holiday during the first and second temple periods. Passover is also called *chag ha-matzot* (the holiday of matzah). During the week of the holiday, observant Jews abstain from leavened bread and eat matzah in its place. On the first night of Passover, Jewish families prepare a special meal and ceremony called a seder, during which the story of the exodus from Egypt is read out loud. (In Israel the seder is conducted on the first night of Passover only. Outside of Israel it is conducted on the first and second nights of the holiday.) During the seder, matzah, a roasted egg, and a roasted shank bone are placed on the table. Other foods including horseradish and bitter herbs, also play a role in the ceremony. Participants are required to drink four cups of wine during the seder meal. Passover ritual and symbolism is thus intimately connected with food and eating.

Since the mid-nineteenth century, the *New York Times* has described Passover observance in New York. The feature of the holiday most frequently mentioned is the eating of unleavened bread. Because matzah and other foods are ritually required during Passover, their supply has always been an important concern

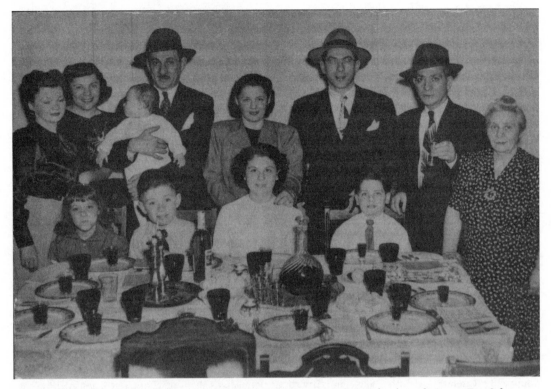

This photograph depicts Sidney and Frances Meda observing Passover with their family on the Lower East Side in 1949. COLLECTION OF THE LOWER EAST SIDE TENEMENT MUSEUM

for the Jewish community. Until the nineteenth century, there was only one synagogue in New York, Shearith Israel, which was the main source of matzah for the small number of Jews in the city. As the Jewish population grew so did the demand for matzah. In 1855, the head of Shearith Israel used matzah consumption to estimate the Jewish population of the city. A *New York Times* article from 1874 notes that there were then "only ten bakers in New York who manufacture the Passover bread; and that they use up over four thousand barrels of flour during the week in preparing matsos. The trade is not confined to this City alone, as the bakers referred to fill orders from Brooklyn, Philadelphia, and many cities outside of the State." In the early twentieth century, matzah production was professionalized and mechanized. On the Lower East Side, A. Goodman and Sons (Goodman's), and Aron Streit (Streit's) opened bakeries to meet the ever increasing demand for matzah driven by Jewish immigration. Manischewitz, which produced matzah in its Cincinnati factory, also sold in the New York market. In 1932, the company opened a second factory in Jersey City, New

Jersey, making it easier to distribute its products on the east coast.

After the late nineteenth century, when large-scale Jewish migration significantly increased the city's Jewish population, matzah and meat were often distributed to poor Jews for the holiday by synagogues and charitable organizations. For example, in 1908 the United Hebrew Communities Charity distributed fifty thousand pounds of matzah to 2,500 families in New York. Passover food was so important that politics were sometimes put aside to provide it—in 1910 Jewish community leaders suspended a boycott against kosher butchers for Passover. Likewise, in 1938 a strike of freshwater-fish workers at Fulton Fish Market was suspended for the holiday season. Even during World War II, the federal and New York City governments attempted to ease kosher meat shortages for the holiday. Increased holiday demand sometimes led to price gouging. To protect consumers, prices were fixed. For example, in 1918 the Federal Food Board fixed poultry and matzah prices for Passover. In 1925 a *Times* headline reported: "Long Island Ducks Break Sale

Record: 39,000 Purchased, Mostly for Use in Pass-over Feast, and Prices Mount." Not until 1995 did the *New York Times* report that Passover price goug-ing seems to have ended, thanks to the concerted efforts of Jewish watchdog groups.

The theme of the Passover holiday, deliverance from oppression, made it symbolically important throughout the twentieth century, for example, during World War II and later for the civil rights movement. Public seders often explicitly addressed these issues.

In addition to the religious and political signifi-cance of Passover, the seder has always been a site of culinary pleasure. Stores throughout New York sell the finest Passover foods. Starting in 1920's Macy's Herald Square store operated a special department for Passover groceries. Asheknazi Jews typically serve gefilte fish, matzah ball soup, potato kugel, brisket, and other specialties for the holiday. Sephardic Jews, unlike their Ashkenazi coreligionists, consider rice and legumes kosher for Passover and, therefore, com-monly include them in their seder meals. Today, seders often include modernized versions of Pass-over classics—for example, chef Dan Barber's Chicken Soup with Rosemary Matzah Balls—and Jewish "foodies" serve meals which combine Ashkenazi, Sephardic, and Middle Eastern dishes and flavors. Some serve dishes unrelated to any Jewish Passover tradition—the 2014 *New York Times* Passover recipes include a hazelnut citrus torte made with quinoa. Passover pasta, made from potato starch, is now quite common. Increasingly, observant Jewish families travel to hotels during the Passover week to avoid having to kosher their homes for Passover. Dining out on Passover is also becoming more common.

See also CHANUKAH; JEWISH; LOWER EAST SIDE; and MATZAH.

Diner, Hasia. *A New Promised Land: A History of Jews in America*. New York: Oxford University Press, 2003.
Moore, Deborah Dash, ed. *City of Promises: A History of the Jews of New York*. New York: New York University Press, 2012.

Ari Ariel

Pastrami

Pastrami is a Romanian-origin, spice-cured smoked beef brisket, often served sliced on rye bread as a hot sandwich. It is an iconic food of most Jewish delis, particularly in New York City, where pastrami as we know it today originates.

The dish came to New York City with the influx of Jewish immigrants from Romania to the United States in the late nineteenth and early twentieth cen-turies (the overwhelming number of immigrants from Romania at the time were Jewish). Romanians had learned the curing technique for *pastramă*, as it was known in Romanian, from the Turks, who for centuries indirectly ruled the nascent country until 1878. The dish most clearly linked to Roma-nian *pastramă* is Turkish *pastırma*, an air-dried cured meat (originally made with camel, goat, or lamb meat). Although perhaps partly apocryphal, the story goes that roving Turkish army men traveled to and throughout Romania by sustaining themselves with the salt-cured *pastırma* which they pressed under their saddles to further the curing process: in Turk-ish and in Romanian etymology a variant of "pastir" means to press.

Romanians added wood and smoke to the mix, and, in general, they preferred the readily available mutton or pork in Romania. However, among Jewish populations, many of whom were if not strictly kosher at least traditionally observant, most lamb, mutton, and all pork products were verboten. For Romanian Jews, therefore, goose, and, when available, beef, were the meats of choice for *pastramă*. The navel or brisket cut was (and continues to be) the cut of choice owing to its marbling and its fibrous toughness which kept the cost of the meat low, but which also lent well to slow curing and robust spicing. Before refriger-ation, the cured meat could be kept for days if not weeks.

In Lower Manhattan, and specifically in the Ro-manian-Jewish stomping ground known as "Little Rumania" (according to the spelling of the time), the first Romanian butchers and modest restaurants starting serving sliced goose *pastramă* by the end of the nineteenth century. Goose was readily available and its meat fatty enough to sustain the curing. But as the price of beef lowered and its availability grew with the expansion of the cattle industry in the United States during the first decades of the twentieth cen-tury, beef "pastrami" began to serve as the norm. Some have speculated the vowel change created a more Americanized sound, particularly because it rhymes with salami.

While American pastrami may have originated with Romanian restaurants and Jewish delis in Lower

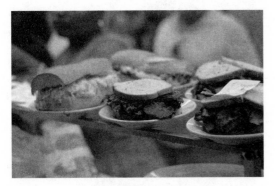

Pastrami is a salt-cured beef made from a brisket cut. At Katz's Deli it is smoked, sliced, and served on rye bread. KATZ'S DELICATESSEN

Manhattan, the dish as we know it today—served on caraway-seeded rye bread with yellow mustard—only became widely popularized in the early years of the twentieth century when Jewish delis, such as the long and still-operating Katz's Deli on Houston Street, started serving it. See DELIS, JEWISH and KATZ'S DELICATESSEN. The German-influenced pan–Eastern European Jewish delicatessens led to the coalescence of Romanian pastrami on German or Russian rye bread with mustard. It was at this time that the pastrami sandwich became not just a Romanian delicacy but a mainstay of Jewish deli menus across the city—and eventually the country.

The growth of the wheat industry in the United States also played a significant role in affecting this development of the pastrami sandwich. *Pastramă* in Romania was (and still is) served on its own, accompanied perhaps by pickled cucumbers and cabbage coleslaw on the side, as continues to be the tradition in most Jewish delis in North America. Serving pastrami on bread was a distinctly American innovation (rather than bread the Romanian staple is a cornmeal-type bread or porridge known as *mămăligă*). In the United States the expansion of the wheat, and, in turn, bread industry in the twentieth century led to the wide availability of not only commercial bread, but commercially sliced bread. By the early midcentury pastrami served on sliced bread became the norm.

With time, and further intercultural fusion, variations such as pastrami sandwiches with melted cheese and sauerkraut became popular, in addition to the classic unadorned sandwich. In fact, the popularity of the pastrami sandwich could not be outmatched: it came to symbolize the Jewish deli. And, as Jewish deli food became iconic not just for Jewish immigrants and their children, but for all New Yorkers, so, too, did pastrami. In his New Year's column on December 30, 1960, the eminent *New York Times* restaurant critic Craig Claiborne suggested preparing crowd-pleasing dishes such as Welsh rabbit, Swiss fondue, or beef pastrami. See CLAIBORNE, CRAIG.

In was also during the postwar period that advances in food technology meant pastrami could be commercially produced in factories on a large, unprecedented scale. The curing and smoking processes were altered or even replaced with chemical processes and additives that sped up the manufacturing and prolonged shelf life, allowing pastrami to be produced in vastly greater quantities, while also rendering the pastrami itself more uniform in texture and flavor.

Machine-sliced meat—as opposed to the original hand-cut—began to take over the cutting process during the postwar period as well. Thus, as pastrami became increasingly popular, and the sizes of the sandwiches grew with American taste towards towering proportions, Jewish delis took advantage of advances in food technology and began serving pastrami that had been at least partially factory-produced and mechanically prepared. Before serving, the meat could be steamed on site and sliced rapidly to keep up with demand. With the exception of a few delis, by the end of the postwar period, handmade pastrami—much like the commercially produced bread it was served on—was a thing of the past.

In the second decade of the twenty-first century, however, handmade pastrami—cured and smoked on site—has experienced a small revival in New York City and across North America with new wave, artisanal Jewish delicatessens that revel in nostalgia. It is as close to the original Romanian Jewish *pastramă* as New York has seen in over one hundred years.

Claiborne, Craig. "Food Welcoming 1961." *New York Times*, December 30, 1960.
Sax, David. *Save the Deli: In Search of the Perfect Pastrami, Crusty Rye, and the Heart of the Jewish Delicatessen.* Boston: Mariner, 2010.

Lara Rabinovitch

Pastry Shops

See BAKERIES.

Peddlers

See STREET VENDORS.

Pépin, Jacques

With New York as his base, Jacques Pépin has taken his culinary ambassadorship to all corners of the United States. He has combined techniques acquired over a half-century as a professional cook, and writing skills that have produced a host of cookbooks, some of them considered landmarks. And his television cooking shows on PBS have educated millions. He is considered by colleagues to be one of the finest craftspeople of all cooking teachers.

Born December 18, 1935, in Bourg-en-Bresse, France, Pépin and his two brothers worked for his mother, Jeannette, a self-taught cook as she opened a series of small restaurants in the gastronomically rich city of Lyon after World War II. At the age of thirteen, Pépin left the family business to embark on a formal apprenticeship at the Grand Hotel de L'Europe in his hometown of Bourg-en-Bresse. Still in his teens, Pépin moved to Paris to work at the Meurice and then the Plaza-Athénée, under renowned chef Lucien Diat. Pépin was assigned to serve as personal chef to three French heads of state, the last being Charles de Gaulle. Eager to expand his knowledge, Pépin immigrated to New York in 1959, speaking no English, and intending to stay for only a year or two.

He was welcomed by chef Pierre Franey into the kitchen of Le Pavillon, considered one of Manhattan's finest restaurants. He soon became friends with culinary luminaries like James Beard, Julia Child, and Craig Claiborne, often cooking with them. While working full time, Pépin passed a high school equivalency test, and earned both a bachelor of arts and a master's degree in French literature at Columbia University. While at Le Pavillon, two different patrons courted Pépin to work for them: the family of presidential candidate John F. Kennedy, and restaurant and motor lodge entrepreneur Howard Johnson. Pépin accepted Mr. Johnson's offer to work in research and development rather than becoming White House chef.

During his ten years at Howard Johnson's, Pépin learned about mass production, marketing, food chemistry, American food taste, and how to write lucid, detailed recipes, a skill few professional chefs possess. He left Howard Johnson's to open his own restaurant, La Potagerie, a trendy Manhattan soup restaurant that was soon a big success. But in 1974 Pépin had a near-fatal car accident, suffering severe injuries that left him unable to keep up the grueling pace in the kitchen.

The event was the catalyst that propelled him into cookbook writing and teaching, traveling the country forty weeks a year at a time when America was ripe for cooking classes. He wrote two groundbreaking step-by-step books on classic French culinary techniques, La Technique (1976), and La Méthode (1979), books that earned him a place in the James Beard Foundation's Cookbook Hall of Fame for their "substantial and enduring impact on the American kitchen."

To date, Pépin has authored twenty-seven books, and has contributed numerous articles to leading food publications and newspapers, including the New York Times.

Starting in 1989, he began shooting television shows for station KQED in San Francisco and has since filmed ten series of twenty-six shows, teaming with his daughter Claudine for several of the series, and ultimately with his longtime friend Julia Child for "Julia and Jacques Cook at Home." He has won a daytime Emmy Award, and more James Beard Awards for his shows and books than anyone else.

In October 2004, Pépin received France's highest civilian honor, the French Legion of Honor. He is also the recipient of two of the French government's highest honors: he was named a Chevalier de L'Ordre des Arts et des Lettres in 1997 and a Chevalier de L'Ordre du Mérite Agricole in 1992. He has also been awarded several honorary doctoral degrees by various U.S. universities.

To reinforce the importance of cuisine in culture, Pépin teamed with Julia Child to develop and teach a groundbreaking masters degree program in gastronomy at Boston University. In 1988, he became dean of special programs at the French Culinary Institute (now the International Culinary Center). While Pépin has acknowledged that most people think of him as the quintessential French chef, he has stated that he considers himself a New Yorker more than anything else. He praised the city for its scope of different cuisines, and says he has reflected these influences in his books and in his teaching.

See also CHILD, JULIA and FRENCH CULINARY INSTITUTE.

Fenzl, Barbara Poole. "Happy Birthday, Jacques." *Food Forum Quarterly* (1Q 2006).

Pépin, Jacques. *The Apprentice: My Life in the Kitchen.* New York: Houghton Mifflin, 2003.

Warner, Scott. "Pépin, Jacques." In *The Oxford Encyclopedia of Food and Drink in America,* 2d ed., edited by Andrew F. Smith. New York: Oxford University Press, 2012.

Scott Warner

Pepsi-Cola

Pepsi-Cola was created in New Bern, North Carolina, but the Pepsi-Cola Company went bankrupt in 1922. It was resurrected by New Yorker Roy C. Megarel, a Wall Street broker. During the Depression, the company again went bankrupt, but in 1931 it was acquired by Charles Guth, who was also president of Loft, Inc., a New York candy company that also operated soda fountains. Guth restructured Pepsi, giving himself 80 percent of the shares. He moved the entire operation to Long Island City, New York. Guth directed chemists employed by Loft to reformulate Pepsi, and they came up with a new formula that omitted pepsin, which had been a key ingredient in the original Pepsi-Cola (hence its name). See SODA FOUNTAINS.

In 1933, Guth made a brilliant marketing move: he started selling 12-ounce bottles of Pepsi for the same price (a nickel) as Coke's 6-ounce bottle. His test market was Baltimore, where it quickly became evident that this price point was irresistible to Americans in the throes of the Depression. With Pepsi skyrocketing, Guth took the new pricing nationwide. Within two years Pepsi had generated a $2 million profit and become America's second-largest soft drink company. In 1934, Pepsi-Cola began buying up bottling operations throughout the United States. Two years later it opened a new bottling plant in Long Island City, Queens. The plant's 147-foot red neon "Pepsi-Cola" sign on top of the plant was visible from Manhattan's Upper East Side. The sign was considered an eyesore, but over time it became a symbol of Long Island City's past.

In 1935, Charles Guth resigned as president of Loft, Inc. to devote his energies full-time to Pepsi, where he was president and general manager. Loft's executives sued Guth, claiming that he had used their firm's staff, resources, and facilities to restart Pepsi, and that the successful Pepsi-Cola Company should really belong to Loft, Inc. In a landmark decision in 1939, the state court ruled that Guth had failed fiduciary responsibilities to Loft. He was removed as president of Pepsi but stayed on as general manager while the verdict was appealed. Guth lost the appeal in 1941 and was then dismissed from his position at Pepsi. The two companies were combined, but the new management spun off the Loft candy stores from the Pepsi-Cola Corporation. Pepsi-Cola shares were first listed on the New York Stock Exchange in 1941.

World War II had a dramatic effect on the soft drink industry. Pepsi-Cola's overseas operations were disrupted. Sugar rationing was imposed in the United States early in 1942, drastically curtailing soft-drink production. See WORLD WAR II. After the war, with sugar again plentiful, Pepsi had a hard time competing with Coca-Cola, which had flourished during the war thanks to its government contracts. Pepsi moved its headquarters to midtown Manhattan in 1948, but continued its bottling operation in Long Island City.

After the war Americans faced inflation, and Pepsi had to raise its prices; sales lagged further. See POST–WORLD WAR II (1945–1975). By 1950, the company

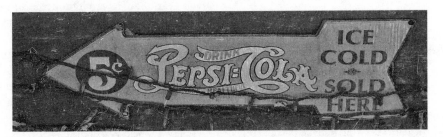

An old Pepsi-Cola sign, encouraging customers to drink its "healthful" beverage. During the Great Depression Pepsi-Cola was rescued from bankruptcy by Charles Guth, who was the president of Loft, Inc., a New York candy company. Guth moved all of the operations to Long Island City. DON O'BRIEN

was almost forced to declare bankruptcy for a third time. Alfred N. Steele and other former Coca-Cola executives were hired to rejuvenate the operation. Steele launched a highly successful advertising campaign, which came to the rescue. Steele married movie star Joan Crawford in 1954, and she lent glamour to Pepsi's image by always having a bottle of Pepsi on hand when she did press conferences and interviews.

Throughout the 1950s, Pepsi continued to expand abroad, particularly into Latin America and Europe. During the 1960s, Pepsi-Cola introduced several new products, including Mountain Dew and Diet Pepsi. In 1965, Pepsi bought Frito-Lay, Inc. and renamed the new corporation PepsiCo. Corporate headquarters moved from Manhattan to Purchase, New York, in 1970, although the soda continued to be bottled in New York City.

Pepsi-Cola closed its bottling plant in Long Island City in 1999, but its iconic "Pepsi-Cola" sign was saved and restored. In 2013, it was reconstructed in front of an apartment complex built on the site of the old bottling plant. It remains one of the most familiar landmarks along the East River.

See also LOFT'S CANDY STORES; QUEENS; SODA; and SODA "BAN".

Capparell, Stephanie. *The Real Pepsi Challenge: How One Pioneering Company Broke Color Barriers in 1940s American Business.* New York: Free Press, 2008.
Smith, Andrew F. *Drinking History: Fifteen Turning Points in the Making of American Beverages.* New York: Columbia University Press, 2012.
Stoddard, Bob. *Pepsi: 100 Years.* Los Angeles: General Publishing Group, 1999.

Andrew F. Smith

Perrier

In 1976, Bruce Nevins, president and part owner of Perrier's U.S. distribution company, headquartered in New York, decided to reposition Perrier as a health and fitness drink through a massive marketing and public relations campaign that would promote Perrier simultaneously to the public and to distributors. Nevins launched an advertising campaign in the spring of 1977 with a hefty television budget. Perrier sponsored the New York City Marathon beginning in November 1977, donating a substantial sum to the race organizers and supplying 7,500 bottles of

Perrier for the runners, along with shorts and shirts bearing the Perrier logo. This was just the beginning of a promotional effort that soon changed the entire bottled water industry and created a new product category. Within a decade, New Yorkers everywhere—at work, at play, at home, or on the road—could be seen clutching their ever-present plastic bottles of brand-name water. Before the ad campaign was launched, Perrier sales generated $500,00 annually. Three years later, sales exceeded $5 million. This campaign was one of the most successful in advertising history.

See also WATER, BOTTLED.

Smith, Andrew F. *Fifteen Turning Points in the Making of American Beverages.* New York: Columbia University Press, 2012.

Andrew F. Smith

Peter Luger's

Peter Luger's Steak House in Williamsburg, Brooklyn, is the only surviving New York restaurant launched by a nineteenth-century German immigrant. Carl Luger brought his family from Donau, Germany, in 1879 and settled in Brooklyn. Eight years later Luger opened a café, bowling alley, and billiard hall at Driggs Avenue and Eighth Street in Williamsburg. It quickly became a favorite in the neighborhood, which was then mostly German. When Carl died, his son Peter Luger jettisoned the bowling alley and billiard hall and renamed the restaurant "Peter Luger's Steak House." The Williamsburg Bridge opened in 1903, and the following year the restaurant was moved to its current location at 178 Broadway, right across from the new bridge. The offerings were simple and straightforward: tomato and onion salad, porterhouse steak, and French fries.

Like most restaurants, Peter Luger's made considerable portions of its profit from the sale of alcohol. In 1922, in the early years of Prohibition, it was raided by the police, and its cellar was emptied of wine and liquor. Peter Luger challenged the confiscation, claiming that the wine was for his personal consumption. (It was legal to possess and drink wine, provided you did not sell or distribute it.) The wine was not returned. See PROHIBITION.

The two World Wars hurt German restaurants in America, and as many German-Americans moved away from New York City, most of the old German-owned restaurants closed. The popular Brooklyn steakhouse survived, but after Peter Luger died in 1941, his son, Frederick, took over, and the restaurant declined until it was finally put up for auction in 1950. Peter Luger's was acquired by Sol Forman, a former patron who owned a factory across the street. Peter Luger's nephew, Carl Luger, who had been the chef, became a part owner. Forman knew little about restaurants, but he transformed Peter Luger's into New York City's most popular steakhouse.

One of the first things that Carl Luger did was to create an actual menu—the restaurant's first ever—and expand its offerings to include shrimp cocktail, creamed spinach, and German fried potatoes, as well as desserts including tarts, cheesecake, and apple strudel. Fish was added to the menu in the 1980s. A bacon appetizer and a lamb chop entrée were added in the 1990s. The offerings now include Caesar salad, prime rib, pot roast, chicken, and the "Luger-Burger."

Peter Luger's has been consistently rated as one of New York City's finest steakhouses.

See also GERMAN; NEW YORK STRIP STEAK; RESTAURANTS; and WILLIAMSBURG.

Fussell, Betty. *Raising Steaks: The Life and Times of American Beef.* Orlando, Fla.: Harcourt, 2008.
Grimes, William. *Appetite City: A Culinary History of New York.* New York: North Point, 2009.

Andrew F. Smith

Pickles

Pickling was introduced to New York by the European settlers who originally founded the colony. But pickles as we think of them today—cucumbers pickled in a brine of vinegar and spices—were popularized in New York City by German and Eastern European immigrants on the Lower East Side. It was the Ashkenazi Jews who settled by the hundreds of thousands on the Lower East Side who introduced the dill pickle to New York City and the United States at large, and solidified New York's position as the nation's pickle capital.

The Big Pickle

Pickled cucumbers and other vegetables were a central part of the diet of Jews in Eastern Europe, adding some interest to a bland diet of bread and potatoes. Before the era of refrigeration, pickling was an important means of preserving fresh food. During the fall months, Ashkenazi housewives would begin the process of pickling cucumbers, cabbage, carrots, tomatoes, and other vegetables in large enough quantities to get them through the cold winter months.

In the late nineteenth century the Lower East Side was the city's pickle district, home to hundreds of manufacturers selling pickles from pushcarts as well as brick-and-mortar shops. Eighty of these businesses were on Essex Street, nicknamed "pickle alley." Producers brined pickles according to their own recipes, competing with each other for the local and national trade. See JEWISH and LOWER EAST SIDE.

Guss' and the Lower East Side Pickle Wars

By the end of the twentieth century, there was only one pickle vendor left on the Lower East Side: Guss' Pickles. Located on the first floor of a tenement building on Essex Street, Guss' sold a variety of pickles—sours, half sours, and new pickles as well as pickled tomatoes, peppers, mushrooms, and other vegetables—from barrels on the sidewalk in front of the shop. Guss' drew people to the Lower East Side from all over the city and country. The shop was featured in the 1988 movie *Crossing Delancey*, in which an Upper West Side woman falls in love with a Lower East Side pickle man.

Isidore Guss, the original owner, died in 1975 and his family sold the business to Harold Baker. In 2001, Baker's son Tim went into business with Andrew Leibowitz, a co-owner of United Pickle in the Bronx

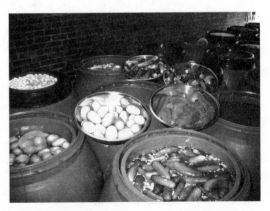

The Pickle Guys is kosher-certified and hearkens back to the old pickle district by selling pickled cucumbers, tomatoes, garlic, olives, mushrooms, beets, string beans, and a host of other pickled items from barrels in a tenement shop on Essex Street. COURTESY PICKLE GUYS

and a supplier to Guss' Pickles. In 2002, Guss' lost their lease and moved to Orchard Street. Meanwhile, Baker and Leibowitz opened a new branch of Guss' in Cedarhurst, New York. In 2004, Baker sold the Lower East Side branch of Guss' to Patricia Fairhurst. These actions began a legal feud, known as the Pickle Wars. Leibowitz claimed the rights to sell the Guss' name and recipes. Baker disagreed and denied Fairhurst the right to use the Guss' name on the Orchard Street store. A lawsuit ensued and when it was settled in 2009, Fairhurst lost the right to the name. She closed shop on Orchard Street and opened Ess-a-Pickle in Brooklyn. She now operates Clinton Hill Pickles, in Brooklyn, and Leibowitz's Guss' Pickles operates out of Cedarhurst.

Today's Pickle Alley

But the pickle wars did not spell the end of pickle production and sale on the Lower East Side. In 2002, when Guss' moved to Orchard Street, long-time Guss' employee Alan Kaufman opened his own shop on Essex, along with some of his co-workers from Guss'. Kaufman's shop, The Pickle Guys, is currently operating on Essex Street, with an annex on Coney Island Avenue in the Kensington section of Brooklyn, a neighborhood with a large Orthodox Jewish population. Like Guss', The Pickle Guys is kosher-certified and hearkens back to the old pickle district by selling pickled cucumbers, tomatoes, garlic, olives, mushrooms, beets, string beans, and a host of other pickled items from barrels in a tenement shop on Essex Street. As Passover approaches, the Pickle Guys grind fresh horseradish on the sidewalk in front of the shop, armed with a gas mask. Like their forebears on the Lower East Side, the Pickle Guys ship nationwide.

Since 2001, the Lower East Side Business Improvement District has hosted the Lower East Side Pickle Festival in the neighborhood every fall, featuring over twenty vendors from New York and elsewhere, participating in demonstrations of pickles from around the world.

Artisanal Pickles

Today, as small-batch producers open artisanal food shops in New York City (and especially in Brooklyn), New York is experiencing a pickle revival. Companies like Brooklyn Brine, McClure's Pickles, and Jacob's Pickles are joining older businesses like United Pickles and The Pickle Guys in returning New York to the center of the nation's small-batch pickle production. Today's New York pickle scene also reflects the influx of new generations of immigrants bringing their own pickling traditions such as Korean kimchi and South Asian achar. See KIMCHI.

Bahrampour, Tara. "Let There Be Pickles." *New York Times*, August 26, 2001.
"The History of Pickles in New York." Lower East Side Tenement Museum. http://www.tenement.org/pickle.
Ralph, Talia. "A History of the Lower East Side Pickle Wars." *Food52*, October 11, 2013. http://food52.com/blog/8520-a-history-of-the-lower-east-side-pickle-wars.

Cindy R. Lobel

Picnics

The words "Gotham" and "picnic" are linked to Washington Irving and James Kirk Paulding's satirical magazine *Salmagundi* (1807). See IRVING, WASHINGTON. "Gotham," a name for New York meaning "Goat Town," was an instant hit, but "picnic," a buzzword meaning "silly," flashed and went south. The joke was that "picnic silk-stockings" worn by fashionable women on the muddy streets of Manhattan illustrated that nudity was the rage. Perhaps, it still is, but now picnic is a ubiquitous word that has come to mean the leisure activity usually associated with enjoying an outdoor meal with friends or family. As adapted by writers and artists, the picnic is integrated into the city's cultural history, character, and attitude. Incubation, however, was slow, and though the word was subterranean, people picnicked whenever and wherever it was convenient. Menus varied according to taste, style, and means, but the standard (then as now) is that *any* totable food (hot or cold) is picnic food.

It was thirty-one years before James Fenimore Cooper highlighted an outing he pretentiously referred to as "a rustic fete" in *Home As Found* (1838). It was another two decades before New York magazines began featuring picnic scenes and Homer Winslow was chosen to lead the way. *Harper's Weekly* commissioned a series of picnic scenes with such generic titles as *Picnic by Land*, *Picnic by Water*, and *A Picnic in the Country*. In 1869, *Appleton's Journal* paired Homer's *Picnic Excursion* (1869) with an anonymous essay claiming that picnicking is the natural

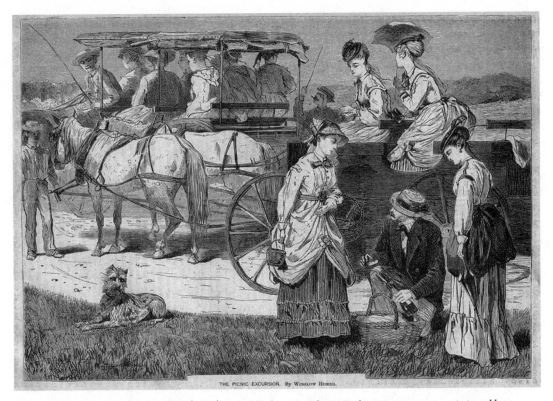

THE PICNIC EXCURSION. By WINSLOW HOMER.

Winslow Homer's *The Picnic Excursion* (1869) was part of a series of New York picnic scenes commissioned by *Harper's Weekly*, with such generic titles as *Picnic by Land, Picnic by Water*, and *A Picnic in the Country*.

birthright of Americans, as if written in the Declaration of Independence or Constitution: "What the full requirements of a picnic may be admits to some range of opinion, but the great charm of this social device is undoubtedly the freedom it affords. It is to eat, to chat, to lie, to talk, to walk, with something of the unconstraint of primitive life...." Ignoring the idea of "primitive picnicking," (a constant myth), Homer's picnic is genteel: a group of suitably dressed middle-class men and women in a wagon waiting for a companion to open a bottle of wine, or perhaps Homer's favorite, rum. Comically, a small terrier looks askance at him.

Four years later, Claude Tavernier's "The Picnic Season" was the front-page illustration for *The Daily Graphic* (1873). Depicting what must have been common, Tavernier shows picnickers boarding a Hudson River steamer and traveling north to Jones' Wood, a commercial picnic ground, where they eat, dance, romance, play games, sing, play music, and climatically, get into a drunken brawl. When it rains, exhausted picnickers return by the light of the moon. This was a socially adopted picnic pattern, so much

so that thirty-one years later, when the *General Slocum*, a paddlewheel ferry en route to Long Island, burned in the lower East River, one thousand picnickers were killed. The city mourned. Charles Ives tried to express the grief in his music but abandoned the project.

Of New York's great parks, Manhattan's Central Park and Brooklyn's Prospect Park are most famous for picnics, but painters and writers have incorporated places from all five boroughs. Adolf Dehn's painting *Spring in Central Park* (1941) shows a happy couple spreading a blanket on the new grass, but there is neither food nor drink. E. L. Doctorow's picnic in his novel *City of God* (2000) takes place somewhere near the Sheep Meadow where paper bags are filled with deli sandwiches and soft drinks. Bernard Waber's *Lyle the Crocodile* (1965) tells the tale of a crocodile who lives with the Primms, on East Eighty-Eighth Street, and picnics in nearby Central Park where he feeds pigeons that flock around him having a picnic of their own.

The Prospect Park picnics of heroine Sophie Zawistowska in William Styron's *Sophie's Choice* (1979) are troubling because she is trying to forget her experience in Auschwitz. She seems happy, but she is not. The salami, bratwurst, Braunschweiger, sardines, hot pastrami, lox, bagels, and pumpernickel she buys at a Flatbush Avenue deli only mask her anguish. Alan J. Pakula's film adaptation (1982) repositions the park picnic, and Sophie, Nathan, and Stingo sprawl on a Prospect Heights South porch roof where they drink wine from long-stemmed glasses. (After all, it is Brooklyn.) On another scale, what-you-see-is-what-you-get in Jacqueline Woodson's happy children's story in Prospect Park. *We Had a Picnic Sunday Last* (1997) boasts a menu of fried chicken, ham, sweet corn, cinnamon bread, cranberry muffins, sweet potato pie, peach cobbler, yams, potato salad, salad, cornbread, homemade ice cream, and a store-bought cake.

Other New York City picnics find their way into the mix. The zaniest is John Sloan's *Arch Conspirators* (1917), a picnic atop the Washington Square Arch, where a group built a fire to make tea, dined on hot dogs, and drank wine and spirits. It was a zany night in January, after which they signed a manifesto declaring Greenwich Village a republic.

The most nostalgic are Alfred Kazin's *A Walker in the City* (1951), a coming-of-age memoir, and Laura Shaine Cunningham's memoir *A Place in the Country* (2001). Kazin never forgets the scene in Forest Park, Queens, so alien to his apartment in Brownsville, Brooklyn, in which he sees "a clearing filled with stone picnic tables." "*Nothing*," he writes, "had ever cried out such a welcome as those stone tables in the clearing—saw the trees in their dim green recede in one long moving tide back into dusk, and gasped in pain when the evening rushed upon us before I had a chance to walk that woodland through." There is no food at Kazin's picnic because it registers in his imagination as an ideal vision. Cunningham builds on the memory of picnicking with her mother somewhere in a Bronx park where she ate soft white-bread sandwiches and fruit packed in a paper bag. Cunningham was four or five and remembers the experience as being "romantick." (Though anyone who has eaten soft white-bread sandwiches knows better.)

At the beach, the most joyous picnic is John Sloan's *South Beach* (1905) testifying to a very happy lunch of steamed crabs and hot dogs eaten without benefit of plates or cutlery. The funniest picnic is Mable Dwight's congested vision of *Coney Island Beach* (1932) in which a dour grandmother watches as a mother repositions a crying toddler's diaper. Food seems everywhere, the toddler's bottle with a nipple, a soda bottle with a straw, hot dogs, and ice cream. The most jumbled is Reginald Marsh's *Coney Island Scene* (1932) in which members of the Brooklyn Roosevelt Club fall after posing in a human pyramid. If there is food, it is lost in the crowd. The most somber is George Hooker's *Coney Island* (1948), a scene under the boardwalk that combines a picnic with a descent from the cross. Without benefit of a blanket, food, or drink, a mournful Mary, in a blue bathing suit, cradles a dead Jesus in bathing trunks. Only in New York, only at Coney Island.

Among the most iconic NYC picnics, the most magical is Faith Ringgold's *Tar Beach* (1988), an illustrated story about a rooftop picnic [tar beach] in Washington Heights, the menu for which is fried chicken, peanuts, soda, iced tea, and beer. For the grittiest picnic, there is Richard Pantell's painting *Backyards* (2001), a scene in a Queens backyard where a family sits at a wooden picnic table surrounded by buildings and junk: a truck, an automobile, and a clothesline full of drying wash. It's either early spring or late fall, for the trees are bare, but the hearty picnickers are taking in the city air in their meager garden, but what they eat is unknown. Finally, for a commuters' picnic, Rosanne Wasserstein's "Picnic in the Station" (1995) is a poetic image of a woman standing in the great lobby of Grand Central Terminal drinking coffee and eating donuts from a paper bag.

Levy, Walter. *The Picnic: A History*. Lanham, Md.: Rowman & Littlefield/AltaMira, 2014.

Irving, Washington, and James Kirk Paulding. *Salmagundi; or, the Whim-Whams and Opinions of Launcelot Langstaff, Esq., and Others*. In *The Complete Works of Washington Irving*, edited by Bruce Granger and Martha Hartzog. New York: Twayne, 1977.

Walter Levy

Pizza

While consumed today across the globe, pizza's accurate history and current definition remain elusive. Centuries of evolution have transformed it from its earliest incarnation into something almost unrecognizable to our pizza-loving ancestors. The grains used evolved from ancient coarse grains to refined white flour but the technique of baking dough over direct high heat was the precursor to modern pizza. In what is today's Italy, the Neolithic nomads, northern Etruscans, and southern Greeks all contributed to pizza's evolution and complexity by introducing dough kneading, employing ovens, adding yeast, and increasing the seasoning. The eighteenth-century Neapolitans, however, perfected the ancient flatbread and created pizza closely resembling what we think of today. Pizza folklore begins with the heralded story of King Ferdinando I and Queen Maria Carolina, Marie Antoinette's sister. Some folkloric explanations for pizza's popularity attribute the queen sharing her "common tastes" and love of plebeian pizza with the people. Yet varying folklore attributes the king himself for loving pizza much to the chagrin of the sophisticated queen. Through building a pizza oven in the palace, the king and queen elevated pizza's humble status. It was in 1889 however, under the reign of King Umberto I of Savoia and Queen Margherita, that pizza transformed into what we think of today. Legend states that a local pizza chef, Raffaele Esposito, in an act to impress and pay tribute to the king and queen, added mozzarella to the commonly consumed tomato and basil recipe. The pizza colors—red, white, and green—conjured up the Italian flag and the legendary pizza took on the name pizza Margherita that it still holds today.

In the late nineteenth century, as southern Italians, primarily from Sicily and Naples, immigrated to the United States and in particular, New York City, they brought pizza with them, often selling pies in small grocery shops next to dry goods, staples, and produce. However, the first stand-alone American pizzeria in New York City (and first in the United States) did not open until 1905. Gennaro Lombardi's idea for a pizzeria, while novel in New York, was modeled after pizzerias throughout Italy. Because pizza production required an expensive wood-fired oven as well as ample space to prepare and stretch the dough, few Italians made pizza at home. Instead, it was made at small outdoor stalls until around 1830, when the first documented pizzeria opened in Naples with wood-burning ovens and some seating. Lombardi's was originally located in Manhattan, at 53½ Spring Street at the northern edge of Little Italy. After closing for several years, it reopened in a larger space at 32 Spring Street. One of New York's oldest restaurants, Lombardi's still maintains a loyal following with New Yorkers and tourists alike. Originally,

Lombardi's, along with other neighborhood pizzerias, catered exclusively to New York's southern Italian immigrants looking for recognizable comfort food from home. These restaurants saw their markets grow following World War II, when returning GIs having served in Italy sought out pizza and other Italian food at home. See ITALIAN; LITTLE ITALY; and LOMBARDI'S.

The coal brick oven pizza that the GIs enjoyed in New York City, while similar to Neapolitan pies eaten in Italy, evolved to meet New York taste preferences. Mirroring the post–World War II economic boom, and glorifying excess and abundance, pizzas too grew in size. Economically fragile Italian immigrants, acculturating to New York life, embraced a lifestyle with an increased emphasis on meat, a feeling of "more than" and a way to distance themselves from previous hunger. Thus New York pizzas were transformed from the previous thin, light, and delicate Neapolitan pizza enjoyed in Italy to a thicker-crust pie heavily laden with cheese, meat, and myriad toppings.

Although Lombardi's enjoys the status as the first New York pizzeria, several competitors soon emerged. Antonio Totonno Pero, Lombardi's original *pizzaiolo* (pizza chef), left Lombardi's in 1924 and opened his own pizzeria, Totonno's in Coney Island. Totonno's, still a family-owned business in Coney Island, closed briefly for fires in 1997 and again in 2009. A victim of Hurricane Sandy, the pizzeria closed for five months in 2012 but is once again open for business with Totonno descendants running the store. Lombardi's and Totonno's set the stage for other classic and still existing New York pizzerias. John Sasso opened up John's Pizza in 1929 originally on Sullivan Street in the West Village. A few years later, after losing a lease, John's moved around the corner to Bleecker Street where it still serves coal-fired pizzas from the original Sullivan Street oven. Pasquale "Patsy" Lancieri and his wife Carmela opened up Patsy's in 1933 in East Harlem—an Italian American enclave. During the 1950s and 1960s, Patsy's became a celebrity haunt for entertainers including Frank Sinatra, Tony Bennett, and Dean Martin; for Yankee baseball greats Joe DiMaggio, Yogi Berra, and Phil Rizzuto; and for politicians beginning with Mayor Fiorello LaGuardia through Mayors Rudy Giuliani and Mike Bloomberg. The pizzeria claims that Francis Ford Coppola used Patsy's as inspiration for the *Godfather* films and the restaurant was used in several other film shoots.

The "fathers" of New York pizza all claimed to have their own secret recipes and taste profiles, yet all original New York pizza share similar traits. New York pizza is cheesy, gooey, with a high, dense border and medium-thick crust, and can be bought by the slice, or whole. New Yorkers for the past several decades enjoy the tradition of arguing over which is the "real" Ray's pizza among the myriad "Rays" pizzerias—all vying for rights to the name. There was Rays Pizzeria of Prince Street that closed recently, Original Rays, Famous Rays, Famous Original Rays, and Ray Bari. Most pizza is topped with mozzarella cheese, tomato sauce, and selected extra toppings. Pizza ordered without additional toppings is considered "plain," "regular," or "cheese." New York pizzas come in 14-, 16-, or 18-inch diameters but are most often ordered by the slice. The traditional method for eating pizza by the slice is to fold it in half lengthwise and eat it while holding in one hand. While New Yorkers are proud of this feat, New York City Mayor Bill De Blasio was vilified in local newspapers for eating pizza with a knife and fork. Pizzerias today generally use deck ovens powered with gas, although some still employ coal or brick ovens, which both conjure up early pizzeria days and help achieve a desirable charred crust. According to the economic law known as the "pizza principle" or the "pizza connection," the price of a New York slice correlates with the current cost of a one-way New York subway fare. As the subway fare has increased rapidly since 1980, New Yorkers test the Pizza Principle with alarming accuracy.

New Pizza Generation

In recent years, New York City has experienced a pizza renaissance as it embraces pizza produced the way New Yorkers did during the early twentieth century. Abandoning gas ovens for their coal and brick alternatives, substituting fresh mozzarella for industrial cheese, and replacing thick, heavy dough with thin, delicate crusts, artisan pizza chefs cater to a new generation of pizza aficionados. A few newcomers ushered in the New American pizza movement, including sustainably committed Franny's Brooklyn pizza restaurant, which opened in 2005, and Roberta's, in Bushwick, Brooklyn. Roberta's uses ingredients sourced from its adjacent farm and Jim Lahey's Co (short for company) which opened in 2009.

Shortly thereafter, Paul Giannone, an engineer by training but enthusiastic pizza hobbyist made his passion his career when he opened Paulie Gee's in Greenpoint, Brooklyn. Fans flocked to Paulie Gee's to partake of his bacon-inspired fare. With outposts in Williamsburg, Brooklyn, Manhattan's Bowery, and Midtown, Forcella Pizzeria features *montanara*, a flash-fried pizza concept from his native Naples, Italy. Even New York restaurateur Danny Meyer recently entered the designer pizza market with the opening of Marta which serves esoteric combinations including okra and lamb sausage. Even as New York City continually embraces new high-end, artisan pizzas adorned with Brooklyn-grown kale, imported burrata, Brussel sprouts, and duck confit, nothing remains as iconic as the time-honored tradition of walking down a street holding a classic New York slice folded in half.

See also PIZZERIAS and ROBERTA'S.

Berg, Jennifer, and Cara De Silva. "Pizza." In *The Encyclopedia of Food and Culture*, edited by Solomon H. Katz and William Woys Weaver. New York: Scribner, 2003.
Haberman, Clyde. "Digging Deep for a Slice of the Pie." *New York Times*, June 21, 2005.
Levine, Ed. *Pizza: A Slice of Heaven*. New York: Rizzoli, 2010.
Romer, Elizabeth. *Italian Pizza and Hearth Breads*. New York: Clarkson Potter, 1987.
Sloman, Evelyne. *The Pizza Book: Everything There Is to Know about the World's Greatest Pie*. New York: Times Books, 1984.

Jennifer Schiff Berg

Pizzerias

"Pizza as the world knows it was invented in New York City, not Naples. Here, in 1905, Gennaro Lombardi opened America's first pizza parlor," proclaims Robert Sietsema, restaurant and food writer for Eater.com and formerly of the Village Voice.

Is that New York chauvinism speaking or historical truth? According to historian and author Carol Helstolsky, pizza went from being "strictly Neapolitan to being Italian-American and then becoming Italian." And, indeed, the style of pizza that became popular around the world—a large round pie slathered with tomato sauce and mozzarella cheese and sliced into triangles—was the style that originated in New York at Lombardi's pizzeria at 53½ Spring Street.

Background

Pizza, a small, plain version of what we know today, was sold by street vendors in Naples as an inexpensive food of the poor—*cucina povera*—and was little known outside of the south of Italy. Pizzerias existed in Naples in the eighteenth century, but without tables. The pizzeria was basically a stand where one could purchase the meager meal or snack, rarely larger than a hand with little or nothing on it. Proprietors might add a table or two if space allowed, but pizza was most often purchased and consumed in the street.

Tomatoes found their way into Italian cuisine in the late seventeenth to early eighteenth centuries, but they were not commonly used on pizza until the early nineteenth century, according to the Associazione Verace Pizza Napolitana (Authentic Neapolitan Pizza Association). The sweet San Marzano tomatoes of the region were favored by the *pizzaioli* (pizza makers) as a topping for their pizza. Still, this tomato was not known outside of Naples.

Pizza found its way to the United States toward the end of the nineteenth century with the wave of poor southern Italian immigrants who baked it at home or bought it from enterprising street vendors.

Gennaro Lombardi, from Naples, was a grocer on Spring Street and was the first to receive a license to sell pizza out of his grocery store. He had all the necessary ingredients in his store and employed a baker from Naples, Antonio Pero, nicknamed Totonno. Business was so brisk that tables were added so patrons could enjoy their pizza on the spot. Immigrants from Naples, factory workers on their lunch break, and families looking for a cheap meal made up the steady clientele. See LOMBARDI'S.

By the late 1920s, Lombardi's was an important gathering spot in what became known as "Little Italy." Its coal-fired, terracotta oven was huge and could hold fifteen pizzas at once. The serving size was increased and the toppings were applied more generously, giving birth to the American name "pizza pie."

At the same time, many of the pizza makers who trained at Lombardi's left to open their own pizzerias, and the trend took off around New York City. Of the more famous, Antonio Pero opened Totonno's in Coney Island, and John Sasso opened John's on Bleecker Street. Pasquale Lancieri came on the scene in 1933 and opened Patsy's in the Italian community of East Harlem. All four remain in operation today,

and Lombardi's is credited with creating what Helstosky calls "the New York pizzeria phenomenon."

The pizza craze spread through the boroughs of New York City and, unlike in Naples, it also spread beyond the city environs. Throughout Northeastern cities such as Boston (Santarpio's in 1933) and New Haven (Pepe's in 1925) and cities in New Jersey, where there were large populations of southern Italian immigrants, pizzerias sprang to life. And they had a new vitality as restaurants and taverns. Even Lombardi's cashed in on the restaurant concept in 1930, when he started offering a few other simple dishes.

Changing Tastes

In the land of abundance, tinned and fresh tomatoes were available, cheese was plentiful, and anchovies found their way on top, along with sausage, pepperoni, and peppers. The crust got thicker and pies became larger—large enough to share, thus inspiring the "pizza party."

New York made the pizzeria popular, and soon it became a fixture in states far and wide, but it was a far cry from its predecessor. Stacked gas-fired steel ovens enabled pizza makers to serve a large crowd of hungry eaters in less time.

One feature that made New York pizza different was the offering of pizza by the slice. One could buy a whole pie or get just one slice for the ultimate fast food. It once again became an inexpensive snack or meal. Ben's Famous, Original Ray's, Joe's, or Sal & Carmine's to name just a few—all New Yorkers pledge allegiance to their favorite go-to neighborhood pizza joint. Several establishments, notably Ray's and Patsy's, became recognizable brands, and legal battles ensued over the proprietorship of these names.

By the time pizzerias were hitting their stride, big business moved in to mass produce the pizza-in-a-box commodity that the world has come to know. Pizza Hut, Domino's, Papa John's, Little Caesars, and their competitors all had less to do with pizzerias than volume and fast food. But New York, once again the innovator, is making strides to reverse that trend.

The age of artisan pizza is supplanting the quick and uniform pie. Places where one sits down to enjoy a drink and a well-crafted, wood-oven-fired facsimile of a Neapolitan pizza—some with innovative toppings—have been gaining traction over the past few years, but don't look to these establishments for a slice to go. This is pizza gone full circle. Some of the best of Gotham's reigning joints, according to the websites Eater.com, Gothamist.com, GrubStreet.com, and TimeOutNY.com, are Roberta's, Kesté, Di Fara, Motorino, Coals, Lucali, Denino's, Zero Otto Nove, Don Antonio by Starita, Co., Franny's, Rubirosa, and Speedy Romeo. And the four original pizzerias—Lombardi's, Totonno's, John's, and Patsy's—are not to be forgotten. They still top the NYC list.

See also ITALIAN; LITTLE ITALY; PIZZA; and ROBERTA'S.

Buonassisi, Rosario. *Pizza: The Dish, the Legend.* Willowdale, Canada: Firefly, 2000.
Helstosky, Carol. *Pizza: A Global History.* London: Reaktion, 2008.

Linda Pelaccio

Plaza, The

The Plaza Hotel, at the corner of Fifth Avenue and Fifty-Sixth Street, overlooking Central Park, is the home of the iconic drinking and dining spaces The Oak Room and The Oak Bar. The Plaza stands on the site of an earlier, smaller Plaza Hotel, built in 1880, which in turn occupied land that was originally a skating pond, where the Astor family indulged in winter sports. In 1905 the old building was torn down and rebuilt, and the new Plaza opened on October 1, 1907, as an opulent grand hotel. The hotel has changed hands many times and is currently owned by Fairmont Hotels & Resorts.

Over the course of more than a century, an array of on-premises dining rooms have come and gone. The 1910s and 1920s brought The Grill Room. In the 1930s, The Persian Room lured cafe society types. The 1940s brought The Rendez-vous, while the 1950s introduced The Edwardian Room, a look back to the hotel's earlier days. The 1960s welcomed Trader Vic's (one of the first theme eateries of the city) and The Oyster Bar, a nod to less formal dining. In the 1970s, trendy boîte Green Tulip welcomed a younger generation, while the 1990s introduced Gaugin, a restaurant-cum-discotheque.

Yet The Oak Room has been a near constant. It started life as The Men's Bar, opening in 1912. Paneled in the finest oak, it was a male-only sanctuary until (like many bars) it closed for the duration of Prohibition. See PROHIBITION. It reopened in 1934, now called The Oak Room. It still was considered a men's sanctuary; women were permitted only after 3:00 p.m. It was not until 1969—after a much-publicized protest by the National Organization for Women—that the barriers finally were dropped and women were welcomed to The Oak Room for lunch as well.

The dark wood-paneled room itself is little changed since The Men's Bar days. Designed by architect Henry Hardenbergh as a bar in austere German Renaissance style, everything in the room was given a German drinking theme, including faux wine casks carved into the woodwork, paintings of three famous German castles, and coats of arms from German families. For a short period, The Oak Room also featured a water fountain in the center of the room.

Meanwhile, the adjacent Oak Bar was established in 1945. From 1912 until Prohibition, it was an unnamed barroom space next to the much grander Oak Room. During the Prohibition years, the bar was removed and the space was leased to brokerage firm E. F. Hutton to use as office space. When Conrad Hilton took over The Plaza in 1943 and found that they still occupied the prime space overlooking the park, he moved the brokerage firm to a mezzanine space. The Oak Bar opened in 1945, adorned with murals of old New York painted by Everett Shinn, a student of Degas.

The Oak Room and Oak Bar were closed for refurbishment between 2002 and 2007 and reopened in time to celebrate The Plaza's one hundredth anniversary. The Oak Room closed yet again in 2011, after a series of rowdy parties held by nightlife impresarios then operating the space raised objections by long-term hotel residents. The Oak Room currently is used as a private event space. According to The Plaza's website, The Oak Bar "will be re-opening shortly and live up to its iconic reputation as a New York City institution."

Batterberry, Michael, and Ariane Batterberry. *On the Town in New York: A History of Eating, Drinking and Entertainments from 1776 to the Present.* New York: Scribner, 1973.
Gathje, Curtis. *At The Plaza: An Illustrated Guide of the World's Most Famous Hotel.* New York: St. Martin's, 2000.

Kara Newman

Polish

There has been a long and vibrant history of Polish cuisine in New York City since the turn of the twentieth century due to a strong Polish diaspora throughout the city, focused particularly in Manhattan, Brooklyn, and, more recently, Queens.

The abundance of Poles in New York City can be traced back to three major waves of Polish immigration to the United States. The first and most substantial group came to the United States seeking opportunity, arriving at the turn of the twentieth century. This wave was referred to as *za chlebem*, which translates to "following the bread," as many had the intention of only staying in New York long enough to earn sufficient money to be able to return to Poland, although ultimately many settled in the United States. The second wave was approximately forty years later, around the time of World War II; they came to escape the tense political and economic situation pervading in Poland at that time. The final and smallest wave was spurred by Poland's deteriorating economy in the mid-1980s.

The first wave was the largest, bringing Poles (as well as some Ukrainians and Russians) to New York City, with the majority of them settling in the Lower East Side and East Village. Sadly this community has dwindled but the remnants can be seen by the few remaining restaurants of the "borshcht belt," the name for the collection of Polish, Ukrainian, and Russian restaurants created by culinary entrepreneurs who came over in the first wave. Despite this, Polish-owned Russ & Daughters is still going strong. See RUSS & DAUGHTERS.

There are now "Polonias," communities of Polish immigrants and American-born Poles, all over New York City, the most concentrated of which is in Greenpoint, Brooklyn. Although gentrification and the resulting increase in rent prices have been instrumental in the decision of many residents to return to Poland, the Polish spirit of the neighborhood is still very much apparent. Greenpoint is full of local stores with signs in their windows that proudly proclaim "mówimy po polsku" (Polish is spoken here) and the food in the area reflects the residents' gastronomical heritage.

Butchers have kielbasa, a heavily-seasoned air-dried sausage, and fresh sausages hanging from the ceiling and smoked pork loin, bacon, and other pork products behind the counter. Polish bakeries litter the streets selling rye bread; *babka*, a yeasted sweet bread served at Easter that also happens to mean "grandmother" in Polish; *makowiec*, a poppyseed pastry roll; and *pączki*, small, deep-fried flattened circles of dough with sweet filling. They are traditionally served on Fat Thursday (*Tłusty Czwartek*), the last Thursday before Lent, although many Polish treats that are served for religious holidays are enjoyed all year round.

Polish restaurants offer standard Polish fare, such as the *pierogi*, steamed or fried dumplings filled with meat, potatoes, cheese, or sauerkraut; fruit fillings are used for dessert pierogi. *Bigos*, a hunter's stew made of meat and sauerkraut, is another favorite and *gołąbki*, minced meat, onions and rice wrapped in boiled cabbage leaves, is delicious.

Also prevalent is *barszcz*, the tart soup that is better known as Russian borscht. However, unlike the Russian variety, Polish *barszcz* is not always red and beetroot is not necessarily the dominating flavor. *Barszcz czerwony* is the red variety and is often served with mushroom-stuffed dumplings called *uszki*. The vegetarian version of this soup is traditionally served at Christmas Eve dinner, *wiglia*. *Barszcz biały* is the white soup, which is made with fermented wheat and the broth from boiled *biała kiełbasa* (white sausage) and it is often eaten on Easter Sunday morning. It is very similar to *żurek*, a sour rye soup, which is sometimes served in a crusty bread bowl.

Polish restaurants are not just limited to Greenpoint. Polish cuisine can be found in Manhattan and Queens and you can even enjoy Polish food in true New York style, from the aptly named Old Traditional Polish Cuisine food truck. If you would rather sit down, it's back to Greenpoint, where Christina's, a Polish-American diner, serves hearty Polish-American classics or Królewskie Jadło, a restaurant guarded by a suits of armor outside the front door, are good places to start.

See also HUNGARIAN; RUSSIAN; and UKRAINIAN.

Falkowitz, Max. "A Tour of the East Village's Borscht Belt Restaurants and Lunch Counters." Serious Eats, February 26, 2014. http://newyork.seriouseats.com/2014/02/best-eastern-european-restaurants-diners-lunch-counters-east-village-polish-ukrainian.html.

Fertitta, Naomi. *New York: The Big City and Its Little Neighborhoods.* New York: Universe, 2009.

Hauck-Lawson, Annie, and Jonathan Deutsch. *Gastropolis: Food and New York City.* New York: Columbia University Press, 2009.

Asia Lindsay

Pop-Up Restaurants

Pop-ups are dining spaces set up temporarily—sometimes for just a single evening or up to months—often in nontraditional dining spaces and advertised via social media or only to a select group of guests. Pop-ups showcase a chef's food expression at a specific moment and are generally themed or centered on a particular ingredient or ethnic cuisine. Mystery is often involved, as some restauranteurs, such as Scott Conant, have used pop-ups as a way to launch a new outlet with the dining location only disclosed at a selected time to those who book a table through an online reservation app. The term "pop-up restaurant" is first attributed to chef Ludovic Lefebvre who saw circus tents along a California highway one day. "What if I could do a restaurant circus," he told *Esquire* in 2011. "Go from city to city. Like a band on tour." He then opened "Ludo-Bites," in 2007, a series of temporary eateries located around Los Angeles.

The "summer of the pop-up" arrived in New York in 2011 when steep retail space costs and increasing operating expenses during an economic downturn drove over a dozen chefs to open pop-up restaurants in the city. Among the first were television's Top Chef alumni Dale Talde who set up *Bodega*, a one-night only project staged in a space on the Bowery, and chef John Fraser, who opened *What Happens When*, a seven-month-long project on Cleveland Street that cycled through four "movements" or menu changes with the seasons—it closed earlier than originally planned due to complications with its liquor license. But just as the phenomena began to gain steam, with a pop-up food court opening on the High Line, *New York Times* writer Neil Genzlinger objected to the term's overuse, contending it had achieved "hipster status—that is, with that word, merely using it labels you a shameless bandwagon-jumper."

"Williamsburg has become the de facto epicenter of pop-up nation in this town, whether it's because experimenting without fear of failure is part of living in this 'hood or the fact that starving artists need more creative dining outlets," noted *Village Voice* food writer Bill Lyons in 2013. Brooklyn Flea and other weekend city markets have provided a space for a host of pop-ups that sometimes later open food stalls at such venues as Williamsburg's Smorgasburg. See SMORGASBURG.

What started out an underground, "guerrilla" movement, showcasing emerging chefs, food-truck operators looking to expand into brick-and-mortar spaces, and restaurant sous chefs wanting to flex some of their own culinary muscle, has now turned into a trendy way for established celebrity chefs to attract a younger generation of patrons. For instance, Momofuku Milk Bar took advantage of the shuttered Madison Square Park Shake Shack outlet for the winter season in 2015 and offered their signature "birthday cake truffles and crack pie slices." Chefs also like pop-ups since check averages tend to be higher than at typical restaurants as diners are more willing to pay for a special, once-in-a-lifetime type of experience.

Some acclaimed out-of-towners, including Chicago's Grant Achatz from Alinea, have recreated their restaurants in New York spaces with pop-ups, temporary versions that, at times, have replicated the original experience down to the number of seats in the dining room and the execution of the courses.

Chefs are also using pop-ups to raise funds and awareness for their favorite causes—often in their existing restaurant spaces but for selected special events. For instance, Blue Hill put on a series of dinners in 2015 called wastED. Guest chefs were instructed to "cook epic meals using food waste." More established venues such as museums have used the pop-up concept to promote exhibits with the addition of food to attract patrons. Some chefs have teamed with large retailers to open miniature versions of their restaurants for a limited time, such as chocolatier Jacque Torres opening a "hot chocolate pop-up bar" in Saks Fifth Avenue in 2015.

And because New York continues to be the center of the media world, advertisers have appropriated the term pop-up, using it to attract media coverage and gain word-of-mouth for food marketing events. In the fall of 2014, Eight O'Clock Coffee and Warner Bros. partnered to open Central Perk, on Lafayette Street, a replica of the cafe in the hit sitcom Friends, to celebrate its twentieth anniversary. Even the NFL got into the act, opening a pop-up in a Times Square hotel during the Super Bowl in 2014, partnering with Danny Meyer's Union Square Events. The eatery, called Forty Ate, had ample televisions and was decorated with forty-seven Super Bowl rings and busts of "Superbowl royalty," including Joe Montana and Terry Bradshaw.

The pop-up concept is even being franchised with the launch of The Dinner Lab, where guests pay a membership fee to access pop-up meals priced between $60 and $80 and offer direct feedback to the chef.

Fussman, Carl. "In Praise of the Temporary Restaurant," *Esquire*, October 10, 2011.

Genzlinger, Neil. "Invasion of the Pop-Ups: Time for a Smackdown." *New York Times*, August 12, 2011.

Hayes, Janice Leung. "Pop-Up Restaurants: A Brief History." *South China Morning Post*, June 6, 2013.

Henninger, Danya. "Are Pop-Up Restaurants Worth the Hype?" Zagat.com, August 6, 2014. https://www.zagat.com/b/philadelphia/are-pop-up-restaurants-worth-the-hype.

Lyons, Bill. "Our 10 Best Pop-Up Restaurants in New York." *Village Voice*, June 17, 2013.

Melnick, Jordan. "New Restaurant Trend Really Pops with Diners." *QSR Magazine*, April 2011.

Dan Macey

Port Richmond

See STATEN ISLAND.

Post–World War II (1945–1975)

New York City's culinary scene suffered for nearly three decades as a result of the two World Wars, Prohibition, and the Depression. During the twenty years after World War II ended in 1945, the city's foodscape enjoyed a period of rapid growth and evolution. Food was plentiful, particularly after all wartime restrictions ceased in 1947. Many New Yorkers had traveled during and after the war, and they had come to appreciate foreign and exotic foods. Three major trends emerged in the postwar period: Restaurants revived and flourished; immigrants flooded into the city, bringing new foods and foodways; and food journalism emerged as an art form.

The number and diversity of New York City restaurants expanded rapidly after World War II. The Horn & Hardart automats, with an affordable menu that welcomed the working person, expanded to fifty outlets in the city by 1950. By this time, most had been converted from nickel-in-the-slot vending operations into cafeterias. See AUTOMATS and VENDING MACHINES. But the advent of fast-food chains, such as White Castle and later Burger King and McDonald's, ate away at their business.

At the high end, the Colony and Le Pavillon, restaurants on New York's fashionable Upper East Side, only grew more popular during the postwar period, and they served as incubators for the city's up-and-coming chefs and restaurateurs. Their success inspired a host of restaurants serving a variety of regional French cuisines, as well as Escoffier's classics. Lutèce opened in 1961, with chef André Soltner at the helm. For more than three decades, Lutèce was considered one of the finest restaurants in America. Sirio Maccioni, who started as a waiter at the Colony in 1956, opened Le Cirque with Jean Vergnes in 1974. See COLONY CLUB; LE CIRQUE; LE PAVILLON; and LUTÈCE. New types of restaurants emerged during the 1950s. Restaurant Associates launched specialty and theme restaurants, such as the Hawaiian Room at the Lexington Hotel (Polynesian, complete with hula dancers), La Fonda Del Sol (South American), Zum-Zum (a chain of cafés specializing in German sausages), Quo Vadis (French and Italian), the Hudson River Club, Tavern on the Green in Central Park, The Four Seasons, and Windows on the World in the World Trade Center. See RESTAURANT ASSOCIATES.

Puerto Rican immigration to New York turned into a flood after World War II. Puerto Ricans settled predominantly in the northeastern part of Manhattan, which is known as "El Barrio" or Spanish Harlem. In El Barrio, Puerto Ricans strived to maintain their food habits. In the 1950s Puerto Ricans owned and supported food stalls in the covered food market that they baptized "La Marqueta," where they sold traditional Caribbean foods. See PUERTO RICAN.

The city's Chinese immigrant population also increased after World War II. In 1958, the city had more than three hundred Chinese restaurants, of which thirty were in the Times Square area alone. By 1960, only fifty of the city's nearly six hundred Chinese restaurants were located in Chinatown. Refugees flooded into the city during and after World War II. See CHINESE COMMUNITY.

When Congress passed the Immigration Act (1965) there was a major shift in immigration patterns. Hundreds of thousands came to the United States from Africa, Asia, and Latin America. Each immigrant group brought its food culture to New York, and city restaurants, spice markets, bodegas, grocery stores, coffee shops, and delis benefitted from the influx of culinary professionals from around the world. As new groups of immigrants, such as Greeks, Puerto Ricans, West Indians, and Koreans, moved into the city, many found running a "deli" (in its New York City sense—a small neighborhood grocery offering some prepared foods as well as packaged items) proved an excellent entry point. Deli owners from newer immigrant groups often include their native favorites alongside tuna sandwiches and potato salad; for instance, Korean American–owned delis frequently sell kimchi and other Asian specialties, while West Indian proprietors offer savory turnovers called "patties." Greek immigrants to New York opened coffee shops. Japanese immigrants introduced New Yorkers to sushi and other Japanese delicacies. Indian, Pakistani, and Bangladeshi immigrants opened spice shops and grocery stores. West Indian newcomers became street vendors and others started up restaurants. West African immigrants moved into the grocery delivery business. Pizza had been eaten by many Italian Americans during the early twentieth century, but after World War II, New York–style pizza became one of the city's (and America's) favorite foods. See KIMCHI; PIZZA; SUSHI; and COFFEE SHOPS.

Supermarkets continued to expand in New York during the 1950s and 1960s. A&P remained America's largest food retailer until 1975, when it ran into financial reversals, as did other large chains in the city. This decline was largely due to increased competition. Small grocery stores, bodegas, and delis cut into supermarket business, as did larger supermarkets outside of the city that were accessible by car. See A&P and SUPERMARKETS.

Food journalism was one reason that New York's culinary scene took off after World War II. Previously, food articles in magazines and newspapers had simply supplied recipes and helpful hints; features were often thinly veiled (or overt) promotions for new food products and the latest kitchen equipment. But as the twentieth century rolled on, some newspaper food writers became extremely popular and influential. Clementine Paddleford, a Kansas native with a degree in Industrial Journalism, became the food editor at the *New York Herald Tribune* in 1936. By the early 1950s her columns reached 12 million readers. See PADDLEFORD, CLEMENTINE.

At the *New York Times*, Jane Nickerson held a similar post until her retirement in 1957. Craig Claiborne, who had trained at L'Ecole Hôtelière in Lausanne, Switzerland, was hired to take her place. Claiborne invited some of America's top chefs and cookbook authors, including Pierre Franey, René Verdon, Jean Vergnes, and Jacques Pépin, to cook in his home kitchen. Claiborne noted down their recipes and comments as they prepared a meal, and presented the recipes in his newspaper columns. Claiborne continued to write for the *New York Times*

on and off for the next thirty-five years. See CLAIBORNE, CRAIG and NICKERSON, JANE.

Another prime player in postwar food journalism was not a newcomer, but the well-established *Gourmet* magazine, which Earle MacAusland had launched in January 1941. He knew little about culinary matters, so he hand-picked an editorial staff of experts. They included Pearl Metzelthin, author of *The World Wide Cook Book: Menus and Recipes of 75 Nations* (1939), and Louis de Gouy, a New York chef, restaurateur, and cookbook author who became the magazine's "Gourmet Chef." MacAusland also hired James Beard, who had just published his first cookbook, *Hors D'oeuvre and Canapés* (1940). The distinguished food writers M. F. K. Fisher, Clementine Paddleford, and Joseph Wechsberg, among others, were early contributors to *Gourmet*. Other magazines, such as *The New Yorker*, also contributed to New York's postwar culinary revolution.

See also BEARD, JAMES; DE GOUY, LOUIS P.; FRANEY, PIERRE; GREEK; *GOURMET*; JAPANESE; KOREAN; *NEW YORK TIMES*; *NEW YORKER*; and RESTAURANTS.

Batterberry, Michael and Ariane Batterberry. *On the Town in New York: The Landmark History of Eating and Entertainments from the American Revolution to the Food Revolution.* New York and London: Routledge, 1999.
Grimes, William. *Appetite City: A Culinary History of New York.* New York: North Point, 2009.
Hauck-Lawson, Annie, and Jon Deutsch, eds. *Gastropolis: Food & New York City.* New York: Columbia University Press, 2008.

Andrew F. Smith

Power Breakfasts and Power Lunches

Although the evening meal gets most of the attention among restaurant-goers, New York City also has a long tradition of "power breakfasts" and "power lunches," business-oriented meals at which the city's power players meet and close deals.

Robert Tisch, of the family that owns the Loews Regency Hotel at Park Avenue and Sixty-First Street, is credited with coining the phrase "power breakfast" in the 1970s. During that decade, Tisch and Wall Street investment banker Felix Rohatyn worked with the mayor to help save New York City as it teetered on the edge of bankruptcy.

At the time, Tisch resided in the hotel. According to Loews chairman Jonathan Tisch:

"My father said, 'Let's meet at the Regency, it's easy for me, I'll just take the elevator.'" Some say the Loews has continued as a prime site for meetings over coffee and eggs due to its location, an easy conduit between the affluent Upper East Side, where many power brokers live, and the offices of Midtown.

Of course, the power breakfast has been around long before the Loews hotel, even if it wasn't called as such. For example, the Plaza Hotel claims an early version in the sanctuary of its all-male Men's Café, where influential guests would have included Mark Twain and Diamond Jim Brady, who might have started their day with pig knuckles and mutton chops to fortify for the discussions at hand.

While the power breakfast is about the efficiency of taking meetings before arriving at the office, the power lunch is exactly the opposite: a leisurely midday meal for businessmen whose status freed them from the confines of a strictly enforced lunch hour.

The term "power lunch" first appeared in Esquire in 1979, in a story about the Grill Room at the Four Seasons restaurant in New York. But the event itself had been thriving ever since lunch became the meal tied most closely to the ticking clock of the workday.

The template for power lunch was set in the 1830s by Delmonico's, where sophisticated cooking, ostentatious décor, and a prime location in the business district proved to be a powerful combination; hundreds of imitators sprang up over the years. Unlike breakfast meetings, alcohol often was (and still is) part of the equation, as in the fabled "three-martini lunch" of the 1960s and 1970s.

Several key elements are common to both "power" meals: a luxurious, often pricey setting, proximity to other powerful individuals, and often, a degree of privacy so deal-making conversations won't be overheard. These meals tend to be all about the power, but rarely about the food.

See also BUSINESS LUNCH and FOUR SEASONS.

Cardwell, Diane. "Coffee and Eggs, Movers and Shakers." *New York Times,* June 5, 2005.
Gathje, Curtis. *At The Plaza: An Illustrated History of the World's Most Famous Hotel.* New York: St. Martin's, 2000.
"Lunch Hour NYC." New York Public Library Exhibitions. http://exhibitions.nypl.org/lunchhour/exhibits/show/lunchhour/power.

Kara Newman

Pre-Columbian

Like other northeastern North American peoples, the Lenape Indians who lived in and around the Lower Hudson Valley possessed a Neolithic (late Stone Age) culture belonging to the so-called "Late Woodland" phase of Native American prehistory. Thus they lacked any technology for making metal cooking pots or knives. Aside from stone and clay, all culinary equipment was drawn from the animal and vegetable kingdoms—for instance, horn, bone, hides, sinews, clamshells (which made good skinning knives or scrapers when the edge was sharpened), wood, bark, reeds, and plant fibers.

Nearly all foods were wild products of local soils and waters. These were hunted or gathered at different times of the year through a partly mobile way of life that saw bands of a few dozen (at most a few hundred) people traveling between temporary encampments to take advantage of some seasonal ripening period or migration throughout a range of several dozen square miles. At the same time, the Lenapes made some use of settled agriculture based on the three great cultivated crops—corn, beans, and squash—natives of the Mesoamerican tropics that are thought to have been widely disseminated to eastern North America by about 1000–1200 C.E.

This people enjoyed a natural resource unparalleled on the East Coast: the southern half of the Hudson River. It is a huge fjordal estuary created during the last Ice Age. The advancing ice sheet deepened and widened the gorge of an existing river, bringing Atlantic Ocean tides more than 150 miles inland to the foot of Cohoes Falls (where the Mohawk River empties into the Hudson) and allowing easy travel by canoe between all points from the ocean to the falls.

The river, along with many local ponds and wetlands also left by the glacier, provided the Lenapes of the Lower Valley with a richer, more varied, and more annually sustained supply of both saltwater and freshwater fish and shellfish than any other Northeastern people. In spring they harvested great numbers of migrating shad, striped bass, and sturgeon from the Hudson. The coastline also yielded many species of roundfish and flatfish as well as mussels, oysters, scallops, hardshell and softshell clams, lobsters, blue crabs, shrimp, and (from Long Island Sound) salmon. This extraordinary bounty made the Lenapes somewhat less dependent on sedentary agriculture than inland neighbors like the Mohawks and Senecas. See FISHING.

On land, virtually every edible plant or animal of the region was exploited. The Northeastern woodland habitat was really an intricate patchwork of habitats. Those in our region included extensive hardwood forest ranges dominated by the American chestnut (since ravaged by blight) along with several species of oak and hickory, dwarf pine barrens, stands of tall white pine, swamps, expanses of open ground where lightning-ignited wildfires had destroyed trees, and even the only true prairie east of Ohio (today's Hempstead Plains on Long Island). Each of these supported its own special animal and plant populations.

The animal resources of the Lower Valley, on both the eastern and western sides, ranged from black bear (much valued for its fat) and white-tailed deer to raccoon, beaver, rabbit, and other small mammals. The water environments supported both shore birds and seasonal migrations of waterfowl including whistling swans and several species of duck and goose. The most important land bird, the American wild turkey, was chiefly hunted in fall, the season when both furred and feathered game was fattest and most flavorful.

Nearly any available wild plant might be eaten, though many required patient processing before cooking. People gathered tree nuts including several kinds of acorns, many roots and tubers (from Jerusalem artichokes to cattail roots), the seeds from some kinds of chenopods, the leaves and shoots of many plants (gathered in spring when they were young, tender, and pleasant tasting), and various berries and small fruits (including both white and red fox grapes).

The absence of iron pots limited cooking methods to boiling, searing, ember roasting (with or without a protective wrapping of leaves), and fire roasting. Simple clay pots could be used for the first, but the only vessels that stood up to repeated use were wooden tubs hollowed out from logs and filled with water, to which cooks then added small rocks heated red-hot in the fire. Heated flat rocks served as searing or grilling surfaces, and roasting in front of an open fire was generally done on spits or racks made from thin branches or stout twigs. Ember roasting was a favorite way of preparing parched corn, as well as maize cakes wrapped in leaves. On some occasions large communal meals were steam-cooked, clambake style, in pits heated with rocks.

The only means of preserving food was by drying, with or without exposure to wood smoke. Salt was never used in the process, and white colonists were surprised to find that the local people did not eat it. They did, however, have a taste for many flavorful animal and vegetable fats, often produced by boiling the source in water and removing the congealed fat once the liquid had cooled.

Before cooking, dried meat or fish might be pounded fine (for faster cooking and more thorough softening) in either a wooden mortar or a hollowed-out rock used as a grinding surface. Pounding and grinding were also well-known ways of breaking down tough plant fibers and reducing corn kernels to meal. (A hard, dense flint corn was the only variety then known in the region.) Some plants might receive further precooking treatment through soaking or boiling in water, or a solution of lye made from wood ashes, to remove bitter or poisonous juices.

Despite these valuable fragments of knowledge, a severe lack of historical records makes it impossible to reconstruct a clear, detailed picture of any "cuisine" predating European arrival in the greater New York area. The unique, irresistible advantages of the river, the coast, and the harbor for inland and overseas commercial traffic unfortunately inspired European colonists to expunge the local civilization from our region more efficiently than from any other site on the Northeast Coast. Our knowledge of Lenape foodways is thus destined to remain at least as dependent on guesswork as concrete insight.

Cantwell, Anne-Marie, and Diana diZerega Wall. *Unearthing Gotham: The Archaeology of New York City.* New Haven, Conn.: Yale University Press, 2001.

Mendelson, Anne. "The Lenapes: In Search of Pre-European Foodways in the Greater New York Region." In *Gastropolis: Food and New York City,* edited by Annie Hauck-Lawson and Jonathan Deutsch, pp. 15–33. New York: Columbia University Press, 2009.

Russell, Howard. *Indian New England before the Mayflower.* Hanover, N.H.: University Press of New England, 1980.

Van der Donck, Adriaen. *A Description of the New Netherlands.* Edited by Thomas F. O'Donnell. Syracuse, N.Y.: Syracuse University Press, 1968.

Anne Mendelson

Pretzels

The history of pretzels is far longer than the history of New York. Legend has it that pretzels were invented by a medieval monk, probably in Italy. The monk shaped the soft dough into the shape of arms crossed in prayer. He would hand them out to children as a reward for learning their prayers. Other legends place the pretzel's origins in France and in Germany. The earliest recorded images of pretzels appear as an emblem in the crest of German bakers' guilds in the twelfth century. Certainly by that point, pretzels were identified as a German culinary treat.

Pretzels were probably introduced to the Americas by German immigrants to Pennsylvania. These Pennsylvania Dutch settlers came from the Palatine and settled in Pennsylvania in the eighteenth century. They baked the twisted concoctions and sold them throughout the countryside. Even today, Pennsylvania is the center of pretzel production in the United States; 80 percent of the pretzels produced in the country come from the Keystone State. Julius Sturgis opened the first commercial pretzel bakery in 1861 in the town of Lititz, in Lancaster County, Pennsylvania. Sturgis is believed to have developed hard pretzels, a variety that kept longer than the traditional soft pretzel, and so was more feasible as a marketable product.

Soft pretzels have been sold on the streets of New York since the early nineteenth century. The tradition of street peddling of food dates all the way back to New York's beginnings as a Dutch port. But in the nineteenth century, newer immigrants, especially Germans and eventually Eastern Europeans began to dominate the peddling trade. Various food items were peddled on the streets of New York, including all kinds of fruits and vegetables, oysters and clams, hot corn, and pretzels, carried around in a basket or box suspended from the vendor's neck or strung along a stick. German restaurants and beer gardens, which began to proliferate in New York beginning in the 1840s as German immigrants flooded into the city, also offered pretzels on their menus. See BEER GARDENS; GERMAN; and STREET VENDORS.

By the twentieth century, pretzels became a standard offering on the ubiquitous New York City hot dog cart. Still today, large soft pretzels are sold from carts around the city, especially in Manhattan. New York–style soft pretzels are different from their Philadelphia counterparts, which are long and narrow, more of a bowtie shape than the figure-eight New York style pretzel. New York pretzels also are generously (some might say profusely) salted, unlike traditional Philadelphia-style pretzels.

Street pretzels cost two dollars and up depending on where the cart is located. Most of the carts sell pretzels from a central distributor, such as J & J Snack Foods, Corp., located in Pennsauken, New Jersey. Many food critics deride these pretzels as "just pretzel-shaped bread." *New York Times* food writer Julia Moskin declared New York street pretzels to be "tasteless as 'Jersey Shore,' dry as a vacant lot in August, tough as a water bug."

In the last few years though, there's a pretzel revival occurring in New York. Artisanal pretzel shops like Sigmund's and Bronx Pretzel Company are making pretzels by hand from tested recipes, hearkening back to the earlier tradition of German-style pretzels in New York. These artisanal pretzels are dipped in a lye solution before being baked in the oven in order to give them the dark brown, crusty outside that distinguishes them from the more bready soft pretzels sold on the street carts. In their offerings, these new pretzel masters are going beyond the standard pretzel twist. At its East Village bar, Sigmund's offers "classic" pretzels but also truffle cheddar, cinnamon raisin, feta olive, and churros pretzels as well as pretzel sandwiches. Sigmund's is owned and run by Lina Kulchinsky who worked as a pastry chef at Bouley and Danube before entering the artisanal pretzel field. Sigmund's also runs a pretzel cart outside of the Metropolitan Museum of Art. The Bronx Pretzel Company—run by Alexis Fauci who tried countless pretzel recipes and consulted with German pretzel bakers before settling on her current recipe—produces pretzel rolls, bacon pretzels, and pretzel calzones. They sell primarily at farmer's markets and specialty shops throughout the New York City region. And Pelzer's Pretzels offers Philadelphia-style pretzels—twisted into a compact shape—from its shop in Crown Heights. Like their nineteenth-century predecessors, New York's increasingly ubiquitous beer gardens also feature pretzels, some made locally and some imported from Germany.

Coe, Andrew. "New York's Best Pretzel Is Made by an Italian in the Bronx." Serious Eats, May 2, 2014. http://newyork.seriouseats.com/2014/05/good-bread-best-pretzel-bronx-baking-company.html

Moskin, Julia. "Making Soft Pretzels the Old-Fashioned Way." *New York Times*, May 25, 2010.

Settembre, Jeannette. "A Pair of Philadelphians Are Bringing Their City's Style of Pretzels to Brooklyn." *New York Daily News*, December 11, 2013.

Upton, Emily. "The History of Pretzels." Today I Found Out, June 2013. http://www.todayifoundout.com/index.php/2013/06/the-history-of-pretzels.

Cindy R. Lobel

Prison Food

Nineteenth-century engravings in the New York Public Library's collection depict rows of imprisoned men enjoying breakfast on Blackwell's Island. Before it was Roosevelt Island, it was Blackwell's Island, a prison and a "lunatic asylum." Infiltrating Blackwell's Island on assignment from *New York World* editor Joseph Pulitzer, investigative reporter Nellie Bly recounts her first meal on Blackwell's Island:

> Placed closed together all along the table were large dressing-bowls filled with a pinkish-looking stuff which the patients called tea. By each bowl was laid a piece of bread, cut thick and buttered. A small saucer containing five prunes accompanied the bread.... I tried the bread, but the butter was so horrible that one could not eat it.... Very few were able to eat the butter. I turned my attention to the prunes and found that very few of them would be sufficient. I tasted [my tea], and one taste was enough. It had no sugar, and it tasted as if it had been made in copper. It was as weak as water.

In examining the living conditions for prison inmates and asylum patients, Nelly Bly's *Ten Days in a Mad-House* (1887) discusses the food there vividly and at great length: "I cannot tell you of anything which is the same dirty, black color. It was hard, and in places nothing more than dried dough. I found a spider in my slice, so I did not eat it. I tried the oatmeal and molasses, but it was wretched, and so I endeavored, but without much show of success, to choke down the tea."

Bly's investigation prompted one of the earliest instances of prison reform in New York (and American history): a grand jury investigation, which resulted in an $850,000 (nearly $22 million today) increase in the budget for New York's Department of Public Charities and Corrections.

Blackwell's Island was just one site for New York City's prisons. New York's criminals, indigents, and "undesirables" have been interned on several islands, in the heart of Manhattan, and on boats and barges moored in the East River. (Even Ellis Island, so long known as the welcome room to generations of Americans, later became a detention center for German and Italian enemy aliens during World War II.)

Of these, perhaps no institution remains quite so infamous as Rikers Island, which thanks to numerous police serials is virtually synonymous with imprisonment in New York City. (A close second is the ominously nicknamed "Tombs.") A meal card from the mid-1930s boasts that "The feeding facilities of the Institution are capable of serving 2,500 inmates three times daily. This is one of the most important and active departments of the institution."

Rikers also boasts the requisite online counterpart of any New York culinary institution: a Yelp profile, with reviews to rival Ms. Bly's. One describes the food at Rikers as "unsuitable for consumption by feral pigs." For the adventurous, another Yelper recommends chicken night, typically on Thursdays.

The provider of all those memorable oily Beefaroni stews, rainbow bologna sandwiches, Thursday night chicken dinners, and bony, white hot dogs is Aramark Foodservices Corp., which holds contracts with six hundred prisons across the United States. On more than one occasional Aramark has been sued for providing substandard food, including "disregard for food temperatures, food being served on rotted trays, rotten or undercooked meat being served, insects in vegetables, and workers not wearing proper protective gear during food preparation and handling" (*Wilson Pagan, et al. v. Westchester County, et al.*).

During Nellie Bly's time, bread, gruel, and molasses were all standard components of the New York prison diet. (New York State Correctional facilities still feature a similar menu item, the "loaf.") In its Roosevelt Island incarnation, Blackwell's Island now houses condos, not criminals, but New York still has a prison population to feed. Rikers Island hosts an inmate population of roughly fourteen thousand, all of whom must be fed three squares a day.

In 2003, measures taken toward improving efficiency consolidated prison kitchens and maximized oven sizes: a single oven can cook up to 6,900 chicken dinners. But for all of these innovations, the challenges encountered by Nellie Bly remain: inmates still report food that is unfit for human consumption, and food that they can't keep down.

Bly, Nellie. *Ten Days in a Mad-House*. New York: Ian
L. Munro.

Gopnik, Adam. "Rikers High." *New Yorker*, February 19,
2011.

"Mid-1930s Rikers Island Penitentiary Images."
CorrectionHistory.org. http://www.correctionhistory
.org/rikerspenmontages2_files/frame.htm.

"To Save the City Money, Rikers Supersizes It." *New York
Times*, July 27, 2003.

Wynn, Jennifer. *Inside Rikers: Stories from Inside the
World's Largest Penal Colony*. New York: Macmillan,
2001.

Alexis Zanghi

Prohibition

Prohibition was a nationwide constitutional ban on the manufacture, sale, and importation of alcoholic beverages that began in 1920 and ended in 1933. It was launched by the Eighteenth Amendment to the U.S. Constitution, which prohibited "the manufacture, sale, or transportation of intoxicating liquors within, the importation thereof into, or the exportation thereof from the United States and all territory subject to the jurisdiction thereof for beverage purposes." In 1919, Congress passed the National Prohibition Act, commonly called the Volstead Act, which defined "intoxicating" as any beverage containing more than 0.5 percent alcohol. The enforcement provisions of the law targeted producers and distributors, but not consumers. Prohibition went into effect in January 1920. In New York City, Prohibition ushered in a unique period in the city's history.

Few New Yorkers ever thought Prohibition would become the law of the land, but the movement to abolish alcohol in America had been gaining support since the late nineteenth century. New Yorkers were strongly opposed to Prohibition because, among other things, liquor was an important business in the city. An 1897 survey of Manhattan found a ratio of one liquor distributor to every 208 residents. The Anti-Saloon League, a national Prohibition advocacy group, considered New York City the "liquor center of America."

The major flaw in Prohibition was the near-impossibility of its enforcement. The federal government had allocated only $4.75 million for enforcement. The Eighteenth Amendment had given concurrent enforcement power to the federal and state governments, but the federal government hired only 1,500 enforcement agents nationally, of whom only 129 were assigned to New York City.

To support the federal agents, the New York State Legislature passed the Mullan-Gage Act on April 5, 1921, making violations of the Volstead Act also violations of state law. It required state and local police to enforce the federal law. During the first two months that the law was on the books, four thousand New Yorkers were arrested for violating it, but fewer than five hundred were indicted, and only six were convicted. None received jail terms. The failure of the Mullan-Gage Act cleared the way for speakeasies to flourish, and by 1922, there were an estimated five thousand of them in New York City. When Al Smith, an ardent opponent of Prohibition, became governor in 1923, Mullan-Gage was repealed. From that time on, city police generally declined to arrest anyone on liquor-related charges, provided that distributors and drinkers did not flaunt their activities.

The speakeasy, typically located in a dark, stuffy basement or back room, became the main conduit for illegal alcohol sales. Customers were eyeballed through a peephole in the door, and admitted only if the guard approved. Speakeasies catered mainly to the middle class. The liquor they served was pricier than pre-Prohibition booze, and notoriously bad: it was occasionally toxic and usually tasted revolting. Imported alcohol was available, but only at extremely high prices, and a lot of what was sold as imports was actually domestic bootleg liquor poured into fancy bottles with fake labels. In one year alone, 625

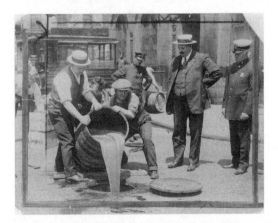

New York City Deputy Police Commissioner John A. Leach (right) watching agents pour liquor into the sewer following a raid during the height of Prohibition, circa 1921. LIBRARY OF CONGRESS

New Yorkers died from ingesting poisoned alcohol, and another 1,295 died from alcohol-related causes.

Wealthier New Yorkers were less affected by the Volstead Act, and throughout Prohibition they could easily secure any alcoholic beverages they desired. The urban middle class had the speakeasies. It was the working class that suffered most from the strictures of Prohibition. Their main alcoholic drink was beer, which was almost unobtainable during Prohibition. Brewing required bulky equipment, while whiskey making could be—and famously was—accomplished in a space as small as a bathtub. Beer was also bulkier to transport than spirits. Distilled spirits were readily available, but working-class New Yorkers could not afford them.

By the late 1920s, alcohol production was in high gear as thousands of illegal stills cranked out hard liquor for anyone who had the cash to buy it. Organized crime stepped in to centralize the manufacture, distribution, and retail sales, and money and power flowed to the crime syndicates. As federal agents took home only about $1,800 per year, and New York City policemen made even less, they were easy marks for hefty bribes. Liquor manufacturers and distributors bribed agents, policemen, judges, and other city leaders, and corruption in New York City reached new heights.

In 1929 New York's police commissioner estimated that the city had thirty-two thousand speakeasies—twice the number of establishments (both legal and illegal) that served alcohol prior to Prohibition. Others said that the commissioner's estimate was far too low—that there were at least one hundred thousand speakeasies in the city. It was estimated in 1930 that U.S. alcohol consumption was about the same as before Prohibition.

Opponents of Prohibition began to make themselves heard. In 1929 Pauline Sabin, a wealthy and politically well-connected New York socialite (who was known to serve cocktails in her home), formed the Women's Organization for National Prohibition Reform. In less than a year, it had more than one hundred thousand members; by 1931, its membership had reached three hundred thousand, and by November 1932 there were more than 1.1 million members.

When the stock market crashed in 1929, and the nation's economy collapsed, Americans blamed the Republicans, who had controlled Congress since 1919 and the presidency since 1921. President Herbert Hoover made a terrible showing in the 1932 election, and the Democrats swept into power with large majorities in both houses of Congress. President Franklin Delano Roosevelt, formerly the governor of New York, pledged to get the economy moving again.

He had his work cut out for him: Federal coffers were empty, almost 25 percent of the American workforce was unemployed, and income tax revenue was down. Roosevelt and his allies presented the repeal of Prohibition as a means of generating revenue. Reinstating the excise tax on liquor was thus one argument for ending Prohibition. Others argued that repeal would restart industries that had once employed hundreds of thousands of Americans. It seemed likely that repeal would also help put an end to the burgeoning crime generated by the illegal production and sale of alcohol. On February 20, 1933, the U.S. Congress proposed and approved the Twenty-First Amendment to the Constitution, which repealed Prohibition. The Amendment was ratified on December 5, 1933, and the "noble experiment," as it was called, was over. Throughout the country, countless toasts were raised to repeal.

See also BEER; DELMONICO'S; SPEAKEASIES; SPIRITS; and TEMPERANCE MOVEMENT.

Behr, Edward. *Prohibition: Thirteen Years That Changed America*. New York: Arcade, 1996.
Beyer, Mark. *Temperance and Prohibition: The Movement to Pass Anti-liquor Laws in America*. New York: Rosen, 2006.
Kobler, John. *Ardent Spirits: The Rise and Fall of Prohibition*. Boston: Da Capo, 1993.
Lerner, Michael A. *Dry Manhattan: Prohibition in New York City*. Cambridge, Mass.: Harvard University Press, 2007.
Okrent, Daniel. *Last Call: The Rise and Fall of Prohibition*. New York: Scribner, 2010.
Slavicek, Louise Chipley. *The Prohibition Era: Temperance in the United States*. New York: Chelsea House, 2008.

Andrew F. Smith

Public Markets

Cities were founded on government's ability to deliver affordable, appropriate, and safe food to its people, and New York City is no exception. Its earliest markets were established around the ports on the southern tip of Manhattan, where commercial activity and population was concentrated. Ships unloaded produce, fish, dairy, and other goods from Long Island, the Hudson River Valley, and beyond.

In the nineteenth century, the city was granting privately owned buildings license to operate as public markets. These closed or covered buildings were lined with stalls. Fulton Market, for example, was built in the 1820s, with nearly ninety stalls filled with produce, meat, coffee, spices, and fish. Ten years later, vendors petitioned to have the fish vendors removed from the market, due to the smell of the fish, the discarded scales, guts, and heads, and the Fulton Fish Market was built across the street. The working and middle classes alike patronized the public markets, where oyster shuckers and hot-corn girls added to the entertaining environment. See CRIES OF NEW-YORK, THE and FULTON FISH MARKET.

Thomas F. DeVoe, a butcher at the Jefferson Market, wrote *The Market Assistant* (1867), in which he describes every item sold in the city's public markets, underscoring the remarkable breadth of game, poultry, fish and other goods available to New Yorkers. He extolled the virtues of public markets, insisting that while private stores might have had an impressive variety, none had the quality or diversity of public markets. DeVoe also defended public markets from their detractors, who complained about unsanitary conditions, and lack of aesthetic appeal, emphasizing their positive effect on property values. See DEVOE, THOMAS FARRINGTON.

As the city's middle and upper classes moved farther north, or west to New Jersey, New York's Lower East Side became identified with the millions of immigrants who filled its streets.

In the early 1900s, pushcarts lined the streets of the Lower East Side, hawking vegetables, cheese, dry goods, baked sweet potatoes, and fish. Hundreds of thousands earned subsistence wages by operating pushcarts, working long hours in all seasons, and working in symbiosis with the many small shops that benefited from the lively street trade.

Other pushcart vendors were mobile, traveling into bourgeois neighborhoods where they were viewed with suspicion and fear. Servants would stretch household dollars by purchasing vegetables from pushcarts; notions such as buttons or ribbon tempted others. Other pushcarts sold pots and pans, or offered services such as knife sharpening.

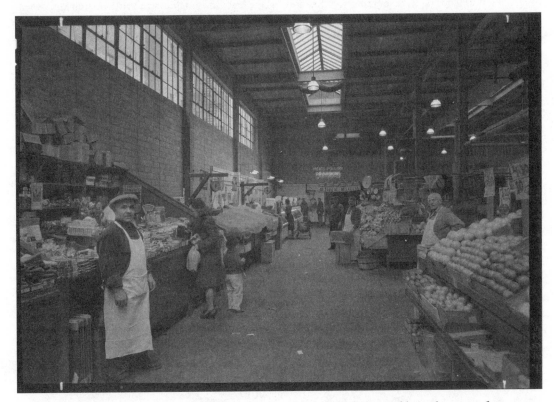

New York City Public Market, First Avenue and Seventy-Third Street, March 1948. Public markets were often chastised for having poor sanitation, but the private vendors offered goods that were unavailable elsewhere in the city. LIBRARY OF CONGRESS

At the turn of the twentieth century, New York had ten public markets housed in large warehouse-style buildings, which were publicly owned and privately managed. They were decrepit, with leaking pipes and refuse piled in the corners. The public markets, located in Lower Manhattan, were left to deteriorate, catering primarily to the poor and working classes. Also in the early 1900s, public debate was fanned by concern over the poor state of New York City's public markets, the lack of a municipal market system, and the resulting high cost of food. Unfavorable comparisons were made to markets in cities such as Paris, Berlin, and Philadelphia, where public funds were invested in gleaming central market halls. World War I cut short discussions about modernization of existing infrastructure. However, a need to regulate food distribution and prevent hoarding and price gouging led to consolidation of markets governance, and the establishment of the Department of Public Markets, Weights and Measures (later called the Department of Markets) in 1917.

By the mid-1930s, the Department of Markets' responsibilities included issuing permits, licenses, managing public markets, inspecting weights and measures, tracking food entering the city, overseeing slaughter facilities, and consumer education. The Bureau of Consumer Services provided price information via a daily radio show on WNYC, as well as classes held at public markets and other sites throughout the city.

Progressives advocated for the removal of pushcarts from the streets, describing them as unsanitary. Mayor Fiorello LaGuardia (in office, 1934–1945) made the containment of pushcarts a priority. With the support of federal funds made available through the Public Works Administration, he initiated the construction of enclosed public markets, beginning in Harlem, where the Park Avenue Market opened to great fanfare in 1936 with more than four hundred stalls. Eventually, nine enclosed markets were built in Manhattan, Brooklyn, and the Bronx. Initially, the markets were successful, filled with throngs shopping for bargains, pushing their way through crowded aisles. Vendors, initially concerned about moving to an enclosed market, grew to appreciate the running water, storage facilities, and the roof over their heads. See LA GUARDIA, FIORELLO.

The enclosed markets were built in neighborhoods where open-air markets had flourished due to a lack of larger-scale grocery stores and self-serve markets, as well as a preference for or habit of shopping at pushcarts. Supermarkets first opened during the 1930s. By the end of World War II, cars, suburbanization, home refrigeration, and a shifting culture of food provisioning meant that daily shopping rounds were replaced by weekly trips to the supermarket. In some neighborhoods, real estate interests pressured to city to turn over land parcels for more profitable use. The Department of Markets scaled back its activities, and was eventually dismantled in the late 1960s. Several enclosed markets were shut down. Some were destroyed, and others were repurposed. Four survive today—Essex Street, Arthur Avenue, Moore Street, and Park Avenue—and are benefiting from a revived appreciation for public markets in New York City.

Postwar suburbanization sped the decline of the city's farmers' markets as well. These "truck" markets, held in the parking lots of the Brooklyn and Bronx Terminal Markets, sold to restaurant owners and hoteliers, grocers and pushcart vendors, but rarely to the general public. When nearby farmland was converted to housing developments, they closed. The appetite for fresh produce was revived in 1976 when the first Greenmarket was held at Union Square with the dual intent of providing farmers struggling to survive in upstate New York with a lifeline, and New Yorkers access to fresh produce in a city where retailers were closing their doors. The Greenmarket was the beginning of what has now been several decades of sustained growth of public markets in various forms, their growth most pronounced in middle-class neighborhoods where they are a valued amenity, as they were nearly two centuries ago.

See also GREENMARKETS and SUPERMARKETS.

Audant, A. Babette. "From Public Market to La Marqueta." Ph.D. diss., City University of New York, 2013.

Bluestone, Daniel. "The Pushcart Evil." In *The Landscape of Modernity: Essays on New York City, 1900–1940*, edited by David Ward and Olivier Zunz, pp. 287–312. New York: Russell Sage Foundation, 1992.

Deutsch, Tracey. *Building a Housewife's Paradise: Gender, Politics, and American Grocery Stores in the Twentieth Century*. Chapel Hill: University of North Carolina Press, 2010.

DeVoe, Thomas F. "The Public Markets: True Value of the Markets to the City." *New York Times*, January 23, 1855.

DeVoe, Thomas F. *The Market Assistant*. New York: Hurd and Houghton, 1867.

"How New York is Fed." *Scribner's Monthly*, October 1877.

Wasserman, Suzanne. "Hawkers and Gawkers: Peddling and Markets in New York City." In *Gastropolis: Food &*

New York City, edited by Annie Hauck-Lawson and Jonathan Deutsch, pp. 153–173. New York: Columbia University Press, 2009.

Babette Audant

Puerto Rican

Throughout the twentieth century, New York City was the main destination of Puerto Ricans who migrated to the United States. As members of the first wave of Spanish-speaking residents in the city, Puerto Ricans played an important role in the creation of the food networks that characterize neighborhoods with a strong Latino presence like East Harlem, the Lower East Side (known as "Loisaida"), and the Bronx. See BRONX; HARLEM; and LOWER EAST SIDE.

These neighborhoods have historically been recognizable by their "bodegas," convenience stores that used to be the main establishments selling Puerto Rican food items. See BODEGAS. "La Marqueta," a market under the Metro North railroad tracks in East Harlem, boomed in the 1950s and 1960s with Puerto Rican vendors selling staples like salted codfish, plantains, cassava, avocados, pigeon peas, and bananas, as well as non-food items like musical records and herbs for traditional medicine and for the practice of Santería.

Today La Marqueta is only a fraction of its former size, but this does not mean that Puerto Rican food has disappeared from the city. In the past few years La Marqueta has been in a process of renovation. Furthermore, many previously hard-to-find foods are now widely available in most neighborhoods. The growth of the Latino population has helped to mainstream Puerto Rican foods. The average New Yorker is now familiar with tostones (flattened fried green plantains) and arroz con pollo (chicken with rice). However, those who actively seek Puerto Rican food beyond these basics are surely to be rewarded with delicious experiences in the city.

Foods

Daily Puerto Rican meals are built around rice and beans and some meat. What gives these common foods a Puerto Rican taste is the use of three ingredients: sofrito, adobo, and achiote. Sofrito is the base of all dishes that are cooked in a wet medium, like beans, soups, and stews. It is a mix of ground onions, sweet peppers, long-leaf cilantro, garlic, and other ingredients chosen by each individual cook. The mix is briefly sautéed at the beginning of the cooking process. Meats of all kinds are not considered properly cooked if they are not first seasoned with a homemade or store-bought adobo, a mix of salt, black pepper, garlic, oregano, and perhaps some lime juice and cumin. The oil or lard used to fry the sofrito is colored with achiote (annatto seeds). The achiote color, the sofrito, and the adobo flavors come together, creating a distinctive effect.

The crowning glory of Puerto Rican cuisine is the transformation of plantains and tubers into many different delicacies. Green plantains are fried and pounded with garlic and seasonings in a wooden mortar and pestle (*pilón*) to form a dome called *mofongo*. In fashionable versions, *mofongo* is shaped like a nest and stuffed with meat or seafood. Ripe plantains are sliced lengthwise to make a layered meat casserole (*piñón*), or a single ripe plantain slice can be wrapped around a ground-meat stuffing, battered with eggs and flour, and fried to make a *pionono*. Grated raw green bananas and plantains, and tubers like cassava, yautía, malanga, and ñames, are used in different combinations to form a dough called masa.

To make *pasteles*, masa is stuffed with a savory meat filling, wrapped in banana leaves and/or paper, and boiled in bundles. Entrepreneurial Puerto Ricans make large quantities of *pasteles* at home to sell to eager customers who do not have the skill or the time to make them but who cannot conceive of celebrating Christmas without them. Another cornerstone of Puerto Rican cuisine is roasted whole pig, plus a number of dishes made with pig intestines. These dishes and an array of fritters are collectively known as *cuchifritos*.

Restaurants

New York City has a wide variety of establishments serving Puerto Rican food. Among the oldest ones are the *lechoneras* and *cuchifritos* shops that can be found in the Bronx and East Harlem. *Lechoneras* like "El Nuevo Bohío," dubbed a "temple to roast pork" by the *New York Times*, specialize in whole roasted pork with golden crackling skin.

Puerto Ricans never abandoned the now trendy "whole hog" way of cooking. For decades, *lechoneras* and *cuchifritos* shops have been serving specialty dishes prepared with all parts of the pig, like *morcillas* (blood and rice sausages). Puerto Rican neighborhoods also have *fondas* serving inexpensive homestyle meals and street food vendors providing tropical fruit ice cream and *piraguas*, which are refreshing shaved ice cones topped with fruit syrups. These traditional foods become more visible during the festivities associated with the Puerto Rican Day Parade that takes place every June.

Newer types of establishments include food trucks, lounges, and pan-Latino restaurants that include Puerto Rican specialties. Some restaurants, notably La Fonda in East Harlem, serve classic Puerto Rican food and also have a broad cultural agenda, like using their walls to showcase the work of Puerto Rican artists. More festive restaurants like Sofrito and Sazón have been known to attract Puerto Rican celebrities like Bronx-born Jennifer Lopez and Supreme Court Justice Sonia Sotomayor.

Chefs

Famous Puerto Rican chefs include Brooklyn-born Daisy Martinez, who has multiple cookbooks and televised cooking shows. Chefs who have defined the new style of cooking in Puerto Rico, like Roberto Treviño, Mario Pagán, and Wilo Benet, have enjoyed the limelight in New York City when participating in cooking competitions on the Bravo and Food Network cable television channels. See FOOD NETWORK. Many well-known Puerto Rican chefs, regardless of where they were born or where they have established their careers, have studied at New York City cooking schools or have trained in some of the most prestigious restaurant kitchens in the city. The food culture of Puerto Rico and New York City have influenced and enriched each other for many decades.

Notwithstanding the prominence reached by many Puerto Rican chefs, there is no doubt that what keeps Puerto Rican cuisine alive and thriving in the city are the little-known neighborhood restaurants and home cooks that lovingly prepare daily meals, and the grateful people that they feed. They refuse to abandon Puerto Rican flavors and have woven them into the fabric of life in New York City.

Benet, Wilo. *Puerto Rico True Flavors*. Baltimore: Read Street, 2010.

Janer, Zilkia. *Latino Food Culture*. Westport, Conn.: Greenwood, 2008.

Ortiz, Yvonne. *A Taste of Puerto Rico: Traditional and New Dishes from the Puerto Rican Community*. New York: Plume, 1997.

Rivera, Oswald. *Puerto Rican Cuisine in America: Nuyorican and Bodega Recipes*. 2d ed. New York: Four Walls Eight Windows, 2002.

Zilkia Janer

Queens

Queens is one of the five boroughs that comprise New York City. It is the largest borough in area, and the second largest (after Brooklyn) in population. Queens is also the most ethnically diverse county in the United States; of its 2.3 million residents, 48 percent are foreign-born, compared to a city-wide average of 33 percent. This large immigrant population and its descendants have played a formative role in Queens' foodways over the past fifty years; although it still remains under the radar compared to Brooklyn, Queens has become increasingly recognized as a destination for foodies over the past few years.

Although the Queens of today is densely populated and heavily urbanized, for most of its existence Queens was a comparatively quiet and rural area. First settled by Europeans in the mid-seventeenth century, it spent the next two hundred and fifty years as a loose collection of towns and farms that was considered part of Long Island. Queens, along with the more distant parts of Long Island, eastern Brooklyn, the lower Hudson Valley, and New Jersey, was a significant source of food for New York City. Produce and dairy products from Queens, as well as oysters and clams from Long Island, traveled west through Queens to Long Island City, where they were sent via ferry to markets in Manhattan. Throughout the nineteenth century, Queens was a major agricultural center for New York City and also a significant agricultural producer for the larger region.

This status started to erode in the mid-to-late nineteenth century, however. Advancements in refrigeration and transportation technology meant that New York City started trading farther and farther afield for numerous types of goods, including perishable foodstuffs. In addition, improvements in infrastructure in the city led the population to start moving to the outer boroughs. The consolidation of the five boroughs into Greater New York in 1898, followed by the opening of the subway in 1904 and the Queensboro Bridge in 1909, paved the way for the urbanization of Queens. Apartment buildings and planned communities began springing up around important transportation hubs in Astoria, Jackson Heights, Woodside, and Forest Hills. Immigrants began moving from Manhattan to Queens, and in some cases new immigrants moved directly to neighborhoods in Queens. By the 1920s and 1930s, different neighborhoods in Queens had developed distinct ethnic identities, with Astoria being heavily Greek, Corona being Irish and Italian, and Forest Hills being heavily Jewish. The rural history of Queens rapidly disappeared, although one of the few remaining traces is the Queens County Farm Museum in Glen Oaks.

As is often the case in New York City, successive waves of immigrants continued to shape and remake their new neighborhoods. In some areas of Queens, the ethnic identity shifted enormously. In Corona, for instance, what had been an Italian and Irish neighborhood became heavily Hispanic after World War II. This shift is visible in the types of restaurants one sees there. A handful of traces of Italian Corona remain, including the famous Lemon Ice King of Corona, which has been in operation since the 1940s, and a few Italian bakeries like Leo's Latticini. But most have been supplanted by Colombian, Dominican, Salvadoran, and Mexican restaurants and groceries,

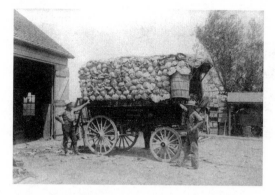

Queens, now one of the most urbanized areas in the nation, was once predominantly farmland. This undated photograph shows the van Siclen farm in Flushing. As agriculture became less important to the community, the van Siclen family turned to banking. QUEENS HISTORICAL SOCIETY

reflecting the demographic shift of the neighborhood.

Astoria continues to be a Greek enclave, full of Greek restaurants and Greek produce stands. The Neptune Diner on Astoria Boulevard epitomizes another contribution Greeks have made to New York's food culture—the ubiquitous diner. The Greek diner, although not as common as it once was, has been a major force in New York City's food culture since the 1940s, when Greek immigrants started establishing restaurants based on the *kaffenion*, a coffeehouse and meeting place common in Greece. See GREEK.

One of the most significant shifts in the food culture of postwar Queens has been the enormous growth of its Asian population. See CHINESE COMMUNITY. In the second half of the twentieth century, spurred by political unrest in their home countries as well as the passage of the Immigration and Nationality Act of 1965, large numbers of Asian immigrants from China, Korea, India, and Pakistan settled in New York, and particularly in Queens. These groups have established communities all over Queens, but are especially concentrated in Flushing, Jackson Heights, and Elmhurst. A 2013 city report found that Flushing was home to 40 percent of New York City's Chinese residents, and the neighborhood as a whole was two-thirds foreign born, compared to about one-third citywide.

The outstanding diversity and the density of particular immigrant groups in Flushing and Jackson Heights are reflected in the food. Flushing has distinctly Korean, Indian, Bangladeshi, Pakistani, and Chinese areas, and each part contains specialty grocers and restaurants for that community's cuisines. See SOUTH ASIAN. Flushing is home to several large banquet halls specializing in dimsum, where the menus are often exclusively in Chinese. Since 2012, Jackson Heights has hosted an annual momo crawl, where participants follow a map throughout the neighborhood and sample Tibetan dumplings from ten different vendors, after which they vote for their favorite. That there are nearly a dozen places to get Tibetan dumplings in a single neighborhood, nestled in between Indian, Pakistani, Korean, Argentinean, Colombian, Dominican, Uzbeki, and Filipino restaurants is a window into the vastness and the diversity of Queens' food offerings. See COLOMBIAN; DOMINICAN; FILIPINO; and SOUTHEAST ASIAN. Everything from yak meat to chicken feet can be found in Queens, without even straying from the 7 train.

Queens has undergone enormous changes over the past century. It has developed from a largely rural area anchored by a few towns to a densely populated network of thriving immigrant neighborhoods, each with their own distinct yet enormously diverse food offerings. The relative affordability of Queens makes it a haven for immigrants, and Queens is also a standout in the number of immigrant-owned businesses, of which many are restaurants, delis, or grocery stores. These businesses anchor their communities, giving immigrants who share a culture a place to reinforce those bonds. But they have also become increasingly attractive to New York City's foodies, who are interested in exploring unfamiliar types of foods and learning about cultures that are not their own, through cuisine. While Queens has a less developed tourist industry than Manhattan or Brooklyn, most guidebooks and tours that do engage with Queens do so on the basis of its food. See WALKING TOURS, CULINARY. The challenge Queens faces in the coming years is how to capitalize on its newfound recognition as a mecca for international cuisine while still remaining a place that provides opportunity and affordability for new New Yorkers.

See also ASTORIA and JAMAICA (QUEENS).

Greater Astoria Historical Society. *Long Island City.* Charleston, S.C.: Arcadia, 2004.

Haller, Vera. "Downtown Flushing: Where Asian Cultures Thrive." *New York Times,* October 1, 2014.

Lewine, Edward. "The Kaffenion Connection: How the Greek Diner Evolved." *New York Times,* May 5, 1996.

Rozeas, Christina. *Greeks in Queens*. Charleston, S.C.: Arcadia, 2012.

Katie Uva

Queens Cocktail

The Queens Cocktail is an obscure cocktail, supposedly named after New York City's borough of Queens. Made with gin, pineapple juice, and sweet and dry vermouths, the drink bears a close resemblance to the Bronx Cocktail, which contains orange juice rather than pineapple.

While the creator of the Bronx cocktail is generally credited as bartender Johnny Solon, he is only one of several who have laid claim to the drink. Among those is Charles A. Beam, whom the *Cincinnati Times-Star* pinpointed in 1899 as originating the Bronx, as well as a cocktail called "the Queen's." A subsequent recipe and instruction for the "Queen's" cocktail also was printed in *Mixer and Server*, Volume 23, a 1914 volume published by the Hotel and Restaurant Employee's International Alliance and Bartenders' International League of America, calling it "an improvement on the Bronx." This version calls for "a small piece each of pineapple and orange," to be carefully placed on either side of a cube of ice in the glass. The drink then is composed of grenadine, dry gin, and both sweet and dry vermouths. "The first one will convince you that a worthy successor of the Bronx has been found," the instructions assure. "The second will do even more. And after that well, you must use your own judgement after that."

The Queen's Cocktail also appeared in *Cocktails: How to Mix Them*, by Robert Vermeire in 1922 with famed bartender Harry Craddock credited as the creator. This variation omits the grenadine. The same recipe—still with the apostrophe in its name—appeared in Craddock's own cocktail book, *The Savoy Cocktail Book* in 1930 and it's the recipe that most bartenders use today. On most modern drink menus, the apostrophe usually is dropped, making it clear that at least the current reference intended is to the New York borough, not royalty.

See also BRONX COCKTAIL.

"Bronx Cocktail." *Cocktail 101* (blog). http://cocktail101.org/tag/queens-cocktail.
Craddock, Harry. *The Savoy Cocktail Book*. Updated ed. London: Constable, 2014.
Vermeire, Robert. *Cocktails: How to Mix Them*. London: Herbert Jenkins, 1922.

Yolanda Evans

Quinby, Moses

See BEEKEEPING.

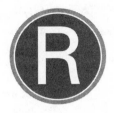

Radio

There are dozens of commercial, public, community, Internet, and satellite radio stations broadcasting from the New York metropolitan area. The first broadcast in New York can be traced to 1907, from an experimental station in the Parker Building then located on Fourth Avenue and Nineteenth Street. On both the AM and FM band, as well as through SiriusXM, the satellite radio service with studios in Manhattan, there is great diversity in content to be found over the airwaves.

While it is not uncommon to hear chefs and other food experts on radio shows, few shows are solely dedicated to food, restaurants, drinking, or eating. Much of the radio programming today is centered on music, talk, and news.

Writer and critic Arthur Schwartz, the "Food Maven," hosted a show from 1992 to 2004 on WOR radio. See SCHWARTZ, ARTHUR. Mike Colameco hosts a syndicated radio show called *Weekend Food Talk* that airs locally on WOR. SiriusXm has a channel dedicated to Martha Stewart that often features food-related content. Anthony Dias Blue, a broadcast personality and wine expert, hosts a segment called the Blue Lifestyle Minute, heard locally on WCBS-AM.

On the public radio station, WNYC, Leonard Lopate often dedicates the last day of the work week to culinary coverage, a segment he calls "Food Fridays." *The Splendid Table*, American Public Media's venerable public radio program hosted by Lynne Rossetto Kasper, broadcasts locally on WNYC.

This is a far cry from the early, so-called golden age of radio (1920s–1950s) when food programs were more easily found. From programs where listeners could call in or send in home recipes to be shared with others, to shows sponsored by companies like General Foods, and Canada Dry soda, many of these food-centric programs were broadcast during the daytime, specifically aimed at homemakers.

Among the popular programs of the time was *Housekeeper's Chat* with Aunt Sammy, a production of the U.S. Department of Agriculture. The host, "Aunt Sammy," known as Uncle Sam's Wife, doled out recipes and cooking tips along with other household advice. A cookbook titled *Aunt Sammy's Radio Recipes* was released in 1927.

The supermarket chain A&P sponsored a fifteen-minute program on NBC called *Our Daily Food*. Another program, *The Mystery Chef*, offered tips for creating a meal on a budget, popular with Depression-era listeners.

Mary Margaret McBride began a radio career on WOR in the 1930s and would later move her household show to other networks throughout the 1940s. On air, she was known for talking about food sponsors while actually tasting items on air.

While some cooking segments and programs aimed at homemakers remained, much of New York's radio programming eventually turned to news, entertainment, sports, and, of course, music.

Perhaps the single largest hub for food and drink broadcasts in New York today is the Heritage Radio Network, an Internet station that emanates from a studio at Roberta's, a pizzeria in the East Williamsburg section of Brooklyn. The station broadcasts a range of culinary broadcasting on topics from urban farming, cheesemaking, beer and home brewing, and more. It is a community-minded station with knowledgeable hosts and a loyal following.

See also HERITAGE RADIO NETWORK and TELEVISION.

Blue Lifestyle website: http://www.bluelifestyle.com.
Bureau of Home Economics, U.S. Department of Agriculture. *Aunt Sammy's Radio Recipes*. Washington, D.C.: U.S. Government Printing Office, 1927. https://archive.org/details/auntsammysradior1927unit.
The Food Maven website: http://thefoodmaven.com/resume.html.
Heritage Radio Network website: http://www.heritageradionetwork.org/about_us.
Mike Colameco website: http://colameco.com.
Rouse, Morleen Getz. "Daytime Radio Programming for the Homemaker: 1926–1956." *Journal of Popular Culture* 12, no. 2 (Fall 1978): 315–357.
WNYC website: http://www.wnyc.org.

John Holl

Railroad Dining

Commuter rail lines played a vital role in the growth of the New York metropolitan region, moving people and goods from the farmlands (later suburbs) to the urban centers, chiefly Manhattan and the New York Harbor. The New York and Harlem Railroad, now known as the Metro-North Railroad Harlem Line, opened in stages beginning in 1832, and connected Lower Manhattan to suburban Harlem, expanding into Westchester County and all the way to White Plains by 1844 as the city expanded. Other rail lines connected the major cities of the Eastern Seaboard. The Long Island Rail Road, for instance, was originally chartered in 1834 to provide daily transit between Brooklyn and Boston, but it was never completed as such because it was superseded by another land route through Connecticut.

In the early decades of rail travel passengers often packed their own meals as there was no on-board dining. Dining options multiplied as passenger lines expanded and train schedules became more reliable. Vendors waited at stations and climbed aboard during scheduled stops to sell sandwiches, drinks, fruit, and other simple fare. Some rail lines employed "news butchers," boys who strode up and down the cars selling newspapers and snacks. The New Haven Railroad, which was incorporated in 1872 and ran from Boston to New York, employed "water boys" to refresh passengers. The ice water was free, but a penny tip was expected. For full meals there were station dining halls, also called "refreshment saloons," often run by the stationmaster's wife. Passengers ate and drank hastily, lest the train depart without them.

One 1857 *New York Times* article reported that "If there is any word in the English language more shamefully misused than any other, it is the word 'refreshment,' as applied to the hurry scurry of eating and drinking at railroad stations."

In the 1860s and 1870s conductors sometimes surveyed the passengers to find out who intended to dine at the next junction and telegraphed ahead to the stationmaster to prepare meals. Still, well-heeled travelers avoided the railroad stations and their sometimes inedible food altogether, instead coordinating their trips to arrive in New York in time to dine at a fine hotel restaurant, such as the Astor House. See ASTOR HOUSE and HOTEL RESTAURANTS.

The Golden Age of Railroad Dining

The era of elegant, even lavish railroad dining did not commence until George Pullman, a young engineer and entrepreneur, formed a partnership with New York Senator Benjamin C. Field in 1857 to build luxurious sleeper cars. The first Pullman sleeper, or "palace car," was ready by 1864. Pullman's next innovation was a "hotel car," a car that offered all of the amenities of a luxury hotel. The *President* went into operation in 1867 with a fully equipped (albeit tiny three feet by six feet) kitchen. A porter doubling as a waiter brought meals directly to the passengers' seats, serving them on folding tables with real glass and silverware and white linens. The quality of the food was good, but dining in the same seat one sat and slept in for days led to restlessness and boredom, and activated class snobbery, since wealthy passengers associated eating where one slept with tenements.

In 1868, Pullman unveiled the *Delmonico*, named after the famous New York restaurant. The name was not an idle boast: it had a dedicated dining car that was considered equal to the finest restaurants of the day. According to historian Jeri Quinzio, "A dinner menu might include up to eighty dishes, from the ubiquitous oysters to wild game, fresh fish, roasts, and a variety of vegetables." See DELMONICO'S.

Dining cars were very expensive to build (the *Delmonico* cost $20,000, nearly four times the average coach car) and required a large staff and specialized equipment to run. Two cooks and four waiters could serve up to forty-eight passengers at once; future dining cars sometimes had upwards of a dozen men on staff. Pullman staffed the cars with freed house slaves, because he believed they would be knowledgeable and deferential to passengers, but also because they were willing to work for less money than white men. Dinner cost around a dollar, which was on par with most upscale restaurants and hotels. It was still not enough to cover the cost of running the car.

Regardless, the pressure to match the competition was such that by the mid-1890s most railroads had dedicated dining cars for long distance travel. Outstanding dining service became a promotional tool. The *Yankee Clipper*, which ran between Boston's South Station and Grand Central Terminal and was operated by the New Haven Railroad, featured stewards in tuxedos, waiters in white suits, and, for many years, a menu consisting entirely of fresh foods—canned foods were banned. Afternoon tea with all of the accoutrements was served on every run.

Ruinous losses, and the emergence of alternative modes of transportation, ended the era of fine rail dining, but well into the twentieth century railroads launched flagship luxury trains that served to make rail travel seem glamorous and exciting. The *20th Century Limited* debuted in 1949, running from New York to Chicago in sixteen hours on the New York Central System. It had glass partitions in the diner, and at night, after the last meal of the evening, the white linens were swapped out for red linens, and the dining car became a nightclub. The *20th Century Limited*'s direct competition, the *Broadway Limited*, which also ran the New York to Chicago route, was completely refurbished in 1972 and remained in operation until 1995. Ads boasted "You pay for first-class meals and get them."

A Long Decline

The Great Depression had a huge impact on railroads. In 1920, Americans took approximately one billion railroad trips, but by 1933 that number had fallen to 435 million. And even before the Depression, railroads were losing money on their dining cars at an unsustainable rate: total dining-related losses ran to $10.5 million in 1925. This forced the railroad companies to consider alternative dining arrangements.

Grill Cars

One change was technology driven: lightweight, cheap, streamlined metal trains came into service in the 1930s. These were the inspiration for the prefabricated metal diners that became popular in New York, New Jersey, and the New England states.

During the Great Depression the hard-hit New Haven Railroad received government funding to subsidize purchase of 205 lightweight, alloy-steel cars, including five dining cars. Delivered in 1937, these "grill cars" offered cafeteria-style seating on benches that ran continuously along both sides of the car, with tables bolted to the floor. Passengers ordered from a service counter, and then sat down with their food tray. There was no oven, only a charcoal grill and steam tables, and various baked goods and cooked meats had to be loaded onto the train from commissaries along the way.

Self-service in theory allowed the railroad to employ fewer people, and to pass the cost savings on to passengers in the form of cheaper menu prices. But passengers—particularly women wearing fashionable high heels—had difficulty carrying their food across a moving platform. Shortly after the first grill car went into service in 1937, the New Haven decided they needed a wait staff after all. "Grill Car Girls" were typically tall and slender, well educated, with minimally a high school diploma and more often a college degree or secretarial schooling. They were very popular with passengers—and they were willing to work for lower salaries than men.

World War II

World War II was actually profitable for the railroads, since passenger and freight traffic increased dramatically. New York was a major port of embarkation, and New York rail lines grappled with the challenge of feeding more passengers while dealing with food rationing. The New York Central urged patience and patriotism: a 1943 ad lay out the challenge by saying "In a kitchen only 6 by 13½ feet, New York Central chefs average more than a meal a minute to meet wartime demands!" One creative solution the New Haven Railroad came up with was to establish "box lunch bars" in Grand Central Terminal. The grill car girls staffed the stands, which could be rolled from platform to platform, allowing passengers to skip the congested onboard cars.

Bar Cars

Bar cars were a popular feature of New York City commuter trains leaving Grand Central from the 1950s to the 1990s. They were precisely what they sound like: traveling bars, where passengers ordered alcohol beverages (usually single serving "nip" bottles to control portion size) and light bar snacks, and fraternized on their ride home from work. Bar cars were a natural evolution from the grill car, which had also served alcoholic beverages. The first dedicated bar car left on an outbound train departing from Grand Central in March 1953 on the New York, New Haven, and Hartford line. These traveling saloons were a big hit during the alcohol-soaked 1950s, when a businessman might have a three-martini lunch and finish out his day with a Bell's Scotch or S. S. Pierce Bourbon (or three) on the ride home to the suburbs.

Despite their popularity, toward the end of the twentieth century the bar cars began disappearing. One issue was seating—as a 2002 *New York Times* article explained, "An average Metro-North train car has about 110 seats, but a bar car has only 28. Even counting customers who stand, bar cars hold a small fraction of what the traditional cars do." Metro-North operated the last bar car in the United States on May 9, 2014, a 7:34 p.m. train from Grand Central Terminal to New Haven.

A New York Tribute to Railroad Dining

The era of fine railroad dining is over, but a tribute to it remains in an unexpected place. On the top floor of Bloomingdales is a restaurant called Le Train Bleu, built in 1979 as a replica of *The Calais-Mediterranée Express*, the French express train with famously blue sleeper cars. Shoppers and train enthusiasts leave their bags on overhead metal storage racks and dine on French bistro fare, surrounded by period-perfect mahogany paneling, Victorian lamps, and green trim.

See also HIGH LINE.

Frattasio, Marc. *Dining on the Shore Line Route.* Lynchburg, Va.: TLC, 2003.
Fuchs, Marek. "Aboard Bar Car, Some Riders Fear Last Call Is Near; A Fight Stirs on Metro-North." *New York Times,* July 29, 2002.
Grant, H. Roger. *Railroads and the American People.* Bloomington: Indiana University Press, 2012.
Quinzio, Jeri. *Food on the Rails: The Golden Era of Railroad Dining.* Lanham, Md.: Rowman & Littlefield, 2014.

Max P. Sinsheimer

Rainbow Room

The Rainbow Room, the restaurant located atop what was the RCA building in Rockefeller Center, opened in October 1934, during the Great Depression and—fortunately—just after the repeal of Prohibition. It was then, and is today, one of the city's most glamorous restaurants. Seating nearly three hundred in a double-height space with unmatched views through twenty-four immense windows, the room was named for an RCA "color organ" that converted musical tones into varying colors projected onto a 41-foot dome above a rotating dance floor. Designed by architect Wallace K. Harrison and interior designer Elena Bachman-Schmid, its style was termed "Streamlined Modern"—not Art Deco as it is called today.

With live orchestras and a café society clientele oblivious to the outside economy, the Rainbow Room was an immediate hit in New York. Big names like Tommy Dorsey, Glenn Miller, Guy Lombardo, Louis Armstrong, and Woody Herman played there. To ensure that everyone had great views and sightlines to the dance floor, the perimeters of the room were terraced, which meant that seated guests were reciprocally on display. They dressed the part, with women in elegant ball gowns, men in tuxedos, and couples ready to prove their prowess on the dance floor.

The Rainbow Room itself was part of a larger complex on the sixty-fourth and sixty-fifth floors of what is now the GE Building. It had various dining and drinking venues, highly coveted party spaces, and the Rainbow Grill, a smaller room that also featured an outdoor terrace. During the day, these rooms comprised the Rockefeller Center Luncheon Club, whose members were tycoons tenanting the building or from nearby offices.

The complex had various operators, including the American News Company, the Brody Corp., and Tony May and Brian Daly. In the 1970s the Rainbow Room began a long decline and in 1985 Rockefeller Center closed it and hired the restaurant consultants, Joseph Baum & Michael Whiteman Company, to plan a thorough $26 million renovation and restoration, and then to operate the 40,000-square-foot complex. These same consultants earlier had created the famed Windows on the World, and success there was immediately repeated at the Rainbow Room where revenues more than doubled. See BAUM, JOE and WINDOWS ON THE WORLD.

At two consecutive nights of grand reopening parties for the Rainbow Room in December 1987, Mayor Ed Koch, Barbara Walters, Liza Minelli, Estée Lauder, the Trumps, and the Helmsleys shared hors d'oeuvres with Rockefeller family members and eight hundred other boldface names.

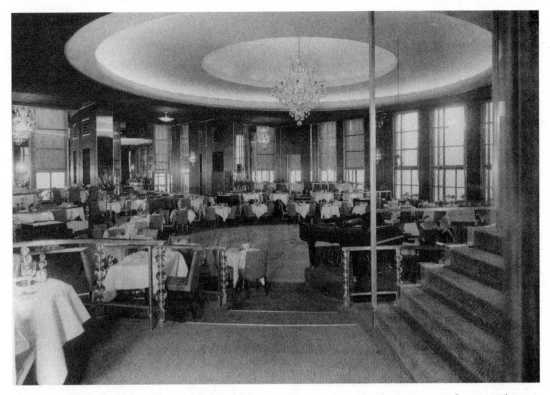

The Rainbow Room restaurant, pictured above, has been a well-known dinner locale since it opened in 1934. This photo was taken April 9, 1941. LIBRARY OF CONGRESS

Lured by high doses of theater and fond memories of marriage proposals and weddings, dancing and romancing with lovers and others, and over-the-top birthday parties, thousands flocked to this historic space along with a new generation of customers. Café society gave way to a more democratically varied clientele. Tuxedos and balls gowns were rare, customers this time opting for what was called "celebration clothing." They came for the spectacular space, for a chance to show off, to experience a bit of history—and to imagine themselves as Fred and Ginger on the dance floor. They sat at tables covered in silver lamé and feasted on chef André Rene's reinvented classics like tournedos Rossini, halibut in a golden balloon, and lobster Thermidor, followed by flaming baked Alaska and frozen pousse-café. See BAKED ALASKA.

Working with architect Hugh Hardy, Baum and Whiteman created a new addition called Rainbow & Stars, a cabaret in the sky with Tony Bennett as the opening act, and the Promenade Bar, where the notion of "Cocktails and Little Meals" got its start, created by consulting chef Rozanne Gold and celebrity bartender Dale DeGroff. This marked the start of America's cocktail revival. See GOLD, ROZANNE and DEGROFF, DALE.

The Cipriani family took over operations in 1999 and effectively closed the room to the public, concentrating instead on more lucrative private parties. They were evicted in 2009 in a dispute with the landlord over unpaid rent and the complex was shuttered for five years while the owner searched, unsuccessfully, for a new tenant. Shrunken to a single floor, redecorated, and reopened in October 2014, it is run by Tishman Speyer Properties, which owns Rockefeller Center. It has been updated technologically but remains elegantly spectacular with an American-inflected menu overseen by chef Jonathan Wright. Although a bar-lounge called SixtyFive is open on weekdays, The Rainbow Room remains closed to the public except for Sunday brunch and Monday evenings.

The Rainbow Room was officially declared a New York City landmark in 2012.

Alexander, Ron. "From Astor to Minnelli, Greetings to the Rainbow Room." *New York Times*, December 10, 1987.

Fabricant, Florence. "65 Floors Up, a Classic Returns." *New York Times*, September 29, 2014.

Giovannini, Joseph. "Rainbow Room: Re-creating the Glamour." *New York Times*, August 7, 1987.

Landmarks Preservation Commission. "Designation List No. 461 LP-2505." October 16, 2012. http://www.nyc.gov/html/lpc/downloads/pdf/reports/2505.pdf.

Rozanne Gold

Random House

Random House, the U.S. division of Random House, the world's largest general interest trade book publisher, is owned by the German multinational, Bertlesmann AG, one of the world's foremost media companies. In 2013, an agreement was made by Bertlesmann and Penguin to merge their respective publishing operations and the result is a consolidated company now known as Penguin Random House. Random House's main U.S. offices are at 1745 Broadway in Manhattan.

Random House USA was founded in 1925 by Bennett Cerf and Donald Klopfer when they purchased The Modern Library, which focused on reprints of classic works of literature.

In 1960, Random House acquired Alfred A. Knopf, Inc. One of Knopf's then young editors, New Yorker Judith Jones, championed a manuscript that at the time seemed unpublishable. Thanks to her keen eye and editorial expertise, *Mastering the Art of French Cooking* by Julia Child, Louisette Bertholle, and Simone Beck, was published in 1961. See CHILD, JULIA; JONES, JUDITH; and KNOPF. Jones and the Knopf imprint brought the works of many culinary luminaries to print including Madhur Jaffrey, Marcella Hazan, Claudia Roden, and Marion Cunningham. See HAZAN, MARCELLA. Knopf continues to publish a well-regarded list of cookbook authors such as restaurateur and television personality Lidia Bastianich and culinary luminaires such as Joel Robuchon and Joan Nathan, among many others. See BASTIANICH, LIDIA.

Jason Epstein, for many years editorial director of the Random House imprint and himself a passionate cook, broke culinary ground by publishing the work of revolutionary restaurateur, chef, and food activist Alice Waters.

In 1988, Random House acquired the Crown Publishing Group, which included the imprint Clarkson Potter, Inc., which publishes best-selling cookbook authors such as Ina Garten, Giada Di Laurentiis, and Martha Stewart.

In 2012, in an expansion of the culinary digital space, Random House acquired the online community and blog TasteBooks, which allows readers and cooks to search, organize, and share individual recipes and recipe collections as well as purchase over ten thousand cookbooks from many publishers.

Garnier, Dwight. "The Meal of His Life." *New York Times*, October 29, 2009.

Moskin, Julia. "An Editing Life, A Book of Her Own." *New York Times*, October 24, 2007.

Random House website: http://www.randomhouse.com/about/history.html.

Carl Raymond

Ranhofer, Charles

Charles Ranhofer (1836–1899) was one of America's greatest restaurant chefs in the nineteenth century. He was born in St. Denis, France, trained as a pastry cook in Paris, and at age sixteen served as personal chef to a prince. Ranhofer immigrated to the United States in 1856. After working in Washington, D.C., and in New Orleans, he returned to Paris in the winter of 1860, making arrangements for royal entertainments at the Tuileries Palace under Emperor Napoleon III.

Two years later Ranhofer settled in New York City, where he managed the kitchen at the Maison Dorée, a fashionable French restaurant on Union Square. He was then hired by Charles Delmonico, owner of the city's most prestigious restaurant, to run the newly opened Delmonico's at Fourteenth Street and Fifth Avenue. For the next thirty-four years (with a three-year gap) Ranhofer dominated Delmonico's and New York City's culinary world. The three-year hiatus occurred when the Fifth Avenue restaurant closed during an economic depression in 1876, and Ranhofer returned to France, where for three years he operated the Hotel American in Enghien-les-Bains.

Ranhofer returned to New York in 1879 to become chef at Delmonico's restaurant at Madison Square, and he remained there until he retired in 1896. In 1894,

Ranhofer published a culinary masterwork, *The Epicurean*—the most comprehensive Franco-American cookbook ever written. In its more than 1,100 pages were 3,500 recipes, for everything from Cream of Cucumber Soup to Saddle of Antelope, Huntress Style. The book detailed the proper furnishing and arrangement of the kitchen and dining room and featured bills of fare for every imaginable event and occasion, including menus for the hundreds of banquets tendered by Delmonico's to famous writers, politicians, presidents, royals, and New York's own upper crust. The average fourteen-course dinner, Ranhofer calculated, should take two hours and twenty minutes—ten minutes per course—to serve and eat, but when necessary the service intervals could be pared down to eight minutes per course so that diners could finish the meal in a mere two hours.

The Epicurean included many of the recipes that made Delmonico's famous, including lobster à la Newberg and baked Alaska. Chefs at fashionable restaurants often flattered the egos of their wealthy patrons by naming dishes after them. As the story goes, in 1876 Ben Wenberg, a shipping magnate who was frequently dined at Delmonico's, showed Charles Delmonico an extremely luxurious way of preparing lobster in a chafing dish. Delmonico put the dish on the menu as "lobster à la Wenberg." For reasons that are lost to history—possibly a falling out between the two men—the name was later changed to lobster à la Newberg.

Leopold Rimmer, who was in charge of one of Delmonico's dining rooms at the time *The Epicurean* was published, bitterly complained that Ranhofer had given "away all the secrets of the house." Rimmer claimed that after the publication of *The Epicurean*, "anyone" could prepare French food. Ranhofer died a year after he retired and was buried at Woodlawn Cemetery in the Bronx.

See also DELMONICO'S and RESTAURANTS.

Parsons, Russ. "Little-Known Cookbook Reveals Early Haute Cuisine." *Los Angeles Times*, February 15, 2000.
Ranhofer, Charles. *The Epicurean*. New York: R. Ranhofer, 1893. Reprint, Mansfield Centre, Conn.: Martino, 2011.
Thomas, Lately [pseud. Robert V. P. Steele?]. *Delmonico's: A Century of Splendor*. Boston: Houghton Mifflin, 1967.

Andrew F. Smith

Rao's

Rao's is a family-owned Italian restaurant in Manhattan's East Harlem neighborhood, founded in 1896 by Charles Rao, an Italian immigrant who purchased a small saloon from the George Ehret Brewery, and named it after his family. See HARLEM. Located at the corner of 114th Street and Pleasant Avenue, near the East River, the relatively small storefront, identifiable by its bright red and white color scheme, is famous for its hard-to-get dinner reservations. Serving southern Italian inspired dishes, meals are served "family style" to the whole table. The restaurant has played a bit part in the annals of the city's organized crime history, as well as serving as a celebrity hangout. The restaurant itself, along with co-owner Frank Pellegrino, occasionally stars on television and in movies.

From its humble beginnings as a bar and grill, Rao's has spawned a mini-culinary empire. Several books inspired by the restaurant's kitchens, penned by Pellegrino and his son, Frank Pellegrino Jr., were published by Random House and St. Martin's Press, along with an album of Italian songs. The restaurant has added locations in Hollywood, and inside the Caesar's Palace Casino in Las Vegas. In 1998, the restaurant expanded into a specialty food business, offering a variety of pastas, canned and jarred vegetables, oils, marinades, and its signature tomato sauce.

Klein, Melissa. "The Mob Murder at Rao's That Was Sparked by a Song." *New York Post*, December 29, 2013.
Rao's Restaurant Group website: http://raosrestaurants.com/our_story.html.
Rao's Specialty Foods website: http://www.raos.com.

John Holl

Rastafari

Rastafari originated in the shantytowns of Kingston, Jamaica, during the 1920s and 1930s. Since then, the movement has grown from its origins into a worldwide entity. Thanks largely to Bob Marley's stardom and Reggae's resounding rhythms, the Rasta message of liberation now reverberates across the globe. In few places is this more apparent than in New York City, home to one of the largest Jamaican populations off the Island.

In essence, Rastafari promotes emancipation from the societal binds of Western culture, or "Babylon." Rastas recognize Babylon as a corrupt force that alienates human beings from their divinely determined pure state. Practitioners reject the economically and politically driven culture of Babylon and opt to cultivate purity as naturalness by growing dreadlocks, avoiding chemical additives, and consuming Ital food.

The term "Ital" derives from "vital." Rastas accept as true that Ital food increases vitality. Given that practitioners eat to generate wellness, they reject the term "diet" on the basis that it includes "die" and instead employ the term "livit" which they derive from "live." Loosely constructed around biblical passages, a Rasta livit aims to insure strength of body and mind.

A proper livit consists largely of fruits and vegetables. Rastas eschew processed, canned, and artificial foods in favor of that which comes from the earth. Ingredients common to the dietary regime include callaloo, coconut, scotch bonnet pepper, tofu, breadfruit, and tamarind. Coconut oil, herbs, spices, and hot peppers flavor popular dishes such as Ital stew, tofu curry, and peas and rice.

Rastas omit white flour, salt, dairy, eggs, alcohol, and most oils from their livit because they believe these ingredients prohibit wellness and hinder spiritual progression. Ingesting dead flesh also pollutes the body; the animals Leviticus prohibits are particularly offensive. However, some Rastas do eat fish smaller than twelve inches in length (anything longer represents for practitioners the cannibalistic forces of Babylon). Others selectively consume chicken, salt, and other restricted goods. Though not all Rastas fully adhere to these strictures, most practitioners and Ital restaurants at least selectively do abide. For example, several establishments in the New York City area season their strictly vegan dishes with salt.

During the 1990s, more than 30,000 Jamaicans immigrated to New York City. As increasing numbers of people of Caribbean descent made the city their home, a Rasta presence developed in the thriving immigrant communities of Brooklyn, Queens, and the Bronx. Ital restaurants opened their doors to meet the needs of growing Caribbean neighborhoods.

Brooklyn, with its significant Caribbean population, offers diners in search of a taste of Ital several options for procuring veggie patties and soursop juice with lime. Strictly Vegetarian and Four Seasons serve the Flatbush area while Scoops and Plates sells Ital food and vegan ice cream in Prospect-Lefferts Gardens.

Veggies Natural Juice Bar, Italfari Health Food and Juice Bar, and Ital Kitchen are located in Crown Heights. Veggie Castle II operates in Richmond Hill, Queens, while the Bronx is home to both HIM Ital Health Food and Vegan's Delight.

The cuisine of Rastafari has profoundly philosophical roots. For practitioners, eating Ital cleanses the body and fosters connection with God, or Jah. Yet the livit's rich Caribbean flavors and healthful preparation appeal to an audience that stretches far beyond Rasta communities to vegans, vegetarians, and New York diners who know that above all else, Ital food is delicious.

See also JAMAICAN.

Barrett, Leonard E. *The Rastafarians*. Boston: Beacon, 1988.
Rosen, Rae, Susan Wieler, and Joseph Pereira. "New York City Immigrants: The 1990s Wave." *Federal Reserve Bank of New York: Current Issues in Economics and Finance* 11, no. 6 (June 2005). http://www.newyorkfed.org/research/current_issues/ci11-6.pdf.

Ariella Werden-Greenfield

Rationing and Food Shortages

See WORLD WAR I and WORLD WAR II.

Raw Food

Raw foods (also known as uncooked or living-food) include fruits, vegetables, grains, nuts, and seeds in their natural state, which cannot be heated above 104–114°F (40–46°C), varying maximum temperature depending on the source. There are variations of the raw diet, ranging from a raw vegan, to raw vegetarian, to raw omnivore; most classify raw vegan as the standard. While the terms "uncooked," "living food," and "raw" are not entirely interchangeable, most associate them to mean the same. A raw diet is typically classified as half to three-quarters of one's diet strictly raw. The attraction of a raw food diet is the belief that cooking foods destroys the nutrients, rendering them toxic.

Raw vegan diets have been used in the treatment for chronic disease, such as heart disease, cancer, and diabetes. Eliminating processed foods and animal-dense meals is thought to reduce one's risk for chronic disease, thus diminishing cholesterol, trans fat, and carbohydrate intake. Numerous studies have been conducted to suggest the benefits of a raw diet in light of chronic disease.

Norman W. Walker spearheaded the juice movement in the 1970s when he wrote *Fresh Fruit and Vegetable Juices: What's Missing in Your Body.* It focuses on improving the body through "juice therapy." Juicing involves separating the fibers of fruits and vegetables from mineral elements and distilled water, thus streamlining the digestive process. Walker also wrote *The Vegetarian Guide to Diet & Salad,* which expands from how to select and assemble raw salads to how to produce the ideal product from a single seed. Walker explains that when food is cooked, the oxygen dissipates and nutrients are not as readily absorbed by the body.

Rynn Berry, who preached a raw diet, explored the upbringing of a few raw-food activists in *Becoming Raw: The Essential Guide to Raw Vegan Diets.* Since 1994, Berry has coauthored the annual *The Vegan Guide to New York City.* Its 2013 edition lists sixteen raw food restaurants and eight raw food boutiques that offer lectures and classes and sell raw snacks, books, equipment and cosmetics. See BERRY, RYNN.

Examples of meals in the raw diet include hearty salads, gazpachos, soaked grains like overnight oatmeal, and fruit smoothies with added supplements like bee pollen, spirulina, and flaxseed, among other options. Foods can also be dehydrated, frozen, or even sprouted.

See also VEGANISM.

Berry, Rynn, and Chris Abreu-Suzuki with Barry Litsky. *The Vegan Guide to New York City.* 19th ed. New York: Ethical Living, 2013.
Davis, Brenda, Vesanto Marina, and Rynn Berry. *Becoming Raw: The Essential Guide to Raw Vegan Diets.* Summertown, Tenn.: Book Pub. Co., 2010.
Stowers, Stacy. "NYC's Best Raw Food Restaurants." CBS New York, April 22, 2014. http://newyork.cbslocal.com/top-lists/nycs-best-raw-food-restaurants.

Lauren Coull

Ray, Rachael

Rachael Domenica Ray (b. 1968) is an Emmy award winning American cook. She is best known for folksy sayings, quick meals, and a media business that includes books, a monthly magazine, several television shows on the Food Network, and one in broadcast syndication. Her business extends to branded products, a pet food line, endorsements, and a charity.

Born and raised in upstate New York, Ray worked with her mother at a number of restaurants, in various positions—from dishwasher to server—before moving to New York City. There, one of Ray's earliest jobs was at the Macy's marketplace where she worked at the candy counter. Later she worked at the specialty food store Agata & Valentina. Her career brought her back to the Albany area where she worked as a cook, buyer, and teacher at a gourmet food store; here she developed meals that could be prepared in thirty minutes. Her first book on that subject was published in 1998.

A television appearance on NBC's *Today Show* catapulted her into her own programs on the Food Network, where she remains a signature star, and eventually syndication. Her daily television show is taped in Manhattan. With a loyal following, she has sold millions of cookbooks and introduced phrases like "Yum-o," "E-V-O-O" (short for extra-virgin olive oil), and "Stoup" (a combination of soup and stew), into household kitchens around the country.

See also TELEVISION.

"Rachael Ray Bio." Food Network. http://www.foodnetwork.com/chefs/rachael-ray/bio.html.
Rachael Ray website: http://www.rachaelray.com/page/about.
Severson, Kim. "Being Rachael Ray: How Cool Is That?" *New York Times*, October 19, 2005.

John Holl

Ray's Pizza

See PIZZA.

Rector, Charles and George

Charles E. Rector (1844–1914) was a renowned New York restaurateur during the early twentieth century. He was born in Lockport, New York; his father owned the Frontier House, a hotel and restaurant in nearby Lewiston. After serving in the Civil War, Rector became a superintendent on a Pullman dining car operating between Philadelphia and Chicago. With borrowed money, in 1884 he opened Rector's Oyster House in Chicago. The first restaurant in that city to serve live oysters (they were shipped from Long Island by train), Rector's became a celebrated seafood house. In 1899, Rector spent $200,000 to launch a second restaurant in New York City. It was an ornately decorated space with an electrically illuminated Greco-Roman façade on Longacre Square (later renamed Times Square). An object of great interest was its revolving door—the city's first. Rector's was one of the city's grand "lobster palaces" but also served other kinds of shellfish as well as meat, poultry, and game. The wine list featured twenty-eight different Champagnes. A French chef, Emil Hederer, ran the kitchen. The restaurant had an orchestra and a small dance floor, where diners could dance between courses.

Longacre Square, a fringe area, was becoming the city's theater district. Rector's catered to the city's social and financial elites and wealthy out-of-town visitors. Spicing up the scene were actors, dancers, and musicians who flooded the lobster palaces late in the evening. Rector's came to be seen as a risqué spot where married men mingled with chorus girls. Among the customers was the corpulent Diamond Jim Brady, famed for the amazing quantities of food he consumed. Rector is reported to have said, "Jim Brady is the best twenty-five customers we have."

George W. Rector (1878–1947) served as an apprentice at his father's restaurants and traveled in France; he claimed to have worked in Paris, at Café Marguery and the Café de Paris, and he also spent time in Bordeaux studying wine. Returning to New York in 1902, he took charge of the dining room at Rector's. In 1909, the Rectors demolished the old place, replacing it with a twelve-story hotel housing a new restaurant, which opened in December, 1910. In 1909 a play by Paul M. Potter, *The Girl from Rector's*, had been a hit on Broadway. A sex farce, it was considered indecent by many and was shut down by the police on the opening night of its out-of-town run. According to an article in the *New York Times*, the play "raised Rector's to the peak of prosperity and popularity." But the restaurant's racy reputation and its association with the hotel drove respectable married men away. Two years later, Rector's went into receivership, but its louche reputation lingered on: The 1913 Ziegfeld Follies featured a number called "If the Tables at Rector's Could Talk."

In 1914, hoping to restore the restaurant's reputation, George started over again at Forty-Eighth Street and Broadway. But Rector found himself facing an even bigger obstacle: Prohibition. Rector's closed for good on New Year's Day in 1919. In his book *The Girl from Rector's* (1927), George Rector blamed Paul Potter and his naughty play for destroying the Rector family business (although apparently he liked the play's title).

George Rector went on to serve as the "Director of Dining Car Cuisine" for a Midwest railroad. He also wrote a weekly column for *Saturday Evening Post*, and several cookbooks, including *The Rector Cook Book* (1928) and *A la Rector's* (1933). During the 1930s, he hosted the radio program, "Dining with George Rector."

See also BRADY, DIAMOND JIM; LOBSTER PALACES; and TIMES SQUARE.

"Era of the Rectors." *New York Times*, November 28, 1947.
Rector, George. *The Girl From Rector's*. Garden City, N.Y.: Doubleday, 1927.
Root, Waverley, and Richard de Rochemont. *Eating in America: A History.* New York: Echo, 1981.

Andrew F. Smith

Red Snapper

See BLOODY MARY.

Reggie! Bar

The Reggie! Bar was a candy bar created in honor of professional baseball player Reginald Martinez "Reggie" Jackson, two-time World Series Most Valuable Player and the most famous clutch performer of his era. It was created and sold by Standard Brands from 1978 to 1980, and by D. L. Clark Candy Co. in 1993.

Early in his career, Jackson expressed interest in playing in New York, and was quoted as saying, "If I played in New York, they would name a candy bar after me." Jackson claims he was joking, but after signing with the New York Yankees in 1977, his agent landed the deal with Standard Brands. For lending his name to the Reggie! Bar, Jackson was to be paid $3 million over ten years.

The candy bar—milk chocolate, peanuts, and caramel—debuted at the Yankees' home opener on April 12, 1978. All 44,667 fans attending received a Reggie! Bar. After Jackson hit a home run, thousands of candy bars were thrown onto the field (Standard Brands executive Roy Cappadocia may have thrown the first bar).

Standard Brands had high hopes, spending $3.5 million to promote the bar, but sales did not meet expectations, and it was discontinued in 1980. It was revived by Clark in 1993, when Jackson was elected to Major League Baseball's Hall of Fame. The new Reggie! Bar (milk chocolate, peanut butter, and peanuts) was given out at Jackson's Hall of Fame celebration at Yankee Stadium on August 14, 1993, and sold commercially, but discontinued shortly thereafter.

See also CANDY.

Coffey, Wayne. "Reggie's Sweet Sensation." *New York Daily News*, July 17, 2007.
Jackson, Reggie, with Mike Lupica. *Reggie: The Autobiography*. New York: Villard, 1984.
Liebig, Jason. "Play Ball!! Baseball's Opening Day Tomorrow!" CollectingCandy.com, April 3, 2012. http://www.collectingcandy.com/wordpress/?p=3062.
Perry, Dayn. *Reggie Jackson: The Life and Thunderous Career of Baseball's Mr. October*. New York: William Morrow, 2010.

Karl Peterson

Reichl, Ruth

Revered and feared by some, thanks to her role as the restaurant critic of both the *Los Angeles Times* (1984–1993) and the *New York Times* (1993–1999), Ruth Reichl has made her mark on the food world.

Ruth Reichl got her start writing about food in 1972 with her cookbook *Mmmmm: A Feastiary*, and, in 1974, dove into the Berkeley dining scene as an owner of Swallow Restaurant, a co-op restaurant that helped define the culinary revolution happening at the time. In 1984, she became the restaurant editor and later food editor for the *Los Angeles Times*, leaving in 1993 to join the *New York Times* as its restaurant critic. Her dual perspective as a restaurateur and as a food writer informed her successful editorship of *Gourmet Magazine* from 1999 to 2009.

Reichl's professional accomplishments include her authorship of a series of memoirs, including *Tender at the Bone*, *Comfort Me with Apples*, and *Garlic and Sapphires*, executive producer for food programming on public television and the Food Network, judge on "Top Chef Masters," and as a lecturer and award-winning journalist. Reichl has also been a passionate advocate for food workers. As Reichl explains: "I feel like we've taken this very strange turn in the sustainability movement. It's very selfish. I want to eat great food, serve my kids healthy foods, and make sure animals are humanely treated. But we have completely neglected the piece that is required to make it all possible—the workers; half the agriculture in this country is done by undocumented workers who live way below the poverty line and are totally exploited."

Reichl is active with the Rural & Migrant Ministry, an ecumenical group dedicated to protecting and lobbying for the rights of farmworkers. She speaks to groups within and outside the food community sharing the plight of these workers and advocating for change and social justice. She says, "How do we get the food movement to the next level? It is clear that we can't go on this way when there are people picking our food and milking our cows who can't afford to eat decently themselves."

See also GOURMET and NEW YORK TIMES.

Parsons, Russ. "Is Fine Dining Ready for a Comeback?" *Los Angeles Times*, March 6, 2013.
Reichl, Ruth. *Tender at the Bone: Growing Up at the Table*. New York: Random House, 1998.
Reichl, Ruth, and Julia Whelan. *Delicious!: A Novel*. New York: Random House, 2014.

Francine Cohen

Restaurant Associates

Restaurant Associates, a subsidiary of Compass Group North America, is a renowned hospitality company based in New York City. Starting with the opening of The Newarker as a fine dining destination at the Newark Airport in 1953, it has transformed from a small company that ran a few lunch counters, working class cafeterias, and airport buffets into a highly imitated company that runs a dizzying array of restaurants in museums, corporate dining rooms, executive suites, conference retreats, parks, and stadiums.

To jump-start The Newarker, Jerome Brody recruited restaurateur Joseph Baum to introduce luxury dining to an airport terminal. See BAUM, JOE. In turn, Baum invested in fine china and furnishing and hired a classically trained Swiss chef, Albert Stockli, to develop the menu. This attention to detail, as well as the spectacle and lavish excess on display at its innovative New York City–themed restaurants, became the hallmark of Restaurant Associates. Baum spent freely to attract leading architects, interior designers, and food consultants like Julia Child, James Beard, and Jacques Pépin. Under his tenure, Restaurant Associates' storied restaurants included the Brasserie, Tavern on the Green, the Forum of the Twelve Caesars, Trattoria, Zum Zum, and La Fonda del Sol, as well as the Four Seasons. Because of his sense of theater and big productions, Mimi Sheraton dubbed Baum the "the Cecil B. DeMille of restaurateurs" in his *New York Times* obituary.

By the end of the 1960s, Restaurant Associates was at the peak of its reputation and began trading as a public company. However, by 1970, thin margins and a plummeting stock price forced Restaurant Associates to merge with Waldorf Systems, a company that concentrated on lower-priced cafeteria operations. Tokyo-based food service conglomerate Kyotaru Co. then acquired the company in 1990. Finally, in 1998, Compass Group USA, the North American division of Compass Group PLC, bought Restaurant Associates. Today, Restaurant Associates operates a portfolio of corporate accounts spanning a variety of industries including publishing and media, advertising, banking and financial, technology, beauty and fashion, sports, law firms, and educational facilities. Moreover, as the manager of several restaurants at prestigious cultural venues, it controls a large portion of the fine dining experience in New York and around the world. For example, in New York City, they operate restaurants and cafes at the Metropolitan Opera House, Avery Fisher Hall, the American Museum of Natural History, the Guggenheim Museum, and the Metropolitan Museum of Art.

See also RESTAURANT GROUPS.

Greene, Gael. "Restaurant Associates: Twilight of the Gods." *New York Magazine*, November 2, 1970.
Grimes, William. "Joseph Baum, American Dining's High Stylist, Dies at 78." *New York Times*, October 6, 1998.
Restaurant Associates website: http://www .restaurantassociates.com/aboutus.

John T. Lang

Restaurant Groups

Hospitality companies and managed restaurant services have been key forces behind many of the restaurants that diners have enjoyed, past and present. In fact, many of those groups have been trailblazers and have had outsized influence on fine dining in New York City. For example, Restaurant Associates transformed itself from a small company, with an airport cafeteria that became a fine dining destination, into a highly imitated enterprise that spawned an array of flamboyant theme restaurants. It is now responsible for the restaurants and cafes in numerous museums, corporate dining rooms, executive suites, conference retreats, parks, and stadiums. Along the way Restaurant Associates and other restaurant and hospitality groups have radically transformed the restaurant business. See RESTAURANT ASSOCIATES.

In the 1950s, two kinds of restaurateurs existed: chain operators and one-of-a-kind fine dining restaurants. Restaurant groups blended those models to conceive new restaurants and set up teams of professionals who could operate more than one location at a time. These groups are important because they control a large portion of the fine dining experience in a particular city, as the managers of several restaurants, often at prestigious venues. Moreover, through their control over multiple properties, the influence of a single chef can be amplified. For example, James Beard, Julia Child, and Jacques Pépin solidified their stature in American culinary lore as menu consultants for Restaurant Associates.

Restaurant groups often start with focus on a particular city or region. In some ways, their sheer presence reflects the importance of place. For example, Stephen Starr now operates more than thirty restaurants, mostly in Philadelphia, that are diverse enough to offer an experience for most budgets, occasions, and food preferences. Lettuce Entertain You Enterprises operates, owns, licenses, or manages more than one hundred establishments throughout the United States but is mostly known for its ventures in and around Chicago. In contrast to place-based models, celebrity chef–driven restaurant groups are a compelling modern model. This is different from a celebrity allowing the use of his or her image to sell food, like Jimmy Buffett's Margaritaville chain or Don Shula's American Steakhouse. Instead, the celebrity chef–driven restaurant group capitalizes on the celebrity and culinary capital of the particular chef.

Wolfgang Puck, who launched Spago in 1982, embodies this trend. The Wolfgang Puck Companies now run more than one hundred fine dining, catering, and quick-casual establishments. Other examples include Daniel Boulud, who owns Feast and Fêtes Catering Company as well as fifteen admired restaurants, seven of which are in New York City. Mario Batali, Joe Bastianich, and Lidia Bastianich's Batali & Bastianich Hospitality Group have more than a dozen restaurants in addition to their partnerships with the Osteria Mozza and Pizzeria Mozza chains. The B&B Hospitality Group also brought Eataly, a large-scale Italian marketplace, to New York and Chicago.

In addition to the groups already mentioned, there are several power players in New York City, each with a distinct focus. The Patina Group, for example, reacquired its restaurant and retail operations from the Compass Group in 2006. Some of Patina's most notable venues now include New York City's Rockefeller Center Ice Rink, Macy's Herald Square, the Grand Tier Restaurant at the Metropolitan Opera, La Fonda Del Sol, and the Brasserie. Since 1985, Danny Meyer's Union Square Hospitality Group has been responsible for some of New York City's most celebrated restaurants, including the Union Square Café, Gramercy Tavern, Blue Smoke, and its chain of Shake Shacks. Also in 1985, restaurateur Drew Nieporent founded the Myriad Restaurant Group and has opened thirty-five restaurants. These restaurants, including Montrachet, Tribeca Grill, Nobu New York City, and Bâtard have drawn critical acclaim as well as attracting celebrity diners and co-owners. See MEYER, DANNY and NIEPORENT, DREW. More recently, chef and owner Tom Colicchio founded the Craft Restaurant Group in 2001 when opening the first Craft Restaurant in New York. Since then, the company has grown to include fifteen New York City locations of the quick-service restaurant 'wichcraft, Craftbar, Colicchio & Sons, and Riverpark as well as Topping Rose House, a full-service luxury hotel and restaurant in the Hamptons. In 2004, David Chang established the New York City–centered Momofuku Restaurant Group, which now includes eight restaurants, a bakery with multiple locations throughout New York City, two bars, a culinary lab, and *Lucky Peach* magazine. See MOMOFUKU RESTAURANT GROUP.

With a prestigious and longstanding reputation for fine dining, New York City can be prohibitively expensive for individual operators to open and run a fine dining restaurant. Restaurant groups and hospitality companies have several advantages over standalone, independent restaurants. By pooling the buying power of all of its restaurants, restaurant groups can get better prices, obtain supplies on more favorable terms, and better manage cash flow. Because of the scale of their purchases, they can make distribution arrangements with national food and restaurant supply distributors, allowing them to maintain consistent quality. Moreover, there is greater continuity between back office operations and executive management functions because business staff can be shared and shifted among and between restaurants. Perhaps most important is the role of financial capital. Banks and investors tend to invest in larger and more established companies. This means that independent restaurants are at a disadvantage and are more likely to be undercapitalized, leading to a greater chance of failure.

This consolidation of food service management and restaurant hospitality can be global in scope. For example, Restaurant Associates and Wolfgang Puck Catering are both subsidiaries of the Compass Group North America, which is a division of the London Stock Exchange–listed Compass Group PLC. Because of their reach, each of these hospitality companies has an outsized influence on fine dining in New York City and throughout the world. This holds true for the style and presentation of food, the marketing of chefs, the standard architecture of restaurant kitchens, and menu design. The standards they set become embraced in their local markets and across their locations as soon as they make a change. Compare this to the slow spread of California cuisine, noted for its fresh, local, and seasonal ingredients. Although this decades-long movement challenged the traditional kitchen hierarchy and the dominance of fine dining, its more egalitarian and informal food scene could be overturned quickly if the hospitality companies decide it would be profitable to go another way. When looking for the next culinary trend or which restaurants have created the most buzz, individual operators may be trailblazers, but they do not and cannot create the market by themselves.

Batali & Bastianich Hospitality Group website: http://bandbhg.com.
Compass Group North America website: http://compass-usa.com.
Craft Restaurant Group website: http://www.craftrestaurantsinc.com/about-us.
Daniel Boulud website: http://www.danielboulud.com.
Momofuku website: http://momofuku.com.
Myriad Restaurant Group website: http://myriadrestaurantgroup.com.
Patina Restaurant Group website: http://www.patinagroup.com.
Restaurant Associates website: http://www.restaurantassociates.com/aboutus.

Union Square Hospitality Group website: http://www
.ushgnyc.com.
Wolfgang Puck Catering website: http://www
.wolfgangpuck.com/catering-events/about.

John T. Lang

Restaurant Letter Grading

Restaurant letter grading came to New York City in July, 2010 under Mayor Michael Bloomberg and Health Commissioner Thomas Farley via legislation added to Article 81, the Food Preparation and Food Establishments article of the New York City Health Code. Specifically, article 81.51 states:

> The Department shall establish and implement a system for grading and classifying inspection results for food service establishments using letters to identify and represent an establishment's degree of compliance with the provisions of this Code, the State Sanitary Code and other applicable laws that require such establishments to operate in a sanitary manner so as to protect public health. The letter "A" shall be the grade representing the highest degree of compliance with such laws. Subject to the provisions of this section, the Department shall provide each operating establishment that it inspects with a letter grade card indicating the establishment's inspection grade, except that no letter grade card shall be provided when the Department orders an establishment closed after an inspection.

The legislation requires that the letter grade be posted prominently in the window of every restaurant in the city (about twenty-four thousand at the time of this writing), but it exempts some establishments such as mobile food vendors as well as institutional cafeterias, soup kitchens, and temporary operations.

Letter grading in New York was modeled after a system implemented in many California municipalities, most notably San Diego, Riverside, and Los Angeles. Advocates for letter grading argue that it simply and prominently communicates important food safety and public health information to the public, thereby holding restaurants to greater accountability in complying with food safety regulations. Before letter grading in New York City, restaurant inspection reports were available on the New York City Department of Health and Mental Hygiene's website or in hard copy after a written request to the department, but not in a particularly user-friendly way and with a lot of tech-

nical language describing the violations. The letter grading system summarizes that information with a single letter.

The legislation passed over the objections of the New York State Restaurant Association and other business groups who argued that the law would hurt business; would be an unethical way for the city to earn revenue via capricious notices of violation resulting in fines and a more frequent inspection schedule; and would oversimplify—and possibly miscommunicate—the complexities of operating a restaurant by summarizing a detailed inspection with a letter grade.

The process involves a system where different violations noted by inspectors have varying point values, based on the potential risk to public health. For example, holding food at an improper temperature counts as a seven-point violation at minimum. A lesser offense, such as a handwashing station being empty of soap, may result in the loss of a point or two. A critical violation that cannot be quickly remedied—for example, a major pest infestation, or a broken walk-in refrigerator resulting in cold food not being held at the proper temperature—may result in the immediate closure of a restaurant until the problem is corrected and the restaurant inspected again.

If a restaurant earns a deduction of from zero to thirteen points, it earns an A upon first inspection. If it earns a B (14 to 27 points) or C (28 points or more but short of closure), the restaurant has the ability to correct the violations and be inspected a second time, unannounced, at least seven days after but typically within thirty days of the first inspection. Upon the second inspection, the restaurant receives its final grade of A, B, or C. Restaurateurs unsatisfied with the grade can dispute it at the New York City Office of Administrative Trials and Hearings Health Tribunal (commonly referred to as "tribunal") and can post a Grade Pending sign until the decision is reached at the hearing.

Foodservice sanitation consultants, who work on behalf of the restaurant, have long been a fixture of the New York City restaurant world but have become more prominent with the implementation of letter grading. The threat of a public display of a B or C—and possible loss of revenue associated with the lower grade—motivates restaurateurs to maintain as high as possible a grade. Consultants help restaurants prepare for inspection, perform third-party mock inspections, and recommend corrective actions to improve and prepare for a real inspection, train employees, and represent restaurants at tribunal.

Critics of letter grading continue to maintain that there is no evidence that it has improved public health in New York City by reducing cases of foodborne illness. At the time of this writing, the New York City Department of Health and Mental Hygiene is preparing a report to address this question.

See also BLOOMBERG, MICHAEL.

"Letter Grading for Restaurants." NYC Health. http://www.nyc.gov/html/doh/html/environmental/food-service-grading.shtml.

Jonathan Deutsch

Restaurant Opportunity Center

The Restaurant Opportunity Center (ROC), which later became Restaurant Opportunities Centers United with local chapters including the founding local, ROC-NY, was formed after the events of September 11, 2001. Many restaurant workers in downtown Manhattan, including more than one hundred at Windows on the World in the World Trade Center, lost their jobs—and many their lives—in the 9/11 tragedy. Windows on the World employee Fekkak Mamdouh and lawyer Saru Jayaraman founded ROC-NY to assist these workers and their families. With the recession that followed, Mamdouh and Jayaraman found themselves supporting additional workers from throughout the city who even before the attack had been struggling with low wages, wage theft, sexual harassment, limited opportunities for advancement and other problems endemic to the restaurant industry.

According to ROC's website and printed materials, "Restaurant Opportunities Center of New York (ROC-NY) is dedicated to winning improved wages and working conditions for restaurant workers and raising public recognition of restaurant workers' contributions to our city." The New York City local has over five thousand members representing a variety of venues and service levels from bars and casual restaurants through fine dining. Members include both kitchen and dining room workers as well as some managers.

Both the local and national ROC seek to accomplish their mission by using a three-pronged strategy: (1) Going after "low-road" employers who use illegal or unfair practices through boycotts, protests, and legal action. This work has yielded millions of dollars in settlements with restaurants. (2) Celebrating high-road employers by promoting their businesses and training and placing workers in these businesses. ROC-NY also operates COLORS, a cooperatively owned high-road restaurant in Manhattan's East Village. (3) Conducting research and lobbying for legislation to improve conditions for restaurant workers such as eliminating the tipped minimum wage, raising the minimum wage as a whole, and instituting paid sick days.

ROC-United was formed in 2007 and ROC locals now operate in New Orleans, Houston, Washington, D.C., Philadelphia, Detroit, Los Angeles, the San Francisco Bay Area, Boston, Miami, and Chicago. There are over thirteen thousand members nationally.

See also RESTAURANT WORKERS.

Jayaraman, Saru. *Behind the Kitchen Door.* Ithaca, N.Y.: ILR, 2014.
Restaurant Opportunity Centers United website: http://rocunited.org.

Jonathan Deutsch

Restaurant Reviewing

As a major culinary and media hub, New York City plays a particularly influential role in shaping national taste through the reviews of its restaurants. Restaurant reviews appear across all media in New York City, from print and Internet publications, to radio and television productions, and even on tiny screens in the back of taxis. The idea that restaurants should be critiqued in the same way as other forms of cultural production did not exist in the United States until the early 1960s. Popular restaurant guides, such as those produced by Duncan Hines in the 1930s and Mobil Oil in 1960, recommended hotels and restaurants to travelers, but did not offer detailed critique of the quality of meals. *Forbes Magazine's Restaurant Guide* covered the New York dining scene in the 1970s but lacked a consistent voice. *Gourmet* magazine ran the "Spécialités de la Maison" column, a roundup of New York City restaurant reviews, from the 1940s until 2006; James Beard was the reviewer. The early reviews were nearly always positive and catered to high-end diners. However, one man is widely credited with developing the modern American form of restaurant reviewing: Craig Claiborne of the *New York Times.* See CLAIBORNE, CRAIG.

The Rise of Restaurant Criticism

Claiborne became the food editor at the *New York Times* in 1957 during a burgeoning restaurant boom. The dining options in New York during the late 1950s were relatively few and expensive. These establishments were generally more concerned with being social hubs for the city's elite than with creating quality cuisine, much less with developing innovative dishes. However, several new and influential establishments, including the Four Seasons, La Caravelle, and Lutèce, raised the quality of food around the city just as the growing middle class was developing a taste for fine food and dining. Claiborne's reviews were the first to offer middle-class diners a window into urban dining from a major publication.

Claiborne debuted his weekly "Directory to Dining" in 1963 with reviews of restaurants in New York City and its suburbs. Claiborne was the first to bring a journalistic approach to restaurant reviewing by using a rating scale of 1 to 4, instituting a policy of three anonymous visits, and refusing to accept free meals or gifts—standards that the *New York Times* still uses today and that have been adopted by many other publications. Claiborne's reviews emphasized food and cooking techniques, guiding readers through the intimidating world of New York dining while cultivating their tastes. As interest in restaurants grew, Claiborne's reviews wielded the power to make a restaurant successful overnight. He continued at the paper as food critic until 1972 and served as the food editor from 1974 to 1986. The *New York Times* continues to devote more resources to its restaurant coverage than any other New York publication.

In the late 1960s, restaurants became destinations in and of themselves, rather than pit stops en route to the theater. They also became a focus of New York counterculture; experimenting with new cuisines and expanding one's taste was one way that people could assert their rejection of establishment culture. Gael Greene, who served as *New York Magazine's* restaurant critic from 1968 to 2000, embraced Claiborne's journalistic approach and added flavors of her own colorful personality (instead of a number scale, she used mouths to rate the "culinary excellence" and hearts for the "total pleasure"). See GREENE, GAEL. Emphasis on the individual diner as part of the larger consumer advocacy trend also played an increasing role in restaurant reviewing in the 1960s and 1970s, as value took on greater importance. Mimi Sheraton, who succeeded Claiborne as restaurant critic of *The New York Times* from 1975 until 1983, embraced this consumer-centered and value-driven culture. See SHERATON, MIMI. Later, Robert Sietsema, the *Village Voice's* restaurant critic for twenty years beginning in 1993, carried on Sheraton's consumer-focused approach, aiming to represent the typical diner in his reviews. Jane Freiman, New York *Newsday's* critic from 1989 to 1995, was another alternative voice to the dominance of the *Times*.

During the 1990s, as New Yorkers became more sophisticated eaters, dining increasingly became a form of entertainment. The lively style of Ruth Reichl's reviews for the *New York Times* (1993–1999) reflected this shift. Reichl was known for fiercely protecting her anonymity by donning many guises while reviewing, and also for attempting to expand the *Times's* coverage; she famously awarded a noodle shop three stars. See REICHL, RUTH. Frank Bruni of the *New York Times* (2004–2009) wrote for an international and culturally diverse audience, most of which would never visit the restaurants he covered. Some of New York's other notable figures include Steve Cuozzo who has been the critic of the *New York Post* since 1998, and Adam Platt at *New York* since 2000. The *Times's* restaurant critic since 2011, Pete Wells, has proven to be an equal opportunist when it comes to negative reviews; he gave unfavorable critiques of both high-end fixture Le Cirque and to Guy Fieri's new American Kitchen and Bar. Many national publications also review New York City restaurants, such as *GQ* and *Bon Appétit*.

The Democratization of Reviewing

The *Zagat Survey* was the first to put restaurant reviewing directly into the hands of consumers by poling diners on their experiences, publishing their quotes and compiling them into ratings. Tim and Nina Zagat first self-published their informal guide to New York City restaurants in 1979 by surveying their friends, and New York City continues to be *Zagat's* largest market. Carrying on the consumer-centric trend that began in 1960s, *Zagat* promoted the idea that "real" diners and not "experts" knew the true value of a restaurant experience. See ZAGAT, TIM AND NINA.

As the New York restaurant scene continued to expand in the 1990s and 2000s, print publications increasingly saw competition from online reviews.

Consequently, some New York publications have followed the national trend and stopped printing restaurant reviews altogether. *Newsday* abandoned its New York City edition in 1995, which had included a review section, and *Gourmet* magazine stopped publishing its monthly restaurant reviews in 2006 after sixty-four years before folding entirely three years later. See GOURMET.

While *Zagat* was the first to express the tastes of the masses, online reviewing made it possible for anyone with an Internet connection to be a critic. Restaurant blogs started to emerge around 2003 and were not bound by any of Claiborne's journalistic standards, but covered a wide range of establishments. While the restrictions of print allow only a fraction of New York's thousands of restaurants to be represented, sites like Yelp, Urbanspoon, and Eater are able to review many more and provide frequent updates. Just as Claiborne opened up new dining worlds for his readers, online reviews expose more people to New York's ever-expanding restaurant scene.

See also BEARD, JAMES; FOUR SEASONS; LE CIRQUE; LUTÈCE; *NEW YORK* MAGAZINE; *NEW YORK TIMES*; RESTAURANTS; RESTAURANT GRADING; and *VILLAGE VOICE*.

Batterberry, Michael, and Ariane Batterberry. *On the Town in New York: The Landmark History of Eating, Drinking, and Entertainments from the American Revolution to the Food Revolution.* London: Routledge, 1999.

Claiborne, Craig. *A Feast Made for Laughter: A Memoir with Recipes.* New York: Holt, Rinehart and Winston, 1983.

Davis, Mitchell. "A Taste of New York: Restaurant Reviews, Food Discourse, and the Field of Gastronomy in America." PhD diss., New York University, 2009.

Dornenburg, Andrew, and Karen Page. *Dining Out: Secrets from America's Leading Critics, Chefs, and Restaurateurs.* New York: Wiley, 1998.

Sietsema, Robert. "Everyone Eats But That Doesn't Make You a Restaurant Critic." *Columbia Journalism Review*, February 2, 2010. http://www.cjr.org/feature/everyone_eats.php.

Adee Braun

Restaurant Row

Restaurant Row, the official designation for Forty-Sixth Street between Eighth and Ninth Avenues, is one of the most visited blocks in Manhattan. When lunchtime and dinnertime roll around, the tourists who throng Times Square and pack Broadway theaters head to this charming block lined with nineteenth-century brownstones and some of the most popular restaurants in New York City. According to the Times Square Business Improvement District, each year, over 12 million theatergoers come to New York to see Broadway shows, and almost all of them arrive early or stay late to enjoy a meal in the neighborhood. The name "Restaurant Row" was made official in 1973 when Mayor John Lindsay dedicated the street and said "Where else in the world, except possibly Paris, could you get sixteen of the best restaurants collected in such a short strip of land?" Many longtime residents point to Lindsay's proclamation as the beginning of the street's, as well as the neighborhood's, gentrification.

Today, Restaurant Row is home to more than thirty eateries, including Becco, owned by the cookbook author and celebrity chef Lydia Bastianich and her son Joe; the Broadway hangout Joe Allen; the eponymous B. Smith's; the New York branch of Paris's Brasserie Athenee; Lattanzi, a bastion of Roman-Jewish cuisine; and Barbetta, the oldest family-owned restaurant in New York City. Other standouts are Bourbon Street, a New Orleans style Cajun eatery; Brazil Brazil, an authentic *rodizio* grill; Sushi of Gari, an upscale Japanese sushi spot; The House of Brews, a beer and burger joint; Sevilla, a Spanish tapas bar; Broadway Joe's, a classic New York steakhouse; and the aptly named Hourglass Tavern, where diners can keep their table until the sand runs out. Other cuisine found on the block includes Italian, French, Thai, Chinese, Greek, and Irish.

See also MANHATTAN and TIMES SQUARE.

Miller, Bryan. "From Casual to Continental Cuisine along the Spruced-up 46th Street." *New York Times*, April 10, 1987.

Mike DeSimone and Jeff Jenssen

Restaurants

Restaurants have been a vital part of New York City life for more than two centuries. The first to open was the restaurant in the City Hotel, built in 1794, and other large hotels followed suit with their own dining rooms, principally serving the hotel guests. Some also had bars. Little is known about the fare served at these early hotel restaurants. Most hotel restaurants operated on the "American plan," which meant that all meals were included in their room charges. Others had restaurants for well-heeled locals, who could come in for coffee, drinks, and meals.

Until the mid-nineteenth century, most New Yorkers went home for midday dinner. As the city grew, and residential areas sprang up far from manufacturing and business districts, lunchrooms opened to serve busy workers. Short-order houses such as Sweeney's and Sweet's, emerged to meet these needs. They typically offered quick service and simple, cheap menu choices. The food was served within seconds of being ordered, and customers, usually dining solo, gulped down their meals in silence and returned to work. Speed of food delivery and moving diners along were the highest priorities.

New York's first golden age of fine dining began in March 1830, when Swiss immigrants John and Peter Delmonico opened "Delmonico & Brother, Restaurant Français." Delmonico's was the city's first stand-alone restaurant and introduced *la haute cuisine française*. It quickly became the city's premier restaurant, catering to the city's elite as well as visiting dignitaries. Delmonico's paved the way for other French restaurants, and by the late 1830s many New York hotel restaurants served French cuisine. See DELMONICO'S and DELMONICO BROTHERS. They served mainly males, and unaccompanied females were not served. Ladies' restaurants, such as Taylor's and Thompson's, emerged in the 1830s.

Faster and more efficient ways of feeding workers continued to develop as the nineteenth century progressed. The Exchange Buffet, which opened in 1885 across the street from the New York Stock Exchange, catered to businessmen on a tight schedule. Customers proceeded down a long buffet of sandwiches, salads, and cakes, tea, coffee, and milk. In 1889, William and Samuel Child opened their first self-service lunchroom on the main floor of the Merchants Hotel. Unlike the Exchange Buffet, they sought a female clientele. They also are credited with introducing the tray to the serving line, so that customers didn't have to juggle dishes in their hands. This restaurant was so successful that the brothers opened more cafeterias—more than a hundred by 1925. By 1929 the city had 786 cafeterias.

In the twentieth century, most lunchrooms were mom-and-pop shops that sold sandwiches, soup, and few other items. By the 1920s, small lunchroom chains began to develop in New York, with only two or three outlets. See LUNCH. These shared a name and were advertised as a "system." Larger chains might have central food preparation and distribution facilities. One of the most successful and long-lived was W. F. Schrafft's, which by 1922 had twenty-two restaurants catering to middle-class women. See SCHRAFFT'S.

By the early twentieth century, Manhattan alone had an estimated five or six thousand restaurants and eating-houses. Some served foreign food, reflecting new waves of immigrants: Chinese, Italian, Hungarian, and German restaurants thrived in New York by the late nineteenth century. See CHINESE COMMUNITY; GERMAN; HUNGARIAN; and ITALIAN. Chophouses, American versions of the English grill-room, were also common.

New forms of restaurants emerged during the late nineteenth century. Louis Sherry opened an elegant place at the corner of Fifth Avenue and Thirty-Seventh Street. Its elaborate décor and its skilled French chefs soon attracted New York's social elite and those who simply loved well-prepared food. See SHERRY'S. After running successful restaurants at two locations nearby and two farther downtown, Thomas Shanley, an Irish immigrant, opened a new, bigger Shanley's in Times Square in 1912. Shanley's drew celebrities from the nearby theaters and his business grew. Shanley is credited with launching New York's first "lobster palace"—an expensive, elegantly decorated establishment that would soon evolve to offer live entertainment such as a floor show, or dancing to a live orchestra. Shanley's and the other lobster palaces served a variety of foods, but lobster was their signature dish. See LOBSTER PALACES and NIGHTCLUBS.

French cookery in New York reached a peak at the beginning of the twentieth century, when hotel restaurants run by French or French-trained chefs—at the Waldorf Astoria, Essex House, and Ritz-Carlton, among others—were among the nation's premier eating places. Affluent New Yorkers also hired French chefs to preside over their household kitchens. See FRENCH; HOTEL RESTAURANTS; RITZ-CARLTON; and WALDORF, THE.

High-end restaurants relied on alcohol sales for much of their profits, so when Prohibition went into effect in 1920, restaurants, particularly lobster palaces and fine dining establishments, were hit hard, and most closed. There were notable exceptions, such as the Russian Tea Room, which was opened by Russian émigrés on Fifty-Seventh Street in 1927; Sardi's, in the Theater District; the "21" Club; and The Colony. See SARDI'S; RUSSIAN TEA ROOM; and "21" CLUB. But even the vaunted Delmonico's fell victim to Prohibition.

By the time the Depression hit in 1931, a variety of foreign cuisines could be found at affordable restaurants and cafés around the city. There were also Jewish restaurants, which served either dairy and vegetarian dishes or meat, but not both, in accordance with Jewish dietary laws. The most famous was the Café Royal, on Second Avenue, then the heart of New York's "Yiddish Rialto." Foreign and ethnic food was and is a defining element in the city's foodscape, and today there are hundreds of different national, regional, and ethnic restaurants to choose from.

When Prohibition ended, in December 1933, the country was in the depths of the Depression and "fancy" restaurants were few and far between. This situation changed when New York hosted the 1939 World's Fair: the eighty-plus restaurants located around the fairgrounds gave New Yorkers a plethora of dining options. See WORLD'S FAIR (1939–1940). Henri Soulé, the maître d'hôtel at the restaurant at the French Pavillon, remained in New York when the Fair ended and opened a restaurant on New York's fashionable Upper East Side in 1941. See SOULÉ, HENRI. Hoping to trade on the restaurant's popularity at the Fair, he named the establishment Le Pavillon. See LE PAVILLON. It survived World War II and remained hugely popular during the 1950s. With Soulé at its helm, Le Pavillon served as an incubator for many of New York's top chefs. French haute cuisine remained the standard for fine dining in New York during the 1960s and 1970s. See HAUTE CUISINE.

Le Pavillon ushered in a second golden restaurant age. New Yorkers became more adventurous about their food. Joseph Baum, who was placed in charge of Restaurant Associates' specialty restaurants in 1955, is credited with popularizing theme restaurants, such as the Hawaiian Room at the Lexington Hotel (Polynesian, complete with hula dancers), La Fonda Del Sol (South American), Zum Zum (German sausage), and Quo Vadis (French and Italian). He also opened the Hudson River Club, Tavern on the Green in Central Park, and The Four Seasons. See BAUM, JOE; FOUR SEASONS; and TAVERN ON THE GREEN.

Baum's approach has influenced many who came after him. The chefs and restaurateurs Drew Nieporent, Daniel Boulud, Danny Meyer, Jean-Georges Vongerichten, Stephen Hanson, and David Chang have followed in his footsteps, designing new restaurant concepts in New York and around the world. See BOULUD, DANIEL; CHANG, DAVID; MEYER, DANNY; NIEPORENT, DREW; and VONGERICHTEN, JEAN-GEORGES. Drew Nieporent, a Cornell hotel management graduate, worked at Tavern on The Green before forming the Myriad Restaurant Group, which operates Tribeca Grill, Nobu New York City, The Daily Burger at Madison Square Garden, and thirty-two other restaurants. Danny Meyer's Union Square Hospitality Group operates the Union Square Café, Gramercy Tavern, and many branches of the Shake Shack, as well as The Modern, Café 2, and Terrace 5, all in the Museum of Modern Art. See SHAKE SHACK and UNION SQUARE CAFÉ. Korean American David Chang opened his first restaurant, the cutting-edge Momofuku Noodle Bar, in the East Village in 2004. He then opened other restaurants in New York and elsewhere and created the Momofuku restaurant group to manage them. See MOMOFUKU RESTAURANT GROUP.

Today New York City's restaurant scene ranges from the glitzy and upper class restaurants to the greasy spoons. Eateries include fast-food chains with cheap eats, small mom-and-pop diners, ethnic establishments run by recent immigrants, and long-established neighborhood cafés, along with the latest white-hot restaurants of the moment.

See also AUTOMATS; CAFES; CAFETERIAS; COFFEE HOUSES; COFFEE SHOPS; and TAVERNS.

Grimes, William. *Appetite City: A Culinary History of New York*. New York: North Point, 2009.
Mariani, John. *America Eats Out: An Illustrated History of Restaurants, Taverns, Coffee Shops, Speakeasies, and Other Establishments That Have Fed Us for 350 Years*. New York: William Morrow, 1991.
Smith, Andrew F. *Eating History: Thirty Turning Points in the Making of American Cuisine*. New York: Columbia University Press, 2009.
Thomas, Lately. *Delmonico's: A Century of Splendor*. Boston: Houghton Mifflin, 1967.

Andrew F. Smith

Restaurant Unions

Labor unions, associations of workers that bargain collectively with employers over employment terms and working conditions, have been a presence in New York City's food and drink industries for more than a century. Most employers fought efforts by their workers to unionize, at least at the beginning, and unions were first successful in higher-end establishments.

Workers in fast-food chains have been less successful in unionizing, although recent labor strategies have broadened organizers' goals to include a national campaign to increase the minimum wage for all workers, regardless of union membership.

Labor unions originated in Germany in the nineteenth century and were brought to the United States with politically leftist German immigrants. In New York City, German waiters organized the first culinary unions in the 1880s under the Knights of Labor, a fraternal organization whose initial goal was to improve the lives of workers through education and cooperation with employers. When cooperation failed, the more radical wing of the Knights organized strikes. These earliest efforts were short lived, and the Knights collapsed in 1888. Some of its members joined the newly formed American Federation of Labor, led by Samuel Gompers, a Jewish immigrant from London who worked in cigar factories in New York City. The American Federation of Labor focused on economic gains, rather than politics and structural change, supporting the Chinese Exclusion Act (1882) and other anti-immigrant legislation that many workers saw as the best path to a decent wage.

In 1891, some of the radical waiters who had joined the American Federation of Labor petitioned it to charter the Hotel and Restaurant Employees National Alliance. The New York chapter became Local 1, but it was an uncomfortable fit as the petitioning members' socialist beliefs did not accord with the American Federation of Labor's "work with capitalism" ideology. By 1911, Local 1 had fewer than two thousand members (primarily bartenders) and had raised dues to a scandalously high $65, with few waiters and cooks in the membership.

On October 29, 1911, the International Hotel Workers Union was formed in New York City to represent cooks and waiters. The International Hotel Workers Union was initially headed by Joseph Dommers Vehling, a German immigrant who thought litigation against abusive employers and education were the solution to the working man's plight. This relatively conservative approach was soon tested when several International Hotel Workers Union members were fired from the Belmont Hotel for participating in the May Day parade. Vehling reluctantly went along with agitators' demands for a strike. Meticulously timed at 7:15 p.m. on May 8, 1912, union stewards blew whistles in each of the Belmont's dining rooms, apologized to the tuxedoed patrons, and explained

that the waiters were striking. Half of the waiters walked out, and by noon the next day, the hotel was virtually empty. The success of the Belmont strike, and of a threatened strike on May 9 at the Waldorf Astoria, launched a tumultuous six weeks, when membership in the International Hotel Workers Union mushroomed from several hundred to nearly sixteen thousand. Waiters and cooks at leading hotels and restaurants staged (or ominously threatened) strikes. Management promised higher wages, a weekly day off, and other improvements, except, significantly, recognition of the union and the right of workers to collectively bargain.

While various negotiations were taking place, the International Hotel Workers Union was faced with challenges from more extreme factions. In 1905, the Industrial Workers of the World (also called the Wobblies) had been founded with the explicitly socialist goal of creating an international workers' commonwealth. Wobbly leader Big Bill Haywood and socialist labor activist Rose Pastor Stokes supported the restaurant workers' strikes, but when the International Hotel Workers Union declared victory on June 25 and called off further strikes, Haywood and Stokes withdrew their support, considering the gains inadequate. The most vociferous of the trade-unionist strikers, who had sided with Haywood and Stokes, found themselves blacklisted, a cautionary lesson to other workers.

The next chapter in the labor battle came quickly in the fall of 1912, when some of the hotels and restaurants cut back on the concessions they had granted in June. At 2:00 p.m. on December 31, the International Hotel Workers Union called a surprise strike against all reneging establishments for New Year's Eve, to begin at 7:00 p.m. The short notice was to prevent establishments from hiring scabs for the year's busiest night; however, with such short notice, the strike was poorly organized and many employees failed to walk out. The Wobblies swooped in to exploit this International Hotel Workers Union debacle, organizing strikes in early January, but this time the hoteliers were better prepared. Using the Wobblies' Socialist image as a justification to react violently, they physically beat strikers and intimidated others. The Wobblies escalated, publicly calling for workers to "harmlessly" adulterate food with excessive salt or otherwise make the food "unsafe." This threat to food's purity backfired as customers were offended and crossed picket lines to dine. The demoralized workers went back to work on January 31, 1913, with no new rights or benefits, leaving commentators to conclude that Vehling's labor movement had been highjacked by "the Reds."

Other attempts to organize hotel and restaurant workers occurred in 1918, 1929, and 1934. But it was not until 1938, after the passage of the Wagner Act in 1935, which made it legal to join a union, that an effective, citywide hospitality union took root, representation that continues in selected segments of New York City's food and drink industries. Local 6 of the Hotel Employees and Restaurant Employees was formed in anticipation of the 1939 World's Fair, to make sure that labor unrest would not mar the expected tourism; it continues to represent culinary and other workers in the city's hotels. Representing workers in cafeterias, executive dining rooms, restaurants, sports arenas, and other food venues in New York City and its environs is Hotel Employees and Restaurant Employees Local 100. Recent statistics place its membership at 250,000.

New York's food workers are also represented by organizations outside of the traditional labor unions. Restaurant Opportunities Center United was launched by workers displaced from Windows on the World after the terrorist attacks of September 11, 2001. Its mission is to improve the working conditions of low-wage food workers not by pushing them into unions but by calling attention to abusive labor practices and encouraging boycotts. Once an establishment feels the economic pinch, the Restaurant Opportunities Center helps the workers negotiate better wages, healthcare, and other benefits that are traditionally part of union contracts without some of the perceived negatives of union membership.

Unionization battles in New York City have influenced debate on national policy. On November 29, 2012, approximately two hundred workers at New York City fast-food outlets went on a one-day strike demanding a $15 hourly wage and the right to unionize without retaliation. The strike received wide publicity and became the impetus for a nationwide series of short strikes among fast-food workers. The movement has become known as Fast Food Forward. Funded in part by the Service Employees International Union, Fast Food Forward is credited with spearheading the current national argument over what a "living wage" should be in twenty-first-century America.

See also FAST-FOOD WORKERS STRIKES and RESTAURANT WORKERS.

Dubofsky, Melvyn. *When Workers Strike: New York City in the Progressive Era.* Amherst: University of Massachusetts Press, 1968.

Finnegan, William. "Dignity: Fast-Food Workers and a New Form of Labor Activism." *New Yorker,* September 15, 2014.

Kimmeldorf, Howard. *Battling for American Labor: Wobblies, Craft Workers, and the Making of the Union Movement.* Berkeley: University of California Press, 1999.

Kuttner, Robert. "A More Perfect Union: New York's Local 6 Shows How Organized Labor Can Survive and Thrive in the Service Economy." *American Prospect,* November 28, 2011.

Zillman, Claire. "Fast Food Workers' $15 Demand: How Aiming High Launched a Social Movement." *Fortune,* December 4, 2014.

Cathy K. Kaufman

Restaurant Workers

With over 200,000 workers, restaurant workers comprise one of the largest and fastest-growing private sector workforces in New York City. As New Yorkers have continued to eat out with increasing frequency, even during times of economic crisis, the New York City restaurant industry has grown rapidly, maintaining jobs even as other sectors have declined. The New York City restaurant industry produces $8 billion in revenue annually. These statistics mirror the industry's prowess nationally; with over 10 million workers, the restaurant industry is one of the largest and fastest-growing sectors in the country, with tremendous potential to provide millions of people access to family-supporting jobs.

Despite its size and potential, the restaurant industry is the lowest-paying employer in both New York City and the nation. Every year, the U.S. Department of Labor releases a list of the ten lowest-paying jobs in America, and every year, restaurant occupations make up six or seven of the lowest-paying jobs, with the two absolute lowest-paying jobs in America being restaurant occupations. The industry is also the largest employer of minimum wage workers.

Approximately 20 percent of the jobs provide livable wages—jobs held largely by servers and bartenders in fine dining restaurants, who can earn more than $100,000 a year. Unfortunately, severe occupational segregation by race results in these jobs being held almost exclusively by white men. New York City's restaurant industry is more heavily immigrant than the industry nationally. Seventy-five percent of New York City restaurant workers are immigrants, and it is estimated that approximately 40 percent of New York City restaurant workers are undocumented. These workers are rarely found in the industry's coveted livable-wage jobs.

The National Restaurant Association (NRA), the industry's national trade lobby, and its New York affiliate, the New York State Restaurant Association have fought to keep the minimum wage for all workers as low as possible, and in particular wages for tipped workers. Restaurant workers and their advocates have fought to raise this wage in New York State, so that the wage for tipped workers will increase to $7.50 per hour as of December 31, 2015. Employers are obligated by law to ensure that tips make up the difference between the minimum wage for tipped workers and the overall minimum wage, but this law is sparsely enforced. A recent U.S. Department of Labor investigation found that 83 percent of all restaurants investigated engaged in some form of wage or tip theft.

Living off tips can be extraordinarily unstable economically. Servers suffer three times the poverty rate of the rest of the U.S. workforce and use food stamps at double the rate of the rest of the U.S. workforce. In New York City, servers' median wage, including tips, is $9.22. Even worse, advocates have found that forcing women to rely on customer tips for their income subjects them to the worst sexual harassment of any industry in the United States. Restaurant workers file sexual harassment complaints to the U.S. Equal Employment Opportunity Commission at five times the rate of all other workers. With the customers paying their income rather than their employer, women must tolerate inappropriate behavior from customers, and are encouraged by managers to "show more cleavage" or sexually objectify themselves in order to sell more food and earn more tips. This kind of objectification contributes to harassment from customers, coworkers, and management.

Until recent legislation passed ensuring all workers paid sick days, 90 percent of New York City restaurant workers have reported not having paid sick days, and approximately two-thirds have reported cooking, preparing, and serving while sick, with implications for the city's public health. Sixty percent of workers report having been burned on the job, and 36 percent report having been cut.

Despite these challenges, many New York City restaurant workers take great pride in their work and seek to advance up a career ladder as in other professions. Although the industry has extremely high rates of turnover, many New York City restaurant workers do not leave the industry for other occupations, but instead stay in the industry for their lifetimes, moving from restaurant to restaurant continuously seeking better wages and working conditions. Many New York City restaurant workers say that they would like to be paid and treated as the professionals that they are.

Restaurant workers in New York City have led the national movement to change their industry. The Restaurant Opportunities Centers (ROC) United is a national restaurant workers' organization that was founded in New York City by restaurant workers displaced from the World Trade Center after the 9/11 tragedy, and has grown to include thirteen thousand restaurant worker members in thirty-two cities nationally. In 2012, New York City fast-food workers organized by the Service Employees International Union (SEIU) and New York Communities for Change initiated a series of national strikes of fast-food workers. In these ways, New York City restaurant workers have been leaders in changing conditions for restaurant workers nationwide.

See also FAST-FOOD WORKERS STRIKES and RESTAURANT UNIONS.

American Community Survey, 2012. Calculations by the Restaurant Opportunities Centers United (ROC-United), based on Steven Ruggles et al., *Integrated Public Use Microdata Series: Version 5.0* [Machine-readable database]. Minneapolis: Minnesota Population Center, 2010. https://usa.ipums.org/usa.

Bureau of Labor Statistics. "Characteristics of Minimum Wage Workers, 2013." *BLS Reports*, March 2014. http://www.bls.gov/cps/minwage2013.pdf.

Jayaraman, Saru. *Behind the Kitchen Door.* New York: Cornell University Press, 2013.

Restaurant Opportunities Center of New York. "Behind the Kitchen Door: Pervasive Inequality in New York City's Thriving Restaurant Industry." 2005. http://rocunited.org/roc-ny-behind-the-kitchen-door.

Restaurant Opportunities Centers United. "Burned: High Risks and Low Benefits for Workers in the New York Restaurant Industry." 2009. http://rocunited.org/burned-2009.

Restaurant Opportunities Centers United. "Tipped Over the Edge: Gender Inequality in the Restaurant Industry." 2012. http://rocunited.org/tipped-over-the-edge-gender-inequity-in-the-restaurant-industry.

Saru Jayaraman

Reuben Sandwich

The Reuben sandwich—layers of corned beef, Swiss cheese, sauerkraut, and Russian or Thousand Island dressing on rye or pumpernickel—was invented in New York by Arnold Reuben (1883–1970), a German-Jewish immigrant.

Reuben opened a small restaurant and delicatessen on the Upper West Side around 1908. He took to naming special sandwiches for the actors who frequented his place after the theater. Around 1914 he created the "Annette Seelos Special" for one of Charlie Chaplin's leading ladies. Seelos's namesake sandwich was made with ham, cheese, turkey, coleslaw, and dressing. The Annette Seelos Special was a clear antecedent of the now-famous Reuben sandwich.

Arnold Reuben later opened a restaurant on the Upper East Side. The first located print reference to a "Reuben sandwich" is in a 1927 newspaper article describing the restaurant's specialty sandwiches. The following year, Reuben moved to 6 East Fifty-Eighth Street, where he expanded the business, now called "Reuben's Restaurant and Delicatessen." Along with sandwiches, the menu featured duck, red cabbage, apple pancakes, chopped liver, matzo-ball soup, borscht, chow mein, and cheesecake. (Reuben said that he devised the cheesecake recipe in 1928, using Breakstone's cream cheese while others were still using cottage cheese; he claimed that it was the first New York–style cheesecake.) See CHEESECAKE and DELICATESSENS.

Reuben's restaurant continued to attract celebrities from the 1920s onward. In 1933, in the midst of the Depression, a newspaper reported that he spent $100,000 "flossing up his two sandwich shops," which had grown "to a national institution." In 1937, the Duke of Windsor visited Reuben's restaurant to dine with celebrities and to enjoy "a Reuben Sandwich." Newspapers all over the country reprinted these articles about Reuben and his unusual sandwiches with their celebrity names.

Reuben never named a sandwich after himself; he left that to others. Recipes for "Reuben sandwiches" began appearing in newspapers across America in 1939. The first-located recipe for a "Ruben" (*sic*) in a cookbook appeared in Joseph Oliver Dahl's *Menu Making for Professionals in Quantity Cookery* (1941). The ingredients were "Rye Bread, Switzerland Cheese, Sliced Corn Beef, Sauerkraut, Dressing." The book was intended for chefs, cooks, and managers of

"Hotels, Restaurants, Clubs, Schools, Fountains, Tea-rooms, Resorts, Camps, Cafeterias, Hospitals and Institutions." Dahl's recipe standardized the formula for the Reuben sandwich, which thereafter became a staple in restaurants in New York and other cities.

In 1942, Arnold Reuben opened the Turf Restaurant in the Brill Building, on Forty-Ninth Street and Broadway. The Brill building was the Mecca for songwriters and musical acts in the 1940s and 1950s, and many musical celebrities ate at the very popular restaurant. In 1964, Arnold Reuben sold his business to a Harry L. Gilman. Reuben died six years later.

In 1956, the Reuben sandwich was entered into a contest by a cook at the Blackstone Hotel in Omaha, Nebraska. It won first place and the sandwich received renewed visibility. It remains on many deli and restaurant menus today.

See also CHEESECAKE; JEWISH; LINDY'S; RESTAURANTS; and TIMES SQUARE.

Batterberry, Michael, and Ariane Batterberry. *On the Town in New York*. New York: Routledge, 1999.
Dahl, Joseph Oliver. *Menu Making for Professionals in Quantity Cookery*. Stamford, Conn.: J. O. Dahl, 1941.

Andrew F. Smith

Reynolds, Alvah Lewis

See CREAM CHEESE.

Ritz-Carlton

Wealthy society in the late nineteenth century associated luxury and fine dining with Swiss hotelier César Ritz and the Ritz-Carlton Hotel Company. The company operated London's Ritz and Carlton Hotels as well as the Parisian Ritz, and the restaurant kitchens were managed under the discerning eye of chef Auguste Escoffier. The company wanted to expand to North America, whose sophisticated travelers were eager for comparable cisatlantic elegance. Negotiations between the hotel company's vice president, William Harris, and Robert W. Goelet, a scion of New York's Gilded Age real estate magnate Robert Goelet, resulted in financing that allowed construction to begin in 1908 on the fourteen-story building on Madison Avenue at Forty-Sixth Street. The hotel opened on December 15, 1910, under Harris's executive management with a special press dinner devised by Escoffier, who was brought from England to supervise the opening of this and another Ritz-Carlton branch hotel in Pittsburgh. The menu included caviar with blinis, green turtle soup, lobster, foie gras, saddle of lamb, squab, and soufflé "Walkyrie." Different wines were paired with each course, and the meal concluded with a vintage 1865 Denis Mounié cognac. Although the initial public relations campaign claimed that the hotel would not be catering exclusively to millionaires, there was an unmistakable aura of affluence, with a construction budget of $2.1 million and furnishings coming in at an additional $500,000.

The original hotel had several dining rooms: an elegant, oval-shaped room with pale green walls, echoing the architectural form favored by the Adam brothers in Georgian England; the Palm Room; and a basement Grill Room. By 1912, the Ballroom and Crystal Room were added for larger fêtes and, thereafter, the Japanese Garden room and a rooftop garden. The hotel's permanent chef was Louis Diat, who had worked for Ritz in both Paris and London. Diat would remain at the helm of the Ritz-Carlton's kitchens until the hotel closed in 1951. See DIAT, LOUIS.

One social change that the Ritz-Carlton helped usher in was tolerance of smoking by women. While a few restaurants had made exceptions for "ladies" smoking in the company of their husbands, the Ritz policy was more broad minded: women of any social class (assuming they could afford the tab) were permitted to smoke, with no (further) damage to their reputation. In the words of its first manager, Harris, "American women know best what is the correct thing to do in a public restaurant, and I would never dream of posing as an 'arbiter of etiquette.'"

This discreet solicitousness was a hallmark of the Ritz experience. Both food and service were famous for the attention given to detail: green coffee beans were roasted daily; a fish tank in the commissary held live fish in a tank, ready to be dispatched when ordered; ice creams were made in-house, as was the charcuterie; a confectionary kitchen made bonbons that were presented as gifts to guests. The kitchens were staffed with between 120 and 150 cooks, and the lush service meant that the kitchens were never a source of serious revenue for the hotel. With Prohibition, the Depression, and the rationing brought on by World War II, the original Ritz-Carlton could not survive.

The brand and the association with elegance have endured, however. In 1999, after many changes of hands, the financially troubled Hotel St. Moritz on Central Park South was acquired by a development group working with a restructured Ritz-Carlton Hotel Company. It has been refurbished and renamed and now offers the Star cocktail lounge and Auden Bistro. In 2001, the Ritz-Carlton Battery Park opened, with 2West Restaurant. But neither, to quote Fred Astaire, is "puttin' on the Ritz."

"Big New Hotel Under Way." *New York Times*, September 3, 1908.

Diat, Louis. "The Ritz in Retrospect." *Gourmet*, January 1951.

Haley, Andrew P. *Turning the Tables: Restaurants and the Rise of the American Middle Class, 1880–1920.* Chapel Hill: University of North Carolina Press, 2011.

Cathy K. Kaufman and Thei Zervaki

Rizzoli

Rizzoli started life in New York City in 1964 as a tony bookstore located at 712 Fifth Avenue, a magnificent turn-of-the-century building designed by architect Alfred Gottlieb. The bookstore was the first American venture of Italian media entrepreneur and filmmaker Angelo Rizzoli. In 1974, he launched Rizzoli New York, a publishing imprint that focused on beautifully produced books in the areas of fashion, interior design, art, architecture, photography, and cuisine and the gastronomic arts. Now part of the RCS Media Group, Rizzoli continues to publish stylishly illustrated books and to distribute works published by other prestigious international houses, such as France's Flammarion and Australia's Hardie Grant, both noted for their extensive culinary libraries.

Among the many culinary and gastronomic works published by Rizzoli are classics such as (the reissued) *Great American Cookbook* by Clementine Paddleford (originally published in the 1960s as *How America Eats*); (the reissued) *La Cuisine: Everyday French Home Cooking* by Françoise Bernard, France's mid-twentieth-century grande dame of home cooking and the French equivalent of Julia Child; and several of Carlo Petrini's works about the slow food movement. Notwithstanding these heavyweights, the Rizzoli's imprint is best known for lavishly illustrated works, many by lesser-known authors and chefs, that are more about the photography and sensual text than the recipes.

But the heart and soul of Rizzoli's has been the romance of its real estate: the original shop was largely gutted in the 1990s to make way for an office tower, although the façade remains and houses part of the chic Henri Bendel store. Before the gutting, Rizzoli's was used as a location for the motion pictures *Falling in Love* (1984) and *Manhattan* (1979). In 1985, Rizzoli's main branch relocated to 31 East Fifty-Seventh Street, a six-story building replete with chandeliers, gracefully decorated vaulted ceilings, rich woodwork, and huge windows: to browse books at Rizzoli's was to lose oneself in reverie in an elegant Renaissance Revival townhouse. Unfortunately, real estate development led to the demise of this flagship location in April 2014, notwithstanding a spirited public protest and unsuccessful last-minute effort to protect the space with a landmark designation.

Predictions of the death of Rizzoli's are premature. In 2014, Rizzoli published *How to Eataly: A Guide to Buying, Cooking, and Eating Italian Food*. The book is part of a tie-in with the Eataly mega-emporium, which includes a small "Rizzoli" bookshop with over four hundred titles devoted to Italian gastronomy. But fans of the independent, elegant old Rizzoli's can rejoice: like a phoenix, a new Rizzoli's is slated to open in 2015 at 1133 Broadway, Manhattan, in the refurbished St. James Building. Dating from 1896, it promises to revive some of the cachet of Rizzoli's previous real estate.

Moss, Jeremiah. "Rizzoli Inside." *Jeremiah's Vanishing New York* (blog), April 10, 2014. http://vanishingnewyork .blogspot.com/2014/04/rizzoli-inside.html.
Rizzoli New York website: http://www.rizzoliusa.com.
"Rizzoli International Publications." Issuu.com. http:// issuu.com/rizzoli.

Cathy K. Kaufman and Thei Zervaki

Roberta's

The *New York Times* writer Sam Sifton referred to Roberta's as "a rural-urban-hippie-punk food Utopia," soon after it opened in 2008. But Roberta's has matured into much more than a hipster hangout known for its wood-fired Neapolitan-style pizza.

Roberta's is a pizzeria, bakery, and restaurant in a gritty part of Bushwick, Brooklyn, dominated by factories, warehouses, and a hipster gentrification movement. It was started by musicians Chris Parachini and Brandon Hoy and chef Carlo Mirarchi in a former garage of cinderblock, and it has evolved into a unique American dining establishment. Noted for its food as well as a hipster scene, even Manhattanites cross the bridge or take the L train to Brooklyn to sample the pizza and the well-executed, creative dishes that garnered two stars from the *New York Times*.

The décor is definitely DIY-style—a *GQ* blogger once likened it to "1970s punk ski chalet"—encompassing communal tables, hard wood benches, mismatched chairs, and strings of Christmas lights. But don't be fooled: it's all about the food. Fare includes housemade charcuterie, sausage, and mozzarella, as well as pastas, roasted meats, and vegetables—and of course, plenty of pizza. Meanwhile, a rooftop garden to grow greens and herbs for the restaurant's use has attracted the attention of legendary California chef and locavore Alice Waters.

Out back behind the storage containers that house the Heritage Radio Network (ground zero for food-centric podcasts) are the tiki bar, the bread oven, and a new, state-of-the-art catering kitchen with a twelve-seat dining room called Blanca, where Mirarchi serves a multicourse tasting menu four nights a week. See HERITAGE RADIO NETWORK.

Fancy fare aside, the pizzas still reign at Roberta's, making up about 60 percent of the food orders. And they are considered some of the best in New York.

See also BUSHWICK and PIZZERIAS.

Sifton, Sam. "Reviewing Roberta's." *New York Times*, August 23, 2011.

Linda Pelaccio

Rodale, Jerome Irving

Jerome Irving Rodale was born the son of a grocer in New York City on August 18, 1898. His father emigrated to the United Sates from Poland. His entrepreneurial spirit was evident in his many and varied interests. He was an accountant, author, playwright, businessman, and most noted as a pioneer of the organic farming movement in the United States. He began his professional life as an accountant, and worked for the Internal Revenue Service. While in his twenties, he changed his name from Cohen to Rodale, which was derived from his mother's maiden name, Rouda. In 1923, he and his brother started Rodale Manufacturing, a company that specialized in making electrical wiring devices. In 1930, they moved their company from New York to Emmaus, Pennsylvania. At that time, he also established a publishing business, which eventually grew into one of the largest independent publishing houses in the world. He continued to write on a variety of subjects and published his *Pay Dirt: Farming and Gardening with Composts* in 1945, among many other books.

In 1940, after studying the farming ideas of Lady Eve Balfour and Sir Albert Howard, and realizing that much of the nitrogen previously used as fertilizer was used to make explosives during World War II, he purchased sixty-eight acres of land in Emmaus, Pennsylvania, where he could experiment with soil enrichment. Born into a family with congenital heart problems, he had an avid interest in promoting healthy lifestyles, and theorized that there was a connection between human health and the nutritional quality of the soil in which food is grown. He nurtured the soil on his land by using composting methods without the aid of chemical fertilizers or pesticides. Intent on sharing his positive results with the public, he established *Organic Farming & Gardening* magazine in 1942 (later renamed *Organic Gardening*, and referred to as "OG"). He coined the term "organic" to mean pesticide-free. In 1947, he established the Soil and Health Society, which was a precursor to the current Rodale Institute, which is an entity devoted to studying the link between healthy soil, healthy food, and healthy people. J. I. Rodale started *Prevention Magazine* in 1950, as a way to communicate his findings for disease prevention. He wanted to shift the research from treating diseases to preventing them. The first issue was entirely devoted to the subject of polio. Some of his positions were questioned by the scientific community because he presented reader evidence and testimonials as accepted research. Some of his claims resulted in disputes with the American Medical Association, and the U.S. Food and Drug Administration.

J. I. was married to Anna Anderson in 1927 and remained so until his death from a heart attack in 1971, which occurred during his appearance on the *Dick Cavett Show* in New York City. The couple had three children, Robert, Nina, and Ruth. J. I. Rodale is buried in Northwood cemetery in Emmaus, Pennsylvania.

Gross, Daniel. *Our Roots Grow Deep: The Story of Rodale.* Emmaus, Pa.: Rodale, 2008.
Rodale A. "The Rodale Dream: 50 Years of Love." *Prevention* 52, no. 9 (September 2000): 275.
Rodale website: http://www.rodaleinc.com.
Yang, Eleanor. "J. I. Rodale." *The (Allentown) Morning Call*, January 1, 2000.

Rosemary Trout

Rooftop Garden

What began as the green roof movement—an endeavor to replace standard roofing materials with material for growing grass and plants on flat city roofs—has evolved into an urban farming movement. Green roofs provide better insulation, decreased environmental heat pockets, reduced wastewater runoff, and many other benefits. Growing food on city roofs takes this a step further by offering viable alternatives to environmentally challenging supply chain issues, and by providing opportunities for underserved communities to participate directly in the local food movement.

New York City has an estimated 40 square miles of rooftop space in Manhattan alone. Internationally-acclaimed programs such as The Earth Institute at Columbia University, located in West Harlem, have made New York City a model for the use of viable rooftop space. Through the support of such programs, New York City has become a leader in urban farming, with three commercial rooftop farms in existence as of October 2014, including Brooklyn Grange (the world's largest rooftop farm), Gotham Greens, and the Whole Foods Rooftop Greenhouse, with more in the planning and approval stages.

Several New York City restaurants and hotels, including Bell Book and Candle, Rosemary's, the McKitrick Hotel, and the Waldorf Astoria, maintain productive rooftop gardens where they grow produce for use in their restaurants, in keeping with their commitments to serving local products. Community organizations such as Hell's Kitchen Farm Project and Eagle Street Rooftop Farm are also using rooftop gardens to educate schoolchildren and underserved communities about fresh produce and urban farming.

See also URBAN FARMING.

Mandel, Lauren. *Eat Up: The Inside Scoop on Rooftop Agriculture.* Gabriola, British Columbia: New Society Publishers, 2013.
Miller, Mark J. "A Farm Grows in Brooklyn—On the Roof." *National Geographic*, April 29, 2014.

O'Brien, Miles, and Jon Baime. "Green Roofs: Ingenuity Sprouting from the Rooftops." *Science Nation*, June 21, 2010. http://www.nsf.gov/news/special_reports/science_nation/greenroofs.jsp.

Spector, Kaye. "10 Urban Farming Projects in New York City." *EcoWatch*, November 8, 2013. http://ecowatch.com/2013/11/08/urban-farming-projects-new-york-city.

Annette Tomei

Ruggerio, David

See TELEVISION and TELEVISION, PUBLIC.

Rum

The history of rum is woven throughout the history of the North American and Caribbean colonies. Rum is a distillate made from sugarcane juice or molasses, a byproduct of the sugar-making process. It arose in the Caribbean, shortly after European settlement there, and it quickly became popular with European gentry and American colonists.

New York City, like New Amsterdam before it, has never truly been a rum town, not even in the colonial era. The colonies most famous for rum were Massachusetts and Rhode Island, which, at the peak of the rum trade, had dozens of distilleries between them.

Rum was sold and imbibed in Gotham, but not at the quantities seen in New England. Rum was, however, distilled within the boundaries of current-day New York. The first rum distillery in North America was on what is now Staten Island, opening in about 1640. Though it initially made applejack, it was producing rum by about 1664. By the 1720s, New York had about sixteen rum distilleries. Among the distinguished New York families that owned distilleries were the Livingstons, the Lefferts, and the Pierreponts.

Rum, however, shows up in the minutes of the town court of Newtown, a community in what is now Queens County. In a case from 1680, for example, arbitrators settled a debt in part by asking the debtors to pay a quart of rum in recompense for the debt.

Among the contributing factors to the American Revolution were several acts of the British Parliament, many of which levied taxes upon the importation from non-British colonies of molasses, sugar, and their byproducts, including rum. The Molasses Act of 1733 (which was rarely enforced), the Sugar Act that followed in 1764 (that actually lowered the tax on imported molasses and sugar but set strict enforcement provisions), and the Stamp Act a year later caused widespread protests in the colonies and led directly to the Stamp Act Congress, held in New York City in October 1765.

The anger is easy to understand: rum was often a form of wages in the colonies. Adam Smith, writing in 1773, notes that in "the province of New York...ship carpenters [earn] ten shillings and sixpence currency, with a pint of rum worth sixpence sterling."

In August 1776, just before the Battle of Long Island (also known as the Battle of Brooklyn or the Battle of Brooklyn Heights), George Washington wrote a letter from his headquarters on Broadway, near Bowling Green, as British forces began to occupy Staten Island, and the British Navy filled the waters surrounding Manhattan and Long Island. Washington commissioned the Commissary General to deliver "to the Colonel of each regiment, Rum in the proportion of half a pint to a man."

Though rum was America's spirit in the colonial era, it fell from favor after the Revolution, as distillers chose to focus on native crops, instead of imported sugar. Apple brandy and rye whiskey became popular in the nascent United States, taking European spirits and adapting them with homegrown crops. As America expanded west, however, farmers discovered how easy it was to make whiskey using another native plant: maize.

Rum entered a long decline in American drinking after the revolution, largely because of import taxes and due to whiskey's extreme popularity. What made it popular again was national prohibition, which began in 1920 with the passage of the Volstead Act. Rum had ceased to be an international beverage prior to Prohibition, and it was enjoyed primarily in the Caribbean. After the Volstead Act took effect, however, wealthy Americans started flying to Cuba and other Caribbean islands to enjoy what they saw as an exotic beverage. Pan American Airways joined forces with Bacardi to promote tourism in Cuba, offering flights between Miami and Havana.

During Prohibition, boats would dock off the coasts of Brooklyn, Long Island, and New Jersey, at the federally defined twelve-mile limit. Fishing boats would creep out, evading the eyes of the Coast Guard, load up with crates of scotch, Canadian whisky, and rum, and bring them to shore, where they eventually made their way to the speakeasies of New York City. See PROHIBITION.

Rum's popularity since the repeal of Prohibition has ebbed and flowed, but it's popular enough now to have spawned two rums distilled in Brooklyn.

The administration of Governor Andrew Cuomo has spearheaded a number of new laws aimed at easing the restrictions against distilling beverage alcohol in the state. Prior to Prohibition, New York State counted hundreds of distilleries within its borders. Prohibition, of course, forced them all to shutter. Thanks in part to the Cuomo administration's initiatives, however, New York now has dozens of liquormakers and the number grows every year. See SPIRITS.

In East Williamsburg, Brooklyn, Bridget Firtle's The Noble Experiment is making Owney's Rum, named for Owen "Owney" Madden, a bootlegger and rum-runner in Prohibition-era New York. Van Brunt Stillhouse in Red Hook, Brooklyn, also makes a rum called Due North.

Curtis, Wayne. *And a Bottle of Rum*. New York: Crown, 1996.
Fitzpatrick, John C., ed. *The Writings of George Washington from the Original Manuscript Sources, 1745–1799*. Vol. 5: *May 1776-August 1776*. Murrieta, Calif.: U.S. History Publishers, 2007.
Simonson, Robert. "New York Distilling History, Before the Current Boom." *Off The Presses* (blog), June 6, 2011. http://offthepresses.blogspot.com/2011/06/new-york-distilling-history-before.html.

Michael Dietsch

Runyon, Damon

Damon Runyon (1880–1946), newspaperman and author of the short stories collectively known as *Guys and Dolls*, was born in Manhattan, Kansas, but found his true home and unique voice in Manhattan, New York.

Runyon was raised in Colorado and followed his father into the newspaper business when he was just fifteen. His name was originally Alfred Damon Runyan, but when a misprint turned Runyan into Runyon, he adopted the change. Later, he dropped Alfred. After working on several different newspapers, he moved to New York in 1910 to work for Hearst's *New York American*. There he wrote about everything from boxing matches to murder trials to New York

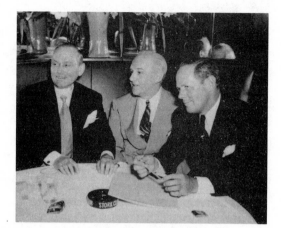

Damon Runyon, Walter Winchell, and Sherman Billingsley (left to right) at the Stork Club in New York, which was owned by Billingsley. Runyon was a newspaperman and the author of *Guys and Dolls*, whose stories used food to reveal character and ethnicity. AP IMAGES

nightlife. He was one of the star reporters of the day and later became a successful short story writer.

Runyon spent much of his time listening to and observing the clientele at Lindy's on Broadway. In his stories it became "Mindy's," the delicatessen where his characters met, talked, and ate Hungarian goulash, gefilte fish, strudel, and cheesecake. For years, Lindy's and Damon Runyon were inextricably linked in the public consciousness. See LINDY'S.

Runyon used food to reveal character and ethnicity. The gamblers, grifters, showgirls, and gangsters who populated his stories ate sturgeon sandwiches on rye or spaghetti, tripe à la creole, or beef stew. Runyon's characters were sympathetic or comic rather than dark or threatening. His writing style, which became known as Runyonese, was notable for his use of 1920s and 1930s underworld slang, some of his own creation, and his near-exclusive use of the present tense. He called the guys Nicely-Nicely, Dave the Dude, and Izzy Cheesecake; the dolls were Mazie Mitz, Dream Street Rose, and Myrtle Marigold. It was a golden era of short story writing, and his were among the most popular. Many of his stories inspired musicals and films, among them *Little Miss Marker*, *The Lemon-Drop Kid*, and most famously, *Guys and Dolls*.

When Runyon died, his ashes were taken up in a plane and strewn over midtown Manhattan.

See also MOVIES and NOVELS.

Breslin, Jimmy. *Damon Runyon*. New York: Ticknor & Fields, 1991.
Runyon, Damon. *Guys and Dolls and Other Writings*. Introduction by Pete Hamill. New York: Penguin, 2008.

Jeri Quinzio

Russ & Daughters

Although the venerable Lower East Side "appetizing" store Russ & Daughters opened in 1914, its history begins in 1907 when Joel Russ, then twenty-two, immigrated to New York City from Stryzow, in the Austrian-Hungarian Empire (now part of southern Poland). Following his marriage a year later to Bella Speier, a fellow recent Jewish immigrant, the couple opened their initial store on Orchard Street, selling salt-cured salmon and herring. In 1920, they moved the J. Russ National Appetizing Store to their still-current location at 179 East Houston Street.

Joel and Bella's three daughters, Hattie, Anne, and Ida, began working in the family business after school and on the weekends, starting in 1924. To honor their children, in 1933 the parents changed the name of the appetizing business to Russ & Daughters. It is believed to be the first time that a business was named after daughters.

Each of the daughters married: Hattie to Murray Gold, Ida to Murray's friend Max Pulvers, and Anne to Herb Federman. At some point, each of the daughters and their husbands worked at the store alongside the founders until Bella died in 1958 and Joel died in 1961.

As the daughters moved away from New York's Lower East Side and eventually retired, the third generation assumed the helm. Practicing attorney Mark Russ Federman and his wife Maria joined the family business in 1978. Meanwhile, the neighborhood surrounding Russ & Daughters experienced major cultural shifts. During the tumultuous 1970s in New York City, the economy floundered, crimes escalated and the once-vibrant Jewish population largely left the Lower East Side, replaced by a growing Latino population from Puerto Rico and then the Dominican Republic. Much of the Jewish population and Jewish-owned-and-operated businesses left the Lower East Side, but Russ & Daughters remained one of the few that stayed committed to the neighborhood.

Under Mark Federman's tutelage, the store that once solely employed Jewish immigrants catering to the exclusively Jewish clientele hired Herman Vargas and Jose Reyes, local Lower East Side residents. Herman Vargas began as a prep cook, then candy counter man, and eventually assumed a management role. Jose Reyes also began in the kitchen, yet rapidly became a famed lox slicer and permanent fixture. In hiring staff from the Hispanic community but retaining the Jewish-style food offerings, Russ & Daughters increased their customer base to reflect the evolving neighborhood demographics yet continued to nurture a loyal Jewish clientele. This change allowed Russ & Daughters to be both a local neighborhood store and an iconic New York City destination, earning a spot on the National Register of Historic Places.

Russ & Daughters now has a fourth generation working at the store, including former chemical engineer Joshua Russ Tupper and cousin Niki Russ Federman. In 2014, the legacy expanded to include the Russ & Daughters Cafe on Orchard Street—not far from the site of the original store. In 2014, celebrating their one hundredth year, Russ & Daughters' legacy was immortalized in a documentary, *The Sturgeon Queens*.

See also APPETIZING STORES.

Cohen, Julie, dir. *The Sturgeon Queens*. DVD. Los Angeles: Seventh Art Releasing, 2014.
Federman, Mark Russ. *Russ & Daughters: Reflections and Recipes from the House that Herring Built*. New York: Schocken, 2013.

Jennifer Schiff Berg

Russian

There are at least three stories to tell about Russian food in New York City. All are grounded in the different waves of immigration that have brought to New York many hundreds of thousands of people from areas that were under Russian political control in the nineteenth and twentieth centuries. The story starts in imperial Russia, which extended well beyond contemporary Russia's recognized boundaries, reaching into areas of Poland and the Baltic states of Estonia, Latvia, and Lithuania (these, collectively, were known as the Pale of Settlement), the Ukraine, and many of the eastern republics.

The first major wave of immigrants involved Jews leaving the Pale of Settlement in the period 1881–1914. Tsarist policy required that most Jews live in

the Pale, and the policy escalated to a forcible relocation program to the Pale after 1882. The Jews were re-
sented by local peasants, and pogroms swept through
the Pale, triggering an exodus that some estimate as
high as 1.5 million people to New York City.

Settling first in the crowded tenements of the
Lower East Side south of Grand Street and then spilling over into Brooklyn, especially Brownsville, and
Harlem, many of these Jews did not identify specifically with Russia but felt part of a pan–Eastern European, Ashkenazi culture. Many were unskilled or
semiskilled workers who found work selling street
food to their neighbors and coreligionists. Other than
modest linguistic shifts, the food of this first wave of
immigrants is similar to that of most other Jews on
the Lower East Side. The appetizing and dairy stores,
such as the Polish Russ & Daughters, and the delis,
such as Katz's, sold the herring, salmon, fresh cheeses,
and cured meats that were familiar to all Eastern European Jews, albeit that the foods were now much
more plentiful, especially the relatively cheap meat.

Remembering "company" meals prepared by his
immigrant mother during his childhood in Brownsville in the 1920s, Alfred Kazin described tables
groaning with gefilte fish, pickles of all sorts, "khalleh"
bread for the Sabbath, chopped liver, followed by
chicken soup with dumplings and noodles, then meatloaf, chicken, prunes, and sweet potatoes cooked in
an open pie, fruit compotes, brown nut cakes, all
finished by "a samovar of Russian tea." For daily meals,
rather than the enriched challah, pumpernickel and
rye breads (some flavored with caraway), bagels, and
bialys were popular. Bialys are thought to originate
from nineteenth-century Bialystok, a time when the
Polish city was under Russian control. Kossar's Bialystoker Kuchen Bakery, on Grand and Essex Streets,
founded in 1936, still bakes what are regarded as New
York's best bialys.

The next wave of emigration brought many aristocratic and bourgeois Russians to New York in the
wake of the 1917 Revolution. Often known as the
white émigrés, this group tended to be Russian Orthodox Christians and imported the more elegant
culinary traditions of the tsarist Russian elites to New
York. It is no coincidence that the Russian Tea Room
opened in 1927 under the direction of expatriate
members of the Imperial Ballet to offer a taste of
home for these well-to-do political exiles. See RUSSIAN
TEA ROOM. The extravagant traditions launched by
these émigrés continue, not only in the long-lived

Russian Tea Room but also in Manhattan restaurants
with evocative names such as the Firebird (now
closed), Onegin, and Mari Vanna. They all present
foods of the privileged: caviar, vodka, champagne,
and chicken Kiev, the last being a dish invented in
Moscow in the early twentieth century, according to
Russian food historian William Pokhlebkin.

Following World War II, another wave entered,
many of whom escaped the Soviet Union or were expatriate Russians in Eastern European countries that
had fallen under the political shadow of the Soviet
Union. These immigrants might be Jewish, Christian,
or secular and mainly settled in the Little Odessa section of Brighton Beach, although some established
a community in the East Village. In the East Village,
restaurants, butchers, and food stores with names
such as the Kiev and Little Odessa operated through
the late twentieth century until they were priced out
by the neighborhood's increasing gentrification.
A few remnants of the earlier Russian culinary culture remain. The ever-popular Ukrainian restaurant
Veselka, opened in 1954, maintains a twenty-four-
hour kitchen. It boasts making three thousand pier-
ogis (piroshki in Russian) every day, twenty-five hundred potato pancakes every week, and five thousand
gallons of borscht (the beautiful magenta soup based
on beets and other vegetables, sometimes enriched
with meat) every year. A newer spot, Oda House,
brings Georgian cuisine to the neighborhood, while
the menu of the Uncle Vanya Café, on West Fifty-
Fourth Street, reads like an encyclopedia of Russian
cuisine, serving traditional pickled mushrooms, herring, blini, vareniki (potato dumplings), pelmeni
(meat dumplings), stroganoff, golubtsy (stuffed cabbage), and kulibiaka (a complex dish of salmon
wrapped in pastry).

A lively Russian community remains in areas of
Brighton Beach, Manhattan Beach, and Sheepshead
Bay in Brooklyn as well as in Rego Park and Forest
Hills in Queens. In Brooklyn, in addition to more
elegant restaurants such as Mednyi Chainik, there
are nightclubs, such as the Tatiana, with flashy, Las
Vegas–style floor shows and mountains of smoked
fish and grilled meats, all washed down by bottles of
vodka placed on the tables. Although an important
cultural symbol for émigrés before the fall of the
Soviet Union, the garish extravagance continues to
attract audiences. Other suggestions for Russian
dining and distinctive dishes can be found in online
guides like Serious Eats. One need not venture to the

far ends of Brooklyn to shop for Russian ingredients, although magnificent Russian markets can be found in Brighton Beach and Sheepshead Bay. Mail order is available from Moscow on the Hudson, with products from "Kremlin caviar" and herbal remedies to Orthodox Easter decorations.

See also BAGELS; BIALYS; BRIGHTON BEACH; EASTER; JEWISH; and LITTLE ODESSA.

Binder, Frederick M., and David M. Reimers. *All Nations Under Heaven: An Ethnic and Racial History of New York City.* New York: Columbia University Press, 1995.

Diner, Hasia. *Hungering for America: Italian, Irish, and Jewish Foodways in the Age of Migration.* Cambridge, Mass.: Harvard University Press, 2001.

Falkowitz, Max. "A Tour of the East Village's Borscht Belt Restaurants and Lunch Counters." Serious Eats, February 26, 2014. http://newyork.seriouseats .com/2014/02/best-eastern-european-restaurants-diners-lunch-counters-east-village-polish-ukrainian .html.

Godinez, Walter. "The World in NYC: Russia." New York International, December 2, 2014. https://nyintl.net/ article/russians_in_new_york_nycs_russian_neigh-borhoods.

Hedges, Chris. "Where Soviet Emigres Finally Let Loose." *New York Times,* August 11, 1990.

Cathy K. Kaufman

Russian Tea Room

Six minutes and twenty-three seconds from Lincoln Center and slightly to the left of Carnegie Hall (as the old radio ads famously put it) stands the Russian Tea Room, a glittering temple of Russian cuisine that, like Mother Russia herself, has weathered numerous regimes yet remains a bastion of power, pomp, and *pelmeni.* Founded in 1926 by émigrés from the Russian Imperial Ballet and run in the early days by ballerina Albertina Rasch, the Russian Tea Room started life as a simple pastry shop at 147 West Fifty-Seventh Street before moving in 1927 to its present location at 150 West Fifty-Seventh Street. Original owner Jacob Zysman sold the establishment in 1932 to Sasha Maeff, who installed a real kitchen and, upon repeal of Prohibition, a long bar, turning the tea room into a full-fledged restaurant serving such specialties as *shashlik, coulibiac,* and borscht.

In 1946 Sidney Kaye bought the Russian Tea Room (with partners, whom he bought out in 1955), ushering in a golden—and green and crimson—era

for the restaurant. Brass samovars glinted above blood-red leather banquettes. Christmas tinsel and red ornaments hung year-round from the Art Deco chandeliers—a joke at first, but soon a defining feature. Eclectic artwork adorned the holly-green walls. Vodka flowed freely and patrons downed mounds of caviar, the restaurant serving more than 2,600 pounds of the delicacy in an average year.

But it was the people—musicians and moviemakers, agents and impresarios, dance legends and showbiz stars—that made the place crackle. Zero Mostel, pretending to be a waiter, would naughtily offer diners "peasant under glass." Rudolf Nureyev, soon after his defection from the Soviet Union, declared that the Russian Tea Room was what he liked most about America, "because there I know I will not be poisoned!" So at home here was George Balanchine that he was allowed into the kitchen to cook his own meals. Over the years, he'd dine here with his succession of ballerina wives, among them Maria Tallchief, whom he met at the Russian Tea Room in 1942 when she was still a teen. Madonna had a brief stint here as a hatcheck girl in the late 1970s before being fired for her risqué attire. And in 1982 Dustin Hoffman famously fooled his agent (Sydney Pollack) in a classic scene from *Tootsie* filmed in one of the Tea Room's power booths. Hoffman, in character even between takes, went so far as to use the ladies' room throughout the shoot.

Faith Stewart-Gordon, actress-wife of Sidney Kaye, presided over the Russian Tea Room for nearly three decades following her husband's death in 1967, fêting celebrities, launching a weekly cabaret, narrating the radio ads that soon became a Russian Tea Room trademark. In 1982 she famously held out when developer Harry Macklowe sought the air rights to the RTR property to complete the Metropolitan Tower; hence the narrow townhouse that houses the RTR is now sandwiched between two towering skyscrapers.

The merry yet elegant days of Stewart-Gordon's reign came to an end when she sold the place to Warner LeRoy in 1995. The showman behind Tavern on the Green shuttered the celebrity clubhouse on New Years Day 1996 and went on to pour $32 million into renovations. When the restaurant finally reopened in 1999, the first-floor dining room was still recognizable. But critics and clientele alike decried the "appalling" theme-park décor of the new banquet halls upstairs, a kitschy Czarist fantasy complete with a 15-foot aquarium in the shape of a juggling

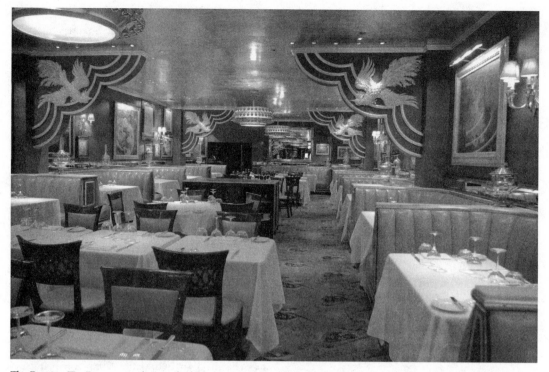

The Russian Tea Room, once known for live music and its celebrity clientele, is now a popular tourist attraction. The eclectic artwork adorning holly-green walls, and Christmas tinsel and red ornaments hung year-round from the Art Deco chandeliers, makes for a distinctive interior. © RUBENSTEIN, PHOTO BY MARTYNA BORKOWSKI

bear, filled with live sturgeon (since replaced with more attractive parrotfish).

The old regulars failed to return to this glitzier version of their beloved Tea Room, and LeRoy's declining health, crippling debt, and the effects of September 11 delivered fatal blows. On July 28, 2002, the year after LeRoy's death, the fabled but now bankrupt Russian Tea Room abruptly closed its doors. The next day, singer Judy Collins, a Russian Tea Room regular since her Carnegie Hall debut in 1962, lamented in a *New York Times* op-ed the loss of this "ante-room to all the glamour and gifts, sizzle and pulse, art, intelligence and determination of [New York City]."

An era truly seemed to be ending when the place was scooped up by the U.S. Golf Association, which dreamed of turning it into a golf museum. Fortune intervened and in late 2006, under the ownership of real estate mogul Gerald Lieblich and his RTR Funding Group, the Russian Tea Room reopened. Nowadays, the samovars and butter-filled chicken Kiev remain, though tourists outnumber locals, and celebrity sightings are few and far between.

Regimes change, regulars defect, reviewers alternately praise and pan. But through it all, the Russian Tea Room remains a New York City icon, just steps to the left of Carnegie Hall, and firmly ensconced in the heart of the Big Apple.

See also RUSSIAN and TEAROOMS.

Collins, Judy. "Goodbye to Buttery Blini." *New York Times,* July 30, 2002.
"Sidney Kaye, Host to Celebrities at Russian Tea Room, is Dead." *New York Times,* August 8, 1967.
Stewart-Gordon, Faith. *The Russian Tea Room: A Love Story.* New York: Simon & Schuster, 1999.

Meryl Rosofsky

Sailhac, Alain

French-born chef Alain Sailhac headed some of the most elite restaurant kitchens in New York City before joining the French Culinary Institute (now the International Culinary Center). His career encapsulates the changing trajectories of training for professional cooking in late-twentieth-century New York.

Sailhac's career followed the vocational path of French cooks and chefs in the mid-twentieth century: he was born in Millau, France, and at age fourteen apprenticed in his hometown at the restaurant Capion. His culinary education was completed in kitchens in Paris, Greece, and Guadeloupe, before he came to New York City in 1965 to work as chef de cuisine at Le Mistral and Le Manoir. He returned to Paris to cook in several prestigious hotels before accepting a position as executive chef at L'Hôtel Royale in New Caledonia and thereafter at Chicago's Le Perroquet. In 1974, he made New York his permanent home, running the kitchen of Le Cygne. In her December 20, 1977, *New York Times* review, Mimi Sheraton awarded the restaurant four stars, calling it "a triumph of haute cuisine."

Sailhac left Le Cygne in July 1978 to become executive chef at Le Cirque, a post he held until 1986; in 1984, the restaurant would garner three stars from the *New York Times*. Thereafter, Sailhac ran the kitchen at the historic 21 Club, served as culinary director to the Plaza Hotel, and consulted for the Regency Hotel. In 1991, he joined the International Culinary Center as dean of culinary studies, where he played a key role in developing the school's student-run restaurant, L'École. He became executive vice president of the International Culinary Center and then dean emeritus. He was named the 1997 Chef of the Year by Les Maîtres Cuisiniers de France and was awarded the Chevalier du Mérite Agricole. He married Arlene Feltman-Sailhac, the director of Macy's De Gustibus, in 1992.

See also FRENCH CULINARY INSTITUTE and LE CIRQUE.

"Alain Sailhac." *Chef's Story*. Heritage Radio Network. http://www.heritageradionetwork.org/archives?search=Alain+Sailhac.
"Chef Alain Sailhac of the International Culinary Center—Biography." StarChefs.com, August 2010. http://www.starchefs.com/cook/chefs/bio/alain-sailhac.

Cathy K. Kaufman

Salisbury Steak

See HAMBURG STEAK.

Saloons

The popularity of the "saloon" grew with the expansion of the United States from the East Coast into the western frontier. The towns that developed along the railroad routes and cattle drive trails offered few amenities to those living in them, or passing through. One of the amenities sure to be found in even the most basic settlement was a place to drink beer and spirits.

These establishments were often nothing more than a wood plank placed on top of two empty beer barrels under a tent or in a crude structure. Beer and spirits were served to an all-male clientele. Female companionship was provided for a price. These basic drinking establishments were known as "saloons," a word derived in the early eighteenth century from French *salon*, and from Italian *salone*, meaning "large hall." By the late 1850s, the term "saloon" had begun to appear in directories and common usage as a term for an establishment that specialized in beer and liquor sales by the drink, with food and lodging offered in a few. In American cities, including New York, saloons allowed only male patrons and were usually owned by one of the major breweries.

In *The Encyclopedia of Chicago*, Perry R. Duis notes that "Brewers purchased hundreds of storefronts, especially on the highly desired corner locations, which they rented to prospective saloonkeepers, along with all furnishings and such recreational equipment as billiard tables and bowling alleys." Not only were saloonkeepers businessmen with ties to breweries, they were usually well-connected politically. Politics was a natural sideline for saloonkeepers because of the social nature of the business. In neighborhoods where literacy was low, they offered a place for the exchange of information about employment and housing. A savvy saloon keeper could turn his access to resources into votes by providing a safe for valuables, a newspaper for the literate, and a bowl on the bar for charity collections.

On busy streets and downtown, the saloon provided a rest stop. And in all areas of the city, the purchase of a drink meant a free "lunch," usually only cold foods, but competition could make some food spreads more elaborate than others.

In the early twentieth century, the New York social activist Jacob Riis chronicled the effects of saloons on New York City: "I tried once to find out how the account stood, and counted to 111 Protestant churches, chapels, and places of worship of every kind below Fourteenth Street, 4,065 saloons." He also notes that the number of saloons for each tenement building in Lower Manhattan was impressive. "Below Fourteenth Street were, when the Health Department took its first accurate census of the tenements a year and a half ago (1899), 13,220 of the 39,390 buildings classed as such in the whole city."

Of particular interest to Riis was the traditional "rushing the growler," sending boys to the local saloon for a bucket of beer for home consumption. He notes that every saloon had a sign hung prominently declaring that "No Child Shall Be Served," however, "I doubt if one child in a thousand, who brings his growler to be filled at the average New York bar, is sent away empty-handed, if able to pay for what he wants."

His belief in the value of temperance, if not outright Prohibition, can be read into the following observation: "Fostered and filled by the saloon, the 'growler' looms up in the New York street boy's life, baffling the most persistent efforts to reclaim him. There is no escape from it; no hope for the boy, once its blighting grip is upon him. Thenceforward the logic of the slums, that the world which gave him poverty and ignorance for his portion 'owes him a living,' is his creed, and the career of the 'tough' lies open before him, a beaten track to be blindly followed to a bad end in the wake of the growler." His anti-saloon sentiment would find satisfaction with the arrival of national Prohibition.

Chroniclers of the Volstead Era noted that "The traditional saloon was declining many years before Prohibition. The automobile took patronage from what was clearly a pedestrian-streetcar institution. Nickelodeons competed for nickels. Increasing numbers of employers demanded abstinence during the workday. Finally, World War I brought not only an attack on anything that seemed remotely German but also a temporary ban on brewing." Newspapers reported that "Prohibition killed the legal saloon in 1920, but over three thousand city speakeasies and dozens of suburban roadhouses, many of them once village taverns, serviced the demand for more secret illegal drinking. When Prohibition ended in 1933, the word 'saloon' became a less desirable moniker and drew the attention of reformers of all sorts and so it virtually disappeared from the public vocabulary. Owners instead chose the name 'cocktail lounge' or 'tavern.'"

See also PROHIBITION and TAVERNS.

Ade, George. *The Old-Time Saloon: Not Wet—Not Dry, Just History*. New York: Long & Smith, 1931; reprint, New York: Old Town Books, 1993.

Burns, Ken, and Lynn Novick, dirs. *Prohibition*. 3 DVD set. Culver City, Calif.: PBS Home Video, 2011.

Riis, Jacob. *How the Other Half Lives: Studies among the Tenements of New York*. New York: Scribner, 1890.

Peter LaFrance

Salvation Army

The nation's first soup kitchens appeared in the late nineteenth century, and among them was the Salvation Army, a Christian mission founded in London that expanded across the Atlantic to New York City in 1880. One of the first Salvation Army shelters in the country to provide food assistance was the "Rescue Home for Fallen and Homeless Girls," which opened in October 1886 in Brooklyn, and offered donations of food to needy women and girls. In 1891, the Salvation Army opened the first dedicated food and shelter refuge in the United States—a low-cost lodging house for men in Greenwich Village. They opened a similar shelter for women in the Bowery shortly after. Within ten years, they had forty-four missions across the country, aiding cities' poorest communities. Unlike other low-cost lodging houses, the Salvation Army was driven by a Christian mission to save souls and provide food and shelter at little or no cost. Their missions were called "corps," and served as community and religious centers. During this time, many corps in New York City offered one-cent meals to the needy. One of their Christmas dinner menus from 1911 includes "soup, celery, cold slaw, turkey with dressing and cranberry sauce, mashed potatoes, fruits, candy, nuts, mince pie and coffee."

Through the Great Depression, the Army operated shelters and kitchens where clients were offered bread, soup, meat loaf, and pies, and could sit at wooden tables. Mindful of the importance of self-respect, Army staff often had clients work in exchange for their meal. It is estimated that the Salvation Army provided social services, including food, to up to a full 20 percent of the homeless population affected by the financial disaster.

It was during World War I that the Salvation Army first began famously distributing doughnut to soldiers. Two female Salvation Army aid workers, ensign Margaret Sheldon and adjutant Helen Purviance, who wanted to serve something sweet to soldiers in the trenches, started serving doughnuts with coffee. Often called "doughnut lassies," the women served thousands of doughnuts a day, frying just seven doughnut at a time, sometimes in soldiers' helmets, using an empty wine bottle for a rolling pin. These Salvation Army volunteers are credited with introducing Americans to the doughnut, a pastry of European origin previously unknown to the States. The Army continued making doughnuts in the United States after the war, celebrating "National Doughnut Day" (the first Friday in June) as a fundraiser for the Army and a way to raise awareness about their work.

Currently, the Salvation Army operates soup kitchens in twenty of its New York City corps, and thirty-six locations distribute grocery vouchers and food packages to the city's needy. Almost one in five New York residents rely on food assistance from organizations like the Salvation Army. Every year, the Salvation Army Greater New York Division alone provides food for almost six hundred thousand people in New York City's five boroughs.

See also HUNGER PROGRAMS and DOUGHNUTS.

Booth-Tucker, Frederick St. George De Lautour. *The Salvation Army in the United States: Annual Report, A.D. 1899.* New York: Salvation Army Printing and Engraving Department, 1899.

Booth-Tucker, Frederick St. George De Lautour. *Light in Darkness: Being an Account of the Salvation Army in the United States.* New York: Salvation Army Printing and Engraving Department, 1902.

Krondl, Michael. *The Donut: History, Recipes, and Lore from Boston to Berlin.* Chicago: Chicago Review Press, 2014.

Salvation Army of Greater New York website: http://ny.salvationarmy.org/GreaterNewYork.

Sandall, Robert, Archibald Raymond Wiggins, and Frederick Coutts. *The History of the Salvation Army.* 6 vols. London: Thomas Nelson, 1947–1955. Reprint 1979.

Allie Wist

Samuelsson, Marcus

Marcus Samuelsson was born in 1970 in Ethiopia and raised in Sweden. When Samuelsson was three years old, he, his sister, and mother were diagnosed with tuberculosis; his mother passed away from the disease. Marcus and his sister were adopted in 1973 by a Swedish couple and raised in Gothenburg, Sweden. Summers spent in Smögen, Sweden, were Samuelsson's earliest culinary encounters, beginning at age six. His grandmother taught him the art of baking, meatball making, and pickling. His adoptive father and uncles took him on fishing excursions and taught him how to cure and preserve the catches.

At age fifteen, Samuelsson enrolled at culinary vocational school Ester Mosesson in Gothenburg; he graduated second in his class. In 1989, he worked in the kitchen of Gothenburg's Belle Avenue restaurant. He then apprenticed for six months at Victoria-Jungfrau in Switzerland's tony Interlaken region, followed by an apprenticeship for Georges Blanc in France. He was offered at full-time gig, but he witnessed a cook degrade and physically assault an underling the day of the job offer, and he turned it down. "It was this very old-school European environment where the chef was screaming in your ear. Every week, people got fired because they were one minute late or they had dirt on their shoes.... I threw up every day before work. That's just what I did to cope," Samuelsson recounted to *Bloomberg Businessweek* in 2014.

In 1991, Samuelsson came to the United States to apprentice for eight months at Scandinavian restaurant Aquavit. He left for a yearlong stint cooking on a cruise ship, and returned to Aquavit in 1994 to work under executive chef Jan Sendel. Eight weeks after Samuelsson returned, Sendel passed away unexpectedly from a heart attack. Samuelsson was appointed as his successor in May, 1995. Samuelsson nabbed the James Beard Foundation's Rising Chef Award in 1999. The chef wrote *Aquavit and the New Scandinavian Cuisine*, a coffee table–worthy cookbook, in 2003.

Samuelsson opened Riingo, an Asian fusion eatery, in 2004 in Midtown East along with Nobu alum Johan Svensson and Tomoe Sushi alum Shigenori Tanaka. Riingo got mixed reviews—a two-star writeup from the *New York Times*'s Amanda Hesser, and a scathing takedown by *New York*'s Adam Platt—and closed in 2012, long after Samuelsson had left its kitchen. In 2006, Samuelsson's second tome, *The Soul of a New Cuisine: A Discovery of the Foods and Flavors of Africa* was released.

His next restaurant, Merkato 55, followed in early 2008, serving up pan-African cuisine in a high-gloss Meatpacking District setting. Frank Bruni gave the restaurant a tepid one-star review, while sites like Eater repeatedly ragged on Merkato 55 for the year and a half it was open. "I shouldn't have done [African cuisine] in a club environment, I shouldn't have taken on a rent that forced us to sell more liquor. I shouldn't have taken on those [business] partners," Samuelsson told the *Daily Beast* in 2012.

Samuelsson's biggest solo hit happened in 2010 with the debut of Red Rooster, located in Harlem at 125th Street and Lenox Avenue and dishing up American comfort grub with Swedish and African inflections. "The restaurant may not be the best to open in New York City this year (though the food is good). But it will surely be counted as among the most important," the *New York Times*'s Sam Sifton wrote of Red Rooster that year. "It is that rarest of cultural enterprises, one that supports not just the idea or promise of diversity, but diversity itself.... The dining room has some of the energy and excitement you can find in the best of Keith McNally's restaurants. Everyone seems to be there, making the scene." Samuelsson's executive chef at Red Rooster, Andrea Bergquist, had held the same role at Merkato 55.

The chef cooked President Barack Obama's inaugural state dinner with the prime minister of India in 2009 at the White House, crafting a primarily vegetarian dinner inspired by First Lady Michelle Obama's vegetable garden. That year his next book, *New American Table*, hit shelves. In 2010, he launched an online magazine, *Food Republic*, chronicling global food culture. He also gained further exposure as the winner of season two of *Top Chef Masters*, a cooking competition show on Bravo that pitted successful chefs against each other in weekly culinary challenges, that same year.

His next restaurant, the speakeasy-esque Ginny's Supper Club, opened in the basement of Red Rooster in 2012. That same year, his memoir, *Yes, Chef* hit bookshelves. "*Yes, Chef* is written with sparkle and grace," lauded the *New York Times* in a review of the chef's "beautiful memoir." Also in 2012, Samuelsson turned out a third restaurant, American Table Café and Bar, housed in Lincoln Center's Alice Tully Hall; an outpost opened in Stockholm, named American Table Brasserie and Bar, shortly after.

Samuelsson continued his Swedish expansion with the March 2013 opening of Kitchen and Table in Uppsala, Sweden, following the 2012 opening of Norda in Gothenburg. He also opened Uptown Brasserie in JFK Airport's Terminal 4 in May 2013. Samuelsson has also lent his name to Marc Burger, located in Macy's outposts in Chicago and Costa Mesa, California. In 2014, Samuelsson released *Marcus Off Duty: The Recipes I Cook At Home*. He was also a mentor on the second season of *The*

Taste, a cooking competition series on ABC, in 2014.

See also AFRICAN AMERICAN and HARLEM.

Bernstein, Jacob. "Marcus Samuelsson Talks New Memoir: 'Yes, Chef.'" *Daily Beast*, July 2, 2012. http://www.thedailybeast.com/articles/2012/07/02/marcus-samuelsson-talks-new-memoir-yes-chef.html.
Samuelsson, Marcus. *Yes Chef: A Memoir*. New York: Random House, 2013.
Sifton, Sam. "Red Rooster Harlem." *New York Times*, March 8, 2011.
Suddath, Claire. "Cruise Ships, Meatballs, and President Obama: An Interview with Marcus Samuelsson. *Bloomberg Businessweek*, February 13, 2014.

Alexandra Ilyashov

San Gennaro, Feast of

The Feast of San Gennaro is an annual street fair held along Mulberry Street in Little Italy over a two-week period each September. Started by Italian immigrants in 1926, today's festival is a vastly expanded form of what was originally a one-day Neapolitan holiday honoring San Gennaro, the patron saint of Naples. The festival hearkens back to Little Italy's days as a major Italian enclave, and although the demographics of the neighborhood have shifted considerably since its founding, the festival still stands as a celebration of Italian heritage, and Italian food.

Features of the festival include rides, games, and street vendors selling prepared foods, jewelry, t-shirts, and small crafts. The focal point of the Feast, however, is the food. Many of the stands and vendors are centered on Mulberry Street, but festivities extend for a few blocks on either side. Festivalgoers wend their way past dozens of Italian restaurants, many of which offer outdoor seating during the feast. Most people, however, patronize the numerous food stands. As the Feast has grown in popularity and exposure over the years, standard street fair offerings have multiplied, and now range from daiquiris to mozzarepas (two grilled cornmeal patties served with melted cheese in the middle) to roasted corn. But Italian food dominates. Many stands sell baked pastas, eggplant or chicken parmesan, as well as hot or sweet Italian sausage topped with peppers and onions.

There are also less commonly known Italian foods available, like pork braciole and arancini. In parts of Italy, braciole are called *involtini*, or "little bundles." They consist of grilled or pan-fried thin cuts of meat, most commonly pork, and then rolled around a filling typically made of cheese and breadcrumbs. Arancini, or "little oranges," are fried balls of risotto that have a filling in the center typically consisting of ground meat or peas and tomato sauce. There are also many varieties of seafood available at San Gennaro, including shrimp cocktail, baked clams, fried oysters, and especially fried calamari—batter-coated deep-fried squid.

Many sweets are also sold at the festival—dozens of flavors of gelato, cannoli, and old-fashioned Italian confections like *torrone*, a large, hard brick of white nougat filled with nuts. Among the most popular desserts there are *zeppole*, deep-fried balls of dough. More recent twists on the *zeppole* include deep-fried oreos and deep-fried candy bars, which have become ubiquitous at the feast.

When it started in 1926, the Feast of San Gennaro anchored a neighborhood dense with Italian immigrants and their descendants. Little Italy had so many Italians in such a small geographic area that different streets became sub-enclaves, with the Sicilians living mostly on Elizabeth Street, Neapolitans on Mulberry, and Calabresi on Mott. That the Feast of San Gennaro, which is specifically a Neapolitan holiday, focuses on Mulberry Street, is a reflection of this breakdown.

By the 1930s, Italian immigration had declined and the Italian presence on the Lower East Side had started to erode. Italians moved to the outer boroughs and later, many moved to Long Island or New Jersey. Today, Little Italy is about 8 percent Italian, which is about the same percentage as the city as a whole. Compared to neighboring Chinatown, which according to the 2000 census was about 63 percent Chinese, Little Italy can no longer be considered an immigrant enclave.

Yet the Feast of San Gennaro remains an important gathering place for Italian Americans. Despite complaints about noise and inadequate sanitation, and despite several shifts in management over the years, the Feast of San Gennaro has been held every year since 1926. The Feast has become more expansive, and no longer focuses on Neapolitan culture or Neapolitan food, and now offers dishes from other parts of Italy, as well as a large array of street food with an Italian American stamp, like meatballs and pizza.

While photo booths and t-shirt stands have proliferated, the Feast is also still firmly anchored in religious tradition. The Church of the Most Precious Blood, the local Catholic church that houses the statue of San Gennarro, is a focal point of the Feast. On September 19, San Gennaro's Feast Day, after a celebratory mass, the statue of San Gennaro is carried from the church through the festival. In recent years, the Feast has hosted about a million visitors a year and donated about $100,000 a year to New York City charities, Catholic schools, and youth organizations.

See also LITTLE ITALY and STREET FAIRS.

"About San Gennaro." Figli di San Gennaro website: http://www.sangennaro.org/about.htm.
Asian American Federation of New York. "Neighborhood Profile: Manhattan's Chinatown." 2003. http://www.aafny.org/cic/briefs/Chinatownbrief.pdf.
Tonelli, Bill. "Arrivederci, Little Italy." *New York Magazine*, September 27, 2004.

Katie Uva

Sardi's

Sardi's has been a fixture in the heart of the theater district since its founding in 1921 as "The Little Restaurant" by Vincent Sardi and his wife, Eugenia. Six years later it was renamed "Sardi's" and moved down the block to its current location at 234 West Forty-Fourth Street. See TIMES SQUARE. Sardi's always catered to the area's theater professionals, offering a discounted menu to actors, working or not—a tradition that continues. Sardi's son, Vincent Jr., was even known to seat his favorite actors in proximity to the most influential producers, shrewdly encouraging some pre-Internet networking.

When the Volstead Act forced the closure of established restaurants whose business depended on strong wine and liquor sales, the lavish Delmonico's collapsed, but "dry" Sardi's survived. See PROHIBITION and DELMONICO'S. It was only after Prohibition that the first-floor's "Little Bar" was installed. All the while, Sardi's built its culinary reputation on a Continental menu, popularizing the term "Continental cuisine." To avoid being identified as an "Italian" restaurant with possible ties to organized crime, Sardi,

who was trained in England, modified traditional recipes to encompass other European cuisines. Here, for example, cannelloni is served not in pasta shells, but wrapped in French crêpes. While still offering some of Eugenia's original recipes (such as the "Shrimp Sardi"), the menu is eclectic, changing with the seasons, and even adapting to health-conscious culinary trends.

The Sardi reputation for casually elegant, old-world food service is carefully maintained by co-owners and co-managers Max Klimavicius, Vincent Jr.'s long-time protégé, and Sean Ricketts, Sardi's grandson. Despite increased competition for today's theater clientele, Sardi's—where the idea for Broadway's Tony awards first emerged—remains a favorite. Seated in a warmly appointed dining room on red leather banquettes, surrounded by caricatures of some 1,200 theater luminaries, its iconic appeal only improves with age.

Grimes, William. "Vincent Sardi Jr., Restaurateur and Unofficial 'Mayor of Broadway,' Dies at 91." *New York Times*, January 5, 2007.
Riedel, Michael. "Life of the Sardi's." *New York Post*, January 31, 2007.
Rothstein, Mervyn. "A Life in the Theatre: Max Klimavicius." Playbill.com, April 25, 2007. http://www.playbill.com/features/article/a-life-in-the-theatre-max-klimavicius-140343.
Squires, Kathleen. "Secrets of Sardi's." NewYork.com, July 25, 2013. http://www.newyork.com/articles/restaurants/secrets-of-sardis-26969.

Jane L. Smulyan

Sashimi

See SUSHI.

Saunders, Audrey

Bartender Audrey Saunders is best known to New Yorkers as the proprietor of Pegu Club, a SoHo bar that opened in 2005. Pegu, named for a storied, late-nineteenth century British officers' club in Burma, is also noted for helping repopularize gin and for bringing forth such cocktails as the Gin-Gin Mule and Earl Grey MarTEAni.

Saunders grew up in Long Island and moved to Manhattan in 1985, where she took classes in French technique at Peter Kump's cooking school (now the

Institute of Culinary Education). She started bartending at the Waterfront Ale House in 1996, but her career really took off after she took a seminar at New York University the following year with legendary mixologist Dale DeGroff, who became her mentor. In 1999, Saunders and DeGroff opened Blackbird on East Forty-Ninth Street, where they worked side by side. After Blackbird, Audrey became the bar manager at chef Waldy Malouf's Beacon Restaurant, and then went on to become the beverage director of the Tonic Restaurant.

Saunders joined the Carlyle Hotel in December, 2001, in the role of beverage director, for the much-acclaimed reopening of the legendary Bemelmans Bar. There, she developed a beverage program that earned the Carlyle a global reputation for cocktails. At the same time, Saunders also became well-known among the small but burgeoning New York mixology community.

When Pegu Club opened in 2005, the new cocktail renaissance still was in early days, and few bars focused on craft cocktails. In addition to bringing once-forgotten pre-Prohibition classics back to the bar, Pegu was particularly influential in setting new standards for bar service: fresh-squeezed juices, beautiful glassware, attention to ice quality and uber-attentive barkeeps became hallmarks. In addition, self-proclaimed "cocktail mom" Saunders has been noted for nurturing generations of future mixologists. Many of the best-known bartenders around the United States honed their skills at Pegu.

Although Saunders has since relocated to Seattle, through Pegu Club and the legions of bartenders that have moved through that bar, her legacy in New York cocktail culture remains firmly intact.

See also DEGROFF, DALE.

Schrambling, Regina. "Audrey Saunders of Pegu Club is a Mixed-Drink Matriarch." *Edible Manhattan*, January 2013.

Kara Newman

Saveur

Saveur magazine was founded in 1994 by Dorothy Kalins (with Chris Hirsheimer and Colman Andrews) under the slogan "savor a world of authentic cuisine." Adam Sachs, who took over as the magazine's editor-in-chief in late 2014, describes the origins of the magazine as a conscious "contrast to what was beginning to be celebrity-chef culture."

Saveur magazine places ingredients in sharp focus and puts food first with single ingredient special issues ("The Beauty of Butter"), thorough histories of foods ("A Complete History of the Donut"), and a strong emphasis on international cuisines and foodways. In one *Saveur* recipe, readers are encouraged to use as many as one hundred cloves of garlic for a single chicken. Until 2011, it had yet to run a single restaurant review.

Describing itself as a food and travel magazine—not just a food publication—*Saveur* has been particularly notable for focusing on food cultures around the world (including what it describes as "forgotten pockets of culinary excellence" in the United States), including culinary tools, techniques, food history, and heritage. It provided a window to international cuisines at a time when most other publications did not, and before the Internet provided easier access to restaurants and recipes from around the world. The magazine has been influential in encouraging writers and readers to view broader culture through a food-focused lens, and encouraging narrative journalism in food.

Based in midtown Manhattan, *Saveur* also has positioned itself as an integral part of New York's food community. Its annual summer barbecues, begun in 2009, have hosted thousands of foodies, and dozens of master chefs from across the city. And it remains a valiant champion of up-and-coming chefs and restaurateurs from across all five boroughs—acting as a window to the world for New York's vibrant food culture.

"Chicken with 40 Cloves of Garlic." *Saveur*, October 2, 2010.
Ermelino, Louisa. "Growing Up Italian in New York's South Village." *Saveur*, September 4, 2014.
"Saveur Launches Restaurant Reviews, James Oseland Explains." Eater.com, February 15, 2011. http://www.eater.com/2011/2/15/6697259/saveur-launches-restaurant-reviews-james-oseland-explains.

Alexis Zanghi

Scandinavian

Scandinavian settlement in New York occurred largely in the nineteenth and twentieth centuries, and many established themselves in the shipyards in Bay Ridge, Brooklyn. Although few remain today, in the 1950s and 1960s this area of the borough was home to the largest congregation of Norwegians outside of Oslo. A store called Nordic Delicacies remains in Bay Ridge and continues to sell largely Norwegian products, one of the few remnants of a bygone era. What used to be known as Little Norway has colloquially been renamed Little Hong Kong. See BAY RIDGE.

Scandinavian people have generally had a simple relationship to their food. It has only recently been elevated from a source of sustenance to a source of enjoyment. Because of this, there have been few Scandinavian restaurants in New York, but that has changed drastically in the last decade.

Founded in Sweden in 1943, IKEA, the largest furniture retailer in the world, contains a Swedish food market as well as a restaurant in each of their stores, and has been one place for Swedish expats to go for a taste of home. Restaurant Castelholm, in the Parc Vendome Apartments on West Fifty-Seventh Street, opened in 1936 and served traditional Swedish smorgasbord. Restaurant Aquavit opened in 1987, with the new concept of a fine dining room as well as a more casual separate café. The fine dining room serves an international cuisine based on Scandinavian flavors, while the café serves traditional Swedish food. The restaurant garnered culinary recognition in the mid-1990s with Marcus Samuelsson at the helm. See SAMUELSSON, MARCUS.

With the inception of New Nordic Cuisine in 2004, several Scandinavian restaurants opened in New York City within a very few years. These restaurants were rooted in the concept of New Nordic Cuisine, and opened to widespread acclaim. New Nordic Cuisine is based on traditional cooking techniques such as pickling, smoking, salting, and purity of products. The idea stems from a manifesto initiated by Rene Redzepi and Claus Meyer, cofounders of the lauded Restaurant Noma in Copenhagen, Denmark.

New Nordic Cuisine has had an immense following among chefs all over the world, many of them in New York. What started out as hype has become a trend with staying power. There is a sort of bipolarity that exists in the Scandinavian influence on the New York food scene between the traditional and the new Nordic Cuisine.

Smith, Andrew F. *The Oxford Companion to Food and Drink*. New York: Oxford University Press, 2007.

Gordinier, Jeff. "A Nordic Quest in New York." *New York Times*, February 18, 2014.

Eirik Osland

Schaller & Weber

Schaller & Weber is a German deli and butcher shop located on Eighty-Sixth Street and Second Avenue, in the heart of the Yorkville section of Manhattan. Yorkville is one of several neighborhoods that was home to a large German population in the late nineteenth and early twentieth centuries, and when it opened in 1937, Schaller & Weber was just one of numerous businesses in the area offering German food. Germans first came to New York City in large numbers in the 1830s and 1840s, mostly settling in an area of the Lower East Side that was soon known as Kleindeutschland, or "Little Germany." Subsequent generations moved out of that neighborhood to a handful of enclaves around the city, including

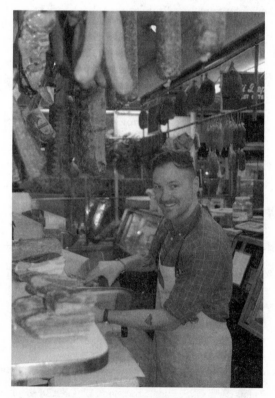

A butcher at Schaller & Weber, the Upper East Side German deli and butcher shop, slicing twice-smoked bacon. SCHALLER & WEBER

Yorkville. The German population peaked in New York City around the turn of the twentieth century, with more than a half-million German New Yorkers.

After the middle of the last century, however, German immigration to New York declined steadily. German New Yorkers became a smaller percentage of the population, and their descendants assimilated and dispersed throughout the city. By 2006, descendants of German immigrants composed about 3.5 percent of the city's population, with very few notably German enclaves surviving. Yorkville's businesses reflected this shift; where there had once been dozens of German bakeries, restaurants, and delis in Yorkville, now only a handful remain, one of which is Schaller & Weber.

Schaller & Weber sells typical deli fare such as chicken and mustard, but it specializes in specifically German items like spatzle, a wide range of cured and uncured meats, as well as brands imported from Germany. Meats are a particular specialty, and New Yorkers can find such offerings as Bockwurst, a pale Bavarian sausage; Pinkelwurst, a northern German sausage made with pork, beef, oats, and onions; and twice-smoked bacon.

Despite changing demographics in the neighborhood, and long-term disruption due to the construction of the Second Avenue subway, Schaller & Weber continues to thrive, a cherished neighborhood specialty store and a reminder of Yorkville's German history.

See DELIS, GERMAN and KLEINDEUTSCHLAND.

Duchnowski, Jillian, and Howard Manthei. *Yorkville.* Charleston, S.C.: Arcadia, 2014.
Nadal, Stanley. "Germans in New York." In *The Encyclopedia of New York City*, edited by Kenneth Jackson. New Haven, Conn.: Yale University Press; New York: New-York Historical Society, 1995.
Schaller & Weber website: http://www .schallerweber.com.

Katie Uva

School Food

The serving of a midday meal in New York City public schools originated with mid-nineteenth-century charities. Founded by Charles Loring Brace and a group of social reformers in 1853, the Children's Aid Society provided free meals to schoolchildren

as part of its broader efforts to reduce underage vagrancy and crime in Manhattan. This model would be echoed by many other organizations into the first half of the twentieth century. Mabel Kittredge's New York School Lunch Committee was the first to focus exclusively on school food as a primary method of reform. In 1908 it started serving lunches at PS 51, an elementary school on West Forty-Fourth Street. In these early years, lunch contents often included calorie-dense, enriched foods that could provide sustained energy. According to their records, meals included a hot soup, bread, and a modest dessert such as sweet crackers or cake.

Charitable organizations, and later the Board of Education's school lunch managers, often found themselves competing with street vendors for customers. Everything from waffles to pickles and candy apples could be had for a few pennies just outside the school grounds. Gathering around the carts and sitting together in the new lunchrooms both offered children the chance to socialize with friends, but most of them preferred to eat outside. For Progressives inspired by Upton Sinclair's *The Jungle*, waging war against these unhygienic, unregulated food providers necessitated government involvement. See SINCLAIR, UPTON. In January 1919, the Board of Education allocated $50,000 (around $700,000 in

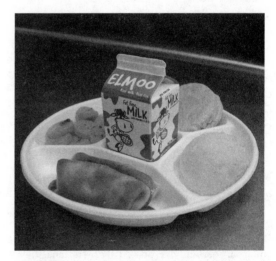

A lunch served to New York City students: sliced turkey with country gravy, orange-roasted carrots, mashed potatoes, a biscuit, and a carton of milk. Although this is a holiday lunch, it is still representative of the quality and portion size of meals served in New York public schools. NEW YORK SCHOOL OFFICE OF SCHOOL FOOD

2015 money) to study the feasibility of implementing a citywide, nonprofit school lunch program. One year later the board allocated an additional $50,000 and began lunch service at selected schools. The program targeted poor immigrant neighborhoods with large numbers of children suffering from malnutrition, with the higher aim of not only preventing starvation but also of teaching modern American food knowledge to children and their parents. Menu items from a 1923 Board of Education menu book included stewed tomatoes with breadcrumbs, cream of bean soup, Italian spaghetti with onion and tomato sauce, succotash, baked salmon, American cheese sandwich, and cocoa. Each suggested daily menu had approximately twelve hundred calories and included the option of serving an additional cup of milk and a bar of unsweetened chocolate or a wrapped candy, a clear attempt to both provide calcium and meet the sweet-tooth needs of the student population in a clean, sanitary manner.

During the Great Depression and its aftermath, school lunch programs across the country expanded with Works Progress Administration funding. See DEPRESSION FOOD. Following federal health and safety food-service guidelines, meals consisted of a hot dish or soup, bread and butter sandwich, and fruit for dessert. The New York City Child Nutrition Project served lunches prepared in two central kitchens to over one hundred thousand students in over seven hundred schools on a daily basis.

After World War II, a national campaign to provide a permanent form of public food assistance for schoolchildren took hold, bringing together those concerned with promoting proper nutrition with farmers and government representatives looking for ways to utilize surplus commodity crops. Led by senators Allen Ellender (Louisiana) and Richard Russell (Georgia), the National School Lunch Program became law in 1946. Although a federal program, states and local constituencies were responsible for the organization and management of their own lunch programs. The purpose of this program, "to protect the health and well-being of the nation's children," certainly resonated with the charities and municipal organizations that had been working toward this goal in New York City for almost a century. As with the Works Progress Administration monies, the Board of Education used the new federal funds to expand the lunch program and offer free or reduced-price lunch to all students who qual-

ified. A key component of this expansion during the postwar period was the Central Kitchen facilities in Long Island City.

The rapidly growing population in general meant that schools in particular needed new facilities for both traditional teaching as well as feeding students. Expanding suburban school districts in Long Island, Westchester, or New Jersey could build new facilities, but in New York City space remained at a premium. Schools that did not have kitchens or cafeterias for on-site food preparation relied on truck deliveries from the Central Kitchen to feed their students. By September 1963, the Central Kitchen distributed nearly 290,000 lunches daily to over six hundred elementary, junior high, and high schools—triple the amount of meals from twenty years earlier. With facilities to prepare full meals from scratch, sandwiches remained reliable standbys for their convenience of assembly and variety of fillings that met the federal dietary requirements. Popular varieties included peanut butter, egg salad, cheese, cold baked beans, and hot dogs. By 1967 reports estimated that students ate over 75 million school lunches over the course of the academic year, and by 1976 the New York City Board of Education ranked as the sixty-third-largest food service organization by volume, coming in ahead of White Castle and Trans World Airlines.

With few exceptions, New York City has led national protocol in school food trends from the postwar period through the present. In the early 1970s, meal packs—frozen meals from corporate vendors that were reheated on site—made their way into city lunchrooms. They helped with an increasingly tight budget but proved unappetizing to students. Critiques of school food have persisted since the introduction of these frozen convenience foods that meet nutrition requirements but tend to lack in taste. Food critic Mimi Sheraton referred to a bulk-convenience piece of fried chicken as "steamy and musty" in her 1976 *New York Times* article "Lunches for Pupils Given Poor Marks." Convenience foods prevailed as the student population continued to grow while budgets shrunk. The school lunch menu for October and November 1976 at PS 22R on Staten Island featured pizza, sloppy joes, hamburgers, sliced bologna, applesauce, French fried potatoes, coleslaw, and sliced peaches among other options. These heavy, high-sodium foods defined the cafeteria experience for generations of New Yorkers.

Vending machines and other forms of "competitive foods" became a fixture on campuses in the 1970s, their contents echoing the ebb and flow of public opinion as the fried snacks of the 1980s came to share space with apple slices in the new millennium. Providing another needed source of revenue and increased food options for children, corporations including Coke, Pepsi, Hershey, and Mars all bid on exclusive vending rights in New York City schools. Although the U.S. Department of Agriculture regulated the nutritional content of the federally subsidized meals, food sold for profit outside of the cafeteria was not subject to these nutritional standards and dietary guidelines. In 2002, the city began an extensive campaign to better children's health by improving school lunches and competitive food options, including removing soda from vending machines, reducing sodium and increasing fiber content, eliminating deep fryers, and replacing canned vegetables with fresh and frozen options. Although ultimately successful, the program came under fire in 2012 when it was discovered that the healthier options brought the calorie content below the U.S. Department of Agriculture's minimum requirements from prior to the Healthy Hunger-Free Kids Act of 2010. See SODA and VENDING MACHINES.

Lunch tray contents reflect how our understanding of health and nutrition has changed over the years. Whole grains and vegetables mandated on 2014 lunch trays have replaced the bread and butter sandwiches of 1910. Grow To Lean NYC: The Citywide School Garden Initiative, a subsidiary of GrowNYC, supports on-site gardens at over three hundred schools, and the School Lunch office of the Board of Education offers free food programs throughout the year, including a free, mobile summer meals program. School food in the new millennium is more diverse than at the turn of the last century but serves the same purpose: to nourish all of Gotham's children.

Claiborne, Craig. "Report Card on Meals: Test Finds Food Nutritious, Bland and More…" New York Times, September 27, 1963.
Levine, Susan. School Lunch Politics: The Surprising History of America's Favorite Welfare Program. Princeton, N.J.: Princeton University Press, 2008.
Nestle, Marion. "Soft Drink 'Pouring Rights': Marketing Empty Calories." Public Health Reports 115, no. 4 (July/August 2000): 308–319.
New York City Board of Education, Works Progress Administration. Workbook for School Lunch Workers.

Vol. 1: Working Instructions for Workers of the New York City Works Progress Administration Child Nutrition Project. New York: New York City Board of Education, Works Progress Administration, 1942.
New York Public Library. "Lunch Hour NYC." http://exhibitions.nypl.org/lunchhour/exhibits/show/lunchhour.
Poppendieck, Janet. Free for All: Fixing School Food in America. Berkeley: University of California Press, 2010.

Shayne Leslie Figueroa

Schrafft's

Schrafft's, the restaurant chain that became a New York dining institution, originated in 1861 as a Boston candy company. Its founder, William F. Schrafft, initially made gumdrops and candy canes. By 1897, when salesperson Frank G. Shattuck joined the company, it was producing such excellent chocolates that Shattuck was convinced Schrafft's could compete in New York. A year later, he opened a Schrafft's candy shop at Thirty-Eighth and Broadway. His sister Jane joined him as manager and suggested they sell ice cream and lunch items as well as chocolates. When that proved successful, Shattuck opened other shops. By 1923, he had purchased the business and owned seventeen shops in New York and five elsewhere. At its peak, the chain stretched from New England to Florida and included restaurants, motor inns, catering businesses, frozen foods, and a food service business in addition to its chocolates.

Shattuck believed Americans wanted "one hundred per cent quality without any fancy foreign names," according to a May 19, 1928, New Yorker profile, and that is exactly what Schrafft's served. It specialized in such homey dishes as egg salad sandwiches with the crusts cut off, cheese bread, and chicken à la king, along with indulgences like butterscotch sundaes. Most shops included a candy counter and a soda fountain as well as table service. Some boasted a bar.

A perfectionist, Shattuck insisted on the finest foods from suppliers and consistent quality from cooks. He required that Schrafft's waitresses, who wore black dresses with pristine white collars, cuffs, and aprons, undergo a neatness inspection every morning. In a departure from then-current practice, Shattuck provided paid vacations and profit sharing. He also employed women as managers, possibly

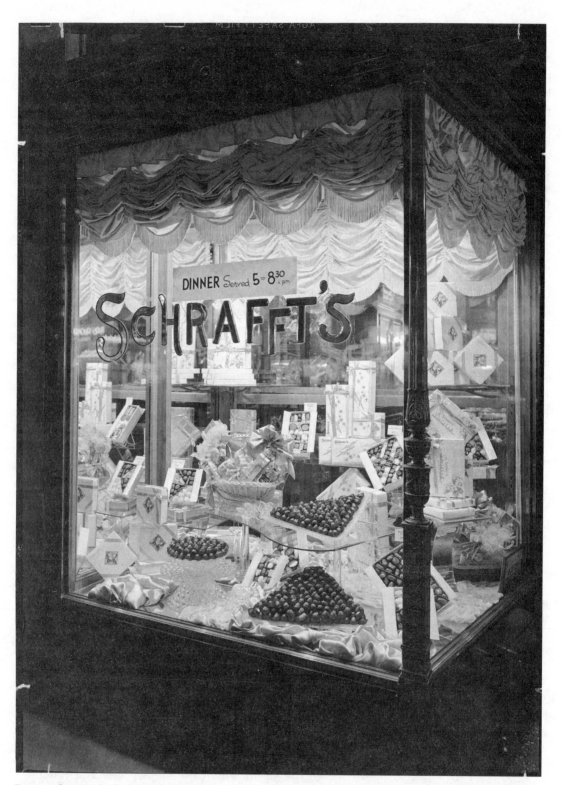

Evening photograph of a Schrafft's window display, April 13, 1929. Schrafft's began as a Boston candy company before becoming an iconic restaurant chain. Most of the high-volume, low-price restaurants also included a candy counter and a soda fountain. MUSEUM OF THE CITY OF NEW YORK

because of the example set by his sister. His employees rewarded him with loyalty; a tenure of twenty or thirty years with the firm was typical.

Schrafft's attracted many female customers, whether because of its reassuring food and respectability or (as some said) because women could sip a martini at Schrafft's while their children sipped sodas. In numerous cartoons, *New Yorker* artist Helen Hokinson fondly caricatured the pleasingly plump ladies who lunched at Schrafft's in their frilly hats. Filmmakers set scenes in Schrafft's, and writers including Mary McCarthy, James Thurber, and Neil Simon sent their characters to Schrafft's.

The Shattuck family owned the company for more than fifty years, but in 1967 they sold it to Helme Products, Inc., a tobacco, candy, and snack foods company. In an attempt to counter declining sales and adapt to changing times and tastes, the company ran trendy ads including a psychedelic television spot created by Andy Warhol. It was no use. The company was sold and broken into various divisions. Not even its famed chocolates could save it. On March 10, 1981, the *New York Times* reported that Schrafft's owner Gulf & Western was shutting down operations.

Today, there is a Schrafft's ice cream shop in Las Vegas, and in Boston the landmark red Schrafft's sign still crowns the former candy factory, now an office complex. But in New York, where it was once part of the fabric of the city, Schrafft's is only a faded memory.

See also CANDY.

Marton, Renee. "Schrafft's." In *The Oxford Companion to American Food and Drink*, edited by Andrew F. Smith. New York: Oxford University Press, 2007.
Slomanson, Joan Kanel. *When Everybody Ate at Schrafft's.* Fort Lee, N.J.: Barricade, 2006.

Jeri Quinzio

Schultz, Dutch

See BOOTLEGGERS.

Schwartz, Arthur

Arthur Schwartz is a walking encyclopedia of New York food, particularly of New York Jewish food.

His four-decade tenure in New York and the subject of one of his eight books, *Arthur Schwartz's New York City Food: An Opinionated History with Legendary Recipes* (2004), explain how this "walking encyclopedia" earned his title.

Arthur Schwartz started as a food editor at *Long Island Newsday* in 1969 and subsequently served as the restaurant critic and executive food editor of the *New York Daily News* from 1979 to 1996. While working at the *News*, he contributed to various radio shows before hosting his own, *Food Talk with Arthur Schwartz* on WOR Radio from 1992 to 2004.

Schwartz's cookbooks cover a range of topics, from New York's cuisine to the intricacies of Italian cooking. *Naples at Table: Cooking in Campania* (1998) established Schwartz as an expert in the field, so much so that the *New York Times* called him "an ambulatory Google on matters Italian." See ITALIAN. The International Association of Culinary Professionals named his 2004 treatise on New York food Cookbook of the Year and awarded *Arthur Schwartz's Jewish Home Cooking: Yiddish Recipes Revisited* Best American Subject Cookbook of 2008.

Although he writes and teaches extensively—the New York Association of Culinary Teachers named him Cooking Teacher of the Year in 1996—Schwartz is most visible as a media personality. His daily radio program earned him the Award of Excellence in Electronic Media from the International Association of Culinary Professionals in 1998, and he hosts *The Breakfast Club* on an NPR affiliate in Connecticut. Since bringing his brand to television in 1988 as the food critic on Fox network's local morning show, *Good Day New York*, he has appeared on the Food Network, on *The Martha Stewart Show*, and in documentaries on New York street food for Japanese public television (2004) and Al Jazeera (2008) and participated in programs about immigrant food in America, including one about the history of the bagel. In addition, Schwartz is a sought-after lecturer, consultant, and memoirist of New York's foodways.

Pfefferman, Naomi. "A Bissel Taste of Big Apple's Best." *Jewish Journal*, May 12, 2005.
Prial, Frank J. "'Food Talk' Host Departs Amid Some Talk of Static." *New York Times*, September 1, 2004.
Reynolds, Jonathan. "FOOD; the Real Thing." *New York Times*, May 23, 2004.

Rozanne Gold

Scribner's

Today an imprint of Simon and Schuster, Scribner's was founded in Manhattan in 1846 by Charles Scribner originally as an independent publisher of religious books. As the nineteenth century progressed the publishing house expanded and began to publish magazines in addition to books. The popular magazine *Scribner's Magazine* published the work of fresh new writers, many of whom became house authors for the company.

Under the leadership of Charles Scribner II the house continued to expand its list, which in the early twentieth century included the works of some of the greatest American writers of the period, including Edith Wharton, Henry James, Ernest Hemingway, Thomas Wolfe, and Ring Lardner. Notably, Charles Scribner's and Sons published F. Scott Fitzgerald's first novel, *This Side of Paradise*, under the guidance of famed editor Maxwell Perkins.

In 1997, through the acquisition of the defunct Bobbs-Merrill publishing company, Scribner published a new edition of the acclaimed American classic cookbook *The Joy of Cooking* by Irma Rombauer and Marion Rombauer Becker. The classic cookbook had not been revised since 1975 yet has remained the bestselling of all the book's editions. Scribner enlisted veteran cookbook editor Maria Guarneschelli, who, along with Rombauer's grandson, created a revised and ultimately controversial edition.

Rather than a mere updating of the same recipes from the earlier editions, this new edition included new specially commissioned recipes reflecting more contemporary food trends. Kitchens had evolved dramatically since the previous editions of the book, and the new edition included methods and recipes using food processors and microwave ovens, now common in home kitchens. Furthermore, the publisher added ingredients that were quickly becoming staples in modern American kitchens including a wider variety of vinegars, rice, peppers, and spices than had been available to home cooks. Recipes included many more selections from international cuisines such as Latin, Thai, Indian, and Vietnamese.

In 2006, this controversial edition was reedited for the seventy-fifth anniversary edition, which included forty-five hundred recipes, a simpler voice, and several sections that had been deleted in the previous edition. This seventy-fifth anniversary edition of the classic remains in print.

Since becoming an imprint of Simon and Schuster, Scribner has continued to publish the work of renowned cookbook writers and culinary authors. The Scribner list includes books by Harold McGee, Shirley O. Corriher, Bobby Flay, Patricia Wells, Michael Ruhlman, Rick Bayless, Jasper White, Daniel Boulud, and Lynne Rossetto Kasper.

"About Scribner." Simon & Schuster. http://imprints .simonandschuster.biz/scribner/about.
"All about Joy." Joy of Cooking. http://www .joyofcooking.com/all-about-joy/all-about-joy.
O'Neill, Molly. "It's a New 'Joy,' But Is It the Old Love?; The Cookbook Now Speaks in a Corporate Tone." *New York Times*, November 5, 1997.

Carl Raymond

Second Avenue Deli

See DELIS, JEWISH.

Seinfeld

See TELEVISION.

Seltzer

Originated in Niederselter, Germany, in the eighteenth century, seltzer began as naturally carbonated, mineral-filled water. Indeed, the word "seltzer" derives from "Selters," the name of a German town renowned for its mineral springs. When Eastern Europeans, many Jewish, immigrated to the United States in the nineteenth century, a sizeable population settled in New York, bringing along a thirst for seltzer.

The heyday of the seltzer delivery trade lasted from the 1920s to the 1960s, reaching around one thousand seltzer men at its peak. By the 1960s, around five hundred seltzer men delivered from six or so factories in New York. By the early 1980s, twenty-two seltzer men remained. The old-fashioned glass bottle, delivered to one's doorstep, can still be procured from an ever-shrinking handful of seltzer men, all of whom source from a single remaining bottler.

Gomberg Seltzer Works in Canarsie, Brooklyn, is the sole New York seltzer factory still in operation, founded in 1953. It is currently run by third-generation owner Kenny Gomberg and Kenny's brother-in-law, Irv Resnick, and fewer than ten seltzer men fill their bottles with the factory's handcrafted, highly carbonated wares. "Good seltzer should hurt the back of your throat," Gomberg said in the 2012 PBS documentary *Seltzer Works*.

In addition to being savored solo, seltzer was commonly used in egg creams, often combined with Fox's U-Bet syrups. In the 1930s, seltzer was dubbed Jewish champagne, a moniker also used to refer to Dr. Brown's Cel-Ray soda. See DR. BROWN'S SODA and EGG CREAMS. Seltzer was also called *belchwasser* in German or *grepes-wasser* in Yiddish because of the drink's digestive aid properties.

The mid-twentieth century seltzer man's gig involved socializing with customers, plenty of heavy lifting, and a hefty salary. "The seltzer bottles were extremely valuable, the routes were very lucrative," third-generation seltzer man Walter Backerman told the *Jewish Week*. "When I was born in the 1950s my father was making anywhere from $300 to $400 a week, which was more than the doctors, probably more than the president of the United States."

Today's remaining seltzer men still pack wooden crates with ten 26-ounce glass seltzer bottles, often sourced from Czechoslovakia and Austria circa the nineteenth century. To make the exceptionally effervescent drink at Gomberg's factory, local tap water is triple-filtered through charcoal, sand, and paper, then chilled to 43°F to further the water's carbon dioxide absorption. The filtered water is pumped into a carbonator containing a duo of paddles that beat the water with 60 to 80 pounds per inch of carbon dioxide gas, and the carbonated water is then pressured into a six-head siphon filler.

Seltzer in plastic bottles can be found in any New York deli or supermarket, but purists eschew it. Store-bought seltzer did indeed hurt Gomberg's business over time, as did "the moving to Florida of many of the old customers." Another alternative to hand-delivered seltzer, SodaStream, gained name recognition and popularity for its at-home carbonation systems in the United States in the early twenty-first century. The company had already been a hit in Australia and England in the 1970s and 1980s but did not see sales take off stateside until going public in 2010. America is currently SodaStream's biggest market.

In 2012, Alex Gomberg, great-grandson of Gomberg Seltzer Works founder Mo Gomberg, started a delivery service, Brooklyn Seltzer Boys, with his father and uncle. The youngest Gomberg focuses his clientele on restaurants, in lieu of traditional home deliveries, as a modern take on the family business.

See also SODA.

Brooklyn Seltzer Boys website: http://www .brooklynseltzerboys.com/seltzer-factory.
Joseph, Barry. "Time in a Bottle." *Jewish Week*, January 2, 2013.
Kilgannon, Corey. "Seltzer Man Is Out of Action, and Brooklyn Thirsts." *New York Times*, September 25, 2009.
Koenig, Leah. "The Next Generation of 'The Seltzer Man.'" *Jewish Daily Forward*, July 17, 2013.
Pollak, Michael. "That Old Celery Fizz." *New York Times*, October 14, 2011.
Rothman, Joshua. "Should Coke and Pepsi Be Worried about SodaStream?" *New Yorker*, February 26, 2013.
Wharton, Rachel. "Schlepping Seltzer." *Edible Brooklyn*, January 20, 2010.

Alexandra Ilyashov

Sex and Food

Food and sex: two basic human appetites, and a handful of sensuous locations have popped up on the island of Manhattan welcoming guests interested in contemplating sex while they drink and nosh. Some of these locales are unique to New York City, while others are outposts of larger chains.

The Museum of Sex, or MoSEX, opened at 233 Fifth Avenue at East Twenty-Seventh Street in 2002. Edible souvenirs from the museum's gift shop have included packaged Dirty Fortune Cookies and the Sea Grape Lickable Massage Candle, but the museum fare ventures beyond sexy snack food. The first eatery at MoSEX was called OralFix Aphrodisiac but has been replaced by the revamped and newly named Play. The Café/Den/Bar operates beyond museum hours, and its black-and-white photographs and faintly suggestive menu (under the heading "Playing Around" is a list of espresso-based drinks) set a gently sexy tone. The museum explores and displays diverse sexual interests and identities, and the compound's presence overall has paved the way for additional Manhattan sex and food experiences.

Veering far from the MoSEX feel is Manhattan's own branch of the Hooters franchise. Originally located at 211 West Fifty-Sixth Street and now on West Thirty-Third Street near Penn Station, the chain prides itself on its down-to-earth atmosphere and attractive waitresses. A beloved buffalo wings recipe, beer, and the hostesses' busts at Hooters have kept loyal customers and tourists supporting the brand since the first location opened in Florida in 1983. A recent development at the Manhattan location is a wine selection ranging from Woodbridge Moscato to Robert Mondavi Private Selection Chardonnay. Regardless of their draw to the scene, patrons may now sip wine while their eyes wander.

Far less obvious but perhaps more universally appealing is Max Brenner, serving up all things chocolate and therefore sexy. Brenner opened his first U.S. location in the Union Square area in 2006. This chocolate heaven with a full lunch and dinner menu features seasonal items inspired by childhood treats (i.e., Shaken Chocolate Milk), while also piquing customers' curiosities with the short but intriguing Chocolate Aphrodisiacs drink menu. The "Satisfaction Guaranteed" contains milk chocolate, caramel liqueur, and Castries peanut liqueur.

Chef "Fed" Federer, a Swiss-trained, Michelin-starred chef, first came to the aid of a handful of New Yorkers intending to explore the wonderful world of aphrodisiacs in 2010 by creating an exclusive supper club. The business expanded to the Sex on the Table Cooking School, offering small, hands-on classes in 2013, with the mantra of culinary and sexual seduction being the art of making the senses work in unison. Those who wish to sample Chef Fed's creations in the privacy of their own homes may obtain products from his food line.

Sex on the Table takes on new meaning at Cheetahs Gentlemen's Club and Restaurant in Midtown, which has a full menu featuring fine dining and body sushi. Also known as *nyotaimori*, the body sushi experience involves a naked woman rolled out into a room, her bare skin artfully decorated with sushi. For $250 each at a minimum of four people per party, guests can enjoy unlimited sake and sushi delivered on the Cheetah stripper of their choice. Whether considered intimate, entertaining, or utterly dehumanizing, this exists on the more extreme end of the spectrum of public-sex-related culinary experiences. When it comes to the most easily identifiable sexy food experiences in Manhattan, little is duplicated, allowing them each to exist on unique and therefore sustainable ground for a wide range of both open-minded and disapproving yet curious patrons.

Dennis, Kelly. "The Hegelian Implications of the Museum of Sex; or, Does MoSex Mean No Sex?" *Art Journal* 65, no. 2 (2006): 8–22.
Sex on the Table website: http://www.sxculinary.com.
Tucker, Reed. "Sex on a Plate: At the Museum of Sex Restaurant, There's Plenty of Naughtiness on the Menu." *New York Post*, February 14, 2014.

Emerald Mitchell

Sex and the City

Eating and drinking played an important role in the groundbreaking HBO series *Sex and the City*, initially running from 1998 until 2004. Large chain restaurant openings, Magnolia Bakery, and the go-to diner were the stages for Carrie Bradshaw's complex relationship with New York. It showed the cosmopolitan, sophisticated, urban life of women drinking and talking about their relationships. It paid tribute to New York as an eater's paradise, but it also played a large role in the city's dining scene by influencing where people went. The show explores the theme of food as status as well as the upper-class wealthy bubble they live in. Whenever Carrie threw back a candy-colored Cosmopolitan or a Manhattan, issuing advice to make room for her own personal dilemmas, she was often at the hot new restaurant.

The signature drink of the show was the Cosmopolitan, and it was fitting for the show's portrayal of four successful women. The series was considered an endorsement of the single female's sexual freedom, made possible by their professional success. Cocktail culture, being out on the town and in the fine dining scene, took precedence over everything.

The women embrace the message that being in the right place demonstrates how powerful they are. Even when their relationships or humiliation knocks them down, they can get dressed to the nines and dose themselves with cocktails. The New York social scene was characterized by eating out and running into everyone worth knowing. In the "Old Dogs New Dicks" episode, an unfortunate encounter with her on-again-off-again boyfriend Big (then more off than on) has Carrie complaining about the coincidence and asking why there is not another restaurant opening that night.

Sex and the City was responsible for putting some restaurants on the map, and not just for diehard fans of the show and tourists. Magnolia Bakery can credit the show for Magnolia fever. See MAGNOLIA BAKERY. When the hit series took off, Bleecker Street had not been the epicenter of bohemian life for a while, but thanks to the overwhelming publicity from the show Magnolia Bakery became a sensation. Magnolia Bakery is now an international empire and the quintessential stop for *Sex and the City* tourists who long to reenact moments of their beloved show.

While the surroundings mostly highlight see-and-be-seen locations and these women's New Yorker cosmopolitanism, the show also pokes fun at their white, upper-middle-class social circle. In the "No Ifs Ands or Butts," episode, when Samantha dates a hip-hop executive of color whose possessive sister chefs at a southern fusion restaurant, her boyfriend's sister sends Samantha her territorial message with Mississippi mud pie. When she and Samantha fight at the club, Samantha makes her feelings known when she says "your okra wasn't all that." These women were informed about food but not prepared for its inseparable links to culture.

Carrie famously said she keeps shoes in her oven because she was out looking fabulous instead of being domestic. Dining out was a symbol of sociability, while dining in suggested isolation and failure (unless Miranda's boyfriend made enchiladas or Aiden made fajitas). This was especially true of episodes featuring a depressed Miranda. In the "What's Sex Got to Do With It?" episode, Miranda self-medicates with Monsieur Payard's éclairs and considers graduating to a cake until a snooty waiter tells her how expensive a cake is. As Miranda's social life dwindles, in the episode "Cock-A-Doodle Do" she routinely orders the same takeout order from a Chinese restaurant. The woman laughs over the phone, signaling to Miranda that she's shaming her for being pathetic. Even though New Yorkers rely on the convenience of takeout and the wide selection, for Miranda, ordering in too much is a defeat. When Carrie is single, she too stays in and orders greasy Chinese takeout as her "pattern."

See also TELEVISION.

Bushnell, Candace. *Sex and the City*. New York: Grand Central, 1996.

Moker, Molly. "Tour the Top 25 'Sex and the City' Locations." Fodor's Travel, March 15, 2014. http://www.fodors.com/news/nyc-top-25-icon-3018.html.

Ashley Hoffman

Shake Shack

Shake Shack's history began with a Chicago-style hot dog cart that Danny Meyer's Union Square Hospitality Group set up in Madison Square Park as an effort to bring in funds to support the Madison Square Park Conservancy's first art installation in 2001. The cart was such a success that, in 2004, the restaurant group was allowed to open a permanent kiosk in the park. See MEYER, DANNY.

Shake Shack mimicked roadside burger stands and instantly generated long lines of people waiting for such standbys as Angus beef burgers, flat-top hot dogs, the vegetarian 'Shroom Burger, Thousand Island–inspired Shack Sauce, and freshly made, rotating flavors of frozen custards. Customers ate at metal tables and chairs in Madison Square Park. In 2005, Peter Meehan reviewed the restaurant for his *New York Times* $25 and Under column, writing "the salty, meaty little burgers swaddled by potato rolls are so good that Shake Shack is swarmed with diners willing to wait twenty minutes or more to order, then wait again while the burgers are griddled to order from morning to night." One of the appeals of Shake Shack has been the high-quality ingredients, including 100 percent all-natural, freshly ground beef and custards made from hormone-free dairy and real sugar. In 2014, the frozen, crinkle-cut fries were revamped in certain locations with fresh, hand-cut fries. Notorious for the endless line snaking around the park, the Shake Shack website launched the "Shack Cam," to give potential customers real-time estimates of line length.

Meyer's Union Square Hospitality Group has opened Shake Shacks in Manhattan, Brooklyn, and Queens. In 2014 there were several locations on the East Coast, as well as overseas in London, Moscow, and the Middle East. That year, to celebrate Shake Shack's ten-year anniversary, celebrity chefs such as Daniel Boulud, April Bloomfield, and David Chang created exclusive specialty burgers, for which customers waited on even longer lines. See CHANG, DAVID; BLOOMFIELD, APRIL; and BOULUD, DANIEL.

Collins, Glenn. "The Accidental Empire of Fast Food." *New York Times*, December 15, 2009.

Meehan, Peter. "$25 and Under: Shake Shack." *New York Times*, September 7, 2005.

Roberts, Daniel. "David Chang Broke All the Rules." *Time*, September 26, 2013.

Shake Shack website: http://www.shakeshack.com.

Andrea Lynn

Shanley, Thomas

See RESTAURANTS and LOBSTER PALACES.

Sheraton, Mimi

New York–based journalist, food writer, and culinary historian Mimi Sheraton has published influential cookbooks, restaurant guides, and memoirs, along with thousands of articles on numerous topics, but she is mainly remembered as possibly the single most important restaurant critic of the twentieth century. From 1976 to 1983, her restaurant reviews for the *New York Times* were devoured by countless readers who were as interested in hearing what she had to say as they were in the restaurants themselves.

A native of Flatbush, Brooklyn, Sheraton was born as Miriam Helene Solomon on February 10, 1926. The elder child of relatively secular parents from an Orthodox Jewish background, her mother, Beatrice, was the daughter of Eastern European immigrants, while her father, Joseph, came to America at the age of one. Her parents called her "Mimi" from an early age, which they pronounced "mimmy"; from college onward, people assumed that her name was pronounced "me-me," and she has pronounced it that way herself ever since. Beatrice was an expert home cook who believed in analyzing and evaluating every dish on the table, while Joseph was a dealer in wholesale fruits and vegetables who taught her that flavor was far more important than appearance and size— principles Mimi would maintain as a restaurant critic, where she frequently tore into restaurants that concentrated on flashiness and plating at the expense of taste. Her mother did not keep kosher, mixing meat and dairy and serving both pork and shellfish, but was steeped in the traditions of Ashkenazi Jewish cooking, as Sheraton recounted in her 1979 book *From My Mother's Kitchen: Recipes and Reminiscences*. Central and Eastern European food would be the

focus of five of Sheraton's books, including *The Bialy Eaters* (2002) and her classic *The German Cookbook* (1965), which has remained in print since its publication.

As Mimi's father objected to her going away to college, she matriculated at New York University's School of Commerce, majoring in marketing with a minor in journalism. In her sophomore year, just after VJ Day, she married returning serviceman William Schlifman, and they moved into an apartment in Greenwich Village. Her new husband wanted to change their last name to Shelby, which Mimi did not like, so she suggested "Sheraton" as a compromise. Needing and wanting to work, she took a job as an advertising copywriter during the day, while completing her degree at night. The marriage itself lasted less than a decade, partly because of her desire to keep working, though she kept the name "Sheraton." Years later, in her 2004 memoir *Eating My Words*, she wrote that she wished that she had returned to the name "Solomon" after her divorce.

As a woman working in advertising in the 1940s, she was assigned to accounts like jewelry and furniture, which led to her taking a job writing for *Good Housekeeping* about interior design. Sheraton became a certified professional decorator to give herself credibility and then moved to *Seventeen* magazine to become their home furnishings editor and subsequently their food editor as well. After a brief stint as a managing editor for a new supplement at *House Beautiful*, she quit and spent the next twenty years writing freelance, mostly but not exclusively about food. In 1955, she married Richard Falcone, then a merchandise manager at Gimbels and later a tableware importer, with whom she would have one son, Marc. The marriage lasted until Falcone's death in 2014. She started writing restaurant reviews for *Cue* and *The Village Voice*, traveling around the world and studying at the Cordon Bleu in Paris. During this time, she published her first two cookbooks and worked as a consultant for Restaurant Associates. Her investigative food articles for *New York* magazine got her hired as a food reporter at the *New York Times* in 1975, just as they were expanding their food coverage. On the strength and popularity of her investigative pieces and blind taste tests, the *Times* promoted her to critic.

During Sheraton's seven and one-half years as America's most famous restaurant reviewer, she endeavored to remain strictly anonymous at the restaurants she visited: donning wigs, eyeglasses, and various disguises; never making reservations in her own name; not allowing herself to be photographed; refusing public appearances; and insisting that the people she dined with not call her "Mimi." Yet, paradoxically, readers felt that they knew her because she brought them into her experiences. Staunchly scientific, she told her readers about her methodology: describing the precautions she took, never accepting free meals, and always paying with cash or a friend's credit card. (The restaurant expenses were considerable, amounting to $95,000 during her last year at the *Times*.) She even discussed the problems she had with her weight resulting from having to dine out at least fourteen times every week, which wound up being one of the factors that led her to quit the *New York Times* and regular reviewing.

While Mimi Sheraton was certainly not the first restaurant critic to dine anonymously (it was standard practice at the *New York Times* when she started there), she was the first to draw back the curtain on just how differently individual patrons may experience the same restaurant. Unlike other types of newspaper critics, a restaurant critic is reviewing dishes prepared expressly for one table, meaning that if a critic is recognized, her or his food may be entirely different from what is prepared for ordinary patrons. Despite Sheraton's disguises, she was occasionally recognized, and she punctiliously reported the differences between how she was treated when she was recognized and when she was not. Rare out-of-date photos of her were posted inside some restaurants to encourage staff to look out for her; one waiter admitted to her that he was promised a bonus of $250 every time he spotted her. Sheraton visited each restaurant at least three times (and up to twelve before publishing a review), attempting to taste nearly every dish on the menu by dining with friends whose plates she would sample.

Sheraton championed excellent and unpretentious food, ranging from the classical French cuisine at Lutèce (her favorite restaurant) to the Italian American food served at the now-famous Rao's, which she discovered and to which she gave three stars even though it was then an obscure eight-table neighborhood eatery. Her tenure coincided with both the expansion of ethnic restaurants in New York, which she eagerly explored, and the development of nouvelle cuisine, which she generally distrusted for its emphasis on presentation rather than flavor. A declared

enemy of restaurants that she saw as trendy and overpriced, she admitted to being subjective in her tastes but claimed to be "objectively subjective"— that is, free from outside influences. An attempt by the then deputy managing editor Arthur Gelb to get her to change a review was the final straw that led Sheraton to quit the *Times* for good in 1983.

Not wanting to return to regular restaurant criticism, she subsequently signed contracts with magazines including *Time, Vanity Fair,* and *Condé Nast Traveler,* for which she wrote extended pieces such as a review of airline food in business class on eleven different airlines. She would go on to explore international interests in her cookbook *The Whole World Loves Chicken Soup* (1995), which won the James Beard and International Association of Culinary Professionals Awards, as well as the massive *1,000 Foods to Eat Before You Die* (2015).

See also NEW YORK TIMES and RESTAURANT REVIEWING.

Sheraton, Mimi. *Eating My Words: An Appetite for Life.* New York: William Morrow, 2004.
Sheraton, Mimi. *From My Mother's Kitchen: Recipes & Reminiscences.* Rev. ed. New York: HarperCollins, 1991.

Marc P. Levy

Sherry's

Operating between 1881 and 1919, Sherry's was a major player in New York's fine dining scene of the late nineteenth and early twentieth centuries. It rivaled such institutions as Delmonico's, especially among younger New Yorkers of wealth and prestige. See DELMONICO'S.

Louis Sherry, the founder and proprietor of Sherry's, worked his way up from a busboy at the Brunswick Hotel to become one of the most famous restaurateurs in turn-of-the-twentieth-century Gotham. Sherry moved from the Brunswick to running the Hotel Elberon on the Jersey shore for two summers. There, he made the acquaintance of wealthy businessmen and financiers. They helped him gain a foothold back in the city as a caterer to the Gilded Age elite. Sherry made a name for himself not only for the quality of his food but for the spectacles he created at high-society dinner parties. As Sherry himself put it, "One of the secrets I learned was that nothing goes further with dainty people than dainty

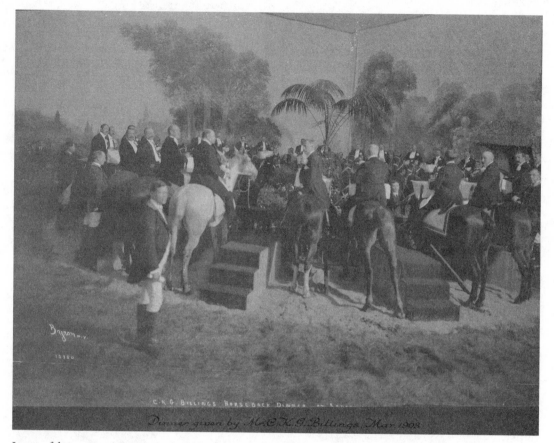

In one of the most notorious examples of the excesses of the Gilded Age, Chicago millionaire C. K. G. Billings celebrated becoming president of the New York Equestrian Club in 1903 by hosting a horseback dinner at Sherry's, where he had the ballroom floor covered with sod and hay strewn about. Billings's thirty-six guests were served dinner on horseback by waiters outfitted in equestrian garb. MUSEUM OF THE CITY OF NEW YORK

decorations". While Sherry had operated an ice creamery and confectionery for several years, it was in 1889 that he opened his first large-scale restaurant and ballroom, on Fifth Avenue and Thirty-Seventh Street. There, he introduced a 5:00 p.m. tea, which drew society ladies, and his restaurant became a go-to spot for New York society in the 1890s.

In 1897, after Delmonico's moved to Fifth Avenue and Forty-Fourth Street, Sherry opened a new restaurant on the opposite corner, designed by famed architect Stanford White. This move reflected the growing predominance of Times Square as the city's central entertainment district at the turn of the twentieth century. See TIMES SQUARE. For the next two decades, Delmonico's and Sherry's battled for the title of New York's finest and most opulent dining establishment.

Sherry's became famous in New York City and beyond for its food and lavish entertainments. In the late nineteenth century, wealthy New Yorkers began to host parties in the grand ballrooms of Sherry's and Delmonico's rather than at home. Louis Sherry wowed them with his over-the-top productions. The most notorious of these was the 1903 horseback dinner hosted by Chicago millionaire C. K. G. Billings to celebrate his assuming the presidency of the New York Equestrian Club. Sherry converted his ballroom into a country estate for the occasion, the floor covered with sod and hay strewn about. Billings's thirty-six guests were served dinner on horseback by waiters outfitted in equestrian garb. The press had a field day over the Billings dinner, deriding the event as a shining example of the excess and wastefulness of the Gilded Age elite. See GILDED AGE.

Sherry's closed in 1919, like many restaurants a victim of Prohibition (and, according to Sherry, the bolshevism of his waiters, who had participated in a large and famous strike in 1912). Sherry opened a small confectionery and catering shop on Park Avenue and Fifty-Eighth Street. In subsequent years, the Sherry name would live on in the labels of his line of delicacies (caviar, olive oil, foie gras) and the Sherry-Netherland Tower, built in 1927.

Batterberry, Michael, and Ariane Batterberry. *On the Town in New York: The Landmark History of Eating, Drinking, and Entertainments from the American Revolution to the Food Revolution.* 2d ed. New York and London: Routledge, 1998.

Grimes, William. *Appetite City: A Culinary History of New York.* New York: North Point, 2009.

Hungerford, Edward. *The Story of Louis Sherry and the Business He Built.* New York: William Edwin Rudge, 1929.

Cindy R. Lobel

Sichuan

See CHINESE COMMUNITY.

Sinclair, Upton

Upton Sinclair (1878–1968) was born in Baltimore but moved to New York to attend Columbia University in 1897. He began writing while still in college, living off dozens of articles, stories, and books.

Sinclair became involved in socialist activities—influenced by Jacob Riis's 1890 muckraking *How the Other Half Lives.* A leftist magazine, *Appeal to Reason,* hired him to write an exposé of working conditions in a Chicago meatpacking plant owned by Philip Danforth Armour. His article created an uproar that only intensified when it was published in the form of a novel, in 1906, as *The Jungle.*

Every year since 1879, the U.S. Congress had considered—without effect—legislation to monitor food safety. The public uproar created by *The Jungle* caused a huge drop in meat sales, so President Theodore Roosevelt empowered the Neill-Reynolds Commission to investigate conditions in the nation's food industry. Its findings (and public pressure) provided the stimulus to enact the Pure Food and Drug Act of 1906, the Meat Inspection Act.

Sinclair used *The Jungle*'s royalties to found an experiment in communal living—Helicon Hall, in

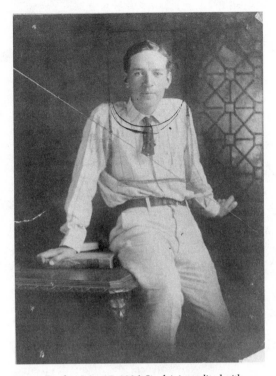

Upton Sinclair, May 29, 1906. Sinclair is credited with garnering attention for the working and sanitary conditions in Chicago meatpacking plants through his 1906 exposé *The Jungle.* The attention caused the government to intervene in the meat industry. LIBRARY OF CONGRESS

Englewood, New Jersey—that failed when its building burned in 1907. He later focused his prolific output on exposing corruption and defending significant lost causes, writing about slavery, the Sacco and Vanzetti trial, the Teapot Dome scandal, as well as ethical living and vegetarianism. He published—under his own name and various pseudonyms—at least eighty books (autobiography, his collected letters, nonfiction, novels). He also produced countless articles, essays, poems, and reviews.

Sinclair had intended *The Jungle* to be an exposé of the packing plants' terrible working conditions but was disappointed to learn that the public was more concerned about the quality of the foods produced there. Looking back, he lamented that he had "aimed at the public's heart, and by accident hit it in the stomach."

Harris, Leon. *Upton Sinclair: American Rebel.* New York: Crowell, 1975.

Sinclair, Upton. *My Lifetime in Letters.* Columbia: University of Missouri Press, 1960.

Sinclair, Upton. *The Jungle.* New York: Heritage, 1965.

"The Month: Notes and Comments." *Westminster Review,* New York: Leonard Scott, 1906.

Gary Allen

Slang

New York City has an abundant legacy of slang words and phrases related to food and beverages. Many either originated in the city or have close associations with its culinary culture. These expressions have enlivened speech for centuries, and many have remained in popular use.

According to lexicographers Barry Popik and Gerald Cohen, "Big Apple," the city's nickname, was first popularized as a reference to New York City in the 1920s by John J. Fitz Gerald in the horse racing column he wrote for the *New York Morning Telegraph.* In the 1970s, the term was picked up by the New York Convention and Visitors Bureau to promote the city. See BIG APPLE.

Some terms emerged to describe the habits of worldly, chic New Yorkers. The "Algonquin Round Table" (a play on King Arthur's Round Table) referred to the literary and journalistic lights—Robert Benchley, Dorothy Parker, Alexander Woollcott, and others—who gathered for meals and witty conversation at the Algonquin Hotel between the two world wars. See ALGONQUIN ROUND TABLE. About the same time, the term "cafe society" came to describe the sophisticated New Yorkers who frequented the city's fashionable supper clubs. A night spot with the same name flourished just off Sheridan Square in Greenwich Village from 1938 through 1948; Billie Holiday debuted the controversial song "Strange Fruit" at Café Society in 1939. The term was further popularized by the movie *Café Society,* released in 1939.

Street vendors have been common in New York for most of its history and have been given many monikers. Irish women who sold apples during the early twentieth century were called "Apple Marys" or "Apple Annies." The Frank Capra movie *Lady for a Day* (1933) centers on a Times Square apple vendor called "Apple Annie." Italian ice cream vendors were known as "hokey-pokey men." The source of the term is not known, but it may have arisen from an Italian phrase containing the word *poco* (meaning "a little").

The terms "breadlines," "soup lines," and "soup kitchen," meaning places where free food was dis-tributed to the poor and unemployed, were common in New York City during the nineteenth and twentieth centuries. Even amid great abundance, soup kitchens still operate in New York City in the twenty-first century. See BREADLINES.

Drinking Places and Beverages

A number of slang terms emerged for drinking establishments. "Rum shop," "grog shop," "grog mill," and "groggery" were early names for low-down establishments that sold a variety of alcoholic beverages. Later, those that catered to the lower classes were also called "gin mills." Bars that sold whiskey were referred to as "skee joints." Bowery saloons were called "distilleries," and those that served particularly toxic concoctions were called "morgues." Places that served cheap red wine were called "red ink spots" or "red ink joints."

The term "saloon" was initially used in New York to mean a high-class drinking establishment, but the phrase quickly came to denote a lower-class place. Many saloons sold beer in "growlers," which initially were two-quart buckets. Going to a saloon for a bucket of beer was termed "rushing the growler." See SALOONS.

If a customer got out of line in a bar or saloon, he could be removed from the premises by a "bouncer." Drinkers who were not choosy about their companions were susceptible to being "slipped a mickey" or a "mickey fin"—a drugged drink that could knock them unconscious.

More upscale drinking establishments were sometimes referred to as "night spots," "watering places," "watering holes," and "watering spots." A small, unassuming bar might be called a "hole in the wall." During Prohibition (1920–1933), "speakeasy" referred to any place that sold illegal alcoholic beverages. Many well-to-do New Yorkers never thought that Prohibition applied to them; they threw "cocktail parties" at home from the 1920s on. When Prohibition ended, drinking establishments called "cocktail lounges" emerged. See COCKTAIL LOUNGES; PRO-HIBITION; and SPEAKEASIES.

Drugstores served soda beverages from the early nineteenth century on, and a wide vocabulary developed around them. A person who made beverages was called a "soda jerk." Many soda fountains also sold "egg creams," soda drinks that include neither eggs nor cream. See SODA FOUNTAINS.

Coffee has been an important beverage to New Yorkers since the early nineteenth century. The city was the nation's center for coffee bean importing, and a New York City inventor manufactured the first mechanical coffee roaster. Special terminology has grown up around ordering coffee: in New York City (and hardly anywhere else), "regular coffee" means coffee with milk. See COFFEE.

Eating Places and Foods

New Yorkers have consumed "quick food," particularly at lunch, since the early nineteenth century, giving rise to an entire category of slang. Early colloquial names for dishes included "a plate of Siamese twins" (fish balls), "woodcock" (pork and beans), "boned turkey," "corduroy" and "West Broadway" (hash), "Irish goose" (codfish, baked or boiled), and "a plate of Tennessee" (hot cornbread). Twentieth-century diner lingo includes "axle grease" (butter), "throw it in the mud" (add chocolate syrup), and "pin a rose on it" (add onion to the dish).

Oysters were common in New York Harbor and the surrounding waters. They were sold in vast quantities in "oyster cellars," "oyster houses," and "oyster bars." Many establishments were on the "Canal Street plan," which meant that you could eat as many oysters as you liked for twelve cents. Others sold oysters from "floating houses," which preserved live oysters for several days by placing them in baskets in the cellar and attic of the oyster boat. See OYSTERS and OYSTER BARS.

During the late nineteenth and early twentieth centuries, some of the city's finer restaurants were known as "lobster palaces." They were expensive, were elegantly decorated, and sported live entertainment, such as orchestras, dancing, and floor shows. They served a variety of dishes, but lobster was their signature dish. Cheaper eateries were called "sawdust joints" or "sawdust places" because sawdust on the floor made it easy to sweep up spills (or, some suggest, blood). Truly lowdown cafes were called "dumps," "cockroach joints," "mulligan joints," or "slop houses." The terms "hash house," "hashery," and "hash joint" referred to a wide variety of cheap eating houses that served much more besides hash—none of it fine cuisine. The cook in such a place was called a "hash-slinger." See LOBSTER PALACES.

Ethnic restaurants also acquired nicknames. Small Italian restaurants, usually located in cellars, were called "spaghetti joints." Chinese restaurants were called "chop suey joints." See CHOP SUEY JOINTS. Kosher restaurants that did not serve meat were called "dairy restaurants." "Black-and-tans" were establishments where both African Americans and whites congregated.

The term "hot dog" may not have originated in New York, but the concept—placing a sausage on a bun—likely did. These were initially called "Coney Island sausage sandwiches," "hot Coney Islands," "Coney Island dogs," or just "Coneys" for short. During the early twentieth century, "chili parlors," which sold chili con carne, emerged in New York. If you put the chili on a hot dog, it became a "chili dog." See HOT DOGS.

"Quick food" or "quick lunch" places, such as cafeterias, buffets, and smorgasbords, specialized in speedy service. Cheap restaurants called "automats" used mechanical food dispensers rather than waiters to serve customers. The restaurant walls were lined with rows of small windowed hatches behind which plates of food were displayed. The customer deposited coins in a slot, turned a knob, and the little door popped open. The automat machines were called "slots," a reference to gambling slot machines. See AUTOMATS.

Deli Slang

German immigrants imported European specialty foods—wines, brandies, meats, and cheeses—and from 1868 sold them in stores called delicatessens. German Jewish immigrants also opened delicatessens. Some, such as Russ & Daughters, Barney Greengrass, and Zabar's, became "appetizing" stores, specializing in smoked and pickled fish, dairy products, and perhaps accessories such as pickles, dried fruit, and nuts. Smoked and brined salmon is one of the most popular offerings. In New York City it is called "lox" (from the Yiddish *lax*, meaning "salmon") and is usually served on a bagel spread with cream cheese. A customer ordering just a little cream cheese asks for a "schmear." See APPETIZING STORES.

An alternative to a bagel is the "bialy" (named for the city of Bialystok, now in Poland, which was predominantly Jewish in the late nineteenth century), a chewy, flat roll that is best eaten hot from the oven. Bialys are similar to bagels but are not boiled before baking. Instead of a hole, the bialy has a depression in the middle, which is filled with onions, garlic, or other seasoning. See BIALYS.

The word "delicatessen" was shortened to "deli" during the 1950s and acquired a more general meaning as a small neighborhood grocery store. As new groups of immigrants—Italians, Greeks, Puerto Ricans, West Indians, Chinese, and Koreans—moved into the city, many found that deli ownership proved an excellent entry point. While some traditional delis have survived, most sell a general line of packaged and prepared foods. Deli owners from newer immigrant groups, though, often include their native favorites—for instance, Korean American–owned delis frequently sell kimchi, while West Indian proprietors offer savory turnovers called "patties." See DELIS, GERMAN and DELIS, JEWISH.

New food slang pops up in New York all the time. Recent additions include the Italian American word "gavone" (from the Italian *cafone*), meaning a greedy, sloppy eater; another Italian word, *agita*, means indigestion or heartburn (or anxiety or anguish); and a "cronut" is a combination of the doughnut and the croissant, devised by pastry chef Dominique Ansel at his eponymous SoHo bakery.

See also CHINESE COMMUNITY; CRONUT; EGG CREAMS; IRISH; and ITALIAN.

Allen, Irving L. *City in Slang: New York Life and Popular Speech*. New York: Oxford University Press, 1993.
Barry Popik website: http://www.barrypopik.com.

Andrew F. Smith

Slow Food

Slow Food International is a nonprofit organization dedicated to preserving local food traditions, protecting biodiversity, and providing an alternative to fast-food culture. It emerged out of the protest movement that accompanied the opening of the first Italian McDonald's outlet near the Spanish Steps in Rome in 1986. The protest leader was Carlo Petrini, an Italian who believed that the industrialization of food was standardizing taste and leading to the loss of thousands of local and regional foods. Following the protests, Petrini founded Slow Food in Bra, Italy, and in 1989 delegates from fifteen countries met in Paris and signed the Slow Food manifesto, stating their opposition to fast food and their support for local culinary traditions. The organization's international headquarters are in Bra, Italy.

Slow Food International's affiliate in the United States is Slow Food USA, a nonprofit educational organization founded in Brooklyn by Patrick Martins. Martins had spent two years in Italy working with Petrini in Bra. When Martins returned to New York in 2000, he began organizing an American affiliate to Slow Food International. Slow Food USA's four major program areas are biodiversity, including the Ark of Taste, which is "a living catalogue of delicious and distinctive foods facing extinction"; children and food; convenings (local, national, and international gatherings); and food communities. In 2003, Martins teamed up with Ben Watson to publish *The Slow Food Guide to New York City: Restaurants, Markets, Bars*.

In 2001 Heritage Foods USA was founded as the marketing arm of Slow Food USA's Ark of Taste project, which connects consumers with purveyors of endangered foods, from sustainably raised rare-breed beef to pawpaws, an indigenous American tree fruit. Its major focus was on heritage turkeys. By 2004 Slow Food USA had grown to more than eleven thousand members and 130 chapters. Slow Food USA spun off Heritage Foods USA, and Martins left to direct the new business, which is based in Brooklyn. (He also started the Heritage Radio Network.)

In 2008 Slow Food USA sponsored a conference called Slow Food Nation, which celebrated traditional and sustainable foods. The conference was organized by restaurateur Alice Waters, who is also vice president of Slow Food International, and Anya Fernald, a sustainable food expert. It was held in San Francisco and was attended by an estimated fifty thousand, including many New Yorkers.

Slow Food USA has thrived since its founding. As of 2014, it had a membership of twelve thousand members divided into 140 local "convivia." It is dedicated to preserving endangered foodways (such as dwindling animal breeds and heirloom varieties of fruits and vegetables), celebrating local food traditions, and promoting artisanal products. It advocates economic sustainability and biodiversity through educational events and public outreach programs.

Slow Food USA's local chapter is Slow Food NYC, founded in Manhattan in 1998. It has six major programs: Urban Harvest, which teaches city children about the benefits of good food; the Snail of Approval, awarded to producers, purveyors, and artisans of authentic and sustainable food and drink in the city; Slow U., a series of educational sessions where participants discuss the food revolution and activist efforts to improve the food chain (with tastings); SFNYC Book & Film Club, which connects people at book events and discussion groups; and The Slur, a bimonthly "happy hour" gathering for members and officers. Slow Food NYC also sponsors or cosponsors events, such as the NYC Sustainable Farm to Restaurant Producer Summit, which brings together local farmers, chefs, and food distributors.

See also HERITAGE RADIO NETWORK.

Martins, Patrick, and Ben Watson. *The Slow Food Guide to New York City: Restaurants, Markets, Bars.* White River Junction, Vt.: Chelsea Green, 2003.
Moskin, Julia. "New Leader for Slow Food USA." *New York Times,* January 8, 2013.
Slow Food New York City website: http://www.slowfoodnyc.org.
Slow Food USA website: http://www.slowfoodusa.org.

Andrew F. Smith

Smilow, Rick

Rick Smilow, the president and owner of the Institute of Culinary Education since 1995, has overseen the transformation of that cooking school from its six cramped teaching kitchens, catering to a small cadre of aspiring professionals and enthusiastic amateurs, to a state-of-the-art educational facility in downtown Manhattan offering programs in the culinary and pastry arts, culinary management, hospitality management, and recreational classes.

Smilow was born in 1956, in Annapolis, Maryland. He earned an MBA in marketing from the Kellogg School of Management at Northwestern University in 1978. Smilow's early culinary experiences were unorthodox for someone who would eventually spearhead a culinary school: he was a brand manager for Nabisco (1984–1988) and thereafter the founder and president of Wag Tail Limited, a line of gourmet pet foods (1988–1994). His entrepreneurial appetite whetted, he purchased the Institute of Culinary Education (then known as Peter Kump's New York Cooking School), where he significantly expanded the size and range of offerings. The industry has recognized the scope of his accomplishment with the 2011 International Association of Culinary Professionals Award of Excellence for Entrepreneur of the Year. Smilow is the author, along with Anne E. McBride, of *Culinary Careers: How to Get Your Dream Job in Food* (2010).

Beyond his business acumen, Smilow has devoted substantial energies to charitable activities. He is (as of 2015) a board member of City Harvest and a former director of the Careers Through Culinary Arts Program (2000–2011). He also participates in or supports philanthropic organizations whose impact is felt outside of New York City, such as the Third World–oriented Action Against Hunger. Smilow brings the Institute of Culinary Education's physical space and people together to aid in disaster relief, holding fundraisers after events such as the 2004 Indian Ocean tsunami, Hurricane Katrina in 2005, and, closest to home, 9/11. As the Twin Towers were smoldering, visible from the school's windows, Smilow halted classes to empty the refrigerators and allow students and faculty to cook for emergency responders and survivors.

See also CAREERS THROUGH CULINARY ARTS PROGRAM (C-CAP) and INSTITUTE OF CULINARY EDUCATION.

"Biographical Sketch—Rick Smilow." http://www.iacp.com/documents/AOE_2011_Smilow.pdf.

Cathy K. Kaufman

Smoked Fish

The smoking of fish and meat goes back millennia. Smoking, salting, drying, and pickling were methods used to preserve foods before the advent of refrigeration. The Dutch colonists, who settled along the coastline of "Breukelen," brought their Old World traditions of fish preservation and began drying, salting, and smoking the local fare the sea served up to them: herring, eels, and oysters. See COLONIAL DUTCH. The British added their own preferences: mackerel, halibut, and "finnan haddie" (smoked haddock). By the last half of the eighteenth century, thanks to the completion of the transcontinental railroad, freshly caught Pacific Ocean salmon submerged in huge casks of heavy salt brine were being shipped from the Pacific Northwest to the ports of New York, much of it to be transshipped to Europe. Some of that salmon stayed in New York and found its way to the German delicatessens of the Lower East Side. It was known as "lox," from the German word *lachs,* meaning "salmon." Some of the lox was smoked; this was known popularly as "smoked lox" and, more technically correct, as "smoked salmon."

Later, with the advent of refrigerated rail transportation, large amounts of Atlantic Ocean salmon were imported from Canada, bathed in a milder salt brine, smoked, and identified as "Nova Scotia."

Poor Man's Food

Smoked fish had always been a poor man's food. For the price of a nickel beer in the saloons of the Lower East Side you could get a free lunch that included pickles and smoked fish. In the early 1860s ships were leaving New York Harbor with smoked fish among the provisions for the Union Army. American relief efforts to the Island of Puerto Rico following a devastating hurricane in 1899 included smoked fish along with rice and beans. By the early 1900s New York newspaper columns targeting the female homemaker provided recipes for smoked fish and extolled its virtue as a tasty and economical alternative to the much preferred fresh fish.

A greater appreciation for smoked and pickled fish came with the German immigration to the Lower East Side in the mid-1800s. The Germans were familiar with smoked fish from their delicatessens in Europe and recreated the same type of "delicacy" shop in New York, where smoked fish was sold alongside smoked meats and cheeses. The large wave of Eastern European immigration to New York's Lower East Side began in 1880 and for the most part displaced the earlier German settlers, who moved their "Kleindeutschland" along with their delicatessens and groceries to the Yorkville section of the Upper East Side. See DELIS, GERMAN and KLEINDEUTSCHLAND. Because of Jewish dietary laws (*kashruth*) the "appetizing store" was created where, instead of selling all manner of smoked, cured, and pickled meat, fish, and dairy products together in one shop as the Germans had done, the Eastern European Jews could buy smoked, salted, and pickled fish products along with the appropriate dairy accompaniments of butter, sour cream, and cream cheese. The Eastern European Jews became the largest consumers of smoked fish in New York.

Retail/Wholesale

By the 1920s the Jews predominated not only in the retail sale of smoked fish through their appetizing stores but also in the import, preparation, and distribution of smoked and pickled fish products through ownership of the smokehouses. In New York City, "smoked fish" became a Jewish industry. Through the 1920s, 1930s, and 1940s several attempts were made to control supply, labor unions, and prices through coercion, extortion, and violence. Investigative commissions were convened by the state of New York, resulting in fines and jail time for several smokers, union officials, and distributors. By the 1950s consolidation of the industry had begun. Some smokers relocated to other parts of the country. Some just closed their doors. Those that remained were engaged in fierce competition for customers. Today, three smokehouses remain in New York City.

Changing Tastes, Changing Lifestyles

Smoked fish had traditionally been eaten with some carbohydrate to counterbalance its saltiness; this was usually large chunks of rye or pumpernickel bread slathered with butter. By the 1930s bagels and bialys became the breads of choice to house smoked fish and cream cheese became the method of holding it all together. The "bagel and lox" was born and, along with other smoked and pickled fish items, became the mainstay of the Sunday brunch enjoyed by the newly affluent second-generation Jews of New York. But smoked and pickled fish products remained largely "Jewish food," with ceremonial value rather than widespread appeal. See BAGELS; BIALYS; and BRUNCH.

In the 1980s there was a sea change in people's regard of what they ate and where that food came from. There would be newspaper sections devoted to food and dining, magazines all about food, and then a food network, with nothing but food shows twenty-four hours a day, seven days a week. Each one of these media outlets competing for an audience and advertisers was focused on scooping the next big thing in food. At the same time there was renewed interest in what was perceived as "authentic." This usually meant ethnic. And in the world of ethnic authenticity there was smoked fish. It was sold, presented, and eaten directly. No transformational recipes were needed. It was clear that smoking fish was no longer just about preservation; it tasted good. No longer was smoked fish to be regarded as simply ethnic food with waning interest from its own cultural audience. It was now embraced by the rest of the world. The humble herring had become haute cuisine. The bagel and lox had gone from Delancey Street to Main Street.

What had been thought of as common, even disdained, is now on the menus of fancy restaurants and first-class airlines. What used to be a relatively cheap food item has become expensive, this largely the result of depletion from overfishing and lack of conservation. Across the country the Sunday brunch has become a national pastime and now often includes smoked sturgeon omelets with crème fraîche and smoked salmon Benedicts. In New York City the Sunday brunch continues as a tradition, a gathering of family and friends with an abundant array of smoked fish: whitefish, sturgeon, sable, trout, and, of course, bagels and lox, accompanied by freshly squeezed orange juice, piping-hot coffee, and the *New York Times*. Along with hamburgers, hot dogs, and pizza, New Yorkers and New York–centrics have placed bagels and lox in the pantheon of quintessentially New York foods.

See also APPETIZING STORES and LOX.

Diner, Hasia R. *Hungering for America: Italian, Irish, and Jewish Foodways in the Age of Migration*. Cambridge, Mass.: Harvard University Press, 2001.

Durham, T. R. "Salt, Smoke, and History." *Gastronomica* (Winter 2001): 78–82.

Federman, Mark Russ. *Russ & Daughters: Reflections and Recipes from the House that Herring Built*. New York: Schocken, 2013.

Marks, Gil. "Lox." In *Encyclopedia of Jewish Food*, pp. 369–371. Hoboken, N.J.: Wiley, 2010.

Ziegelman, Jane. *97 Orchard: An Edible History of Five Immigrant Families in One New York Tenement*. New York: HarperCollins, 2010.

Mark Russ Federman with Hannah Petertil

Smorgasburg

Smorgasburg is an outdoor food market on the Brooklyn waterfront that occurs on Saturdays and Sundays, seasonally. Started in 2011 by Jonathan Butler and Eric Demby, the duo who founded The Brooklyn Flea in 2008, Smorgasburg grew from fewer than a dozen vendors to hosting around one hundred rotating small businesses each day, with ten thousand to fifteen thousand daily visitors.

Smorgasburg grew out of the popularity of the handful of food vendors who the founders invited to set up shop at The Brooklyn Flea. When high consumer demand became clear for this small-batch and often innovative approach to food and drink—and when the founders had to start turning away otherwise qualified applicants because of space—Demby and Butler decided to start a food-focused version of The Brooklyn Flea and dubbed it Smorgasburg, in part after Williamsburg, where they first found available space. See WILLIAMSBURG. This newly available marketplace for food and drink vendors corresponded with the rising interest in thoughtfully sourced and prepared foods, and the narrative of Brooklyn being a profitable and supportive place to start a small business. Brooklyn became known as a place where food businesses could get their start, with relatively affordable space and opportunities to sell their product with low overhead. Smorgasburg became an important resource for these new entrepreneurs to launch, with a number making the jump to brick-and-mortar locations.

Smorgasburg has continued to grow in popularity, with two locations a week and a full roster of vendors interested in selling at each location. This unique outdoor food market has also inspired Butler and Demby's next project, which is an indoor beer hall and food court in Brooklyn's Crown Heights neighborhood, the first of its kind in the borough. However, the outdoor food market ethos is still strong, and the founders continue to expand, hosting Smorgasburg events in various places around the city.

Robbins, Liz. "Kings of Small Batch Empire in Brooklyn." *New York Times*, October 27, 2012.

Suzanne Cope

Snapple

The beverage company Unadulterated Fruit Juices, which would famously boast that its products were made "from the best stuff on earth," was founded in 1972 by three New York men: Leonard Marsh (1933–2013), his brother-in-law Hyman Golden (1923–2008) and childhood friend Arnold Greenberg (1932–2012). Marsh, the son of Russian Jews, and Greenberg grew up together in the Brownsville section of Brooklyn, once home to many Eastern European immigrants. Golden, the son of a Romanian window washer, was raised in Middle Village, Queens.

The three men held a variety of jobs before hitting the beverage jackpot. Marsh sold eggs. Golden worked as a business broker before partnering with Marsh to launch a window-washing business. Greenberg worked at his father's East Village deli, located on First Avenue near St. Mark's Place, selling lox, herring, and pickles. By the 1950s, he was running it.

As the East Village neighborhood changed, with hippies replacing the Eastern European Jews, Greenberg turned the deli into a health-food store. In 1972, the three men each chipped in $6,000 to launch Unadulterated Fruit Juices, which sold organic drinks to stores like Greenberg's. Marsh would later admit that he knew "as much about juice as about making an atom bomb."

The venture was part-time at first. Marsh and Golden kept the window-washing business. Even though it was one of the first beverage companies to offer drinks made with natural ingredients, Unadulterated Fruit Juices did not do particularly well initially. "Then one day we woke up," Marsh once said. "We realized we had a business."

One of the company's early products was a carbonated apple juice, from which the name "Snapple" was derived—a combination of "snappy" and "apple." In 1980, when the company started calling itself Snapple, its founders had to pay $500 to a Texas man who already owned the name.

The carbonated apple drink proved problematic. "When it first came out, we sold 500 cases," Greenberg told the *New York Times* in 1994. "The next month, we sold 500 more cases and got some calls from distributors. 'You've changed your formula,' they said. 'This Snapple's tasting better and better.' Then one day in our warehouse, the tops of the bottles started shooting off. Bang! Pop! We found out it was fermenting. We'd made Champagne."

The founders' naiveté proved to be an asset when it came to Snapple's biggest success: a line of bottled iced teas launched in 1987. The recipe for a lemon-flavored variety was developed with the help of a tea vendor and a bottler. One of the reasons it tasted better than other brands was that it was made without preservatives and brewed and bottled hot, a novelty in the industry at the time. Other iced teas on the market were packed cold in cans and often tasted tinny as a result. Snapple tea was also sold year-round, in contrast to other bottled teas that hit shelves only in the summer. "Tea was around for many years. We made it better," Marsh said.

Snapple sales skyrocketed. In 1991, the company was forced to move from its Brooklyn headquarters to larger digs in Valley Stream, Long Island. The founders hardly let success go to their heads. Marsh

and Golden still shared an office until the company moved again in 1994. That year, sales of Snapple and its more than fifty flavors topped $674 million, up from just $4 million ten years earlier.

One of the company's key drivers in the early 1990s was its advertising. Snapple was promoted on Howard Stern's and Rush Limbaugh's radio shows, and the outfit produced several TV spots, including a 1991 ad featuring Ivan Lendl. In 1993, Snapple partnered with ad agency Kirshenbaum & Bond to launch a wildly popular campaign featuring Wendy Kaufman, the "Snapple Lady." Kaufman was an actual employee in Snapple's order department and had taken it upon herself to answer fan mail that arrived at the headquarters. As a love-struck teenager, Kaufman had mailed a fan letter to Barry Williams, who played Greg on *The Brady Bunch*, and was crushed when she never received a response. Snapple built an ad campaign around Kaufman answering real letters from real customers, including a TV commercial that dispatched former New York Mayor Ed Koch to Kentucky to set straight a man who'd written to say that Snapple was "perhaps the only good that has ever come out of New York." Kaufman's strong Long Island accent and sunny personality made her an instant star. She appeared on late-night talk shows and toured the country on behalf of the drink. Kaufman said she was getting three thousand letters a week by 1996, when the campaign was canceled.

One of the byproducts of the company's explosion was a string of damaging rumors—some laughable—perhaps created by rivals. One story claimed Snapple was anti-abortion. Another said it supported the Ku Klux Klan because its bottles were printed with a *k* enclosed in a circle (actually the sign for "kosher"). Snapple hired private investigators but never discovered the source of the whisper campaigns.

In 1994, Quaker Oats bought Snapple for an astonishing $1.7 billion. The three Snapple founders each made more than $127 million. Sales, however, soon slowed, and three years later, Quaker dumped the beverage company for just $300 million. The *Los Angeles Times* called the original deal "one of the worst flops in corporate-merger history." In 2002 Snapple was sold to Cadbury Schweppes for $1.45 billion. It is now part of a spin-off company called Dr Pepper Snapple Group, based in Texas.

In 2003 Snapple announced a controversial five-year, $166 million deal to become the official beverage of New York City. The company gained exclusive rights to place vending machines in municipal buildings, including public schools, police stations, and sanitation depots. The deal called for Snapple to pay the city $8 million a year for five years, as well as another $13 million a year, depending on sales. Snapple would also put $12 million a year into ads to promote the city. The partnership was called hypocritical by some, considering it was championed by a mayor, Michael Bloomberg, who was on a mission to combat obesity and would later attempt to ban sugary drinks over sixteen ounces. In the end, the deal proved to be a disaster. Bloomberg had projected that a million cases of Snapple would be sold each year. Only fifty thousand were sold the first year and seventy thousand the second. In 2005 the partnership was reworked after sales in city buildings fell 93 percent below projections. The new deal was valued at just $33 million.

See also TEA and SODA.

Chawkins, Steve. "Leonard Marsh Dies at 80; Cofounder and Former CEO of Snapple." *Los Angeles Times*, May 25, 2013.

Winters, Patricia. "Snapple Secret: Friendship." *New York Daily News*, March 21, 1994.

Reed Tucker

Soda

Soda has been and continues to be one of New York's most popular drinks, ever since it was first sold in the early nineteenth century. Who precisely sold the first soda in the city has been debated, but most sources credit Benjamin Silliman, a Yale chemistry professor. Silliman and a partner purchased costly soda-making equipment in 1809 and opened two retail soda-water outlets, one at the City Hotel, near Trinity Church on Broadway, and the other at the Tontine Coffee House at Wall and Water Streets (the New York Stock Exchange first met on the second floor). Silliman sold soda or seltzer (plain carbonated water) freshly made on the premises. In 1819 a traveler in the city observed that ice-chilled soda water, a "pleasant and healthful drink," was sold "on every street corner" in the summer and that some were sold at soda shops in Greenwich Village. Despite the popularity of the novel beverage, its production could be difficult and dangerous: the carbonation was produced under high pressure using

sulfuric acid. Workers could be seriously burned by the acid, and containers of charged soda water sometimes exploded. Despite the risks involved in making it, soda water continued to be an important part of the city's beverage menu.

John Mathews, who had worked in the soda industry for several years in England, immigrated to New York in 1832. He had learned how to make and build carbonating machinery from Joseph Bramah, a British inventor. Mathews introduced a new "apparatus for charging water with carbon dioxide gas" that was much safer than the old method. He supplied carbonated water to vendors but also manufactured and sold the charging apparatus. From that point on the American soda industry rapidly expanded. Because of his influential role, Mathews is considered the "father of American soda water."

During its early years, "soda" was simply plain carbonated water, served refreshingly cold. This changed in the mid-nineteenth century, when some vendors began selling a spicier version of soda called "ginger pop." The identifying sign of these vendors depicted two men "dueling" with bottles instead of pistols, with a cork and a stream of liquid flying forth from each bottle like a bullet from a gun.

Plain soda was cheap at two cents per glass; flavored soda cost a nickel, which was still affordable to virtually all New Yorkers. On Wall Street stood Delatour's soda-water stand, which during the summers dispensed soda water and mineral water to long lines of customers.

The late nineteenth century saw the birth of the soda fountain. These were originally installed in restaurants, drugstores, and department stores, but soon there were stand-alone fountains, which typically sold a variety of soda flavors and ice cream. The two were soon combined into a perennial favorite, the ice cream soda.

Soda fountains offered a wide selection of flavors, made by mixing soda with syrups. One New York City fountain offered thirty-two different syrups, eight kinds of mineral water, and plain soda water. Another reportedly had three hundred flavors. Aside from flavorings, other ingredients were added to soda to make specialty fountain drinks: a popular one during the 1880s was made with chocolate syrup, cream, and raw eggs.

The temperance movement threw its support behind soda fountains, which the anti-alcohol faction saw as more desirable alternatives to bars, saloons, or taverns. By 1891, the city had more soda fountains than it had bars.

"Jewish Champagne"

By comparison to other groups, most immigrant Jews drank little alcohol, and bars and saloons languished in neighborhoods where Jews settled. As an alternative, two companies owned by Jews began manufacturing soda water, which the immigrants found an acceptable substitute for European mineral waters. By 1899 the Lower East Side, the heart of Jewish New York, had twenty soda shops. When the Sugar Trust's activities increased the price of sugar, Jewish soda manufacturers switched over to bottling seltzer (plain soda water), referred to as "Jewish champagne" and labeled the "staple beverage of Yiddish New York." By 1907 there were more than one hundred Jewish seltzer manufacturers in the city. The water was bottled in glass, with a metal siphon that maintained the carbonation until the water was dispensed. A Brooklyn candy-store owner, Louis Auster, has been credited with inventing one of the city's iconic beverages, the egg cream. Despite its name, which suggests the richer drink described above, this classic fountain beverage contains only soda water, milk, and chocolate syrup.

Pepsi-Cola

Pepsi-Cola was widely promoted and sold in New York beginning in the early twentieth century. Loft's, a chain of candy stores, acquired a chain of soda fountains that sold Coca-Cola. Loft's president, Charles Guth, requested a wholesale discount from Coca-Cola, but he was turned down. When Pepsi-Cola went bankrupt during the Depression, Guth acquired the company and moved its operations to New York City. He had Pepsi's formula modified to his liking and then canceled his contract with Coca-Cola and relaunched Pepsi. A large Pepsi bottling plant was built in Long Island City, with corporate headquarters located in Manhattan. The headquarters moved out of Manhattan to Purchase, New York, in 1970; the bottling plant closed in 1999.

Soda Regulation

Soda has remained one of New Yorkers' favorite beverages, sold in supermarkets, bodegas, restaurants, and fast-food operations and dispensed from vending machines throughout the city. For decades, offices, hospitals, and other public institutions were equipped with soda machines. In the early 1990s, cash-poor New York City schools began selling "pouring rights" to large soda companies, which then supplied vending machines and snack bars with their products. By the early twenty-first century, 80 percent of the city's high schools and half of its elementary schools sold sugary sodas. During the early twenty-first century, sugary soda was identified as a major contributor to the U.S. obesity epidemic. Since about half of adult New Yorkers and almost 40 percent of the city's public elementary and middle school students are obese or overweight, sugar-sweetened sodas were removed from machines in public schools and other public institutions in 2005, replaced by beverages supplied with Snapple-brand beverages. This was done in hopes of reducing obesity and controlling the rising incidence and cost of diet-related chronic diseases (estimated at $2.8 billion annually in New York City in 2013).

In 2010, as part of a larger campaign against obesity in New York City, Mayor Michael Bloomberg proposed that the Supplemental Nutrition Assistance Program (SNAP, formerly known as "food stamps") exclude soda and other sugared drinks from the food purchases it covers. The proposal was rejected by the U.S. Department of Agriculture, which runs the program.

In yet another attempt to fight the rising tide of obesity in New York City, in 2012 the city's Board of Health approved Mayor Bloomberg's proposal to limit the size of sugared drinks to no more than sixteen ounces when the beverages were sold at movie theaters, restaurants, mobile food carts, and sports arenas. The city's health commissioner, Thomas Farley, predicted that this regulation could help New Yorkers "avoid gaining some 2.3 million pounds a year." The soda and fast-food industries countered by forming a lobbying group, New Yorkers for Beverage Choices, to challenge the regulation. Theaters complained that they would lose an estimated 20 percent of total profits on their refreshment sales. Others pointed out that the regulation did not apply to grocery stores, where anyone could still buy soda in a one- or two-liter bottle. The fast-food industry complained that necessary adjustments to their drink-dispensing equipment would cost millions of dollars, thereby cutting into profits. The regulation was challenged in court and struck down by a judge, who called the regulation arbitrary in that it applied only to certain beverages in certain retail settings. The decision was appealed, but the lower court's decision was upheld.

See also EGG CREAMS; JEWISH; LOFT'S CANDY STORES; PEPSI-COLA; SELTZER; SODA "BAN"; SODA FOUNTAINS; and TEMPERANCE MOVEMENT.

Smith, Andrew F. *Drinking History: Fifteen Turning Points in the Making of American Beverages.* New York: Columbia University Press, 2012.
Stoddard, Bob. *Pepsi: 100 Years.* Los Angeles: General Pub. Group, 1999.

Andrew F. Smith

Soda "Ban"

The title of this article is a pejorative reference to New York City Mayor Michael Bloomberg's proposal in 2012 to restrict the size of sugar-sweetened beverages sold in specific restaurants and stores—those under city jurisdiction—to sixteen ounces or less. City officials called their proposal the Sugary Drink Portion Cap Rule and intended it to apply to drinks containing more than twenty-five sugar calories in eight ounces. Although customers could order as many sixteen-ounce servings as they wished, opponents quickly framed the proposal as a "ban."

The proposed rule logically followed a series of city campaigns aimed at encouraging New Yorkers to reduce consumption of sugary drinks as the first line of defense against obesity. Health Department posters and videos illustrated the amount of sugar in sodas, how soda sugars are converted to fat in the body, the number of miles that must be walked to compensate for soda calories, and the link between large soda portions and amputations resulting from type 2 diabetes. The city also tried—but failed—to obtain permission from the U.S. Department of Agriculture to restrict sales of sodas to participants in the Supplemental Nutrition Assistance Program (formerly food stamps).

City officials were convinced that the health risks associated with excessive soda consumption were well established, and they knew that soda sizes had increased in recent years. Just one sixteen-ounce soda contains the entire amount of sugar—fifty grams or twelve teaspoons—appropriate for an entire day.

Because sugar-sweetened beverages are highly profitable, and larger sizes even more so, the Cap Rule elicited fierce opposition. The soda industry trade group, the American Beverage Association (ABA), mounted a massive public relations campaign to convince New Yorkers that the "ban" was an expression of "nanny-state" politics and an infringement on freedom of choice. The ABA funded an ostensibly grassroots "front" organization to oppose the rule. It paid volunteers to collect signatures on opposing petitions; put signs on delivery trucks ("Don't let bureaucrats tell you what size beverage to buy"); ran advertisements on television, in movie theaters, and on airplane banners; and sent mailings to homes with instructions about how to protest.

The city argued that it had the authority to enact such public health measures if its mayor-appointed Board of Health agreed, which it did in September 2012. The rule was to go into effect six months later, which gave the ABA time to organize a coalition of community organizations to join it in petitioning the state Supreme Court to stop the Cap Rule or declare it unconstitutional. Indeed, the court blocked the rule one day before it was to go into effect, terming it "arbitrary and capricious" because it applied only to places under city jurisdiction (and, therefore,

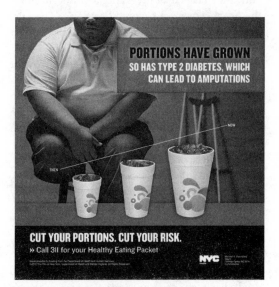

NYC.gov poster showing the growing volume of beverage containers over time, illustrating the connection between larger soda sizes and type-2 diabetes. This campaign came under criticism when the "amputee" turned out to be Photoshopped from a stock photo. NYC.GOV

not to grocery stores, bodegas, or convenience stores, which are under the jurisdiction of the New York State Department of Agriculture and Markets) and set no limits on refills.

The city appealed, but the State Appellate Court confirmed the injunction in July 2013. It ruled that the City Council, not the mayor's Board of Health, had the authority to pass such rules. In June 2014, the State Appeals Court agreed. Thus, what started out as a legal challenge to the Cap Rule ended up as a challenge to the question of whether the city's Board of Health has the authority to pass regulations designed to protect the health of its citizens.

Why had the mayor not gone to the City Council for approval? He knew that the majority of City Council members, who had been lobbied heavily—and sometimes supported—by soda companies, would oppose it. City officials believed that the Board of Health did have the necessary authority and would be an easier route.

Funding by soda companies explains some of the otherwise surprising opposition to the rule. While it is understandable that the National Restaurant Association and the New York State Association of Theater Owners would oppose the rule, it is less obvious why community groups such as the New York State chapter of the National Association for the Advancement of Colored People and the Hispanic Federation did so. Although they argued that the rule was discriminatory, paternalistic, and damaging to minority-owned small businesses, they for years had accepted generous donations from Coca-Cola and PepsiCo.

While the legal challenges were in progress, the city eventually organized an impressive collection of medical, public health, and minority community groups to support the rule, but these efforts came too late to counter public opposition. In retrospect, the rule might have survived challenges more easily if the city had organized widespread public support from the start by linking the measure to broader efforts to serve the health needs of low-income New Yorkers.

Despite this setback, reducing the size of sugary drinks has much traction. Soda sales are declining in the United States, and soda company officials are well aware that serving sizes must be reduced. Soon after the demise of the Cap Rule, the seven-and-one-half-ounce mini-cans became the most important driver of soda sales in North America.

See also BLOOMBERG, MICHAEL and PEPSI-COLA.

Confessore, Nicholas. "Minority Groups and Bottlers Team Up in Battles over Soda." *New York Times*, March 12, 2013.

Nestle, Marion. *Soda Politics: Taking on Big Soda (and Winning)*. New York: Oxford University Press, 2015.

New York City Department of Health and Mental Hygiene. "Sugary Drink Portion Cap Rule: Fact vs. Fiction." http://www.nyc.gov/html/doh/downloads/pdf/cdp/sugary-drink-facts.pdf.

Vartanian, Lenny R., Marlene B. Schwartz, and Kelly D. Brownell. "Effects of Soft Drink Consumption on Nutrition and Health: A Systematic Review and Meta-Analysis." *American Journal of Public Health* 97 (2007): 667–675.

Marion Nestle

Soda Fountains

"Soda fountain" refers to both the mechanism that dispenses soda water and the establishment where it is installed. In the pre–air conditioning and refrigeration age, the cold carbonated water that flowed from these machines was a true wonder. Thousands of soda fountains dotted New York City between the mid-nineteenth and twentieth centuries that quenched the thirsts of drinkers from every social stratum.

Naturally carbonated water has been used as a health tonic since ancient times. European scientists first developed the process of artificially carbonating water in the eighteenth century. Soda water continued to be a popular health drink commonly served in pharmacies. Early fountains were small countertop contraptions connected by tubes to a carbonating machine that was chilled with ice.

One of the first people to popularize soda water beyond its medical usage was Benjamin Silliman, a Yale chemistry professor who was inspired to spread mineral water to the masses after a trip to a Saratoga Springs spa in 1806. He first sold carbonated water to a New Haven apothecary, and then he set his sights on New York City, where in 1809 he opened the Tontine Coffeehouse on Wall Street and installed a fountain at the City Hotel. Both fountains were operated by a manual pump and did not always provide uniform carbonation. One of Silliman's later rivals was John Matthews, who developed and sold a sophisticated fountain in the 1830s that used sulfuric acid and marble chips that he originally

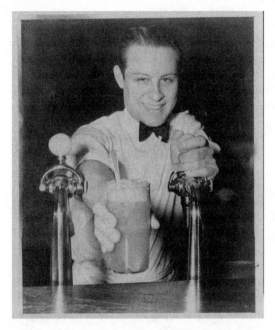

A "soda jerk" passing ice cream soda between two soda fountains, December 19, 1936. The froth on top of the drink is a chemical reaction from the salt in the ice cream that made ice cream floats so popular. STAFF PHOTO BY ALAN FISHER / LIBRARY OF CONGRESS

purchased from the construction site of Saint Patrick's Cathedral. Matthews continued to improve his models for years, and by the 1860s he was running a large soda fountain factory on Twenty-Sixth Street and First Avenue.

As more soda parlors popped up around the city, some began offering flavored syrups. By the end of the century there were hundreds of different varieties available, such as celery tonic, ginger, nectar, pepsin, sarsaparilla, root beer, and champagne. Customers could add fruit, phosphates, egg, malted milk, or *koumyss* (a fermented milk beverage) to their drinks. Soda jerks, as the fountain operators were known, entertained customers as they theatrically mixed up their concoctions. Establishments vied for attention by purchasing the latest elaborately decorated fountain or hulking spectacle. The largest fountain measured 40 feet long and was built for a Riker's drugstore at Sixth Avenue and Twenty-Third Street.

By the end of the nineteenth century there were an estimated fifty thousand to sixty thousand soda fountains across the United States in 1895, mostly in urban areas. Though soda water could still be purchased at almost any drugstore, most sales were for nonmedicinal purposes. In New York, soda fountains were also found in hundreds of department stores, haberdasheries, confectionaries, hotels, and restaurants and soda was even dispensed by sidewalk vendors. Two of the busiest fountains were at pharmacies near the Brooklyn Bridge, where soda water was made all day and night.

Soda fountains were particularly popular with women as they could not dine at restaurants without a male companion. Some parlors even advertised directly to women, like Huyler's, a popular New York City chain that promoted their fountains as "the shrine before which the Vassar girl bows down in worship." As a clean and wholesome alternative to the speakeasy, the number of soda fountains in New York City swelled during Prohibition. Establishments responded by expanding their menus to include light meals and, increasingly, ice cream—an addition that would later play a role in the downfall of soda fountain culture.

Ice cream sodas had become popular after the Civil War, and by the end of the nineteenth century they were soda fountain staples, along with sundaes. More ice cream was sold at soda fountains than at ice cream parlors. After World War II, soda fountains were still found in most drugstores, but as people moved out of the cities and into the suburbs, a culture of highways and fast-food chains replaced the neighborhood soda parlor hangout. Ice cream could now also be easily purchased at supermarkets and stored in home freezers. By the end of the 1960s the bottled soft drink market had exploded, marking the final chapter of the soda fountain era. Today soda fountains are seeing a small revival in New York City at restaurants such as the Brooklyn Farmacy & Soda Fountain in Carroll Gardens, Bubby's in TriBeCa, Fort Defiance in Red Hook, and Northern Spy Food Co. in the East Village.

See also EGG CREAMS; SELTZER; and SODA.

Funderburg, Ann Cooper. *Chocolate, Strawberry, and Vanilla: A History of American Ice Cream*. Bowling Green, Ohio: Bowling Green State University Popular Press, 1995.

Funderburg, Anne Cooper. *Sundae Best: A History of Soda Fountains*. Bowling Green, Ohio: Bowling Green State University Popular Press, 2002.

Quinzio, Jeri. *Of Sugar and Snow: A History of Ice Cream Making*. Berkeley: University of California Press, 2009.

Adee Braun

Soda Water

See SELTZER and SODA.

Sokolov, Raymond

Raymond Sokolov has been a writer, journalist, cookbook author, and restaurant critic. Born August 1, 1941, in Detroit, Michigan, his interest in journalism blossomed at age ten, when he was interviewed following his precocious victory in a spelling bee. He was educated at Harvard, writing for *The Crimson* and spending summers in the early 1960s eating his way through Europe. He was deep into his doctoral research in Homeric Greek when, in 1965, he was offered a position as a correspondent in *Newsweek*'s Paris bureau. There he published his first piece of food journalism, a review of Robert Carrier's *The Connoisseur's Cookbook*. Returning to New York in 1967, he continued writing for *Newsweek*'s culture desk until he was hired by the *New York Times* to replace the venerable Craig Claiborne as the paper's food editor in 1971.

Sokolov lacked formal training in cookery and had no obvious qualifications to step into Claiborne's shoes. Befitting that politically turbulent era, he shook up the New York culinary world with his restaurant reviews and editorial choices. He found many of New York's classic French restaurants mediocre but was thrilled by the unfamiliar cooking of immigrants arriving in the wake of the 1965 Immigration and Nationality Act, especially the fiery cuisines of Sichuan and other mainland Chinese provinces. Breaking away from the *Times*'s Eurocentric bias, he awarded the paper's coveted four-star rating to Hunam, a Midtown spot preparing Hunan cuisine. Sokolov also wrote provocatively about serious issues in the guise of food writing, sampling prison food on site after a food riot sparked the deadly 1972 Attica uprising and taste-testing eleven dog foods (along with his pooch) while reporting that Americans spent four times more on commercial food for Fido than for Baby. Shortly thereafter, he was fired. Looking back, Sokolov called the *Times* an "inappropriate perch for an intellectual child of the sixties with a scornful view of the New York food scene and its class-bound standards."

Sokolov's subsequent career matched his polymath interests: for twenty years he wrote A Matter of Taste, a monthly gastro-ethnographic column for *Natural History*, the journal of the American Museum of Natural History. His essays deconstructed the culinary code of nouvelle cuisine, reported on American regional cookery, explored botanical exotica, and unraveled the gastronomic ramifications of the Columbian Exchange. Even when employed in nonculinary posts, including as founding editor of the Leisure and Arts page for the *Wall Street Journal*, a position he held until 2002, he never left food entirely: he published several cookbooks and works of culinary history, among them *The Saucier's Apprentice* (1976), *Why We Eat What We Eat* (1991), *With the Grain* (1996), and *The Cook's Canon* (2003). From 2007 to 2010, he traveled throughout the United States and Europe, writing restaurant reviews for the *Wall Street Journal*. Sokolov now resides in New York's Hudson River Valley.

See also AMERICAN MUSEUM OF NATURAL HISTORY; CLAIBORNE, CRAIG; and NEW YORK TIMES.

Sokolov, Raymond. *Steal the Menu: A Memoir of Forty Years in Food*. New York: Knopf, 2013.

Cathy K. Kaufman

Soltner, André

André Soltner was the chef at Lutèce from 1961 to 1994, during which time it became known as the finest French restaurant in America. See LUTÈCE. Born in the Alsace region of France in 1932, Soltner was discovered in 1961 at Chez Hansi in Paris, where he had recently been promoted to head chef, and was lured to America by Lutèce's original owner, André Surmain, who was looking for an exciting chef for his new restaurant, located in a gray townhouse at 249 East Fiftieth Street in Manhattan. Four years later, Surmain made Soltner a partner in the restaurant as promised (Soltner had threatened to quit otherwise), and in 1972 Soltner bought out Surmain, ushering in Lutèce's greatest era and winning a fourth star from the *New York Times*.

In a New York restaurant scene that was largely dominated by restaurateurs, Soltner was a traditional chef-owner who cooked in the kitchen while his wife Simone ran the front of the house. They lived above the restaurant and were there for every service. On Sundays, Monday lunch, and the entire month of August, while Soltner was away, Lutèce was closed. Much beloved by his staff, his customers, and other chefs, Soltner was famous for never raising his voice in the kitchen. Modest but stubborn, he turned down all offers to open additional restaurants, make commercial endorsements, or host a cooking show. Soltner explained that his place was in Lutèce's kitchen or going into the dining rooms, always in his chef's white and high toque, to chat with customers, make suggestions, and take orders.

More interested in taste than in presentation or innovation for its own sake, Soltner cooked traditional French and Alsatian cuisine, presented classically but simply. His focus was on getting the best and freshest ingredients, locally sourced if possible, and it was his promise to buy fresh fois gras that led Ariane Daguin to found D'Artagnan. Soltner sold Lutèce in 1994, the vast majority of his staff (nearly all of whom had worked under him for many years) left with him, and the restaurant limped along for another decade before closing. Soltner became the dean of classic studies at the French Culinary Institute (now the International Culinary Center), where he has taught and mentored young chefs for over twenty years. With Seymour Britchky, he is the author of *The Lutèce Cookbook* (1995).

"Chow Time: Mimi Sheraton and Andre Soltner on What's Changed since Lutèce." Capital New York, January 4, 2011. http://www.capitalnewyork.com/ article/culture/2011/01/1078267/chow-time-mimi- sheraton-and-andre-soltner-whats-changed-lutece.
Schrambling, Regina. "A Chef in Full: Soltner Beyond the Kitchen." *New York Times*, December 8, 2000.

Marc P. Levy

Soulé, Henri

Henri Soulé (1903–1966) reestablished French haute cuisine in New York City through his Manhattan restaurant, Le Pavillon. Born in Saubrigues, in southwestern France, in 1903, Soulé began his restaurant career as a busboy at the Hotel Continental in Bayonne and then as a waiter at Hotel Mirabeau, where he became captain. After stints at London's Trocadero Restaurant and elsewhere, in 1933 he became the manager and chief of staff at the Café de Paris. Charles Drouant, owner of Café de Paris in Paris and several other restaurants, was asked to organize and run the restaurant planned for the French Pavilion at the 1939 World's Fair in New York. Drouant asked Soulé to serve as its general manager. When Le Restaurant du Pavillon de France opened on May 9, 1939, it attracted a wide audience. Americans found the authentic French cuisine a revelation, and the *New York Times* called the restaurant "an epicure's delight."

When the restaurant closed for the winter in October, World War II had started in Europe. Soulé returned to France, where he joined his unit in Bordeaux. In early 1940 he was demobilized and sent back to New York to reopen the French Pavilion restaurant. When it closed for good on October 27, 1940, France was occupied by the German army. Most of those who had come from France to cook and serve at the restaurant decided not to return home at that time.

Once the World's Fair had ended, it occurred to Drouant to open a restaurant in New York City. He sought investors, one of whom may have been Joseph P. Kennedy, father of the future president John F. Kennedy. When Drouant decided to go back to France, Soulé took over. He found a suitable location on New York's fashionable Upper East Side, and hoping to attract the patrons he had served at the World's Fair, he named the establishment "Le Pavillon." Soulé was joined by many of his former colleagues, including Pierre Franey, who had been the *poisson commis* (assistant fish cook).

Soulé invited the rich, famous, and powerful to the restaurant's opening on October 15, 1941. Le Pavillon was an unqualified success from the beginning, even as the United States entered the war less than two months later. Franey enlisted in the U.S. Army and helped liberate France. He returned to rejoin the staff at Le Pavillon and moved steadily up the ranks, becoming executive chef in the early 1950s.

New York's wealthiest and most prominent citizens—Astors, Cabots, Kennedys, Rockefellers, and Vanderbilts—were regulars at Le Pavillon. The autocratic Soulé made a virtue of snobbery. Under the guise of protecting the sensibilities of his refined customers, he refused entrance to anyone who did not meet his standards. Soulé is also thought to have coined the term "Siberia," referring to the tables closest to the kitchen (the least desirable in most restaurants). Buoyed by the success of Le Pavillon, in October 1958 Soulé opened La Côte Basque, a slightly more casual alternative to Le Pavillon.

Then came 1960, an unfortunate year for Le Pavillon. The economy slumped, affecting the restaurant's bottom line. Soulé ordered a staff reduction at Le Pavillon, but Franey refused to dismiss anyone from his *brigade de cuisine*. Newcomer Jacques Pépin, a rising star who had been at the restaurant for just eight months, joined Franey in his protest, and the two walked out, forcing Le Pavillon to close temporarily, though it opened later with a new staff. (In a dramatic shift, both Franey and Pépin went to work for the Howard Johnson's restaurant chain, where the money was better and the hours less onerous.) Chef Roger Fessaguet left Le Pavillon as well, becoming executive chef at La Caravelle, owned by Fred Decré and Robert Meyzen.

When Soulé died in 1966, Craig Claiborne eulogized him as the "Michelangelo, the Mozart and Leonardo of the French restaurant in America." Le Pavillon survived a few years after Soulé's death. Though it was replaced by other fashionable French restaurants, adherence to Escoffier's precepts was no longer de rigueur. Chefs forged new paths, taking inspiration from other cuisines and creating novel variations on the classics. Soulé's greatest achievement, according to Claiborne, was his nurturing of chefs, restaurateurs, and other individuals who were influential in America's fine dining scene.

See also CLAIBORNE, CRAIG; FRENCH; HAUTE CUISINE; LE PAVILLON; and WORLD'S FAIR, 1939–1940.

Batterberry, Michael, and Ariane Batterberry. *On the Town in New York: The Landmark History of Eating, Drinking, and Entertainments from the American Revolution to the Food Revolution.* New York and London: Routledge, 1999.
Claiborne, Craig. "In Classic Tradition, Henri Soule had Towering Standards in Pursuit of Gastronomic Perfection." *New York Times,* January 28, 1966.
Kuh, Patric. *The Last Days of Haute Cuisine: America's Culinary Revolution.* New York: Viking, 2001.
Wechsberg, Joseph. *Dining at the Pavillon.* Boston: Little, Brown, 1962.

Andrew F. Smith

Soul Food

See AFRICAN AMERICAN; HARLEM; and SYLVIA'S.

Soup Kitchens

See HUNGER PROGRAMS.

South and Central American

United States immigration laws curtailed the arrival of South and Central Americans until the mid-1960s, when the Immigration Act of 1965 reversed legislative restrictions that had existed since 1924. In 2013, a U.S. Census poll estimated that Latinos made up 28.6 percent of New York City's population. Dominicans

and Puerto Ricans who claim Caribbean heritage account for a large percentage of that group concentrated primarily in Manhattan and the Bronx. The predominance of Caribbean Latinos is reflected in the food landscapes of those boroughs and throughout the city where "Spanish food" and "Spanish restaurants" abound and are synonymous in New York parlance with the flavor profiles and food of these two groups. Mexican immigrants, who represent the Latino majority throughout the rest of the country, make up the third largest Latino ethnic group throughout the five boroughs and have a less conspicuous influence on the palates of New Yorkers than in cities like Chicago and Los Angeles. The remainder of the Latino population in New York is made up of immigrants from every country in Central and South America and these groups have tended to settle in Queens.

Though showcased to varying degrees in grocery stores and restaurants around the city, nowhere is the culinary diversity and presence of Central and South American people better represented and more concentrated than Queens. In the neighborhoods of the city's most culturally, ethnically, and linguistically diverse borough you can take a culinary tour of Central and South America, finding restaurants, food trucks, and food carts that allow exploration of flavors and ingredients from Mexico to Chile and back again. Throughout the borough it is possible to find tacos, tortas, and varieties of tamales from across both regions, and pastries from Argentina and Uruguay, as well as Paraguayan and Surinamese restaurants. In Corona, Elmhurst, and Jackson Heights, a large number of people from every Central American country, as well as Colombians, Peruvians, Ecuadorians, and Mexicans mingle, making those neighborhoods the perfect place to sample different interpretations of chicken and rice, tamales, or other masa-based dishes. Corona is also the location of Tortilleria Nixtamal, which makes and sells fresh tortillas and prepared masa and whose products can be found in stores throughout New York City.

Argentina, Chile, and Brazil are represented in Jackson Heights, Woodside, Sunnyside, and Astoria. In fact, the only Chilean and Paraguayan restaurants in the city are found in Sunnyside and Astoria, respectively. Argentinian and Brazilian churrascarias (restaurants traditionally serving only grilled meat and a few complimentary sides popular in Brazil, Argentina, Paraguay, and Uruguay) can be found throughout Astoria. Little Brazil in Astoria along Thirty-Sixth

Street is a wonderful place to eat and shop in Brazilian grocery stores and produce markets for popular products from Brazil, Argentina, Uruguay, and Paraguay.

In Woodside, Mi Tierra grocery store carries a wide array of products from all over Central and South America. Food trucks and carts serving street foods abound in Jackson Heights. They are a long-standing tradition in Central and South American countries, and a host of them serve tamales, *elotes* (corn on or cut from the cob served with condiments including chile powder, lime juice, cheese, and mayonnaise), tropical fruit juices, ices and ice creams from the regions, grilled meats, and other small bites. Finally, there are bakeries from Argentina and Uruguay serving pastries and cakes: the Argentinian Rio de la Plata Panaderia and Confiteria, known for dulce de leche cakes and empanadas, and Uruguayan La Nueva Bakery, which sells *alfajores,* sandwich cookies made of cornstarch or finely ground manioc flour and filled with dulce de leche, and *arrollados*, a rolled cake commonly filled with dulce de leche, alongside sandwiches and savory dishes.

Richmond Hill's Little Guyana is home to Guyanese of South Asian descent as well as a number of Guyanese restaurants, bakeries, and grocery stores that sell spices and other ingredients used in South Asian Guyanese cooking. Richmond Hill is also the home to immigrants from Suriname and the only Surinamese restaurants in the city.

As immigration from Central and South American countries to New York City continues to grow, so too will the culinary landscape of Queens and the rest of the city. These immigrants will contribute new flavors and ingredients to the city's already diverse ethnic mix.

See also CARIBBEAN and QUEENS.

Lynn, Andrea. *Queens, A Culinary Passport: Exploring Ethnic Cuisine in New York City's Most Diverse Borough.* New York: St. Martin's Griffin, 2014.
Peralta, Marlene. "Latinos in Queens: Much Diversity, Little Political Clout." Voices of NY, September 16, 2014. http://www.voicesofny.org/2014/09/latinos-queens-much-diversity-little-political-clout.
Semple, Kirk. "Take the A Train to Little Guyana." *New York Times,* June 8, 2013.
Torres, Andrés. "Latino New York: An Introduction." *NACLA Report on the Americas,* Winter 2013.
U.S. Census Bureau. "New York (city)/New York." Quick Facts. http://quickfacts.census.gov/qfd/states/36/3651000.html.

Rachel Monet Finn

South Asian

The earliest archival trace of South Asian food in New York is among a group of itinerant merchants selling textiles between Chittagong in East Bengal, New Orleans, and New York at the end of the nineteenth century. They established the first settlements often in black neighborhoods, replete with cafes, restaurants, cookshops, and tea shops. Harlem may have been home to East Coast America's first Indian restaurants directed toward its own community, which did not leave any trace in print (and could only be recovered by interviews with the aged children of the original inhabitants). Arguably, the place that served more Indian meals than any other in Manhattan by the early twentieth century was at the four-story building at 100 West Thirty-Eighth Street, home of the segregated British Merchant Sailors' Club for Indian Seamen, which had a mess hall that seated eighty people and in the first year served 198,200 meals.

The first visible Indian restaurant, established in 1913 in New York City, was named Ceylon India Inn on Eighth Avenue and Forty-Ninth Street, where it became a center of Indian nationalist activity. But the owner, K. Y. Kira, sought to reorient its focus from inside the community to outside it—as was becoming common with the demand for ethnic food among a new Anglo-American middle class.

By the 1920s the locus of the discussion of Indian food shifted to the takeover of the Royal British Navy by "little brown men"—often called "lascars"—who ate rice and curry onboard ship. In a 1925 article in the *New York Times,* John Carter explained that "the shift of economic forces during and since the war [World War I] has left little of her British character, save the

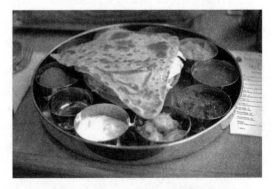

A South Indian lunch tray at Saravana Bhavan, in the Kips Bay area of Manhattan. JONATHAN MCINTOSH

officers, who are English." He complained that the religion of these new entrants to shipping "demands that they shall eat no meat unless it has been slaughtered in accordance with the prescribed ritual. The diet of Indian Moslems consists of mutton, curry and rice: rice, curry and mutton ad infinitum." There were other perverse problems with these Orientals, Carter continued, specifically their propensity to contract strange ailments from curses and such others and promptly die from them, to the great inconvenience of the captain. Although paid lower wages, to Carter it was not clear that Orientals were cheaper to run a shipping line because a crew of "fifty British will handle a vessel for which seventy lascars would be hardly enough. Moreover, Orientals, for all their philosophies of Nirvana and of indifference to death, nearly always grow panic-stricken in an emergency, with corresponding risk to vessel and cargo." It is these lascars who, on jumping ship, would give us the first chain of cheap curry houses in the Western metropolis.

It appears from the frequency of discussion about curry in the course of World War II that media coverage of the Indian national movement led by Mahatma Gandhi, requirements of a low-protein wartime diet (with its flavor challenges), and exposure to the taste of Allied Indian troops conspired to put curry on the American palate, at least of gastronomes and journalists such as Jane Holt of the *New York Times*. She often worked in conjunction with the Civilian Defense Volunteer Office (with an interest in civilian nutrition, especially vitamin deficiency) and trade organizations such as the Spice Trader's Association. Where Holt left off, Jane Nickerson continued, in her News of Food column, announcing the "first direct shipment of curry powder since the war" to arrive from Madras on September 7, 1946, and informing us that "the East India Curry Shop [is] a restaurant that probably serves the most 'authentic' curries in town."

Richard Huey, who sang the hit "Bloomer Girl," opened Aunt Dinah's Kitchen in 1935, which served southern fried chicken, barbecue, Mexican chili, sweet potato pie, and East Indian curry. The 1939 Works Progress Administration guide to New York City listed four "East Indian Restaurants." The four Indian restaurants listed in the *Manhattan Telephone Directory* by 1949—the earliest reference in a telephone directory to a cluster of Indian restaurants in New York—are India Bengal Garden, India Prince, India Rajah, and India Restaurant. By the late 1940s advertisements for Indian restaurants such as India's Garden Inn proliferated in the pages of the African American *New York Amsterdam News*. The 1956 edition of *Menu: The Restaurant Guide of New York* identified three Indian restaurants serving curries, samosa, shish kebab, and rijsttafel.

That pattern of a few places with mixed reviews continued into the 1970s. The 1978 edition of *Mary Waldo's Restaurant Guide to New York City and Vicinity* lists nineteen Indian and Pakistani restaurants. The *New York Times* had more than one hundred articles on Indian food in the 1970s compared to thirteen in the 1960s. It was in the 1980s that Indian food decisively moved from the category of the exotic, rare, and subcultural to the ubiquitous and the numbers began to shift from Queens to Manhattan. By 1989, Dawat, perhaps the best Indian restaurant in New York City at that time, pulled itself into gastronomic discourse by claiming that it served "The 'Haute' Cuisine of India... under the culinary supervision of Madhur Jaffrey, who has been called, 'the finest authority on Indian cooking in America' by Craig Claiborne." It managed to say all that in its tiny advertisement in the *NYNEX Yellow Pages*. Through the decade of the 1990s the *New York Times* carried three hundred articles on Indian food compared to 1,264 on Italian, 840 on Chinese, 368 on Japanese, and 316 on Mexican, adding Indian to the regular repertoire of the ethnic American restaurant.

Most of the three hundred–odd Indian restaurants today, with names such as Mughal Raj, Tandoor, Taj, Baluchi's, and Bombay Grill, serve northern menus. Many of these restaurants are owned by Pakistani and Bangladeshi immigrants and can be classified by price and offerings as cheap curry houses—with an average price of entrées at $11.21 (average of all the restaurants with prices on their menu), appetizers at $5.21, and desserts at $3.50, for a total meal for one at $18.56 in 2014. About one-fourth of these eateries are clustered in half a dozen neighborhoods, such as on Sixth Street between First and Second Avenues (about a dozen restaurants) and Murray Hill (about two dozen eateries on Lexington Avenue between Twenty-Sixth and Thirty-First Streets) in Manhattan. In the borough of Queens there are concentrations in Jackson Heights on Seventy-Fourth Street between Roosevelt and Thirty-Seventh Avenue (about two dozen) and Richmond Hills (about half a dozen). In the borough of Brooklyn there are a handful of Pakistani places on Coney Island.

In contrast to the cheap curry house, there is a small selection of expensive Indian restaurants with named chefs—such as Devi, Tulsi, Ada, Amma, Junoon, and Tamarind—which are owned by expatriate Indians and Americans. These are sometimes the only Indian restaurants with a wine list that can get past the threshold of thirty-dollar entrées. New York City audiences continue to expect cheap Indian food and are often unwilling to pay for the necessary skilled labor and local and sustainable ingredients that have become de rigueur in upscale American restaurants.

Celebrity restaurateur Danny Meyer and Chef Floyd Cardoz, whose Indian-influenced haute cuisine restaurant Tabla closed in 2010 after twelve years, have noted that it was the first restaurant in their chain that would take a hit in a downturn because rich patrons were unwilling to pay top dollar for Indian food when the economy tightened. Between the ubiquitous cheap curry house and the rare thirty-dollar-entrée elite restaurant, Café Spice found a niche for a while with interesting lunch thalis for about twenty dollars. But they had to close their establishment on University Place in Lower Manhattan, squeezed between the recession and rising rents. Subsequently, they have learned to specialize in supplying Whole Foods and university cafeterias with prepared meals. That mid-market space is still relatively lightly populated by Indian restaurants, but a number of fast casual concepts are preparing to move into the twelve-dollar to fourteen-dollar lunch model popularized by Chipotle (these potential indie chains are self-consciously modeling themselves after it), with ambitions of serving "California-style Indian cuisine." Two concepts, one by Hasnaian Zaidi, a young Stanford-trained entrepreneur of Pakistani heritage with a microchain of restaurants named Tava-Indian coming out of Silicon Valley, and another by Basu Ratnam, Phil Suarez, and Jean-Georges Vongerichten named Inday, are hoping to spread the gospel of fast casual Indian food (without being too Indian) in the mid-market niche. At the same price point a solid southern Indian tiffin concept is Saravana Bhavan. Indian-style wraps and dosas have spawned a small genre of interesting fast casual concepts such as Hampton Chutney, Tiffin, and Thelawala.

New subregional South Asian cuisines—Sri Lankan, southern Indian, northeastern Indian—beyond the usual Punjabi, Mughlai, and Bangladeshi food, are beginning to be available in New York City. Excellent string hoppers and lamprie can be tasted at San Rasa on Staten Island and Sigiri in the East Village. Dosas, *uttapams*, and *vadas* can be conveniently acquired around Murray Hill (Manhattan) or Jackson Heights (Queens). New chains such as Saravana Bhavan have become the standard to beat for a crispy dosa or a cruchy *vada* with a spicy coconut–curry leaf–mustard dip. Gujarati vegetarian thalis, Chettinad mutton *kothu parotta*, Kolkata-style Bengali food, and Indian Chinese Hakka flavors are becoming familiar to Anglo foodies. Most interestingly a shift toward a Nepali labor force in Indian eateries and non-Indian restaurants, such as Japanese *ramen-yas*, is opening up the next phase of the ethnic succession, first in toil and then hopefully in taste.

The northern rim of the Himalayas, from Kashmir to the northeast of India and the extra-Indian domains of Nepal and Bhutan, are coming into view in the diaspora as some of the fastest-growing populations. Tara Niraula of the New School, who studies Nepali immigration, estimates that there are about twenty thousand Nepalis in Queens who are undercounted in the American Community Survey (estimated at under four thousand in New York City and 86,528 in the United States in 2011). Along with the swelling number of Nepali migrants, elements of Newari cuisine of the Kathmandu Valley, such as *sukula* (air-dried meat), bamboo shoots, *gundruk* (pan-fried fermented mustard leaves), minced buffalo liver with spices, along with various vegetable curries and rice, are becoming accessible in places such as the Woodside Café in Queens and Café Himalaya in the East Village. Yelp listed thirty-one self-described Himalayan restaurants (including Nepali, Bhutani, and Tibetan) in 2014.

This is a promising turn away from the Indian heartland. The northern rim and the peninsular edge of South Asia, which is where most South Asians live, have been barely visible in the cultural representation of the region, swamped by images from the Indo-Gangetic valleys and the northern-oriented taste of tandoori rotis, naans, dal makhni, channa masala, aloo gobi, samosas, butter chicken, raita, and other such canonical dishes, which are undeniably delicious but overexposed.

See also LITTLE INDIA and SOUTHEAST ASIAN.

Bald, Vivek. *Bengali Harlem and the Lost Histories of South Asian America*. Cambridge, Mass.: Harvard University Press, 2013.
Carter, John. "Little Brown Men Carry Britain's Flag." *New York Times*, August 30, 1925.

Cheshes, Jay. "The Chipotle Effect: How Chefs Are Reinventing Fast Food." *Wall Street Journal*, February 6, 2015.

Nickerson, Jane. "News of Food." *New York Times*, September 7, 1946.

NYNEX. *Manhattan Yellow Pages: Manhattan Area Code 212.* New York: NYNEX, 1988–1989, p. 1481.

van Gelder, Robert. "Introducing the 'I Got a Song' Man." *New York Times*, October 22, 1944.

Krishnendu Ray

Southeast Asian

For many Southeast Asian immigrants who have settled in New York City, the issue of food has gone beyond feeding the marginalized enclave and building "mom and pop" livelihoods to that of seeking their own identity on their own terms. On the forefront of this recent trend to "mainstream" their food are first-generation Asian Americans and newly arrived immigrants from a higher educational and socioeconomic level in their home countries—most of whom now look at the city as their own turf and are confident in staking a claim in the constantly evolving New York City restaurant scene.

The strategy of the contemporary generation is quite simple: run a small and flexible operation, open in a venue requiring less capital (pop-ups, food trucks, kiosks, carts) in spaces with less expensive rent, focus on a specific food type, and let one's culinary roots provide inspiration for new flavors, ingredients and spicing. Strange flavors are embedded in the comfort of the familiar such as sandwiches, soups, spring rolls, and noodles. The difference is that it is the Asian chef now putting his or her own stamp on a "reimagined and reconstructed" cuisine found only in New York City.

Num Pang, the Cambodian-owned sandwich chain, which has expanded to six locations in Manhattan, is a compelling case in point. In 2008, the *New York Times* wrote about the shrinking Cambodian community in the city. Faced with violence where many have settled in the Bronx and a bleak future in the city, many decided to seek employment opportunities elsewhere. The following year, an enterprising Cambodian chef, Ratha Chaupoly, opened his first sandwich shop near Union Square. The concept of a Cambodian version of the Vietnamese banh mi was an instant success. Freshly baked semolina loaves filled with pulled pork, fresh herbs, and a Cambodian slaw laced with his house dressing is one example which successfully instructs the diner that Cambodian food is easy to comprehend and friendly to the non-Asian palate.

Southeast Asian food in New York City comes from a disparate group of cultures transplanted from a subregion of Asia located south of China and east of India. Through the past few decades, there has been uneven representation in the city of cuisines coming from the three major areas of this region: the peninsula known as the Southeast Asian mainland, including Myanmar (Burma), Laos, Thailand, Vietnam, Cambodia, Malaysia, and Singapore, as well as the two archipelagos on the east and south of the mainland, the Philippines and Indonesia.

The immigrant communities that settled in the city in the latter part of the twentieth century came for different reasons. The 1962 military coup in Burma put in place a repressive regime that pushed out families to set up new and challenging lives in a city that had its equally harsh and dangerous side. The U.S. involvement in the French Indochina War (Vietnam War) brought an influx of refugees from Vietnam, Cambodia, and Laos in the 1970s and 1980s. A decade later, the Asian fiscal crisis of 1996 brought in a wave of Thais, Indonesians, and Malaysians whose once stable economies were now threatened by a fiscal meltdown felt throughout the world.

Southeast Asian Culture and Food as Exotica

Toward the end of the twentieth century, New York, a global city, gave rise to celebrity chefs and restaurateurs along with their high-profile architects whose designs gained brand status to attract a high-end market. In the mid-1980s, the restaurateur Brian McNally opened Indochine, which became a fashion industry hub. Using Vietnam as a cultural starting point, he designed a space with walls painted with lush green palms overlooking black and red rattan lounge chairs in the waiting area to give an illusion of a tropical French colonial oasis in the middle of industrial NoHo. Rolls of vegetables and shrimp wrapped in rice paper, dumplings, and some skewered chickens along with cucumber chili martinis were enough to convey a sense of Vietnamese food.

A decade later, David Rockwell, who designed and built Nobu in TriBeCa, created the iconic Vong for the Alsatian star chef Jean-Georges Vongerichten. The chef had spent several years in Thailand, and his knowledge of a hundred and fifty Asian spices (according to the restaurant's press release) conveyed some authenticity to his Thai-inspired French American cuisine. See THAI.

Both restaurants gained international status, sprinkling stardust on anyone lucky to snag a table on a given night. In the case of Indochine, it was a moment when two cultures on opposite ends of a power spectrum (two former archenemies of a divisive war) were forced to share the same space in unequal terms. And as Vong's star finally dimmed and closed in 2009, it would be the last time such a powerful combination of east and west would be tried again with great success, fanfare, and longevity.

The Persistence of Culture

The flavors of Southeast Asian cuisines are regional, and the nuanced distinctions are found in how spices and herbs are used. All cultures use rice as a staple. Salt is mostly derived from fermented fish sauce and pastes. India brought fiery curries to Myanmar, Thailand, Malaysia, and Indonesia, with the Philippines remaining a holdout in the use of spice, chilies, and curry mixtures, preferring the cooling effect of sourness flavored with garlic and onions. See FILIPINO.

All of these are reflected in the food that is served in restaurants in New York City. Vietnamese restaurants serve pho, the broth and noodle staple of the north; the tiny plates of dimsum from Hue; and the caramelized grilled meats from Ho Chi Minh City. Myanmar's national dish is *mohinga*, a fish-based broth with noodles and vegetables, topped with fried shallots and peanuts.

Malaysian and Singaporean restaurants serve a sampling of *laksas* (curried noodle soups made from a paste pounded with shallots, dried shrimp, and *belacan*, a fermented shrimp paste) and dishes that they share with Indonesia: *rendang* (braised beef in galangal, ginger, and coconut milk), satays (skewered beef or chicken in peanut sauce), and *rojak* (fruit salad with sweet and sour sauce made with palm sugar and fish sauce).

Northern Thai/Lao Food in Ascendance

The most interesting and intriguing development is the growing visibility of Lao food. In the past, most Lao restaurateurs positioned themselves as either Thai or Vietnamese for business purposes. But they are now putting their food on the map through Zabb Elee in Elmhurst, which has established another branch in Manhattan. Zabb Elee (which means "deliciously spicy" in Lao) is listed as northern Thai. The owners are from the province of Roi Et, which was formerly part of Laos before Thailand took over in the early 1900s. Known also as Isan or Esan cooking, the traditional Lao dishes on the menu are papaya salad, Lao soup, and *larb* (ground meat salad) flavored by *pla dek*, river fish fermented in cooked rice and salt. Laotians do not have curries or use coconut milk in their cooking. Flavors come from fresh ginger, galangal, lemongrass, chilies, and Laotian cilantro. Their iced dessert, called *nam kang sai*, uses palm seed, coco jelly, glass jelly, croutons, grenadine, condensed milk, and shaved ice. A standout dessert, not listed on the menu, is the black sticky rice porridge with longan cooked in coconut milk, salt, and sugar.

It is a myth that the original flavors of a cuisine can only be found in the home countries of immigrant groups. Memory in transplanted spaces can oftentimes be more reliable with the effort to preserve flavors and cooking methods. Both home cooking and restaurants will always be rich sources of stories and information about the individuals who build new lives in New York City. The flavor profiles of the Southeast Asian expatriates will persist as a source of their own humanity and identity in the constantly changing landscape of Gotham.

Ray, Krishnendu. "The Immigrant Restaurateur and the American City: Taste, Toil and the Politics of Inhabitation." *Social Research* 81, no. 2 (Summer 2014): 373–396.

Satler, Gail. "New York City Restaurants: Vernaculars of Global Designing." *Journal of Architectural Education* 56, no. 3 (2003): 27–39.

Shaftel, David. "Little Cambodia, Growing Still Littler." *New York Times*, January 20, 2008.

Amy Besa

South Street Seaport

See FULTON FISH MARKET.

Speakeasies

The most popular usage of the word "speakeasy" refers to the illegal drinking establishments that came to be as a result of the passage of the Eighteenth Amendment to the U.S. Constitution, which paved the way for the National Prohibition Act, also known as the Volstead Act. January 17, 1920, was the first day of national Prohibition on the sale and production of alcoholic beverages.

Prohibition eliminated the saloons of New York City and replaced them with often well-hidden places where beer and booze were openly served. These were called "speakeasies."

This was not the first time the word "speakeasy" had entered the popular vocabulary in the United States. At the end of the nineteenth century six states had already gone "dry." *Merriam-Webster's Collegiate Dictionary* (eleventh edition) defines it as a word originating in 1889 as "a place where alcoholic beverages are illegally sold." The term is reported to have originated with saloon owner Kate Hester, who ran an unlicensed bar in the 1880s in McKeesport, Pennsylvania.

After the advent of Prohibition, the number of speakeasies boomed, particularly in New York. Before Prohibition there were fifteen thousand legal drinking establishments in New York City. During Prohibition the number of drinking establishments more than doubled to over thirty-two thousand, all of them illegal. The exact count will never be known since these illicit outposts usually were well hidden. However, the New-York Historical Society maintains that "official" estimates ranged from twenty thousand to one hundred thousand establishments, including more than half a dozen managed by Texas Guinan, Manhattan's most famous speakeasy hostess. One of the most ostentatious speakeasies was The Mansion, found at 27 West Fifty-First Street in "a former banker's idea of the Lycee Palace."

The types of venues varied widely, from tiny rooms hidden in the back of restaurants, shops and private homes, to large, glitzy pleasure palaces with live music and dancing. Some of the more notable speakeasies that could be found on Manhattan included Jack & Charlie's, at 21 West Fifty-Second Street (today 21 Club), The Bath Club was at 35 West Fifty-Third Street (today the Museum of Modern Art), Zum Brauhaus sat at 239 East Eighty-Sixth Street in Yorkville (today a furniture store). In the introduction to Al Hirschfeld's *The Speakeasies of 1932* (2003), Pete Hamill notes that "From the beginning, millions of citizens felt that the national movement to make drinking illegal was directed at the cities in general and New York in particular."

This erosion of the respect for government and the legal system had a long-lasting effect on the American national psyche, ushering in a general cynicism and distrust. Many cities proudly proclaimed that they were the nation's wettest.

The growth of New York City speakeasies had two unintended but significant effects on everyday life in New York City. Before Prohibition, most "respectable" women would not be welcome in a public bar. Once Prohibition went into effect, women as well as men began flocking to speakeasies, like George's Place (507 Lexington Avenue), which Hirschfeld says was known for patrons who were "women in their late thirties, who learned to drink ten years ago."

The other significant change in social norms came with the introduction of "black-and-tans," integrated cabarets and nightclubs, usually in black neighborhoods and usually featuring the leading African American jazz musicians. Racial barriers disappeared at the Catagonia Club and Club Ebony. The African American magazine *The Messenger* called the black-and-tan "America's most democratic institution," where "we see white and colored people mixed freely. They dance together not only in the sense of both races being on the floor at the same time, but in the still more poignant and significant sense of white and colored people dancing as respective partners." New York's *Amsterdam News* noted that "The nightclubs have done more to improve race relations in 10 years than the churches, white and black, have done in 10 decades."

The restaurant industry incorporated jargon that reflected the speakeasy when it adopted the term "eighty-sixed," as in "That dish has been eighty-sixed." The origins of that cryptic phrase can be traced to the corner of Bedford and Barrow Streets in New York's Greenwich Village, where Chumley's was tucked away discreetly. Chumley's was a popular Manhattan speakeasy that opened in 1922 on the site of a former blacksmith shop. Police would reportedly warn owners to "eighty-six" everyone out the back door (86 Bedford Street) while the police or federal agents raided the place. For unknown reasons law enforcement would always enter through the Pamela Court entrance.

Other establishments began their storied history as speakeasies, including The Stonewall, now famed as a gay haven. See STONEWALL INN. One of the last enduring speakeasies that can truly lay claim to the title is the Ear Inn on Spring Street. This three-story building was completed in 1812 and was owned by an African American man named James Brown, who ran a tobacco shop on the ground floor. Five years later, Brown closed the tobacco shop and opened a tavern, which, because of its location only a few feet from the Hudson River shore, became very popular among sailors and longshoremen. The establishment changed hands numerous times before publican Thomas Cloke sold it on the eve of Prohibition.

During Prohibition the ground floor was a speakeasy, while the upstairs changed from a boarding house to a headquarters for smugglers and a brothel. When Prohibition was repealed, the bar was reopened as The Green Door, with a neon sign that read "BAR." In the late 1960s the neon tubing that formed the front of the "B" in the sign failed, leaving an "E" which has survived to this day.

Prohibition ended in 1933. When the need to procure liquor and drink secretly vanished, so did most speakeasies.

In the early twenty-first century, along with the resurgence in cocktail culture, a number of speakeasy-style bars opened their doors for the first time, such as Please Don't Tell. This near-hidden East Village bar, modeled on the Prohibition-era speakeasies, opened in 2007, including a secret entrance through a phone booth. This is only one of the new breed of modern bars that features the traditional cocktails developed before Prohibition. The added allure of having to know exactly where to go to find the places that specialize in "mixology" has created a market for pubs, bars, and taverns hidden from sight in a similar way as the speakeasies of Prohibition. In short, in New York the speakeasy has survived.

See also PROHIBITION; SALOONS; TEMPERANCE MOVEMENT; and "21" CLUB.

"Bootlegging." *Dictionary of American History*. 2003. Encyclopedia.com. http://www.encyclopedia.com/topic/bootlegging.aspx.

Hirschfeld, Al. *The Speakeasies of 1932*. Milwaukee, Wis.: Glen Young, 2003.

Lerner, Michael A. *Dry Manhattan: Prohibition in New York City*. Cambridge, Mass.: Harvard University Press, 2007.

Okrent, Daniel. *Last Call: The Rise and Fall of Prohibition*. New York: Scribner, 2010.

Paterson, Boo. *The Greatest Speakeasies in New York City*. New York: Boo York City, 2014.

"Speakeasy." *Dictionary of American History*. 2003. Encyclopedia.com. http://www.encyclopedia.com/topic/Speakeasy.aspx.

Peter LaFrance

Spirits

New York's tipplers have always brought a variety of distilled spirits to the table, whether imported or made to preserve the bounty of local orchards and farmland. In addition to beer, cider, and wine, which have a relatively lower alcohol content, distilled spirits have been an integral part of life in Europe for centuries. Alcohol was used to lubricate business transactions and commemorate social occasions, and it was considered to have medicinal properties as well.

European settlers brought varied liquors (particularly brandy) and fortified wines such as port and Madeira with them, but in general imported spirits were only available to the wealthy. Many immigrants fermented and distilled spirits for personal consumption from whatever fruits, grains, and flavorings were readily available.

Dutch colonists, who settled the region around present-day New York beginning in the 1600s, opened the first commercial distillery in New Amsterdam: William Kieft, the Dutch director general of the colony, set up a still on Staten Island in 1638, producing brandy. (According to some accounts, the distillery also made rum, applejack, and whiskey from corn and rye.)

The most common spirit in colonial times was rum. New England's trade with the West Indies provided molasses, which spurred rum production in New England's coastal towns. Rum was made, sold, and imbibed in New York but not in the massive quantities seen in New England. See RUM.

In the New York area, fruit brandies were a staple. Colonists planted apple and other fruit trees shortly after their arrival in America. In addition to making apple-based ciders and pear-based perries, those fruits were distilled—and apple brandy was among the most consumed spirits. Applejack (apple brandy aged in oak barrels) also flourished across the river in New Jersey as early as the 1690s. By the 1800s, production of "Jersey lightning" flourished in the mid-Atlantic states, with copious amounts also made in the New York area.

While some colonial-era distillers surely were motivated by the abundance of local fruit and the need to find a way to preserve and profit from harvests, another strong motivator was the fact that wines and spirits imported from Europe were taxed.

In terms of consumption, early Americans favored alcoholic beverages over alternatives such as water of variable safety and perishable milk. Beer, cider, and distilled spirits were considered more wholesome and were readily available. Many of these spirits were undoubtedly rough and strong, so it is no coincidence that many colonists favored mixed drinks, ranging from possets (made with spiced hot milk, similar to eggnog) to rum-based punches. See COCKTAILS.

Although whiskey (made from grains, particularly wheat, rye, and corn) had long been available in New York and elsewhere in colonial America, it took on increased prominence in the mid-1800s. An influx of Scottish and Irish immigrants began in the late seventeenth century, bringing the whiskey-making traditions of their homeland along with them. Unlike rum, which was dependent on imported molasses, whiskey could be made with American-grown grains. Further, Americans spilling into rural areas such as western Pennsylvania, Maryland, Virginia, and the Carolinas found that their corn and rye were cheaper to ship to market in the form of whiskey than as grain. As high tariffs and strained trade relations with Great Britain cut off supplies of West Indian molasses, crippling rum production, in 1802, the whiskey excise tax was repealed, making whiskey not only plentiful but affordable.

In the early 1800s, New Yorkers and other Americans enjoyed a whiskey glut, something that many would come to find objectionable. Notes Thomas Pegram in *Demon Rum* (1998, p. 10), "whiskey and cider stood supreme as the national beverages. Yet a nationwide drinking binge launched the temperance movement." See PROHIBITION.

As German immigrants entered the country in large numbers in the 1840s, they established breweries. Before long, beer supplanted whiskey as the national (and state) beverage. See BEER.

Today, New York enjoys a rich and varied drinking culture. Nearly every conceivable type of spirit is imported and sold in the city—indeed, many liquors are available in New York City before they are rolled out in other areas of the country. In addition, a recently revitalized urban distillery culture means that an array of spirits, primarily whiskey and gin, are now produced within city limits, including some products that are available only in New York.

See also DISTILLERIES.

Lerner, Michael A. *Dry Manhattan: Prohibition in New York City*. Cambridge, Mass.: Harvard University Press, 2012.
Pegram, Thomas R. *Battling Demon Rum: The Struggle for a Dry America, 1800–1933*. Chicago: Ivan R. Dee, 1998.
Prial, Frank. "One Family's Story: Apples to Applejack." *New York Times*, May 4, 2005.
Smith, Andrew F. *Drinking History: Fifteen Turning Points in the Making of American Beverages*. New York: Columbia University Press, 2013.

Kara Newman

Spotted Pig

See BLOOMFIELD, APRIL.

St. Patrick's Day

Observed and held annually on March 17 to honor the patron saint of Ireland, St. Patrick's Day is a citywide celebration most publically marked by a parade along Fifth Avenue. St. Patrick's Day celebrations in New York are documented since at least the mid-eighteenth century, when colonial newspapers posted announcements that Irish colonists would gather at certain taverns to mark the day. In the 1760s, the *New York Mercury* reported a celebration of the playing of "fifes and drums, which produced a very agreeable harmony." In the first half of the nineteenth century, various marches started at local parish churches, terminating at "Old" St. Patrick's Cathedral on Mott and Prince Streets. Starting in the 1890s, the contemporary parade took shape. It begins at Forty-Fourth Street and marches up Fifth Avenue, passes St. Patrick's Cathedral, and terminates at Seventy-Ninth Street. The parade is broadcast locally on the WNBC television network.

However, the revelry of the day extends far beyond the parade route and is most keenly felt inside the city's countless bars, restaurants, and taverns, where, as the expression goes, everyone is Irish for the day. Two of the most notable, historic Irish bars in New York are McSorley's and the White Horse Tavern, while Paddy Reilly's Music Bar, which features live Celtic music, claims to be the only all-Guinness draft bar in the world. See MCSORLEY'S OLD ALE HOUSE and WHITE HORSE TAVERN.

Guinness, the iconic dry stout, produced by the Dublin-based brewery, which is owned by Diageo, is the unofficial drink of the day. It is immediately recognizable by its dark color and cascading pour from nitrogenated tap lines that results in a creamy white head atop. Served in a tulip-shaped glass and logoed with an Irish harp, the brewery says it should take 119.5 seconds to pour a perfect pint, a custom thrown out the window on a day where 13 million pints are sold around the world. Other beverages, such as Jameson whiskey (owned by Pernod Ricard) and Bailey's Irish Cream (owned by Diageo), are also popular. The three are combined to create a drink known as a "car bomb." Smithwick's ale is also regularly available and consumed en masse.

In 2014, Guinness waded into political waters by withdrawing its sponsorship for the city's parade. The company cited an "inclusionary policy" that prevented openly gay marchers from identifying their sexuality or displaying signs to the same effect.

Also associated with the holiday is corned beef and cabbage, found on countless restaurant menus, with the two main ingredients piled high in grocery stores. March remains the single biggest month for cabbage out of the year, despite being a year-round crop. The holiday is also the biggest time of year for the cut of beef. While synonymous with the Irish, the meat and vegetable dish took root in America during the eighteenth century, where the salted beef was inexpensive and cabbage was both affordable and abundant. During March it is also common for bakeries, coffee shops, and restaurants to offer soda bread, a quick bread leavened with baking powder, lightly sweetened, and usually containing currants and caraway seeds. Certain bagel shops will also use Kelly green food coloring in their products for a festive touch. Irish breakfasts, complete with blood pudding and grilled tomatoes, are often specials to steel one for the drinking ahead.

See IRISH.

McNamara, Robert. "Colorful History of the St. Patrick's Day Parade." About.com. http://history1800s.about .com/od/entertainmentsport/a/stpatparade.htm.
Morris, Craig. "How Corned Beef and Cabbage Became a Holiday Staple." *USDA Blog*, March 15, 2013. http://blogs.usda.gov/2013/03/15/how-corned-beef-and-cabbage-became-a-holiday-staple.
Southall, Ashley. "Guinness Withdraws Sponsorship of Parade." *New York Times*, March 17, 2014.
Tam, Ashely. "Your NYC St. Patrick's Day Irish Food Itinerary." Serious Eats, March 13, 2014. http://newyork.seriouseats.com/2014/03/st-patricks-day-best-irish-food-nyc.html.

John Holl

Stadium Food

Watching New York professional teams compete may well be a spectator sport, but ever since a 1924 article in the *New York Times* called fans "voracious consumers of refreshments," feeding the city's spectators has been big business. Harry Stevens is considered the father of modern-day concessions, credited with first bringing food to the bleachers at the Polo Grounds in 1894. He hired up to 250 "white-coated salesmen-waiters" for each game, and they hawked refreshments up and down the stadium steps, allowing fans to eat at their seats without missing a play.

Stevens, who came to New York via Ohio and England, started out selling mostly ham and cheese sandwiches and hard-boiled eggs as early as 1864. While hot dogs were first reportedly sold via pushcarts outside of ballparks in the late 1800s, Stevens pioneered selling frankfurters inside sporting events, noting that "one touch of the frankfurter made the whole world kin." At the counters in the rear of the Polo Grounds, he said, "you would find a prominent banker eating a frankfurter and drinking a glass of beer and beside him would be a truck driver doing precisely the same thing." See HOT DOGS and NATHAN'S FAMOUS. Stevens is also credited with turning popcorn and peanuts—then considered circus or carnival foods—into ballpark staples.

Stevens's concession business, which at one time or another supplied food to Yankee Stadium, Madison Square Garden, Meadowlands Sports Complex, and Shea Stadium, was sold to food service giant Aramark in 1994. Legends Hospitality Management, a firm owned by the New York Yankees, the Dallas Cowboys, and the private equity firms Goldman Sachs and Dallas-based CIC Partners, bought the Yankees' concession business in 1998. Legends, which has operated concessions at both minor and major league stadiums, including Angels Stadium in Anaheim, California, had $53 million in concession sales in 2013 at Yankee Stadium, making food sales at Yankee Stadium the top in major league baseball. Aramark continues to hold the concession business at CitiPark Stadium, where the Mets play.

Except during Prohibition, when ginger ale, sarsaparilla, and near-beer were peddled, beer has always been a big part of the sporting fan experience, especially since many teams were owned or sponsored by breweries. The one-time Yankee's slogan "a dog and some brew, chase away the blues" epitomized the connection. New York–based brewery Knickerbocker was long associated with the New York Giants baseball team at the Polo Grounds, Schaefer with the old Brooklyn Dodgers at Ebbets Field, and Rheingold

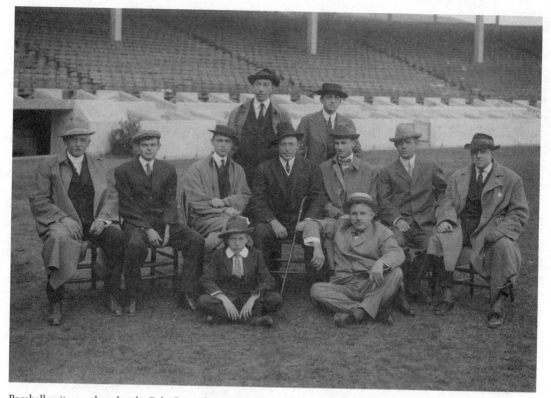

Baseball writers gathered at the Polo Grounds in 1911. Seated on the ground is concessionaire Harry M. Stevens, who is credited with first bringing food to the bleachers at the Polo Grounds, and his son Hal. PACH BROTHERS STUDIO/ NATIONAL BASEBALL HALL OF FAME LIBRARY

with the Mets. Beer was first served in thick glasses, later paper cups, and more recently plastic souvenir cups often emblazoned with a sponsored logo alongside a favorite team player. See BEER and BREWERIES.

For much of the twentieth century, stadium food concessions offered a limited selection of food—hot dogs, fries, nachos, chicken fingers, peanuts, and Cracker Jacks—and were fairly standard throughout professional sports since they were mostly served by a few large food-service companies. "Considering that New York is renowned for its exquisite culinary delights, the food selection at Yankee Stadium is a major disappointment," claimed the authors of *The Ultimate Baseball Road-Trip* (2004). Some efforts to broaden and improve the offerings started in 1995 when the Yankees brought in Mike's Deli, which anchored the Arthur Avenue Market in the Bronx, to introduce neighborhood flavors inside the ballpark. Mike's offered similar menu items as his Arthur Avenue shop: Italian sandwiches, Caesar salads, meatballs, and Parmigiana. Over at Shea, knishes were offered

but were referred to in one *Times* review as "leaden" and described as being able to "choke a python." See KNISH. Pizza rolls followed, as did chicken tenders in most sports venues.

While the sheer numbers of mouths to feed at sporting events has limited what can be realistically served in minutes, the large stadium food suppliers have more recently teamed with upscale restaurant chains to produce signature items tailored to a new generation of somewhat more sophisticated and demanding American fans who crave unique flavors. Hamburgers have long been a second-tier food at most stadiums since health regulations forced the meat to be overcooked, but Danny Meyer's Shake Shack, installed at the Met's new Citi Field Park in 2009, has given the wiener some real competition. Meyer's firm also operates an outlet of his Blue Smoke barbecue joint as well as a taqueria and Belgian fry stand at Citi Field. See SHAKE SHACK. Shrimp po'boys and crab cake sandwiches are offered at the Catch of the Day stand run by Esca's Dave Pasternack. One food hold-

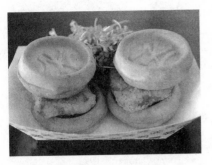

Yankee Stadium's fried chicken and waffles offered during the 2014 season. NEW YORK YANKEES

over that made the cut at the new Citi Field from old Shea Stadium is Mama's sandwich from Queens-based Leo Latticini.

In 2009, when the new Yankee Stadium opened, the team touted "over 250 culinarians working in 17 kitchens" preparing food "from scratch" that included a "steady program of celebrity chefs preparing signature dishes in the club area, à la minute dining in restaurants and suites, a candy wall . . . with an ever-changing mix of new and classic treats and a pastry kitchen that featured home-made gelato." Lobel's steak sandwiches at Yankee Stadium consistently rank among the best ballpark foods.

Over the river at Metlife stadium, opened in 2010 and home to both the Jets and the Giants, chefs hired from Delaware North Companies Sportservice have tried to boost the culinary selection. The Meadowlands New Jersey venue brings a variety of more local flavors via Home Food Advantage portable stands that offer Asian noodles, gyros, tacos, grilled cheese sandwiches, sushi, Campbell's soups, and meatball sandwiches made from a recipe from head chef Eric Borgia's grandmother.

The Barclays Center, which opened in 2010 in Brooklyn, is the home of the Brooklyn Nets basketball team and, starting in 2015, the New York Islanders hockey team. Food service is overseen by Chicago-based Levy Restaurants and emphasizes the stadium's connection to the neighborhood with fifty-five local Brooklyn vendors. Fat, saucy Sicilian slices are offered at an outpost of Gravesend Pizza. Battered and fried fish tacos are available at Calexico's two stands. Peppery white cheddar bratwurst can be had at Michelin-starred chef Saul Bolton's Brooklyn Bangers & Dogs. And Fatty 'Cue's brisket-topped mac and cheese and pulled pork banh mi are offered at two sites inside the arena. Top food props at the site belong to

Habana Outpost's gooey, pulled-pork-stuffed Cubano sandwich.

The renovation of Madison Square Garden, which was completed in 2013, added some serious food talent to the home of the New York Rangers hockey team, the New York Knicks basketball team, and a variety of concerts and other performance entertainment. "Since the whole world is changing, given the appreciation for better food, why wouldn't people want wonderful food in an arena?" chef Jean-George Vongerichten told the New York Times. And as of 2015, fans can pick up a chicken sandwich from Jean-George; a "pizzaiolo" sausage with sweet peppers, tomatoes, and onions from Andrew Carmellini; smoked brisket on a potato bun from chef Elizabeth Karmel's Hill Country; or a burger made from a blend of brisket, short rib, and chuck meat topped with bacon jam from Drew Nieporent's Daily Burger. See VON-GERICHTEN, JEAN-GEORGE and NIEPORENT, DREW. Also available are lobster rolls from Aquagrill, hefty pastrami sandwiches from the Carnegie Deli, and kosher food including chicken taquito dogs and knishes from Carlos & Gabby's. And even though stadium food has come a long way from boiled hot dogs and peanuts, the Yankees, Mets, and Jets all continue the tradition of allowing fans to bring their own food "as long as items are brought in a clear plastic grocery-style bag."

"Ball Fans Must Eat." New York Times, April 13, 1924.
Adams, Bruce, and Margaret Engel. Fodor's Ballpark Vacations. New York: Fodor's Travel, 1997.
Chapman, Francesca. "Aramark Swallows Harry M. Stevens." Philadelphia Daily News, December 13, 1994.
Collins, Glenn. "At Madison Square Garden, It's Hey Getcher Lobster Roll." New York Times, September 20, 2011.
Miller, Bryan. "Ballpark Dining." New York Times, August 10, 1990.
Pahigian, Josh, and Kevin O'Connell. The Ultimate Baseball Road-Trip. Guilford, Conn.: Lyons, 2004.

Dan Macey

Starbucks

Starbucks, the coffee mega-chain, was not born in New York City. The company started in Seattle in 1971 as a specialty coffee bean importer and whole-bean roaster, and the main affiliation to New York City is the company's chief executive officer, Howard Shultz. Shultz was born in July 19, 1953, in Brooklyn, New York. He grew up in the Canarsie Bayview

Houses of the New York City Housing Authority with his two siblings, and he went to the Canarsie High School. Schultz attended the Northern Michigan University and graduated in 1975 with a degree in communications. He worked at Xerox Corporation and Hammarplast before he joined Starbucks Coffee Company as the marketing director in 1982. In August 1987, Schultz acquired Starbucks assets from the original Starbucks management team for $4 million that he raised from investors and changed its name to Starbucks Corporation. Along with the six stores in Seattle it opened fifteen new ones in 1988. Starbucks made its jump to the East Coast and opened its first store in Manhattan in March 1994 at Eighty-Seventh Street and Broadway, the company's largest store at the time. The *New York Times* expressed Manhattanites' anticipation for grande-size lattes with articles the likes of "Starbucks to Taste New York, at Last." The second store opened in August 1994 at First Avenue and Seventy-Fifth Street.

Starbucks in New York

Starbucks is known for aggressively expanding and for opening stores in very close proximity to each other. In pricy Manhattan Starbucks followed the same strategy and opened stores sometimes seemingly next door to each other. The *I Quant NY* blog states that half of Manhattan is within four blocks of a Starbucks. The company was criticized for its corporate techniques designed to dominate the coffee market, but in reality more specialty coffee shops entered the market as a result of Starbucks' influence, successfully competing with the mega-chain retailer.

Crain's New York stated in 2011 that there were 256 stores in New York City, 194 of which were in Manhattan. At the time, Starbucks was the number three national chain in New York by number of outlets. As of December 31, 2013, there were 212 Starbucks stores in Manhattan. The numbers keep changing as new stores open and old ones close.

In 2007, Starbucks announced its first partnership with a New York celebrity chef and restaurant owner, Marcus Samuelsson. Samuelsson created two new coffee blends and two pastries for the company.

Starbucks in Brooklyn

The first Starbucks in trendy Williamsburg, popular with hipsters and artistic crowds, opened in July 2014 to a mixed reception. It is located at 405–409 Union Avenue. Local residents have resisted the idea of the chain's move in the area, showing their preference for independent specialty coffee retails.

See also COFFEE and COFFEE SHOPS.

Fabricant, Florence. "Food Notes." *New York Times*, August 31, 1994.
King, Harriet. "Starbucks to Taste New York, at Last." *New York Times*, October 7, 1993.
Kramer, Louise. "SUITS: He Probably Makes a Mean Skim Latte." *New York Times*, September 2, 2007.
Schonfeld, Zach. "Williamsburg Coffee Shops Aren't Afraid of the Big Bad Starbucks." Newsweek, July 23, 2014.
Schultz, Howard, and Dori Jones Yang. *Pour Your Heart into It.* New York: Hyperion, 1997.
Wellington, Ben. "Half of Manhattan Is Within 4 Blocks of a Starbucks." *I Quant NY* (blog), April 17, 2014. http://iquantny.tumblr.com/post/82964955696/half-of-manhattan-is-within-4-blocks-of-a-starbucks.

Thei Zervaki

Startups

People thought Empire Mayonnaise was some sort of early April Fool's Day joke when it opened in 2012. Brooklyn, home to a growing number of too-precious farm-to-table restaurants and handmade crafts, was getting its own store selling nothing but artisanal mayonnaise. But a joke it was not: the store opened in a small space in Prospect Heights, selling rosemary, sriracha, and black garlic flavors of mayonnaise for about seven dollars a jar. People stopped thinking of it as a parody store quickly: the products became a hit and are now found in Whole Foods and Dean & DeLuca, showing just how ripe a place New York City has become for innovative food startups. (Incidentally, the shop was the butt of a joke in a 2014 episode of *Saturday Night Live*, where modern-day New York street thugs talk about picking up their favorite flavor of mayo.)

That was the product of the early 2000s, which kicked off a wave of food innovation in New York City not seen since the days of seltzer delivery and the invention of the egg cream. See EGG CREAMS. Entries in the startup food scene in New York of late often begin with a simple home recipe—mayonnaise or pickles, for instance—grow a small following, and then develop into a free-standing business. Or sometimes it is in the form of a company that wants to revolutionize an industry, from coffee roasting to chocolate to ingredients for your dinner.

The Brooklyn Flea Effect

One of the most successful incubators for food businesses has been the Brooklyn Flea, a hodgepodge mix of antiques, handmade goods, and local food that started in Fort Greene in 2008. It quickly became a testing ground for people to try out new food concepts, many of which expanded into brick-and-mortar businesses. Asia Dog, for instance, had a small stand at the Flea, selling its pork belly and banh mi–inspired hot dogs. It eventually expanded to other events, such as Central Park concerts, before opening a full store on the Lower East Side in 2011.

People's Pops started selling its naturally made frozen treats crafted out of produce purchased from the Union Square farmers' market at the Flea in 2008, with flavors such as watermelon-basil and sweet rhubarb. It quickly went from three hundred popsicles a week to twelve hundred. The company also took that huge demand and expanded it into a permanent storefront in 2012 in Park Slope. The Brooklyn Brew Shop started selling its homebrew kits at the Flea in 2009. Two years later it published a beer-making book, and not long after its do-it-yourself beer kits were available in stores across the country. Liddabit Sweets started peddling its artisanal candies in the early days of the Flea. In 2014 it got its own permanent shop and commercial kitchen, after already getting distribution in several stores and markets.

The Flea itself has been a success story. It expanded to a second location in Williamsburg and in 2011 added Smorgasburg, a food-only version of the Flea that attracted big crowds of tourists and Manhattanites from across the river on weekends. See SMORGASBURG. It also partnered with Whole Foods to bring a new vendor each month into the SoHo store, along with other products. In 2014, it opened a sort of permanent version of Smorgasburg in Crown Heights, called Berg'n, that features food and beers from local vendors.

Food Fever Hits New York

McClure's Pickles was one of the biggest success stories from New York's food community in the early 2000s. See PICKLES. Brothers Joe and Bob McClure started making the crisp, carefully spiced pickles in

2006, using their grandmother's recipe. The recipe was a hit, and they eventually expanded into offering Bloody Mary mix and potato chips. See BLOODY MARY. Though they produce their products in Detroit (where Joe lives), they keep offices in Brooklyn, and their products can be found in bodegas and stores citywide. They now share a space in the eight-acre Pfizer building in South Williamsburg with other success-story food startups: Brooklyn Soda Works, Steve's Ice Cream, People's Pops, and chocolate maker Madecasse.

The early successes to come out of the New York startup scene were tech companies that revolutionized whole industries: microblogging platform Tumblr, location-based social network FourSquare, and crowdfunding site Kickstarter, to name a few. But since then others have taken technology and mixed it with what is on your dinner plate. In 2010, two Harvard Business School graduates set up a website for a subscription beauty product sample delivery service called Birchbox, based in New York. It is now a multimillion-dollar company with operations in Belgium and Spain, offering snack-sized mulled wine kits, vinegar cruets, and single-origin sipping chocolates.

That subscription model spawned other similar services. In 2012, two friends realized that their busy schedules were not leaving room for decent meals, so they created Plated, a service that lets users select from a menu of meals and delivers an all-in-one box to their door with all the fresh ingredients. Blue Apron launched in 2012, providing a similar service, out of the Brooklyn Navy Yard, which has become a startup hub.

Farmigo started in 2009 as an online shopping hub for farmers' markets. In 2014 it expanded its mission into becoming a hub for helping other food startups. It began hosting Food Hacker events, where successful food entrepreneurs from across the city gather to share stories of their accomplishments.

New Yorkers have begun to treat chocolate seriously too. The blog *Grub Street* gives Mast Brothers, based in Brooklyn's Williamsburg neighborhood, credit for pioneering the "single-origin, bean-to-bar, and stratospheric cacao content," borrowing from Eurocentric practices. They have inspired other chocolate startups: Long Island City–based Gnosis Chocolate, which makes raw chocolate and was founded by a holistic health counselor; Red Hook, Brooklyn–based Cacao Prieto, which imports cacao pods from a family farm in the Dominican Republic and ships the beans to Brooklyn; and a handful more that make chocolate seem like a very adult treat.

New York has been behind cities like San Francisco and Portland when it comes to the so-called third-wave coffee (high-quality, artisanal) movement. But it has caught up in recent years with spots like Café Grumpy (the shop that became the Cheers to the HBO show *Girls*), which opened a coffee shop and roastery in the then-desolate Greenpoint neighborhood in 2005, and Gorilla Coffee, which expanded its carefully sourced, locally roasted operation from a small shop in Park Slope in 2002 to a pour-over bar around the corner, with eventual plans to open a 4,000-square-foot roasting plant and coffee bar in Gowanus.

Booze

It is strange to think about now, but it was not too long ago that people considered Brooklyn's alcohol scene long dead. See BEER. The borough was home to loads of breweries that all disappeared by the end of the twentieth century. It was not until Steve Hindy decided to open Brooklyn Brewery in 1988 that the suds came back and big time. Brooklyn Brewery beers are now found across the world, and an outpost of the brewery opened in Sweden. See BROOKLYN BREWERY. Sixpoint Brewery opened in 2004, and Kelso followed in 2006. By 2007 state liquor laws had relaxed, and a distillery boomlet began in New York City, the first of its kind since Prohibition. The first was Kings County Distillery, making craft whiskey and moonshine. More than twenty distilleries opened in the city in the first five years. See DISTILLERIES.

The Rise of Coworking

The spirit of collaboration that has created such a vibrant cultural scene in the city has expanded its influence into the startup realm with the rise of coworking spaces. The spaces—shared offices, production facilities, or just basic infrastructure—facilitate innovation and new projects, especially for small companies that could not afford their own free-standing space just yet. For example, in Brooklyn's Sunset Park, you will find Industry City, a one-hundred-year-old, sixteen-building complex of former distribution and shipping centers that is becoming a hub of activity. MakerBot, the pioneering three-dimensional printing company that was founded in Brooklyn, was one of the first tenants of the space, and more followed in droves, representing a variety of industries,

including lots of food—chocolatier Liddabit Sweets opened its first permanent factory and location there in 2014, and several other food ventures that need shared kitchen space to get started are moving in too. See SUNSET PARK.

"People want to make things again," Industry City's chief executive officer Andrew Kimball says. "There are new technologies and a real consumer interest in locally made products. That has led to an explosion of demand for space, and the creation of communities in which these innovators are next to each other."

Correia, Margarida. "Popsicles in Hot Demand in Brooklyn." *New York Daily News*, September 20, 2009.
Kaysen, Ronda. "Food Start-Ups Find a Home in Brooklyn." *New York Times*, March 27, 2012.
Leland, John. "90 Proof New York." *New York Times*, December 27, 2013.
Robbins, Liz. "Kings of a Small-Batch Empire in Brooklyn." *New York Times*, October 27, 2012.

Tim Donnelly

Staten Island

Staten Island is the third-largest borough by land area yet has the lowest population, which gives much of the island a more suburban feel than most of New York City. The first European settlers on Staten Island—the Dutch, followed soon by English, French Huguenots, Germans, and enslaved Africans—were farmers and fishermen. The population of the island remained small until the beginning of the nineteenth century, when the settlers rebuilt their towns after years of British occupation during the Revolution. Manufacturing of various kinds—especially shipbuilding and beer brewing—joined farming, fishing, and oystering in the nineteenth century as Staten Islanders catered to the rapidly growing populations of Manhattan, Brooklyn, and northern New Jersey. The island has always attracted a wide range of immigrants, as it still does today, and they have all brought their food cultures with them. Some of these—Italian pizza and ices, German baked goods and beer—have lengthy histories, and others—Sri Lankan, Mexican, and Russian, for example—are recent arrivals. See ITALIAN; GERMAN; MEXICAN; and RUSSIAN.

Staten Island was located on an important road system linking the Middle Atlantic, through New Jersey, to Long Island and New England. Goods and people traveled across the Arthur Kill (a narrow

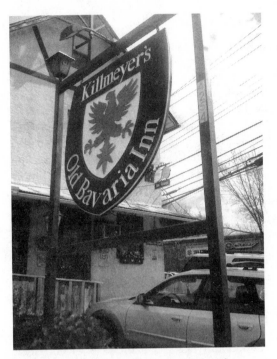

Killmeyer's has been around since 1859, when the neighborhood was a German factory town. It is the oldest bar on Staten Island, and one of the oldest in New York City. COURTESY KILLMEYER'S OLD BAVARIAN INN

tidal strait dividing Staten Island and New Jersey) to Port Richmond and then made their way by boat, light rail, and wagons to Manhattan and Brooklyn. Staten Island's population grew from four thousand after the Revolution to almost seventy thousand in 1900, fueled by waves of European immigrants—Germans, Irish, Italians, Greeks, and Eastern Europeans—who flocked to the ever-increasing jobs in local industries, bringing their foodways. Much of the North Shore of Staten Island, linked by regular ferry service to Manhattan after the Civil War, became increasingly urban and supported several thriving breweries—Bechtel, Bachmann, and Eckstein, among others—that specialized in a distinctive German lager. See BEER and BREWERIES. Germans chose this area for their breweries because of the abundant natural springs, cool caves to store the beer casks in, and easy access to the Manhattan market and the seaport. Prohibition dealt a crippling blow to this important sector of the local economy. Rubsam and Horrmann's, the largest of the brewers, was the only one to recover and continue into the 1950s. Given the importance of German immigrants to the island's history, it is

not surprising that Killmeyer's Old Bavarian Inn, which opened in 1859 to cater to German factory workers on the South Shore, may be the Island's oldest continuously operating tavern. Appropriately, it is a great place for enjoying large steins of draft beer, waitresses in dirndls, and classic sausages and sauerkraut.

Oysters were an important source of income for many Staten Islanders, dating back to the first Dutch settlers, who adapted the oystering traditions of the local Lenape tribes. With the rapid growth of the New York and global markets for oysters during the nineteenth century a large free black community developed on Staten Island to meet the demand. See OYSTERS. Settling in a community they eventually called Sandy Ground (named for the sandy soil where they also grew strawberries for the New York market), Staten Island became an important stop on the Underground Railroad for African Americans fleeing the South between the abolition of slavery in New York in 1827 and the end of the Civil War. The abundant oyster beds surrounding the island (most of New York Harbor) suddenly collapsed in the early twentieth century as a result of overfishing and pollution.

Migration from Brooklyn and other parts of New York increased rapidly after the Verrazano Narrows Bridge was completed in 1964, and the former farming villages of Staten Island were developed into large tracts of suburban housing. Nonetheless, the eleven-acre Decker Farm, the oldest continuously working farm in New York City (since 1810, when the Decker family acquired it), still produces pumpkins, tomatillos, and a variety of other crops for sale at the local Greenmarket. It is now part of Historic Richmondtown, where several important historic buildings have been restored and opened to the public. Visitors may also enjoy cooking demonstrations on the open hearth of a nineteenth-century farmhouse kitchen at the Guyon-Lake-Tysen House in Historic Richmondtown.

Now over one-third of the residents of Staten Island identify as Italian American, so Italian eateries of many kinds can be found all over the island. Denino's Pizzeria, routinely mentioned on the short list of "Best Pizza in New York City," was founded in 1937. Renowned for a pizza with a slightly thicker, softer crust than other classic New York pies, Denino's has spawned many imitators, claiming loyal fans from far beyond the tri-state area. Not too far from

Denino's, Ralph's Famous Italian Ices began in 1928 when Ralph Silvestro began selling ices from a truck. He opened his first store in 1945, and the various specialty flavors of ices and ice cream attract crowds to the neighborhood all summer long and during the winter as well. Recent Italian immigrants to Staten Island are relieved to find high-quality imported ingredients—artisanal pastas, fine olive oils, cheeses, salumi, anchovies, Christmas and Easter cakes, and other delicacies—at the three branches of Pastosa and many other Italian American pork stores. Pastosa is justly famous for its store-made mozzarella and various kinds of ravioli and tortellini, some of the best in all of New York City.

Recent waves of immigrants from Asian countries, Liberia, Albania, the former Soviet Union, and South America continue to enrich the borough's food culture. Immigrant day laborers from Mexico have flocked to the Port Richmond neighborhood since the 1990s, where a lively Mexican and Latin American food scene is developing, from bakeries to restaurants to small grocery stories and bodegas. There are Polish and Pakistani food festivals at the Snug Harbor Cultural Center every summer. See POLISH. And a Little Sri Lanka has developed near the ferry terminal in the St. George neighborhood, where the first Sri Lankan restaurant in the United States opened in 1995. Now the growing Sri Lankan community supports a small but exciting collection of restaurants, and food stores offer masala dosas, string poppers, and newspapers from home in both Tamil and Sinhalese.

Staten Island is the fastest-growing borough in New York City, and much of that growth is driven by immigrants arriving from all over the world. Just as in the rest of the five boroughs, these immigrants bring their food cultures, open restaurants and food stores, and contribute to an ever-changing tapestry of diverse eating and drinking experiences for the community.

Gold, Kenneth, and Lori Weintrob, eds. *Discovering Staten Island: A 350th Anniversary Commemorative History*. Charleston, S.C.: History Press, 2011.

Kurlansky, Mark. *The Big Oyster: History on the Half Shell*. New York: Random House, 2006.

Lobel, Cindy. *Urban Appetites: Food and Culture in Nineteenth-Century New York*. Chicago: University of Chicago Press, 2014.

"Staten Island Breweries." Staten Island History.com. http://www.statenislandhistory.com/staten-island-breweries.html.

Alison A. Smith

Steak Tartare

Steak tartare, traditionally comprised of minced, chopped, or ground raw beef tossed with raw egg yolk, capers, onions, and chopped parsley, first cropped up on menus at chic hotels in France at the beginning of the twentieth century. By the 1920s, the protein-packed dish was dubbed "beefsteak à l'Américaine," as mentioned in notable French chef Auguste Escoffier's 1921 culinary guide, though its connection to the United States is unknown. Besides high-quality beef, the dish required sauce tartare, then made of pureed hard-cooked egg yolks, vinegar, chives, and oil, which is widely believed by historians to be steak tartare's true namesake. "Beefsteak à l'Américaine" debuted in 1926 at Joseph Niels's Brussels restaurant Le Canterbury. However, by 1938, sauce tartare was nowhere to be found in the steak tartare recipe in *Larousse Gastronomique*, which consisted of raw ground beef topped with a raw egg.

"The vogue for steak tartare really started after the Second World War, in the 1950s," French food historian Patrick Rambourg told the *New York Times* in 2005 after steak tartare had become popular throughout France and Belgium in the second quarter of the twentieth century. But Americans did not have a taste for the dish until travel to Europe became popular postwar. It arrived in New York in the mid-twentieth century. Later on, a scene in the 1987 film *Wall Street* featured the ruthless financier Gordon Gecko (played by Michael Douglas) initiating a young stockbroker (Charlie Sheen) into rich living by ordering steak tartare at the 21 Club. See "21" CLUB. Contemporary chefs have tinkered with the classic slew of ingredients, with common modern-day additions that include Worcestershire sauce, Tabasco sauce, shallots, chives, scallions, pickled gherkins, and mustard—or, in the version at Les Halles, when Anthony Bourdain was the chef: a bit of ketchup.

Late twentieth-century versions of the dish, some faithful to traditional preparations and others flaunting innovative revisions to the classic recipe, can be found at Balthazar, Odeon, Estela, Takashi, M. Wells Dinette, Prune, and Employees Only. Also pleasing the palettes of raw meat enthusiasts in New York in recent years are versions made with lamb, including dishes at The Cannibal, Empellon Cocina, and Dover.

Druckman, Charlotte. "A Recipe for Steak Tartare, Family Style." *Wall Street Journal*, September 5, 2014.

Sietsema, Robert. "Some Like It Raw: 11 Tasty Downtown Tartares." Eater NY, February 21, 2014. http://ny.eater.com/maps/some-like-it-raw-11-tasty-downtown-tartares.

Smith, Craig. "The Raw Truth: Don't Blame the Mongols (or Their Horses)." New York Times, April 6, 2005.

Strand, Oliver. "Steak Tartare Is the Dish of the Moment: A New Generation of Chefs Reinterprets the Classic." Vogue, November 3, 2014.

Alexandra Ilyashov

Steingarten, Jeffrey

Jeffery Steingarten is a respected food critic based in New York City. In 1989, when Steingarten left his career as a corporate lawyer to indulge his love for food and become the food critic of *Vogue* magazine, his first assignment was for Anna Wintour, the then infamous editor-in-chief at *House and Garden*. She requested a 4,200-word piece on microwaved fish. It was not an assignment he took lightly, and he requested twelve microwave ovens to get the job done properly. He got three. When Wintour left *Home and Garden* to become the editor at *Vogue*, Steingarten followed her to become the food critic at *Vogue*. His only stipulation was that he would get the same salary as a New York City plumber. Wintour, not commonly known to give in to demands, complied.

Steingarten, according to an article in the *Guardian*, immediately understood "the awesome responsibilities of his post" and vowed to become completely omnivorous. "If he could not overcome his dislike of say, anchovies and desserts in Indian restaurants, his aversion to blue food (excluding berries) and kimchi (the national pickle of Korea) then he would, he felt, be like the art critic who couldn't abide yellow."

This mantra gave rise to his first book, *The Man Who Ate Everything* (1997), and the sequel, *It Must Have Been Something I Ate* (2002). In a career as a food critic that spans more than twenty-five years, he has become a leading man in his genre, having won a *National* magazine award and a dozen James Beard awards and further garnered many more nominations. See JAMES BEARD AWARDS.

In 1994, his writing on French gastronomy earned him the title of Chevalier in the Order of Merit by the Republic of France. Steingarten's pieces have also been featured in the *New York Times*, *Men's Vogue*, and *Slate magazine*. He is a frequent judge and contributor on the Food Network programs *Iron Chef America* and *The Next Iron Chef*. See FOOD NETWORK.

Steingarten, Jeffrey. *The Man Who Ate Everything*. New York. Vintage, 1997.

Steingarten, Jeffrey. *It Must Have Been Something I Ate*. New York. Vintage, 2002.

Eirik Osland

Stella D'oro

Stella D'oro is a brand of Italian cookies and crackers that originated in the Bronx. Italian immigrant couple Joseph and Angela Kresevich established the company there as the Stella D'oro bakery in 1932. When they expanded in 1950, their Kingsbridge factory became a neighborhood mainstay until 2008 when production ceased there. A related yearlong strike associated with declining working conditions at Stella D'oro became a touchstone for conversations about workers' rights and waning industry in postindustrial New York City.

Stella D'oro quickly became known for its breadsticks, breakfast treats, cookies, and toasts. Long before biscotti were trendy, Stella D'oro sold the coffee biscuits—hard ones called "toast" and soft ones called "sponge"—in flavors like anisette and almond. They also had a large line of cookies, including Swiss Fudge, Margherite, and Almond Delight.

While the cookies (and their creators) were Italian, Stella D'oro's dairy-free recipes made them popular with kosher Jews in New York and beyond as they could be eaten alongside both meat and dairy meals. The Swiss Fudge cookies are sometimes called "shtreimels," after the fur hats that some wear on the Sabbath.

In 1950, the company moved into a new factory in the Kingsbridge section of the Bronx. An Italian restaurant was attached. The Stella D'oro factory became an informal landmark in Kingsbridge, the smell of cookies baking an olfactory fixture of the neighborhood—cinnamon and ginger at Christmastime, licorice when the anisette cookies were baking, almond at other times.

In 1965, Joseph Kresevich died and Phil Zambetti, Angela Kresevich's son from a previous marriage, took over the business. Zambetti ran a worker-friendly company, and he was a much-loved leader. Under his aegis, Stella D'oro expanded its markets to other locales including Chicago, Boston, San Francisco, and Florida. Stella D'oro's unionized workers received a generous benefits package including sick leave, a pension plan, and paid vacation days. Since the Stella D'oro factory eschewed mass-production machinery (cookies were made by hand or on improvised machines), its cookie makers were skilled and enjoyed considerable job security and longevity. Employees stayed at the company for decades.

In 1992, with Zambetti retiring, his sons decided to sell the company to RJR Nabisco, which in 2000 was itself purchased by Philip Morris (with Kraft Foods under its aegis). At this point, Stella D'oro was a very profitable company, a $64 million a year business with 575 employees nationwide. At its Bronx plant, it employed 138 workers from twenty-two countries.

Under Kraft, the Stella D'oro brand lost its originality. Workers' vaunted position within the company declined and ingredients were changed, resulting in a lower-quality product. Kraft also briefly removed the pareve (kosher) designation from the cookies, introducing a milk-based chocolate. This move garnered letters of protest from Orthodox rabbis and, more importantly, led to declining sales. Kraft resumed the kosher designation, but Stella D'oro sales continued to slide, falling by more than half in the span of a few years.

In 2006, Kraft sold the company to leveraged buyout firm Brynwod Partners. After the workers' contract expired in 2008, Brynwood implemented cuts to wages and benefits, prompting the workers to strike. After the strike had dragged on for more than eleven months, the National Labor Relations Board ordered Brynwood to reinstate the workers, pay them retroactively, and begin a round of collective bargaining. In response, Brynwood announced plans to close the facility. They sold the brand to the Lance Company, which moved operations to Ohio in October 2009. Stella D'oro workers and their allies attempted to force the company to keep the Bronx plant open, holding demonstrations and rallies and appealing to local politicians. The protestors framed their battle as part of a larger fight to protect workers' wages and the loss of industrial jobs in New York, especially the Bronx. Despite these efforts, the factory closed down and the smell of freshly baked cookies in the Bronx ceased after sixty years.

Today, the Lance Company produces Stella D'oro's signature breadsticks, Swiss Fudge, and biscotti out of its plant in Ashland, Ohio. The Kingsbridge Stella D'oro plant was demolished in 2012.

See also BAKERIES; BRONX; and ITALIAN.

Berger, Joseph. "Of Milk and Cookies, or How Orthodox Jews Saved an Italian Recipe." *New York Times*, January 12, 2003.

Frazier, Ian. "Out of the Bronx: Private Equity and the Cookie Factory." *New Yorker*, February 6, 2012.

Cindy R. Lobel

Stonewall Inn

Stonewall, located at 53 Christopher Street, is a historical bar where a riot occurred that sparked the gay liberation movement in the United States. At the time of Stonewall's opening in 1966, serving alcohol to openly gay men and women was illegal as it marked the space as a disorderly house. Stonewall was owned by Tony Lauria, a member of the Genovese crime family. He paid off the police so that they would look the other way and allow him to operate the bar. Many of the bars that served gay patrons were owned by members of the Mafia, who saw a market among gay New Yorkers and who could work with the police to allow them to run illegal operations.

Stonewall gained a reputation as a safe environment. It was less likely to be raided than other bars that catered toward homosexual patrons. In 1968, the *Gay Scene Guide Quarterly* advertised the spot this way: "53 Christopher Street, One of the most active spots in town currently. Very crowded on weekends. Casual." The bar drew a mix of people including transgender people, teenage boys, and lesbians. There was no running water, and bartenders washed glasses in vats of water.

Police raids were common, to give the appearance of law enforcement, but often no arrests were made. Typically patrons ran away at the first sign a raid was happening. But June 28, 1969, was different. At approximately 1:20 a.m., eight detectives from the First Division pushed through the door and ordered the approximately two hundred patrons who were inside to line up and produce identification. Allegedly, they made homophobic remarks about the patrons.

People have different accounts about the actual moment that set the rebellion off, but several first-hand accounts point to the moment when a lesbian dressed in stereotypically male clothing complained that her handcuffs were too tight. Reportedly, in response police hit her with a baton and threw her into the car. She yelled out to the crowds that had spilled out onto the street, "Why don't you guys do something?"

Allegedly, this was the call to action. The patrons sang and danced in kick lines like the Rockettes and screamed epithets at the police as they loaded hand-cuffed patrons into their van. People chanted and threw coins, cans, bottles, and bricks from a construction site nearby. Those who were part of the riots explained that their response was a result of built-up resentment for the discrimination that finally boiled over the surface that night. Everyday hate crimes and injustices had finally piled too high. Some of the patrons' tactics were violent, and they also sang about gay power. Several patrons were injured, and four police officers were hurt.

After that night, the media coverage brought more crowds out. Rioting and street fighting continued for three days. Homosexuals were encouraged by the resistance and walked hand in hand for the first time in public with loved ones of the same sex. This was a landmark moment that garnered media attention, which is why some people refer to as the birth of gay pride. Overnight "celebrities" from the infamous night posed for pictures and led choruses about gay power.

A story in the *Village Voice* led to more riots and protests because people felt the reporting was degrading. The account of the night stated that police raided the Stonewall Inn because it was an unlicensed club, not because of homophobia. *Time* magazine called being gay "a serious and sometimes crippling maladjustment," deciding that homosexual living was "without question shallow and unstable." But the fact that there was newfound visibility and discussion encouraged a surge in empowerment within the gay community to challenge damaging stereotypes, championing the causes of the "homophile movement" (Gay Activists Alliance, Gay Liberation Front, and North American Conference of Homophile Organizations).

Three months after the rebellion, the Stonewall Inn closed because its reputation was compromised by the associated uprising. On June 28, 1970, people came to Stonewall to commemorate the one-year anniversary. Christopher Street Liberation Day was the first ever pride celebration in history, and it is celebrated around the world today. New York's Gay Pride Parade occurs every year on the anniversary of the Stonewall rebellion and passes by the Stonewall Inn.

In the 1970s and 1980s, a bagel sandwich shop occupied the space, then a Chinese restaurant, and then it became a shoe store. In 1990, a bar called "Stonewall" opened in the space. Christopher Street saw a resurgence of gay bars in the subsequent decade. The Stonewall Inn was added to the U.S. National Register of Historic Places in 1999 and named a National Historic Landmark in 2000.

There is running water at the gay bar now, and gay marriage is legal, but you do not need to be inside to dress like a drag king or hold hands with someone of the same gender. Now there is partying to house music, and a welcoming atmosphere prevails. They have drag queen shows, karaoke, male dancers, and lesbian go-go dancers. They serve taps, mixed drinks, and bottled beers.

See also GAY BARS and POST–WORLD WAR II (1945–1975).

Bonanos, Christopher. "A Photographic Look at the Birth of Gay Pride." *New York*, June 24, 2014.
Duberman, Martin. *Stonewall*. New York: Penguin, 1993.
Stonewall Inn website: http://www.thestonewallinnnyc.com/StonewallInnNYC/HOME.html.
Stuart, Tessa. "Full Moon Over the Stonewall: Howard Smith's Account of the Stonewall Riots." *Village Voice*, June 27, 2014.
"Then & Now: Stonewall Inn Through the Years." *American Experience*. PBS.org. http://www.pbs.org/wgbh/americanexperience/features/then-and-now/stonewall.

Ashley Hoffman

Stork Club

The Stork Club was one of New York City's most famous nightspots. It was opened in 1929 on West Fifty-Eighth Street by the former bootlegger Sherman Billingsley, whose friends supplied his establishment with adequate amounts of alcohol during Prohibition. See PROHIBITION. Regularly raided by city, state, and federal agents, the club was shut down in 1931, but it reopened after a move to East Fifty-First Street. When Prohibition ended in 1933, the Stork Club was among the first establishments in the city to receive a liquor license. Billingsley moved the club to 3 East Fifty-Third Street, where it became a hangout for socialites, film stars, power brokers, radio personalities, newspaper columnists, showgirls, and racketeers, all of whom flocked to the club to drink, eat, and dance. Frequent celebrity attendees included Lucius Beebe, Jackie Gleason, Walter Winchell, Frank Sinatra, Lucille Ball, Judy Garland, Orson Welles, Ethel Merman, Ernest Hemingway, Jack Benny, and Theodor Geisel (creator of "Dr. Seuss"), to name a few. Goings-on at the club frequently found their way into the next morning's newspaper columns, which was a perfectly good reason for the publicity-hungry to show up.

The Stork Club served good food, and its drinks were famous. Syndicated journalist and writer Lucius Beebe published *The Stork Club Bar Book* in 1946, and Sherman Billingsley published *The Stork Club Cookbook* in 1949 (reprinted in 2009). Those who frequented the Stork Club and other fashionable nightclubs, such as the Copacabana, El Morocco, Toots Shor's, the 21 Club, and the Latin Quarter, came to be known as "Café Society," a term popularized by Lucius Beebe.

The Stork Club's popularity declined during the late 1950s, and it suffered from serious labor issues, including a four-year strike by two labor unions. It closed in 1965 but was not forgotten. A 1945 film titled *The Stork Club* featured Betty Hutton as a hat-check girl at the club who saves the life of a drowning man. Books and more recent movies about the heyday of New York City nightclubs often mention it.

See also "21" CLUB.

Blumenthal, Ralph. *Stork Club: America's Most Famous Nightspot and the Lost World of Café Society*. Boston: Little, Brown, 2000.
Stork Club website: http://storkclub.com.

Andrew F. Smith

Street Fairs

The famed urbanist Jane Jacobs wrote in her book *The Death and Life of Great American Cities* that when a city successfully "mingles everyday diversity of uses and users in its everyday streets," its residents can "thus give back grace and delight to their neighborhoods instead of vacuity." Jacobs might have been talking about the diversity on display in New York City during the warm months, when residents can find a street fair most weekends. The city is full of street festivals like the Atlantic Antic or the Italian-centric Feast of San Gennaro, but the regular weekly affairs share a common DNA seen all across the city. There you will find vendors hawking a wide variety of ethnic foods, including *pupusas* (corn tortillas with soft cheese filling), Jamaican roti, vegan Caribbean soul food, and New York City staples, from pizza baked in portable wood-fired ovens to locally

brewed beer. They are usually a mix: part carnival, part block party, and part community outreach.

For the biggest collection of doubles (chickpea sandwiches on fried bread), Jamaican roti, and other Caribbean street food, walk along Eastern Parkway in Brooklyn for the annual West Indian Day Parade every Labor Day. It is one of the loudest, most colorful parades in the whole city—and the best place to find nutcrackers, which are incredibly boozy fruit juice concoctions sold on the sly along the route. See CARIBBEAN; JAMAICAN; and WEST INDIAN DAY PARADE.

The Ninth Avenue International Food Festival claims to be the largest, oldest food festival in the city. It shuts down the street in Manhattan's Hell's Kitchen every May to assemble a global sampler platter of cuisines from Italy, Poland, Greece, Spain, Thailand, and more. See NINTH AVENUE FOOD FESTIVAL.

While the average street fair in New York City usually contains the same combination of tchotchke stands, bounce houses, and local vendors, a handful stand out far above the rest. The annual Atlantic Antic, usually at the end of September, stretches a mile down Brooklyn's Atlantic Avenue, where restaurants and shops have spread their wares into the street since 1974. It is sometimes described by New Yorkers as the only worthwhile street fair. It is certainly the only one referenced in a song by the Beastie Boys, who rhymed "So I'm out pickin' pockets at the Atlantic Antic / And nobody wants to hear you cause your rhymes are so frantic."

While cars and pedestrians battle on the Manhattan roads most of the year, three consecutive Saturdays in August, seven miles of streets become clear of cars for Summer Streets. People can walk, run, bike, and take part in activities along the way. The city turns tunnels into art projects and offers up activities like zip lining over the usually car-clogged streets, even though it is only for a few early hours every year.

You will find something similar on Bedford Avenue every June, where Williamsburg Walks takes over the neighborhood's main drag and fills it with grassy patches, life-sized Scrabble, and art projects. It is part of the Northside Festival, which brings hundreds of musicians and bands—both big names and up-and-coming local groups—to the neighborhood, sometimes to set up a stage on the street. See WILLIAMSBURG.

Fort Greene's colorful Afro-Caribbean vibe goes on display every Memorial Day weekend at the DanceAfrica Bazaar, which involves more than two hundred vendors offering African, Caribbean, and soul foods, crafts, and fashions outside the Brooklyn Academy of Music.

For one of New York City's most festive, and oldest, traditions head to Little Italy in September for the Feast of San Gennaro, billed as New York's biggest and longest-running religious festival. See LITTLE ITALY and SAN GENNARO, FEAST OF. Since it was first held in 1926 as an annual celebration of the patron saint of Naples, it has grown from a one-day affair to an eleven-day celebration. It is full of music, wine, and carnival games. But the "feast" part of the name is serious business. San Gennaro is a Shangri-La for the hungry, where you will find traditional fare like *zeppole* and sausage and peppers. Look further and you will find plenty of unique delicacies, such as roasted hazelnuts on a string or *torrone* (pronounced TUH-ro-nay), a soft nougat made from honey, sugar, egg whites, and roasted nuts.

Scores more street festivals are scattered throughout the year. The London Terrace street fair in Chelsea, for instance, is a big stoop sale that, according to the blog *Chelsea Now*, is always "gloriously bereft of funnel cakes, overpriced lemonade, threadbare sheets, and tube socks of dubious aesthetic value."

Two celebrations take over city streets for Bastille Day. See FRENCH. One is on East Sixtieth Street on the three blocks between Fifth and Lexington Avenues, featuring crepes, cheeses, macaroons, and patisserie treats, along with accordion music and dances. The other takes over several blocks on Brooklyn's Smith Street, where patrons are given the chance to drink Lillet cocktails outdoors while playing pétanque (a French version of bocce) or just listen to music from the Francophile Bar Tabac.

The Hester Street Fair began in 2009 and echoes a generations-old Lower East Side street vendor tradition. See STREET VENDORS. Each spring—usually opening in April and closing in early October—the fair sets up where Hester Street meets Essex, on the site of Manhattan's original pushcart market. The fifty vendors offer up locally made goods and grub from hit eateries, including lobster rolls from Luke's Lobster and Mexican food from Oaxaca Tacos.

Jacobs, Jane. *The Death and Life of Great American Cities.* New York: Random House, 1961.

Litvak, Ed. "Hester Street Fair Announces Opening Day Lineup." *The Lo-Down*, April 16, 2013.

"London Calling: 'Terrace' Street Fair Set for Sept. 28." *Chelsea Now* (blog), September 12, 2013. http://chelseanow.com/2013/09/london-calling-terrace-street-fair-set-for-sept-28.

Miller, Stephen. "Summer Streets and (Mostly) Car-Free Central Park: Same As Last Year." *Streetsblog NYC* (blog), June 19, 2014. http://www.streetsblog.org/2014/06/19/summer-streets-and-mostly-car-free-central-park-same-as-last-year.

Tim Donnelly

Street Vendor Project

In 1998, as a lark before heading off to law school, Sean Basinski made burritos and sold them from a street cart in midtown Manhattan. The hours were longer and the workload was more grueling than he had imagined. But Basinski's fellow vendors had it even harder: most, he found, were immigrants with poor English-language skills and little understanding of their legal rights and responsibilities. Three years later, as a newly minted lawyer, Basinski founded the Street Vendor Project, which operates under the nonprofit Urban Justice Center.

Street Vendor Project members—who sell all sorts of goods in New York, not only food but also flowers, T-shirts, artwork, even emergency umbrellas—pay annual dues. In exchange they receive access to loans and small-business training, legal representation before the city's administrative courts, and assistance in such matters as negotiation of fines and recovery of confiscated property.

To help clarify "the complicated, and sometimes unfair, rules that govern street vending" in the city, the organization collaborated on a concise multilingual guide, distributed to Street Vendor Project members and nonmembers alike. "Vendor Power!," which illustrates the most commonly violated rules in clear diagrams, also includes text in Bengali, Chinese, Arabic, and Spanish as well as English.

The Street Vendor Project has made repeated public calls to increase the number of vending permits, which with few exceptions have been capped for decades, and to open more streets to vending. By far, however, the project that attracts the most attention is the Vendy Awards, an annual street-food competition and fundraiser first held in 2005. See VENDY AWARDS. Since then the Vendy Cup has been awarded to makers of German sausages, Sri Lankan dosas, Middle Eastern shawarma, and Salvadoran pupusas—but never, yet, burritos.

See also FOOD TRUCKS and STREET VENDORS, REGULATION OF.

Center for Urban Pedagogy. "Vendor Power! A Guide to Street Vending in New York City." http://welcometocup.org/file_columns/0000/0012/vp-mpp.pdf.

Horn, Jordana. "Vendor Defender." *Pennsylvania Gazette* (May/June 2010).

Street Vendor Project website: http://streetvendor.org.

Dave Cook

Street Vendors

Vendors have sold their wares on New York City's streets since colonial days, providing food and drinks such as bread, seafood, fruit, nuts, vegetables, and milk. In the early years, vendors played a crucial role in providing city dwellers with water. The vendors drew water from springs farther north on the island and brought it down twice daily by wagon.

City officials tried to regulate street vendors as early as 1691, passing an ordinance forbidding the vendors from operating until two hours after the public markets opened. In 1707 the authorities tried to ban street vendors entirely, but they did not succeed at this virtually impossible task. See PUBLIC MARKETS.

Waves of European immigrants flooded into New York beginning in the 1830s. Street vending was a logical occupation for these newcomers, since they did not need to be skilled in a trade or fluent in English; if they operated within their own communities, they could do business in their native language, stocking exactly the merchandise they knew their countrymen would want. And the city relied on street vendors: the population increased from 391,000 in 1840 to 2.5 million in 1890, and the traditional food-shopping venues—retail grocery stores and public markets—were hard-pressed to meet the demand. Pushcart vendors could also charge less for their goods than rent-paying shop owners or market stall-holders.

In an effort to control the positioning of vendor carts, which often clogged the streets, city officials began requiring pushcart vendors to relocate every thirty minutes. The law was pretty much ignored, but when a police officer came into view the vendors would move their carts into a circle just a few yards away. In crowded quarters filled with new immigrants, such as the Lower East Side, the law was very difficult to enforce. See LOWER EAST SIDE.

The city also tried to manage street vendors by creating open-air pushcart markets, which forced vendors into specific areas. The first was established on Hester Street in 1886, but the most popular pushcart venue was Paddy's Market, which covered both sides of Ninth Avenue between Thirty-Fifth and Forty-Second Streets and sometimes drew as many as two hundred vendors. The Irish, Italian, French, Middle Eastern, and Greek vendors sold produce, bread, meat, fish, poultry, spices, coffees, and teas. But these open-air markets did not prevent other vendors from operating on busy streets.

When the City Bureau of Licenses was created in 1863, vendors were required to be licensed. This action had the strong support of food retailers, such as grocery store and restaurant owners, who felt that street vendors took away their business and that pushcart-clogged streets and sidewalks discouraged their customers. But rather than complain openly about the competition, business owners argued that the congestion made it difficult for emergency vehicles, such as fire engines, to navigate the city.

Pushcart vendors were subject to condemnation in the press. One newspaper account claimed that vendors picked up their produce from the refuse on docks, in railroad yards, and at auctions and wholesale markets, where broken boxes and rotten food were discarded. The produce was often small and substandard, and it was sold in unsanitary conditions, wrote more than one journalist.

These exposés led the city to examine vendor problems. The Pushcart Commission, appointed in 1906, studied the trade and found that Jewish, Italian, and Greek immigrants made up 97 percent of the more than four thousand legal pushcart vendors. The Italians sold fruit and vegetables, the Greeks sold fruit and ice cream, and the Jews—the largest group—sold a much broader selection of foods and beverages. See JEWISH; ITALIAN; and GREEK. They mainly worked on the streets of Manhattan and in the Jewish neighborhoods of Brooklyn, such as Brownsville. The commission found that many pushcart vendors were compelled to bribe police, other city officials, and store owners in order to remain in place. If the payoffs did not materialize, arrests often followed. In 1904 alone more than five thousand vendors were arrested for obstructing sidewalks and streets and for failure to move their stands every thirty minutes, as then required by city ordinance. Arrests were made for some unusual reasons, for example, a complaint that a whistle on a peanut cart bothered the congregation of a local church. The commission found little evidence of health issues with the food sold by the vendors. In fact, fewer problems were ascribed to street vendors than to grocery stores. Since street vendors had no place to keep unsold stock, they bought their produce, fish, or meat daily, in small quantities, whereas grocers placed large orders and kept the food in the store for longer periods of time. Also, contrary to what merchants claimed, the commission found that open-air vendor markets increased business for local stores. See GROCERY STORES.

For all of its research, the commission offered few solutions to the problem of congestion on the streets and sidewalks of New York, and during the next few years the number of vendors increased dramatically. In 1913 the city designated vending areas, such as streets with access to the Manhattan, Williamsburg, and Brooklyn Bridges, in hopes of reducing the number of vendors in Manhattan.

The U.S. Department of Agriculture did another study of New York street vendors in 1925. It found that the ethnic makeup of the trade had changed: 63 percent were Jewish, mainly immigrants from Eastern Europe, 32 percent were Italian, and the rest were German, Irish, African American, or others. An estimated one million Manhattanites were dependent on these vendors for all or part of their food supply. Like the Pushcart Commission, the Department of Agriculture found few sanitary problems with New York City street vendors—they still received fewer violations from the Health Department than did grocery stores and stalls in large markets. The main exception, according to the report, was fish. Sold from pushcarts, it was a "menace to health." The report recommended that sanitary conditions be strictly enforced to protect food from flies, dust, and insects. This was especially important for foods that were typically not washed after purchase, such as candy, breadstuffs, pretzels, dried fruit, and shelled nuts.

The next challenge to vendors was the arrival of automobiles in the city. Vendors who operated in the streets caused traffic delays, especially during rush hours. In 1918 the city declined to issue any more licenses and began to strictly enforce existing laws, so many vendors went into other trades or moved out of the city. During the 1920s, reporters lamented the loss of the city's iconic street vendors, such as those selling hot tamales, apples, pretzels, hot dogs, and hot corn.

But the number of street vendors exploded when the Depression hit. In 1930 an estimated 7,900 vendors plied the city's streets, and as the economy worsened, many more appeared on the scene. Vendors, many unlicensed, again clogged the streets, often selling defective products and preying on unsuspecting tourists, which did nothing to improve the city's image. In the 1930s, the city, led by Mayor Fiorello La Guardia, built enclosed markets in an effort to remove what LaGuardia called the "pushcart evil" from the streets of New York. Four of these markets remain today, including Essex Street Retail Market and Arthur Avenue Retail Market. See LA GUARDIA, FIORELLO; ESSEX STREET MARKET; and ARTHUR AVENUE.

Throughout the twentieth century, changes in immigration patterns continued to alter the ethnic composition of street vendors and their offerings. The Immigration and Nationality Act passed Congress in 1965 and the Immigration and Reform Act passed in 1986 loosened restrictions on immigration from Asia (particularly China), the Caribbean, Central America, and Africa, and these immigrants came to dominate the trade.

New York City's mayors continued their attempts to control street vendors, requiring them to pay for permits from the health department. Food vendors must list and describe the foods they intend to sell and agree to collect and remit sales tax. As the number of permit seekers exceeds the number of available permits, they are distributed by lottery. During the 1990s, Mayor Rudolph Giuliani tried to eliminate vendors from more than a hundred streets; he also tried, unsuccessfully, to force them into pushcart markets. Current restrictions keep carts at least ten feet from a crosswalk and twenty feet from building doorways.

Pushcart vendors allow the average New Yorker (and the curious tourist) to sample different ethnic foods, such as *coco helado* (coconut water ice) in Latino neighborhoods and button-sized Hong Kong–style teacakes in Chinatown.

Hot dogs, however, are the preferred food for street vendors. They are precooked, relatively inexpensive, and easy to prepare. Pushcarts just need warm water to keep the hot dogs ready, buns, and condiments. See HOT DOGS. Carts also sell soda and other goodies. The average vendor nets between $14,000 and $16,000 per year, according to street vendor advocacy groups.

Motorized vending vehicles plied New York City streets as early as the 1920s. Since the 1930s Good Humor ice cream trucks have lured children with their jingling bells, and beginning in the 1950s soft-serve ice cream vans, such as Mister Softee, lurked near schools and playgrounds, their siren song a maddeningly repetitious recorded jingle. Beginning in the late 1990s, food trucks began to proliferate around New York. Some of the pioneers of this resurgence sold coffee and/or desserts, but they were soon joined by others offering ethnic specialties: Chinese dumplings, Belgian waffles, Wiener schnitzel, fish tacos, and Roman-style pizza. Coming full circle, artisan ice cream makers now park their pastel vans in upscale neighborhoods—with nary a jingle to distract from the enjoyment of their pricey treats.

Today there are an estimated twenty thousand licensed and unlicensed street vendors in New York City. They tend to be immigrants and people of color. Most work long hours for relatively low pay. In 2001 Sean Basinski launched the Street Vendor Project to advise vendors and help them overcome challenges. It is a project of the Urban Justice Center, a nonprofit organization that provides legal representation and advocacy to marginalized groups of New Yorkers. The Street Vendor Project launched the street food cook-off and the Vendy Awards in 2005; these are given to the operators of the city's finest food carts and trucks. At the awards ceremony, held on Governor's Island, attendees stand in long lines to sample the finalists' offerings.

See also CRIES OF NEW-YORK, THE; IRISH; PUBLIC MARKETS; STREET VENDORS, REGULATION OF; STREET VENDOR PROJECT; and VENDY AWARDS.

Kraig, Bruce, and Colleen Taylor Sen. *Street Food around the World: An Encyclopedia of Food and Culture.* Santa Barbara, Calif.: ABC-CLIO, 2013.
Vandenberghe, Tom, Jacqueline Goossens, and Luk Thys. *New York Street Food: Cooking & Traveling in the 5 Boroughs.* Tielt, Belgium: Lannoo, 2013.

Andrew F. Smith

Street Vendors, Regulation of

Regulation of vendors on the island of Manhattan is older than New York itself. In 1641 New Amsterdam, Native Americans and "country people," as the Dutch colonists called them, brought fish and corn to the public, outdoor marketplace—but on a haphazard schedule, until officials designated Monday as market day. See COLONIAL DUTCH.

During the centuries since, regulations on street vendors have tended not simply to manage their activities under the rubric of "public order" but to curtail them. When interests of landowners and more established merchants have been balanced against the rights of vendors to earn a living, even at a subsistence level, usually the vendors have not gotten good weight.

Repeated rationales have emerged: vendors unfairly compete with brick-and-mortar businesses; they block streets that should be devoted solely to the smooth flow of traffic; they are dirty and unseemly, reduce the local quality of life, and lower the value of real estate. Vendors have even been accused of being too noisy. Their cries, called out to attract buyers, were outlawed by New York in 1908, to little effect. (More recently, a similar complaint has been leveled at the Mister Softee ice cream jingle.) See CRIES OF NEW-YORK, THE.

All of these reasons may have figured in the reforms of Fiorello La Guardia, who became mayor in 1934. See LA GUARDIA, FIORELLO. Pushcarts, which sold both food and merchandise, had been regulated since the 1880s, first by a rule that required them to "move along," later by attempts to isolate them in designated streets. But as the city grew, the ranks of pushcarts grew with them. Sixty outdoor pushcart markets operated across the city at the height of the Depression, an image that did not comport with plans for the 1939 World's Fair and the portrait of a refined, modern New York.

Funded by New Deal redevelopment money, La Guardia directed the construction of nine indoor markets, including the Essex Street Market, to clear the streets of pushcarts, while closing all but seventeen of the sixty outdoor markets by the end of 1939. See ESSEX STREET MARKET. His administration also sharply reduced the number of pushcart permits. The new, indoor markets could accommodate only a fraction of the displaced vendors, forcing many to go on relief or to operate outside the law.

Subsequent generations of street-food vendors have found that the supply of permits still falls far short of demand. Permits were capped during the administration of Ed Koch, who became mayor in 1978 on a law-and-order platform, and with few exceptions have not been increased in decades, enabling a large black market. Koch's successors Rudolph Giuliani, who closed off many streets to vending, and Michael Bloomberg, who raised fines dramatically, also tipped the balance against vendors. See BLOOMBERG, MICHAEL. Moreover, the regulatory web is notoriously tangled. In New York, street-food vendors are regulated not by a single agency but by at least seven: the Departments of Health, Consumer Affairs, Sanitation, Environmental Protection, Finance, and Parks, as well as the New York Police Department.

One outdoor realm of food vendors, however, continues to receive the city's blessing: farmers' markets. The Greenmarkets, founded in 1976 and numbering more than fifty, are the best known. See GREENMARKETS. In 2008 Mayor Bloomberg supplemented their ranks by permitting one thousand "green carts" that sell fresh fruits and vegetables. The permits are valid only in underserved neighborhoods, but they do offer some additional food vendors the opportunity to grow and thrive.

See also FOOD TRUCKS and STREET VENDORS.

Basinski, Sean. "Hot Dogs, Hipsters, and Xenophobia: Immigrant Street Food Vendors in New York." *Social Research: An International Quarterly* 81, no. 2 (2014): 397–408.

Bluestone, Daniel. "The Pushcart Evil." In *The Landscape of Modernity: New York City 1900–1940*, edited by David Ward and Olivier Zunz, pp. 287–314. Baltimore: Johns Hopkins University Press, 1997.

Wasserman, Suzanne. "Hawkers and Gawkers: Peddling and Markets in New York City." In *Gastropolis*, edited by Annie Hauck-Lawson and Jonathan Deutsch, pp. 153–173. New York: Columbia University Press, 2008.

Dave Cook

Streit's

See MATZAH.

Sugar Refining

Sugar refining has been an important part of New York City since colonial times when partly refined cane sugar was imported and converted into pure sugar. Sugar refineries operated in the city by the early seventeenth century. Several refineries operated in New York, and refining was one of the most important industries in the city. Refineries were the largest buildings in the city by the beginning of the American Revolution. During the war, British authorities closed the refineries and used the space for housing American prisoners of war. When the war ended in 1783, the city's sugar refineries quickly rebounded.

The city's most important sugar refining company was founded in 1807 by William Havemeyer, an immigrant from Bückeburg, Germany. He had learned the art of sugar refining in London and had come to New York in 1798 under contract from a British refining company to run its sugar factory on Pine Street, in Lower Manhattan. Nine years later, Havemeyer and his brother William opened their own sugar refinery in a small building on Vandam Street.

The Havemeyers' refinery was just one of many operating in the city at that time. New York's port facilitated shipping of raw sugar from the Caribbean and Louisiana, and partially refined cane syrup had been shipped there from the West Indies since the early eighteenth century. New York refineries converted the juice into solid forms, the most common being eight- to ten-pound cone-shaped "loaves." New York itself had a large market for sugar, and the city's road, canal, and, later, train connections allowed refined products to be transported easily to points north, south, and west.

The Havemeyers' business flourished, and their children and grandchildren expanded it in subsequent decades. In 1857 the Havemeyers moved from Manhattan across the East River to South Third Street in Williamsburg, where they built what would become the world's largest and most technologically advanced sugar refinery. Initially, it processed thirty thousand pounds of sugar per day, but this gradually increased as additional facilities were built.

The company continued to expand, frequently entering into partnerships with other refiners. In 1863 the company was reorganized as Havemeyers & Elder. By 1872, New York processed 59 percent of the sugar imported into America. Fifteen years later, this had risen to 68 percent. The Williamsburg refinery burned down in 1882, but it was quickly reconstructed with an even greater production capacity. By the 1890s the Brooklyn plant was refining twelve hundred tons of sugar daily.

There were many other sugar refiners operating in New York City and Brooklyn. As a result of mass production, the price of sugar continued to decline, and in 1882 the refiners tried to fix prices in the city. After this attempt failed, in 1887 Havemeyers & Elder and seven other sugar industry leaders formed the Sugar Trust. Dominated by the Havemeyers, the trust was intended to lower production in order

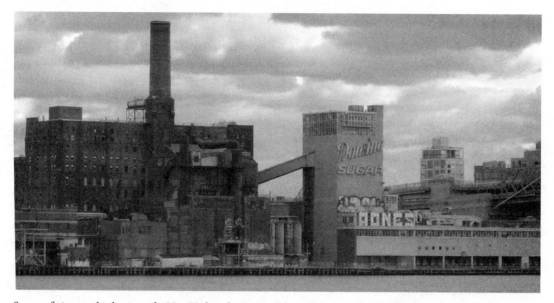

Sugar refining was big business for New York in the nineteenth century. By 1887, New York processed 68 percent of the sugar imported into the United States. The large Domino sugar refinery in Williamsburg—the last one in New York City—closed in 2004. BEYOND MY KEN

to raise prices and increase profits for all the companies. The trust was taken to court and in 1891 was declared illegal by the New York State Supreme Court. The Havemeyers sidestepped the judgment by incorporating as the American Sugar Refining Company in New Jersey, while keeping their headquarters on Wall Street. Inefficient plants were closed, while others were combined, and the American Sugar Refining Company did manage to fix the price of refined sugar.

Historically, sugar was sold in bulk. The American Sugar Refining Company was among the first to package various forms of sugar for retail sale. Packaged sugar cubes and granulated sugar in bags were available by 1879. In the 1880s the American Sugar Refining Company's package labels claimed that the contents were completely pure (in contrast to what might be scooped from an open barrel in a grocery store). In 1898 the company created Eagle brand of granulated sugar and Crystal Domino Sugar (small tablets of solid sugar). Both were sold in five-pound packages. To promote its consumer products, the company launched a very successful advertising campaign, placing ads in newspapers and mass-circulation magazines. The American Sugar Refining Company also supplied individually wrapped paper packages of sugar to finer restaurants under the Domino brand

name. It was originally made in rectangular pieces similar to dominoes.

By 1907 the American Sugar Refining Company and its Domino brand controlled 97 percent of all refined sugar production in the United States. The company was challenged in federal court and in 1921 lost a major antitrust case. Although its control of sugar production declined to 32 percent and for a time it ceased to dominate American sugar refining, the American Sugar Refining Company's sales rebounded in the 1920s and 1930s.

With the outbreak of World War II, the transport of sugar was disrupted. Sugar rationing went into effect in March 1942, and the American Sugar Refining Company barely survived the war. After the war, New York City's sugar refining industry declined. City refineries were closed as more efficient—and less costly—factories were built elsewhere.

The American Sugar Refining Company went through several name changes, becoming Amstar in 1966. In 1988 Amstar was acquired by the British sugar giant Tate & Lyle and renamed Domino Sugar Corp. Tate & Lyle sold Domino Sugar to the Florida Crystals Corporation and the Sugar Cane Growers Cooperative of Florida in 2001, and Domino Sugar was renamed Domino Foods, Inc.

The large Domino sugar refinery in Williamsburg—the last one in New York City—closed in 2004. The property is being redeveloped, and preservationists hope that at least one building, with the proportions of a one-pound box of sugar and emblazoned with "Domino Sugar" in yellow neon letters, will survive.

See also HAVEMEYER FAMILY and WILLIAMSBURG.

Havemeyer, Harry W. *Merchants of Williamsburgh: Frederick C. Havemeyer, Jr., William Dick, John Mollenhauer, Henry O. Havemeyer*. Brooklyn, N.Y.: Havemeyer, 1989.
Smith, Andrew F. *Sugar: A Global History*. London: Reaktion, 2015.
Warner, Deborah Jean. *Sweet Stuff: An American History of Sweeteners from Sugar to Sucralose*. Washington, D.C.: Smithsonian Institution Scholarly Press, 2011.

Andrew F. Smith

Sunset Park

Sunset Park is a predominantly ethnic working-class neighborhood in southwest Brooklyn. Located just south of Brooklyn's Park Slope and the Greenwood Cemetery, north of Bay Ridge, due west of Borough Park, plummeting downhill to the New York Bay, Sunset Park has large Chinese, Mexican, and Indian communities, as well as Hispanic, Scandinavian, Italian, and Irish populations. Settled first by Native Americans and later by the Dutch in the 1600s, the intervening centuries saw the neighborhood dominated by the British, then Irish, Norwegian, and Finnish waves of immigration. Once an agricultural area, Sunset Park later became the focus of a lively port trade along the Upper New York Bay. As the shipping trades dwindled in the later part of the twentieth century, many of the original Scandinavian community began to flee to the suburbs, and the neighborhood then saw an influx of immigration from Mexican, South and Central American, and Chinese and South Asian communities.

This neighborhood is the go-to culinary destination for those seeking some of the best Asian, Mexican, and Hispanic cuisines that New York City has to offer. There are more street food vending carts per capita in Sunset Park than in any other neighborhood in New York City, and a variety of sit-down restaurants, ranging from palatial dimsum parlors to barebones taco stands.

The section of Fifth Avenue running south from Sixty-Fifth Street toward Greenwood Park—also referred to as Little Latin America—is peppered with Mexican, South, and Central American businesses, taquerias, and bodegas selling tamarind candles, tomatillos, Jaritos sodas, and other Mexican staples. Tacos, whether *carne asada, lengua* (a brisket-like beef tongue), or *carnitas* (fried pork), abound. Probably the best Mexican sandwiches in New York City can be found here, including tortas (pressed heros with jalapeño, sliced avocado, queso blanco, mayo, lettuce, and meat) and *cemitas* (chipotle pepper, onion, refried beans, papalo leaf, Oaxaca cheese, avocado, and meat inside a sesame egg bun). Other specialties include red *pozole*, and *pollo en pipián verde*, a specialty of Puebla, where many residents in Sunset Park's Mexican community can trace their heritage. Nearby are Puerto Rican, Dominican, Colombian, Salvadoran, Peruvian, Nicaraguan, Honduran, and Ecuadorian cuisines. See DOMINICAN; MEXICAN; and PUERTO RICAN.

Sunset Park has the fastest growing Chinese population in New York City and rivals Manhattan and Flushing, Queens, in terms of the quality and variety of Asian cuisines available. Eighth Avenue between Sixty-Fifth and Fortieth Streets in Brooklyn defines the rough boundaries of Brooklyn's Chinatown, featuring regional Chinese cuisines including Hunan, Cantonese, and Sichuan styles. See CHINESE COMMUNITY. The grocery and superstore Fei Long extends the length of a football field down Sixty-Fourth Street, and includes every type of Chinese fruit and vegetable imaginable, as well as fish, meats, dry goods, and a food court. Bubble teahouses and cheap, tasty dumpling shops dot the streetscape of Eighth Avenue, alongside dollar stores and fishmongers hawking their catch. Southeast Asian fruits such as durian, rambutan, and jackfruit can be found, in tandem with a rich primer of Asian greens and vegetables, such as bok choy, gai lan (Chinese broccoli), snow pea shoots, yard-long beans, and bitter melon.

Malaysian, Vietnamese, and Thai cuisines are also strong dining choices in Sunset Park, boasting authentic flavors (although most restaurants are Chinese-owned). At Malaysian restaurants such as Banana Leaf, Randang Village, and New Belachan, one can sample tongue-curling *asam laksa* soup, soured from lemongrass and screw pine (pandanus) leaves; *mee goring*, egg noodles with potatoes in savory squid paste; or *nasi lemak*, a smorgasbord of coconut rice, curry chicken, tart vegetable pickle, refreshing cucumbers, eggs, and *belachan* (the fermented fish paste that gives Malaysian food its unique funk). While bahn mi is the go-to at Vietnamese sandwich shops such as Ba Xuen, sit-down restaurant Thanh Da heats up the regional fare with their specialties *bo bun Hue*, a beef noodle soup from the Central Vietnam region of Hue, and *bun rieu*, a crab paste, tomato, and vermicelli soup.

Many residents who have formerly lived in neighborhoods in Manhattan or Park Slope, Brooklyn, are now migrating to Sunset Park due to a wealth of brownstones and apartments available at more affordable rates. Chain stores are increasingly finding Sunset Park more attractive as well, with small businesses giving way to Dunkin' Donuts, CVS, and Papa John's Pizza, sometimes ironically setting up shop alongside longtime neighborhood businesses. As this history of the neighborhood implies a long-standing tradition of diverse change, it pays to savor the mosaic of flavors currently available in this panoply of cuisines.

See also BROOKLYN.

DiGregorio, Sarah. "Our Ten Best Sunset Park Restaurants." *Village Voice*, March 26, 2010.
Mishan, Ligaya. "A Soup Saved from the Cold—Hungry City: Yu Nan Flavour Garden in Sunset Park, Brooklyn." *New York Times*, January 23, 2014.
Sietsema, Robert. "Pampazos and Pozole at Sunset Park's Xochimilco." *Village Voice*, April 15, 2009.
Sietsema, Robert. "Banana Leaf: Here's Your Skanky Wallop." *Village Voice*, November 16, 2011.

Sherri Machlin

Supermarkets

Supermarkets, with their one-stop-shopping experience, have been in existence for less than one hundred years. Before supermarkets sold a vast array of goods under a single roof, shoppers in New York City and across the country procured foodstuffs from a combination of public markets, street peddlers, and small stores dedicated to specific products, such as meat, produce, and baked goods.

New York City has been home to a fair share of supermarket history. The Great Atlantic & Pacific Tea Company, Inc. (A&P), which still operates more than three hundred stores across the country, is widely recognized as the first chain grocery store. Founded by George F. Gilman and George H. Hartford, the original A&P opened in New York City in 1859 at 31 Vesey Street, where it sold tea, coffee, and spices. Additional stores opened throughout the city and by 1881, A&P was the first chain to operate one hundred stores in sites across the United States.

New York City has also been home to grocery chains that began as brotherly ventures. Cyrus, Frank, and Charles Jones opened their first store—originally called the Jones Brothers Tea Co.—in 1872 in Scranton, Pennsylvania. Later renamed Grand Union, the store expanded from Scranton to eastern Pennsylvania, Michigan, and New York, eventually building a headquarters and warehouse in Brooklyn. Like A&P, Grand Union experienced incredible growth. By 1912, the chain operated two hundred stores across the country, and by 1931, more than seven hundred stores.

Similarly, brothers Charles and Diedrich Gristede opened their first small grocery store in 1888 at Forty-Second Street and Second Avenue. Fifty years later, the brothers' business operated more than 150 stores. There are currently more than thirty Gristede's stores throughout Manhattan, Westchester, and Brooklyn. Started by Nathan Glickberg in 1933 as a family venture, Fairway markets began as a fruit and vegetable stand and now operate a number of stores throughout the city.

By the 1920s, chain grocery stores, like A&P, as well as Kroger and Piggly Wiggly, proliferated in many American cities, offering a wider array and more consistent supply of goods at lower prices. The supermarkets of the 1930s, however, offered a new combination of retail services. These included self-service design, a transactional process in which customers no longer ordered their items from a clerk but instead roamed the aisles of inventory themselves, as well as economies of scale with lower prices, more options, and larger volume sales. Customers exuberantly flocked to new supermarkets in great numbers. The opening day of a new supermarket served as a local festival of consumption, routinely characterized by long lines, large crowds, giveaways, and a frenzied excitement.

New York boasted the first supermarkets. In 1930, Michael J. Cullen opened the first King Kullen store on Jamaica Avenue in Queens. Compared to smaller chain grocery stores, King Kullen offered greater convenience and lower prices. Shoppers enthusiastically embraced King Kullen and by 1936, more than a dozen stores marked Long Island's foodscape.

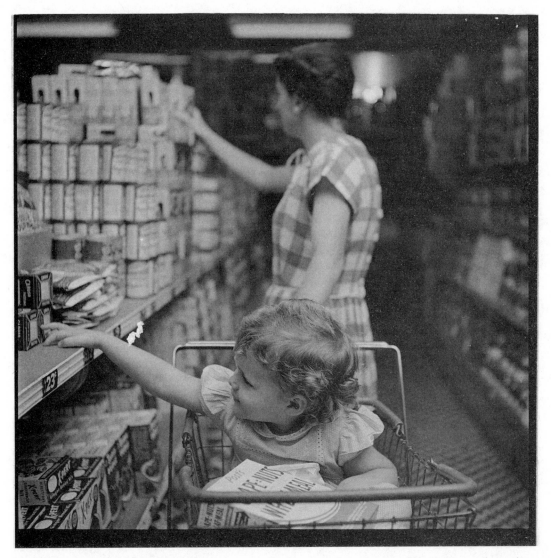

A child in a carriage with her mother in the supermarket. Supermarkets made shopping for groceries easy for mothers, as they brought together a wide variety of decently priced food items in a single location. This photo was taken by Stanley Kubrick for *Look* magazine, 1946. © SK FILM ARCHIVES/MUSEUM OF THE CITY OF NEW YORK.

Today, King Kullen operates thirty-eight stores in the area.

After opening their first grocery store in 1932 at Eighty-Third Street and Lexington Avenue, Nicholas D'Agostino Sr. and his brother Pasquale relocated to Seventy-Seventh Street and Third Avenue in 1938, where they operated another of New York's first supermarkets. A marvel to shoppers, they sold meat, dairy, produce, baked goods, and additional food products all in one store. In the 1950s, the brothers' business was also one of the first in New York City to incorporate shopping carts and frozen food cases.

D'Agostino's currently operates twenty-six stores in New York and Westchester.

In many U.S. cities, supermarkets revolutionized how food was purchased and consumed, often tied to a pervasive car culture. In New York City, however, a variety of food retailers have continued to share market space, including not only grocery stores and supermarkets, but also specialty markets, delis, greengrocers, convenience stores, discount warehouses, wholesale clubs, co-ops, health-food shops, and produce carts. Today, New York City boasts more grocery stores per square mile than elsewhere, but fewer stores per capita, which can result in crowds and lengthy lines. Although New York City grocery stores may offer specialty items, the stores are usually smaller than suburban ones and, due to space constraints, they tend to offer fewer options overall. Furthermore, despite higher prices, city grocery stores often turn lower profits than suburban locations due to high retail rents. New Yorkers also shop differently. With smaller kitchens and low car ownership, they trek to neighborhood grocery stores with bags or hand-carts in tow about three times per week, more than the national average of twice per week. Although options abound, New York City's current food retail environment in many ways mirrors the days before the rise of the supermarket.

See also A&P; FAIRWAY; GROCERY STORES; KING KULLEN; and WHOLE FOODS.

Belasco, Warren, and Roger Horowitz, eds. *Food Chains: From Farmyard to Shopping Cart.* Philadelphia: University of Pennsylvania Press, 2009.
Deutsch, Tracey. *Building a Housewife's Paradise: Gender, Politics, and American Grocery Stores in the Twentieth Century.* Chapel Hill: University of North Carolina Press, 2010.
Mayo, James. *The American Grocery Store: The Business Evolution of an Architectural Space.* Westport, Conn.: Greenwood, 1993.

Emily J.H. Contois

Supplemental Nutrition Assistance Program (SNAP)

Most commonly known as "food stamps," the Supplemental Nutrition Assistance Program (SNAP) has been part of New York City's arsenal against hunger for decades. Food insecurity has been part of many New Yorkers' experience, whether as recent immigrants to the United States, as starving artists new to the city, or as resident working poor and welfare recipients. While earlier measures to address food insecurity were largely private—bread lines and food pantries run by churches, charities, and philanthropists—government-administered food assistance has existed in New York City for nearly a century.

In 1933, President Franklin D. Roosevelt enacted an early antecedent of SNAP to alleviate crushing food insecurity as part of his one hundred days legislative program. In 1939, another, state-based food relief program was begun in Rochester, New York, and soon spread to New York City. In 1967, as part of President Lyndon Johnson's War on Poverty, the food stamp and Women, Infants, and Children programs were initiated. In the early 2000s this program was renamed SNAP. Recipients stopped receiving actual paper stamps and began using electronic benefits transfer cards.

Today, nearly 20 percent of New York City residents (1.7 million of 8.4 million) receive some form of SNAP. And New York City residents comprise two-thirds of all Empire State residents currently receiving SNAP.

Administered by the city's Human Resources Administration, food stamp enrollment occurs in New York City at a rate much higher than the national average as wage earners have faced persistent unemployment and stagnant wages alongside rapidly escalating and nearly completely unchecked costs of living. However, some reports (most notably the city's Independent Budget Office) suggest that this trend is abating.

But SNAP dollars are not just a lifeline for recipients—they form a significant component of New York's food economy. Farmers' markets, such as GrowNYC, not only accept SNAP but offer incentive programs, encouraging SNAP recipients to spend their dollars at the farmer's market and offering cash bonuses for doing so. See GROWNYC. And the vast network of independent bodega owners and small grocery chains that dominate low-income and gentrifying areas also rely on SNAP monies for their income. In fact, such establishments are so reliant that when cuts were made to SNAP in 2013, one bodega owner told the *New York Daily News* that he had to let two employees go for lack of business. See BODEGAS.

In 2012, New York City, at the directive of Governor Andrew Cuomo (and over the wishes of then-mayor Michael Bloomberg) ceased its policy of fingerprinting SNAP recipients. (Bloomberg also sought to ban the application of food stamp monies to sugary sodas.) At the time, New York City was one of two cities that fingerprinted SNAP recipients, a policy initiated in 1996 by Mayor Rudolph Giuliani and continued by Bloomberg. See BLOOMBERG, MICHAEL.

New York's reliance on SNAP persists even as menu prices escalate throughout all five boroughs. For much of New York, $36 is the price of an entrée—or even a glass of wine—at any number of restaurants profiled in this volume, and indeed, such items can go for a great deal more than $36. But for one in five New Yorkers, it represents a week's worth of meals. Similarly, a tasting menu for two at Thomas Keller's Per Se is $642, while the monthly food stamp allotment for a family of four is $632.

This harsh disparity is fast becoming a defining factor of New York City. And for many New Yorkers, an electronic benefits transfer card is just as vital as a MetroCard. See HUNGER PROGRAMS.

Byrne, John Aidan. "It's Not Working: Nearly 2 Million New York City Residents on Food Stamps." New York Post, April 14, 2013.

Hine, L. W. "Bowery Mission Bread Line on a Cold Winter Night." New York Public Library Digital Collections. http://digitalcollections.nypl.org/items/510d47d9-a98e-a3d9-e040-e00a18064a99.

Hu, Winnie, and Kim Severson. "Cut in Food Stamps Forces Hard Choices on Poor." New York Times, November 7, 2013.

Rodriguez, Cindy. "Cuomo Ends Controversial Policy of Fingerprinting Food Stamp Recipients." WNYC News, May 17, 2012. http://www.wnyc.org/story/210148-cuomo-ends-fingerprinting-food-stamp-recipients/.

Slattery, Dennis, and Corrine Letsch. "Food Stamp Cuts Hurt New York City Stores as Customers Spend Less on Groceries." New York Daily News, March 17, 2014.

Ulla, Gabe. "The 14 Most Expensive Tasting Menus in America." Eater.com, January 28, 2013. http://www.eater.com/2013/1/28/6489897/the-14-most-expensive-tasting-menus-in-america.

U.S. Department of Agriculture, Food and Nutrition Service. "A Short History of SNAP." http://www.fns.usda.gov/snap/short-history-snap.

Alexis Zanghi

Sushi

Sushi, one of the most common foods served in New York City's restaurants in the twenty-first century, is a relatively recent addition to the city's culinary repertoire. Its arrival dates to the late 1950s, when Japanese businessmen flocked to New York, opening overseas offices for Japanese companies. These professionals demanded authentic, high-quality Japanese food, not the made-up American dishes identified as "Japanese," and they could afford the best. Japanese chefs and sushi masters were brought over to prepare the food their compatriots craved.

As upscale Japanese restaurants opened, manned by sushi professionals, their Japanese customers invited American colleagues to try the novel cuisine. Japanese food is complex and subtle, but what received the most attention was sashimi—sliced filets of raw fish—and sushi—vinegared rice topped with raw fish (among other things). Before that time, most New Yorkers had not had the opportunity to eat raw fish.

Interest in Japanese food, especially the raw fish preparations, began to grow in the 1960s, when Craig Claiborne, the New York Times's food editor, first wrote about it. Two years later he cautioned that raw fish was probably still "a trifle too 'far out' for many American palates." But by 1965 Claiborne described New York City as "a metropolis with a growing public enthusiasm for the Japanese raw fish specialties, sashimi and sushi." Two years later, he noted that "gastronomically there has been no phenomenon in recent years to equal the proliferation of Japanese restaurants, East Side, West Side and up and down the town." By 1970, Claiborne proclaimed sushi and sashimi haute cuisine in their own right, noting that New Yorkers had taken to them "with what could be regarded as passion." See CLAIBORNE, CRAIG.

Sushi's newfound visibility and prestige was upheld by subsequent Times food critics. Mimi Sheraton first reviewed the restaurant Hatsuhana in 1978. She tasted raw tuna from the sushi bar, and gave the restaurant two stars. Sheraton reviewed Hatsuhana again in 1983 and gave it four stars—the first time the New York Times had awarded a Japanese restaurant such an honor. Restaurant reviews helped popularize sushi, and more and more New Yorkers were willing to try it. Hatsuhana lives on, joined by many other distinguished sushi purveyors including Masa, Sushi Yasuda, Blue Ribbon Sushi, Kurumazushi, Sushi Seki, and Sushi of Gari.

The sushi served in inexpensive restaurants and sold in grocery stores and delis is usually made with smoked tuna prepared in Southeast Asia. Smoking preserves the fish, so it can be sold weeks or months later with relatively little deterioration. The smoking also fixes the tuna's bright red color, and it acquires no obvious smell from the process.

Today, virtually every community in New York City has at least one—and often many—establishments where sushi is sold. People of all backgrounds also grab sushi packs for a quick office lunch, or they save up to indulge in an omekase, or "chef's choice" high-end sushi-bar dinner. Some are very expensive. Masayoshi Takayama, owner of Masa, charges up to

$500 for a single sushi dinner (not including tax, tip, or beverages).

See also JAPANESE and RESTAURANTS.

Corson, Trevor. *The Story of Sushi: An Unlikely Saga of Raw Fish and Rice*. New York: Harper Perennial, 2008.
Smith, Andrew F. *American Tuna: The Rise and Fall of an Improbable Food*. Berkeley: University of California Press, 2012.

Andrew F. Smith

Sweet'N Low

Sweet'N Low is an artificial sweetener manufactured by the Cumberland Packing Corporation in Brooklyn, New York. Derived from saccharin, the sugar substitute was created in 1957 by Ben and Marvin Eisenstadt.

Ben Eisenstadt ran a cafeteria on Flushing Avenue at Cumberland Street, across from the Brooklyn Navy Yard, during World War II. When the war ended, in 1945, his business quickly declined, so he sold the cafeteria's contents and began packaging individual tea bags. Eisenstadt had long been appalled by the open sugar bowls used to sweeten tea, considering them unsanitary. His wife, Betty, suggested he use the tea bag machines to place sugar in individual packets, the way it would place tea in individual bags. The plan worked. Eisenstadt pitched the idea to sugar companies, but since he had failed to apply for a patent, the companies simply copied the idea without paying him royalties.

Eisenstadt continued to package sugar under the name Cumberland Packing Corporation. His eldest child, Marvin, joined the business in 1956 after receiving a degree in chemistry from the University of Vermont. Together, father and son tried to package

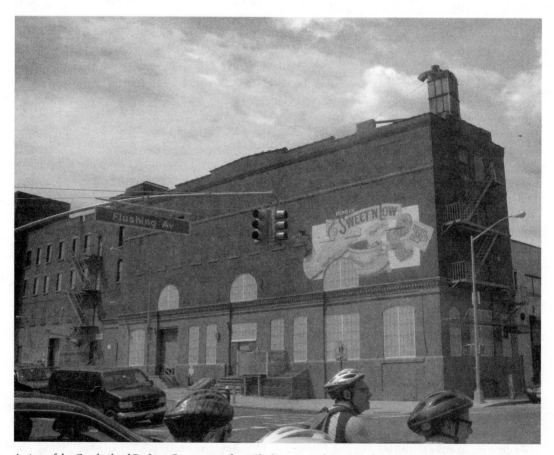

A view of the Cumberland Packing Corporation from Flushing Ave, where Sweet'N Low is packaged, along with many other individually packaged, single-serving products. JIM HENDERSON

numerous items. Among their successes were the soy sauce packets still popular with Chinese take-out.

Using Marvin's chemistry knowledge, the pair took interest in saccharin, an artificial sweetening agent first produced in 1878. Until that time, it was available only in liquid or tablet form, and was typically reserved for diabetics and the obese. They found that mixing powdered saccharin with dextrose, cream of tartar, and calcium silicate created a long-lasting, low-calorie sugar substitute. Having learned from Ben's previous error, the Eisenstadts were careful to patent their creation before bringing it to market. They chose the color pink to stand out from the other packets that might be in a sugar bowl, and took the name from Ben's favorite song, "Sweet and Low" by Joseph Barnby, which in turn had been derived from a poem by Alfred, Lord Tennyson. The trademark patent—number 1,000,000—registered the name and the curvy, musical-staff logo. With weight reduction the rage at the time, the concept was an instant hit. It soon faced competition from other low-calorie sweeteners, such as aspartame (marketed as Equal in a bright blue bag).

In 1977, a study suggested that saccharin caused bladder cancer in male rats. Congress passed the Saccharin Study and Labeling Act, allowing the continued sale of Sweet'N Low, but requiring it to carry a warning label. The cancer claim was eventually discredited, and the label was removed in 2000.

In 1994, Marvin Eisenstadt was indicted for tax fraud. In his 2006 memoir *Sweet and Low: A Family Story*, Rich Cohen, disinherited grandson of Ben Eisenstadt, alleged that Marvin had hired a member of the Bonanno crime family to provide illegal campaign contributions to Senator Alfonse D'Amato. Federal prosecutors denied that claim.

Cumberland Packing Corporation is still based out of its original Brooklyn location. It also manufactures Sugar in the Raw, Nu-Salt, and Butter Buds, among other substitutes.

Cohen, Richard. *Sweet and Low: A Family Story*. New York: Farrar, Straus and Giroux, 2006.

Thomas, Robert McG., Jr. "Benjamin Eisenstadt, 89, a Sweetener of Lives." *New York Times*, April 10, 1996.

Keith Williams

Swiss

See DELMONICO BROTHERS; DELMONICO'S; and CHALET SUISSE.

Sylvia's

The average restaurant doesn't have a long life span—maybe three to five years if they make it past the first one. Sylvia's, at 328 Malcolm X Boulevard near 127th Street in Harlem, has been in business since 1962.

The restaurant was founded by Sylvia Woods, well known today as the Queen of Soul Food. Woods was an ambitious teenager determined to leave the poverty of the South Carolina cotton fields of her youth behind her when she moved to New York to join her mother, who had already moved there for better work opportunities. At first she worked in a hat factory in Queens and in the 1950s was a waitress for ten years at a small Harlem luncheonette (six booths and fifteen stools) known as Johnson's. When its owner retired, Woods bought the place for $20,000 with help from her mother, who mortgaged the family farm to do so. Woods renamed it "Sylvia's."

Over the years, the restaurant, located around the corner from the Apollo Theater, spread out to include an entire block. Famed for its southern soul food, Sylvia's became known as the meeting place for Black America. Filmmaker Spike Lee used the restaurant as a location for his 1991 film, *Jungle Fever*.

It has served pretty much the same food since its inception. Generations of civil rights activists, national and local politicians, celebrities, singers, busloads of tourists, and just plain folk from the neighborhood have come there for the meat loaf in Sylvia's special sauce, the southern fried chicken, the sweet potato pie and candied yams that characterize its menu. These days, however, less heart-stopping dishes like salads topped with grilled salmon, herbed baked eggs, and vegetable platters can be ordered there as well. But they're not the reason people come to Sylvia's.

Sylvia's has always been a family affair, involving not only Woods's childhood sweetheart and husband, Herbert Woods—they met when she was eleven and he was twelve and both were working in the fields—but also their children (two sons, Van and Kenneth Woods, and two daughters, Bedelia and Crizette). Their children and grandchildren now own and operate the much-expanded restaurant, which has grown to include an entire block and can seat more than 250 people.

Woods retired when she was eighty. In 2012, when she was eighty-six, Wood died at her home, just hours before the then mayor of New York Michael

Bloomberg was to give her a medal commemorating the fiftieth anniversary of her restaurant at a gala reception at Gracie Mansion. Her husband Herbert died in 2001.

The success of the restaurant led to a catering service, a banquet hall, a line of packaged soul products, including her bottled hot sauce and cornbread and pancake mixes, sold nationally, and two cookbooks: the 1992 *Sylvia's Soul Food: Recipes from Harlem's World Famous Restaurant* (written with Christopher Styler) and the 1999 *Sylvia's Family Soul Food Cookbook,* (written with Melissa Clark). The Sylvia and Herbert Woods Scholarship endowment distributes four-year partial scholarships to children of and around the Harlem Community.

See also HARLEM and WOODS, SYLVIA.

Fox, Margalit. "Sylvia Woods, Soul-Food Restaurateur is Dead at 86." *New York Times,* July 20, 2012.
Sandoval, Edgar, Michael J. Feeney, and Helen Kennedy. "Queen of Soul Food Sylvia Woods Dies at 86." *New York Daily News,* July 19, 2012.

Judith Weinraub

Syrian and Lebanese

Beginning in the 1880s, tens of thousands of immigrants from Greater Syria (today the countries of Syria, Lebanon, Palestine, and Jordan) settled in Lower Manhattan, in an area known as Little Syria. See LITTLE SYRIA. Many also settled in what was then known as the South Ferry neighborhood of Brooklyn. These early immigrants were mostly Christian but included Muslims, Druze, and Jews. The Syrian and Lebanese community was prominent in the textile industry in New York from the 1890s through the 1930s and made important contributions to Arabic-language publishing worldwide. It also established some of the first Arabic-speaking Christian congregations in the United States. These entrepreneurial immigrants opened dozens of grocery stores and restaurants, making a lasting impact on the Arab food scene in New York City.

Nearly a century before hummus became available in every grocery store, Syrian and Lebanese immigrants opened restaurants in Lower Manhattan. By 1908 there were more than fifty such restaurants and grocery stores, catering mainly to an Arab immigrant clientele. These early restaurants and cafes often did not have formal names and were known only by their location or proprietor. In the 1920s, after Syrian- and Lebanese-owned restaurants started attracting more non-Arab visitors, many adopted more "exotic" names, like The Sheik, The Arabian Inn, and the Egyptian Rose Restaurant, reflecting the portrayal of Arabs in Hollywood movies and popular culture.

To date, the majority of Arab or Middle Eastern cuisine nationwide is Levantine. Syrian and Lebanese immigrants were the first to open successful restaurants, serving kibbeh, hummus, falafel, stuffed grape leaves, shish kabob, and *baqlawa* (baklava). Later, immigrants from other Arab countries built on this success and continued to offer these dishes, which had become Middle Eastern restaurant staples. There is still a prominent Syrian and Lebanese presence in the Arab American food community in New York City, notably Sahadi's on Atlantic Avenue. The Sahadi family has been in the food business in New York since the 1890s. Pistachios are also part of the legacy of the Syrian and Lebanese community in New York. One of the first and largest importers of pistachios, which are native to Turkey, Iran, and Syria, was an Armenian immigrant family from Greater Syria, the Germacks, who had a large operation in Lower Manhattan in the 1920s. The Germack family continues to import and roast pistachios in Detroit.

The legacy of these early Syrian and Lebanese restaurants in Lower Manhattan and Brooklyn survives through the diverse array of Arabic restaurants that have graced, and continue to grace, Atlantic Avenue: from the first Sudanese restaurant, Wadi Halfa, that opened in 1971 to the numerous Yemeni and Egyptian restaurants of the 1980s and 1990s. Often, these new restaurants opened in the same locations as previous Syrian- and Lebanese-owned establishments, sometimes maintaining the same name.

See also ARAB COMMUNITY; EGYPTIAN; FALAFEL; HALVA; and HUMMUS.

Khater, Akram Fouad. *Inventing Home: Emigration, Gender, and the Middle Class in Lebanon, 1870–1920.* Berkeley: University of California Press, 2001.
Younis, Adele L., and Philip M. Kayal. *The Coming of the Arabic-Speaking People to the United States.* Staten Island, N.Y.: Center for Migration Studies, 1995.

Matthew Jaber Stiffler

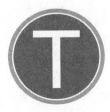

Tavern on the Green

Tavern on the Green (Sixty-Seventh Street and Central Park West) is housed in an 1870 structure built to hold Central Park's sheep. It has been in operation since 1934. After the sheep were sent to Brooklyn's Prospect Park, a restaurant was opened in the space, one which featured a large dance floor, outdoor seating, and even then the iconic trees wrapped in white lights. When Joe Baum's Restaurant Associates took over the reins in 1962, Tavern on the Green began its true ascent into celebrity, becoming a destination spot for tourists and New Yorkers alike. See BAUM, JOE and RESTAURANT ASSOCIATES.

In 1974 Warner LeRoy (grandson of one of the founders of Warner Brothers Studios and son of the producer of *The Wizard of Oz*) spent two years and $10 million to reopen Tavern on the Green. Diners in the new glass-enclosed Crystal Room, bursting with Tiffany glass and Baccarat chandeliers, now marveled at a garden of illuminated animal-shaped topiaries. Former *New York Times* restaurant critic Pete Wells wrote that in its heyday, Tavern on the Green was a "wedding cake palace as imagined by a six year old princess with a high fever." The restaurant teemed with celebrities and can be seen in films such as *Ghostbusters* and *Wall Street*.

Tavern on the Green was known as a "special occasion" destination yet struggled to win critical praise for its food. In the 1990s, however, Patrick Clark, one of the nation's highest-profile African American chefs, won applause for lifting the culinary standards of the establishment. Despite being one of the nation's top-grossing restaurants, bankrolling the sprawling property amid an economic recession was a challenge.

In 2009 the company filed for Chapter 11 bankruptcy protection, and the New York City Department of Parks and Recreation did not renew the site's operating license. The restaurant's opulent fixtures were auctioned off, and the stripped-down palace was used as a gift shop and visitors' center. Private investors reopened the restaurant in 2014. The Crystal Room had been torn down, and 2014 saw three different executive chefs at the helm. New Yorkers now hold their breath waiting to see the fate of this storied attraction.

"Tavern on the Green." NYTimes.com. Updated December 9, 2009. http://topics.nytimes.com/top/ reference/timestopics/organizations/t/tavern_on_ the_green/index.html.
Wells, Pete. "A Celebrity Steps Back into the Spotlight," *New York Times*, June 24, 2015.

Claire Stewart

Taverns

A tavern is an establishment that sells alcoholic beverages and often food. Almost as soon as there were Dutch settlers on Manhattan there were taverns. Many of the early taverns provided lodging.

The first tavern on Manhattan Island was the Staat's Herberg (City Tavern) at Coentes and Pearl, built in 1642. The importance of the Staat's Herberg was such that it was used as New Amsterdam's and then New York's city hall until 1812, when the present city hall was finished.

Taverns flourished because of demand as well as lax licensing regulations. Each social group in the city had a tavern where it chose to gather. Visiting

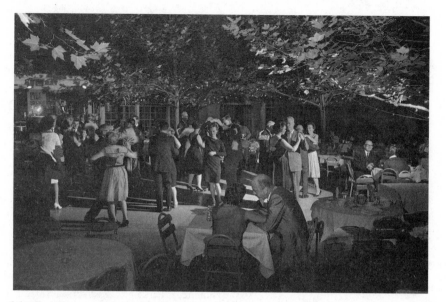

Dancing and drinks at Tavern on the Green in the 1960s. It was a popular destination, with its large dance floor, outdoor seating, and iconic trees wrapped in white lights. JOHN MURVACKI/*NEW YORK TIMES*/REDUX

farmers gathered at Sergeant Litschoe's tavern. The soldiers and rough sort gathered at the White Horse Tavern. Sailors and apprentices drank at the Blue Dove. When revolution was in the air the Liberty Boys drank and plotted at Montayne's Tavern. The Bull's Head Tavern became a meeting place for cattlemen to share a bit of gossip. The first Tammany Club in New York City met in Martling's Tavern.

From the first settlement to today, taverns have been where New Yorkers meet, debate, and overindulge. Apartment living fosters a demand for a place to socialize. In the nineteenth century, taverns provided immigrants a place to speak their native tongue as well as learn English. Taverns also provided ways to communicate with the old country through letter writers who would send messages back to hometowns. Alcoholic beverages were, of course, consumed in great quantities. All sorts of financial transaction also made the tavern an important part of society as most tavern customers had little faith in bankers. The following taverns and their historical significance are listed according to age.

Fraunces Tavern, located in the financial district (54 Pearl Street, corner of Broad Street), is New York's earliest tavern and is still in operation today. It is considered to be Manhattan's oldest surviving building and has been listed on the National Register of Historic Places since 1977. See FRAUNCES TAVERN.

The Ear Inn, at 326 Spring Street, is a three-story building completed in 1812, the home of a black man named James Brown. In 1817 Brown opened a tavern that was very popular among sailors and longshoremen. During Prohibition the ground floor was a speakeasy, while the upstairs changed from a boarding house to a headquarters for smugglers to a brothel. When it reopened in 1977, there were restrictions to changing signage on historic buildings. The owners painted over part of the "B" on the old neon sign, creating the "EAR Inn," in homage to a music magazine with the same name published upstairs.

The Stonewall Inn, at 53 Christopher Street (between West Fourth Street and Waverly Place), was built between 1843 and 1846 as a stable. The building became a restaurant in 1930 and remained so until it was gutted by a fire in the mid-1960s. The Stonewall Inn is now one of the most famous gay bars in the United States, the site of the Stonewall riots in 1969. See STONEWALL INN.

Though some claim the ale house was founded in 1854, municipal records deem it impossible. Whatever the year, it is certain that McSorley's has some of the oldest urinals still in public use in New York City, dating back to 1911. Famous patrons have included Abraham Lincoln, Teddy Roosevelt, and E. E. Cummings, who referred to McSorley's as "snug and evil" in a 1923 poem, "Snug and Warm Inside

McSorley's." Until 1970 women were not allowed in the bar, an attitude reflected by their former motto "Good Ale, Raw Onions and No Ladies." See MC-SORLEY'S OLD ALE HOUSE.

Pete's, "the tavern that O. Henry made famous," dates back to 1829, though it was not operated as a bar until 1864. As was the case for most of the other pubs, Prohibition meant business as usual, though its brief status as a flower shop was one of the more creative covers. It lies in the Gramercy Park Historical District, though it has not been specifically designated as a New York City landmark.

The Landmark Tavern, 626 Eleventh Avenue (corner of Forty-Sixth Street), originally built in 1868, was on what was then the waterfront, before Twelfth Avenue was built over with landfill. During its speakeasy days, the establishment was frequented by gangster, actor, and Hell's Kitchen resident George Raft.

Old Town Bar joined the Union Square neighborhood in 1882. It survived Prohibition by becoming a speakeasy under the name Craig's Restaurant, where patrons hid their booze in compartments underneath their seats. At first, Old Town served only men at the bar, with an upper dining room for families. Old Town is known as a literary bar—Frank McCourt, Billy Collins, and Nick Hornby are among the writers who frequented the high-ceilinged establishment.

Opened in 1880, The Whitehorse Tavern was first a longshoremen's bar. In the 1950s it became a literary hangout. Among its many acclaimed patrons were Dylan Thomas, Michael Harrington, author and political organizer Dan Wakefield, Jim Morrison, Hunter S. Thompson, and John Ashbery. See WHITE HORSE TAVERN.

Dating back to 1884, P. J. Clarke's was named after its second owner, Irish immigrant Patrick J. Clarke, who bought it in 1912. Johnny Mercer wrote his song "One for My Baby" on a napkin at P. J. Clarke's. Buddy Holly proposed to his wife there. It is has also served as the location for numerous films, including *The Lost Weekend, Annie Hall,* and the television series *Mad Men.* See P. J. CLARKE'S.

See also SALOONS and SPEAKEASIES.

Chappelle, George S. *The Restaurants of New York.* New York: Greenberg, 1925.
Lathrop, Elise. *Early American Inns and Taverns.* New York: Tudor, 1926.
"Stonewall." National Historic Landmarks Program, National Park Service, 2008.

Peter LaFrance

Tea

Known in China as *ch'a* and derived from the *Camellia sinensis* plant, tea is thought to have been discovered about 2700 B.C.E. by Emperor Shen-Nong. The beverage was also imported from India, Indonesia, and Ceylon, as Sri Lanka was then known, and played an important role in New York.

Portugal became Europe's first importer of tea in 1557, with The Netherlands in 1610 commencing trade in what they initially deemed medicine. Intimates of Louis XIV started the fashion of adding milk to tea in 1636. Introduced into England by the mid-1600s, tea's popularity soared after 1662 when King Charles II married the Portuguese infanta Catherine de Braganza, whose dowry included access to Portugal's Asian ports, enhancing the East India Company. As the royals were confirmed tea drinkers, it became the chic beverage for English high society.

With the Portuguese, Dutch, French, and English vying for control and bringing diverse traditions to the New World, tea influenced colonial development and lifestyle. In 1642, the Dutch West India Company built "Aunt Metje Wessells Tavern," serving traders and ship captains journeying regularly to *Nieuw Amsterdam.* A decade later the first city hall was located in a nearby converted tavern. After Peter Stuyvesant's 1647 inauguration, he attempted to regulate the quality of taverns. See TAVERNS. In New Amsterdam, Dutch courtesy required accommodating the tastes of each guests by offering several types of tea brewed in different pots accompanied by sugar, saffron, and peach leaves.

Sold by the Dutch and French, tea was generally free of import tax. In 1670, a Massachusetts advertisement noted the availability of expensive Hyson green tea and black Bohea tea, composed of shreds of pekoe and soughing. Colonists who could not afford imported beverages sometimes imbibed Native American substitutes, such as sage and black teas.

By the 1680s with names oftentimes connoting political allegiances, numerous New York coffeehouses modeled on European precedents emerged. Such establishments functioned as venues for merchants, magistrates, and businessmen engaged in trials, city council meetings, or private dealings, while providing newspapers and usually serving coffee, tea, and chocolate. Special meeting rooms distinguished coffeehouses from taverns. The former were used daily by regular customers, whereas the latter were patronized for social purposes and by visitors seeking lodging. See COFFEEHOUSES.

In the late 1600s, tea was considered a rare, exotic, expensive novelty but, nevertheless, quickly became America's favorite hot beverage. Men drank it during breakfast, women at an afternoon tea table, and both in the evenings. New York silversmiths wrought original designs for sterling teapots.

Although in 1730 a writer in the *New York Gazette* proclaimed it injurious, tea was transformed from health tonic to a rite of hospitality. Women's enjoyment of afternoon parlor tea parties reflected social status and upheld their husbands' position. Guests at such events brought their own teacups, saucers, and spoons. Hostesses proudly displayed sets designed en suite with wood handles and lid knobs, creamer, and sugar bowl. For serving tea, occasional tables the size of a large tray were introduced, designed to be used in front of or between chairs.

In the 1750s and continuing afterward, interest in tea was manifest. Vauxhall Gardens contained a tea garden. Spring Gardens advertised the best green tea served between 3:00 and 6:00 in the afternoon, as did Newfoundland, which additionally listed a hot loaf, and the Tavern in the Field provided afternoon tea and coffee. The Corporation of New York erected a tea water pump over a desirable spring, and the Common Council enacted "a law for the Regulating of the Tea Water Men in the City of New York." Tea leaves could be purchased at shops throughout the colonies.

During the reign of Queen Anne, who preferred tea over ale for breakfast, new forms for serving the beverage evolved, such as the pear-shaped Queen Anne–style teapot. Sugar bowls and tongs, milk and crew pitchers, teaspoons, and tea caddies were often placed on rotating, tilt-top tables until Chinese-influenced American Chippendale furnishings became popular with the elite.

Slightly prior to the American Revolution with its concomitant tea boycott, one-third of all colonists consumed between 1.2 million and 2 million pounds of tea yearly, with most inhabitants drinking it twice a day. Then patriots ceased relishing this once permitted beverage. The Continental Congress lifted the ban on selling tea prior to the signing of the Declaration of Independence, while prohibiting buying it from the East India Company.

With the signing of the Treaty of Paris on September 3, 1783, tea drinking, tea parties, and tea balls regained their previous élan. Shortly thereafter, the United States began to acquire tea directly from Canton, China. By 1789, more American ships sailed to China than any other country except Great Britain.

In the middle of the nineteenth century, American publications extolled "tea for ladies" and romanticized Chinese, Indian, and Sri Lankan plantations. Many Americans began drinking tea as an iced beverage, especially the trendsetting lemon version termed "à la Russe."

By 1860, there were sixty-five specialty tea stores in Gotham. George F. Gilman and George H. Hartford, importers of tea among other products, sold tea in their shop as well as through the mail. Three years later, their business was renamed the Great American Tea Company. By 1865 they owned five New York retail shops. With the completion of the intercontinental railroad in 1869, tea from Asia was shipped to San Francisco and delivered by train throughout the United States. The company's name became the Great Atlantic and Pacific Tea Company, or A&P. In the 1870s, A&P was the largest distributor of tea. See A&P.

Before the turn of the century, tea consumption hit a peak, with Americans consuming an average of 1.56 pounds of tea yearly, which within a decade declined to an average of one pound. Late-nineteenth-century tearooms offered an alternative to exclusively male saloons. Largely owned, operated, and frequented by women, these lunchrooms became a popular venue, falling out of favor after the repeal of Prohibition in 1933. Interest in tea resurged in 1952 when Lipton introduced the four-sided tea bag. The rise of herbal teas and bottled and canned iced teas in the decades that followed also helped spark fresh interest among tea drinkers.

See also TEAROOMS.

Smith, Andrew F. *Drinking History: Fifteen Turning Points in the Making of American Beverages.* New York: Columbia University Press, 2013.

Ukers, William H. *All About Tea.* 2 vols. New York: Tea and Coffee Trade Journal, 1935.

Michele Kidwell-Gilbert

Tea Party

Although the drama of the Boston Tea Party is considered an iconic event leading up to the American Revolution, New York had its share of "tea party" events as well. British Parliament imposed a variety of taxes, under which America's colonists chafed. Beginning in 1733, this included the Molasses Act, the Sugar Act, and, the following year, the Stamp Act, requiring that printed material be produced on official stamped paper. The Sons of Liberty famously protested, "No taxation without representation." By 1765, merchants boycotted British goods and signed the Non-Importation Resolutions.

Meanwhile, Parliament's Townshend Acts introduced duties on imports including tea. As a result, rejecting tea became an honorable symbol. In 1770 the Battle of Golden Hill occurred in wheat fields that the Dutch called Golden Hill, and that April Townshend duties were repealed, except a threepence tax on tea, creating a black market. Parliament passed the Tea Act in 1773, enabling the East India Company to export to chosen distributors and bypass taxes rendered to Britain.

On September 27, Great Britain dispatched to various cities seven ships containing underpriced East India Company tea. New Yorkers reacted, declaring obnoxious "tea commissioners and stamp distributors." Merchants passed a resolution thanking London ship captains who would not allow their vessels to transport East India Company freight subject to duty. A Sons of Liberty meeting held at city hall denounced the tea trade monopoly as "public robbery."

On November 23, the first shipment arrived in Boston. As for New York, the *Nancy*, brimming with tea, had been driven off course, so Gotham's "action against the tea" occurred that April.

New York's Sons of Liberty held a tea protest meeting at city hall, attended by several thousand colonists, to discuss how to handle their expected shipment of tea. Their formal opposition included the following:

1st. Resolved, that whoever shall aid or abet, or in any manner assist, in the introduction of tea from any place whatsoever, into this colony, while it is subject, by a British Act of Parliament, to the payment of a duty, for the purpose of raising a revenue in America, he shall be deemed an enemy to the liberties of America.

2d. Resolved, that whoever shall be aiding, or assisting, in the landing, or carting of such tea, from any ship, or vessel, or shall hire any house, storehouse, or cellar or any place whatsoever, to deposit the tea, subject to a duty as aforesaid, he shall be deemed an enemy to the liberties of America.

3d. Resolved, that whoever shall sell, or buy, or in any manner contribute to the sale, or purchase of tea, subject to a duty as aforesaid, or shall aid, or abet, in transporting such tea, by land or water, from this city, until the 7th George III, chap. 46, commonly called the Revenue Act, shall be totally and clearly repealed, he shall be deemed an enemy to the liberties of America.

4th. Resolved, that whether the duties on tea, imposed by this Act, be paid in Great Britain or in America, our liberties are equally affected.

5th. Resolved, that whoever shall transgress any of these resolutions, we will not deal with, or employ, or have any connection with him.

Parliament responded with the Coercive Acts, which patriots termed Intolerable Acts. In response New York's Colonial Assembly created the Committee of Correspondence, facilitating communications between colonies.

Encountering numerous storms including one in early April, driven off course to the island of Antigua, with eighty Scots lost at sea, the *Nancy*, commanded by Captain Benjamin Lockyear, docked at Sandy Hook on April 18. Lockyear was informed that he was not permitted to unload his vessel, sail for Murray's Wharf near Wall Street, or visit the custom house. With a fifteen-man vigilance committee organized by the Sons of Liberty appointed to enforce these decisions, the consignee further suggested Lockyear return to London with his cargo. He agreed to these instructions and was subsequently treated as a hero. A cheering crowd greeted him at his lodging house, and a band playing "God Save the King" accompanied his escorted return to his vessel as he prepared to return the controversial tea shipment to England.

Other ships were not as accommodating. On the day after, the *London*, which during the preceding December had unloaded and replaced tea in Charleston, arrived at Murray's Wharf. Discovering its captain had lied about eighteen tea chests aboard the ship, angry colonists in face paint dumped its cargo.

Given the incessant adverse legislation emanating from Parliament, the quest for independence was inevitable. New York patriots functioned in the forefront of the struggle against Great Britain, which culminated in the Revolutionary War. Had there been a president from New York in the early federal period, perhaps the unfolding of events might have been transcribed differently.

See also TEA.

Burrows, Edwin G., and Mike Wallace. *Gotham: A History of New York City to 1898.* New York: Oxford University Press, 1999.

Stokes, I. N. Phelps. *The Iconography of Manhattan Island, 1498–1909: Compiled from Original Sources and Illustrated by Photo-Intaglio Reproductions of Important Maps, Plans, Views, and Documents in Public and Private.* 6 vols. New York: Arno, 1967. First published 1922.

Michele Kidwell-Gilbert

Tearooms

Tearooms made their debut in New York City in the late 1890s. The small, feminine eating places serving light lunches and afternoon tea marked a transition in the city's status hierarchy that brought women of high social status into public prominence both as entrepreneurs and as consumers.

In 1896 Ellin Lowery and Enid Wilmerding took the bold step of establishing one of the city's first tearooms, known simply as the Afternoon Tea Room. Located on Fifth Avenue near the Waldorf Hotel, it mimicked a fine home with flowered satin wallpaper, Irish lace, rare china, cut glass, and old family silver.

A short time later other tearooms opened in the same area. One of them, The Fernery, grew out of a florist shop run by two women on the Social Register. The Waldorf turned its Palm Room, which had been a men's bar, into a tearoom, creating a space where respectable women could venture unescorted. Tearooms were quickly becoming standard features of top hotels such as The Plaza and luxury restaurants such as Sherry's.

The early tearooms kept a low profile with inconspicuous signs and restful interiors. They gained prestige by attracting women of society. Soon there would be tearooms for working women and middle-class shoppers, but the elite origins of New York's tearooms continued to set the tone. Miss Tipton's, in the Eighteenth Street shopping district, advertised, "Patronized by the Best People." The food served in tearooms was delicate and dainty. In the early years of the twentieth century, biscuits, chicken salad, and wine jellies were preferred over steaks, chops, and other hearty dishes served in what tearoom fans called "ordinary restaurants."

The fashionability of Fifth Avenue tearooms inspired a countercultural reaction among Greenwich Village women, who created tearooms in their own offbeat style. Ramshackle and bare, often with ceilings painted in bright colors and drawings scrawled on walls, they became centers for an emerging youth culture. They have been documented in the photographs of Jessie Tarbox Beals.

Tearooms were especially plentiful in the Village, so much so that an article in the June 1922 issue of *Vanity Fair* titled "The Four Social Zones of Fifth Avenue" characterized Fifth Avenue at Eighth Street as "the District of Batiks, Art Students, Tea-Rooms, and free verse poets." Greenwich Village tearooms were notable in the 1920s not only for their dismissal of bourgeois notions of décor but also for their inventive names at a time when most restaurants went by their owner's name. A 1922 sampling reveals The Purple Pup, the Vermillion Hound, T.N.T., and the Green Witch.

Tearooms reached their peak of popularity as novel and female-friendly eating places in the 1920s. Yet only about ninety-four tearooms appeared in the 1924 guidebook *Rider's New York City*. Undoubtedly some were left out, yet it is clear that the social significance of tearooms as eating places catering mostly to women—a customer segment many restaurants wanted to win—far exceeded their numbers. *Polk's Trow's New York Directory*, 1924–1925, listed over 6,900 restaurants in greater New York City but only about 125 tearooms.

By the 1930s women had become frequent patrons of restaurants of all types, so much so that there was something of a backlash against the feminine impact on dining. The author of a 1931 article called "Food for the Eye" joined with a prominent New York restaurateur to chide women for the prevalence of "comic salads of ingredients chosen principally because of their improbability" and "baked meats garnished with incongruous and disgusting fruits." During the Depression the number of tearooms in New York grew somewhat, but they lost considerable cachet. Some areas were overcrowded with them, particularly side streets in the East Forties and Fifties. With the end of Prohibition tearooms vied to increase male patronage and raise check averages. The Village's Jumble Shop, for instance, began serving cocktails and added steaks, chops, and stews to its menu. African American tearooms in Harlem often served as community centers and were already accustomed to serving men.

The life of a tearoom was often brief, but a few persisted far beyond the peak in the 1910s and 1920s, even as women were welcomed into most restaurants. The Schrafft's chain was notably successful. The long-lived Mary Elizabeth's took over the space at 291 Fifth Avenue formerly occupied by the Afternoon Tea Room of 1896 and went on to become an institution. The Bird Cage tearoom in the Lord & Taylor store won many faithful patrons, as did the Kirby-Allen, named for its two female proprietors, which ended its fifty-year run in 1973.

Eating establishments serving afternoon tea made a small comeback in the 1990s and persist into the present. However, the era of "ladies' restaurants" such as tearooms has clearly ended.

See also COFFEEHOUSES; HOTEL RESTAURANTS; LUNCH; and SHERRY'S.

"Glimpses of New York Tea Rooms." *Tea Room and Gift Shop* (November 1923): 5–7.

McCulloch-Williams, Martha. "Tea Rooms, as Conducted in New York." *Good Housekeeping* (December 1906): 594–600.

Sherwin, Louis. "Food for the Eye." *Forum and Century* (June 1931): 341–346.

"Tea Rooms Spreading Here." *The Sun*, September 16, 1906.

Ware, Caroline F. *Greenwich Village, 1920–1930*. Boston: Houghton Mifflin, 1935.

Whitaker, Jan. *Tea at the Blue Lantern Inn: A Social History of the Tea Room Craze in America*. New York: St. Martin's, 2002.

Jan Whitaker

Television

For more than sixty years, New York City television stations have aired food-related shows. They have fallen into four major categories: how-to cooking, travelogues, food history, and science-related programs.

Stations began experimenting with how-to cooking shows during the early 1940s. James Beard, a trained actor and opera singer, hosted a series of fifteen-minute programs called *I Love to Cook!* for NBC in 1946; they aired after a variety show, *Elsie Presents*, introduced by a puppet version of Borden's Elsie the Cow. Beard was awkward and ill at ease in front of the camera, and the program was discontinued, but television programmers liked the idea, and other cooking shows soon followed. Restaurateur and cooking school owner Dione Lucas hosted the first national thirty-minute cooking show on CBS in 1948. Her programs, *To the Queen's Taste* and later *Dione Lucas's Cooking Show*, focused on French food, but her stern and somewhat forbidding presentation made French cookery seem complex and difficult.

It was Julia Child's *The French Chef* that launched food television as we know it. Taped in Boston on WGBH, the series aired in 1963 on New York's public television station WNDT (later renamed WNET). The show influenced many New Yorkers, who have acknowledged that their interest in food dates to watching those programs. Following Child's lead, other chefs, restaurateurs, and food personalities took to the airwaves, and cooking shows appeared on both commercial and public television stations. *Joyce Chen Cooks* was first broadcast on WNDT in 1966. Three years later *The Galloping Gourmet*, starring Graham Kerr, was first broadcast in New York. While none of these programs were produced in New York, they all influenced the New Yorkers who watched them.

The continuing popularity of cooking shows culminated in the creation of the cable television Food Network in 1993 in New York City. At first it focused on instructional cooking shows—colloquially referred to as "dump and stir" programs. They were relatively inexpensive to make and formulaic in their construction, as many such programs had already aired on other television stations. However, the network's programming continued to expand.

By 2001 the Food Network was reaching 75 million households, including some of the most affluent TV viewers in America. In 2010, the Food Network launched the Cooking Channel. Bobby Flay, owner of New York's Mesa Grill, hosted shows on the Cooking Channel.

By 2013, the Food Network was being watched in 96 million homes—virtually every American home that had a cable or satellite TV hookup—and its website had 7 million users monthly. Its national headquarters is located in Chelsea Market at 75 Ninth Avenue in Manhattan.

Many New York restaurateurs, chefs, and culinary personalities developed and hosted cooking programs on various television channels. These include

Sara Moulton (*Cooking Live, Cooking Live Primetime,* and *Sara's Secrets*), Mario Batali (*Multo Mario*), and Rachael Ray (*Rachael Ray, 30 Minute Meals, Rachael Ray's Tasty Travels, $40 a Day,* and *Rachael vs. Guy: Celebrity Cook-Off*).

New York's culinary scene also appears in many cable television programs. The HBO show *Treme* includes a chef, Janette Desautel, played by Kim Dickens, who tests her mettle in New York. The series featured New York restaurants, including Tom Colicchio's Craft, Eric Ripert's Le Bernardin, and David Chang's Momofuku Ko and Ssäm Bar. Rocco DiSpirito and his restaurant, Rocco's, featured in NBC's six-part reality soap opera *The Restaurant.* One episode of CUNY's *Asian American Life* series hosted by Ernabel Demillo featured the Brooklyn Kitchen in Williamsburg.

New York chef David Ruggerio starred in the twenty-six-part WNET series *Little Italy with David Ruggerio,* which explored the garlic-scented world of Italian American cooking. New Yorker Burt Wolf has hosted many PBS food-related series, such as *What We Eat and Why, What Are They Eating?,* and *Holidays.* New York chefs David Chang and April Bloomfield have starred in the PBS series *The Mind of a Chef.* The third season in 2014 is narrated by New Yorker Anthony Bourdain. New York restaurateur Lidia Bastianich has starred in many PBS series, including *Lidia's Italy, Lidia's Family Table, Lidia's Italian-American Kitchen, Lidia's Italian Table,* and *La Cucina di Lidia.* Hosted by cookbook author and chef Mike Colameco, *Colameco's Food Show* showcases New York City's chefs and restaurants, from the upscale Per Se, Le Bernardin, and Daniel to the places that make the best fried chicken, noodles, hot dogs, sandwiches, and burgers.

The film series *Appetite City,* which started in 2011, is hosted by William Grimes on NYC Life (Channel 25). It delineates the history of New York City through its iconic foods, markets, and restaurants. Episodes include "Fine Dining," "Diners," "Street Food," "Green Markets," "Oysters," "Chinatown," "Delis," and "Soul Food."

Some television programs have popularized New York foods. The Magnolia Bakery on Bleecker Street, for instance, was featured in *Sex and the City* and in many other films and television series. A *Seinfeld* episode popularized black and white cookies; another episode introduced viewing audiences to "the Soup Nazi," who required high regimentation of his patrons.

The Soup Nazi was modeled on Ali Yeganeh's restaurant Soup Kitchen International, on West Fifty-Fifth Street. Likewise, New York City's food and beverage scene, especially the Manhattan cocktail, during the 1960s was popularized in the AMC series *Mad Men,* which ran from 2007 to 2015.

See also BASTIANICH, LIDIA; BATALI, MARIO; BEARD, JAMES; CHELSEA MARKET; COOKIES; FOOD NETWORK; GRIMES, WILLIAM; HAZAN, MARCELLA; KATZ'S DELICATESSEN; LUCAS, DIONE; MAD MEN; MOULTON, SARA; RAY, RACHAEL; and SEX AND THE CITY.

Collins, Kathleen. *Watching What We Eat: The Evolution of Television Cooking Shows.* New York: Continuum, 2009.

Salkin, Allen. *From Scratch: Inside the Food Network.* New York: Putnam's, 2013.

Andrew F. Smith

Television, Public

For more than fifty years, public television in New York has aired culinary programs. Channel 13, WNET, was New York City's public broadcast station. It is the parent of WLIW, Long Island's public television station, and since 2008 it has operated NJTV, New Jersey's public station. All three stations can be viewed in New York City.

In 1962 WNET was created as WNDT, which stood for New Dimensions in Television. The name was changed in 1970, after a merger with National Educational Television. Since 1963 Channel 13 has aired cooking shows, such as Julia Child's *The French Chef. Joyce Chen Cooks* was first broadcast on WNDT in 1966. While these programs were not produced by WNET, they influenced New Yorkers who watched them. Food writer Michael Pollan, for instance, watched *The French Chef* on WNET as a child, and in 2009 he wrote that "whenever people talk about how Julia Child upgraded the culture of food in America, I nod appreciatively. I owe her."

Burt Wolf, also a New Yorker, hosted several PBS food-related series, such as *What We Eat and Why, What Are They Eating?,* and *Holidays.* Chefs David Chang and April Bloomfield, both chef-owners of Manhattan restaurants, were featured in the PBS series *The Mind of a Chef.*

New York restaurateur Lidia Bastianich has starred in many PBS series, including *Lidia's Family Table, Lidia's Italian-American Kitchen, Lidia's Italian Table,* and *La Cucina di Lidia*. Other food-related shows on WNET include *Martha Stewart's Cooking School*, *A Chef's Life*, and *Eat! Drink! Italy! With Vic Rallo*.

Mike Colameco's Food Show, which began its fourteenth season in 2014, has showcased New York City's restaurateurs such as Daniel Boulud, Thomas Keller, Gabrielle Hamilton, Dan Barber, Eric Ripert, Alain Ducasse, and April Bloomfield and restaurants from upscale Per Se, Le Bernardin, and Daniel to the places that make the best fried chicken, noodles, hot dogs, sandwiches, and burgers. Also, WNET has produced its own food programming. Beginning in 1997, New York chef David Ruggerio starred in a twenty-six-part series, *Little Italy with David Ruggerio*, which took an affectionate look at Italian American food. The WNET website has previews of past and present shows and recipes from them.

Create TV is a commercial-free television network owned by American Public Television. It distributes the best of public television's how-to programs. Its cooking shows include *New Scandinavian Cooking*, *Simply Ming*, *America's Test Kitchen from Cook's Illustrated*, and *Lidia's Italy*. Its programs are regularly shown on WNET, NJTV, and WLIW.

Finally, NYC Media, channel 25, the official broadcast network of New York City, airs several food-related programs, such as *Firehouse Kitchen*, *Food and Drink with Time Out New York*, *Food Curated*, *Healthy Soul*, and *Frankie Cooks*.

See also BARBER, DAN; BASTIANICH, LIDIA; BLOOMFIELD, APRIL; RESTAURANTS; and TELEVISION.

Create TV website: http://createtv.com.
NYC Media website: http://www.nyc.gov/media.
Pollan, Michael. "Out of the Kitchen, Onto the Couch." *New York Times Magazine*, July 29, 2009.
WNET website: http://www.wnet.org.

Andrew F. Smith

Temperance Movement

The New York Temperance Society, which advocated complete abstinence from all alcoholic beverages, was founded in 1829 by Robert M. Hartley, a New York City merchant. He was motivated by the belief that the city's high child mortality rate was caused by spoiled or tainted milk, largely from dairy cows being fed spent brewery mash.

Hartley circulated tracts, published exposés, spoke to large audiences, and gained widespread support. The campaign that Hartley launched eventually succeeded in closing many city dairies that produced "swill milk." See MILK, SWILL. This may or may not have affected child mortality, but it certainly had little effect on alcohol consumption.

Temperance advocates faced one very serious problem—there were few nonalcoholic alternatives to bars and saloons. Temperance and other groups funded the construction and maintenance of "ice-free" drinking fountains, particularly in public parks, and sent water wagons around the city where people could drink water for free. Temperance advocates also encouraged restaurants to offer glasses of water to patrons when they sat down, a custom that continues today.

To draw business away from bars and saloons, the Church Temperance Society, an Episcopal Church group, bought a lunch wagon in 1893. They sold "late-night lunches" for ten cents. It was so successful that the society bought more wagons. By 1898 New York City had eight temperance wagons that annually supplied 230,000 meals. The society used the net profits from the wagons to construct free water fountains in the tenement districts of New York.

A step up from the free public water fountains were the soda fountains. Plain soda was cheap, and virtually everyone could afford it. Soda water stands dispensed drinks to long lines of customers during the summers. Soda fountains competed to offer the most flavor selections. One offered thirty-two different syrups, eight kinds of mineral water, and soda water. By 1891 New York had more soda fountains than it had bars, and the number of soda fountains increased during the early twentieth century. Soda fountains increasingly attracted younger New Yorkers. See SODA FOUNTAINS.

Temperance coffeehouses, or "temperance drinking saloons," and tearooms were other alternatives to the ubiquitous bars and taverns. At a coffeehouse, respectable businessmen could socialize without being subjected to the temptations of beer, wine, or whiskey. Tearooms attracted women, who increasingly joined the city workforce beginning in the late nineteenth century. Women could enjoy an alcohol-free lunch in tearooms, and their number increased during the early twentieth century. By 1925 New York City reportedly had eight thousand tearooms. See COFFEEHOUSES and TEAROOMS.

New York State temperance advocates succeeded in their fight for legislation in 1896, when the state legislature passed the Raines law, which banned liquor sales on Sundays. But the law had a substantial loophole: alcohol could legally be sold with meals in any hotel with more than ten rooms. Within months, hundreds of "Raines hotels" had opened (many of them were also brothels). Some bars and taverns began opening again on Sundays, but the authorities usually turned a blind eye, provided that they kept a low profile. A survey of Manhattan and Bronx saloons in 1908 found that 5,000 of the 5,820 legal saloons served alcohol on Sunday. See SALOONS.

The movement to abolish alcohol use nationwide steadily gained support throughout the nineteenth century. Some cities and counties upstate supported prohibition, but the people of New York City were firmly against it. Liquor was an important business in the city: an 1897 survey found a ratio of one liquor distributor to every 208 Manhattan residents. Saloons were also an important source of support for the Tammany Hall political machine, which had controlled city government since 1854.

During the early twentieth century, many well-to-do New Yorkers had been persuaded to support a ban on alcohol. The Anti-Saloon League, the main national lobbying organization for prohibition, set its sights on New York City, the "liquor center of America." The league's literature cited statistics indicating that every week 75,000 quarts of gin, 76,000 quarts of brandy, 100,000 quarts of champagne and wine, 498,000 quarts of whiskey, 33 million quarts of domestic beer and ale, and 300,000 quarts of assorted other alcoholic beverages were consumed in New York City. As the city's population was only 4.7 million, it was clear that New Yorkers—and people visiting the city for the sole purpose of drinking—were downing a tremendous amount of alcohol. Few New Yorkers ever thought Prohibition would become the law of the land, which it did in 1920.

See also BARS; PROHIBITION; and SODA.

Lerner, Michael A. *Dry Manhattan: Prohibition in New York City*. Cambridge, Mass.: Harvard University Press, 2007.

Andrew F. Smith

Tenement Museum

The Lower East Side Tenement Museum presents New York's immigrant past through a blend of family narratives and everyday objects, or artifacts. The most important of these artifacts is the nineteenth-century tenement at 97 Orchard Street that houses the museum. On "exhibit" at the Tenement Museum are the building's original wooden stairwell, narrow hallways, and cramped living quarters. Six of the building's apartments have been reconstructed to depict the day-to-day lives of families that once lived in the tenement. A central focus of those lives was the challenge of putting food on the table. The Tenement Museum treats food as another kind of historic artifact, using it to further elucidate immigrant life, both past and present.

The Tenement Museum owes its existence to a pair of lucky accidents. In 1935 the landlord of 97 Orchard chose to close off the building's upper floors rather than comply with a new building code. The tenants were evicted on short notice, the apartments left empty and untouched for over fifty years. In 1988 Ruth Abram and Anita Jacobson, the museum's founders, were scouting for office space for an immigrant history project when they happened on 97 Orchard, a slice of immigrant New York inadvertently preserved.

The first structures in New York built for multiple families, tenements began to appear on the Lower East Side in the first half of the nineteenth century. The building at 97 Orchard Street is a five-story brick tenement built in 1863 when the Lower East Side was a neighborhood of German artisans and shopkeepers. At the time of construction, it had twenty-two apartments and space for two street-level businesses. Comprised of three small rooms, each apartment covers a total of 325 square feet.

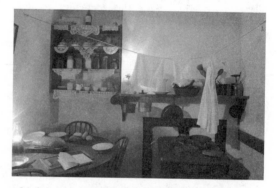

A kitchen at the Tenement Museum on 97 Orchard Street. There was no refrigeration or running water available in most tenements, and foods were therefore limited to those that could be stored at room temperature and did not run the risk of spoiling. TENEMENT MUSEUM

Kitchens—which were originally windowless—were equipped with coal-burning stoves but no running water. Instead, water for cooking and cleaning was retrieved from a pump in the tenement yard. In the absence of refrigeration, perishables were stored on window ledges or fire escapes but only in cold weather. At other times of the year, tenement homemakers commonly shopped once and even twice a day, buying just enough for the next meal. A major renovation to 97 Orchard in 1905 included the installation of indoor plumbing and gas lines. By this time, the Lower East Side was a predominantly Russian Jewish neighborhood of pushcart markets and sweatshops. Living on Orchard Street, directly above a pushcart market, homemakers had easy access to a wide variety of fruits and vegetables, baked goods, and dry goods, all at rock-bottom prices.

Over the course of its lifetime 97 Orchard has withstood the wear and tear of over seven thousand residents. Successive attempts to refurbish the building's interior are apparent in the many layers of peeling paint, tattered wallpaper, and worn linoleum that the museum has left "as is." Like the rings on a tree, those layers evoke a sense of movement through time. From Germans to Irish to Russians and Italians, the immigrant families profiled by the museum likewise reflect the neighborhood's evolving demographics and, by extension, its ever-changing food culture. For example, in the 1860s 97 Orchard was home to a German beer saloon owned by John and Caroline Schneider. While John tended to saloon patrons, Caroline cooked for them. Among her specialties were dishes like stewed pig knuckles, herring, and potato salad, food offered to any customer who paid for a five-cent glass of lager. Jumping ahead to the 1910s, Fannie Rogarshevsky—like many tenement homemakers of the period—took in boarders. As a kind of mini-landlady, she provided both a bed and home-cooked meals, serving foods like gefilte fish and stuffed cabbage, among other Eastern European Jewish staples. Separated by roughly fifty years, these two immigrant entrepreneurs exemplify the changing ways that women used their cooking expertise to earn a living.

The preservation of native foods and food traditions was a priority common to all immigrant groups. To meet their culinary needs, immigrants established networks of food importers, shopkeepers, and tradespeople. For Jewish immigrants that network included kosher butchers. Museum visitors can meet the Lust-gartens, proprietors of a kosher butcher shop once located at 97 Orchard that was the target of rioters. In 1902, Jewish women protesting the high price of kosher meat marched through the streets of the Lower East Side, stopping to smash butcher shop windows along the way. The Lustgartens' store was one casualty of the women's frustration.

The Tenement Museum has developed several food-themed programs. Walking tours lead guests on culinary tasting excursions of the Lower East Side that highlight the neighborhood's cultural and gastronomic diversity. In the evenings, visitors can experience sit-down tastings of neighborhood fare in the museum's private dining room. In a free program designed for recent immigrants, guests participate in a baking workshop devoted to challah, the Sabbath bread once prepared by Fannie Rogarshevsky. The focus on past foodways gives new immigrant families an opportunity to consider their own food traditions and to see their migration experiences along a historic continuum. More broadly, in keeping with the founders' original mission, the museum uses food to create bonds of understanding between people of divergent backgrounds—whether immigrants or not—promoting tolerance amid diversity.

See also LOWER EAST SIDE.

Dolkart, Andrew S. *Biography of a Tenement House in New York: An Architectural History of 97 Orchard Street.* Sante Fe, N.M.: Center for American Places, 2005.
Ziegelman, Jane, *97 Orchard: An Edible History of Five Immigrant Families in One New York Tenement.* New York: Harper, 2010.

Jane Ziegelman

Thai

Thai cuisine is known for its contrast of flavors and texture and its variety of preparation methods. In New York City it is easy to find both traditional and contemporary Thai food.

Typically, a Thai meal consists of five elements: rice, vegetables (both raw and cooked), a curry dish, a fried dish, and a stir fry, along with sauces and dips. Some of the most popular ingredients typical of Thai food are lemongrass, kaffir lime leaves, coconut milk, garlic, shallots, peppers, fish sauce, chilies, and palm sugar, which adds sweetness to spicy dishes. Thai cuisine is inclusive of most fish, meat, shellfish, and poultry, with rice and noodles as staples served in or with most dishes. Vegetables that often appear in Thai dishes include eggplant, tomatoes, mushrooms, bean sprouts, cabbage, cucumbers, potatoes, and various types of squash. Pineapple, winter melon, durian, rambutan, papaya, and mangosteen are some of the fruits that appear in both sweet and savory dishes.

The Thai community, which began emigrating from Thailand in the 1960s, is spread all over New York City, with more than half making their homes in several neighborhoods in Queens, including Elmhurst, Jackson Heights, and Woodside. As such, Thai restaurants are spread throughout the boroughs. Publications such as *Time Out New York* and the *Village Voice* as well as the *Zagat Survey* frequently publish lists of the best Thai restaurants in the area. Popular and notable ones include SriPraPai and Ayada in Queens; Song, Am Thai Bistro, and Pok Pok NY in Brooklyn; and Zabb Elee, Somtum Der, Kin Shop, and Larb Ubol in Manhattan.

At these and other local Thai restaurants, customers will find dishes popular in America, including chicken satay, curry dishes, rice dishes, noodle soups, pad thai, and more innovative ones like jackfruit and sparerib curry, curry paste–spiked burgers, sweet potato chiang mai, tempura fries, and noodles with sweetbreads.

Markets where Thai ingredients are available include the Bangkok Center Grocery in Chinatown, the Asia Market Corporation, Kalustyan's, and the Hong Kong Supermarket. Customers shop for ingredients for weekday meals and for special celebrations and holidays, including Asalha Puja, Loy Krathong Festival, and Songkran, which is Thailand's New Year.

See also SOUTHEAST ASIAN.

Asian American Federation. "Profile of New York City's Thai Americans: 2012 Edition." http://www.aafny .org/cic/briefs/thai2012.pdf.
"Best Thai Food in New York." *Time Out*, January 6, 2015.
Feldman, Zachary. "The 10 Best Thai Restaurants in NYC." *Village Voice*, October 1, 2013.

Tracey Ceurvels

Thanksgiving

Thanksgiving—now celebrated on the last Thursday of November—is one of the most important American holidays. It is typically celebrated with a big dinner that traditionally includes turkey, stuffing (dressing), cranberry sauce, sweet potatoes, and pie (pumpkin, mince, and apple). Early American colonists celebrated community days of thanksgiving in response to specific events, such as a military victory, a good harvest, or a providential rainfall. New England's Puritans were particularly enamored of thanksgivings, which to them were solemn religious occasions spent in church. By the late eighteenth century, days of thanksgiving revolved around a family dinner eaten after a church service.

When New York City was the capital of the United States, President George Washington proclaimed October 3, 1789, a day of "national Thanksgiving," but the tradition was not continued by succeeding presidents. During the early nineteenth century, many New Englanders moved to New York, introducing the city to the New England version of the holiday, with all its culinary trappings plus local fare, such as doughnuts and crullers. In 1830 New York was the first state outside of New England to declare Thanksgiving a state holiday.

Well-to-do New Yorkers often celebrated Thanksgiving by sharing their bounty with the city's poor and hungry. On Thanksgiving Day in 1846, the Ladies' Home Mission of the Episcopal Church offered Thanksgiving dinner for the poor of Five Points, a slum district in what is today Chinatown. It continued to do this for decades. In 1850, the Ladies Home Missionary Society of the Methodist Episcopal Church served hundreds of turkey dinners to the indigent. This tradition of feeding the poor continues today, with many New Yorkers (usually including the mayor) putting in some time in a soup kitchen or other public food program—or by donating to organizations that serve the city's less fortunate.

It was not until 1863, in the midst of the Civil War, that President Abraham Lincoln declared the last Thursday in November a national day of thanksgiving. In response, George W. Blunt, a member of New York's Union League Club, was moved to propose sending a holiday feast to Union soldiers and sailors in Virginia—"poultry and pies, or puddings, all cooked, ready for use." The Union League Club appealed to hotel operators, restaurateurs, bakers, and affluent private individuals to roast quantities of turkeys and chickens—twenty or more, if they could manage it—and send them to a central location so that they could be shipped south to the troops.

Delmonico's, the city's most luxurious restaurant, contributed thousands of stuffed and roasted turkeys,

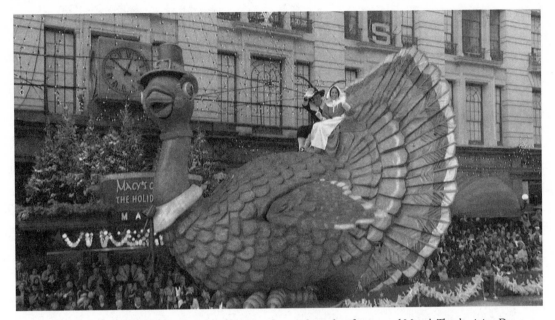

Two people dressed as pilgrims ride the signature turkey float in the eighty-first annual Macy's Thanksgiving Day Parade, November 22, 2007. AARON CAMPBELL

which were packed up and sent by train, ship, and wagon to Virginia. In only three weeks, the Union League Club had collected more than $56,500, which it used to buy 146,586 pounds of poultry, most of it from the Fulton Market. The market donated its $3,386 profit back to the fund. Another 225,000 pounds of poultry was received as contributions, along with enormous quantities of the other Thanksgiving dinner components. The project gave a boost to Northern morale, as the *New York Herald* proclaimed: "A people in the midst of a bloody war, having tens of thousands of soldiers in the field, and war ships studding every sea, yet every day expanding into greater commercial importance, and celebrates its national elections, feasts, and holidays with peace and harmony."

In addition to the family gathering and feast, Thanksgiving has come to be the traditional day for featured football games. In 1876, the newly formed Intercollegiate Football Association scheduled a championship game in New York City on Thanksgiving Day. This may or may not have been the first game played on Thanksgiving, but it created a tradition that is still observed. For many households, especially after the advent of radio and television, the football games changed the focus of the holiday. As early as 1893, a *New York Times* editorial stated that Thanksgiving should be renamed as it no longer had

any religious content; "football day" was mentioned as a possible alternative.

The Macy's Thanksgiving Day Parade was started by the store's employees on November 27, 1924. The parade stepped off on 145th Street in Harlem and ended in front of the Macy's store in Herald Square. Hydrogen-filled (today helium-filled) balloons were introduced in the late 1920s, and they became the event's signature attraction. Traditionally, the last float of the parade carries Santa Claus, marking the official start of the Christmas shopping season. Millions of visitors and television viewers watch the giant character balloons as they are marched down the avenues. The restaurants along the parade route that are open are fully booked, but most New Yorkers opt for viewing the parade on TV before sitting down to eat Thanksgiving dinner at home.

Because of the vast waves of immigration that have arrived in the city, not all New Yorkers celebrate Thanksgiving with traditional American fare. Many substitute or add dishes that reflect their culinary heritage, creating a fusion feast. In Chinatown, Thanksgiving is a traditional day for weddings as many restaurants are closed, their banquet rooms booked far in advance.

See also CIVIL WAR and DELMONICO'S.

Baker, James W. *Thanksgiving: The Biography of an American Holiday*. Durham: University of New Hampshire Press, 2009.

Smith, Andrew F. *Starving the South: How the North Won the Civil War*. New York: St. Martin's, 2011.

Smith, Andrew F. *The Turkey: An American Story*. Urbana: University of Illinois Press, 2006.

Andrew F. Smith

Theater and Food

New York City's world-class culinary scene is closely rivaled by its world-class theater scene—and there are virtually countless productions where the two worlds meet. Since the early twentieth century (and perhaps even since the mid-nineteenth), food in New York theater productions has appeared as a projectile; then, with the advent of realism, as something integral to the story, where it would be prepared and sometimes consumed in a dramatic context; and then, as an adjunct to an immersive production. (This last example is distinct from "dinner theater" where the audience gets "dinner and a show" and which is more likely to be found outside of the city.)

The first food on an uptown New York stage may have been the pie-in-the-face thrown at William Hammerstein's Victoria Theatre in the golden age of vaudeville. More recently, Blue Man Group has continued the slapstick tradition, using food to entertain and provoke. In *Tubes*, they stuff their cheeks with "marshmallows" (cream cheese, in fact); they chomp down on breakfast cereal for percussive effect; they daintily ingest Twinkies, then shock the audience when the "creamy filling" (pureed bananas) spurts out of their chests. It may be no small coincidence that two of the group's founding members acquired some of their food savvy while working for New York caterer Glorious Foods.

Realism in drama was a reaction to the lighter American fare (or even the melodramas) typical of the early New York stage. Playwright Eugene O'Neill

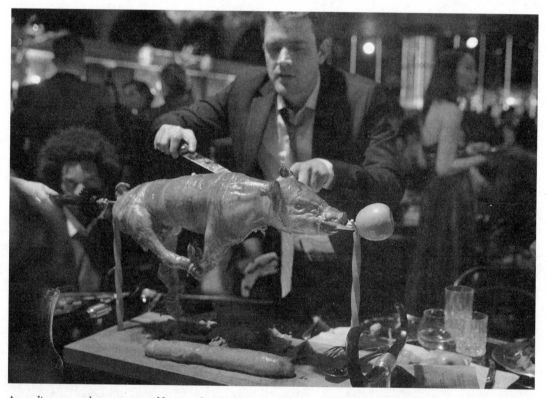

An audience member carves a suckling pig during the dining portion of the "Queen of the Night'" show in the restored Billy Rose's Diamond Horseshoe nightclub in the basement of the Paramount Hotel, January 22, 2014. "Queen of the Night" is an immersive theater experience including acrobatic acts, striptease, physical contact, and lavish dining. SARA KRULWICH/*NEW YORK TIMES*/REDUX

was one of its first and greatest proponents. In his sole comedy, *Ah, Wilderness!* (1933, but set in 1906), the entire second act takes place around the family dining table where a four-course meal is served to and eaten by the cast: soup, fish, vegetables, and lobster ("You don't get any dessert or tea after lobster, you know"). Was real food used? Most likely the food was edible, but it is also likely that the "fish" was made of bread. Prop masters have to be creative to be "realistic." When Carol Channing portrayed Dolly Levi in *Hello, Dolly!* (1964), the "dumplings" she consumed each night at the Harmonium Gardens (inspired by Manhattan's historic Lüchow's) were actually small cotton-candy spheres—spun and molded backstage before each performance.

By 2003, however, when Theresa Rebeck and Alexandra Gersten-Vassilaros's post-9/11 dinner-party play *Omnium Gatherum* (a Pulitzer Prize finalist), was produced off-Broadway, the five-course onstage meal (prepared off-site) was very real. In fact, "The whole meal has been designed by Bobby Flay." Chef Alfred Portale of Gotham Bar and Grill supervised the nightly preparations: a vegetable amuse-bouche, wild salmon, roasted lamb, salad, and a custard dessert. In the second (and final) month of its run, Flay served as chef, introducing some new dishes as well. The script was adapted accordingly.

That same year, playwright and former *New York Times Magazine* food writer Jonathan Reynolds presented his off-Broadway memory play *Dinner with Demons*, in which he prepared a five-course meal—on stage and in full view of the audience—while talking about the role of food in our lives, his life, and what it was like to grow up with his late parents, the titular "demons." In a fully functional electric kitchen (complete with a working sink), he nightly prepared a deep-fried fourteen-pound turkey (in a custom-built acrylic fryer), potato soufflé, braised cardoons, tomato sorbet, and apple pancakes. Although audiences could savor the appetite-inducing cooking aromas, New York State food-preparation certification laws prevented Reynolds from sharing his creations with them—much to the benefit of the backstage crew.

By requesting a "voluntary offering" or by presenting gratis, the sole actors in some off-off-Broadway productions have been able to (legally) present their food-centric plays, preparing a meal and serving it to the audience in such pieces as Ed Schmidt's *The Last Supper* (performed in his Brooklyn apartment,

2002) and Elke Solomon's *A Tavola: A Performance* (Judson Memorial Church, 2013).

And then there are the immersive shows, where audiences pay not only the price of admission but also the price of a meal—and even to be part of the production. These range from the gastronomically basic, improv-based *Tony n' Tina's Wedding* (originally performed in 1988, with a Greenwich Village "wedding" and a baked ziti reception) to the over-the-top gastronomy and circus-like spectacle of 2014's *Queen of the Night* (at the Paramount Hotel's Diamond Horseshoe), where audience members may interact with the performers and dine on lobster, oversized ribs of beef, or even a roast suckling pig still on the spit—some paying more than five hundred dollars for the privilege.

To see the creative range of ways food and theater have shared the spotlight in New York City is to understand that the two are not likely to be teased apart any time soon. It is a tradition of more than a hundred years' standing—and, by perpetually reinventing itself, one that shows no signs of aging.

Bloom, Ken. *Broadway: An Encyclopedia.* 2d ed. New York: Routledge, 2004.

Fabricant, Florence. "Food Takes Center Stage, with Chefs in the Wings." *New York Times,* October 8, 2003.

Isherwood, Charles. "A Circus of Intimate Sensation." *New York Times,* February 2, 2014.

Prideaux, Tom. "What a Hello for Dolly: Carol Channing Carries Off a Musical and Feats of Fake Eating." *Life* (April 3, 1964): 107–113.

Simonson, Robert. "Theater: A Show in Which the Turkey's the Thing." *New York Times,* December 14, 2003.

Witchel, Alex. "On Stage and Off." *New York Times,* December 13, 1991.

Jane L. Smulyan

Thomas, Jerry

Jerry Thomas, a bartender in New York during the nineteenth century, is noted for writing one of the first known manuals for bartenders. Thomas was born "on or around November 1, 1830," according to historian David Wondrich's biography of the bartender, in Sackets Harbor, New York. At sixteen, he began life as a New Haven barkeeper and joined up with the navy shortly thereafter. At the age of nineteen, he settled in San Francisco during the height of the Gold Rush, becoming a bartender in a saloon in nearby Downiesville, California.

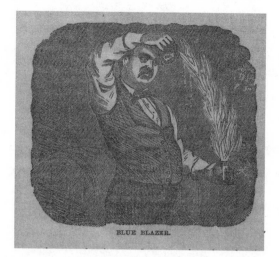

BLUE BLAZER.

An artist's rendition of Jerry Thomas, author of one of the first bartending handbooks, mixing his signature drink, the Blue Blazer. The cocktail consists of blended whiskey, boiling water, powdered sugar, and a bit of lemon zest. DAVID WONDRICH, PERSONAL COLLECTION

By 1852, Thomas decided he had had enough of El Dorado and headed back east, eventually landing in New York City. In 1858, he became principal bartender at the Metropolitan Hotel, a large and fashionable establishment on the corner of Prince Street and Broadway, at the time the heart of the city's shopping district.

Over the next eighteen years, Thomas would become America's most famous bartender, embodying the bravado and showmanship of the mixologist archetype of the day, "a sporting character of wide experience and infinite jest" (Wondrich, 2007, p. 26). For example, his signature drink was the blue blazer, which involved lighting whiskey on fire and passing it back and forth between two mixing glasses, creating an arc of blue flame.

During his time at the Metropolitan, he also did something that no other American bartender had ever done: he wrote a cocktail book, *How to Mix Drinks, or The Bon-Vivant's Companion* (alternately titled *The Bar-Tender's Guide*), first published in 1862. In general, bartenders regarded their recipes as trade secrets, and few ever committed their formulas to paper, let alone printed them to share with others.

At the height of the Civil War, Thomas returned to San Francisco for two years—ostensibly to avoid being drafted into military service—returning in 1865. After that, he operated saloons in various locations with his brother George. By 1876 they closed

their final bar, ending Jerry Thomas's turn as a star, although he continued to work in bars in and around New York City. He died on December 14, 1885, at the age of fifty-five.

See also MIXOLOGY.

Wondrich, David. *Imbibe! From Absinthe Cocktail to Whiskey Smash, a Salute in Stories and Drinks to "Professor" Jerry Thomas, Pioneer of the American Bar.* New York: Perigee, 2007.

Kara Newman

Three-Martini Lunch

The three-martini lunch became associated with New York City in the 1950s and 1960s, when sales and advertising executives famously gathered to discuss business matters over long lunches lubricated with martinis. The martini of choice for these occasions was the "silver bullet," consisting of six ounces of gin and just a drop of vermouth, served "straight up" (without ice) and topped with a thin strip of lemon peel. In this corporate culture, martinis served "on the rocks" (with ice) were frowned upon, as were vodka martinis. Olives were also unwelcome as they displaced too much alcohol.

The "three-martini lunch" became infamous in 1977, when President Jimmy Carter complained bitterly about the "$50 martini lunch," a deductible business expense that he thought should be disallowed. This expression somehow evolved into the "three-martini lunch"—a phrase that Carter claims never to have uttered. Carter did call for the Internal Revenue Service to remove the tax deduction for such business expenses. Letters published in the *New York Times* and other newspapers defended the practice.

Carter's "puritanical" attack elicited a flurry of jokes, cartoons, and editorials. Former presidential candidate Barry Goldwater, for instance, quipped, "None of us had a three-martini lunch until Carter was elected." Corporate culture was changing in the 1970s, and by the time Carter attacked the three-martini lunch it was already on the way out. The phrase was revived in the award-winning AMC television series *Mad Men*, launched in 2007. The series, set in the 1960s, revolved around the fictional character of Don Draper, a Madison Avenue advertising executive. Martinis figured large in his lifestyle. Popular though the program was, it did not return the traditional three-martini lunch to New York's corporate culture.

See also BUSINESS LUNCH; COCKTAILS; *MAD MEN*; MARTINI; and TELEVISION.

Conrad, Barnaby, III. *The Martini: An Illustrated History of an American Classic.* San Francisco: Chronicle, 1995.
Della Femina, Jerry. "The Heyday of the Three-Martini Lunch." *New York Times Magazine*, October 28, 1989.
Edmunds, Lowell. *Martini, Straight Up: The Classic American Cocktail.* Rev. ed. Baltimore: Johns Hopkins University Press, 1998.

Andrew F. Smith

Times Square

Times Square has bustled with interesting food history from its 1902 inception, attracting a tasty hodgepodge of highfalutin, low-down, stand-up, and sit-down culinary delights over many decades. Of all New York's dining destinations and restaurant rows, it is Times Square that arguably has hosted the widest mix of high-end and low-cost food in close proximity.

In the early 1900s and 1910s, most Times Square food options catered to theatergoers and guests at middle- and upper-class hotels such as the Astor (1905) and the Knickerbocker (1906). The market for fine dining was so strong that the larger hotels, notably the Astor, ran restaurants that became destinations unto themselves. Collectively, the Astor's ballrooms could provide lavish dinners to up to eleven hundred people, and everything from the prices to the clientele was decidedly upper crust. Thanks to the New York Public Library's Buttolph Menu collection, we know that a breakfast banquet at the Astor in 1906 included grapefruit, *bouillon en tasse*, roast squab on toast, beet salad, lobster à la Newberg, *filet de boeuf mignons sauté*, ice cream, and coffee. See HOTEL RESTAURANTS.

Beginning in 1908, restaurants touted as "lobster palaces," such as Murray's Roman Gardens (Forty-Second Street), Café de l'Opera (Forty-First Street), and Rector's (Broadway at Forty-Fourth Street), ushered in a peculiar new brand of upwardly mobile dining, with decadent portions and spectacular décor but no society connections needed. A short-lived trend of the early twentieth century, lobster palaces enabled middle-class New Yorkers from any background, be they Ellis Island immigrant or native-born, to splurge on a Times Square feast. See LOBSTER PALACES. The Murray's décor was really over the top, with

Roman statuary and Egyptian motifs enveloping customers as they gorged themselves on lobster and other delicacies. At Rector's in 1913, frog legs and fried scallops cost a dollar, while the large broiled lobster ran three dollars and fifty cents. The menu notes that those wanting only bread and butter had to cough up ten cents per person, leaving at least some space, in theory, for poorer New Yorkers.

Adding to this mix in 1912 was the Horn & Hardart "automat" at Broadway and Forty-Sixth Street. For only a nickel in the food dispensers, patrons could partake of soups, sandwiches, pastry, pie, and doughnuts, usually baked or cooked fresh daily at Fiftieth Street and Eleventh Avenue. It was open twenty-four hours a day, seven days a week and blew apart conventional notions of respectable sit-down dining, so it is not surprising that this automat, along with nearby Childs, became a site of "raucous gatherings by homosexual men and prostitutes" in the wee hours of the morning. Some of the more notable mentions of this automat are in the play *The Odd Couple* (1965), the film *That Touch of Mink* (1962), and *Gentlemen Prefer Blondes* (Broadway 1949, film 1953). Although best known for its food dispensers, it did have made-to-order options and, of course, seating. See AUTOMATS and CHILDS.

Times Square visitors who wanted to rub shoulders with actors, or at least see their famous caricatures on the wall, would have gravitated to Sardi's Restaurant (1927). On Forty-Fourth Street just west of Broadway, Sardi's stands out as a Broadway hangout, the site of many opening-night parties, and the only known restaurant in Times Square with a separate, more affordable menu just for actors. Also opening in the 1920s but relocating several times throughout its Times Square tenure, was the storied Lindy's. Frequented by Mafiosi in the 1950s and chronicled in the stories of Damon Runyon as the barely disguised Mindy's, Lindy's was best known for its delicious cheesecake. See SARDI'S and LINDY'S.

Given the overcrowded pressure cooker environment of Times Square, some venues offered very little or no seating, in the style of Nathan's Famous Hot Dogs, Elpine Drinks, Orange Julius, and Nedick's. Elpine gained fame in *The Sweet Smell of Success* (1957), when Tony Curtis's character scarfed down a hot dog and juice beneath the iconic, smoke-ring-emitting Camel cigarette sign. See NATHAN'S FAMOUS and NEDICK'S.

Beyond the 1950s, eateries went from bare bones and rough to bleak and possibly dangerous. At Nathan's in the 1970s and 1980s, the hamburgers, fries, onion rings, and broiled lobster rolls were no great hazard, but the grimy deli counter in the poorly ventilated basement was reportedly touch and go. Even worse, it was apparently too close for comfort to the restrooms, and the entire downstairs drew a homeless population. Although they were popular among Times Square's growing Latino and African American demographic, these affordable establishments were also feared by some as symbols of "urban crisis."

Fine dining was down but not out in the 1980s as it got a jolt from the expensive, rotating restaurant atop the gargantuan Marriott Marquis hotel in 1986. Even as this and other expensive restaurants arrived, cheap standbys held strong, especially on Forty-Second Street between Seventh and Eighth Avenues. Amid X-rated marquees, affordable "greasy spoons" such as Tad's Steakhouse and Blimpie's remained in reach for those priced out of the "The View" at the Marriott.

Most recently, Times Square has gotten chain or theme restaurants such as Olive Garden and Hard Rock Café, raising concerns that its wonderful weirdness could be swallowed up by bland, tourist-oriented outlets. Considering, however, that food on the go is still kicking at kiosks such as Rickshaw Dumplings and Nuchas, and that the district's quirky theatricality still sings at sites like Ellen's Stardust Diner (with a singing waitstaff since 1987), it is unlikely that Times Square food will ever match that of a mall foodcourt. As long as there are purveyors willing to innovate or cram kitchens and counters into impossibly small spaces, one can hope that Times Square's peculiar culinary flavor will remain distinctive.

Peretti, Burton W. *Nightclub City: Politics and Amusement in Manhattan.* Philadelphia: University of Pennsylvania Press, 2007.

Sagalyn, Lynne B. *Times Square Roulette: Remaking the City Icon.* Cambridge, Mass.: MIT Press, 2001.

Timothy R. White

capitalize on its fame, he began to plan a Toffenetti for Manhattan. When it opened in 1940 (it stood for three decades), the gargantuan restaurant had a thousand seats and offered food around the clock. Eventually, according to an article in the *New York Times*, it averaged three thousand meals a day.

Fame, however, came not simply from its size and offerings but also from Toffenetti's singular gift for turning a phrase. An Italian immigrant inspired by traditional American food, he enrolled in Northwestern University's School of Commerce to learn to better promote it. Study of stimulus response theory and exploration of what he called the "psychology of happy eating" gave him what he sought. Long before we called it "menu speak" (descriptions meant to whet the appetite and sell dishes), he was practicing it and became a virtuoso. His menu, wrote the *New Yorker*, is a "prose masterpiece that inevitably excites the salivary glands."

Early on he advertised "Delicious Hot Roasted Juicy Sugar-Cured Ham Sandwich liberal in size with Pickle," a description that greatly increased trade, but he went on to depictions much more imaginative and ornate. Potatoes, a specialty, were described as "Rough Skin but Tender-Hearted, from the Lava Beds of Idaho, Product of Millions of Years of Evolution." Spaghetti was "a hundred yards of happiness," served with a sauce "made from a treasured recipe of old discovered by Mrs. Toffenetti in the archives among the ruins of the ancient castle of the Count of Bonpensler in Bologna." Strawberry shortcake was called the "tonic of spring." Toffenetti loved his food so much that he once said it required a poet laureate to describe it. Lacking someone else to do the job, he did it himself.

Grimes, William. *Appetite City: A Culinary History of New York.* New York: North Point, 2009.

"The Talk of the Town." *New Yorker*, April 8, 1944.

Cara De Silva

Toffenetti, Dario

Dario Toffenetti was the proprietor of what he dubbed "the busiest restaurant on the world's busiest corner." The restaurant was Toffenetti, and the corner was Broadway and Forty-Third Street. Already well known for his eateries in Chicago, the move to Times Square developed from participation in the 1939 New York World's Fair. His venture there was popular, and to

Tofutti

Tofutti is a brand of tofu-based kosher, dairy-free, lactose-free products, created by New York restaurateur David Mintz in the 1980s. Originally, the company's focus was nondairy frozen desserts, but as time has passed, Tofutti has created nondairy versions of many products, including frozen pizza and cream cheese.

In the late 1970s, David Mintz was owner of Mintz's Buffet, a New York City glatt kosher restaurant. See JEWISH. Many customers asked for ice cream for dessert, but he could not offer it because Jewish law forbids serving dairy within a certain time after eating a meal that included meat. Looking for an alternative to dairy-based ice cream he read about tofu in a wholesale food magazine. Curious, he bought some in New York's Chinatown. See CHINESE COMMUNITY.

Initially, Mintz was unimpressed by tofu, but he persisted in experimenting with it, sensing its potential. In time, he successfully incorporated it into some savory dishes, such as quiche and beef stroganoff; however, a tofu-based frozen dessert was more of a challenge. This came only in 1981, when with the help of Ruben Rapaport (now director of product development for Tofutti) he created Tofutti and began selling a soft-serve version in New York City.

During the 1980s, Tofutti experienced great success. Its appeal was not limited to observant Jews. Strict vegetarians, people with dairy allergies and lactose intolerance, and people wishing to avoid ice cream's cholesterol and saturated fats all found Tofutti an enjoyable alternative.

At first, Tofutti was sold mostly in the New York Metropolitan area. But after making a public offering in 1983, the company started selling the frozen dessert in pint-sized hard packs in a variety of flavors and made an agreement with Häagen Dazs to distribute Tofutti in several eastern states. Expansion led the company to relocate from Brooklyn to a larger facility in Rahway, New Jersey, in 1984. In 1985 the company's stock was traded on the American Stock Exchange, and in 1986 the company received a patent for Tofutti.

With success came challenges. Competition from other nondairy frozen desserts meant stagnant revenues as the decade closed. Moreover the public became somewhat suspicious of Tofutti's status as a "health" or "diet" food. While protein-rich and cholesterol-free, Tofutti was higher in calories than conventional ice cream.

Mintz responded by hiring Francis Mullin as the company's new president. Mullin oversaw increasing exports of Tofutti, developing a lower-calorie version of Tofutti, cross-promoting with Diet Coke and Lean Cuisine, and developing new products such as Tofutti Cuties (Tofutti ice cream sandwiches). The company cut its workforce and moved to a smaller facility in Cranford, New Jersey, in 1989.

In 1992 Tofutti recorded its first profit in seven years. New products developed during the 1990s included Sour Supreme, imitation cheese slices, pizza, and potato pancakes. Tofutti Cuties was the company's bestseller, being ranked eighteenth out of 124 ice cream sandwiches on the market, according to A. C. Nielsen.

Eftimiades, Maria. "Tofu Innovator Dreams of New Creations." *New York Times*, February 19, 1989.
Grant, Tina. *International Directory of Company Histories (Book 64)*. St. James, Mo.: St. James, 2004.
Londin, Louise. "Soy Delis—Mintz's Buffet." *Soyfoods*, no. 5 (Summer 1981).
Shurtleff, William, and Akiko Aoyagi. *Tofutti and Other Soy Ice Creams: The Non-Dairy Frozen Dessert Industry and Market*. Lafayette, Calif.: Soyfoods Center, 1985.

Karl Peterson

Tontine Coffee House

See COFFEEHOUSES.

Tootsie Roll

The invention of the Tootsie Roll, a perennial American favorite, is credited to a New York City confectioner named Leo Hirschfeld. Hirschfeld, an immigrant from Laupheim in southern Germany, arrived in Brooklyn in 1888. Two years later he moved to Manhattan where he became a salaried employee of Stern & Saalberg, a food manufacturer. The company's major product was "Bromangelon," a flavored powder for making jellied desserts. Advertisements for Bromangelon featured a character called "Tattling Tootsie"—who may have been named for Hirschfeld's little daughter Clara, nicknamed "Tootsie." While at Stern & Saalberg, Hirschfeld invented a number of machines, several for candy making. He eventually became vice president of the company.

In September 1908 Stern & Saalberg launched a new confection that Hirschfeld had developed: a small, log-shaped chocolate caramel called the "Tootsie Roll." Unlike other penny candies, each Tootsie Roll was individually wrapped. The following year, the company launched a major advertising campaign, and Tootsie Rolls quickly became a national favorite. In 1917 Stern & Saalberg was renamed the Sweets Company of America. Hirschfeld left the firm around 1920 to become a part owner of another candy company, Mells Candy Corporation. He died two years later.

The Sweets Company eventually extended its original Tootsie Roll line to include Tootsie Nut Rolls, Tootsie Kisses, and Tootsie Caramels. In 1931, the company introduced the Tootsie Pop, a spherical lollipop with a chocolate caramel center. During the Depression the company ran into financial troubles, and it was eventually acquired by Joseph Rubin & Sons of Brooklyn. In 1938, the Sweets Company of America moved its manufacturing facility to Hoboken, New Jersey.

During World War II, Tootsie Rolls found a place in soldiers' ration kits, because the candy could survive extremes of heat and cold. After the war, the company was one of the first to target its advertising toward children by sponsoring such popular television shows as *The Mickey Mouse Club, Howdy Doody, Rin Tin Tin,* and *Rocky & Bullwinkle*.

The Sweets Company of America was renamed Tootsie Roll Industries in 1966. Today it is headquartered in Chicago.

See also CANDY.

Candy Professor website: http://candyprofessor.com.

Andrew F. Smith

Torres, Jacques

Jacques Torres, also known as "Mr. Chocolate," was born in Algiers, Algeria, on June 14, 1959. His family moved to the small village of Bandol, in the south of France, where he entered a pastry apprenticeship at age fifteen. In 1980, he began working with Michelin two-starred chef Jacques Maximin at the iconic Hôtel Negresco on the French Riviera, and on his days off he attended school, earning a master pastry chef degree. By 1983, he was teaching pastry classes in Cannes, and in 1986 he became the youngest person to win the title Meilleur Ouvrier de France Pâtissier, a grueling challenge of pastry prowess.

Torres came to the United States in 1988 to work as Corporate Pastry Chef at the Ritz-Carlton Hotel Company. He moved to New York City to head the pastry kitchen at Le Cirque in 1989, where he would remain the executive pastry chef for eleven years. While there, he hosted a fifty-two-episode public television series, *Dessert Circus with Jacques Torres,* and his first cookbooks, *Dessert Circus* (1997) and *Dessert Circus at Home* (1998), flowed from these programs. A three-year series on the Food Network,

Chocolate with Jacques Torres, followed. He joined the faculty of the French Culinary Institute in 1993 and designed the school's "classic pastry arts curriculum" in 1996. He is now dean of pastry arts.

Torres left Le Cirque in 2000 to open his first artisanal chocolate factory and shop, in Brooklyn's DUMBO neighborhood. Patrons can see the chocolates being made through the factory windows. Torres now has seven outlets scattered across Manhattan and Brooklyn, identified by their brown awnings ornamented with a stylized cacao pod. He is the author of *Jacques Torres' Year in Chocolate: 80 Recipes for Holidays and Celebrations* (2008). He has won many awards, among them the 1994 James Beard Foundation Pastry Chef of the Year.

See also FOOD NETWORK; FRENCH CULINARY INSTITUTE; and LE CIRQUE.

"Chef Jacques Torres, MOF." Jacques Torres Chocolate (website). http://www.mrchocolate.com/news/about/chef-jacques-torres-mof.
"Jacques Torres." Biography.com. http://www.biography.com/people/jacques-torres-20928983.

Cathy K. Kaufman

Trader Joe's

Trader Joe's is a privately held specialty grocery chain founded in 1958 in the Los Angeles area by Joe Coulombe. Originally called Pronto Market, the first outlets were convenience stores; they suffered when the 7-Eleven chain moved into the California market. In 1967 Coulombe changed the focus of the stores to provide more sophisticated foods not easily found in neighborhood grocery stores. He introduced the stores' distinctive Polynesian motif and called the rebranded venture Trader Joe's, a riff on the famous Trader Vic's bar at the Plaza Hotel. In 1979 Coulombe sold the chain to a private German company, although Coulombe remained with the company until 1987. After he left, new management expanded the Trader Joe's brand into a nationwide chain.

Trader Joe's opened its first store in Manhattan on March 17, 2006, at 142 East Fourteenth Street, and additional stores opened in Queens (2007), Brooklyn (2008), and Manhattan's Chelsea and Upper West Side neighborhoods (2010). Trader Joe's is not a conventional grocery store: it stocks far fewer choices, averaging roughly four thousand different items, compared to the fifty-thousand or more items in a typical full-service grocery store. What distinguishes Trader Joe's is its budget-conscious "foodie" appeal, made possible because most of its products are produced under its private label. Many of its foods are partially prepared, such as precut vegetables, simmer sauces, and frozen entrées. From tropical trail mixes to Greek-style yogurt and gluten-free coconut flour, Trader Joe's products appeal with unique and jolly packaging as well as clever marketing in its monthly mailed brochure *The Fearless Flyer*, and point-of-sale advertising, often written by employees in each store, is tailored to appeal to local, urbane shoppers.

But Trader Joe's cheerful looks and low-cost items do not come without opposition. The company's branded products are bought or imported directly from producers whose names are never stated, and it refuses to disclose where the organic products under its label come from. Uneven selection, items that disappear and reappear on the shelves, and an overall corporate secrecy are part of the company's culture. Stingy with the media, Trader Joe's executives seldom give interviews: a rare exception was made for *New York Times* reporter Julia Moskin, who wrote one of several *Times* articles in advance of the opening of the first New York City outpost. Nonetheless, Trader Joe's enjoys what many describe as a cult-like following.

One of Trader Joe's most famous innovations has been its "Two Buck Chuck," bargain basement–priced wine produced by Bronco Wine Company under the Charles Shaw label. Debuting in California at $1.99 per bottle in 2002, the prices have since gone up. The Trader Joe's Wine Store on East Fourteenth Street (a shop separate from the main grocery store, as required by local ordinance) sells an array of wines, including "Two Buck Chuck" (now priced north of three dollars) as well as more prestigious bottles veering toward the twenty-dollar price point.

See also GROCERY STORES and SUPERMARKETS.

Llopis, Glenn. "Why Trader Joe's Stands Out from All the Rest in the Grocery Business." Forbes.com, September 5, 2011. http://www.forbes.com/sites/glennllopis/2011/09/05/why-trader-joes-stands-out-from-all-the-rest-in-the-grocery-business.

Moskin, Julia. "For Trader Joe's, a New York Taste Test." *New York Times*, March 8, 2006.

Ramirez, Anthony. "A Tiki Room with Aisles of Discounts Makes Its City Debut." *New York Times*, March 18, 2006.

Thei Zervaki and Cathy K. Kaufman

Trans Fat Elimination

In December 2006, the New York City Board of Health passed an amendment to the city's Health Code to include Section 81.08, which restricted artificial trans fats served in food service establishments to 0.5 grams per serving. Natural trans fats in products from ruminant animals were not restricted because of lack of consensus about their health impact and the small amounts found in food. Artificial trans fats, found in products like shortening, margarine, snack foods, baked goods, fried items, and fast food, made through the process of partial hydrogenation of oils, were in the food supply for nearly one hundred years. Partial hydrogenation increased the shelf life of oils, changed them to solid textures good for baking, and were an inexpensive alternative to solid animal fats. However, the fat was also implicated in heart disease, a leading cause of death in New York City, and other health concerns, and the safety of artificial trans fats had been debated for decades.

In the 1990s a few influential studies confirmed the harm of the fat, and the Center for Science in the Public Interest, a consumer advocacy group, petitioned the U.S. Food and Drug Administration to add artificial trans fats to food labels. The federal ruling was implemented in 2006; however, restaurant foods had no nutrition label. The growing importance of food eaten away from home in American culture made restaurant food an important source of artificial trans fat. The New York City ordinance addressed this gap.

The restriction became known as a "ban" and made national headlines quickly. Although many culinary purists stated they never used products containing artificial trans fats, fast-food operators, bakers, and doughnut makers did. Margarine and shortening were also important to kosher bakers and restaurateurs who served soul food. Industry trade groups, such as the New York City chapter of the New York State Restaurant Association, protested the ordinance as unnecessary government interference that limited the choice of restaurateurs and consumers. However, public testimony showed New York City consumers and public advocates supported the ordinance, as did many food businesses such as Sylvia's, the landmark soul food restaurant in Harlem and the Waterfront Alehouse in Brooklyn and Manhattan. Some, like the B. R. Guest restaurant group, saw it as beneficial to their guests and assisted with the ordinance. The city set up the Trans Fat Help Center with the

New York City College of Technology to aid businesses in making the change, and the two phases to implement the ordinance ended in 2008. The ordinance required operators of food-service establishments to read and save food labels for inspections to look for foods containing artificial trans fat, and violations carried a fine of two hundred to two thousand dollars. Most New York City food businesses quickly complied, and distributors assisted in finding acceptable alternatives.

The ordinance was the first public health measure in New York City targeting restaurant and ready-to-eat food to reduce food-related chronic disease. Although controversial, other similar policy efforts, like calorie labeling for menus and limits to sugary beverage sizes, were more hotly contested. In November 2013, the Food and Drug Administration proposed to remove artificial trans fats as a food additive from the Generally Recognized as Safe (GRAS) list. In June 2015 after a long period of public comment they finally did remove trans fats from the GRAS list, and gave food manufacturers three years to comply by removing partially hydrogenated foods from their products.

See also BLOOMBERG, MICHAEL; MENU LABELING; and SODA "BAN."

Johnson, Kimberly-Elizabeth. "A Social History of the New York City Trans Fat Policy." PhD diss., Syracuse University, 2014.
Jacobson, Michael F. "Petition for Rulemaking to Revoke the Authority for Industry to Use Partially Hydrogenated Vegetable Oils in Foods," May 18, 2004. http://cspinet.org/new/pdf/trans_fat_petition_may_18.pdf.
Notice of adoption of an amendment (§81.08) to article 81 of the New York City health code. New York City Department of Health and Mental Hygiene, 2005. http://www.nyc.gov/html/doh/downloads/pdf/public/notice-adoption-hc-art81-08.pdf.

Kimberly-Elizabeth Johnson

Trillin, Calvin

Calvin Trillin, born December 5, 1935, is an American humorist and longtime New Yorker who has written extensively on the subject of food. Born in Kansas City, he attended Yale University and served two years in the U.S. Army. He began writing for the *New Yorker* magazine in 1963 and has been a resident of Greenwich Village ever since. See GREENWICH VILLAGE. In addition to contributions to the *New*

Yorker and *The Nation,* Trillin has published twenty-eight books, including the *Tummy Trilogy,* which incorporates three earlier books on food: *American Fried; Alice, Let's Eat;* and *Third Helpings.* He has also appeared in two off-Broadway one-man shows and has made appearances in film and television.

While widely considered one of today's foremost writers on food, Trillin does not consider himself to be a food writer. As Dianne Jacob writes in *Will Write for Food* (2005), "[Trillin] adamantly refuses to describe his work as food writing. He calls it 'writing about eating,' and doesn't distinguish it from any other nonfiction. He insists he is not a cook, has no culinary knowledge, and does not rate food."

Whatever may be the appropriate label for him, food is frequently at the heart of Trillin's work. The cuisine of his native Kansas City and Jewish specialties such as bagels are frequently the stars of his stories, but Galician peppers, Lunenburg sausage, Cajun boudin, Ecuadorian ceviche, and many other enticing foods make appearances in his writing. On the way to discovering that next great meal, Trillin encounters all that surrounds the taco stands and barbecue joints he loves so well.

The recipient of the 2012 Thurber Prize for American Humor, Trillin has, as part of the New Yorker Festival, given an annual food tour of Lower Manhattan for the last fourteen years, which begins in Greenwich Village and wends southward to Manhattan's Chinatown. Given the limited space and once-a-year conditions of the tour, tickets are highly prized among New York's foodies.

See also NEW YORKER.

Farmer, Ann. "35 Lucky, and Hungry, Diners Eat and Walk with Calvin Trillin." *New York Times,* October 5, 2008.
Plimpton, George. "Calvin Trillin, the Art of Humor No. 3." *Paris Review,* no. 136 (Fall 1995).
Trillin, Calvin. *The Tummy Trilogy.* New York: Farrar, Straus & Giroux, 1994.

Karl Peterson

Tschirky, Oscar

Swiss immigrant Oscar Tschirky (1866–1950) was renowned in New York City during his fifty-year reign over the restaurants at the Waldorf, and then the Waldorf Astoria, Hotel. The day after arriving in New York City in 1883, he took a job as a busboy at the Hoffman House, a popular hotel on Broadway and Twenty-Fourth Street. He later waited tables at Delmonico's, eventually becoming the manager of the restaurant's catering department. Tschirky joined the staff at the new Waldorf Hotel, located on Fifth Avenue at Thirty-Third Street, two months before it opened in 1893. (In 1897 the adjoining Astoria Hotel would be combined with the Waldorf into a single entity, the Waldorf Astoria.)

Tschirky's management skills helped launch the Waldorf's several restaurants. He took charge of its private dining rooms, which became the favorite haunts of the city's most famous residents and visitors. The financier J. P. Morgan, the actress Lillian Russell, and the multimillionaire gourmand Diamond Jim Brady were frequently seen there. Tschirky took note of the favorite dishes and drinks of his important guests, enabling him to host them with unparalleled personal service. His performance in the Waldorf's dining rooms led to his promotion to hotel steward, with responsibility for supplying all provisions, supervising all food preparation, and managing all restaurant staff, which included thirty-five chefs and six hundred others.

The hotel's restaurants served French cuisine, and Oscar, as he was known (because, as he said, most Americans could not pronounce his last name), proclaimed that the food served at the Waldorf was equal to that offered at the finest restaurants in Paris. Tschirky compiled menus and recipes from his chefs into *The Cook Book of Oscar of the Waldorf* (1896). It includes many recipes created at the hotel, such as the Waldorf salad. See WALDORF SALAD.

Tschirky innovated some practices that were later adopted by other restaurants. Unlike the menus at many other New York City haute cuisine restaurants, the Waldorf's were in English, although a bilingual (French and English) menu was available on request. Tschirky also simplified the Waldorf's menus. Other temples of fine dining had ridiculously large *cartes* listing a thousand items or more. Tschirky pared down the offerings and even decreased the number of courses. Other city restaurants soon followed suit.

In January 1907, the Waldorf Astoria made a bold move, posting an announcement that "Ladies without escort will be served in the restaurants at any hour." This contravened an unwritten rule that single women who entered its restaurants would basically be ignored. The finer city restaurants had always "discouraged" solo female patrons. (This policy, of course, was suspended when it came to wealthy women who were known at the restaurants.) There was strong public opposition to the Waldorf's new policy, and the hotel yielded to it, but the door had been opened, and gradually restaurants began to change their attitude toward women who wished to dine alone.

In 1929 the owners of the Waldorf Astoria sold the building to make way for the construction of the Empire State Building. They relocated to a full-block site on Park Avenue, building a massive new hotel of unprecedented luxury. There were three dining rooms, one of which was the Palm Court, which Tschirky served as maître d'hôtel until his retirement in 1943. His memory lives on in the name of the hotel's casual restaurant, Oscar's.

See also DELMONICO'S and WALDORF, THE.

Schriftgiesser, Karl. *Oscar of the Waldorf.* New York: Dutton, 1943.
Tschirky, Oscar. *The Cook Book by "Oscar" of the Waldorf.* Chicago and New York: Werner, 1896.

Andrew F. Smith

Twenty-First Century

Twenty-first-century New York City is a diverse, energetic, and ambitious place. The city is undergoing a continuing economic rebirth, enjoying a new and substantial wave of immigration from various parts of the world, and continuing to benefit from a declining crime rate. All of these factors are reflected in the city's thriving food culture. The volume and diversity of New York's food offerings are immediately apparent to visitors and locals alike. As of 2015, New York City was home to twenty-four thousand restaurants, or one restaurant per 350 residents.

New York has always been a city of immigrants, and each successive group has contributed to the city's foodways. In the twenty-first century, the largest sources of new immigrants to the city are the Dominican Republic and China, followed by Mexico, Jamaica, and Guyana. This represents a significant shift away from the largely European immigration patterns of the nineteenth and early twentieth centuries, and that shift is also visible in the wide availability of East and South Asian as well as South American and Caribbean foods in the city.

Another stream that fuels twenty-first-century New York's food culture is the emergence of the "foodie." A somewhat amorphous and at times controversial term, foodies in essence are food hobbyists, people who pride themselves on their knowledge of food and their willingness to experiment with new foods. Foodie culture supports the extensive gourmet market industry in New York and has given rise to new trends, like food trucks and food festivals such as Smorgasburg and Madison Square Eats, among many others. Food tourism has also become a growing practice in New York for both locals and out-of-towners. Some types of food tourism take the form of annual events, like the Flushing Momo Crawl, while others are a consistent offering from walking tour companies like Big Onion Walking Tours and Urban Oyster or a regular option from established public history institutions like the Lower East Side Tenement Museum.

Despite the enormous energy and innovation surrounding food in New York City, the twenty-first-century city continues to face significant challenges when it comes to food. One of the critiques of present-day New York's food culture is that it exacerbates economic inequalities. While some people in the city eat elaborate gourmet meals on a regular basis and enjoy access to a wide variety of fresh produce, many others in the city struggle to keep food on the table and live in "food deserts," a controversial term for areas where affordable fresh food is not regularly available.

New Yorkers continue to debate whether there is a connection between food deserts and the rate of obesity in the city, but both are issues the city has attempted to respond to over the past decade. In 2008 the administration of Mayor Michael Bloomberg successfully passed a law mandating that chain restaurants in the city display nutritional information on their menus. See MENU LABELING. That same year, the city launched the Green Cart Initiative. The plan was an effort to simultaneously provide low-priced produce to underserved areas and to provide a way for low-income people to gain business experience as cart vendors. A 2014 report from Columbia University found that the initiative showed evidence of accomplishing some of its goals, but the long-term effects remain to be seen. Toward the end of his final term as mayor Bloomberg attempted to regulate soft drinks by proposing a ban on the sale of sodas larger than sixteen ounces. The plan was controversial, heavily opposed by the Pepsi Corporation, and ultimately struck down by the New York State Court of Appeals in 2014. See SODA "BAN."

Another major theme in New York's food culture, and an area that may ultimately bridge New York's gap in income equality, is that of food sourcing and food production. Many New Yorkers have expressed a growing interest in locally sourced,

small-scale food production from both an economic and an environmental standpoint. This shift is visible in several ways. Beekeeping was legalized in New York City in 2010, and by 2012 there were two hundred registered hives in the city and as many as two hundred additional unregistered ones. See BEEKEEPING. There has also been a tremendous growth in farmers' markets in the city, with most of the vendors coming from New Jersey and the Hudson Valley. A 2012 report from the New York State Comptroller's Office noted that there were 138 farmers' markets in New York City. That number represents about one-quarter of all of the farmers' markets in the state of New York as well as a 73 percent increase in the number of New York City farmers' markets since 2006. New York City has worked to make these markets more accessible to low-income residents, and those efforts appear to be bearing fruit. In 2011 New York City farmers' markets did $2.6 million in sales using food stamps, which are now accepted at the majority of farmers' markets. See GREENMARKETS.

The city has also seen a significant increase in community supported agriculture programs over the past several years. In community supported agriculture, participants purchase a share of a weekly or monthly portion of produce, generally collected from several farmers in the tri-state area. Because the produce is delivered directly from farmers to consumers, the programs are often less expensive than retail produce, and many emphasize local sourcing and environmentally sound production methods. See COMMUNITY SUPPORTED AGRICULTURE.

In addition to farmers' markets and community supported agriculture, most of which derive their offerings from New Jersey, Westchester, and the Hudson Valley, there have been developments in urban farming in recent years. A U.S. Department of Agriculture census released in 2012 recorded thirty-one farms in the five boroughs. A research project conducted by the Columbia University Design Lab advocated for the further development of urban farms in the city as a potential benefit both to the environmental health of the city and to the food security of its residents. See URBAN FARMING.

Modern New York City is a site of multifaceted innovation in food. The city's current food culture is diverse but also stratified, reflecting serious inequalities. The issue of food diversity, availability, and sustainability is central to present-day politics in New York and to questions of the city's future.

See also FOOD DESERTS.

Department of City Planning, City of New York. "Mayor Bloomberg, City Planning Executive Director Barth, and Immigrant Affairs Commissioner Shama Release Newest New Yorkers Immigration Report Depicting Important Social and Economic Role of Foreign-Born Residents." Press release, December 18, 2013. http://www.nyc.gov/html/dcp/html/about/pr121813a.shtml.

DiNapoli, Thomas P., and Kenneth B. Bleiwas. "Farmers' Markets in New York City." Office of the State Comptroller, August 2012. http://www.osc.state.ny.us/osdc/farmersmarkets_rpt6-2013.pdf.

Grynbaum, Michael M. "New York's Ban on Big Sodas Is Rejected by Final Court." *New York Times*, June 26, 2014.

Segal, Adi. "Food Deserts: A Global Crisis in New York City." *Consilience: The Journal of Sustainable Development* 3, no. 1 (2010): 197–214.

U.S. Department of Agriculture. "USDA Census of Agriculture: 2012 Census Volume 1, Chapter 2: County-Level Data." http://www.agcensus.usda.gov/Publications/2012/Full_Report/Volume_1,_Chapter_2_County_Level/New_York.

Katie Uva

"21" Club

Often referred to as "21 Club" or "The 21 Club," 21 is notorious for its role as a speakeasy during Prohibition (1920–1933). Located in midtown Manhattan, it is one of the few one-time speakeasy spaces that continues to operate as a bar and restaurant.

The 21 Club was the nearly accidental creation of two college kids from the Lower East Side, Jack Kriendler and his cousin Charlie Berns. During Prohibition, their uncle let them work in his speakeasy on the Lower East Side. The more they worked, the less appealing college seemed. Prohibition had turned New York into a gold mine.

In 1922, the cousins first opened the Red Head (Sixth Avenue, between Fourth Street and Washington Place), which (according to Pete Kriendler, Jack's younger brother) was run as a "jazzy, jivey, good clean fun" kind of place, popular with the fraternity crowd. The cover charge was fifty cents, and patrons drank liquor from teacups, a common practice during the Prohibition years. Three years later, they bought a space across the street, calling it the Club Fronton.

In 1926, Kreindler and Berns moved into Midtown—and a handsome townhouse with an iron gate, at 42 West Forty-Ninth Street, which they named the Puncheon Grotto. Eventually, the space would be razed to make way for Rockefeller Center.

On January 1, 1930, the cousins bought a townhouse at 21 West Fifty-Second Street, on a block already notorious for housing speakeasies, and named it "21" after the address. The club was a success from the beginning, attracting a wealthy and important clientele from café society, politics, and Wall Street. They established a no-press, no-photographers policy—another reason the upper crust liked the place. Conversations between the city's power players could be off the record, credit was extended to guests, and it had a highly masculine, clubby vibe. A professional "greeter" recognized all the "right" guests. The literary elite especially adored Jack, aka "The Baron," whose colorful taste ran to sable-lined overcoats, cutaways, and Havana cigars.

The club was raided only twice. The first time was in 1930, after gossip columnist Walter Winchell was banned from 21 and tipped off federal agents in retribution. The second time was in 1932, when federal agents spent hours at the club searching for the two thousand cases of liquor, apparently hidden behind the cellar door and never found. The liquor out front had already disappeared, after the bartender pushed a button, overturning the shelves behind the bar and sending bottles crashing down an iron grating and into the New York sewage system.

During Prohibition, the private speakeasy club was separated from the public space and hidden behind thick brick walls, which sprang open at the insertion of a long metal wire into a tiny hole that released a catch in the door. That door is still there. However, the basement now houses an extensive wine cellar and private dining spaces. The 21 Club is now owned by the London-based hotel company and luxury adventure travel operator Belmond Ltd.

See also CLUBS; PROHIBITION; and SPEAKEASIES.

Kriendler, H. Peter, and H. Paul Jeffers. *"21": Every Day Was New Year's Eve: Memoirs of a Saloon Keeper.* Lanham, Md.: Taylor, 1999.

West, Richard. "The Power of '21.'" *New York Magazine*, October 5, 1981.

Kara Newman

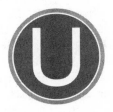

Ukrainian

New York is home to a large population of immigrants from Ukraine, the largest country within Europe. Several enclaves of Ukrainians inside the five boroughs exist, but among the most popular are in Brighton Beach, sometimes referred to as "Little Odessa," and a section of the East Village, often referred to as "Ukrainian Village" or "Little Ukraine." That area lies within the borders of Houston and Fourteenth Streets and Third Avenue and Avenue A and may at one point have housed upward of sixty thousand immigrants. See LITTLE ODESSA.

With a number of social clubs, markets, Ukrainian-specific businesses, and restaurants, the area has retained much of its heritage despite the rapidly changing nature of the city. One of the more popular and enduring Ukrainian restaurants in the East Village is Veselka, which has been serving traditional dishes since 1954 to both regulars and tourists. Common Ukrainian-inspired dishes include kielbasa, borscht, stuffed cabbage, pierogi, and bigos, a stew.

Little Ukraine is the scene of the annual Ukrainian Festival, typically held in May at the Saint George Ukrainian Catholic Church, across East Seventh Street from McSorley's Old Ale House. Food stands and cultural displays are often set up along Taras Shevchenko Place, a small street that connects East Seventh and East Sixth Streets, named after a Ukrainian artist, poet, and writer.

McKinley, Jesse. "Neighborhood Report: East Harlem; Ukrainian Accent Gets Stronger." *New York Times*, November 16, 1997.
Saint George Ukrainian Catholic Schools website: http://www.saintgeorgeschools.org/100101.html.
Ukrainian Institute of America website: http://ukrainianinstitute.org.
"Ukrainians in New York." Brama.com. http://www.brama.com/stgeorge/ny.html.

John Holl

Union Square Cafe

When Danny Meyer's award-winning Union Square Cafe opened in 1985 on East Sixteenth Street near Fifth Avenue, it was one of the first establishments to revitalize the formerly gritty Union Square. Meyer asked architect Larry Bogdanow, who also designed Savoy, Union Pacific, Telepan, City Hall, and the Cub Room, to create a restaurant that was easy, comfortable, and timeless. Bogdanow created an American trattoria with an airy interior that was elegant but casual, with cherry-wood floors and green wainscoting.

In 1988 Michael Romano joined the restaurant as the executive chef, and only a few months later Union Square Cafe received three stars from the *New York Times*. With his classical training and the Union Square Greenmarket nearby, Romano was one of the first chefs to popularize a menu of seasonal, contemporary American cuisine. Some of the most popular dishes over the years included fried calamari with spicy anchovy mayonnaise, bibb and red oak leaf lettuce salad, yellowfin tuna burger, and polenta with blue cheese and walnuts. Desserts, which might include a peach melba sundae, pumpkin cheesecake, or warm chocolate brownie custard with toffee sauce, change seasonally. But one classic always remained on the menu: the banana tart with macadamia brittle and honey-vanilla ice cream.

Union Square Cafe has received many awards, including the James Beard Foundation's Outstanding Service in 1995 and Outstanding Restaurant in 1997. In 1998 and 1999 the *New York Times* awarded it three stars, and the Zagat Survey has named it a favorite restaurant many times since 1998. In 2001 the James Beard Foundation named Romano Best Chef in New York City. It is also well known for its hospitality. In 2005, when Romano became director of culinary development at the Union Square Hospitality Group, Carmen Quagliata took over as executive chef. In October 2013 Romano left the restaurant to run Union Square Tokyo, the Japanese outpost of the restaurant.

In the summer of 2014 Meyer announced that because the landlord asked for a significant increase in rent, the Union Square Cafe would close in December 2015 after more than twenty-five years in the same location. In an article in the *New York Times*, Danny Meyer said, "There's no such thing as a New York restaurant that is immune to real estate."

See also MEYER, DANNY.

"Chef Michael Romano of Union Square Tokyo—Biography." StarChefs.com. November 2010. http://www.starchefs.com/cook/chefs/bio/Michael-Romano.

Grimes, William. "Larry Bogdanow, 64, Dies; Crafted Cozy Restaurants." *New York Times*, June 29, 2011.

Moskin, Julia. "Union Square Cafe Joins Other Victims of New York City's Rising Rents." *New York Times*, June 23, 2014.

Mullen, Matt. "Danny Meyer's Union Square Cafe to Close." *Observer*, June 24, 2014.

Tracey Ceurvels

Upper East Side

The Upper East Side is a neighborhood in the borough of Manhattan bordered by Fifth Avenue to the west, Fifty-Ninth Street to the south, the East River, and Ninety-Sixth Street to the north. Throughout the course of New York's history, the Upper East Side has been the residential neighborhood for the city's wealthy and elite whose businesses may be found in other parts of the city. The area is noted for its major avenues: Fifth, Madison, Park, and Lexington, along which many affluent residents continue to live. Once known as the "silk stocking

district," the densely populated area is considered the home of the highest concentration of wealth in the United States.

The Upper East Side is home to a number of the city's foremost cultural institutions, predominantly museums such as the Metropolitan Museum of Art; the Solomon R. Guggenheim Museum; the Frick Collection; the Cooper-Hewitt, Smithsonian Design Museum; and the Whitney Museum of Art, most of which can be found along the stretch of Fifth Avenue dubbed "museum mile." Famous historical as well as contemporary families who have made the Upper East Side their home include the Astors, the Roosevelts, the Rockefellers, and the Kennedys. See MUSEUM FOOD and COOPER-HEWITT, SMITHSONIAN DESIGN MUSEUM.

In the late 1700s and into the early years of the 1900s, the area was farmland and gardens that serviced the city's markets. With the introduction of the New York and Harlem Railroad in 1837, the area began to commercialize. The development of Central Park in the 1870s brought wealthy residents from the more crowded sections of the city northward, and Fifth Avenue became lined with elegant, palatial residences. After elevated subway lines and the once open railroad tracks were covered to make what is now Park Avenue, residential expansion continued eastward to the East River.

As immigrants poured into the city throughout the course of the nineteenth century, successful German, German Jewish, and Irish residents moved into the newly built homes of the Upper East Side and commuted to their work much farther downtown. Following the tragic fire and river disaster of the passenger boat the *General Slocum* in 1904, many of the city's German immigrants moved northward and settled in the Upper East Side neighborhood of Yorkville. See JEWISH and GERMAN.

Bordered by Seventy-Ninth Street to the south, Ninety-Sixth Street to the north, Third Avenue to the west, and the East River to the east, the neighborhood of Yorkville became a predominantly German enclave and home to butchers, beer and wine merchants, and German restaurants, few of which exist today. Classic meat and butcher shops, such as Ottomanelli (founded in 1900) and Schaller & Weber (founded in 1927), continue to survive. See SCHALLER & WEBER. The Upper East Side's growing Jewish population began to open delicatessens and shops selling pickles, smoked salmon, and other classic Jewish staples. A bit farther west, Eli Zabar's E.A.T., on Madison Avenue and Eighty-First Street, is a modern, upscale iteration of the deli popular in the well-heeled neighborhood. See DELIS, JEWISH and ZABAR'S.

Dining options on the Upper East Side have traditionally skewed toward high-end, expensive restaurants that serve the neighborhood's wealthy residents. A tradition of fine dining that began in the nineteenth century with the establishment of elite men's social clubs as well as extravagant dinners, parties, and balls in private homes continues to the present. The Upper East Side is home to world-famous restaurants such as Café Boulud, The Mark, and JoJo, by chefs Daniel Boulud and Jean-Georges Vongerichten. Other notable chefs with Upper East Side restaurants include David Burke and Lidia Bastianich.

Hotel dining has long been a component of the Upper East Side food scene. The dining rooms of hotels such as the Plaza Athénée, the Pierre, and the Carlyle have drawn diners for many years. See HOTEL RESTAURANTS.

Despite the high-income demographic, the Upper East Side remains diverse, and Second and Third Avenues are filled with smaller, lower-priced dining options including Indian, Thai, Japanese, and Latin cuisines as well as classic all-American bar food alongside Irish pubs. The under-thirty-year-old demographic, while still evident on the Upper East Side, has been moving elsewhere in the city to locations such as the gentrified Lower East Side and Brooklyn. Still, restaurant owners who cater to this crowd are finding success on the Upper East Side, such as Michael Chernow of The Meatball Shop.

See also MANHATTAN and YORKVILLE.

"History." Uppereast.com. https://www.uppereast.com/history.
Kaufman, Joanne. "For Starters, the Upper East Side." New York Times, March 14, 2014.
Ottomanelli Brothers website: http://nycotto.com.
Schaller & Weber website: http://www.schallerweber.com.

Carl Raymond

Upper West Side

The Upper West Side is a neighborhood in the borough of Manhattan bordered on the south by Fifty-Ninth Street, the east by Central Park West, the west by the Hudson River, and the north by 116th Street.

The Upper West Side includes some of New York's most important cultural and educational sites, including the Lincoln Center for the Performing Arts, the American Museum of Natural History, the New-York Historical Society, and Columbia University. See AMERICAN MUSEUM OF NATURAL HISTORY; NEW-YORK HISTORICAL SOCIETY; and COLUMBIA UNIVERSITY. The Lincoln Center complex at Sixty-Fifth Street and Broadway includes the constituent organizations the Metropolitan Opera, the New York Philharmonic, Lincoln Center Theater, New York City Ballet, and the Juilliard School. Major religious institutions include the Cathedral of St. John the Divine, Riverside Church, and the Jewish communities of Shearith Israel and Ansche Chesed.

The area now known as the Upper West Side was settled by Dutch immigrants in the mid-seventeenth century and was known as *Bloemendal*, a well-known name in New York in its Anglicized form, "Bloomingdale." Throughout the eighteenth and nineteenth centuries, the area was rough and rocky, populated by wealthy merchants who built homes and farms as an escape from the crowded masses of Lower Manhattan.

As Manhattan continued its progression northward, the character of the Upper West Side began to change, particularly by 1900. The expansion of the subway line in 1904 brought the New York City transit system as well as waves of Manhattanites to the Upper West Side. As New York's population moved in, enticed by the increased space and affordable prices, a mixture of immigrant groups flooded the area. So many African American and Caribbean immigrants flocked to the area just south of Sixty-Seventh Street that the neighborhood became known as "San Juan Hill," a tribute to the soldiers lost during the Spanish–American War. By the 1960s this area had filled with tenement buildings, which were razed to make way for the construction of Lincoln Center.

The post–World War II years brought waves of Eastern European and Caribbean immigrants to the Upper West Side, and while many thought of the area as predominantly Jewish, there were, in fact, groups of Russians, Dominicans, Cubans, Haitians, Puerto Ricans, and Ukrainians. This cultural mix, combined with the area's cultural institutions, have contributed to the diversity of the Upper West Side today. See RUSSIAN; DOMINICAN; CUBAN; PUERTO RICAN; and UKRAINIAN.

The Upper West Side has been home to some of the city's most beloved as well as influential restaurants and food retailers throughout its development. Amsterdam Avenue's Barney Greengrass, a seafood retailer and the self-proclaimed "sturgeon king," has been in business since 1908 and now includes a restaurant along with the eponymous retail store. See BARNEY GREENGRASS. Citarella, located on Broadway at Seventy-Fifth Street with additional locations in Manhattan and on Long Island, opened its doors as a premier seafood retailer in 1912, and the business continues today with fresh seafood, imported specialties, and its own line of branded products. Fairway Market on Broadway and Seventy-Fourth Street had its beginnings as a small fruit and vegetable market started by Nathan Glickberg in 1933 and today is a major grocer with nine locations in the city. See FAIRWAY MARKET. Zabar's has been a fixture on the Upper West Side for imported food, coffee, and smoked salmon since its founding in 1934. See ZABAR'S. In recent years, national chain retailers such as Trader Joe's and Whole Foods Market have entered the area. See TRADER JOE'S and WHOLE FOODS.

Fueled by its diverse population, the Upper West Side has long been an attraction for restaurant lovers searching for a variety of cuisines. Many Latin, Asian, and Italian establishments along with classic American can be found lining Amsterdam and Columbus Avenues. Higher-profile restaurants featuring celebrity chefs can be found as well. Time Warner Center at Fifty-Ninth Street boasts Thomas Keller's Per Se, and the Trump Hotel Central Park includes Jean-Georges Vongerichten's three-Michelin-starred flagship Jean-Georges, as well as the more casual Nougatine and Terrace. See VONGERICHTEN, JEAN-GEORGES. Audiences attending Lincoln Center performances may dine on the center's campus at Lincoln Ristorante, under Jonathan Benno, or choose from a variety of cuisines such as Daniel Boulud's Mediterranean-inspired Boulud Sud and his charcuterie-based Bar Boulud, classic and creative Chinese cuisine at Michael Tong's Shun Lee West, Terrance Brennan's Picholine, and Gabriel Aiello's eponymous Gabriel's. See BOULUD, DANIEL. A longtime favorite of the Upper West Side was Café des Artistes located in a historic artists' residence at 1 West Sixty-Seventh Street. After closing in 2000 and remaining empty for several years, the space has reopened under new ownership as Il Leopardo,

maintaining its famous diaphanously draped wood nymphs done by Howard Chandler in 1934. Café Fiorello is a Lincoln Center postperformance haunt, with performers staggering in, and is famous for its pizza and antipasto buffet featuring more than thirty vegetables with additional seafood options.

A classic Upper West Side favorite is the French bistro-style Café Luxembourg, which was opened in 1983 by restaurateur Keith McNally. Other chefs and restaurateurs who have made the Upper West Side their culinary home include Bill Telepan (Telepan) and Tom Valenti (Ouest, among other ventures).

In addition to the growing, small ethnic cafes and restaurants that stretch northward on Broadway and the avenues, the Upper West Side contributes to New York's food scene with multiple Greenmarkets managed by GrowNYC including locations on Broadway and Sixty-Sixth Street at Tucker Square and on Columbus Avenue and Seventy-Ninth Street at the Museum of Natural History. See GREENMARKETS and GROWNYC.

The Upper West Side borders on Central Park, which has long been a favorite destination for al fresco foodies. Visitors bring picnics and outdoor fare to enjoy before the Public Theater's free Shakespeare in the park performances at the Delacorte Theater or during outdoor performances of opera, classical, and popular music on the Great Lawn.

See also MANHATTAN.

Waxman, Sarah. "The History of the Upper West Side." NY.com. http://www.ny.com/articles/upperwest.html.

Carl Raymond

Urban Farming

Urban farming is the cultivation of crops and animal husbandry within and on the fringe of a metropolitan area. The integration of farming into urban life provides direct food distribution to urban consumers, reduces urban ecological impacts, and utilizes urban resources such as vacant land, organic waste, water runoff, and labor power. Urban food production may be found in a variety of locations, including backyard, patio, and rooftop gardens; commercial operations; vacant lot cultivation; institutional gardens (e.g., schools, hospitals, and prisons); and community gardens. Diverse agricultural practices and purposes are key features in the development, resiliency, and sustainability of urban farming. Urban farming helps to build food justice through subsistence production, provides income-generating opportunities for the urban poor and working-class communities, and fosters urban sustainability. New York City is a leader in urban farming, itself part of a broader food movement emerging throughout the United States.

During the late nineteenth century Queens and Kings were the most important agricultural counties in the United States. The two future city boroughs led the country in farm value, yield per acre, and farm output and served as a breadbasket to the rapidly growing cities of New York (then only on Manhattan) and Brooklyn (contemporary downtown Brooklyn). The two urban centers provided nearby farmers with ready access to large markets, abundant natural fertilizers in the form of organic waste produced by people and animals, and an ample supply of labor in the form of newly arrived immigrants, many of whom had agrarian backgrounds.

The first true period of urban farming in New York City unfolded during World War II, when the American home front was dotted with "victory gardens." Supported by the federal government, victory gardens were cultivated by groups and individuals to supplement food rations and to free up industrial production for the war effort while simultaneously serving as a display of patriotism. According to the *New York Times*, an estimated 450,000 victory gardens existed within New York City at the height of the war.

Today, urban food production may be found in a variety of locations throughout New York City and includes various processing, marketing, and service activities. Most food production in New York City occurs within community gardens, many of which emerged in the late 1970s and 1980s as grassroots efforts to address urban abandonment through the productive uses of vacant lots. Indeed, New York City today has more community gardens than any other city in the United States.

Today's increase in urban cultivation is inspired by a growing interest in food politics throughout the United States. Although New York City's food production occurs mostly in community gardens, the expansion of urban farming in New York City is driven by the development of market-oriented urban

farms that produce fruits, vegetables, eggs, honey, and other products for sale. In large part the growth of market-oriented urban farming may be interpreted as an attempt to "scale up" urban agriculture, an effort to move beyond gardening as a hobby in the deliberate effort to produce greater quantities of food for wider distribution.

At times community gardens and urban farming are largely indistinguishable forms of urban cultivation—particularly as oriented toward producing food in the city. As Edie Stone, a longtime urban farming advocate and former director of Green-Thumb, New York City's community gardening program, the largest support agency of its kind, explains, "the distinction between urban farms and community gardens is largely false." Most community gardens in New York City, Stone notes, "always focused on food production." Community gardens, however, are mostly cultivated for self-consumption, whereas urban farms produce for a wider distribution.

Although the different urban farming projects in New York City have specific goals, aims, and practices, all articulate a critique of the conventional food system and use urban farming as a tool to address those various problems. In addition to hundreds of community and school gardens, notable examples of urban farming in New York City include community farms such as East New York Farms, Added Value, bk farmyards, Bed Stuy Farm, and Hattie Carthan Community Farm, all in Brooklyn, as well as La Finca dal Sur in the Bronx. Commercial farms in New York City include Eagle Street Rooftop Farm in Brooklyn and two firms that operate multiple rooftop farm sites in Brooklyn and Queens: Brooklyn Grange and Gotham Greens. These farms produce fruits, vegetables, eggs, and honey for sale at farmers' markets, on-site farmstands, and through community supported agriculture programs to restaurants and stores. Most of the farms are open to the public for tours and host volunteer workdays. In addition to producing local, organic food for urban consumers, farms in New York City prioritize the educational opportunities created through farming the city.

Urban farming is expanding throughout New York City and is beginning to enjoy support from political leaders astute to the potential benefits of its practice. To fulfill its promise, urban farming needs to be fully embraced, understood not simply as a temporary fad driven by bourgeois food tastes.

Rather, to be truly transformative, urban farming must be viewed as an integral and permanent part of the city.

See also COMMUNITY SUPPORTED AGRICULTURE; VICTORY GARDENS; and WORLD WAR II.

Cohen, Nevin, Kristin Reynolds, and Rupal Sanghvi. *Five Borough Farm*. New York: Design Trust for Public Space, 2012.

"Freedom Gardens Are Lagging in City." *New York Times*, May 15, 1948.
Hodgson, Kimberly, Marcia Campbell, and Martin Bailkey. *Urban Agriculture: Growing Healthy, Sustainable Places*. Chicago: American Planning Association, 2011.
Weissman, Evan. "Brooklyn's Agrarian Questions." Special issue, *Renewable Agriculture and Food Systems* 30, no. 1 (2015): 92–102.

Evan Weissman

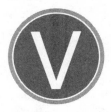

Veganism

Although the concept of veganism, a diet free of any animal products, has been around since the turn of the nineteenth century, the term "vegan" was coined much later, in 1944, when Donald Watson took the beginning and end of the word "vegetarian" and spliced them together, cofounding the Vegan Society in the United Kingdom as well in the process. Initially slow to gain popularity, the diet, philosophy, and lifestyle have now become mainstream in New York.

Veganism in New York City can be traced back as far as 1833, when Asenath Nicholson published America's first ever "veg(etari)an" cookbook in collaboration with Sylvester Graham, better known for inventing graham flour and the graham cracker. The book, *Nature's Own*, featured some recipes with dairy, but both Nicholson and Graham strongly advocated against its use. In the book, Nicholson states, "Good bread, pure water, ripe fruit and vegetables, are my meat and drink *exclusively*." In 1837 Graham started his first vegan journal, the *Journal of Health and Longevity*, which he distributed in New York.

Soon after, Roswell Goss opened the Graham Boarding House at 63 Barclay Street, Manhattan. It was the first completely vegan guesthouse. Goss stated that "its table is supplied with the best Vegetables & Fruits that can be procured, excluding entirely Animal Food and stimulants of all kinds."

In the 1840s, Dr. John Burdell became New York's first vegan dentist, working closely with Graham, Nicholson, and William Andrus Alcott (Louisa May Alcott's uncle) to promote the animal-free lifestyle. The year 1850 saw the inaugural meeting of the American Vegetarian Society, at Clinton Hall. It was America's first secular vegetarian society; they continued to have meetings until 1922.

Soon others jumped on the bandwagon, with Russel Thacher Trall publishing America's first completely vegan cookbook in 1874. *The Hygeian Home Cook-Book; Or, Healthful and Palatable Food without Condiments* contained recipes "without the employment of milk, sugar, salt, yeast, acids, alkalies, grease, or condiments of any kind."

Up to this point, health was the leading philosophy behind veganism. Animal rights was not a motivating factor until 1892, when Henry S. Salt published *Animals' Rights Considered in Relation to Social Progress* in London, with the New York edition following suit in 1894. It was the first instance of animal rights being considered explicitly in the United States.

From then on the vegan movement has grown in New York and rapidly so in recent years. Prominent contemporary members of the vegan community include Victoria Moran, founder and director of Main St. Vegan Academy, an organization that trains people as vegan lifestyle coaches, and Rynn Berry, New York's best-known vegan food historian and author of *The Vegan Guide to New York City*, who passed away in 2014.

Thanks to the efforts of these tireless advocates of the vegan lifestyle, veganism is so well known now that celebrities have joined the community, with perhaps Beyoncé and Jay-Z's much-hyped twenty-two-day vegan diet in 2014 being the most notable case. Other famous New York vegans include Bill Clinton and Famke Janssen.

The abundance of cheap vegan restaurants in the city has made it an easy dietary choice no matter your budget. The diverse range of vegan food available

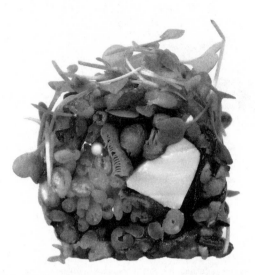

The Mighty Mushroom roll from Beyond Sushi, a vegan alternative to conventional sushi. The roll consists of two different kinds of mushrooms, with six-grain rice instead of white rice and tofu instead of seafood, and is wrapped in arugula rather than seaweed laver. BEYOND SUSHI

reflects the international face of the city. It spans the usual suspects, such as Indian, Italian, and Chinese cuisine, as well as more niche tastes, such as Peruvian and kosher cuisine, diner food, sushi, bakeries, and even ice cream parlors. Some stalwarts of the New York vegan scene include Angelica's Kitchen, the Blossom franchise, and Pure Food & Wine, which is also raw. Vegan food can also come to you; one of New York's most successful food trucks, the Cinnamon Snail, is completely vegan.

New York has its fair share of vegan art. Famous examples include *Tofu on Pedestal in Gallery* (2002), a piece of tofu in water, by Jonathan Horowitz. Art critic Ken Johnson of the *New York Times* described it as "a quiet, quasi-religious plea for dietary change." The exhibition also included portraits of two hundred famous vegetarians.

Vegan food and fashion events occur frequently across the city to add to the seventy-odd exclusively vegan restaurants. Retail shops such as Vaute Couture and MooShoes offer edgy, cruelty-free fashion, and Joshua Katcher's men's fashion line, Brave Gentleman, is making strides in men's animal-free fashion. Vegan wedding dresses are even available in the city. Although the vegan scene is centered in Manhattan, the monthly Vegan Shop-Up caters to a Bushwick cli-

entele, and restaurants serving vegan food can be found in all five boroughs.

Being vegan also opens doors to the city's thriving vegan community. New York has the largest vegan and vegetarian MeetUp group in the United States, gathering every few weeks for food-based activities and to talk all things vegan. In true New York fashion, vegetarianism and veganism even have their own festival. The Veggie Pride Parade stops traffic once a year, and the NYC Vegetarian Food Festival is a popular draw.

See also BERRY, RYNN; GROWNYC; and TOFUTTI.

Berry, Rynn, Chris Abreu-Suzuki, and Barry Litsky. *The Vegan Guide to New York City*. Brooklyn, N.Y.: Pythagorean, 2013.
Happy Cow: The Healthy Eating Guide (website). http://www.happycow.net.
Smith, Andrew F., ed. *The Oxford Encyclopedia of Food and Drink in America*. 2d ed. New York: Oxford University Press, 2012.

Asia Lindsay

Vending Machines

Coin-operated vending machines have been an important part of New York's culinary scene since the late nineteenth century. These mechanical devices made it possible to sell food and beverages twenty-four hours a day without the need for a store or a sales force.

Vending machines were developed in Europe in the late nineteenth century. Beginning in 1888, the Thomas Adams Gum Company began selling gum in vending machines on New York City's elevated train platforms. See GUM. The Stollwerck Brothers, the largest chocolate manufacturer in Europe, acquired the contract for gum and chocolate dispensers on subways, and by 1906 these vending machines generated two thousand dollars per day in gross sales. By 1926 there were more than ten thousand machines on subway and elevated train platforms. Other operators set up penny-in-the-slot gum, peanut, and candy machines in other locations around the city.

The vending machine principle was also at the heart of automats, which dispensed more substantial food. In December 1902 James Harcombe opened the first automat in New York. Through a coin-operated system it sold sandwiches, pies, coffee cake, cookies, pudding, hot dogs, vegetables, and side dishes that were displayed in glass compartments so that customers could see what they were getting. Heated or refrigerated compartments were used to keep food hot or cold. Empty compartments were filled by workers who prepared food behind the row of machines. To compete with traditional table-service restaurants, the automat offered a wild assortment of lavish dishes, including lobster à la Newberg, a luxurious dish popularized by Delmonico's beginning in the 1870s. For beverages, there was a choice of coffee, beer, wine, and cocktails. Despite widespread promotion, the restaurant closed about 1907. The Horn & Hardart chain opened its first New York automat in 1912, and within a few years, the company operated fifteen automats in the city. During the Depression, when cheap meals were in great demand, they expanded to fifty outlets. See AUTOMATS.

During Prohibition (1920–1933), refrigerated soda machines became common in New York. The dispensers were made in the city by the Sodamat Company, which also established "sodamats" in several locations in New York. Each of these arcades had from twenty to thirty-six machines, each dispensing a different soft drink—including root beer, orangeade, and loganberry juice—into a paper cup, with ice. Advertisements for the sodamat claimed that the beverages were provided within eight seconds after the coin was dropped in. And they certainly caught on: one sodamat in Coney Island reportedly served more than seventeen thousand beverages in a single day and 170,000 in its first month.

Canned soft drinks were first available in vending machines in the 1960s. As of 1981 some of the contraptions could even talk to their customers. Five years later, the first machines that accepted credit and debit cards were introduced. Wireless transmission between the devices and warehouses began service in 1993. By the twenty-first century these systems collected consumer data, monitored needs for resupply, tracked sales trends, and reported issues with the machine.

In 2009 Coca-Cola Company introduced the "freestyle" machine, a touchscreen soda fountain, which features more than one hundred different flavors of Coca-Cola beverage products. These machines have been set up in several McDonald's locations and other chains in the city.

After World War II, coin-operated food machines also became ubiquitous in New York City schools, selling snack foods, including soda, candy, chips,

cookies, and doughnuts. During the 1970s, vending machines in New York City schools were assailed as too-convenient sources of empty calories, but it was not until 2003 that sugary sodas and other junk foods were banned from schools. Vending machines on school grounds were limited to dispensing bottled water, low-fat snacks, and 100 percent fruit juices. Some even dispense fresh fruit and other nutritious foods.

See also CANDY; COFFEE; SCHOOL FOOD; and SODA.

Segrave, Kerry. *Vending Machines: An American Social History*. Jefferson, N.C.: McFarland, 2002.
U.S. Business and Defense Services Administration. *The Automatic Vending Machine Industry: Its Growth and Development*. Washington, D.C.: U.S. Government Printing Office, 1962.

Andrew F. Smith

Vendy Awards

First presented in November 2005 in a cramped, unheated street cart storage space in the East Village, the Vendy Awards have grown into a sprawling outdoor celebration of New York's best street food. In a festival atmosphere, competitors prepare their dishes for judges and attendees. Proceeds benefit the Street Vendor Project, which provides legal assistance and advocacy for vendors of food and merchandise. See STREET VENDOR PROJECT.

Only a single award—the Vendy Cup, for best overall—was presented in that initial year. Hallo Berlin, a purveyor of German sausages manned by an émigré born in East Berlin, beat out a Sri Lankan–born dosa maker, a Middle Eastern seller of sliced lamb sandwiches and platters, and a Greek American vendor of grilled chicken. The four finalists, selected from about two hundred vendors nominated by the public, all operated from food carts, though Rolf Babiel—who had peddled wursts for more than twenty years—was successful enough to already have opened a beer garden in Hell's Kitchen. All four sold savory items, and all did business in Manhattan, three of them in or near Midtown.

By 2009 the event, dubbed by Mario Batali as "the Oscars of food for the real New York," had taken on a showtime character. At the fifth Vendy Awards, eleven vendors and more than one thousand attendees flocked to the grounds outside the Queens Museum of Art. Sunny weather, live music, and all-you-could-drink beer, wine, and soda helped compensate for long lines. (Even so, the event website counsels attendees, "Please wear comfortable shoes.... standing in line is part of the Vendy—and street food—experience.") The event's egalitarian nature kept spirits lively, too. Except for the Vendy Cup, all awards were determined by popular vote. They still are.

Eight vendors that year, including all four finalists in a new category for best dessert, drove to the event in food trucks, many decked out with splashy, professionally produced graphics. (Another brought belly dancers instead. He did not win.) Several finalists, among them the winner of another new category, rookie of the year, employed social media such as Facebook and Twitter to drum up support. However, though the event site was within walking distance of Roosevelt Avenue—famous for its dense population of street-food vendors, many of them recent Spanish-speaking immigrants—nine finalists did the bulk of their business in Manhattan.

Continued growth led to a change of venue the following year to the event's current home, on Governors Island. Additional Vendy events have also been held in Philadelphia, Chicago, New Orleans, and Los Angeles. Trucks have lost their preeminence, while a best-of-market category has been added to honor vendors from the likes of Hester Street Fair and Smorgasburg. See SMORGASBURG. Across all categories, the fare of many recent finalists would have been at home at that first Vendys. Other dishes, such as a ramen burger whose "bun" consists of fried noodles, have been wildly reimagined.

Whether their menus are traditional or inventive, almost all recent finalists display social media smarts, many in concert with a formal business plan. The odds would seem to favor the newer, the nimbler, and the investor ready. Yet for the five events from 2009 to 2013, four Vendy Cup winners were longtime veterans of the ball fields at Red Hook, a Brooklyn venue that built its fame on old-fashioned word of mouth.

See also FOOD TRUCKS.

Bowen, Dana. "In a Battle of Street-Food Vendors, the Wurst Wins." *New York Times*, November 11, 2005.

Vendy Awards website: http://www.vendyawards .streetvendor.org/newyorkcity.

Zimmer, Erin. "A Look at the 2009 Vendy Awards." Serious Eats, September 27, 2009. http://newyork .seriouseats.com/2009/09/a_look_at_the_2009_ vendy_awards.html.

Dave Cook

Vichyssoise

Vichyssoise is a silky chilled potato-leek soup created by French chef Louis Diat (1885–1957) in 1917 for patrons of the Ritz-Carlton, then at Madison and Forty-Sixth Street. Diat claimed that he first made vichyssoise to refresh the Ritz's summer guests dining on the hotel's hot rooftop. He was inspired, he said, by childhood memories of his mother's simple hot leek and potato potage, which he and his brother would spike with cold milk on warmer days. As a very young man Diat had worked as the soup chef under Auguste Escoffier at the Ritz in both Paris and London before coming to New York in 1910 to lead the New York Ritz-Carlton's kitchen.

Although distinctly American, the roots of vichyssoise are in classic French leek and potato soups like the ones in the *Royal Cookery Book* by Jules Gouffé (1869) and Escoffier's *Le Guide Culinaire* (1903). To make the modern classic American vichyssoise, first sliced leeks and onion are sautéed in butter, and then sliced potatoes are added with water or chicken broth. The soup is simmered until the potatoes are very soft, then it is strained and returned to the pot with some combination of milk, half and half, and light and heavy cream, depending on the version. After a brief simmer, it is chilled. Diat's original recipe called for half milk and half "medium" cream at this stage, with the addition of heavy cream once the soup is cold. Most recipes for the classic version include a chive garnish, but James Beard also laced his with nutmeg and cayenne.

Creator Diat christened his soup *crème vichyssoise glacée* after the renowned spa town Vichy, forty miles from his boyhood home in central France. Vichyssoise is not pronounced "vishy-SWAH," as some Americans do, but rather "vishy-SWOZ." In a story reminiscent of the 2003 "freedom fries" incident, after World War II politically conscious chefs temporarily redubbed the soup *crème gauloise glacée*, since the city of Vichy was associated with the Nazi-controlled French regime during the war.

At the request of the soup's fans, beginning in 1923 Diat began to serve vichyssoise year-round. He later authored several cookbooks and included a recipe for it in *Cooking á la Ritz* (1941), including a version with a cup of tomato juice added to every three cups of soup.

Vichyssoise became wildly popular in New York, especially in the mid-twentieth century, and subsequently its fame spread across the country. The soup is no longer as ubiquitous on menus as it once was—and is not on either of the menus for the Ritz-Carlton's current New York City locations—yet vichyssoise holds its own on Manhattan menus to this day. Although you can still find the classic version here and there, it is more likely to be updated. Usually it is lightened somewhat, with less cream or no cream at all, or enriched with fresh herbs or vegetables, like the carrot version that has been offered at Lafayette Café in NoHo or the one with a watercress cremeux and lovage oil at Bar Boulud at Broadway and Sixty-Fourth Street.

See also RITZ-CARLTON and DIAT, LOUIS.

Beard, James. *James Beard's American Cookery*. Boston: Little, Brown, 1972.

Koenig, Leah. "The Lost Foods of New York City: Vichyssoise." *Capital New York*, January 3, 2013.

O'Neill, Molly. *The New York Cookbook*. New York: Workman, 1992.

Schwartz, Arthur. *Arthur Schwartz's New York City Food*. New York: Stewart, Tabori & Chang, 2004.

Stradley, Linda. "Classic Vichyssoise Soup Recipe." What's Cooking America. http://whatscookingamerica.net/Soup/VichyssoiseSoup.htm.

Jennifer Brizzi

Victor's Café

Víctor del Corral had limited restaurant experience in America and little formal education but plenty of gumption. Back in his native Guanabacoa, Cuba, he had owned a small restaurant called Café Carral, followed by the restaurant Sonia in Havana, named after his only daughter. These were simple cafeterias specializing in a limited array of traditional Cuban foods and featuring some of the generic Spanish dishes by then so popular in Havana.

Del Corral left Cuba for the United States in 1956 in search of opportunities for his family in the midst of the growing conflict between Fidel Castro's insurgents and President Fulgencio Batista's government. He settled on New York's Upper West Side with the help of relatives, and his wife Eloína Ruíz de Ugarrio and his daughter Sonia joined him a year later, in July 1957. Surviving an initial period of hardship and isolation, del Corral worked as a dishwasher and waiter at local restaurants, saving every penny to open his own business. He spent hours looking at an old and decrepit building, once home to a veterinarian clinic, on the corner of Seventy-First Street and Columbus Avenue from the windows of his apartment, dreaming that one day it would be his. Soon it was: he claimed to have opened his small cafeteria-style restaurant, with twenty-six chairs and twelve banquettes, at this site for $2,900 in cash.

Del Corral managed the place and did the daily shopping, becoming a familiar figure in every wholesale market selling tropical products in the Bronx and Spanish Harlem. Because there were few butchers who knew how to cut beef and pork Cuban-style in those days, del Corral did all the butchering himself, taking pride in cutting the best *palomilla* (a thin top sirloin filet) in town. In turn his wife Eloína became the pastry chef, moving the whole baking operation across the street to the couple's apartment. She would lower freshly made pastries, flans, and puddings in a basket to Víctor, who waited on the street below. During mango season, the whole family worked night and day, peeling and slicing ripe mangoes for freezing to use throughout the year in creamy *batidos* (milk shakes).

By the 1980s, it was clear that the Columbus Avenue location was too small to support del Corral's dogged determination to conquer Manhattan. Taking a financial risk, he bought a building on 236 West Fifty-Second Street in the heart of the theater district. After a costly remodeling job, he opened the largest, most ambitious Cuban restaurant in the city, Victor's Café 52. The *New York Times* critic Mimi Sheraton found fault with foods that had lost the charm and purity of the early days. A major revamping of the menu, a more careful and attractive food presentation, and a new look for the interior grounded in Cuban aesthetics in the late 1980s and early 1990s offset the setback. On the menu, Cuban classics like del Corral's fabulous black beans continued to shine together with excellent beef dishes like the *palomilla*, the iconic *ropa vieja*, a few innovations rooted in Cuban and Latin American cooking, and a tender and juicy Argentinian skirt steak with chimichurri, which Victor's Café helped popularize. It was Victor's Café that put the Cuban mojito on the map, starting a craze for this seductive Cuban drink in the United States that is still going strong.

Though his daughter managed the restaurant and del Corral had become a wealthy entrepreneur, he continued to control the purchase of many key ingredients, from carefully selected black beans from colder regions in the United States (which he considered superior to beans grown in warmer climates) to prime beef sourced in Kansas to the freshest Florida red snapper and stone crab. During this period, Víctor's Café cemented its reputation as the preferred meeting place for Cuban artists, musicians, sport figures, and politicians in New York, and it was not uncommon to spot famed movie and theater actors like Richard Chamberlain sitting quietly in a corner eating Cuban food.

In 1971, at the height of the Columbus Avenue restaurant's success, del Corral commissioned a bas-relief from Cuban sculptor Arturo Martín, a San Alejandro Art School graduate, to be placed by the Seventy-First Street entrance of the restaurant. It is a sugar harvest scene showing a young shirtless sugarcane cutter (*machetero*), standing next to a cart carrying sugarcane pulled by two oxen. In 2012, after del Corral's family had sold the Columbus Avenue restaurant and the building that housed it, the relief was scheduled for dismantling by new owners planning to turn the place into a trendy nightclub. A vigorous campaign by concerned neighbors and preservationist groups such as Landmark West and the Historic District Council protected it for posterity.

Víctor del Corral died in 2006 at the age of eighty-four. Now managed by Monica Zaldívar, Víctor's granddaughter, the restaurant remains a family-owned business. Catering to a mixed clientele of theatergoers, stars, as well as Cubans and Latin Americans from all walks of life, the restaurant has not lost its appeal.

See also CUBAN.

Kilgannon, Correy. "A Dispute Erupts over the Fate of a Mural." *New York Times*, February 26, 2012.

Presilla, Maricel. *Celebrating Cuban Cuisine: In Commemoration of Victor's Café 52 25th Anniversary.* New York: Privately printed, 1987.

Presilla, Maricel. "Cuban American Food." In *The Oxford Encyclopedia of Food and Drink in America*, edited by Andrew F. Smith, Vol. 1, pp. 357–359. New York: Oxford University Press, 2004.

Maricel E. Presilla

Victory Gardens

During World War II, as part of the total war effort, the federal government urged civilians to grow "victory gardens" to offset the large volume of American food diverted to the military and allied countries. Victory gardening reached its peak in 1943 as three-fifths of the U.S. population produced more than 8 million tons of food, some 40 percent of the fresh produce consumed that year. New York City residents participated in sizeable numbers, cultivating four hundred thousand victory gardens on six thousand acres of land. Their 1943 cumulative harvest was estimated at 200 million pounds of food, valued at $30 million. Tomatoes were the most popular crop, followed by beans, beets, carrots, lettuce, and Swiss chard.

The city's Parks Department provided preliminary plot inspection service to citizens in order to determine an appropriate fertilizer regimen. But unlike Chicago and San Francisco, New York City would not make provisions for gardening on public land. The federal government had discouraged urban gardening efforts at the outset of the war, and the city administration generally maintained that stance. State, private, and volunteer agencies picked up the slack to provide New Yorkers education and assistance, including establishing a telephone line to answer gardening questions and sponsoring demonstration meetings on winter storage methods. New York University, Columbia University, and the New School all offered courses on victory gardening. The *New York Times* published regular columns to educate victory gardeners. Many institutions sponsored training courses for victory garden leaders, including the Manhattan YMCA, the Brooklyn Academy of Music, and the Staten Island Museum. The Brooklyn Botanic Garden held lectures on such topics as "Testing the Soil," "Planning Gardens," "Ordering Seeds," and "Maintenance Spraying" and created a 40-by-10-foot model victory garden on its grounds.

New York City retail establishments facilitated and capitalized on the victory garden movement. Macy's flagship Manhattan store on Thirty-Fourth Street offered free lectures and films and distributed a free twenty-two-page *Victory Garden Guide* to customers who signed its *Victory Garden Pledge Book*. Items for sale included seeds, seed-starting pots, raspberry seedlings, sheep manure, garden lime, hoses, and wheelbarrows. Bloomingdale's held courses sponsored by the American Women's Voluntary Services. The Abraham & Straus department store opened the Victory Garden Center, which offered lectures. The Gertz department store in Jamaica, Queens, held the Victory Harvest Fair and awarded war bonds to the most impressive harvests.

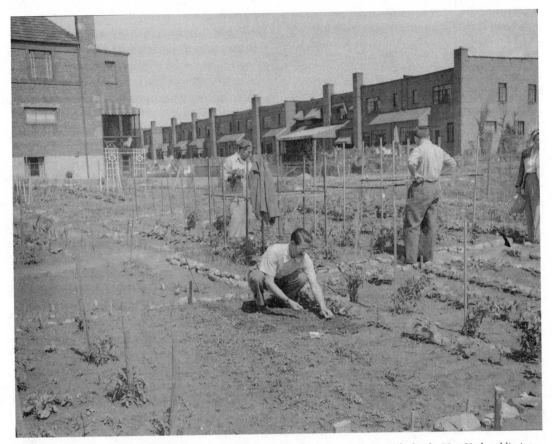

Victory gardening at Forest Hills, Queens, June 1944. The victory gardens were cared for by the New York public, in order to be able to send food to the soldiers fighting in World War II. LIBRARY OF CONGRESS

Notable New York City victory garden locations included the Charles Schwab estate on Riverside Drive in Manhattan, Rockefeller Center, the rooftop of a Children's Aid Society building, a large swath of undeveloped Brooklyn land owned by Fred C. Trump (the father of Donald Trump), and the City Patrol Corps headquarters in Woodhaven, Queens.

See also URBAN FARMING and WORLD WAR II.

Bentley, Amy. *Eating for Victory: Food Rationing and the Politics of Domesticity*. Champaign: University of Illinois Press, 1998.

Lawson, Laura. *City Bountiful: A Century of Community Gardening in America*. Berkeley: University of California Press, 1995.

U.S. Department of Agriculture, Conference Committee Personnel. National Defense Garden Conference Washington, D.C., December 19–20, 1941. http://naldc.nal.usda.gov/naldc/catalog .xhtml?id=CAT31030763&content=pdf.

Daniel Bowman Simon and Amy Bentley

Village Voice

The *Village Voice* has put itself at the center of New York City's multitextured food and bar scene almost since it launched in 1955. And a lot of that time was spent in those bars itself. The paper, considered the grandfather of the nation's alt-weekly market, was originally located in Sheridan Square, near the White Horse Tavern, the bar where Dylan Thomas famously had his last of many drinks before he died. The *Voice*'s staffers were regulars there, including Seymour Krim, a *Voice* writer whose collected work, *Views of a Near-Sighted Cannoneer*, contributed to the launch of the new journalism movement of the late 1960s. See WHITE HORSE TAVERN.

The *Voice* was founded in 1955 by Ed Fancher, Dan Wolf, and author Norman Mailer, who wrote that he wanted it to "give a little speed to that moral and sexual revolution which is yet to come upon us." It began by covering news in Greenwich Village and expanded to become a vanguard of the city's bohemian spirit of the time, with serious emphasis on arts coverage, cultural criticism, and food writing. See GREENWICH VILLAGE. The paper would eventually become a free staple found in bars and coffee shops around the city.

As bohemian tastes shifted in the city, so did the paper's focus. Recalling the Village's heavy drinking in the postwar era, *Voice* contributor Michael Harrington wrote in 1972, "Bohemia could not survive the passing of its polar opposite and precondition, middle-class morality. Free love and all-night drinking and art for art's sake were consequences of a single stern imperative: thou shalt not be bourgeois."

Eschewing the bourgeois of the city's dining scene became the trademark for the *Voice*'s most famous food critic, Robert Sietsema. Sietsema joined the paper in 1993 and remained an anonymous critic, able to report accurately on the dining offerings without bias from the waitstaff (in photos and videos, he often appeared wearing a horned devil mask). Unlike other critics who focused on the white tablecloth, au courant dining of Manhattan, Sietsema preferred the treasures of the far-flung neighborhoods of the outer boroughs, from classic Italian joints to unique Yemeni cuisine.

His favorite story for the paper, he told the *Jewish Daily Forward* in 2013, was a 2008 exposé called "Iron Chef Boyardee," ripping the American version of the television show *Iron Chef* (filmed in Chelsea) for being a big pile of bogus kitchen magic. "As the taping progressed, we felt more and more like we were viewing the scene in *The Wizard of Oz* when Toto pulls aside the curtain and the wizard's tricks are revealed," he wrote.

After the paper was sold to Phoenix-based New Times media in 2005, it faced steady circulation declines and staff turmoil. It came to a head in 2013 when it axed its longtime quiver of critics: Sietsema, gossip and nightlife critic Michael Musto, music critic Robert Christgau, and theater critic Michael Feingold.

In recent years, the paper has focused its food coverage largely on its website, with its *Fork in the Road* blog focusing on openings, food industry news, food events, and more. But its annual Best of NYC list is still a staple of the print edition, rounding up a coveted list of titles including Best Bartender, Best Whiskey Bar, and Best French Fries. It branched out into hosting its own food event in 2007, Choice Eats, an annual chef showcase of usually more than fifty restaurants chosen by the paper's critics. In 2010 the *Voice* began hosting Brooklyn Pour, a craft brewery event featuring more than one hundred beers.

Bruinius, Harry. "Norman Mailer, 1927–2007." *Village Voice* (November 6, 2007).

Sietsema, Robert. "Iron Chef Boyardee." *Village Voice* (February 19, 2008).

Batterberry, Michael, and Ariane Batterberry. *On the Town in New York: The Landmark History of Eating, Drinking, and Entertainments from the American Revolution to the Food Revolution*. New York and London: Routledge, 1998.

Jacobson, Mark. "The Voice from Beyond the Grave." *New York* (November 14, 2005).

Rosen, Jody. "X-ed Out: The *Village Voice* Fires a Famous Music Critic." *Slate*, September 5, 2006. http://www.slate.com/articles/arts/music_box/2006/09/xed_out.html.

Frank, Thomas. *The Conquest of Cool: Business Culture, Counterculture, and the Rise of Hip Consumerism*. Chicago: University of Chicago Press, 1997.

Tim Donnelly

Vongerichten, Jean-Georges

Jean-Georges Vongerichten (b. 1957), with eleven restaurants in New York City including his eponymous three Michelin–starred restaurant Jean-Georges in the Trump Tower overlooking Columbus Circle and Central Park, has defined American nouvelle cuisine for New York diners for almost three decades. Born in Alsace, France, Vongerichten studied under such master chefs as Paul Bocuse to hone his classic French skills before falling under the spell of Asian cuisine. His signature fusion of French and Asian techniques pares the heaviness from the French while relying on the intense flavors of market-fresh ingredients to create a lighter, Asian-influenced dining experience.

Vongerichten arrived in New York City in 1986 to operate the dining room at the Drake Hotel on Park Avenue. Under his guidance the menu transitioned from classic French to much lighter fare of his own creation. This change was partly customer driven. Jean-Georges began to notice sauces being ordered on the side and then not eaten. He reasoned that New Yorkers, unlike Europeans, ate most of their meals out, so could not eat heavy, classic French-style meals most days of the week.

To replace the gravies, sauces, and rich flavors of his traditional cooking style using fresh produce, he turned to broths and juices. The resulting lighter dishes were so popular that he now refers to his juicer as the most important appliance in his kitchen.

His first restaurant in New York, JoJo (his nickname as a young boy), opened in 1991 on two floors of a brownstone on the Upper East Side (160 East Sixty-Fourth Street). JoJo immediately garnered a three-star review from the *New York Times* and continues to receive them. Since then, he has opened more than a dozen innovative and well-received eateries in New York City alone. His namesake restaurant, Jean-Georges, in the Trump Towers, opened in 1997 to a four-star review in the *New York Times*. It went on to earn three Michelin stars, one of only seven in New York City to receive such recognition.

Bon Appétit's 2004 Restaurateur of the Year and the successful pioneer of a global haute cuisine franchise, Vongerichten's lighter cuisine has had a great influence on the way New Yorkers dine. He is an award-winning cookbook author whose restaurants—the design, menu, and presentation—are all his vision. In 1990 his *Simple Cuisine: The Easy, New Approach to Four-Star Cooking* became an important cookbook in every young chef's library. His kitchens typically have 150 different herbs and spices, which he combines with market-fresh fruit and vegetables (purchased at the Greenmarket four days a week) to create new and exciting flavor profiles. Whether it is fine dining or casual, fresh, organic, and locally sourced ingredients are the backbone of his menus.

See also BOULEY, DAVID; BOULUD, DANIEL; MEYER, DANNY; and NIEPORENT, DREW.

McInerney, Jay. "Jean-Georges Is Seeing Stars." *New York* (June 27, 2005).
Vongerichten, Jean-Georges. *Simple Cuisine: The Easy, New Approach to Four-Star Cooking.* Upper Saddle River, N.J.: Prentice Hall, 1990.

Richard Frisbie

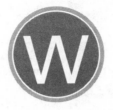

Waldorf, The

In 1893 on the site of his father's mansion at Fifth Avenue and Thirty-Third Street, the millionaire developer William Waldorf Astor opened a thirteen-story hotel designed by the architect Henry Janeway Hardenbergh. Four years later Waldorf's cousin and rival John Jacob Astor IV (who died on the *Titanic*) erected the seventeen-story Astoria Hotel on an adjacent site. The two hotels were joined by a corridor, but they were not merged until 1931 when the renamed Waldorf Astoria became the tallest, largest, and (considered by some) grandest hotel in the world.

In 1929 the decision was made to tear down the hotel and sell the site to the developers of what would become the Empire State Building. The hotel closed on May 3, 1929. The present forty-seven-story building dates from 1931 and was designed by the architects (Leonard) Schultze and (S. Fullerton) Weaver. An art deco landmark, it stretches a full square block from Park to Lexington Avenues between Forty-Ninth and Fiftieth Streets.

Soon an elegant destination and a favorite of high society, the Waldorf was particularly known for its fine dining rooms, which from 1893 to 1943 were run by the legendary maître d'hôtel Oscar Tschirky. See TSCHIRKY, OSCAR. Known as Oscar of the Waldorf, Tschirky set the tone for the food served there: an extensive variety of dishes, some specifically created for the Waldorf (among them eggs Benedict, veal Oscar, and the Waldorf salad—made of apples, walnuts, celery, grapes, and mayonnaise, which has become an American icon), is still served in the hotel's restaurants and can be found in restaurants and hotels all over the world. (Cole Porter brought the Waldorf salad into popular culture in his 1934 song "You're the Top," with the lines "You're the top. You're a Waldorf salad.") See WALDORF SALAD.

Never trained as a chef, Tschirky nonetheless assembled a cookbook "illustrative of the best methods of preparing food at the present day." A 907-page volume, including a lengthy index, the 1896 cookbook is reflective of the tastes of the time and the kind of food served in the hotel's restaurants. Recipes are provided for just about anything the elegant clientele who ate there might want. They range from the simple (chicken pot pie) to the more unusual (lark patties anyone?) as well as all the standards of the day, including soups, canapés, a variety of simple and composed salads, meats, poultry and game, side dishes, garnishes, hot desserts, and puddings. He also provided wine guidance—Sauternes with oysters, claret with entrees, port wine with desserts—as well as an extensive list explaining which foods were in season at specific times of the year. (After his death, Tschirky's menu collection, memorabilia, and papers were donated to Cornell University.) Today, guests at the hotel can eat at three American and classic European restaurants: Peacock Alley, the Bull and Bear Prime Steakhouse, and Oscar's American Brasserie.

The first hotel to offer room service, the Waldorf has welcomed many prominent national and international figures and diplomats, among them the Duke and Duchess of Windsor, Cole Porter and his wife Linda Lee Thomas, and General and Mrs. Douglas (Jean) MacArthur. Jean MacArthur continued to live there until her death in 2000.

In 1945 *Weekend at the Waldorf*, starring Ginger Rogers, was the first major motion picture filmed entirely at a hotel and outside Hollywood studios. In 1957, a suite was created on the thirty-fifth floor of

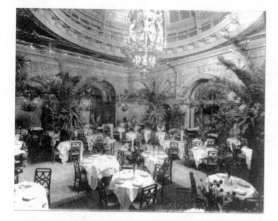

The Palm Garden Dining Room of the Waldorf Astoria Hotel, circa 1902. An elegant destination and a favorite of high society, the Waldorf was particularly well-known for its fine dining rooms, which from 1893 to 1943 were run by the legendary maître d'hôtel Oscar Tschirky. LIBRARY OF CONGRESS

the hotel for Queen Elizabeth II, who was visiting the United States. The official residence of the U.S. ambassador to the United Nations, a suite on the forty-second floor of the Waldorf Astoria Towers with its own private entrance has been home to several former UN ambassadors including Adlai Stevenson, Daniel Patrick Moynihan, Madeleine Albright, and Richard Holbrooke.

Conrad Hilton purchased management rights to the hotel in 1949. In 2014 the Angbang Insurance Group purchased the Waldorf from the Hilton Hotel Corporation for $1.9 billion, making it the most expensive hotel ever sold in the United States. As part of the deal, the Hilton Hotel Corporation will continue to operate the Waldorf under a one hundred–year management contract, and the hotel will undergo a major renovation. The Waldorf was named an official New York City landmark in 1993.

See also HOTEL RESTAURANTS.

"Hotel History." Waldorf Astoria. http://www .waldorfnewyork.com/about-the-waldorf/ hotel-history.html.
Tschirky, Oscar. *The Cookbook, by Oscar of the Waldorf.* New York: Werner, 1896.

Judith Weinraub

Waldorf Salad

In March 1893, maître d'hôtel Oscar Tschirky invented the Waldorf salad for the inaugural dinner at the restaurant of the Waldorf Hotel (the predecessor to the Waldorf Astoria). The three common ingredients in his original recipe, which was published in 1896, are chopped apples and celery mixed into a mayonnaise-style dressing.

Later cooks presented their own incarnations of the Waldorf salad by adding other ingredients and by providing specifics about the mayonnaise. There is even a variation called Emerald salad that replaces the celery with cauliflower.

Walnuts were one of the earliest additions, followed by citrus, in the form of either juice or grated rind, along with grapes or even raisins. Occasionally, the addition of chopped or shredded meat such as chicken or salmon changed it to a light lunch or dinner. The salad was often served on a bed of crisp lettuce. These variations soon appeared on menus and dinner tables across the nation as the popularity of this quintessential New York salad spread.

Oscar Tschirky, who is credited with defining the art of hospitality in New York, created other dishes which went on to become classics of American cuisine, such as lobster Newberg and veal Oscar. Known simply as Oscar of the Waldorf, he presided over dinners for the most powerful and important people in the world, setting the standard for quality, service, and presentation that was quickly adopted first throughout Manhattan and then elsewhere as his fame spread.

But his Waldorf salad had more going for it than his blessing and the cachet of its Fifth Avenue origins, although coming from the posh Waldorf Hotel did not hurt. The combination of crunchy, sweet, and savory ingredients smoothed by a silken mayonnaise was a bold and tasty creation. New York City, and then the nation, embraced it.

Today, Oscar's Brasserie in the Waldorf Astoria serves roughly ten thousand Waldorf salads each year. While the version served at the hotel today is true to the roots of the more than century-old recipe, it has been lightened and jazzed up for modern palates. Instead of mayonnaise, crème fraiche and yogurt whisked with lemon juice and walnut oil provide the dressing. Julienned apples, both Granny Smith and gala, bring a sweet and tart crispness, while similarly julienned celery root lends a crunchy and savory counterpoint. White pepper and finely chopped black truffles lend a piquant and earthy depth to the salad, which is topped with microgreens and surrounded with red grapes and walnuts with a baked-on spiced sugar coating of paprika, cayenne, fennel seed, and coriander. The cost for the 2014 incarnation of Oscar Tschirky's famous Waldorf Salad was fourteen dollars.

See also WALDORF, THE.

Chen, Susannah. "Get the Dish: Waldorf Salad." Popsugar TV, May 13, 2013. http://www.popsugar .com/waldorf-salad-recipe-from-waldorf-astoria-20170230.
Tschirky, Oscar. *The Cook Book, by Oscar of the Waldorf*. New York: Werner, 1896.
Waldorf Astoria website: http://www .waldorfnewyork.com.

Richard Frisbie

Walking Tours, Culinary

New York City is a mecca for guided neighborhood walks where one can taste the city's culinary diversity. Television programs like Anthony Bourdain's *No Reservations* and Andrew Zimmern's *Bizarre Foods America* have tempted the culinary adventurer to seek tongue-tingling thrills. See BOURDAIN, ANTHONY. With low capital requirements and few barriers to entry, there are dozens of tour companies. Most are small businesses or sole proprietorships, although a few are part of larger national or international companies.

Issues of class, ethnicity, assimilation, sustainability, and nostalgia bubble beneath the surface of many of these tours. Some boast of experiencing the "real" New York, valuing the culinary exoticism of immigrant communities in the cheaper outer boroughs over the "touristy" foods that have been diluted in the "melting pot." Other tours, in older, often more assimilated, neighborhoods, highlight the search for "authentic" old New York, ferreting out the "true" deli pickles and bagels that shame the imitators back home. Still others cosset the connoisseur of specific foodstuffs: chocolate, pizza, locally brewed beer, and cocktails all have dedicated tours. The following is a partial introduction to the many options.

Queens, especially the neighborhoods of Jackson Heights and Flushing, is home to many newly arrived immigrants, who continue, as best they can, the street food and small restaurant traditions of their homelands. Local Finds Queens Food Tours (www .foodsofqueensny.com) was founded in 2013 to "seamlessly balance food, history, culture, architecture, and neighborhood attractions." SideTour (www.sidetour.com), a national company, promises to take you "around the world in 80 minutes on

an Astoria food walk." See QUEENS and JACKSON HEIGHTS.

Brooklyn's oldest tour company is NoshWalks (www.noshwalks.com), founded in 2000 by Myra Alperson. One can sample the Turkish, Russian, and Chinese cuisines found in Bensonhurst or the Near Eastern and Central Asian fare prepared by Jewish immigrants in Borough Park. NoshWalks has recently added the Latino delights of the Bronx to its roster. A Slice of Brooklyn (www.asliceofbrooklyn .com) pits a classic pizza match-up: Grimaldi's wood-fired, thin-crusted Neapolitan, eaten under the shadow of the Brooklyn Bridge, against the thick, chewy Sicilian of L&B Spumoni Gardens in Bensonhurst. While not exclusively a walking tour, as participants are ferried about by bus, monitors queue up film clips as one traverses the featured neighborhoods. Movie buffs can disco their best *Saturday Night Fever* or relive *The French Connection*'s car chase while careening under the Brooklyn-Queens Expressway. Not satisfied with Brooklyn's pies? Then try Scott's multiborough pizza bus tours (www.scottspizzatours.com). See BROOKLYN and PIZZA.

Many of Manhattan's food walks veer to the more luxurious and celebrity conscious. On Location Tours (onloctiontours.com) takes visitors to the eateries made famous in *Sex and the City*. New York Chocolate Tours (www.sweetwalks.com) caters to chocoholics: participants sample artisanal chocolates made by some of New York's finest boutique chocolatiers. Among the many offerings through City Foods Tours NYC (www.cityfoodtours.com/newyork/new-york-food-tours-general-info.html) is a Prohibition-inspired cocktail extravaganza haunting some of the Lower East Side's trendy lounges. More traditional is Foods of New York (www.foodsofny.com). Founded in 1999, it walks groups of sixteen to eighteen through the Italian heritage of Greenwich Village and the history of the Chelsea Market, Chinatown, and other Manhattan neighborhoods. See SEX AND THE CITY; TELEVISION; MOVIES; PROHIBITION; and MANHATTAN.

Most larger companies operate in several boroughs. The international Context Travel (www .contexttravel.com), in New York since 2006, offers intimate, bespoke culinary tours in Manhattan and Brooklyn, emphasizing neighborhood histories as well as food. Urban Oyster (www.urbanoyster .com), founded in 2008, offers "multi-sensory experiences…that reveal the stories behind the people and places." Food on Foot (foodonfoottours.com/about.htm), founded in 2009, is unique in that it does not actually include tastings as part of its tours: it escorts participants (or sells information to allow a self-guided walk with discount coupons at selected venues), offering what it calls "an eating tour with some history." Each participant (groups can be as large as thirty-five) buys what he or she may want to eat.

For those who long for cabbie nostalgia, there is Famous Fat Dave's five-borough eating tour (famousfatdave.com). A former cab driver who preferred tips on great food to the monetary kind, Dave Freedenberg designs itineraries for each small group, shuttling clients across town in his decommissioned vintage Checker. In addition to Bourdain's *No Reservations*, Fat Dave has been featured on public television's *Charlie Rose Show*, The History Channel, and others.

See also MAGNOLIA BAKERY.

Bulow, Alessandra. "10 Summer Food Tours in New York City: Plus One Epi Editor's Under-$50 East Village Eating Tour!" Epicurious, June 20, 2014. http://www.epicurious.com/archive/blogs/editor/2014/06/summer-food-tours-in-new-york-city-2014.html.

Colley, Jessica. "10 Fun and Filling Food Tours in New York City." NewYork.com, January 28, 2014. http://www.newyork.com/articles/tours/10-fun-and-filling-food-tours-in-new-york-city-59339/.

Kugel, Seth. "Their Itinerary Is Your Menu." *New York Times*, August 26, 2007.

Cathy K. Kaufman

Washington Heights

Washington Heights, named for the Revolutionary War Fort Washington, is in northern Manhattan, with its southern boundary at 155th Street, stretching from the Harlem River to the east and the Hudson River to the west, and concluding approximately at 193rd Street. It divides into two distinct sections. The eastern, older section grew when the IRT subway line arrived around 1906, while the section west of Broadway developed later, when the IND subway line arrived in the early 1930s. In the early twentieth century the neighborhood was home to many Jewish, German, and Irish families, and by the early 1930s the neighborhood was nicknamed "Frankfurt on the Hudson." The northern area of the Heights east of Broadway later was home to a significant community of Greeks and Armenians, but it is now populated by people from the Dominican Republic. It is often said to be the second largest Dominican "city" after Santo Domingo. See DOMINICAN.

St. Nicholas Avenue—sometimes known as the "Dominican Broadway"—is the commercial spine of Dominican Washington Heights. The area's "Times Square" would be its intersection with 181st Street, where many bus lines converge. Spanish is the area's first language, especially east of Broadway. Bodegas, small restaurants, bakeries, and bars dot many of the blocks, especially between 157th and 165th Streets. Here you can find an abundance of Dominican markets and restaurants. *Mofongo* is one of the signature foods, made up of mashed green plantain, flavored with a range of garlic and other sauces, and topped with seafood, poultry, or other meats. Year-round, but especially in warm weather, Dominican sidewalk food vendors proliferate, offering empanadas and other fried specialties, *majarete* (pudding) and other sweets, and occasionally unusual tropical produce, such as the June plum (also known as Jew's apple). Taco trucks and fresh fruit juice carts are popular along St. Nicholas, and tamale vendors also peddle Mexican and Salvadoran foods. It is typical for the mobile juice vendor to immediately add sugar—lots of it!—after squeezing several fresh oranges into a cup, unless the buyer specifically requests that no sugar be added when making the purchase. Outstanding Dominican food can be found all over, but the best known of these restaurants would probably be El Malecon at Broadway and 175th Street, El Mofongo Café on St. Nicholas Avenue at 183rd Street, and Marisco Centro, a seafood restaurant, on St. Nicholas Avenue at 184th Street.

Other ethnic influences are scattered in Washington Heights: Yeshiva University, the world's oldest Orthodox Jewish institution of higher learning, has been based in the northeastern corner of upper Washington Heights since the mid-1920s. A number of kosher eateries and markets sit close to its campus on Amsterdam Avenue between 182nd and 187th Streets.

The enclave north of 181st Street, west of Broadway, has been dubbed "Hudson Heights" by Realtors, and the food scene here has evolved as the neighborhood has become gentrified. The type of bodega (local market) that was a centerpiece in the Broadway musical *In the Heights* is slowly disappearing, although more can be found in the northernmost and southernmost reaches of the neighborhood, especially along St. Nicholas Avenue and some of the side streets.

Along 181st Street west of Fort Washington Avenue, for example, is a string of relatively new restaurants, many catering to the growing number of professionals in the area. These include Thai, Italian, New American, an upscale Irish bar/eatery, and other cuisines. New Leaf Restaurant & Bar, in a 1930s building designed by the Olmsted Brothers in Fort Tryon Park, is an example of how the neighborhood now draws diners from around the city as a food destination serving (mainly) locally sourced foods. Its setting within the park also makes it attractive for weddings and other private events. But the evolution of the Hudson Heights section is perhaps epitomized by the saga of Frank's Market on West 187th Street. Originally a German-owned meat market when founded in the 1930s, it is now a gourmet market.

Adding to Hudson Heights's eclectic mix are three Salvadoran restaurants scattered between 174th and 187th Streets, two Venezuelan eateries, and two Russian markets, which serve the modest-sized Russian community living in Washington Heights that was established when "refuse-niks" were finally allowed to leave in the 1970s. There are no Russian restaurants however, and many of the prepared foods, including rich cakes and pastries, are brought in from Brooklyn, especially the Brighton Beach and Midwood neighborhoods. See BRIGHTON BEACH.

See also MANHATTAN.

"Hamilton Heights." Harlem & the Heights Historical Society. http://harlemandtheheightshistoricalsociety .org/pages/upper3.htm.
"Washington Heights, Manhattan." Serious Eats. http:// newyork.seriouseats.com/manhattan/washington-heights.

Myra Alperson and Cathy K. Kaufman

Washington Market

Washington Market was the largest public market in New York City throughout the nineteenth and early twentieth centuries. It was established in 1812 by the city's Common Council. The original market took up the block bounded by Washington, West, Fulton (then called Partition), and Vesey Streets on the Lower West Side of Manhattan. The original Washington Market building was a two-story structure. The lower level housed vendors' stalls, and the upper story was used for the Night Watch and other city offices. In 1818, the center market housed fifty-five butchers' stands. Fishermen and country vendors, who came from New Jersey, Staten Island, Manhattan, and Westchester, sold poultry, dairy products, and fruits and vegetables grown on nearby farms from tables in the "country market," a small shed located in the back of the main building. Over the subsequent decades, Washington Market grew to accommodate the growing trade and increased supply entering the city as a result of transportation and technological improvements such as the Erie Canal, ice production, railroads, and steam transportation.

When it opened, Washington Market was part of the city's public market system, which consisted of six public markets regulated by the city government. See PUBLIC MARKETS. The public markets were the source of most of the fresh food sold within the city limits. Washington, like the other markets, serviced residents in its nearby neighborhood. The market system was highly regulated by the city, in part to protect the public health and pocketbook but also in part to protect the trade of the market vendors who paid fees to the city for the privilege of selling in the markets. For this reason, while markets closed and new markets opened to accommodate changing residential patterns in the colonial and early national city, the city government did not approve new markets that were too close geographically to existing markets.

But with the growth of the city and New York's rise as the country's main food distribution center, Washington Market became a major food wholesale market. By the 1850s, the market encompassed five hundred stalls and had spread out to dominate the entire neighborhood around it. An annex, West Washington Market, containing an additional four hundred market stands, was built across the street from the original market house. Market wagons filled the streets and sidewalks on the blocks adjacent to the market house, wholesale grocers and provisions merchants opened warehouses nearby, and food-processing concerns established factories and showrooms in the area. Trains, boats, and wagons delivered fresh fruits, vegetables, fish, seafood, and dairy products to the piers, rail yards, and sheds of the Washington Market area.

In the 1860s, New York butcher and market chronicler Thomas De Voe described Washington Market as "without doubt the greatest depot for the sale of all manner of edibles in the U.S." supplying "many

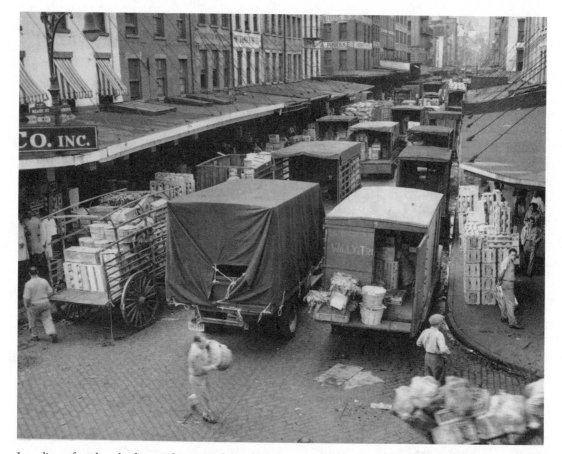

Long lines of trucks unloading produce at Washington Market, 1946. For years, the Washington Market was the largest provider of fresh produce for the city of New York and was also the largest public market, housing hundreds of vendors and taking up several city blocks. LIBRARY OF CONGRESS

thousands of our citizens [and] many of the surrounding cities, towns, villages, hotels, steamers, (both ocean and river) and shipping vessels of all descriptions." According to De Voe, the market offered "almost an endless variety and vast amounts of meat, poultry, fish, vegetables, fruits, &c., which daily concentrate here." See DE VOE, THOMAS FARRINGTON.

By this point, the food landscape in New York City had changed considerably from the early national period. As the city grew geographically, the municipal government ceased establishing new markets. With the exception of Harlem Market, no public market was established above Fourteenth Street after 1830. In 1843, the city government overturned the laws forbidding the sale of fresh meats outside the public markets. Private retailers opened groceries uptown as well. By midcentury then, few individual

householders shopped for their daily necessities at Washington Market. Instead, they patronized private retail groceries near their homes. Washington Market itself turned primarily to a wholesale function. And while the abundance and variety of goods in the market were universally celebrated, the conditions of the market house and its surroundings were universally derided by the press and reformers of the time. Throughout the second half of the nineteenth century, they called for the privatization of Washington and other public markets or for closing them altogether. But Washington Market and the food businesses that surrounded it continued to serve as the nation's principal wholesale food distribution center well into the twentieth century. As late as the 1940s, one-eighth of the nation's wholesale produce passed through New York City, primarily through Washington Market.

By this point, however, Washington Market was losing ground as trucks replaced railcars as the primary transporter of foodstuffs into New York City. The narrow, crowded streets of the Lower West Side became increasingly inhospitable to trade, and in 1962 the city moved its central wholesale terminal market to Hunts Point in the Bronx. See HUNTS POINT. In the late 1960s, the Washington Market house and many of the surrounding buildings were demolished as part of the Washington Street Urban Renewal Plan to make way for modern residences and public institutions such as St. John's University's Manhattan campus and the Borough of Manhattan Community College. Today, the area that once housed Washington Market is TriBeCa, one of the most expensive residential neighborhoods in Manhattan. Many of the old loft buildings that once housed food concerns now offer luxury housing to wealthy New Yorkers. Vestiges of the old Washington Market may still be seen on the engraved cornices of buildings showing the names of the food processors and wholesalers that once filled the neighborhood.

De Voe, Thomas F. *The Market Book: A History of the Public Markets of the City of New York*. New York: Augustus M. Kelly, 1970. First published 1862.

Lobel, Cindy R. *Urban Appetites: Food and Culture in Nineteenth-Century New York*. Chicago: University of Chicago Press, 2014.

Tangires, Helen. *Public Markets and Civic Culture in Nineteenth-Century America*. Baltimore: Johns Hopkins University Press, 2003.

Cindy R. Lobel

Water

Water has always been the most commonly consumed beverage in New York City. Water is also used in cooking and in the production of other beverages, such as brewing, distilling, and soft-drink bottling. In colonial times city dwellers had access to plentiful water from springs, ponds, lakes, and some rivers. (The Hudson, being a tidal estuary, mingles salt and freshwater and is not a suitable source for drinking water.) The exception was the southern tip of Manhattan, where the Dutch first settled. Although the Dutch colonists collected rainwater in cisterns and dug wells, as the city grew there was not enough water to meet their needs. In addition, the need to keep drinking water separate from wastewater—and the

dangers of failing to do so—were only dimly understood. Wells became polluted, and waves of waterborne diseases such as cholera swept the city. See COLONIAL DUTCH.

Residents who could travel north, beyond the city's walls, collected fresh water from springs. Those who could not make the trip themselves could buy spring water from vendors who carted it into the city twice daily.

Under English colonial rule, new wells were systematically dug, and in 1686 a public well system was established. But, as had happened under the Dutch government, problems persisted as the population grew. By the 1780s, wells had become polluted not only with seepage from privies, garbage heaps, and cemeteries but also with effluent from commercial operations such as hatters, dyers, and starch makers. As the city expanded northward, other water sources became unusable or were covered over. Waterborne diseases continued to spread throughout the city. In the summer, when these diseases were rampant, the city's well-to-do left town, heading north into the Catskill Mountains. In 1832 a cholera epidemic killed 3,513 New Yorkers.

The Great Fire of 1835, which destroyed much of the city's commercial center, blazed out of control in part because no reliable water source existed to put out the fire. Calls for a water system befitting the growing metropolis followed. Health and economic concerns (the city's brewers, among others, complained that they needed more fresh water for their operations) finally convinced the city government to embark on a massive project that would bring fresh water to Manhattan via an aqueduct. In a tremendous feat of engineering, the Croton River was dammed north of the city, reservoirs were built, lakes were controlled, and a 41-mile gravity-fed aqueduct, parts of it in underground tunnels, was constructed. The project began in 1837, and when it was completed five years later, the system delivered 36 million gallons of water to the city daily.

On October 14, 1842, New Yorkers celebrated the advent of their new, safe water supply with parades and fireworks. Private houses were connected directly to the system, so homeowners had running water and indoor privies for the first time. The less privileged continued to draw water from public taps for decades to come, but they could at least be confident of its purity. They were also served by public bathhouses. During this same period the city began to construct

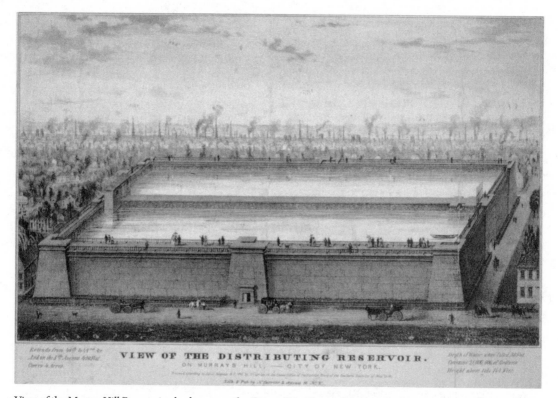

View of the Murray Hill Reservoir, also known as the Croton Distributing Reservoir, a massive above-ground structure that stored water after it was purified and ready for consumption. The New York Public Library's main building was built on the lot where the Reservoir once stood. LIBRARY OF CONGRESS

a waste system that piped raw sewage into the bay, which helped protect some of Manhattan's fresh water (while doing untold damage to the bay).

Once the Croton Aqueduct was completed, New York City's brewing industry thrived. Simultaneous with its growth was the rise of the temperance movement. Temperance advocates faced a difficult question: if New Yorkers were to stop drinking alcoholic beverages, what would they drink? Public water fountains were installed to make available the new city water supply. Later, temperance and other groups funded the construction and maintenance of "ice-free" drinking fountains for public refreshment in parks and elsewhere. Temperance advocates also encouraged restaurants to offer a glass of water to customers when they sat down at a table. See PROHIBITION and TEMPERANCE MOVEMENT.

Within a decade of its completion, the Croton system proved inadequate, and new reservoirs were added to supply the need. The water system infrastructure was modernized again in the early twentieth century. The new Croton system, completed in

1911, bore little resemblance to the original. Land that had once held reservoirs was turned over to the city. The New York Public Library's main building, at Fifth Avenue between Fortieth and Forty-Second Streets, was built on the lot where the Croton Reservoir once stood, and Central Park's Great Lawn is located on the former site of the Receiving Reservoir. See NEW YORK PUBLIC LIBRARY.

In 1898, when the city was consolidated, the system was extended to 1.6 million new residents of Staten Island, Brooklyn, Queens, and the Bronx. Indeed, access to Manhattan's water system was a major argument for consolidation in rival city Brooklyn. In 1905 the state legislature created the public Board of Water Supply with the power to condemn land and build new aqueducts and reservoirs. Construction of a new Catskill Mountain water system began in 1907. Within ten years, water from the Catskills was flowing into New York.

By the time the entire system was completed, in 1926, the city's water requirements had already outpaced the supply. By 1951 New York City was drawing water from the Delaware River. The final component of the Delaware system was put into place in 1964. The Croton system still supplied about 10 percent of the city's needs, while the Catskill and Delaware systems supplied 90 percent.

Since the 1840s, the New York City watershed has enveloped upstate farms, hamlets, and homesteads. Upstate communities and businesses objected to the restrictions imposed on farming, hunting, and hiking in many parts of the city's watershed. The creation of the Environmental Protection Agency, the establishment of strict water quality standards, and the city's financial crisis in the 1970s changed the city's relationship with communities in its watershed. In 1977, the city and upstate communities signed the Watershed Memorandum of Agreement, which balanced the city's needs with those of the people living in the watershed areas. The adoption of new agricultural practices by Catskill farmers reduced the flow of pollution into the reservoir system.

This agreement encouraged the city to ramp up water conservation efforts, including placing meters in private homes and apartments and billing residents for water usage rather than charging a flat rate. Improved leak detection efforts were undertaken. A law was passed mandating the installation of water-saving toilets, showerheads, and other plumbing devices. These efforts greatly reduced water usage.

For years, New York City prided itself on having the largest nonfiltration system in the country. The water delivered to New Yorkers was considered pure; it met all federal and state standards, so it did not have to go through a purification process. However, increased commercial and residential development upstate created serious runoff problems from sewage-treatment plants. Beginning in the 1990s the city again began to buy land around the upstate reservoirs, and new legislation put tighter controls on sewage discharge and new development. But even these new measures were insufficient. In 1993 the federal government required the city to filter Croton water, and in 2008 the Croton system was shut down for construction of a filtration plant under Van Cortlandt Park, the aqueduct's entry point in the northwest Bronx.

Today, the city's water supply system is the most extensive metropolitan water supply network in America. The city's watershed extends 2,000 square miles into upstate New York. Every day it delivers 1.1 billion gallons of water, which courses through

tunnels, pipes, and mains. Many of these conduits date back to the nineteenth century, and the city mains burst fairly often, spewing millions of gallons of water into city streets, homes, and businesses. So far, city officials have found it is easier and cheaper to repair breaks when they occur rather than to replace the entire aging system.

Two major tunnels brought water to the city: Water Tunnel No. 1, completed in 1917, and Water Tunnel No. 2, completed in 1936. Neither tunnel could be inspected or significantly repaired since they opened. In 1970 the city began construction of Water Tunnel No. 3, which will bring water from the Bronx to Manhattan and eventually to Queens and Brooklyn. To date, it has cost the city $4.7 billion and is the largest public works project ever undertaken in New York City. The first section, from the Bronx to Manhattan, was completed in 2013. The next 10-mile section to Queens and Brooklyn is scheduled for completion in 2021.

City water is regulated by the Environmental Protection Agency and local authorities, who annually test almost five hundred thousand samples of city water. New York tap water has won regional and national competitions for the best municipal water.

See also WATER, BOTTLED.

Koeppel, Gerard T. *Water for Gotham: A History*. Princeton, N.J.: Princeton University Press, 2000.
Soll, David. *Empire of Water: An Environmental and Political History of the New York City Water Supply*. Ithaca, N.Y.: Cornell University Press, 2013.

Andrew F. Smith

Water, Bottled

New Yorkers have been drinking bottled water for almost two centuries. It was almost always imported from outside the city, particularly from mineral springs fairly close by. The spa at Saratoga Springs, in upstate New York, had attracted Europeans since well before the American Revolution, and it remained popular throughout the nineteenth and early twentieth centuries. In 1820 Dr. Darius Griswold began bottling water at Saratoga's Congress Springs. He stuck with the business for just a few years before leasing the bottling rights to Dr. John Clarke and Thomas Lynch in 1823. Clarke and Lynch promoted Saratoga Mineral Water, the first commercially successful bottled water in the United States. It was first distributed to New York City and then shipped to other eastern cities. By 1830 Dr. Clarke was shipping twelve hundred bottles of water a day, and by 1856 the company was distributing more than 11 million bottles annually throughout the United States and to foreign countries. As the nineteenth century progressed, more Americans ventured into the business of bottling and selling spring water.

As bottling technology became more efficient, smaller bottles of water for table use became available and affordable for most New Yorkers. In the early twentieth century, New Yorkers also began taking an interest in bottled water from other countries. One early favorite was Perrier, which came from springs at Les Bouillens, a spa in the town of Vergèze in southern France. Testimonials were used to promote the naturally carbonated water, advertised as "The Champagne of table waters", and sales of Perrier skyrocketed.

In 1907 Perrier established an American subsidiary, Great Waters of France, in New York City. The new Perrier distributor began a massive marketing campaign, branding Perrier as a "Luxury from France" and as "The Chosen Table Water of Europe." Perrier could not be imported during World War I, and the Depression made extravagances like imported spring water superfluous.

World War II again stopped all importation of Perrier, and after the war fewer New Yorkers were willing to pay a premium for imported sparkling water, which tasted pretty much like the far cheaper but equally bubbly club soda or seltzer. Consumers also resisted paying for still spring waters, which tasted about the same as New York City's high-quality tap water. Perrier was served in some restaurants but sold in very few stores. Distributors were unwilling to tie up funds in a product that just did not sell.

Decades later, in 1977, Perrier launched another major ad campaign that grabbed the public's attention and sent sales sky-high. It was just the beginning of the bottled water craze. Many other bottled waters were imported, including traditional favorites such as Gerolsteiner and Apollinaris from Germany, Evian from France, and San Pellegrino from Italy. These were later joined by Fiji from the Fiji Islands, Voss from Norway, Ty Nant from Wales, and newer brands from all over the world.

Some of New York's favorite waters are domestic, including Deer Park, originally from a western Maryland spring. Deer Park water was first bottled in 1873 as drinking water for passengers on the Baltimore & Ohio Railroad. In 1966 the B&O sold the operation, which became Deer Park Spring Water, Inc., and the water was marketed primarily in the New York metropolitan area. Poland Spring, from Maine, is New York's top-selling bottled water. Soda manufacturers such as Pepsi and Coca-Cola have brought purified waters (Aquafina and Dasani, respectively) to the market, and today New Yorkers continue to consume large amounts of bottled water.

But some New Yorkers have found problems with the bottled water craze. Environmentalists point out that water is very heavy, and shipping bottles of it thousands of miles (from Fiji to New York, for example), is an unjustifiable waste of energy. Others see the plastic bottles, made from polyethylene terephthalate, as the primary problem. Although New York has a major recycling program, about 90 percent of plastic bottles nationwide end up in landfills, not recycling centers.

In 2008 New York governor David Patterson proposed phasing out the purchase of bottled water for the office's state-owned agencies. Beginning that same year, the City of New York stopped supplying bottled water to its downtown offices and to city-funded events and functions. Instead, water coolers were installed to provide filtered tap water for drinking. Also in 2008 "serial entrepreneur" Craig Zucker started Tap'd NY, a company that sold bottles of New York City tap water (filtered by reverse osmosis) as "an honest and local alternative" to waters imported from thousands of miles away. The bottles bore tongue-in-cheek claims such as "No glaciers were harmed in making this water."

The New York City Department of Environmental Protection took this approach a step further, sending out portable multispigot water fountains that are parked in outdoor locations around the five boroughs during the summer. After the fountain is hooked up to a fire hydrant, New Yorkers can fill up their own bottles with pure, tasty New York City water.

See also PERRIER and WATER.

Gleick, Peter H. *Bottled and Sold: The Story Behind Our Obsession with Bottled Water*. Washington, D.C.: Island, 2010.

Royte, Elizabeth. *Bottlemania: How Water Went on Sale and Why We Bought It*. New York: Bloomsbury, 2008.

Smith, Andrew F. *Drinking History: Fifteen Turning Points in the Making of American Beverages*. New York: Columbia University Press, 2012.

Andrew F. Smith

Waxman, Nach

Nahum "Nach" Waxman is one of the owners of Kitchen Arts & Letters, an Upper East Side bookstore that he opened in 1983. The thirteen thousand books at Kitchen Arts & Letters go far beyond cookbooks. They cover the anthropology of food from the history of farming to molecular gastronomy and what humans did with their food along the way. More than one-third of the books are imported. Periodicals range from *Art Culinaire*, *Saveur*, and *Food Arts* to *Modern Farmer* and *Cherry Bombe*.

The books reflect Waxman's background as a Jersey boy educated at a Hebrew academy in Philadelphia, with a degree in South Asian anthropology from Cornell, and graduate work at the University of Chicago and Harvard. His work as a book editor and love of the physical aspects of book publishing, especially books that require complicated layouts, accidentally led to cookbooks. One of the first he worked on was *Better than Store Bought*.

What Waxman learned after almost two decades in publishing was that he wanted to work for himself. He decided to open a specialty bookstore, and food was beginning to grab the public's interest. In 1983 he opened Kitchen Arts & Letters at 1435 Lexington Avenue, between Ninety-Third and Ninety-Fourth Streets, with seven or eight hundred books.

Waxman always intended Kitchen Arts & Letters to be a gathering place for people in the food industry, and they still account for close to 70 percent of sales. The shop's patrons have always been food giants; Julia Child and James Beard were early visitors. Now they include chefs Jean-Georges Vongerichten, Daniel Boulud, Mario Batali, Dan Barber, and Wylie Dufresne. Customers from all over the world bring tales of new food trends years before they hit the general public.

For years, every couple of weeks Waxman, then-manager Matt Sartwell, and another staff member would brainstorm about new acquisitions, like how to make that new Italian food book differentiate itself from the eight hundred already on the shelf. Often, they tried the recipes in the cookbooks. Anglo-Indian cookbooks are a major interest for Waxman, especially spicy food; so is Jewish food.

Waxman is not just a bibliophile but also a matchmaker. Like a sommelier you trust to recommend the ideal wine you never heard of to accompany your meal, he pairs the perfect book with the right recipient. Many culinary scholars have been the beneficiaries of Waxman's magnanimity when the book they did not know they needed arrived in the mail.

Waxman also collects nineteenth-century advertising trade cards about every type and aspect of food: seeds, stoves, restaurants, candy, baking powder, even farm equipment. His particular interests are medicinal foods like Liebig's Meat Extract and alcoholic patent medicines. In July 2014 Waxman catalogued his collection of six thousand trade cards, donated them to Cornell, and curated an online exhibit.

Kitchen Arts & Letters is for people who love food and books as part of an examined life. On January 1, 2014, Sartwell became the majority owner of the store. Now Waxman concentrates on out-of-print books. In 2014 Waxman and Sartwell compiled and edited the book *The Chef Says: Quotes, Quips, and Words of Wisdom*. Waxman is a member of the James Beard Foundation's Hall of Fame.

See also KITCHEN ARTS AND LETTERS.

Fox, Nick. "Q & A with Nach Waxman." *New York Times*, October 21, 2008.

Linda Civitello

Wechsberg, Joseph

Joseph Wechsberg (1907–1983), the Czechoslovakian-born American food writer, began his career holding not a pen but a violin bow. He hoped to become a great violinist.

But Wechsberg was energetic and curious, and he had a range of jobs after he received a law degree in Prague in 1930: cruise violinist, croupier, and reporter for Czech- and German-language newspapers. It was when he and his wife were unexpectedly stranded in the United States after Hitler's invasion of Czechoslovakia that he was set on the path to his true calling. While adjusting to life in America, he discovered the *New Yorker* and thought he might like writing for it. (Food writing still lay in the future.) Before he was shipped back to Ostrava as an American GI, he was invited to write a story for the *New Yorker* about returning home. It was published in 1943, beginning a relationship with the magazine that lasted from 1943 to 1975.

His beat at the *New Yorker* was European culture, but his heart beat for food. He wrote about great chefs and restaurateurs in France and New York and, in doing so, helped to explain to postwar-generation

Americans what made French haute cuisine the ne plus ultra of the table.

His essay on Fernand Point, owner of Le Pyramide, France's legendary restaurant in Vienne (Isère), is a model of his singular style: excess through restraint. Even the title, "The Finest Butter and Lots of Time," suggests speed in abeyance.

As Americans became the world's most frequent flyers in the 1960s and 1970s, Wechsberg's articles began to appear in numerous American periodicals (*The Atlantic, Bazaar, Esquire, Gourmet, Holiday, Horizon, McCall's, New York Times, New York Times Magazine, Playboy, Saturday Review, Travel & Leisure,* and *Woman's Day*). Reading him was like attending finishing school; in addition to providing a culinary education, he provided Americans with sorely needed savoir faire (e.g., "Some Tips on Tipping" and "Perfect Service" in *Gourmet*). *Gourmet* magazine became his main platform for the larger brief: to expound on the glories of the European table in France and beyond—the Belgian, Czech, German, Hungarian, Italian, Polish, and Swiss traditions. In the 1970s he began writing the magazine's Paris Journal column.

And he began to write books, which gave him ample space to express his admiration for culinary perfection. In *Blue Trout and Black Truffles: The Peregrinations of an Epicure* (1953), he describes the great traditions of dining during the last days of Habsburg rule in Mitteleuropa. In *Dining at the Pavillon* (1962), he describes the mind-boggling combination of talents that Henri Soulé, owner of New York's Le Pavillon, needed in order to operate and maintain the standards of America's temple to French cuisine.

His other food-related books include *The Cooking of Vienna's Empire* (1968) and *Trifles Make Perfection: The Selected Essays of Joseph Wechsberg* (1999), a posthumous essay collection. His essays also appear in *Remembrance of Things Paris: Sixty Years of Writing from Gourmet* (2004) and *Secret Ingredients: The New Yorker Book of Food and Drink* (2007).

See also GOURMET and NEW YORKER.

Joseph Wechsberg website: http://josephwechsberg.com.
"Joseph Wechsberg, 75, A *New Yorker* Writer." *New York Times*, Tuesday, April 12, 1983.
Shawn, William. "Joseph Wechsberg." *New Yorker*, April 10, 1983.
Wechsberg, Joseph. *Blue Trout & Black Truffles: The Peregrinations of an Epicure*. New York: Knopf, 1953.
Wechsberg, Joseph. *Dining at the Pavillon*. Boston: Little, Brown, 1962.

Valerie Saint-Rossy

Weight Watchers

Weight Watchers began in 1962 when Jean Nidetch, a Queens housewife who had struggled with her weight since childhood, gathered a group of friends, hoping to make weight loss stick once and for all. At the time, she had begun yet another diet, a plan designed by the free obesity clinic at the New York City Department of Health. Nidetch and her friends met on a weekly basis in her Queens home to check in, supporting one other through the struggles and successes of weight loss. Within two months the group's membership was still growing, and by October 1962 Nidetch had lost seventy-two pounds, achieving a goal weight of 142 pounds, which she proudly states that she maintained throughout the rest of her life.

Inspired by her long-awaited weight-loss success, Nidetch dedicated her life to motivating others to do the same. She began by sharing her diet plan through informal gatherings, including one at the home of Felice and Albert Lippert. The Lipperts collectively lost one hundred pounds following Nidetch's plan and gained her enthusiasm for the program. With the Lipperts, Nidetch created the "Weight Watchers" name and hatched plans to grow. Nidetch incorporated Weight Watchers in 1963 with herself, her husband, Marty Nidetch, and the Lipperts as the four founding members. They opened the first Weight Watchers operation in Little Neck, New York, in a space above a movie theater. Members paid a three-dollar registration fee and two dollars per week to attend meetings—the same price as to see a movie downstairs. As attendance and demand grew, the Nidetchs and Lipperts opened additional locations in the city and eventually began to franchise across the United States.

Former Weight Watchers followers who had lost weight with the program and kept it off led program meetings. The meetings consisted of private weigh-ins, a lecture by the group leader, and open discussion. Members were taught to avoid foods high in sugar and fat and how to identify which foods were "legal," Nidetch's term for foods permitted on the diet plan. The plan mandated at least one weekly serving of liver and at least five fish servings—though this recommendation was later modified following research on fish and mercury poisoning. Most notably, meetings provided members with social support and a newfound space to share their weight-loss experiences. The formula of diet plan plus in-person group meetings worked for more than just the Lipperts and Nidetchs. By 1967 New York City hosted nearly three hundred meetings a week, as did twenty-five franchise operations in sixteen states across the United States and on multiple continents abroad.

Weight Watchers Inc. expanded not only across the globe but also into members' homes and the aisles of the supermarket. The organization launched a line of diet-approved frozen dinners, which within ten years would expand to a menu of twenty-three different offerings—such as a 140-calorie lunch of flounder and chopped broccoli and a 510-calorie meal of ziti with veal, cheese, and sauce. In addition to food products, Nidetch published the *Weight Watchers Program Cookbook* in 1966 and introduced the *Weight Watchers Magazine* in 1968. That same year, Weight Watchers operated ninety-one franchises in forty-three states and the company's public offering completely sold out. Weight Watchers continued to extend its reach and was operating in forty-eight states and ten countries by 1972.

Weight Watchers members embraced both the program and Nidetch, so much so that seventeen thousand enthusiasts gathered for the company's tenth birthday in 1973, held at Madison Square Garden. Bob Hope entertained members, many of whom waited excitedly in line for Nidetch's autograph. The venue was stocked with snacks especially selected for the occasion: "legal" hot dogs with buns that counted as one slice of bread, a "frosted treat" that counted as eight ounces of skim milk and a serving of fruit, dried apple chips, and sugarless soft drinks. By its fifteenth birthday in 1978 Weight Watchers had expanded into all fifty states and twenty-six countries abroad and was acquired for upward of $70 million by H. J. Heinz Company.

Highly recognizable spokespeople have formed one of the hallmarks of Weight Watchers. Charismatic, funny, noticeably blond, and snappily dressed, Nidetch remained Weight Watchers' spokesperson into the 1980s. Subsequent spokespeople included Lynn Redgrave, starting in 1984, and the Duchess of York, Sarah Ferguson, who became spokesperson in 1997 and remained so for more than a decade. More recent spokespeople include Jenny McCarthy, Jennifer Hudson, and Jessica Simpson.

Just as the face of Weight Watchers has changed over the years, so has the program itself. In 1972, the organization unveiled a new and less restrictive regimen than the original 1963 version. This eating plan added what Nidetch called "the foods that temptation is made of"—like spaghetti, macaroni, potatoes, rice, ice creams, cereals, and mayonnaise—back to the menu. In the 1990s a very popular points-based system revamped the food exchange program. In 1999 Artal Luxembourg, S.A., took ownership of Weight Watchers, launching Weight Watchers Online as a separate company in 2001 and Weight Watchers Online for Men in 2007 with spokesperson Charles Barkley.

Not only popular among members, multiple randomized trials have also found Weight Watchers to be an effective weight-loss program, although, as is true with most weight-reduction programs, keeping the weight off after leaving the program remains a problem. Today, consumers spend more than $3 billion on Weight Watchers–branded products and services and more than one million people across thirty countries attend one of forty-four thousand weekly Weight Watchers meetings.

Hellmich, Nanci. "Weight Watchers Founder Jean Nidetch Shares Her Start." *USA Today*, March 22, 2010.

Ickeringill, Nan. "Weight Watchers, Inc.: They Talk Their Way Out of Obesity." *New York Times*, March 20, 1967.

"Jean Nidetch: The First Weight Watcher." *Entrepreneur*, October 10, 2008.

Nidetch, Jean. *Weight Watchers Program Cookbook*. Great Neck, N.Y.: Hearthside, 1973.

Emily J. H. Contois

West Indian

See CARIBBEAN and WEST INDIAN DAY PARADE.

West Indian Day Parade

Each Labor Day, beginning at approximately 11:00 a.m., the annual West Indian Parade passes through Crown Heights in Brooklyn, New York. Assembling in the streets around Utica Avenue, it passes along several miles of Eastern Parkway to end at the junction of Flatbush and Grand Army Plaza. An estimated two million spectators typically line the broad avenue during this seven-hour extravaganza. New York City's most colorful parade, there is an almost unending stream of dramatically decorated vehicles carrying elaborately dressed revelers, accompanied by noise emanating from steel pans and whistles.

Each float holds a group, a masquerade band (*mas*) or camp, which has spent months preparing for this day. Often working in secret, themes for each float are carefully drawn up by skilled designers. These exotic concepts are translated into elaborate costumes for their king and queen and the many "camp" followers. The focus is to outdo rivals, win approval from the adoring crowds, and carry home the top cash prizes.

The West Indian American Day Carnival (as it is correctly titled) is organized by the West Indian American Day Carnival Association. Permission was first obtained for the parade to be established on Eastern Parkway in 1969. Variations of the event had been held in Harlem since 1916, both indoors and outdoors, but the permit for these was revoked in 1964 after some disruptive incidents. During its time in Brooklyn the parade has been mostly peaceful, carefully monitored by the New York Police Department's Seventy-Seventh and Seventy-First Precincts, which are jointly responsible for the area.

Carnival, beloved by West Indian people, has a complicated birthright, tied as it is to colonialism and religious celebration, as well as being an expression of freedom. Some historians believe the first "modern" Caribbean carnival originated in Trinidad, which still has the largest *mas* in the region. The concept was probably imported by French émigrés from Brazil, where the tradition of carnival on Fat Tuesday goes back to the eighteenth century.

While Jamaican reggae and Haitian *compas* abound, the parade is defined by calypso and soca music from Trinidad. Many of these songs make reference to the Labor Day carnival, including "Gunplay on the Eastern Parkway," "Melee (on the Eastern Parkway)," and "Labor Day in Brooklyn." The carnival is an assertion of Pan-Caribbean pride, bringing together multiracial peoples, demonstrating the vibrancy of the Caribbean. Beginning in late August bodegas and corner stores throughout the boroughs sell flags of every Caribbean nation, flags that will adorn the hoods of cars, be draped from windows, and wrap the bodies of revelers. As Monday morning dawns individuals from this broad ethnic background blend together to create a living montage, a tide of patriotic expression, flowing on to the Parkway.

A multitude of vendors closely line the route, jointly offering almost every conceivable form of West Indian food. The air is filled with the smells and smoke from pans and cooking stoves. Each island is represented by its national dish or favorite food: pepper pot from Guyana, shark and bake from Barbados, ackee and saltfish from Jamaica, *cocina criolla* from Puerto Rico, and accra from Haiti. Other dishes such as oxtail, rice and peas, beans and rice, escoveitch fish, jerked chicken or pork, curried goat, roasted corn, and fried plantain are also ubiquitous. Sugary desserts abound, such as coconut gizzada, grater cake, and carrot cake, along with sorrel, limeade, ginger beer, and punch. There are also hot dogs, spicy Italian sausages, and ice cream for those uninterested in sampling West Indian cuisine. A wide array of vendors sell artwork and trinkets among the jostling crowd.

Besides its importance as a celebration of Caribbean culture, the carnival has a significant economic impact. Not only does it create a ready market for a wide array of small street vendors, it also attracts visitors from far and wide. The New York Visitors Bureau estimates the impact to be around $200,000 annually. The continued success of the event has led other cities in America and Canada to attempt to replicate it, including Miami, Boston, and Toronto. Yet New York's West Indian Day Parade remains the benchmark by which American carnival celebrations are measured. For those wishing an introduction to West Indian cuisine and culture there can hardly be a better place than Eastern Parkway on Labor Day.

See also CARIBBEAN and STREET FAIRS.

"The Birth & Evolution of Trinidad Carnival." Discover Trinidad & Tobago. http://www.discovertnt.com/articles/Trinidad/The-Birth-Evolution-of-Trinidad-Carnival/109/3/32.
"History of Carnival." Rio.com. http://www.rio.com/rio-carnival/history-carnival.
West Indian American Day Carnival Association Inc. website: http://wiadcacarnival.org.

Bill Moore

Whiskey War

See DISTILLERIES.

White Horse Tavern

The White Horse Tavern, located at 567 Hudson Street, on the west edge of Greenwich Village, is one of New York's oldest taverns, dating to 1880. A three-story Victorian building, it is best known as a favorite haunt of intellectuals and bohemians during the 1950s and 1960s, including James Baldwin, Jack Kerouac, Norman Mailer, Anaïs Nin, Hunter S. Thompson,

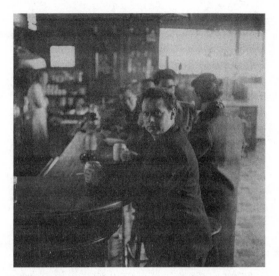

Dylan Thomas, the famous British poet, often frequented the White Horse Tavern on occasions when he visited New York, and famously had his last drink here on November 5, 1953, before falling ill and dying four days later. PHOTOGRAPH BY BUNNY ADLER

the Scottish poet Ruthann Todd introduced Thomas to the White Horse. In *Dylan Thomas in America* (1955) Brinnin describes how quickly Thomas appeared at ease at the tavern: "when he got to the White Horse it was all over... much to the delight of his proprietor, who found his business doubled by the many people—friends and mere 'ardents'—who would assemble there at all hours in the chance that Dylan might turn up."

Thomas loved New York City and visited three more times. On his last visit, in October 1953, his health was poor; he suffered from gout and gastritis and reportedly had periodic blackouts. On October 23 he collapsed after two performances of his drama *Under Milk Wood*. Despite this, he continued drinking heavily. On November 3, returning to the Hotel Chelsea after a night at the White Horse, Thomas reportedly said, "I've had eighteen straight whiskies. I think that's the record!" Many, including the barman at the time, are certain this was an exaggeration. He returned to the White Horse the next day, falling ill enough that the following morning a doctor was called to his hotel room. The doctor injected steroids and morphine on three occasions, which affected his already-troubled breathing (he used an inhaler and had lung issues). Thomas soon fell into a coma and was taken to St. Vincent's Hospital, where he died on November 9. The cause of death was pneumonia. Surprisingly, there was no evidence of cirrhosis, and there is some dispute over whether medical malpractice or hard drinking killed him.

After Thomas's death the White Horse Tavern continued to be an important meeting place for new generations of writers and intellectuals. In her masterpiece *The Death and Life of Great American Cities* (1961), Jane Jacobs wrote of the White Horse Tavern that on winter nights "the doors open, [and] a solid wave of conversation and animation surges out and hits you." Jack Kerouac frequently drank to excess and was bounced from the tavern on a few occasions; a popular story goes that someone scribbled "JACK GO HOME!" on the bathroom wall. The novelist Norman Mailer gathered a regular group of friends at the White Horse every Sunday and supposedly conceived the *Village Voice* with Dan Wolf and Ed Francher there. See VILLAGE VOICE. Bob Dylan played for tips at the White Horse in the early 1960s.

In the late 1960s business slowed, and in 1967 the owner, James Hoffman, sold the White Horse to a friend named Eddie Brennan. Eddie was a long-

James Laughlin, and, most famously, the Welsh poet Dylan Thomas, who consumed his last drink at the White Horse on November 4, 1953, before falling into a coma and dying five days later. Tourists, students, and literary pilgrims pay homage to Thomas by drinking at the White Horse and visiting the Dylan Thomas Room, where his portrait and two plaques memorializing him hang.

The tavern began as a barroom built for a brewery in 1880. Before that time the property had been used variously as an oyster house and a book store. In its early days the White Horse attracted a blue-collar crowd, typically laborers and longshoremen who worked the nearby docks along the Hudson River and afterwards congregated at the spacious bar, built from a single piece of mahogany. During Prohibition the White Horse operated as a speakeasy. See SPEAKEASIES.

By the mid-twentieth century the White Horse Tavern had become a favorite watering hole for visiting British intellectuals and writers; the quiet atmosphere, working-poor regulars, stock ales, and pub fare, including a thirty-five-cent roast beef special, reminded them of their pubs back home. In 1950 the American poet Malcolm Brinnin convinced Dylan Thomas to visit the United States for a well-paid poetry reading tour. Once he arrived in New York,

shoreman for more than a decade until an injury forced a change of careers. He tended bar at the White Horse before scraping together the $10,000 he needed to buy it. He remains the co-owner as of 2015, and relatively little has changed at the tavern. The menu remains standard pub fare: hamburgers, grilled cheese, roast beef sandwiches, shepherd's pie, sausages, French fries, and the like. The scene has changed considerably, though: today you are more likely to find New York University students and locals having a beer than bohemian writers or laborers.

See also GREENWICH VILLAGE and TAVERNS.

Brinnin, John Malcolm. *Dylan Thomas in America*. Boston: Little, Brown, 1955.
"Did Hard-Living or Medical Neglect Kill Dylan Thomas?" BBC Arts, November 8, 2013. http://www.bbc.co.uk/arts/0/24748894.
Kramer, Karen. "Eddie Brennan on Waterfront, White Horse, Dylan Thomas." *The Villager* 75, no. 32 (December 28–January 3, 2005).
Schmalbach, Sarah. "Tavern that Put Poet Under, Finds New Life at 125." *The Villager* 74, no. 29 (November 24–30, 2014).
"The White Horse Tavern: Dylan Thomas' Second Home." *All Things Considered*. WNYC. October 31, 2014.

Max P. Sinsheimer

Whole Foods

Whole Foods is a supermarket filled with artisanal, organic, and local produce with multiple locations throughout New York City. As a major purveyor of alternative foods, the stores are a boon to the many food makers in New York City. For consumers who want (and can afford) the best food money can buy—for either culinary or ethical reasons—Whole Foods is a seven-days-a-week alternative to New York City's Greenmarkets. See GREENMARKETS.

The chain was founded by four natural foods storeowners from Austin, Texas. It was meant to be a supermarket of "hippie foods" that could turn organic and vegetarian foods into a mainstream phenomenon. Natural foods supermarkets existed in big cities like Boston and Los Angeles, but no one had ever tried it in Austin. John Mackey, Renee Lawson Hardy, Craig Weller, and Mark Skiles consolidated their stores into a supermarket with a nineteen-person staff. In September 1980, the first Whole Foods Market opened.

Apart from the foods it carried, the design could have belonged to any modern supermarket—there were proper checkout stands and bright lighting. In order to meet their new sales goals, the founders decided to add coffee, beer, wine, and—most unusual of all in a natural food market dominated by vegetarians—meat to the items sold in stores. By the end of the year, the store had increased its staff to one hundred and was the highest-volume natural foods store in the country. Founder John Mackey later referred to the business model as "conscious capitalism," meaning a focus not only on traditional profits but also on the social and environmental costs of business decisions.

By 1984, Whole Foods was ready to expand. They stayed close to home at first, opening stores in Houston and Dallas, followed by New Orleans. Not all of the new stores were built from scratch. Many were natural foods stores that Whole Foods acquired. By 2000, they owned 117 stores throughout the United States. In 2001, Whole Foods finally came to Manhattan, opening a store in the Chelsea neighborhood at Twenty-Fourth Street and Seventh Avenue.

Today, Whole Foods has eight locations in New York City, with four more set to open by 2016. Their initial growth was steady—the second store in Columbus Circle did not open until 2004. But as the good food movement started to grow throughout the United States, the demand for local, wholesome food rose with it. New Whole Foods continued to pop up throughout Manhattan, reinforcing the spread of gourmet foods, local value-added products, and farmers' market foods outside of the Greenmarkets.

Unlike other large chains, no two Whole Foods locations are ever alike. Their size and shape vary widely: the Chelsea store has about 18,000 square feet, while the Bowery location claims over 75,000 square feet. More importantly, each store (whether in New York or any other city) tries to have unique offerings tailored to the surrounding community. The stores of New York City have everything from bars to bike repair shops, Indian street food to their body product store, Whole Body. When Whole Foods opened their eighth New York City store in Brooklyn (the first location outside of Manhattan) in 2013, they put a working greenhouse on the roof. Run and designed by Gotham Greens, the 20,000-square-foot farm uses an aquaponic system that allows them to grow lettuce and other greens with twenty times less water than other methods of farming. The rooftop greenhouse supplies Whole

Foods Brooklyn as well as other locations throughout the city. Their Gowanus location also has a restaurant and bar called The Roof, where customers can enjoy craft beer and locally made foods.

New York City is a powerhouse when it comes to originating food trends. Whole Foods has tried to capitalize on that reputation by carrying products from local companies and food makers, whether a dairy upstate or a company that bakes snack foods in Brooklyn. Currently, there are three main influencers when it comes to the direction Whole Foods takes throughout New York City. Their "forager" visits popups like Smorgasburg and local businesses to taste new foods and determine whether they will be a good fit for their stores. A "culinary coordinator" tracks food trends and ideas for Whole Foods in-store food venues. Finally, their "regional president" oversees the operations of each store, with duties ranging from real estate development and store design to purchasing and marketing. See SMORGASBURG.

With their model of conscious capitalism, Whole Foods holds a unique place in New York City's food movement. They are willing to embrace new trends and foster local talent as long as it reflects their customers' desires. They will go out of their way to bring in food from local farms as long as New Yorkers buy it. With a consumer base that can choose to order food online, visit the farmers' market, or visit any number of gourmet grocery stores around the city, a rooftop farm is just the beginning of the lengths to which this chain will go to keep them happy.

See also GROCERY STORES and SUPERMARKETS.

"Company Info." Whole Foods Market. http://www.wholefoodsmarket.com/company-info.
Gwynne, Sam. "Born Green." *Saveur*, May 26, 2009.
Paumgarten, Nick. "Food Fighter." *New Yorker*, January 4, 2010.

Tove K. Danovich

Williamsburg

Williamsburg is a neighborhood in northern Brooklyn, bordered to the east by Bushwick, to the north by Greenpoint, to the west by the East River, and to the south by Bedford-Stuyvesant. Originally part of the Dutch settlement of Bushwick, Williamsburg's proximity to the river made it an important location for fer-

rying Long Island's produce across the river to markets in Manhattan. In the 1820s and 1830s, when the construction of the Erie Canal led to explosive growth in New York City, Williamsburg was transformed. While it had been an unincorporated village of just one thousand people in the mid-1820s, thirty years later the town of Williamsburg joined the borough of Brooklyn with a population of thirty-two thousand. In those years it also evolved from a quiet rural area and upper-class vacation spot to a bustling industrial neighborhood, home to numerous European immigrants from Germany and Ireland. Once again Williamsburg's river access shaped the neighborhood. Now its shoreline was dotted with dozens of factories, including oil refineries, glue factories, glassworks, breweries, distilleries, the Pfizer pharmaceutical plant, and the Havemeyer and Elder sugar plant, which was operated by several successive sugar companies into the twenty-first century. See GERMAN; IRISH; and SUGAR REFINING.

The Williamsburg Bridge opened in 1903, spurring the migration of immigrants from Lower Manhattan into the neighborhood. Williamsburg became, in different areas, heavily Polish, Italian, and Jewish. After World War II, a major Hasidic Jewish population moved into the neighborhood, followed in the 1950s and 1960s by Puerto Ricans and Dominicans. Each of these successive waves of immigrants shaped Williamsburg's food culture. Peter Luger Steakhouse was established in 1887, geared toward Williamsburg's then heavily German population, and has operated in the same spot since as well as opening a handful of satellite locations in Manhattan and on Long Island. Joyva, the nation's largest purveyor of halva and other kosher desserts, has been based in Williamsburg since 1907. Bamonte's, an unassuming Italian restaurant on Withers Street, has been in operation since 1900. Dozens of Polish, Puerto Rican, and Dominican restaurants are sprinkled throughout Williamsburg, as well as neighboring Bushwick and Greenpoint. See JEWISH; PUERTO RICAN; DOMINICAN; PETER LUGER'S; HALVA; and BUSHWICK.

In addition to its numerous culinary influences, Williamsburg was for a time an enormously important center of brewing in the United States. In 1900 there were forty-five brewers in Brooklyn, including eleven in heavily German Williamsburg. While brewing had all but disappeared from Brooklyn by the 1980s, the establishment of Brooklyn Brewery in 1996 launched a small revival. Brooklyn Brewery, as well as Sixpoint Brewery and Kelso, are now based in Williamsburg and nearby Greenpoint. See BEER; BREWERIES; and BROOKLYN BREWERY.

By the end of the twentieth century, Williamsburg was undergoing yet another transition. Artists, bohemians, and some young professionals, priced out of Manhattan, had begun to move to the area starting in the 1980s, drawn by the low rents, the diversity, and the fading industrial atmosphere. Soon Williamsburg became the "hot" neighborhood in New York City, and with the influx of newcomers, it began to gentrify. Rents increased, zoning laws began to change, and Williamsburg's food culture also shifted. Dozens of new restaurants opened, emphasizing high quality and often expensive fare. Every type of food can be found in Williamsburg, including rare fusions, like the Jewish–Japanese restaurant Shalom Japan.

Williamsburg has also been a leader in food beyond traditional restaurant settings. Brooklyn Bowl, a bowling alley with a bar and a full menu, as well as Nitehawk Cinema, a dine-in arthouse movie theater, are known for their innovative and ever-changing food offerings. Brooklyn Flea, a company that runs several flea markets on the East Coast, is most known for its markets in Fort Greene and Williamsburg, which feature a wide variety of local food vendors. In 2011 the company also spawned Smorgasburg, a vast weekly food festival full of food trucks and small stands from local businesses. Smorgasburg has grown so popular in recent years that it has become a part of music festivals like AfroPunk and has spread to Crown Heights, where it is called Berg'n, and even as far as Jones Beach on Long Island, where it had its inaugural summer in 2014. See SMORGASBURG.

Williamsburg has become a mecca for people who are passionate about food. The sheer variety of cuisines and the inventiveness with which food is sourced and made there have placed Williamsburg at the forefront of New York's food scene. But for all of its popularity, Williamsburg has also been a source of controversy. Long-term residents complain that their neighborhood has been colonized by hipsters and foodies, and the scene's emphasis on artisanal products, veganism, and organic and local sourcing has been a point of derision. In part, this is an age-old issue of cultural conflict, of the new replacing the old and the old feeling an angry dislocation in response. But there is also the question of access and equality. In a city where so many New Yorkers struggle to afford food and grapple with food deserts, the density of so many kinds of high-quality and often very ex-pensive food in Williamsburg is one ingredient in the ongoing tension in New York City's history of the wealthiest and the most powerful displacing poorer residents.

See also BROOKLYN.

Lederer, Victor. *Williamsburg*. Charleston, S.C.: Arcadia, 2005.
Martin, Brett. "A Scene Grows in Brooklyn." *Bon Appétit*, July 13, 2010.
Sulzberger, A. G. "When Brooklyn Brewed the World." *New York Times*, July 10, 2009.

Katie Uva

Windows on the World

Windows on the World was the quintessential New York restaurant: it took diners to the edge. On the 107th floor of the World Trade Center's North Tower, trend-setting cuisine vied with 90-mile views. It was the most visible restaurant in the world and one of the highest grossing, almost $38 million one year. It lived up to its acronym: WOW.

Born in the bicentennial, 1976, Windows was a Cinderella story. With New York City on the verge of bankruptcy in 1975, critics reviled the Port Authority's $950 million World Trade Center complex, built on the bulldozed site of Washington Market, the country's major fruit and vegetable exchange. See WASHINGTON MARKET.

Windows became the jewel in the crown of spectacular New York restaurants created by consultants Joe Baum and Michael Whiteman and later leased to Hilton International. See BAUM, JOE. The menu by Barbara Kafka and James Beard, executed by French chef André René, went beyond fashionable continental cuisine and broke global ground. The Hors d'Oeuvrerie served *smørbrød* to sushi. At lunch, Windows was a private club with nominal dues, open even to women, unlike other Manhattan clubs at the time. The Grand Buffet ($7.95) contained Madras chicken curry, salumetti, six kinds of herring, and smoked chicken with Moroccan lemon relish. At dinner, the public feasted on quail eggs in tarragon aspic, frog legs in sorrel and cream, and pressed squab tabaka. Swiss pastry chef Albert Kumin, aided by his former Culinary Institute of America student Nick Malgieri, created dessert dazzlers that included a frozen amaretto soufflé.

After the February 26, 1993, bombing in the World Trade Center garage, the Port Authority put the restaurant up for bid again. Baum and Whiteman won again. Dishes like a show-stopping white clam risotto with poached lobster napped in green sauce were the creation of chef consultant Rozanne Gold, now a four-time James Beard Award winner. See GOLD, ROZANNE. In 1996, the new Windows, operated in conjunction with BE Windows Corporation, opened after a $25 million rebuild designed by Hugh Hardy, with graphics by Milton Glaser.

In 1997, Food Network star Michael Lomonaco became executive chef/director. His "American spirit" cuisine reflected America's new pride in its regional, creative, culinary identity: California artichoke salad, pan-fried Catskill trout, rib eye of American buffalo with Vidalia onions, and autumn pumpkin cheesecake. Wild Blue, the more intimate chophouse, served sautéed Hudson Valley foie gras with nectarine and plum compote, and American lamb T-bone chops. In The Greatest Bar on Earth, mixologist George Delgado, inspired by the view, created Ellis Island iced tea and the Lady Libertini martini. On Monday night, September 10, 2001, Dale DeGroff, now known as "King Cocktail," hosted a tequila tasting. See DEGROFF, DALE.

By Tuesday, September 11, 2001, Windows had a $1 million wine collection, and Kevin Zraly's wine school had educated fourteen thousand people. As seventy-nine Windows staff served breakfast to five hundred guests, terrorists flew commercial airliners into the towers.

When the Freedom Tower opened in 2014, there was no upscale restaurant at the top of the downtown skyscraper. The world feels the omission of the restaurant that New Yorkers said put diners close to heaven.

Morabito, Greg. "Windows on the World, New York's Sky-High Restaurant." Eater NY, September 11, 2013. http://ny.eater.com/2013/9/11/6547477/windows-on-the-world-new-yorks-sky-high-restaurant.

Greene, Gael. "The Most Spectacular Restaurant in the World." New York, May 31, 1976.

Linda Civitello

Wine and Winemaking

Although New York City is not a winemaking region, it is well noted for its density of influential restaurants with highly regarded wine lists and wine-focused retailers. That said, New York State is an up-and-coming wine region, with particular attention paid to the Long Island and Finger Lakes areas.

Although early Dutch settlers found wild grapevines growing when they arrived in New York, those high-acidity, low-sugar-content native grapes produced sour, harsh-tasting wine. As a result, vines needed to be brought over from the Old World; the earliest record of an attempt to grow European grapevines in New Netherlands dates from 1642. Those grapes intended for winemaking were planted in what is now Manhattan. Although those vines did not survive, later plantings managed to flourish elsewhere in the state. Eventually it was discovered that vinifera canes could be grafted onto native rootstock.

American colonists tended to make fruit (including grapes) into cider, perry (made from pears), or brandy. Winemaking in America did not thrive until much later (1800s). Until then, wine was imported from Europe, making it expensive and hard to obtain. As a result, it generally was consumed only by the rich and the elite.

A winegrower from southern France, Alphonse Loubat, emigrated to Brooklyn in the 1820s accompanied by several thousand three-year-old grapevines. He planted them on a slope above Gravesend Bay in the old Dutch village of New Utrecht. Of note, he also supplied vines to Nicholas Longworth in Ohio when Longworth was experimenting with European vines to build what would become America's first major commercial wine venture. But both Longworth and Loubat struggled desperately against diseases and bugs unknown in France. Loubat eventually sold his New Utrecht property for building lots and returned to France.

This would become a familiar story for wine in the New York City region; scores of winemakers would bravely try, and fail, to cultivate wine grapes. But eventually, success would be found farther north, in the Hudson Valley region. The Underhill plantation on Croton Point is considered New York's first successful commercial vineyard, planted in the 1820s. The Hudson Valley also is home to the nation's oldest winery, Brotherhood Winery, founded in 1839.

Today, New York's two largest and fastest-growing wine regions are the Finger Lakes and Long Island. Wineries in New York now produce 12 million cases of wine annually, making the Empire State the third-largest wine producer in the country, behind only

California and Washington State, according to a 2014 study conducted by Wines Vines Analytics. New York is a "cool climate" state in terms of grape growing, so the wine styles resemble those of northern Europe more than those of California. Today, a handful of urban wineries exist in Brooklyn and other boroughs, but the grapes are brought in from vineyards outside of New York City.

See also BEER and SPIRITS.

Adams, Andrew. "New York Ranks Third in Terms of Wine Production." *Wines & Vines*, May 12, 2014.

Figiel, Richard. *Circle of Vines: The Story of New York Wine*. Albany: State University of New York Press, 2014.

Pinney, Thomas. *A History of Wine in America: From Prohibition to the Present*. Berkeley: University of California Press, 2005.

Kara Newman

WNET

See TELEVISION, PUBLIC.

Wolf, Burt

See TELEVISION, PUBLIC.

Wolf, Clark

Clark Wolf (b. 1954) is the founder and president of Clark Wolf Company, a New York City–based consultancy providing services to the food, restaurant, and hospitality business. Wolf's involvement with food goes back to his roots in California where, after a period as a waiter, he worked in the burgeoning area of artisanal food retail, including at the Oakville Grocery. In 1982 he moved to New York City and a year later began lecturing to and consulting for specialty grocery stores, opening Clark Wolf Company in 1986.

Wolf has written for *Forbes* and *Cook's* magazines, serves as a contributing authority to *Food Arts*, and is the author of *American Cheeses* (2008) and coeditor of *101 Classic Cookbooks, 501 Classic Recipes* (2012). In 2009 he was inducted into the Who's Who of Food and Beverage in America, and he was the founder of the New York chapter of the American Institute of Wine & Food. See AMERICAN INSTITUTE OF WINE & FOOD.

Recognized by many of his peers as a trend spotter in the world of food, Wolf has acted as consultant to a range of national hotel chains, food and marketing boards, as well as many recognized New York City restaurants such as the Russian Tea Room and Smith & Wollensky. See RUSSIAN TEA ROOM.

His involvement with the New York City food scene is evident not only through his advisement to clients in the hotel and restaurant trade but also via educational initiatives, particularly his relationship with New York University's Department of Nutrition, Food Studies, and Public Health. Wolf has served as chair of the Advisory Board to the department and since 2005 has been the primary organizer and moderator of the Critical Topics in Food series, held at New York University's Fales Library and Special Collections. His involvement in these programs has helped facilitate debate and discussion around all aspects of food—its production, marketing, consumption, and history—and further the importance of food studies as a burgeoning area of both academic and consumer interest. See NEW YORK UNIVERSITY and FALES LIBRARY.

Wolf, Clark. *American Cheeses: The Best Regional, Artisan and Farmhouse Cheeses, Who Makes Them, and Where to Find Them*. New York: Simon & Schuster, 2008.

Charlotte Priddle

Women's Clubs

The women's club movement in Gotham was most visible in the decades between the Civil War and the 1920s, although some women's benevolent and reform associations predated the Civil War. Organized largely by middle-class New Yorkers, these postbellum clubs created a respectable space outside of the domestic sphere for women to learn from one another and share their concerns about the larger world.

Jane Cunningham Croly started Sorosis, the first prominent women's club in Manhattan, in 1868 as a response to the New York Press Club's refusal to initially include women at a dinner for Charles Dickens. It was a female-only club, establishing a homosocial environment for self-empowerment and attracting women from a variety of careers—journalism, law, education, and medicine among them. Controversial topics were kept to a minimum as Sorosis's goal was to create a cordial community of women. Much of the discussion instead revolved around culture and art. The club mobilized New York's restaurant scene, holding its bimonthly meetings at Delmonico's and in the process challenging the etiquette that prohibited women from attending restaurants without escorts. In 1873 Sorosis members spearheaded the creation of the Association for the Advancement of Woman, a national organization undergirded by the assumption that women's unique skills could resolve community problems.

The Brooklyn Woman's Club formed one year after Sorosis, in 1869 at the home of Anna C. Field. It stressed the importance of self-improvement, and its primary goal early on was to create a home for self-supporting women. Interests ranged from studying prisons to creating free kindergartens.

In 1890 Croly helped found the General Federation of Women's Clubs to connect clubwomen across the nation. The federation included clubs beyond those dealing exclusively with literature, shifting the movement's center of gravity from culture to reform. Unlike more radical activists who challenged the gender status quo, however, many clubwomen celebrated men's and women's different responsibilities in society as they discussed and implemented reforms, accepting what historian Karen Blair has called "domestic feminism" and municipal housekeeping. In 1894 women in the Empire State founded the New York State Federation of Women's Clubs and Societies. By the end of the nineteenth century the clubs within New York City dominated this new federation: twenty-nine from Brooklyn and thirty-six from Manhattan out of a total of 186 clubs registered statewide. Nearly a decade later, the New York City Federation of Women's Clubs organized to strengthen the ties between clubs within the metropolis.

Gotham's clubs revolved around an array of themes. At the end of the century, Brooklyn claimed the greatest number of literary clubs within the New York State Federation. Other groups served as alumnae clubs, such as the Associate Alumnae of the Packer Collegiate Institute in Brooklyn, while some focused on helping working-class women. The National Society of New England Women tapped into Americans' growing genealogical interests in the late nineteenth century, restricting membership to those who could trace their roots back to New England. In a two-year time span, its membership leapt from eight to five hundred. A few remained strictly literary clubs, but many branched out into reform as the decades progressed.

A number of New York's clubs connected professional women. The Professional Woman's League, for instance, united the growing number of career women who made Gotham their home. It was one of the first women's clubs in New York to have its own clubhouse. Journalists and writers could participate in the Woman's Press Club, which also provided funds for members in distress, and nurses need only look to the Metropolitan Trained Nurses' Club for professional support.

Of those focused on urban reform, the Woman's Health Protective Association was particularly notable. Started in 1884, its first efforts concentrated on ridding the East Side of the odor emanating from slaughterhouses. It went on to demand a host of other reforms in everything from sanitation to education. The organization's work inspired the creation of Health Protective Associations elsewhere.

Several of these clubs were exclusive, some with daunting waiting lists and byzantine admission policies. At least one went so far as to develop a secret password and handshake to create a bond among members. Perhaps the most highbrow, the Colony Club constructed an elaborate clubhouse first on Madison Avenue and later on Park Avenue, which included everything from a swimming pool to private dining rooms. Members' last names spanned the elite alphabet—from Astor to Morgan to Whitney. The initial membership fee was a steep $150, followed by $100 annual dues.

Club life frequently included luncheons and dinners as well as teas. Some were held within individuals' homes. Other clubs took advantage of Gotham's restaurants, halls, and hotels. The Woman's Press Club, for instance, held Saturday afternoon teas in a room in Carnegie Hall. It also hosted a valentine party, complete with food, music, and creative valentines. The New York State Federation of Women's Clubs and Societies used Sherry's for its initial, organizational meeting. The New York City's Mothers' Club and the Woman's Press Club frequently held meetings at the Waldorf Astoria, and the Eclectic Club regularly hosted luncheons at Delmonico's.

While some club leaders were reluctant to challenge gender norms and Croly herself had originally hoped to keep suffrage and club work separate, women's clubs did create a safe space for female empowerment and thought by promoting a sense of community among women. Ultimately, in 1914, one year before the Empire State's first suffrage referendum and after years of division on the subject, the New York State Federation of Women's Clubs voted to endorse enfranchisement, helping to bring clubwomen's influence to bear on the question of political equality.

See also CLUBS; COLONY CLUB; DELMONICO'S; and GILDED AGE.

Blair, Karen J. *The Clubwoman as Feminist: True Womanhood Redefined, 1868–1914*. New York: Holmes & Meier, 1980.

Croly, J. C. *The History of the Woman's Club Movement in America*. New York: Allen, 1898.

Roberts, Ina Brevoort, ed. *Club Women of New York, 1906–1907*. New York: Club Women of New York Co., 1906.

Scott, Anne Firor. *Natural Allies: Women's Associations in American History*. Urbana: University of Illinois Press, 1991.

Lauren C. Santangelo

Women's Magazines

For sourcing recipes, cooking tips, and household advice, magazines directed at women have long been part of New York's culinary landscape. For decades, women's magazines were dominated by the Seven Sisters, a group of women's service magazines. (Their name came from the Greek myth of the Seven Sisters, Pleiades.) The Seven Sisters included *Better Homes and Gardens* (established in 1922), *Family Circle* (1932), *Good Housekeeping* (1885), *Ladies' Home Journal* (1873, folded in 2014), *McCall's* (1873, which in 2001 was folded into *Rosie* magazine, owned by celebrity Rosie O'Donnell, subsequently shuttered in 2002), *Redbook* (1903), and *Woman's Day* (1937). Most were published in New York City.

To be a food editor at a women's service magazine was a glamorous job. Perks included wonderful luncheons at the newest, best restaurants in Manhattan, with the "required" hat and a pair of white gloves, and junkets at home and abroad. The perks were great, but the salaries were not. Secretaries assisted in answering readers' mail, whether it was a question about how to plan a party, a problem with a recipe, or help finding a lost recipe. Much time was spent selecting just the right dish to be photographed for the editorial pages. Once all the recipes under consideration were made, the dishes were viewed by the photographer, the art director, and the stylist and only the most photogenic chosen for publication.

When the ad market flattened in the 1960s and competition appeared in the form of new magazines that targeted modern women, a shift took place. From 1960 to 1970, sales figures slipped, even though magazines had recharged themselves for a contemporary audience. So-called women's magazines included less food-focused content. At the same time, a growing number of magazines were established that focused exclusively on food but were not necessarily targeted to women alone.

Robert Stein, who edited *Redbook* and *McCall's* from 1965 to 1986 at a time of big changes for women and magazine circulations, kept up with the changes. He felt women were interested in substance that could relate to their lives, including issues like civil rights and peace, and he featured Dr. Martin Luther King Jr., Margaret Mead, Rachel Carson, and Dr. Benjamin Spock. Herbert Mayes, who had engaged Dr. Spock as his family's pediatrician, then brought Spock to *Good Housekeeping*. Stein was the last male editor of a women's magazine, and he considered himself a dinosaur.

Women's magazines must be credited as a "participating forum and democratizing force." Helen Gurley Brown's *Cosmopolitan* promoted the empowerment of women. New York female writers and modern magazine culture raised questions about what it meant to be a woman in the public eye, how gender roles would change because men and women were working together, and how the growth of the magazine industry would affect women's relationships to their bodies and minds.

Ladies Home Journal in 2012 was the first women's magazine to socialize its content, using reader-generated material for most of its articles and columns. As a result, amateur contributors added as much as the professionals to portray women and their life experiences. There was great excitement in 2012 about the *Journal* going into the new media. But some questioned whether this was new or whether it was doing something that had been done in magazines in the past. Actually this was the way women's magazines had been written in America. It was *Ladies Home Journal* that, in the 1890s, changed American magazines from being reader driven to being advertising driven, as we have today.

The *Journal*, with its collaboration of professional editors and amateur reader-writers, folded in 2014, but platishers—a mash-up of "publisher" and "platform"—carry on. *Condé Nast Traveler* opened its website to contributors. *Forbes* had done that a few years previously. The *New York Times* proclaimed that platishers were likely here to stay.

Today women's magazines and food magazines have diverged. Most "women's magazines," especially those targeted to younger women, no longer have any food content at all—and if they do, it is about restaurants and cocktails and culinary travel, not recipes to make at home. But now we see plenty of recipes in family-oriented women's magazines as well as fitness/diet and food magazines. In addition, the role of traditional print magazines has shifted as more recipe content has moved into digital-format apps and mobile content.

Carmody, Deirdre. "Identity Crisis for 'Seven Sisters.'" *New York Times*, August 6, 1990.

Finkel, Rebecca. "The Aging of the Seven Sisters." *Media Life*, July 1999. http://www.medialifemagazine .com:8080/news1999/july99/news1728.html.

Ives, Nat. "Seven Sisters Hold Ground While Newbies Dive." *Advertising Age*, May 14, 2009.

Newman, Judith. "Year of the Woman—Once Ticketed for Decline or Irrelevance, the Seven Sisters Have Recharged Themselves for a Contemporary Audience That Has Timeless Concerns." *AdWeek*, March 29, 1993.

Ward, David. "A Foodie Frenzy: A Taste for Food-Related Coverage Has Helped This Magazine Sector Hold Steady." *Direct Marketing News*, August 15, 2008.

Carol Brock

Woods, Sylvia

Sylvia Woods (1926–2012), born in the small tobacco-belt town of Hemingway, South Carolina, was the founder of Sylvia's, a family business and cultural institution in the Manhattan neighborhood of Harlem. Woods was known by the nickname "The Queen of Soul Food," a moniker prominently displayed across the restaurant awning.

Woods and her husband Joe became New Yorkers during the second phase of the Great Migration—the movement of southern blacks to the North in search of better opportunities and freedom from Jim Crow laws and violence. While "soul food" purveyors in the South were usually rural, small-scale, family operations run out of the living room or back porch, soul food restaurants in the North like Sylvia's could accommodate larger crowds, offering them the foods and atmosphere, smells and company that made them feel a sense of continuity and a little less homesick.

Her first job in a restaurant was shortly after her arrival in New York City at Johnson's Luncheonette in the 1950s. A few years later she bought the luncheonette, and over a fifty-year period she would expand it to encompass the whole block.

While Sylvia's neighbors Amy Ruth's, Miss Maude's Spoonbread, and Miss Mamie's Spoonbread Too as well as Marcus Samuelsson's Red Rooster have all made their mark on the definition and direction of soul food and Harlem's soul food community, Sylvia's long-standing presence speaks to a historical role unmatched by the others. Here, civil rights activists strategized, and a half-century of African American culture creators and creatives made business deals and collaborations that would shape the history of everything from congressional races to the empires of hip-hop moguls. While this is typical for long-held African American restaurants, the powerful position of being in Harlem at a great time of cultural change and historic achievement, from the march on Washington to the presidential election of Barack Obama, amplified Sylvia's as a cultural and culinary center where the issues of the day were consumed and digested right along with fried chicken, collard greens, black-eyed peas, chitterlings, cornbread, barbecued pork chops, peach cobbler, and sweet potato pie. When progressive civil rights activist Reverend Al Sharpton wanted to have a personal summit with conservative Fox News anchor Bill O'Reilly, he took him to Sylvia's.

Restaurants like Sylvia's do more than serve up the staples of soul. They represent regional traditions. New York's Great Migration drew largely from the southeastern seaboard—Maryland, Virginia, the Carolinas, Georgia, and Florida. Sylvia's okra and tomato gumbo, cowpeas and rice, fried whiting, and fish croquettes speak to a specific geography in the history of African American foodways. Sylvia's has also responded to the need of the community for healthier options, from vegetarian collard greens to herb-roasted chicken, fresh fish entrées, steamed vegetables, and lower-sodium offerings. After her death in 2012, the corner in front of her lounge at Lenox Avenue and 127th Street was named Sylvia Woods Way in honor of her career and culinary legacy in Harlem and beyond.

See also HARLEM and SYLVIA'S.

Fox, Margalit. "Food Restaurateur Is Dead at 86." *New York Times*, July 20, 2012.

"Woods, Sylvia." In *African American National Biography*, edited by Henry Louis Gates Jr. and Evelyn Brooks

Higginbotham. New York: Oxford University Press, 2008.

Woods, Sylvia, and family. *Sylvia's Family Soul Food Cookbook: From Hemingway, South Carolina, to Harlem.* New York: William Morrow, 1999.

Michael Twitty

World's Fair (1939–1940)

The New York World's Fair of 1939–1940 was an ambitious undertaking. Its creators, a combination of state and city officials, private businessmen, and heads of industry, hoped to generate an event as successful and prominent as the recent Century of Progress Exposition, which had taken place in Chicago in 1933. As such, the fair was designed on a grand scale, costing millions of dollars and drawing participants from twenty-three states, many major corporations, and nearly two dozen foreign nations.

The fair had many exhibitions and amusements to offer visitors, and most of these reflected one of two major themes: the supremacy of technology and the growing importance of internationalism. Food at the fair promoted these themes as well. While there were certainly plenty of places for fairgoers to have a hot dog or other commonplace snack (Childs, the leg-

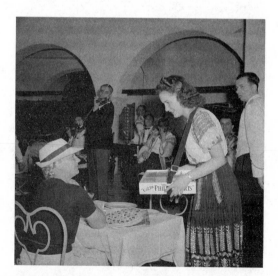

A cigarette girl at the 1939–1940 World's Fair. The fair encouraged visitors to sample cuisines from around the world, with pavilions showcasing the cultures and cuisines of foreign countries. WURTS BROTHERS/ MUSEUM OF THE CITY OF NEW YORK

endary restaurant chain, operated eighty hamburger stands at the site), the fair also encouraged its visitors to sample cuisines from around the world. At the same time, fairgoers were made deeply conscious of their identities as Americans, and the fair urged them to learn about and celebrate the country's increasingly industrial processes of food production and distribution and to allow these processes further entry into their domestic lives in the form of appliances.

Pavilions showcasing the cultures of foreign countries had been a feature of many earlier world's fairs, and the New York World's Fair continued that strategy. The fairgrounds were divided into seven distinct zones, with most of the international pavilions contained in the Government zone. There, visitors were invited to view the displays and sample the foods of countries from Albania to Venezuela. Many of the international pavilions featured their own foods alongside American foods or featured Americanized versions of international foods. However, there were many more traditional offerings, including sukiyaki at the Formosan Tea Room, reindeer at the Finnish Pavilion, and calf brain at the Polish Pavilion.

The breakout hit of the international restaurants was Le Restaurant Français, which sat atop the French Pavilion overlooking the Lagoon of Nations. The restaurant was considered upscale and its cuisine authentic, and it was extremely popular with fairgoers. After France fell to the Nazis during the fair's second season, some of Le Restaurant Français workers, led by maître d' Henri Soulé, remained in New York and opened Le Pavillon, a more permanent version of the restaurant they had operated at the French Pavilion. Le Pavillon remained open for thirty years and played an important role in fostering the American craze for French cuisine during the 1950s.

Alongside the many international food options, American food and foodways were also a significant presence at the fair. In addition to ubiquitous concessions, some food companies had their own pavilions. In fact, food was another zone at the fair, featuring companies like Heinz, whose pavilion was housed inside a large dome topped with an allegorical figure of Perfection; Schaefer, the Brooklyn brewery whose pavilion contained a 160-foot-long bar; and Swift and Co., where fairgoers could watch employees packing bacon.

The Food Zone was anchored by the Food Building, which was an abstract celebration of industrialized food production. Inside, a surrealistic mural depicted flying lobsters, roses growing in a desert, a cauliflower punching an insect, an avocado with jewels inside of it, and a clock running backward inside a tin can. All the images were intended to symbolize the ways in which modern science and technology had allowed humankind to defy and even transcend nature when it came to food production. Visitors received an even more concrete example at the Borden Dairy pavilion, where a machine called the Rotolactor placed cows on a kind of carousel that milked fifty of them simultaneously. Elsie the Cow became a widely recognized logo for Borden and was featured on numerous promotional materials for the fair.

Food was consciously on display at the Food Zone, of course, but it also played a central role in other parts of the fair. Futurama, a ride that took visitors on an aerial trip through the future world of 1960, contained detailed provisions for irrigation, farming, and transporting the food supply from farm to city. In addition to Futurama's large-scale concept of streamlined, automated farms as one ingredient in the vast landscape of the future, other areas focused on more acute aspects of food. The General Electric pavilion featured numerous kitchen appliances to make food preparation more efficient in individual households, and most of the food pavilions offered cookbooks to visitors.

The New York World's Fair of 1939 had several simultaneous goals. It hoped to foster cultural exchange and an understanding among its visitors that the modern world was smaller and more interconnected than ever before. It hoped to promote a heroic view of science and technology as forces for unwavering good and improvement. It also was an unabashedly commercial endeavor, seeking to attract visitors; to get those visitors to part with their money through exhibits, rides, and concessions; and to plant an allegiance to consumerism that would bear fruit for generations. Food was an important tool in carrying out each of these strategies. In a country that was just then beginning to emerge from nearly a decade of want, in a world where food shortages and food crises were a not-too-distant memory, the vision of a world of plenty, aided by science, industry, and international understanding, was deeply compelling.

See also CHILDS; LE PAVILLON; and WORLD'S FAIR (1964–1965).

Azzarito, Amy. "New York Haute Cuisine." Biblion, New York Public Library. http://exhibitions.nypl.org/biblion/worldsfair/fashion-food-famous-faces-pop-culture-fair/essay/essay-azzarito-french-food.
Gelernter, David. *1939: The Lost World of the Fair*. New York: Harper Perennial, 1996.
Morabito, Greg. "A Food Tour of the 1939 World's Fair." Eater NY, June 19, 2012. http://ny.eater.com/archives/2012/06/worlds_fair.php.
Wood, Andrew F. *New York's 1939–1940 World's Fair*. New York: Arcadia, 2004.

Katie Uva

World's Fair (1964–1965)

The New York World's Fair of 1964–1965 was a conscious effort by its organizers to capitalize on nostalgia for the 1939 World's Fair. As a result, the 1964 World's Fair bore many resemblances to the earlier fair. Like its predecessor, the second fair featured a wide variety of international pavilions that showcased the history and culture of foreign nations. As in 1939, in 1964 the fair once again was underwritten by a variety of corporate sponsors, whose pavilions aimed to entertain but also to encourage the public to have unwavering confidence in American business and industry.

In both of these settings, food once again was an effective tool for promoting the fair's ideals. Originally, there was supposed to be a five-story World of Food pavilion stationed immediately inside the main gate. The pavilion would be a massive tribute to American food culture, featuring a model kitchen and fifty exhibitors, including major corporations like Hershey and Pepsi-Cola. But because of funding mishaps, the pavilion was never completed and, in fact, was torn down just two weeks before it was set to open.

This error decentralized the American food presence at the fair. Some corporations, like Hershey, stationed themselves in the Better Living pavilion. Coca-Cola sponsored the "It's a Small World" ride, which later became a permanent fixture at Disney World. Many of the companies that had planned to participate in the World of Food pavilion simply were left out of the fair.

As in 1939, there were plenty of standard concessions scattered throughout the fair. But the 1964 World's Fair was characterized by a new cosmopolitanism and a new affordability. Another major departure from 1939 was that, in part because the dispute with the Bureau of International Expositions meant many European nations did not participate and in part because of global political shifts that had occurred after World War II, the international pavilions and consequently the food offered to fairgoers was not as Eurocentric as it had been in 1939. Africa as a continent had its own pavilion, as did a handful of individual African nations. The Philippines and Thailand were also represented. The fair introduced the cuisines of these regions to many Americans for the first time.

But without a doubt the single most successful culinary offering at the Fair was the Belgian waffle. Originally advertised as the "Bel-Gem Waffle," it had premiered at the Brussels Expo in 1958 and had also appeared at the Seattle World's Fair in 1962. But it took off at the New York World's Fair and has been heavily associated with it ever since, as well as being embraced in America as a street food.

Many have commented on the 1964 fair as a pivotal moment for American culture, the last moment of widespread trust in corporations and technology. Because the culture shifted so dramatically after the fair, it is tempting to be dismissive of its message. But in a way that was perhaps less intentional, the fair did anticipate the future. In its embrace of the culture and foods of the Global South, it reflected the new wave of immigrants that was just beginning to reshape America in the mid-1960s. In its promotion of portable, low-cost, culturally diverse types of food, it introduced a food culture that continues to pervade America today.

See also POST–WORLD WAR II (1945–1975) and WORLD'S FAIR (1939–1940).

Barber, Casey. "The Culinary Impact of the 1964 World's Fair." *Gourmet Live* (blog), January 4, 2012. http://www .gourmet.com/food/gourmetlive/2012/010412/ the-culinary-impact-of-the-1964-worlds-fair.html.
Cotter, Bill, and Bill Young. *The 1964–1965 New York World's Fair*. New York: Arcadia, 2004.
Samuel, Lawrence R. *The End of the Innocence: The 1964–1965 New York World's Fair*. Syracuse, N.Y.: Syracuse University Press, 2010.

Katie Uva

World War I

The First World War (1914–1918) broke out in Europe in July 1914. The war affected New York City well before the United States entered the conflict on April 6, 1917. For decades prior to World War I, Great Britain, Belgium, and Germany had found it more economical to import food than to produce it domes-

tically. When the hostilities broke out, food became central to the countries involved in the fighting. Almost overnight, European nations began ordering unprecedented quantities of food from the United States. Although American farmers stepped up production, food prices rose in the United States, including New York City.

New Yorkers were soon forced to pay record prices for basics such as flour, potatoes, cabbage, onions, carrots, butter, cheese, and poultry. The added expense was a tremendous hardship for the city's working poor, and as prices continued to escalate, hundreds of thousands of New Yorkers faced starvation. On February 19, 1917, an estimated three thousand women in Brownsville and Williamsburg, Brooklyn, rioted to protest inflated food prices, torching peddlers' pushcarts and stands. On Manhattan's East Side, people boycotted high-priced grocery stores. Violence continued throughout February and into March, with thousands of New Yorkers engaging in demonstrations. In March, many poultry dealers closed and launched a boycott of wholesalers as a result of rapid price increases. The demonstrations were easily controlled, but the problem of high prices remained.

To help the city deal with food shortages, public officials encouraged New Yorkers to eat more rice in place of wheat and other grain needed for the war effort and to replace meat with milk or eggs. But most New Yorkers resisted these recommendations. President Woodrow Wilson appointed Herbert Hoover as Food Administrator. Hoover requested voluntary price restrictions but later set prices for basic foodstuffs to prevent war profiteering. In January 1918 Hoover asked Americans to observe one meatless day, two porkless days, and two wheatless days each week. There were voluntary "meatless Tuesdays" and "sweetless Saturdays." Tuesdays and Saturdays were to be "porkless." On all days the public was asked to have at least one completely meatless and wheatless meal. These voluntary restrictions were observed by most restaurateurs and by many New Yorkers.

New York City had a large German American population, some of whom supported Germany before the United States entered the war. A wave of anti-German feeling swept the city. German restaurants and other food-related businesses suffered. Many of the city's breweries and distilleries were German owned. When the United States declared war on Germany on April 6, 1917, opportunistic prohibition advocates denounced the "pro-German brewers and liquor dealers" as "a disloyal combination." Distillers were also labeled "unpatriotic" for using grain needed for the war effort.

Under the circumstances, it was difficult for German Americans in New York to counter these charges. In August 1917 Congress passed the Food and Fuel Control Act (Lever Act), which banned the use of foodstuffs in the production of whiskey and gin for the duration of the war and restricted brewing as a way to conserve grain. Over the objections of most New Yorkers, the U.S. Senate and House passed a national prohibition amendment—the Eighteenth Amendment—in late 1917, although it would not go into effect until three-quarters of the states approved it.

New Yorkers were exhorted to grow and preserve their own fruits and vegetables, and many did. Bakers and homemakers were encouraged to bake bread using at least 20 percent of cereals other than wheat. New Yorkers complied with the request, and soon "Victory Bread" was the only kind available at bakeries, grocery stores, and restaurants. Pastries, cakes, pie, waffles, and other flour-based foods were also required to be made with 20 percent nonwheat flour.

When the war ended in November 1918, New Yorkers rejoiced. Restrictions were eliminated, food prices declined, and except for the brewing and distilling industries, the city's culinary scene regained a semblance of normality. In January 1919 the requisite number of states ratified the Eighteenth Amendment, and national Prohibition became the law of the land a year later. Dining in New York would never be quite the same.

See also PROHIBITION.

Hayden-Smith, Rose. *Sowing the Seeds of Victory: American Gardening Programs of World War I.* Jefferson, N.C.: McFarland, 2014.

Andrew F. Smith

World War II

The Second World War (1939–1945) changed the way New Yorkers ate, both during and after the war. Even before the United States entered the fighting in December 1941, the city's food supply was curtailed: imports from Germany, Italy, France, and other European nations disappeared as the British navy imposed a blockade of Axis-controlled countries. New York families changed their eating habits as even common foods became unavailable. Some people who employed domestic help lost their cooks and other staff

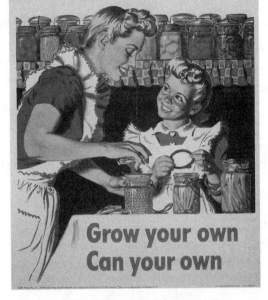

A poster from the Office of War Information. During World War II the shortage of canned goods caused a gardening initiative, encouraging New Yorkers to grow their own food for consumption to save the cans for the soldiers who needed them more. ALFRED PARKER, 1943, OFFICE OF WAR INFORMATION

to the armed forces or war-related jobs and had to become self-sufficient in the kitchen.

The availability of canned goods in grocery stores declined as metal was commandeered for the ongoing military buildup in the United States; metal goods were also being shipped to allied countries. In 1942, canned goods became scarce. To replace canned fruits and vegetables, New Yorkers planted "victory gardens" in parks, in vacant lots, in playgrounds, on rooftops, and in outer-borough backyards. During the war, New Yorkers established an estimated 450,000 such gardens, growing strawberries, asparagus, peas, beets, carrots, lettuce, radishes, broccoli, Swiss chard, corn, onions, cucumber, beans, and many other vegetables. Tomatoes were planted in Rockefeller Plaza, and beanpoles wrapped in leaves and tendrils were visible on penthouses.

During the war, many New Yorkers volunteered for or were drafted into the armed services, and soldiers and sailors from all over the country came through the city on their way overseas. Canteens were set up for military personnel, and female volunteers prepared cakes and sandwiches which were served with coffee, milk, and, when available, fresh fruit. One canteen in Brooklyn served fourteen thousand servicemen in a single month in 1942.

After the United States entered the war, the U.S. Office of Price Administration froze food prices and set up a rationing system. Beginning in January 1942 "Rationing for Victory" went into effect: over time, restrictions were placed on purchases of meat, sugar, coffee, grains, butter, cooking oil, cheese, canned goods, and some other processed foods. There were no restrictions on poultry, organ meats, or fish. Rationing for some foods, such as wheat, which was sent to Europe to feed wartorn nations and refugees, continued until 1947.

The city responded to these culinary changes in unusual ways. German restaurants in Yorkville stopped serving sauerkraut, renaming it "liberty cabbage" to signal their owners' patriotism. Macy's sold baby chicks and rabbits with incubators and instructions on how to raise and prepare the animals for the table. Organizations offered courses on how to feed a family while dealing with rationing. The *New York Times* and other city newspapers published recipes that addressed the new culinary realities.

The lack of beef was a particular problem that was not easily resolved. In October 1942 New York City's mayor, Fiorello La Guardia, declared optional "meatless Tuesdays," asking city hotels and restaurants to voluntarily give up serving beef, pork, veal, and lamb on Tuesdays. Restaurants offered a variety of nonmeat items, such as pancakes, vegetarian cutlets, nut burgers, eggs, and vegetables. Even when meat was available it was organ meats—liver, brains, sweetbreads—not the more familiar choice cuts. Despite La Guardia's request and compliance by many restaurants, the city's meat supply continued to dwindle. In January 1945 La Guardia made meatless Tuesdays mandatory for restaurants and required grocery stores to refrain from selling meat two days a week. See LA GUARDIA, FIORELLO.

Sugar was generally unavailable after the Japanese military occupied the Philippines, although some sugar was imported from the Caribbean during the war. Chocolate, another import, was also in short supply, and most of it was destined for military rations. Salty snacks, such as potato chips and peanuts, became much more popular during the war and remained so when the war ended.

During rationing there was a thriving black market in New York City for flour, spices, wine, and eggs. Some merchants did a lively business in black market foods. As leaders of New York women's organizations told the director of the Office of Price Administration, when wives and mothers could not buy food in grocery stores, they had no choice but to turn to the black market to feed their families.

Another serious problem was the shortage of workers. With men going off to serve in the armed forces, women took their places, and they were soon the majority of the staff in grocery stores and food-production industries. Waitresses outnumbered waiters in restaurants, diners, and other mid-price eateries. Many employees worked overtime, and as there were few consumer goods on the market, they socked away some savings.

The war years were particularly good ones for the city's restaurants. The Horn & Hardart automats thrived, as did cafeterias, such as Childs and Schrafft's. Le Pavillon, a haute cuisine offshoot of the French pavilion at the 1939 World's Fair, was launched in October 1941, and despite food shortages, it flourished throughout the war, becoming one of America's most prestigious restaurants. From 1939 to 1946 restaurant sales in New York quadrupled. When the war ended, restaurant profits soared even more: New Yorkers wanted to reward themselves for the hardships of the previous years, and many had savings that they were eager to spend, now that there was something to spend it on.

See also CHILDS; LE PAVILLON; POST–WORLD WAR II (1945–1975); SCHRAFFT'S; and VICTORY GARDENS.

Bentley, Amy. *Eating for Victory: Food Rationing and the Politics of Domesticity*. Urbana: University of Illinois Press, 1998.

Diehl, Lorraine B. *Over Here! New York City during World War II*. New York: Smithsonian/HarperCollins, 2010.

Andrew F. Smith

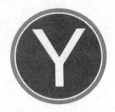

Yiddish Rialto

See RESTAURANTS.

Yonah Schimmel Knish Bakery

The Yonah Schimmel Knish Bakery has stood on Houston Street, between First and Second Avenues, since 1910. The establishment, said to have begun as a pushcart circa 1890, took its name from Yonah (or Yoineh) Schimmel, a Romanian-born teacher of religion and Hebrew who partnered with his cousin, Joseph Berger. From 1912 Berger ran Schimmel's with his wife Rose Berger née Schimmel (the name is written with and without a "c"). Their descendants operated it through the mid-1970s, when, on Sundays the hoi polloi flocked to the then-dilapidated neighborhood to wait in line at the shop. In 1995 the shop was implicated in a loan-sharking scheme.

Actor Fyvush Finkel recorded a Yiddish-language radio ad for Schimmel's in the 1930s, reinforcing the bakery's ethnic appeal. In the 1940s folklorist Nathan Ausubel called it "a landmark, just as recherché as the Stork Club or 21." Artists have immortalized Schimmel's and its iconic yellow and blue sign. Hedy Pagremanski captured it in a 1976 oil painting, accessioned into the collection of the Museum of the City of New York. Max Ferguson painted the shop's portrait in 1993. In 2013 sculptor Randy Hage constructed a highly detailed one-twelfth-scale diorama of the storefront at 137 East Houston Street.

Inside, Schimmel's is a gallery of nostalgia, complete with a dumbwaiter, newspaper clippings, and autographed photos that line the walls. Notebooks on the formica tables harbor the reminiscences of visitors from Germany, France, and Japan. In 2002, the reopening of the neighboring Sunshine Theater signaled the return of knishes as a movie-time snack.

Woody Allen's 2009 comedy *Whatever Works* featured Schimmel's, and Larry David, whose character described knishes as delicious things ("I don't *want* to know what's in them") he has consumed for six decades. In 2015 flavors on offer included potato, kasha (buckwheat groats), cabbage, jalapeno cheddar, and chocolate cheese, in addition to a menu of soups, kugel, and egg creams. The shop is now owned by Alex Wolfson and his daughter Ellen Anistratov, professed relatives of Schimmel who coined the motto "One world. One taste. One knish."

See also KNISH and MRS. STAHL'S KNISHES.

Ausubel, Nathan. "Hold Up the Sun! Kaleidoscope: The Jews of New York," first draft, Works Progress Administration Historical Records Survey: Federal Writers' Project, Jews of New York, New York Municipal Archives, microfilm no. 176, box 7, folder 243, 21–25.

Roberts, Sam. "Celebrating the Freshest 100-Year-Old Knish." *City Room* (blog), *New York Times*, January 13, 2010. http://cityroom.blogs.nytimes.com/2010/01/13/knish.

Yonah Schimmel Knish Bakery website: http://www.knishery.com

Silver, Laura. *Knish: In Search of the Jewish Soul Food.* Waltham, Mass.: Brandeis University Press, 2014.

Laura Silver

Yorkville

Yorkville is a neighborhood on Manhattan's Upper East Side whose boundaries are Seventy-Second

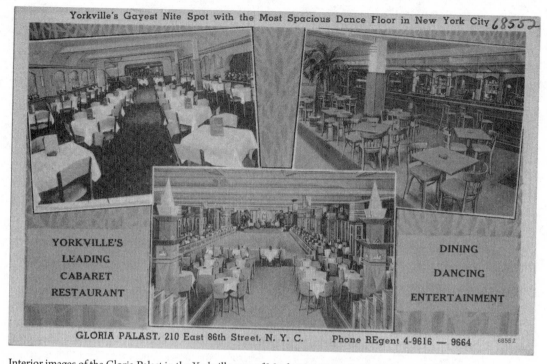

Yorkville's Gayest Nite Spot with the Most Spacious Dance Floor in New York City 6855 2

YORKVILLE'S
LEADING
CABARET
RESTAURANT

DINING
DANCING
ENTERTAINMENT

GLORIA PALAST, 210 East 86th Street, N. Y. C.   Phone REgent 4-9616 — 9664   68552

Interior images of the Gloria Palast in the Yorkville area of Manhattan. It was known for its spaciousness, which was conducive to lively crowds. BOSTON PUBLIC LIBRARY, TICHNOR BROTHERS COLLECTION

Street (south), Third Avenue (west), Ninety-Sixth Street (north), and the East River (east). Historically, Yorkville was an ethnic enclave for German, Irish, Czech, Hungarian, and other Eastern European immigrants. See GERMAN; IRISH; and HUNGARIAN. However, in recent decades, Yorkville's immigrant culture has largely disappeared as longtime residents left the area.

In the last decades of the nineteenth century, German Americans trickled into Yorkville from Kleindeutschland, the Lower East Side enclave where they had settled earlier in the century. See KLEINDEUTSCHLAND. This shift picked up speed in 1904 when the *General Slocum*, a steamship ferry carrying a thousand of Kleindeutschland's residents, sank and most onboard perished. After the disaster, many moved to Yorkville, cementing its place as the center of German American culture in New York City. The newer Eastern European groups followed the Germans' lead and moved to Yorkville as well.

In Yorkville's heyday, the German, Czech, and Hungarian communities all had areas of concentration, where their businesses and cultural centers could be seen. Eighty-Sixth Street was known as "German

Broadway" or "Sauerkraut Boulevard," with German restaurants and delicatessens such as Maxl's, the Bavarian Inn, Kleine Konditerei, Cafe Geiger, and Bremen House peppering the street east of Third Avenue. Every September, the Steuben Parade marched down Eighty-Sixth Street, filled with proud German Americans wearing traditional costumes on floats and riding horses or marching on foot. People would go to Elk Candy for marzipan and to Karl Ehmer's Butcher Shop for bratwurst.

The Hungarians clustered around Seventy-Ninth Street, while the Czechs dominated Seventy-Second Street. They had their cultural landmarks as well, and some of them have survived. For example, the Sokol New York Hall athletic club is still in existence, as well as the Jan Hus Presbyterian Church with its Neighborhood House, a center of Czech social activity. Unfortunately, the restaurants and bars from the earlier decades of the twentieth century are gone, with one exception: that of the Yorkville Coffee Mill, a Hungarian cafe with a secluded patio where goulash and open-faced sandwiches dominate the menu.

Yorkville held perhaps less significance for the Irish since they historically have congregated in several neighborhoods throughout New York City, for example, Five Points (now Chinatown) and Hell's Kitchen. See FIVE POINTS and HELL'S KITCHEN. However, there are still several Irish pubs in Yorkville, including Finnegan's Wake on First Avenue and Dorrian's Red Hand Restaurant on Second Avenue, and until the late 1990s the St. Patrick's Day Parade terminated at Eighty-Sixth Street and Third Avenue, hinting at the area's importance to the Irish American community.

Twenty-first-century Yorkville bears witness to continued attempts to preserve the neighborhood's German and Eastern European heritage in the face of gentrification. In 2007 a proposal put forth by the German American Steuben Parade Committee to change East Eighty-Sixth Street to General von Steuben Way was rejected by the local community board. However, Heidelberg Restaurant (with its lederhosen-wearing waiters) continues to draw fans of German sausages and bock beer. The Czech government–financed renovation of the Bohemian National Hall on Seventy-Third Street includes an upscale restaurant called Hospoda (the Czech word for "pub" or "beer hall"). And Andre's Café and the Yorkville Meat Emporium (aka the Hungarian Meat Market) attract people looking for Hungarian cuisine.

At the same time, restaurants from many other disparate cultures are making a name for themselves in Yorkville. Common cuisines such as Italian, Japanese, and Indian are well represented in the neighborhood. See ITALIAN and JAPANESE. Restaurants featuring less common cuisines can be found there as well, such as Alsatian, Peruvian, Persian, and Argentinian. As for food markets, German butcher Schaller & Weber and German bakery Glaser's Bake Shop are still in operation; however, they now have to compete with mainstream supermarket chain Fairway, as well as a branch of Whole Foods. See FAIRWAY MARKET; SCHALLER & WEBER; WHOLE FOODS; and SUPERMARKETS.

See also MANHATTAN and UPPER EAST SIDE.

Gariti, Elizabeth. "What Happened to Germantown?" Uppereast.com. http://www.uppereast.com/germantown.

Hooker, Richard J. *Food and Drink in America: A History*. New York: Bobbs-Merrill, 1981.

Nadey, Stanley. *Little Germany: Ethnicity, Religion and Class in New York City, 1845–1890*. Urbana: University of Illinois Press, 1990.

"Walking Tour: Czech and Slovak Yorkville." *Slavs of New York* (blog), July 6, 2008. http://nycslav.blogspot.com/2008/07/walking-tour-czech-and-slovak-yorkville.html.

Karl Peterson

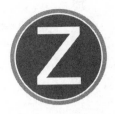

Zabar's

Zabar's iconic orange and white logo, emblazoned across a Broadway block on Manhattan's Upper West Side, has become the symbol of a quintessential New York institution. In eighty years, Zabar's has transformed from neighborhood grocery to New York destination to internationally recognized brand.

The store's history begins in 1921 or 1922, when the first member of the Zabar family, a sister, immigrated to the United States from Ostrapolia, Russia. An immigrant from what is now the Ukraine, Louis Zabar first operated a family grocery store in Brooklyn in the early 1930s. In 1934 he started what is now Zabar's, opening a 22-foot-wide shop along Broadway at West Eightieth Street. In 1936 he was joined by Lillian Teit, from the same Ukrainian village, who would go on to become the matriarch of the Zabar family.

Uniting his business sense with her culinary abilities, the couple first operated a deli in Brooklyn and then moved the business to the Upper West Side. Zabar's slowly grew during the first decade as Louis and Lillian opened up four delicatessen and appetizing stores between Eightieth Street and 110th Street.

In 1950, following Louis Zabar's death, Lillian and her three sons—Saul, Stanley, and Eli—inherited the four stores and sold all but the one on Eightieth Street and Broadway. From that time on, although Zabar's expanded in square footage, sales volume, and offerings, the family elected not to open additional locations, even rejecting David Liederman (of David's Cookies) and his 1985 offer to purchase and turn Zabar's into a national franchise. The original Zabar's occupied one small storefront on Broadway at

Eightieth Street. From 1979 through 1998 the family acquired adjacent storefronts, creating a Zabar's that now occupies eighteen thousand square feet of Manhattan's prime Upper West Side real estate.

Like many entrepreneurial businesses, Zabar's was handed down across generations. However, interestingly, a nonfamily member became a full partner in just the second generation. Murray Klein came to America in 1950, having survived World War II. Elevating from Zabar's janitorial work to business partner during the 1960s, Murray became Zabar's public face, until a few years before his death in 2007.

Over the decades, Zabar's has changed a great deal yet, in some ways, has remained the same. During the early years Zabar's relied on the neighborhood residents, while today much of Zabar's clientele travels from beyond New York City. Through an extensive mail-order business, Zabar's has gained global exposure yet still maintains its liberal Jewish Upper West Side identity, which began in the mid-1950s as upwardly mobile Jews moved into the once Irish Catholic area. Just as the neighborhood was overwhelmingly Jewish, so were Zabar's clientele and employees. During the 1950s Zabar's was staffed exclusively with Jewish employees, and the customer base, virtually all Jewish, came mostly from Manhattan, Brooklyn, or the Bronx. As is typical in New York City, the predominantly Jewish Upper West Side slowly changed its demographic picture and so did the Zabar's clientele and staffing. While Zabar's still has a culturally Jewish allure, few current employees beyond management are in fact Jewish. Behind the counter line, Chinese and Dominican men and women skillfully slice sable, lox, and sturgeon—once the domain solely of Jewish men.

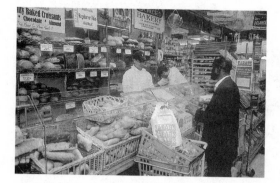

The many options at the breadcounter of Zabar's, on the Upper West Side. PHOTO BY JOE ZARBA

As Zabar's employees and clientele have evolved, so have the offerings. Smoked fish still holds center stage, but now it sits alongside new additions. According to Saul Zabar, some of the traditional food itself has changed. Originally, the lox was salty, but now, to accommodate changing food preferences and health issues, they use a less salty processing technique.

As Zabar's evolved, its status as a New York institution grew, in large part because of the increasing media coverage. The "Malassol Caviar and Beluga Caviar War of 1983" began as the Beluga caviar supply decreased and, unable to meet holiday consumer demand, Zabar's set a price war against the Macy's Cellar, which at the time had cornered the caviar market. Zabar's lowered its price, which in turn forced Macy's to do the same. Prices continued to plummet, with the public appreciating caviar bargains and Zabar's relishing press coverage. This "war" followed an earlier one in 1976 when Zabar's sold Cuisinarts well below market price. Cuisinart, afraid of tarnishing its image, refused to ship to Zabar's unless it increased the price. Zabar's successfully sued Cuisinart. Both the "Beluga Caviar War" and the "War of the Cuisinarts" attracted positive public relations coverage for Zabar's and helped the store garner a larger market share and consumer loyalty.

Zabar's media coverage continually propels the store into the local, national, and global spotlight. Featured in films and television (*You've Got Mail, Friends, Sex and the City, The Colbert Report, Law & Order, Gossip Girl, 30 Rock, Seinfeld*, etc.), Zabar's upholds institutional status. But for Upper West Side residents, Zabar's is theirs. As novelist and cultural critic Nora Ephron once espoused in the *New York Times*, "Zabar's is the ultimate West Side institution. It is messy and middle-class; it gives the impression of disorganization without being disorganized; it gives the appearance of warmth without being truly friendly.... Zabar's perfectly embodies New York's most basic emotion, unrequited love. I love Zabar's more than Zabar's loves me."

See also GROCERY STORES and UPPER WEST SIDE.

Berg, Jennifer Schiff. "From Pushcart Peddlers to Gourmet Take-Out: New York City's Iconic Foods of Jewish Origin, 1920 to 2005." PhD diss., New York University, 2006.

Ephron, Nora. "Eat, Drink, and Be Merry." *New York Times*, November 4, 1984.

Katz, Susan, Murray Klein, Saul Zabar, and Stanley Zabar. *Zabar's Deli Book*. New York: Hawthorn, 1979.

Zabar's. "Our History" (store brochure). New York: Zabar's, 2001.

Jennifer Schiff Berg

Zagat, Tim and Nina

Tim and Nina Zagat are the originators of the Zagat survey, a ranking and aggregation of popular opinions about restaurants. For many years, the Zagat (rhymes with "the cat") survey was best known as a slim, pocket-sized red book, which New Yorkers referred to religiously for restaurant reviews. The Zagat survey has expanded well beyond just New York to international coverage—and well beyond just print format as well.

Tim Zagat grew up in Connecticut and Central Park West and Nina, on Long Island. The couple met at Yale Law School, married, and discovered the joys of French cuisine when, as corporate lawyers, their respective law firms sent them to Paris, where the couple lived for two years.

While in Paris, they discovered France's *Guide Michelin* and created a kind of crib sheet—the genesis of their idea—rating their favorite Paris restaurants for friends. When the couple returned to New York, they created what would become the original Zagat survey, which required participants to fill out a questionnaire evaluating food, décor, and service at each restaurant they had been to in the past year on a 1 to 3 scale. (The current iteration of the survey uses a similar questionnaire.) This system was deliberately similar to the rating system used by Michelin; indeed, quoted in *New York* magazine, Tim Zagat said outright, "I want to create the *Michelin Guide to the United States*."

The Zagat survey started out in 1979 as a mimeographed sheet—evaluating seventy-five restaurants—that Tim and Nina distributed to friends. At a dinner party with friends, one of the guests had complained about the restaurant reviews of a major newspaper. Everyone agreed that the paper's reviews were unreliable. Tim subsequently suggested taking a survey of their friends, who became the core of that first survey.

Although it started out as a hobby, before long it consumed more and more of their spare time and their budget. Eventually, Nina suggested turning the hobby into a business—if not to make real money from it, at least to recoup their expenses. Only seventy-five hundred copies of their first edition—in 1983, rating 317 restaurants—were printed.

At first, the couple published the survey themselves, driving boxes of books to New York bookstores. After a cover story in *New York* magazine in late 1985, sales took off, reaching seventy-five thousand per month the following year.

In 2011 the Zagats sold the guidebook empire for a reported $125 million to Google. They continue to operate the business from Google's New York office.

See also RESTAURANT REVIEWING.

Gardner, Ralph, Jr. "Dishing with the Zagats." *Wall Street Journal*, November 4, 2014.
McMath, Quita. "The Food Spooks: Previewing the Insiders' Guide to New York Restaurants." *New York* (November 25, 1985): 60–74.

Kara Newman

Zeppole

Zeppole, as they are served in New York, are fried, yeast-based fritters, thickly dusted with sugar, about the size of a ping-pong ball. In many New Yorkers' minds they are firmly linked to such Italian American events as Mulberry Street's autumn San Gennaro street festival. The presence of fritters at these occasions is noted as far back as 1903, when a *New York Times* correspondent to East Harlem's festival of the Madonna of Mount Carmel described "Boys at the doors of bakeshops [hawking] 'Pizzarelli caldi'—hot pizarelli [*sic*]. The pizarello is a little flat cake of fried dough, probably the Neapolitan equivalent to a doughnut." It is possible the reporter mixed up the name (there seems to be no other reference to a similarly named fritter). What is certain is that Italians have a tradition of frying dough that goes back to Roman times.

Something called "zeppolle" appear in Bartolomeo Scappi's *Opera* (1570), but here the recipe refers to a sort of sweetened chickpea fritter. By the nineteenth century a Neapolitan understood a *zeppola* (plural, *zeppole*) to mean a ring-shaped fritter made with a hot-water and flour dough. Zeppole di San Giuseppe were a more luxurious variant. This dough was made with choux pastry, and the resulting fried pastry was filled with pastry cream. Italian-American pastry shops still make these for the saint's March 19 feast day. The more common, street-food variety are formed from a thick batter that is essentially thinned pizza dough. Small blobs of this are dropped into fat, forming irregular lumps, which are finally rolled in sugar. They are greasy, slightly chewy, and irresistible when fresh. Much the same dough is used for many sorts of *fritelle* all over Italy. Naples has a savory version occasionally referred to as "zeppole," and Apulia makes a yeast doughnut with the same name. Nonetheless, the "zeppoles" (as Italian-Americans call them) found at New York's street fairs are now as American as pizza and biscotti.

See also DOUGHNUTS and ITALIAN.

Krondl, Michael. *Sweet Invention: A History of Dessert.* Chicago: Chicago Review, 2011.
"Quaint Italian Customs of Summer Festal Days; with Music, Gifts and Feasting the Denizens of Little Italy Pay Their Devotions to the Saints—Curious Phases of the Celebrations." *New York Times*, July 12, 1903.

Michael Krondl

DIRECTORY OF CONTRIBUTORS

Jillian Adams
PhD candidate, Central Queensland University, Victoria, Australia

Ken Albala
Professor of History, University of the Pacific

Kelly Alexander
Culinary instructor, Duke University; Consulting editor, *Saveur* magazine; food contributor to NPR's *The State of Things*

Nicholas Allanach
Director of Academic Operations, The New School

Gary Allen
Empire State College, State University of New York

Myra Alperson
Founder, Noshnews and Noshwalks, and author of *Nosh New York*

Ari Ariel
Assistant Professor and Faculty Coordinator for the Master of Liberal Arts in Gastronomy program, Boston University Metropolitan College

Babette Audant
Departments of Tourism and Hospitality and of Culinary Arts, Kingsborough Community College, City University of New York

Scott Alves Barton
PhD candidate, Food Studies, New York University

Emma Becker
The New School for Public Engagement

Amy Bentley
Associate Professor of Food Studies, New York University

Jennifer Schiff Berg
Clinical Associate Professor of Food Studies, New York University

Amy Besa
Owner, Purple Yam Restaurant (NYC and Malate, Manila), and coauthor of *Memories of Philippine Kitchens*

Warren Bobrow
Mixologist, chef, and writer; editor of culture, *Wild River Review*

Maggie E. Borden
Assistant Editor, Media & Publications, James Beard Foundation

Adee Braun
Freelance food history writer

Jennifer Brizzi
Food writer and cooking teacher

Carol Brock
Founder of Les Dames d'Escoffier International

Linda Amiel Burns
Restaurant entrepreneur, The Symphony Café and One Fifth Avenue Restaurant and Bar

Christine C. Caruso
Social, Behavioral and Administrative Sciences, Hostos Community College, City University of New York

Tracey Ceurvels
Freelance writer

Jim Chevallier
Food historian and author of *Après Moi, Le Dessert* and *August Zang and the French Croissant*

Simone Cinotto
University of Gastronomic Sciences, Turin, Italy

Linda Civitello
Author of *Cuisine and Culture: A History of Food and People*

Andrew Coe
Independent scholar and author of *Chop Suey: A Cultural of Chinese Food in the United States*

Francine Cohen
Editor in Chief/Consultant, *Inside F&B* (www.insidefandb.com)

Gerald Cohen
Professor of Arts, Languages, and Philosophy, Missouri University of Science and Technology

Kristie Collado
Department of Nutrition, Food Studies, and Public Health, New York University

Emily J. H. Contois
American Studies, Brown University

Dave Cook
EatingInTranslation.com

Suzanne Cope
English Department, Manhattan College

Lauren Coull
Nutrition, New York University

Tove K. Danovich
Food and agriculture journalist and editor

Lisa DeLange
Kingsborough Community College, City University of New York

Bob Del Grosso
Department of Hospitality and Sports Management, Drexel University

Cara De Silva
Writer, editor, and food historian

Mike DeSimone
Entertaining & Lifestyle Editor, *Wine Enthusiast* magazine

Jonathan Deutsch
Professor and Director, Culinary Arts and Food Science, Drexel University

Tracey Deutsch
Professor of History, University of Minnesota, and author of *Building a Housewife's Paradise: Gender, Politics, and American Grocery Stores in the Twentieth Century*

Michael Dietsch
Author of *Shrubs: An Old Fashioned Drink for Modern Times*

Carolyn Dimitri
Associate Professor of Food Studies, New York University

Hasia Diner
Paul S. and Sylvia Steinberg Professor of American Jewish History; Director, Goldstein-Goren Center for American Jewish History, New York University

Tim Donnelly
New York Post

Doug Duda
Director of Development, International Association of Culinary Professionals

Carol Durst-Wertheim
Kinsgsborough Community College, City University of New York

Megan Elias
Director, Center for Excellence in Teaching, Learning, and Scholarship, Borough of Manhattan Community College, City University of New York

Meryle Evans
Culinary historian, food and travel writer

Yolanda Evans
Freelance writer

Mark Russ Federman
Owner, Russ & Daughters

Rebecca Federman
Electronic Resources Coordinator, New York Public
Library

Jared Michael Guy Fernandez
MA candidate, Food Studies, New York University

Shayne Leslie Figueroa
Food Studies, New York University

Rachel Monet Finn
Writer, librarian, and food historian

Margaret Fiore
School of Writing, New School for Public Engagement

Polly Franchini
Editor of *Sicily: Culinary Crossroads* and *Puglia:*
A Culinary Memoir

Paul Freedman
Professor of History, Yale University

Richard Frisbie
Freelance writer and owner of Hope Farm Press
Bookshop

J. Anne Funderburg
Author of *Sundae Best: A History of Soda Fountains*

Ramin Ganeshram
Journalist, chef, and cookbook author

Rozanne Gold
Chef, journalist, cookbook author, and international
restaurant consultant

Mackensie Griffin
New York University alumna, Food Studies MA

Annie Hauck-Lawson
Coauthor of *Gastropolis: Food and New York City*

Ashley Hoffman
Senior Features Editor at Abrams Media and freelance
writer for newspapers and magazines

John Holl
Editor of *All About Beer Magazine* and author of
The American Craft Beer Cookbook

Tonya Hopkins
Food and drink writer and author of *Food for the Soul:*
Recipes from Harlem's Abyssinian Baptist Church

Alan Houston
Independent scholar

Alexandra Ilyashov
Fashion News Editor, Refinery29

Zilkia Janer
Professor of Global Studies and Geography,
Hofstra University

Saru Jayaraman
Restaurant Opportunities Centers United

Jeff Jenssen
Entertaining & Lifestyle Editor, *Wine Enthusiast*
magazine

Kimberly-Elizabeth Johnson
West Chester University of Pennsylvania

Cathy K. Kaufman
President, Culinary Historians of New York

Layla Khoury-Hanold
Food writer and blogger

Michele Kidwell-Gilbert
Chair, Archaeology Committee, The National Arts Club,
and Wortham Scholar-Writer, New York Public Library

Chi-Hoon Kim
PhD candidate, Anthropology, Indiana University
Bloomington

Bruce Kraig
Author of *Hot Dogs: A Global History*

Michael Krondl
Food historian and author of *Sweet Invention:*
A History of Dessert

Peter LaFrance
Publisher, BeerBasics.com

John T. Lang
Department of Sociology, Occidental College

Leeann Lavin
Author of *The Hamptons & Long Island Homegrown Cookbook*

Alexandra Leaf
Culinary historian and author of *The Impressionists' Table*

Marc P. Levy
Culinary historian

Walter Levy
Independent scholar

Vivian Liberman
Independent scholar

Asia Lindsay
TEDx screener at TED Conferences

Arthur Lizie
Author of "Food and Communication" in *Routledge International Handbook of Food Studies*; Professor of Communication Studies at Bridgewater State University

Cindy R. Lobel
Assistant Professor, Lehman College, City University of New York

Janice Bluestein Longone
Special Collections, Hatcher Library, University of Michigan

Michele Louis
The New School

Casey Man Kong Lum
William Paterson University

Andrea Lynn
Author of *Queens: A Culinary Passport—Exploring Ethnic Cuisine in New York City's Most Diverse Borough*

Dan Macey
Food stylist

Sherri Machlin
Author of *American Food by the Decades* and *Cooking the Books: A Year in Dishes*

Tawnya Manion
Culinary and Health Program Director, SMART University

Lidia Marte
Department of Sociology and Anthropology, University of Puerto Rico, Río Piedras Campus

Renee Marton
Author and Chef-Instructor, Institute of Culinary Education

Jeffrey A. Marx
Historian of cream cheese, rabbi of the Santa Monica Synagogue

Anne E. McBride
Director of the Experimental Cuisine Collective and coauthor of *Les Petits Macarons: Colorful French Confections to Make at Home*

James McWilliams
Professor of History, Texas State University

Mark McWilliams
English Department, United States Naval Academy

Kristina Mellegard
Culinary arts student

Anne Mendelson
Food historian, cofounder of the Culinary Historians of New York, and author of *Milk: The Surprising Story of Milk through the Ages*

Ted Merwin
Dickinson College

Christopher Mitchell
Adjunct professor of History and Women's/Gender Studies, Rutgers University-Newark, Hunter College at CUNY, and Pace University

Emerald Mitchell
The New School for Public Engagement

Georgette L. Moger
Freelance writer

Bill Moore
PushCartFoods.com

Marion Nestle
Paulette Goddard Professor of Nutrition, Food Studies, and Public Health, New York University

Jackie Newman
Editor-in-Chief, *Flavor and Fortune*

Kara Newman
Spirits Editor, *Wine Enthusiast* magazine

Joanne Nicholas
Writer and editor

Alexandra Olsen
New York University

René Alexander Orquiza Jr.
Lecturer and Assistant Director of Studies, History and
Literature, Harvard University

Eirik Osland
Professional Food Writing, The New School

Linda Pelaccio
Host, Heritage Radio Network

Karl Peterson
Author of *The Dairy Free Traveler* food blog

Hannah Petertil
Editor, Taste Savant

Barry Popik
Etymologist and Consulting Editor for *The Oxford
Encyclopedia of Food and Drink in America*

Lynne Posner
Freelance writer, editor, and food professional

Maricel E. Presilla
Culinary historian, restaurant owner, and author of *The
New Taste of Chocolate: A Cultural and Natural History of
Cacao with Recipes*

Charlotte Priddle
Fales Library and Special Collections, New York
University

Jeri Quinzio
Author of *Food on the Rails: The Golden Era of Railroad
Dining, Pudding: A Global History*, and *Of Sugar and
Snow: A History of Ice Cream Making*

Lara Rabinovitch
Coeditor of *Choosing Yiddish: New Frontiers of Language
and Culture*

Krishnendu Ray
Associate Professor of Nutrition and Food Studies,
New York University

Carl Raymond
Writer, educator, and member of the Culinary Historians
of New York

Timothy C. Ries
Director of Park Services, Friends of the High Line

Peter G. Rose
Independent scholar

Meryl Rosofsky
Department of Nutrition, Food Studies, and Public
Health, New York University

Valerie Saint-Rossy
Food writer and cookbook editor

Lauren C. Santangelo
Princeton Writing Program, Princeton University

Stephen Schmidt
Principal writer and researcher for the Manuscript
Cookbooks Survey

Amanda Schuster
Editor in Chief of The Alcohol Professor and freelance
contributing writer

Arthur Schwartz
Former restaurant critic and Executive Food Editor,
New York Daily News

Aren Seferian
Tufts University

Jessica Sennett
Food Studies, The New School

Melina Shannon-DiPietro
Director of High Line Food & Revenue Founding
Director of the Yale Sustainable Food Project

Laura Silver
Instructor, Department of Food Studies,
New School of Public Engagement, and Research Associate,
Hadassah-Brandeis Institute of Brandeis University

Daniel Bowman Simon
Doctoral Fellow, Food Studies, New York University

Robert Simonson
Journalist and author of *The Old-Fashioned*

Max P. Sinsheimer
Senior Editor, Oxford University Press

Bonnie Slotnick
Owner of Bonnie Slotnick Cookbooks

Alison A. Smith
History Department, Wagner College

Andrew F. Smith
Food Studies Department, The New School

Jane L. Smulyan
Freelance writer

Harley J. Spiller
Museum educator

Claire Stewart
Department of Hospitality Management, New York City College of Technology, City University of New York

Matthew Jaber Stiffler
Arab American National Museum

Alexandra J. M. Sullivan
PhD candidate, Geography/Earth and Environmental Sciences, CUNY Graduate Center, and Manager of Fresh Start Organic Eatery & Market

Marvin J. Taylor
Director, Fales Library Special Collections, New York University

Farha Ternikar
Author of *Brunch: A History*

Annette Tomei
Chef

Esther S. Trakinski
Lawyer and MA candidate, Food Policy and Systems, New York University

Michael Traud
Assistant Teaching Professor and Program Director, Hospitality and Tourism, Drexel University

Rosemary Trout
Culinary Science, Center for Hospitality and Sport Management, Drexel University

Reed Tucker
New York Post

Michael Twitty
Chef, author of the *Afroculinaria* food blog

Katie Uva
CUNY Graduate Center

Domenic Venuto
Independent food writer

Kimberly Wilmot Voss
Nicholson School of Communication, University of Central Florida

Scott Warner
Freelance food writer and President of theCulinary Historians of Chicago

Suzanne Wasserman
Director, Gotham Center for New York City History/ CUNY Graduate Center

Judith Weinraub
Independent writer and editor

Evan Weissman
Department of Public Health, Food Studies, and Nutrition, Syracuse University

Ariella Werden-Greenfield
Feinstein Center for American Jewish History, Temple University

Susan Sarao Westmoreland
Food Director, *Good Housekeeping*

Jan Whitaker
Independent scholar

Timothy R. White
History Department, New Jersey City University

Keith Williams
Freelance writer

Allie Wist
Food Studies Graduate Program, New York University

Khaled Younes
Food writer

Alexis Zanghi
Fellow, Creative Writing, University of Minnesota Twin Cities

Almaz Zelleke
Visiting Assistant Professor, New York University Shanghai

Thei Zervaki
Freelance writer, journalist, and translator

Jane Ziegelman
Author of *97 Orchard: An Edible History of Five Immigrant Families in One New York Tenement*

BIBLIOGRAPHY

General Works about New York City

Allen, Irving L. *City in Slang: New York Life and Popular Speech*. New York: Oxford University Press, 1993.

Anbinder, Tyler. *Five Points: The 19th-Century New York City Neighborhood That Invented Tap Dance, Stole Elections, and Became the World's Most Notorious Slum*. New York: Free Press, 2001.

Burrows, Edwin G., and Mike Wallace. *Gotham: A History of New York City to 1898*. New York: Oxford University Press, 1999.

Cantwell, Anne-Marie E., and Diana diZerega Wall. *Unearthing Gotham: The Archaeology of New York City*. New Haven, Conn.: Yale University Press, 2001.

Diehl, Lorraine B. *Over Here! New York City during World War II*. New York: Smithsonian, HarperCollins, 2010.

Erenberg, Lewis A. *Steppin' Out: New York Nightlife and the Transformation of American Culture*. Chicago: University of Chicago Press, 1981.

Freeland, David. *Automats, Taxi Dances, and Vaudeville: Excavating Manhattan's Lost Places of Leisure*. New York: New York University Press, 2009.

Goodfriend, Joyce D. *Before the Melting Pot: Society and Culture in Colonial New York City, 1664–1730*. Princeton, N.J.: Princeton University Press, 1992.

Haenni, Sabine. *The Immigrant Scene: Ethnic Amusements in New York, 1880–1920*. Minneapolis: University of Minnesota Press, 2008.

Jackson, Kenneth T., ed. *The Encyclopedia of New York City*. New Haven, Conn.: Yale University Press, 1995.

Jackson, Kenneth, and John B. Manbeck, eds. *The Neighborhoods of Brooklyn*. New Haven, Conn.: Yale University Press, 1998.

Jacobs, Jaap. *The Colony of New Netherland: A Dutch Settlement in Seventeenth-Century America*. Ithaca, N.Y.: Cornell University Press, 2009.

Janowitz, Meta F., and Diane Dallal, eds. *Tales of Gotham, Historical Archaeology, Ethnohistory and Microhistory of New York City*. New York: Springer, 2013.

Krohn, Deborah L., and Peter Miller, eds. *Dutch New York between East and West: The World of Margrieta van Varick*. New Haven, Conn.: Yale University Press, 2009.

Mayer, Grace M. *Once upon a City: New York from 1890 to 1910*. New York: Macmillan, 1958.

McKay, Ernest A. *The Civil War and New York City*. Syracuse, N.Y.: Syracuse University Press, 1990.

Mensch, Barbara. *South Street*. New York: Columbia University Press, 2007.

Morris, Lloyd R. *Incredible New York*. New York: Random House, 1951.

Reitano, Joanne R. *The Restless City: A Short History of New York from Colonial Times to the Present*. New York: Routledge, 2006.

Reitano, Joanne R. *The Restless City Reader: A New York City Sourcebook*. New York: Routledge, 2010.

Shorto, Russell. *The Island at the Center of the World: The Epic Story of Dutch Manhattan and the Forgotten Colony That Shaped America*. New York: Doubleday, 2004.

Spann, Edward K. *Gotham at War: New York City, 1860–1865*. Wilmington, Del.: Scholarly Resources, 2002.

Trager, James. *The New York Chronology: The Ultimate Compendium of Events, People, and Anecdotes from the Dutch to the Present*. New York: HarperResource, 2003.

Vanderbilt, Gertrude Lefferts. *The Social History of Flatbush: And Manners and Customs of the Dutch Settlers of Kings County*. New York: Appleton, 1881.

New York City Food Histories

Batterberry, Michael, and Ariane Batterberry. *On the Town in New York: The Landmark History of Eating, Drinking, and Entertainments from the American Revolution to the Food Revolution*. 2d ed. New York and London: Routledge, 1999.

Grimes, William. *Appetite City: A Culinary History of New York*. New York: North Point, 2009.

Hauck-Lawson, Annie H., and Jonathan Deutsch, eds. *Gastropolis: Food & New York City*. New York: Columbia University Press, 2008.

Lobel, Cindy R. *Urban Appetites: Food and Culture in Nineteenth-Century New York*. Chicago: University of Chicago Press, 2014.

Newman, Kara. *The Secret Financial Life of Food: From Commodities Markets to Supermarkets*. New York: Columbia University Press, 2012.

Schwartz, Arthur. *Arthur Schwartz's New York City Food: An Opinionated History and More Than 100 Legendary Recipes*. New York: Stewart, Tabori & Chang, 2004.

Shulman, Robin. *Eat the City: A Tale of the Fishers, Trappers, Hunters, Foragers, Slaughterers, Butchers, Farmers, Poultry Minders, Sugar Refiners, Cane Cutters, Beekeepers, Winemakers, and Brewers Who Built New York*. New York: Crown, 2012.

Smith, Andrew F. *New York City: A Food Biography*. Lanham, Md.: Rowman & Littlefield, 2014.

General Bibliography

Anderson, Will. *The Breweries of Brooklyn: An Informal History of a Great Industry in a Great City*. Croton Falls, N.Y.: Anderson, 1976.

Astor, Jane. *The New York Cook-Book*. New York: Carleton, 1880.

Balinska, Maria. *The Bagel: The Surprising History of a Modest Bread*. New Haven, Conn., and London: Yale University Press, 2008.

Bastianich, Lidia. *Lidia's Italian Table: More Than 200 Recipes From the First Lady of Italian Cooking*. New York: William Morrow Cookbooks 1998.

Bayles, W. Harrison. *Old Taverns of New York*. New York: Frank Allaben Genealogical Co. 1915.

Benepe, Barry, and John L. Hess. *Greenmarket: The Rebirth of Farmers Markets in New York City*. New York City: Council on the Environment of New York City, 1977.

Berry, Rynn, and Chris Abreu-Suzuki, with Barry Litsky. *The Vegan Guide to New York City*. 17th ed. New York: Ethical Living, 2010.

Bluestone, Daniel. "The Pushcart Evil." In *Landscape of Modernity*, edited by David Ward and Oliver Zunz, pp. 287–312. New York: Russell Sage Foundation, 1992.

Brody, Iles. *The Colony*. New York: Greenberg, 1945.

Bromell, Nicolas. "The Automat: Preparing the Way for Fast Food." *New York History* 81, no. 3 (July 2000): 300–312.

Bryson, Lew. *New York Breweries*. Mechanicsburg, Pa.: Stackpole, 2003.

Cahn, William. *Out of the Cracker Barrel: The Nabisco Story, from Animal Crackers to Zuzus*. New York: Simon & Schuster, 1969.

Caldwell, Alison. "Will Tweet for Food: The Impact of Twitter and New York City Food Trucks, Online, Offline, and Inline." *Appetite* 56, no. 2 (April 2011): 522.

Chappell, George Shepard. *The Restaurants of New York*. New York: Greenberg, 1925.

Dearing, Albin Pasteur. *The Elegant Inn: The Waldorf-Astoria Hotel, 1893–1929*. Secaucus, N.J.: Stuart, 1986.

DeGennaro, Jeremiah J. "From Civic to Social: New York's Taverns, Inside and Outside the Political Life of the United States after the Revolution." MA thesis, University of North Carolina at Greensboro, 2008.

DeVoe, Thomas F. *The Market Assistant*. New York: Hurd and Houghton, 1867.

DeVoe, Thomas F. *The Market Book Containing a Historical Account of the Public Markets*. Vol. 1. New York: Privately printed, 1862.

Diehl, Lorraine B., and Marrianne Hardart. *Automat: The History, Recipes, and Allure of Horn & Hardart's Masterpiece*. New York: Clarkson Potter, 2002.

Ducasse, Alain, and Alex Vallis. *J'Aime New York: 150 Culinary Destinations for Food Lovers*. Issy-les-Moulineaux, France, and New York: Alain Ducasse, 2013.

Evans, Meryle R. "Knickerbocker Hotels and Restaurants 1800–1850." *New-York Historical Society Quarterly* 36 (1952): 377–410.

Fifty Recipes on Flavoring by a Famous New York Chef. Richmond, Va.: Sauer [1920s?].

French, Earl R. *Push Cart Markets in New York City*. Washington, D.C.: Agricultural Economic Bureau, U.S. Department of Agriculture, 1925. http://naldc.nal.usda.gov/download/CAT10675911/PDF.

Garrett, Thomas Myers. "A History of Pleasure Gardens in New York City, 1700–1865." PhD diss., New York University, 1978.

Goossens, Jacqueline, Tom Vandenberghe, and Luk Thys. *New York Street Food*. Tielt, Belgium: Lannoo, 2013.

Hutcheson, John C. "The Markets of New York." *Harper's* 35 (July 1867): 229–236.

James, Rian. *Dining in New York*. New York: John Day, 1930.

Levinson, Marc. *The Great A&P and the Struggle for Small Business in America*. New York: Hill and Wang, 2011.

Maccioni, Sirio, and Peter Elliot. *Sirio: The Story of My Life and Le Cirque*. Hoboken, N.J.: Wiley, 2004.

Manzo, Joseph T. "From Pushcart to Modular Restaurant." *Journal of American Culture* 13, no. 3 (Fall 1990): 13–21.

Mariani, John, with Alex Von Bidder. *The Four Seasons: A History of America's Premier Restaurant*. New York: Crown, 1994.

Marx, Jeff. "The Days Had Come of Curds and Cream: The Origins and Development of Cream Cheese in America, 1870–1880." *Food, Culture & Society* 15 (2012): 177–195.

Mendelson, Anne. "To Market, to Market: A Profile of Thomas F. De Voe." *NYFoodStory*, 1 (Fall 2012): 3, 14–16, 18.

Mitchell, Joseph. *McSorley's Wonderful Saloon*. New York: Pantheon, 1992.

"Old New York Coffee-Houses," *Harper's* 64 (March 1882): 481–499.

Ray, Krishnendu. "Exotic Restaurants and Expatriate Home Cooking: Indian Food in Manhattan." In *The Globalization of Food*, edited by David Inglis and Debra Gimlin, pp. 213–226. Oxford and New York: Berg, 2009.

Rimmer, Leopold. *A History of Old New York Life and the House of the Delmonicos*. New York: Privately printed, 1898.

Rose, Peter G., trans. and ed. *The Sensible Cook: Dutch Foodways in the Old and the New World*. Syracuse, N.Y.: Syracuse University Press, 1989.

Sardi, Vincent, and Richard Gehman. *Sardi's: The Story of a Famous Restaurant*. New York: Holt, 1953.

Schriftgiesser, Karl. *Oscar of the Waldorf*. New York: Dutton, 1943.

Schwartz, Arthur. *Arthur Schwartz's New York City Food: An Opinionated History and More Than 100 Legendary Recipes*. New York: Stewart, Tabori & Chang, 2004.

Seiger, Karen E. *Markets of New York City: A Guide to the Best Artisan, Farmer, Food, and Flea Markets*. New York: Little Bookroom, 2010.

Shuldiner, Alec Tristin. "Trapped behind the Automat: Technological Systems and the American Restaurant, 1902–1991." PhD diss., Cornell University, 2001.

van der Sijs, Nicoline. *Cookies, Coleslaw, and Stoops: The Influence of Dutch on the North American Languages*. Amsterdam: Amsterdam University Press, 2009.

Slantez, Priscilla Jennings. "A History of the Fulton Fish Market." *Log of the Mystic Seaport* 36 (Spring 1986): 14–25.

Slomanson, Joan Kanel. *When Everybody Ate at Schrafft's: Memories, Pictures, and Recipes from a Very Special Restaurant Empire*. Fort Lee, N.J.: Barricade, 2006.

Taylor, Denise S., Valerie K. Fishel, Jessica L. Derstine, et al. "Street Foods in America—A True Melting Pot." In *Street Foods*, edited by Artemis P. Simopoulos and Ramesh V. Bhat, pp. 25–44. World Review of Nutrition and Dietetics 86. Basel, Switzerland: Karger, 2000.

Thomas, Lately [pseud. Robert V. P. Steele?]. *Delmonico's: A Century of Splendor*. Boston: Houghton Mifflin, 1967.

Walsh, William I. *The Rise and Decline of the Great Atlantic & Pacific Tea Company*. Secaucus, N.J.: Lyle Stuart, 1986.

Wasserman, Suzanne. "Hawkers and Gawkers: Peddling and Markets in New York City." In *Gastropolis: Food and New York City*, edited by Annie Hauck-Lawson and Jonathan Deutsch, pp. 153–173. New York: Columbia University Press, 2009.

Wechsberg, Joseph. *Dining at the Pavillon*. Boston: Little, Brown, 1962.

Where and How to Dine in New York; the Principal Hotels, Restaurants and Cafés of Various Kinds and Nationalities which Have Added to the Gastronomic Fame of New York and Its Suburbs. New York: Lewis, Scribner, 1903.

White, Charles Henry. "The Fulton Street Market." *Harper's* (September 1905): 616–623.

Williams, Ellen, and Steve Radlauer. *The Historic Shops and Restaurants of New York*. New York: Little Bookroom, 2002.

Zagat Survey. *New York City Restaurants 2009*. New York: Zagat Survey, 2008.

New York City Cookbooks

Alsop, Richard. *The Universal Receipt Book or Complete Family Directory by a Society of Gentlemen in New York*. New York: Riley, 1814.

Appel, Jennifer, and Allysa Torey. *The Magnolia Bakery Cookbook: Old-Fashioned Recipes from New York's Sweetest Bakery*. New York: Simon & Schuster, 1999.

Bradley, Jimmy, and Andrew Friedman. *The Red Cat Cookbook: 125 Recipes from New York City's Favorite Neighborhood Restaurant*. New York: Clarkson Potter, 2006.

Claiborne, Craig. *The New York Times Cook Book*. New York: Harper & Row, 1961.

Clark, Annie. *The New Waldorf Cook Book*. New York and London: Tennyson Neely, 1899.

Federman, Mark Russ. *Russ & Daughters: Reflections and Recipes from the House That Herring Built.* New York: Schocken, 2013.

Greenbaum, Florence Kreisler. *The International Jewish Cook Book.* New York: Bloch, 1918.

Hesser, Amanda. *The Essential New York Times Cook Book: Classic Recipes for a New Century.* New York: Norton, 2010.

Kellar, Jane Carpenter, comp. and ed. *On the Score of Hospitality: Selected Receipts of a Van Rensselaer Family, Albany, New York, 1785–1835. A Historic Cherry Hill Recipe Collection.* Albany, N.Y.: Historic Cherry Hill, 1986.

Lahman, DeDe, Neil Kleinberg, and Michael Harlan Turkell. *Clinton St. Baking Company Cookbook: Breakfast, Brunch & Beyond from New York's Favorite Neighborhood Restaurant.* New York: Little, Brown, 2010.

Lebewohl, Sharon, and Rena Bulkin. *The Second Avenue Deli Cookbook: Recipes and Memories from Abe Lebewohl's Legendary Kitchen.* New York: Villard, 1999.

Lewis, Edna, and Evangeline Peterson. *The Edna Lewis Cookbook.* Indianapolis, Ind.: Bobbs-Merrill, 1972.

Man, Anna. *The Little New York Cook / Die kleine New Yorker köchin.* New York: Verlag von Steiger, 1859.

Meyer, Danny, and Michael Romano. *The Union Square Café Cookbook: 160 Favorite Recipes from New York's Acclaimed Restaurant.* New York: HarperCollins, 1994.

New York Receipt Book. New York: Centaur, 1881.

O'Neill, Molly. *New York Cookbook.* New York: Workman, 1992.

Ranhofer, Charles. *The Epicurean.* New York: Ranhofer, 1894.

Tschirky, Oscar. *The Cook Book by "Oscar" of the Waldorf.* Chicago and New York: Werner, 1896.

Beverages

Berk, Sally Ann. *The New York Bartender's Guide: 1300 Alcoholic & Non-Alcoholic Drink Recipes for the Professional and the Home.* New York: Black Dog & Leventhal, 2006.

DeGroff, Dale. *The Craft of the Cocktail.* New York: Clarkson Potter, 2002.

Grimes, William. *Straight Up or On the Rocks: The Story of the American Cocktail.* New York: North Point, 2001.

Smith, Andrew F. *Drinking History: Fifteen Turning Points in the Making of American Beverages.* New York: Columbia University Press, 2012.

Spoelman, Colin, and David Haskell. *The Kings County Distillery Guide to Urban Moonshining: How to Make and Drink Whiskey.* New York: Abrams, 2013.

Thomas, Jerry. *The Bar-Tender's Guide; or How to Mix Drinks.* New York: Alvord, 1862.

INDEX

Page numbers in boldface refer to the main article on the subject. Page numbers in italics refer to illustrations

A

A. Goodman and Sons (bakery), 451
A. J. Gordon's Brewing Company, 387
A&P, **1–3**, 250
    Cullen at, 155, 319
    D'Agostino competition with, 159
    first chain grocery store, 578
    origins of, 251
    sponsor of *Our Daily Food* radio show, 483
"Abattoirs" (De Voe), 170
ABC Cocina, 168
Abraço Blue Bottle (coffee shop), 129
Abram, Ruth, 594
Abrams, Steve, 367
access to food, 78–79. *See also* food deserts; food insecurity
Accounting for Taste (Ferguson), 135
Achatz, Grant, 466
Acheson, Hugh, 211, 212
Ackerman, Jason, 229
Acme Smoked Fish, 354, 409
Action Against Hunger, 539
Ada (restaurant), 553
Adams, Franklin Pierce, 7
Adams, John, 222
Adams, Thomas, Sr., 255–56
Added Value, 615
Addison, Bill, 187
Adel's (restaurant), 263
Adrià, Ferran, 197, 400
advertising, **3–5**. *See also* marketing
    American Sugar Refining Company, 576
    D'Agostino, 159
    Geo. Winter Brewing Co., 7
    Mallomars, 367
    Nathan's Famous, 405
    Nedick's, 407
    in *New York Amsterdam News*, 552
    Oreos, 436
    Perrier, 636
    Piel Brothers, 71
    Rheingold Beer, 72
    Russian Tea Room, 513
    Snapple, 542
    Tootsie Rolls, 604
    Uneeda Biscuit, 404
    Waxman's collection of advertising trading
        cards, 637
Affordable Care Act (2010), 205
Afghani food, 205
African American(s), **5–7**
    in the Bronx, 77
    catering, 98
    at Chock full o'Nuts, 116
    in commercial kitchens, 106
    food trucks, 219
    gay bars, 236
    Great Migration, 262
    in Harlem, 262–63
    in Hell's Kitchen, 269
    in Jamaica, 302
    oystering on Staten Island, 565
Afro-Caribbean food influence, 5
Afternoon Tea Room, 590
agriculture. *See also* community supported agriculture; farms;
        rooftop gardens; urban farming
    Erie Canal impact on, 195
    Native American, 193
    in Queens, 479, 615
Agriculture, Department of
    Emergency Food Assistance Program, 280
    on food deserts, 214
    organic foods and, 437
    study of street vendors, 573
Ah, Wilderness (O'Neill), 599
Aiello, Gabriel, 614
Ai Fiori (restaurant), 278
Airline Diner, 173
AIWF. *See* American Institute of Wine & Food
Alam, Sayedul, 315
A la Rector's (G. Rector), 492
Albala, Ken, 136, 154
Albanians, 19, 77

Albermarle (hotel), 278
alcohol. *See also* breweries; cocktails; Prohibition; spirits; wine
 and winemaking
 absence in Arab restaurants, 17
 in Easter celebrations, 185
 Five Points, 209–10
 Indo-Caribbean, 290
 Korean, 325
 Little Odessa, 346
 Little Syria, 346
 New Year's and, 411
 in New York movies, 395
Alcott, William Andrus, 617
Alder (restaurant), 179
Aleichem, Sholem, 322
Alejandro, Reynaldo, 153
Alex and Henry's (restaurant), 77
Alfama (restaurant), 249
Alfanoose (restaurant), 201
Al Forno (restaurant), 179
Algonquin Round Table, **7–8**, 87, 536
Alice, Let's Eat (Trillin), 606
Alienist, The (Carr), 433
Alinea (restaurant), 305
All Around the Town (Dyer and Cole), 140
Allen, Beverly, 100
Allen, Gary, 154
Allen, Ida Bailey, **8**
Allen, J. Roy, 341
Allen, Ted, 212
Allen, Woody, 323, 445, 655
Allen & Killcoyne Associates (architects), 182–83
Alleva (dairy store), 160, 345
Alleva, Pina, 160
Alleva, Robert, Jr., 160
Alleva, Robert, Sr., 160
All in the Family (television sitcom), 437
All in the Industry (radio show), 86
"All You Can Hold for Five Bucks" (Mitchell),
 390, 418
Almayass (restaurant), 18
Alperson, Myra, 629
Amazing Adventures of Kavalier and Clay, The
 (Chabon), 433
Amelia award, 154, 271
"America Eats" Project, **8–9**, 414
America Farm to Table (Batali), 37
American Beverage Association, 545
American Beverage Corporation, 179
American Brewing Co., 76
American Cheeses (Wolf), 646
American Chef Corps, 307
American Chicle Company, 256
American Cookery (Simmons), 119, 142, 416
American Craft Museum, 399
American Culinary Federation, 105–6
American Express, 174, 224
American Food (Jones), 313
American Food Writing (O'Neill), 436
American Fried (Trillin), 606
American Guide series (Federal Writers' Project), 8
American Home Foods, 255
American Institute of Wine & Food, **9–10**, 261, 646

American Kitchen Magazine, 287
American Museum of Natural History, **10–11**, 340
 Our Global Kitchen: Food, Nature, Culture (exhibition), 400
American Personal & Private Chef Association, 107
American Place, An (restaurant), 203
American Sugar Refining Company, 266, 576
American Table Café and Bar, 518
American Vegetarian Society, 617
America's Test Kitchen, 315
America's Test Kitchen from Cook's Illustrated (television
 show), 593
America the Beautiful Fund, 48
America Walks into a Bar (Sismondo), 46
Amerikaner, 54
Amiel, Jack, 299
Amma (restaurant), 553
Amy Ruth's (restaurant), 6, 649
Amy's Bread, 31, 68, 108
Anchor Equipment Company, 74
Anderson, Jean, 427
Anderson, Walter A., 224
Andoh, Elizabeth, 154
Andres, Jose, 228
Andre's Café, 280, 657
Andrews, Colman, 197, 521
Angela's Ashes (McCourt), 294
Angelica's Kitchen (restaurant), 618
Angus McInDoe (pub), 294
Animal Crackers, 142, 404
Animals' Rights Considered in Relation to Social Progress
 (Salt), 617
Anistratov, Ellen, 655
Ansel, Dominique, 151, 178
antebellum period, **11–14**
 hotel restaurants, 277–78
Anthora cup, 128
Anthos (restaurant), 245
Anti-Saloon League, 473, 594
Apex Technical School, 260
Appeal to Reason (magazine), 535
Appel, Jennifer, 366
Appetite City (Grimes), 64, 249, 250, 592
Appetite for Life (Fitch), 324
appetizing stores, **14–15**, 311, 537, 540. *See also* Barney
 Greengrass; Russ & Daughters
 in the Bronx, 77
 dairy products, 160
 Jackson Heights, 300
 Lower East Side, 351–52
 lox in, 353
Apple, Raymond Walter, Jr., 422–23
apple brandy, 509
applejack, 557
apple-knocker, 84
Appleton's Journal, 458
Aquavit (restaurant), **15–16**, 518, 522
Aquavit and the New Scandinavian Cuisine
 (Samuelsson), 518
Arab community, **16–17**
 in Bay Ridge, 40
 falafel introduced by, 201
 in Little Syria, 346–47
Arabian Inn (restaurant), 346

Aramark, 472, 559
Arbuckle Brothers Coffee Company, 4
Arcadia (restaurant), 203
Arepejou, Paul, 265
Arirang House (restaurant), 326
Ark Restaurants, 359
Armani Ristorante, 168
Armenians, **17–18**, 315, 630
Armour, Philip Danforth, 535
Arno, Peter, 354
Arnold, Dave, 101, 391
    modernist cuisine, 392
    Museum of Food and Drink, 401
Arons, Andy, 242–43
Arthur Avenue, **18–19**, 77
    Italian restaurants, 295
    public market, 476
Arthur Avenue Retail Market, 19, 76, 230–31, 573
Arthur Schwartz's Jewish Home Cooking (Schwartz), 527
Arthur Schwartz's New York City Food (Schwartz), 527
Arthur's Tavern, 248
artisan production
    bagels, 28
    breads, 31, 68
    cheese, 104
    Edible support of, 188
    New Amsterdam Market and, 409
    pickles, 458
    pizza, 463–64
    pretzels, 471
    SoFi awards for, 202
Artists' Evening at Petitpas (Bellows), 447
Art of Cookery, The (Glasse), 416
"Arts and Traditions of the Table" series
    (Sonnenfeld, ed.), 135, 136
Aschkenasy, Peter, 355
Ashkenazi, Michael, 309
Ashkenazi Jews, 512
Asia Dog, 563
Asia Market Corporation, 596
Asian cuisine
    at Gotham Bar and Grill, 241
    in Sunset Park, 577
Asian fusion, 172, 232, 233
Asian Jewels (restaurant), 172
Asians
    in Harlem, 263
    immigration after 1965, 342–43
    in Jackson Heights, 300–301
    in Jamaica, 302
    in Queens, 480
Asimov, Eric, 200, 423
Asprinio, Stephen, 212
Associazione Verace Pizza Napolitana, 463
Astor, Brooke, 134, 330
Astor, John Jacob, 20
Astor, John Jacob, IV, 627
Astor, William Waldorf, 627
Astor Center, **19–20**
Astor House, **20–21**
    catering to theatergoers, 601
    early menus from, 382
    in haute cuisine, 264

    independent restaurant at, 278
    oysters, 442
    table d'hôte at, 277
Astoria, **21–22**, 479
    beer garden, 47
    Brazilians in, 66
    gay bars, 236
    Greeks in, 245, 480
    Japanese in, 308
    South and Central American food, 550
Astoria Hotel, 627
Astor Liquors, 19
Astor Wines and Spirits, 19
At Home with Magnolia (Torrey), 367
Atlantic Antic, 570
Atlantic Garden, 46–47
Aunt Dinah's Kitchen (restaurant), 552
Aurora (restaurant), 39, 162
Auster, Louis, 189, 544
Australian, **22–24**
Ausubel, Nathan, 322, 655
Automat (Hopper), 274
automats, **24–25**, 204–5, 537, 618–19
    conversion to cafeterias, 92
    Hopper on, 274, 275
    lunches, 357
    in Manhattan, 369
    movies on, 395
    post-World War II expansion, 467
automobiles and street vendors, 573
A Voce (restaurant), 296
awards. *See* International Association of Culinary Professions
    Award; James Beard Awards; Silver Spoon Award;
    Vendy Awards
    Amelia award, 154, 271

B
B. Altman (department store), 168
B. R. Guest restaurant group, 605
B. Smith's, 499
Babbo Ristorante e Enoteca, 36, 249, 296
Babiel, Rolf, 619
Bachmann brewery, 565
Bachman-Schmid, Elena, 486
Backerman, Walter, 529
Back Forty (restaurant), 203
BackPack Program, 282
Backyards (Pantell), 460
Baertschi, Alfred and Clara, 100
Bagatelle (bar), 236
Bagel Bakers Association, 27
Bagel Café, 249
bagels, **27–28**, 2
    bialys compared to, 51
    in brunch menus, 85
    Fabricant on, 199
    Jewish, 309
    lox and, 353
    with smoked fish, 540
Bagels and Yox (comedy), 28
baked Alaska, **29**
Baker, Harold, 457
Baker, Tim, 457–58

bakeries, 2
  on Arthur Avenue, 19
  breadlines at, 239
  in Brighton Beach, 73
  Colombian, 132
  during colonial period, 67
  cookies sold by, 142
  Delmonico's, 165, 166
  Easter foods, 186
  Ellis Island, 192
  English colonial, 193
  French, 227
  German, 67, 237, 321
  Greek, 245
  Indo-Caribbean, 289–90
  industrial, 67
  Jewish, 311
  on Lower East Side, 351
  Polish, 465
  pretzel, 471
  in Queens, 22, 300, 301
  recorded in 1900 census, 67
  ship's biscuits, 30, 67
Baking with Julia (television show), 110
Balance, and Columbian Repository, The, 35
Balance, The (magazine), 390
Balanchine, George, 513
Baldor Specialty Foods, 32
Balducci, Luigi, 252
Balducci's, **32**, 105, 252
Balfour, Eve, 508
Ball Park Franks, 277
Balthazar (restaurant), 68, 334, 566
Bamonte's (restaurant), 643
Banchetti (Messibugo), 416
B&B Hospitality Group, 495
B&H Dairy Restaurant, 189
Bangkok Center Grocery, 596
Bangladeshis, 173, 301
Banglo-Indo-Pak food, 343
Bank Coffee House, 427
Banks, Emily, 72
Banner Smoked Fish, 353–54
Bar Americain, 210
barbecue, 223, 325, 326
Barber, Dan, **33**
  at French Culinary Institute, 228, 260
  on *Mike Colameco's Food Show*, 593
  Passover food, 452
  patron of Kitchen Arts and Letters, 637
Barber, David, 33
Barbetta (restaurant), 499
Bar Boulud, 614, 621
Barbour, Beverly, 75, 338
bar cars, 485–86
Bareburger (restaurant), 259
Barkley, Charles, 639
Barlow, Joel, 103
Barney Greengrass, **33–34**, 537, 614
Baron, Stanley, 45, 70
Barr, Andrew, 126
Barr, Ann, 246
Barricini (chocolate shop), 94, 350

Barry, Dan, 231
bars, **34–35**. *See also* cocktail lounges; gay bars
  at Astor house, 20
  free lunch in, 173
  Greenwich Village, 248–49
  in Greenwich Village, 248–49
  in luxury hotels, 390
  at the Plaza, 464
  speakeasy style, 557
Bar Suzette, 108
Bartenders Guide: How To Mix Drinks (Thomas),
  127, 600
Bartending Agency and School of Mixology, 135
Barthes, Roland, 87
Bartholdi (hotel), 278, 407
Barton's, 94
Baruir's Coffee, 18
baseball and hot dogs, 275, 276
Basinski, Sean, 574
Baskin-Robbins, 288
Bass, John, 315
Bast Brothers Chocolate, 116
Bastianich, Joe, 35, 36, 186, 495, 499
Bastianich, Lidia, **35–36**, 296, 495, 499, 613
  Eataly, 186
  Jones, Judith, and, 313
  and Knopf, 324, 488
  in PBS series, 592
Batali, Mario, 36, **36–37**, 296, 495
  cooking shows, 592
  Del Posto and, 35
  Eataly, 186
  in Food & Wine Classic, 211
  James Beard Award to, 305
  in *Lucky Peach*, 356
  patron of Kitchen Arts and Letters, 637
  on PBS's *Spain ... On the Road Again*, 53
  pizzerias, 248
  on Vendy Awards, 619
Batali & Bastianich Hospitality Group, 495
Bâtard (restaurant), 429, 495
Bath Club, The (speakeasy), 556
Batterberry, Michael and Ariane, **37–39**, 127
  Food Arts, 212–13
  Food & Wine, 211
Battle of Golden Hill (1770), 589
Battle Row, 269
Baum, Joseph (Joe), **39**, 493, 501, 585
  DeGroff and, 162–63
  at The Four Seasons, 221, 222
  La Fonda del Sol, 66
  Lang and, 332
  and Rainbow Room, 486
  Windows on the World, 644
Baum + Whiteman, 39, 240, 486, 487
Bavarian Inn (restaurant), 656
Bayless, Rick, 365, 528
Bay Ridge, **40**, 521
Bay Ridge Food Co-op, 214
Bazooka Bubble Gum, 256
BBQ with Bobby Flay (television show), 218
BCD Tofu House, 325
Beacon Restaurant, 521

Beals, Jessie Tarbox, 590
Beam, Charles A., 481
Beame, Abe, 247
beans
    in Depression food, 170
    English colonial consumption, 194
    Sweet Holy Beans, 175–76
bean-to-bar chocolate. *See* chocolate, craft
Beard, James, **40–42**. *See also* James Beard Awards; James Beard
        Foundation
    Baum and, 39
    Brock and, 75
    on Cannon, 95
    co-founder of Citymeals-on-Wheels, 119–20
    culinary school, 144, 370
    at De Gustibus, 365
    Felidia and, 36
    in The Four Seasons, 221
    friendship with Child, 110
    at *Gourmet*, 362, 468
    haute cuisine and, 265
    Hesses on, 271
    house of, 249
    on hummus, 279
    I Love to Cook! television show, 591
    impact on American cooking, 241
    influence on Kornbleuth, 74
    in Institute of Culinary Education, 290
    Jones, Judith, and, 313
    at Kitchen Arts and Letters, 320
    Kump and, 327
    at La Caravelle, 329
    Les Trois Petits Cochons and, 227
    on Lewis, 340
    on Manhattan clam chowder, 372
    menu consultant for Restaurant Associates, 494
    menu of Windows on the World, 644
    Nickerson and, 428
    papers in Fales Library, 202
    patron of Kitchen Arts and Letters, 637
    Pépin and, 454
    restaurant reviewer, 497
    Vichyssoise, 620
    and word brunch, 84
Beard Birthday Fortnight celebrations, 304
Beard on Food (Beard), 313
Beastie Boys, 570
Beatles, The, 449
Becco (restaurant), 35, 36, 296, 499
Bechtel brewery, 565
Beck, Simone, 110, 488
    Jones, Judith, and, 312–13
    Knopf and, 323
    Kump and, 327
Becoming Raw (Davis, Marina, and Berry), 50, 491
Bedford Cheese Shop, 105
Bedford-Stuyvesant, **42–43**, 97, 178
Bedford-Stuyvesant Campaign against Hunger, 317
Bed Stuy Farm, 615
Beebee, Lucius, 570
Beecher's Handmade Cheese, 105
Beech-Nut, 341
beekeeping, **43–45**, 608

beer, **45–46**. *See also* beer gardens; breweries; microbreweries
        and brewpubs
    beer
        in Staten Island, 565
        colonial Dutch, 133, 262
        during colonial period, 194, 557
        Fourth of July, 223
        German, 237
        German deli and, 164
        Guinness, 293, 558–59
        Indo-Caribbean, 290
        Japanese, 308
        lager, 70
            introduced in beer gardens, 46
        Prohibition and, 474
        sold in growlers, 536
        at sporting events, 559, 560
        stout, 293
Beer: Tap Into the Art and Science of Brewing (Bamforth), 440
beer gardens, 13, **46–47**
    Five Points, 209
    gay, 236
    Kleindeutschland, 237, 321
    La Birreria, 186
    pretzels in, 471
Beer Here: Brewing New York's History (exhibition, NYHS),
        400, 419
Beers Cornell, 302
Belgian waffle, 652
Belin, Pierre, 265
Beling, Stephanie, 217
Belizean Grove (club), 126
Bella Landauer Collection, 419
Bell Book and Candle (restaurant), 508
Bellow, Saul, 433
Bellows, George Wesley, 299, 447
Bellucci, Andrew, 350
Bemelmans Bar, 391, 521
Benchley, Robert, 7, 536
Benedict, Lemuel, 190–91
Benepe, Adrian, 48
Benepe, Barry, **47–48**
    in Greenmarkets, 246–47
    in GrowNYC, 254
    Hess and, 270
Benet, Wilo, 478
Benfaremo, Nicola and Peter, 297
Bengalis in the Bronx, 78
Bengtsson, Emma, 15–16
Benjy's Kosher Pizza Dairy, 201
Bennets, Leslie, 153
Bennett, Helene, 75, 338
Bennett, Tony, 461
Benno, Jonathan, 614
Benny's (restaurant), 450
Ben's Cheese Planet, 160
Ben's Famous (pizzeria), 463
Bensonhurst, **48–49**
    as Italian enclave, 81
    Italian restaurants, 295
Bensonhurst cocktail, 83
Bentley, Amy, 197, 426
Bentley, Gladys, 236

Ber, Ross, 43, 44
Beranbaum, Rose Levy, 202
Berg, Jennifer, 426
Berger, Joe, 280
Berger, Joseph, 655
Berghoff, Stephanie, 154
Berg'n, 563, 643
Bergquist, Andrea, 518
Berlin, Hallo, 619
Bernard, Françoise, 242
Berns, Charlie, 609
Bernstein, Leonard, 269
Berra, Yogi, 461
Berry, Rynn, **49–50**, 491, 617
Bertelsmann AG, 324
Bertholle, Louisette, 110, 488
    Jones, Judith, and, 312–13
    Knopf and, 323
Berz Beez Honey, 43
Besa, Amy, 208
Best Foods, 267–68
Best Loved Recipes of the American People (Allen), 8
Better Homes and Gardens (magazine), 647
Between Meals (Liebling), 340, 341, 418
Beyti Turkish Kabob, 73
BG (restaurant), 168
Bialy Eaters, The (Sheraton), 532
bialys, 5
    with smoked fish, 540
Bialys Bakers Association, 50
Bialys Eaters, The (Sheraton), 50
Bice Group, 167
Bickford's (restaurant chain), **51**
Bidder, Alex von, 222
Big Alice Brewing Co., 387
Big Apple, **51–52**, 536
Big Apple, The (drink), 52
Big Apple Barbecue Block Party, 52
Big Apple Martini, 52
Big Apple Mojito, 52
Big Onion Walking Tours, 608
Bilet, Maxime, 391
Billie Black's (restaurant), 263
Billingsley, Sherman, 569, 570
Billion Oyster Project, 434
Bing Gre Kimchee Pride, 319
Birchbox, 563
Bird Cage (tearoom), 168, 591
Birreria, La (beer garden/brewery), 186
Bishara, Rawia, 40
Bishop, Isabel, 448
Bissinger, Karl, 339
Bittman, Mark, **52–54**, 423
    on Hazan, 267
Bizarre Foods America (television program), 629
bk farmyards, 615
Black, William, 115, 116, 128
black and tans, 537, 556
black and white cookies, **54–55**, 142
    on *Seinfeld*, 54, 142, 592
Blackbird, 521
Black Swan (restaurant), 43
Blackwell's Island, 472

Blair, Karen, 647
Blais, Richard, 212
Blanc, Georges, 63, 518
Blanca (restaurant), 86, 507
Blass, Bill, 141, 330
Bleecker Luncheonette, 249
BLK ProjeK, 78
Block, Adrian, 22
blogs
    Chelsea Now, 571
    Eater, 187
    Food52, 216
    Food Politics, 408
    Fork in the Road, 624
    Grub Street, 563
    Hesser in, 272
    Inquisitive Eater, 410
    I Quant NY, 562
    James Beard Foundation, 307
    on restaurants, 499
Blood, Bones and Butter (Hamilton), 261–62
Bloody Mary, **55**, 5
Bloomberg, Michael, **55–56**
    menu labels, 381, 608
    at Patsy's, 461
    regulation of sodas, 544, 545–46
    restaurant letter grading, 496
    Snapple–New York deal and, 543
    street vendors and, 574
Bloomberg News, 187
Bloomfield, April, **56–57**
    on *Mike Colameco's Food Show*, 593
    in *The Mind of a Chef*, 592
    Shake Shack and, 531
Bloomingdale (neighborhood). *See* Hell's Kitchen
Bloomingdale's, 168, 622
Blot, Pierre, **57–58**, 143, 226, 417
Blount, Roy, Jr., 178
BLT Burger, 259
Blue, Anthony Dias, 483
Blue Apron, 563
blue blazer drink, 34, 600
Blue Dove (tavern), 586
Blue Hill at Stone Barns Center for Food and Agriculture, 33, 466
Blue Hill Restaurant, 33, 249
blue laws, 253
Blue Lifestyle Minute (radio), 483
Blue Man Group, 598
Blue Note, 248
Blue Ribbon Sushi (restaurant), 581
"Blue Skies, No Candy" (Greene), 246
Blue Smoke (restaurant), 386, 495, 560
Blue Trout and Black Truffles (Wechsberg), 418, 637
BLVD Bistro, 263
Bly, Nellie, 472
boarding houses, **58–59**, 617
Boar's Head cold cuts, 164
Bobby Flay's Barbecue Addiction (Flay), 210
Bobby Flay's Boy Gets Grill (Flay), 210
Bobby Flay's Burgers, Fries and Shakes (Flay), 210
Bobby Flay's From My Kitchen to Your Table (Flay), 210
Bobby Flay's Grill It! (Flay), 210

Bobby Flay's Mesa Grill Cookbook (Flay), 210
Bobby Flay Steak, 210
Bobby's Burger Palace, 210
Bocuse, Paul
    Bouley and, 62
    Boulud and, 63
    Claiborne and, 124
    Vongerichten and, 624
Bodega (restaurant), 466
Bodega Association of the United States, 60
bodegas, **59–60**, 98, 229, 252
    Essex Street Market and, 196
    Puerto Rican, 477
    relying on SNAP recipients, 579
Bogdanow, Larry, 611
Bohemian Citizens' Benevolent Society, 47
Bolo (restaurant), 210
Bolton, Saul, 399, 561
Bon Appétit (magazine), 262, 370, 625
Bonavia (restaurant), 35
Bond, James, 243
Bonfire of the Vanities (Wolfe), 433
Boni, Ada, 266
Bon Vivant's Companion, The (Thomas), 162. *See also Bartenders*
        Guide: How To Mix Drinks (*Thomas*)
Booker and Dax, 101, 393
Book of Bread, The (Jones and Jones), 313
BOOM! (exhibit, MOFAD), 401
Booth, Janine, 212
bootleggers, **60–61**, 175
Borchardt, H. W., 163
Borden, Gail, Jr., **61**, 122
Borden Company, 61, 651
Borgatti's pasta, 19
Borgnine, Ernest, 293
Boring, Ty-Lör, 212
Born, Samuel, 80, 94
Born Sucker Machine, 80, 94
Boroughs, William S., 248
Bostonians, The (James), 432
bottled water. *See* water: bottled
Bottom Line (restaurant), 249
Boulder Creek Steakhouse, 40
Bouley (restaurant), 62
    Barber at, 33
    James Beard Award, 304
    Kulchinsky in, 471
Bouley, David, **62**
    Le Cirque, 336
    Montrachet, 429
Bouley Bakery and Market, 62
Boulud, Daniel, **62–63**, 334, 613, 614
    Citymeals-on-Wheels, 120
    hamburgers by, 259
    influenced by Baum, 501
    at Le Cirque, 336, 363
    on *Mike Colameco's Food Show*, 593
    owner of Feast and Fêtes Catering Company, 495
    patron of Kitchen Arts and Letters, 637
    Scribner's, 528
    Shake Shack and, 531
Boulud Sud, 63, 614
Bourbon Street (restaurant), 499

Bourdain, Anthony, 37, **63–64**, 566, 592
    on Eater, 187
    Lucky Peach, 356
    Mind of a Chef, 101
    in *The New Yorker*, 418
    No Reservations, 629
Bourdon, Francis, 24, 204–5
Bower, Richard, 221
Bowery
    gay bars, 235–36
    ice cream sandwiches, 287
    ice cream shops, 288
Bowery Kitchen Supply, 108
Bowery Mission, breadline at, 67, 6
Bowien, Danny, 233
Boy Meets Grill (television show), 211, 218
Brace, Charles Loring, 523
Bradford, Cornelius, 129, 130
Bradshaw, Terry, 466
Brady, Diamond Jim (James Buchanan), 6
    at Café Martin, 348
    eggs Benedict and, 190
    at Gage & Tollner, 235
    at Grand Central Oyster Bar, 243
    at Lüchow's, 355
    at the Plaza, 469
    at Rector's, 492
    at the Waldorf, 607
Brady, Mathew, 4
Bramah, Joseph, 543
Brasserie (restaurant), 494, 495
Brasserie Athenee (restaurant), 499
Braun, H., 311
Bravo television network, 211–12, 478
Brazil Brazil (restaurant), 499
Brazilian, **65–66**, 550–51
bread, **66–68**
    Arab, 17
    Eastern European, 73
    English colonial, 194
    Jewish rye, 31, 67
    pastrami and, 453
    pretzels, 471
    in prison food, 472
    pumpernickel at German deli, 163
    regulations about, 29–30, 67, 133
Bread, Fish, Fruit (Lawrence), 448
breadlines, **68–70**, 6
    Gilded Age, 239
    during Great Depression, 168–69
Breakfast Club, The (NPR), 527
breakfasts. *See also* brunch; power breakfasts and power lunches
    at the Astor House, 21
    diner, 173
    Dominican, 176
    Easter celebration, 185, 186
Breakstone, Isaac, 103, 149
Breakstone, Joseph, 149
Breakstone Brothers Dairy, 149
Bremen House, 656
Brennan, Eddie, 641
Brennan, Terrance, 614
Brenner, Leslie, 63

Brescio, John, 350
Breslin Bar and Dining Room, 56, 57, 278
Brewed in America (Baron), 45, 70
breweries, **70–72**. *See also* microbreweries and brewpubs
  advertising for Geo. Winter Brewing Co., 7
  in the Bronx, 76
  in Brooklyn, 81, 564
  in early Bushwick, 85
  German immigrants and, 558
  late twentieth century, 333–34
  in Manhattan, 369
  during Prohibition, 60
  saloons and, 516
  in Staten Island, 565
  water supply and, 633
  in Williamsburg, 643
brewpubs. *See* microbreweries and brewpubs
Brice, Fannie, 165
Brickman, Sophie, 419
Bride's Cookbook, The (Cannon), 95
"Brigade de Cuisine" (McPhee), 418
Brighton Bazaar, 73
Brighton Beach, **72–74**, 345. *See also* Little Odessa
  Russians in, 81, 512
  Ukrainians in, 611
Briguet, Georges, 265, 369
Brinnin, Malcolm, 641
Britchky, Seymour, 65, 549
British Food (Spencer), 136
British Merchant Sailors' Club for Indian Seamen, 551
Broadway Joe's (restaurant), 499
Broadway Limited, 485
Broadway Panhandler: A Cook's Best Resource, **74**
Broadyke Market, 292
Brock, Carol, **74–75**, 335, 338, 370
Brody, Jerome, 221, 243–44, 493
Bromangelon, 603
Broncanelli, Gino, 295
Bronck, Jonas, 75
Bronco Wine Company, 605
Bronfman, Samuel, 221
Bronx, **75–79**. *See also* Arthur Avenue
  bodegas, 59
  Caribbeans in, 97
  diners, 173
  egg creams, 189, 190
  food desert, 214–15
  food trucks, 219
  Italian restaurants, 295
  microbreweries, 387
  Puerto Ricans in, 477
Bronx Beer Hall, 19
Bronx Brewery, 76, 387
Bronx cocktail, **79–80**
Bronx Flavor (television show), 78
Bronx Pretzel Company, 471
Bronx Tale (movie), 299
Bronx Terminal Market, 78, 284, 476
Brooklyn, **80–82**. *See also* Bay Ridge; Bedford-Stuyvesant;
    Bensonhurst; Brighton Beach; Bushwick; Flatbush;
    Park Slope; Red Hook; Sunset Park; Williamsburg
  after World War II, 314
  Australian restaurants, 23

  as brewing center, 45, 70
  Caribbean in, 97
  Chinese in, 114
  craft chocolate, 117
  diners, 173
  distilleries, 175
  egg creams, 189, 190
  Filipinos in, 207
  food desert, 214–15
  Greenmarkets, 247
  Italian restaurants, 296
  microbreweries, 387
  pickles, 458
  Polish in, 465
  public market, 476
  Russians in, 512
  Starbucks, 562
  urban farming, 615
  walking culinary tours, 629
Brooklyn Bangers & Dogs, 561
Brooklyn–Battery Tunnel, 346–47
Brooklyn Bowl, 643
Brooklyn Bread House, 18
Brooklyn Brewery, 46, 72, 81, **82–83**, 334, 386, 387, 564, 643
  Glaser's design of logo, 4
Brooklyn Brew Shop, 563
Brooklyn Brine, 458
Brooklyn Cacao, 117
Brooklyn chocolate cake. *See* Ebinger's Blackout Cake
Brooklyn cocktail, **83**
Brooklyn Congress of Racial Equality, 187–88
Brooklyn Cookbook, The (Stallworth and Kennedy), 103
Brooklyn Daily Eagle (newspaper), 375
Brooklyn decadence cake. *See* Ebinger's Blackout ake
Brooklyn Eagle, 435
Brooklyn Edible Social Club, 126
Brooklyn Farmacy & Soda Fountain, 190, 547
Brooklyn Flea, The, 541, 563, 643
Brooklyn Grange, 82, 508, 615
Brooklyn Heights, Egyptian food in, 191
Brooklyn Museum of Art, 399, 450
Brooklyn Pour, 624
Brooklyn Roasting Company, 129
Brooklyn Sandwich Society, 126
Brooklyn Seltzer Boys, 529
Brooks, Emily, 141
Brotherhood Winery, 645
Broun, Heywood, 7
Brown, Alton, 29
Brown, Helen Gurley, 648
Brown, Henry Collins, 373
Brown, Henry E., 178–79
Brown, James, 556, 586
Brown, Patricia, 153
Brown, Tina, 417
Browne, Junius Henri, 59
Brownie Corporations, 179
Brownstone, Cecily, 201, 202, 428
Bruke, Harman Burney, 79
brunch, **83–85**, *8*
  bagel and lox, 540
  Easter, 185
  smoked fish at, 541

Brunch at Bobby's (television show), 210, 217
Bruni, Frank, 62, 498
    Hess on, 271
    on Merkato 55, 518
    at the *New York Times*, 423
Brushstroke (restaurant), 62
Bubby's (soda fountain), 547
Buck, Leslie, 128
Budin (coffee shop), 129
Buds (restaurant), 210
buffet/salad bars, 73
Buford, Bill, 37, 324
Bugialli, Giuliano, 296
Bull and Bear Prime Steakhouse (restaurant, Waldorf), 627
bulldozer drink, 84
Bull's Head Tavern, 586
Bun & Burger, 259
Bungalow Bar (food trucks), 218–19
Buonavia (restaurant), 296
Buon Italia, 108
Burdell, John, 617
Bureau of Consumer Services, 476
Burger Bistro, 259
Burger King, 205, 206, 301
Burgess, Anthony, 153
Burke, David, 324, 613
Burke's Complete Cocktail & Drinking Recipes (Burke), 79
Burns, Jabez, 131
Burros, Marian, 88, 423
Bushwick, 81, **85–86**
Bushwick Food Cooperative, 214
Bushwick Initiative, 85
Bushwick Open Studios, 85
Bushwick Review, 86
business lunch, **86–87**. *See also* power breakfasts and power
            lunches; three-martini lunch
    at The Four Seasons, 222
Business Week (magazine), 240
Bustanoby's (lobster palace), 348
butchers, **87–89**. *See also* De Voe, Thomas Farrington
    Easter meats, 185, 186
    French, 226
    German, 232, 237
    Greek, 245
    at Hunts Point, 283–84
    Irish, 232
    Jackson Heights, 300
    Jewish, 311–12
    Polish, 465
    private shops, 12
    on Upper East Side, 612
Butler, James, 251
Butler, Jonathan, 541
Butler Grocery Stores, 251
Butter, Cheese, and Egg Exchange, 137
Butter and Cheese Exchange, 104, 137
Buttercup Bake Shop, 366
Byron, O. H., 373

C
cabbage, 163, 559
Cacao Prieto, 117
Cachapas y Mas (restaurant), 291

Cadbury Schweppes, 542
Café2 (MoMA), 399, 501
Café Boulud, 63, 101, 278, 613
Café Brevoort, 226
Café de La Esquina, 173
Café de l'Opera, 348, 601
Café de Paris, 336–37
Café des Artistes, 249, 332, 614
Café Des Artistes Cookbook, The (Lang), 332
Café des Beaux Arts, 348
Café Figaro, 248, 249
Café Fiorello, 614
Cafe Francis, The (Luks), 447
Cafe Geiger, 656
Café Glechik, 73
Café Grumpy (coffee shop), 129, 564
Café Himalaya, 553
Café Kashkar, 73
Café Lalo, 129
Café Luxembourg, 334, 614
Café Martin, 226, 348, 384
Café Nicholson, **91**
    Fales Library collection, 202
    Edna Lewis and, 6
    Lewis in, 339
Café Ollin, 263
Café Royal, 311, 501
cafés. *See also* coffeehouses
    Australian, 23
    in early Arab community, 16
    Greenwich Village, 248
Café Sabarsky, 399
Café SEA, 168
Café Serai, 399
"Café Society," 536, 570
    "21" Club and, 609
    at Rainbow Room, 486
Café Spice, 553
Cafeteria (Soyer), 448
cafeterias, **92–93**, 500
    Childs and, 111
    fast food, 204
    penny, 363–64
Café Wha?, 248
Caffè Reggio, **93**, 248
Caffè Storico (restaurant), 399, 419
Cage, John, 221
Cahan, Abraham, 311
Calabira sausage shop, 19
Calandra formaggio, 19
California cuisine, 265
Callies, Misty, 261
Cambodians in the Bronx, 78
Cameron, Angus, 313
Canada Dry Bottling Company, 179
Canaday, John, 423
candy, **93–95**
    deep fried candy bars, 161
    Life Savers, 341
candy shops
    Jackson Heights, 300
    Loft's, 349–50
Cann, John, 260

canneries, 442
Cannibal, The (restaurant), 566
cannoli, 31
Cannon, Poppy, **95–96**
Can Opener Cook Book (Cannon), 95
canteens during World War II, 654
Cantor, Eddie, 165
Capote, Truman, 330, 339
car bomb (drink), 559
Carbone, Mario, 296
Cardoz, Floyd, 553
Careers Through Culinary Arts Program (C-CAP), **96**, 539
Carême, Marie-Antonin, 102, 264
Caribbean(s), **96–98**, 550. *See also* Dominican(s)
    in Bedford-Stuyvant, 43
    in the Bronx, 77
    in Crown Heights, 81
    food trucks, 219
    goat meat, 284
    in Harlem, 263
    in Inwood, 291
    in Jamaica, 302
Carlos & Gabby's, 561
Carlton, The (hotel and restaurant), 162
Carlyle Hotel, 521
Carmel, Dalia, 202
Carmellini, Andrew, 336, 561
Carnegie, Andrew, 355
Carnegie Deli, 145, 165, 561
Carnegie Hill Brewing Company, The, 387
Carnivore's Manifesto, The (Martins), 86
Carolina Rice Kitchen, The (Hess), 271
Carpenter, Maile, 180
Carrier, Robert, 548
Carter, John, 551–52
Carter, Susannah, 177
cartoons, 418–19
Caruso, Enrico, 190, 322, 355
Casa Brasil (restaurant), 66
Casa della Mozzarella, 19
Casas, Penelope, 290, 324
Case, Frank, 7
Casella, Cesare, 228
Casey, Kathy, 377
Castelholm (restaurant), 522
Castle Garden at the Battery, 46
Catagonia Club, 556
Catcher in the Rye, The (Salinger), 433
catering, **98–99**
    Great Performances, 244–45
    Hamilton, Gabrielle, in, 261
    Louis Sherry and, 533
Catholics in Jackson Heights, 300
Catholic Welfare Council, 193
Catsimatidis, John, 250–51
Cavallaci, Fabrizio, 93
Cavallero, Gene, 264
CBE Feeds, 240
C-CAP. *See* Careers Through Culinary Arts Program
Cecchini, Toby, 147
Cecil, The (restaurant), 6, 263
Cedar Bar, 448
Cedar Bar (Grooms), 448

Cedar Tavern, 249
Ceglic, Jack, 160–61
Cellar Bar and Grill (Macy's), 365
Cel-Ray, 178–79
Cendrillon (restaurant), 208
Center for Food and Environment, 135
Center for Science in the Public Interest, 605
Central American. *See* South and Central American
Central Park
    impact on Upper East Side, 612
    picnics in, 459, 614
Central Park Casino, **99–100**
Central Perk (restaurant), 466
Century Association, 125
Cercle des Gourmettes, Le, 110
Cerf, Bennett, 488
Ceylon India Inn (restaurant), 551
Chabon, Michael, 433
Chalet Suisse (restaurant), **100–101**
Chalet Suisse (Schlüter), 100
Chalsty's Café (MCNY), 402
Chamberlain, Samuel, 241, 242, 361
Chambord (restaurant), 199
champagne and New Year's Eve, 412
Chang, David, **101**, 325, 392
    on Eater, 187
    at French Culinary Institute, 228, 260
    influenced by Baum, 501
    James Beard Award, 305
    kimchi recipe, 319
    Lucky Peach founded by, 355, 356
    in *The Mind of a Chef*, 592
    Momofuku Restaurant Group, 495
    Shake Shack and, 531
Change Makers (gum), 256
Channelle (patisserie), 301
Chanukah, **101–2**, 350
Chappell, George S., 225
Chardenet, Betty, 224
Charleston Garden (restaurant), 168
Charlie O's (restaurant), 39
charlotte (English), 102–3
charlotte russe, **102–3**
Chateau Gardens (restaurant), 332
Chaupoly, Ratha, 554
cheesecakes, **103–4**
    Junior's, 313–14
    Lindy's, 342
    made with Downsville Cream Cheese, 149
    New York cheesecake, 31
cheesemongers, **104–5**
    dairy stores, 160
    Fairway, 200
    French, 227
    Italian, 295
Cheetahs Gentlemen's Club and Restaurant, 530
chefs, **105–7**, 141, 406–7, 478
    African American, 5–6
    private, **107–8**
Chef Says, The: Quotes, Quips, and Words of Wisdom
    (Waxman and Sartwell, comps. and eds.), 637
Chefs Boot Camp for Policy and Change, 307
Chefs & Champagne events, 306

Chef's Cook Book of Profitable Recipes, The (De Gouy), 162
Chefs de Cuisine Association of America, 106
Chef's Life, A (television show), 593
Chef's Pass, 62
Chef's Story (television show), 261
Chef's Tale, A (Franey), 225
Chelsea Brewing Company, 387
Chelsea diners, 173
Chelsea Market, 88, 105, **108–9**, 358
    Food Network in, 217, 218, 591
Chelsea Market Passage, 274. *See also* High Line
Chelsea Now blog, 571
Chen, Yong, 136
Cherche Midi (restaurant), 352
Chernow, Michael, 613
chestnuts, **109**
Cheung, Chris, 233
chewing gum. *See* gum
Chez Brigitte (restaurant), 249
Chez Lucky Pierre (restaurant), 42
Chez Mouquin (Glackens), 447
Chiclets, 256
Child, Julia, **109–10**
    Beard and, 42
    co-founder of American Institute of Wine & Food, 9
    at De Gustibus, 365
    in Food & Wine Classic, 211
    Hesses on, 271
    home cooks and, 106
    in Institute of Culinary Education, 290
    James Beard Award to, 305, 306
    James Beard Foundation and, 306, 335
    Jones, Judith, and, 312–13
    at Kitchen Arts and Letters, 320, 637
    Knopf and, 323, 324
    Kump and, 327
    in Les Dames d'Escoffier, 338
    menu consultant for Restaurant Associates, 494
    Moulton and, 393, 394
    Pépin and, 454
    television shows
        Bastianich on, 36
        The French Chef, 591
        reruns on Food Network, 217
children
    cupcakes and, 156
    educational programs of MCNY, 402
Children's Aid Society school free meals, 523
Childs (restaurant), **110–12**, 204, 334, 601
    lunches, 357
    paintings of, 448
    at World's Fair, 1939–1940, 650
    during World War II, 654
Childs, Samuel and William, 92, 111, 500
    fast food by, 204
    lunch and, 357
Chilean food in Harlem, 263
China Institute in America, 113
Chinatown, 113, 114. *See also* Five Points
    Chinese New Year, 412
    groceries, 210
    Hess on, 271
    Hopper on, 274, 275

    Kleindeutschland in, 237
    spread into Lower East Side, 352
    Thanksgiving day weddings, 597
Chinatown Ice Cream Factory, 289
Chinese Casino (restaurant), 76
Chinese community, **112–15**
    bakeries, 31
    in Bensonhurst, 49
    doughnuts, 177
    fast food, 205
    in Five Points, 210
    food in Harlem, 262
    Hazan in, 266
    influence of on Jamaican, 303
    Jewish interest in, 311
    Little Italy and, 344–45
    paintings of restaurants, 448
    in Park Slope, 450
    in Queens, 480
    in Sunset Park, 577
Chinese Cooking Classes of Madame Grace Chu, 144
Chinese Exclusion Act (1882), 112
Chinese Food Made Easy (television show), 217
Chinese Restaurant (Sloan), 448
(Memory of a) Chinese Restaurant (Weber), 448
Chipotle Mexican Grill, 205, 553
ChipShop (restaurant), 161, 162
Chipwich, **115**
Chock full o'Nuts, **115–16**, 128, 132, 300, 407
chocolate
    craft, **116–17**, 563
        Loft's, 349–50
        Torres and, 604
    English colonial consumption, 194
    syrup in egg creams, 189–90
    during World War II, 654
Chocolate with Jacques Torres (television series), 604
chocolatiers, 94, 186
Choi, Roy, 220, 319, 325
Choice Eats, 624
chophouses, 500
Chop Suey (Hopper), 274, 275
Chop Suey: A Cultural History of Chinese Food in the United States (Coe), 440
Chop Suey, USA (Chen), 136
chop suey joints, 112, **117**, 537
    Hopper on, 274, 275
CHOW (COLORS Hospitality for Workers) Institute, 206
Christgau, Robert, 624
Christian holidays. *See* Christmas; Easter
Christina's (diner), 465
Christmas, **117–19**
Christmas Carol, A (Dickens), 119
Christopher Street Liberation Day, 568
Christy, Howard Chandler, 332
Christy, Liz, 254
Chu, Grace Zia, 144, 266
Chumley's (speakeasy), 248, 249, 556
Churchill's (lobster palace), 330, 348
Church Temperance Society, 172, 593
Churrasco restaurants, 66
cider, 557
Cimino, Teresa, 373, 374

Cinnamon Snail (food truck), 618
Citarella (grocery store), 200, 252, 614
Citarella, Mike, 252
City Bureau of Licenses, 572
City Farms Markets, 79
City Foods Tours NYC, 629
City Harvest, 215, 280, 281, 370
    research and policy initiatives, 282–83
    Smilow and, 539
City Island, 78
City Island Beer Company, 76
Citymeals-on-Wheels, **119–20**, 246, 429
City of God (Doctorow), 459
City University of New York (CUNY), **120–22**, 121
Civil War, **122–23**, 238
    hardtack, 403
    Thanksgiving dinner for the Union soldiers, 596–97
Claiborne, Craig, **123–25**, 422
    advice to Moulton, 393
    on Baum, 39
    Beard and, 42
    on Chock full o'Nuts coffee shops, 115
    Easter brunch menu, 84
    eulogy of Soulé, 550
    Fabricant on, 199
    on falafel, 201
    on Four Seasons, 221
    Franey and, 224–25
    on Hazan, 266
    Hesses on, 271
    on hummus, 279
    on Japanese food, 581
    Jones, Judith, and, 312–13
    on Katz's Delicatessen, 165
    on La Caravelle, 329
    on Le Pavillon, 337
    on Les Trois Petits Cochons, 227
    on Lewis, 340
    on Lindy's cheesecake, 342
    on Lucas, 354
    on *Mastering the Art of French Cooking*, 110
    on Maxwell's Plum, 377
    and modern form of restaurant reviewing, 497–98
    The New York Times Cookbook, 141
    on pastrami, 453
    Pépin and, 454
    in post-World War II culinary revolution, 468
    replaced at the *New York Times* by Sokolov, 548
    Silver Spoon award to, 213
    on Soulé, 338
    on sushi, 308
    on taco food trucks, 219
    on traditional foods for Chanukah, 102
Clark, Edward, 98
Clark, Melissa, 424, 584
Clark, Patrick, 6, 585
Clark, Robert, 354
Clarke, John, 635–36
Clarke, Patrick J., 445, 587. *See also* P. J. Clarke's
Clarke Group, 445
Clarkson Potter, Inc., 488
Clark Wolf Company, 646
Classic French Cooking (Claiborne and Franey), 224, 225

Classic Italian Cookbook, The (Hazan), 266
Clean Water Act (1972), 209
Clinton. *See* Hell's Kitchen
Clinton, DeWitt, 194, 268
Clinton Fresh Foods, 391
Clinton Hill Pickles, 458
Clinton Street Baking Company, 352
Cloke, Thomas, 556
Club Ebony, 556
Club Fronton, 609
clubs, **125–26**
CNN, 217
Co (pizzeria), 462
Coach House, The (restaurant), 140
coal-pot cooking, 194
Coals (pizzeria), 464
Coca-Cola Company
    bottled water, 636
    free-style vending machine, 619
    at World's Fair, 1964–1965, 651
cocktail, definition, 372, 390
cocktail lounges, **126–27**, 536
cocktails, 34, 35, **127–28**. *See also* Bloody Mary; Bronx cocktail;
        Brooklyn cocktail; Cosmopolitan; Manhattan; Martini;
        mixology; Old-Fashioned cocktail; Queens Cocktail
    at Booker & Dax, 101
    at Cotton Club, 148
    at Dylan's Candy Bar, 182–83
    Grimes on, 249
    Ladies Who Lunch and, 331
    on *Mad Men*, 366
    revival by DeGroff, 162–63
Cocktails: How To Mix Them (Vermeire), 481
coffee, **128–29**, 537
    Armenian, 18
    espresso, 93, 295
    importance in early American diet, 138
    imported from Brazil, 65
    Irish, 293
    third-wave, 564
    Turkish, 17, 346
coffeehouses, 128, **129–31**
    as alternative to bars and taverns, 593
    compared to coffee shops, 131
    tea served at, 587–88
coffee roasters, **131**
coffee shops, 129, **131–32**
    compared to coffeehouses, 129
    Hopper on, 275
    lunches, 357–58
Coffin, Robert Tristram, 241
"Cognitive Cooking with Chef Watson: Recipes for Innovation
        from IBN and the Institute of Culinary Education," 291
Cohen, Gerald, 536
Cohen, Irwin B., 108
Cohen, Leah, 212
Cohen, Rich, 583
Cohn, Harry, 337
Cohn, Selwyn, 178–79
Coit, Henry L., 387
Colameco, Mike, 483, 592
Colbin, Annemarie, 144, 335, 370, 406
Cole, Nat King, 293, 445

Cole, Rosalind, 140
Cole, Thomas, 447
Colicchio, Tom, 101
    on Food Network, 218
    founder of Craft Restaurant Group, 495
    at Gotham Bar and Grill, 241
    influence on Chang, 393
    in *Top Chef*, 212
Colicchio & Sons, 495
Collins, Billy, 587
Collins, Judy, 248, 513, 514
Collins, Peggy, 427
Colombian, **132–33**
colonial Dutch, **133–34**. *See also* New Amsterdam
    cheese, 104
    diet, 262
    doughnuts, 177
    Harlem established by, 262
    leavened bread, 66–67
    market day, 574
    New Year's cakes, 414
    New Year's Day parties, **181–82**, 414
    seafood, 193
    settlers in Brooklyn, 80
    smoked fish, 539
    spirits, 557
    tea, 587
    Upper West Side, 613
    water, 633
colonial period. *See also* Colonial Dutch
    bread, 67
    breweries, 45
    candy making, 93
    corn consumption, 193–94
    corned beef, 145
    German immigration, 237
    lunch during, 356
    newspaper advertisements, 4
    New Year's, 411
    smoked fish, 539
    spirits, 557
    St. Patrick's Day, 558
    tea, 587
    water, 633
Colony, The (restaurant), 334
    haute cuisine in, 264
    Maccioni at, 134, 336
    post-World War II popularity of, 467
    during Prohibition, 500
Colony Club, 125, **134**, 331, 647
COLORS (restaurant), 206
Columbia Hall, 236
Columbia University, **135–36**
    courses on victory gardening, 622
Columbia University Press, 135, **136**, 335
Columbus Park, 210
Comfort Me with Apples (Reichl), 493
Commentary (magazine), 201
Committee to Save Grand Central Station, 243–44
commodity exchanges, **136–38**
Commonwealth Brewing Company New York, 387
community gardening, 215, 615. *See also* GrowNY
    hunger programs and, 281

Community Healthcare Network, 317
Community Kitchen (food pantry), 281
community supported agriculture (CSA), **138–40**, 253, 608
    in Bay Ridge, 40
    farm to table and, 203
    GrowNYC and, 254
    organic food, 437–38
Compleat Housewife, The (Smith), 416
Complete Magnolia Bakery Cookbook, The, 367
computer-generated recipes, 392
ConAgra, 255
Conant, Scott, 466
Coney Island
    Feltman in development of, 206–7
    hot dogs, 205, 275–76
    oysters at, 442
    Pakistani restaurants, 552
Coney Island (Hooker), 460
Coney Island Beach (Dwight), 460
Coney Island Scene (Marsh), 460
confectioners, 30, 94
Confectioner's Art, The (exhibition, American Craft Museum), 399
Congee Village, 352
Connelly, Kate, 211
Connie's Inn, 6
Connoisseur (magazine), 340
Connoisseur's Cookbook, The (Carrier), 548
Conoit, John, 287
Conrad, Joseph, 323
Consolidated Baking Company, 67
Conte, Mike, 397
Context Travel, 629
Continental Baking Company, 156
convenience stores, 252
Convivium Osteria, 233
Cook, Cheryl, 147
Cook and the Gardner, The (Hesser), 271–72
Cookbook for Two (Allen), 8
Cook Book of Oscar of the Waldorf, The (Tschirky), 264, 607, 627
cookbooks, **140–41**
    by Allen, 8
    in antebellum period, 13
    by Claiborne, 224, 225
    collections
        Fales Library, 201–2, 240
        of Margaret Barclay Wilson, 415, 416
        at New York Public Library, 421
        at the New York Public Library, 420
    by De Gouy, 162
    by Diat, 171
    doughnuts in, 177
    by Fabricant, 200
    by Filippini, 166
    by Flay, 210
    on fondue, 100
    Food52, 216
    by Franey, 224, 225
    by Gold, 240
    haute cuisine, 264
    by Hazan, 266–67
    by Hesser, 271–72

cookbooks (*continued*)
Italian, 296
Jewish, 311
by Jones, Judith, 312–13
by Kump, 328
by Lang, 332
by Lewis, 340
by Lucas, 354
by Metzelthin, 241
by Pépin, 454
publishing
by Knopf, 323–24, 488
New York center of, 370
by Ranhofer, 166–67
by Woods, 263
cookbook stores. *See* Kitchen Arts and Letters; Rizzoli
Cookery Book, The (De Gouy), 162
cookies, **142–43**, 287, 414, 567
Cooking à la Ritz (Diat), 171, 362, 620
Cooking at Home (Child and Pépin), 324
Cooking Channel, 217, 218, 416, 591
Cooking for Christmas (Turgeon), 119
Cooking for Mr. Latte (Hesser), 272
Cooking for One Is Fun (Creel), 125
Cooking Light (magazine), 240
Cooking Live (television show), 394, 592
Cooking Live Prime (television show), 394, 592
Cooking Manual of Practical Directions for Economical Every-Day Cookery, The (Corson), 143, 146, 417
Cooking of Vienna's Empire, The (Wechsberg), 638
cooking schools, **143–44**, 370. *See also* Cordon Bleu
Cooking School; Culinary Institute of America;
De Gustibus Cooking School; French Culinary
Institute; Institute for Culinary Education; Natural
Gourmet Cooking School; Natural Gourmet
Institute for Health and Culinary Arts; New York
Cooking School; Peter Kump's New York
Cooking School
by De Gouy, 162
French, 226
by Hazan, 266
James Beard Cooking School, 42
late twentieth century, 333, 335
opened by women, 106
Sex on the Table Cooking School, 530
Cooking School Text Book and Housekeepers' Guide, The
(Corson), 143, 146
Cooking with Master Chefs, 36
Cook It Outdoors (Beard), 41
Cook "n" Scribble, 436
cooks, African American, 5–6
Cook's (magazine), 153, 304, 646
Cook's Canon, The (Cokolov), 548
Cookshop, 135
CookShop program, 282
Cook's Tour, A (Bourdain/television show), 63
cookware stores. *See* Broadway Panhandler
Cool-Brands International, 115
Cooper, James Fenimore, 433, 458
Cooper Hewitt, Smithsonian Design Museum, **144–45**
Feeding Desire: Design and the Tools of the Table 1500–2005
(exhibition), 399–400
Copacabana, 430

Copeland's (restaurant), 263
Coppola, Francis Ford, 345, 461
Corbett, "Gentleman Jim," 243
Cordon Bleu Cook Book, The (Lucas), 354
Cordon Bleu Cooking School (Paris), 354, 370
Core Club, 126
Corkbuzz, 108, 249
corned beef, 294, 559
corned beef sandwich, **145–46**, 165
Cornell University, 281
Corn Exchange, 137
Corona, 479, 550
Corriher, Shirley O., 528
Corson, Juliet, 143, **146–47**, 370, 417
Cortland, Stephanus van, 225
Corton (restaurant), 429
Cosmopolis (DeLillo), 434
Cosmopolitan (Cecchini), 147
Cosmopolitan (cocktail), **147**, 530
Cosmopolitan (magazine), 648
Cosmopolitan Club, 125, 331
Costco Wholesale, 263
Cotheal, Isaac E., 181
Cotton, Ed, 212
Cotton Club, 6, 60, **147–48**, 262, 430
Coulombe, Joe, 604
Council on the Environment of New York City, 48, 254–55.
See also GrowNY
Counter Space: Design and the Modern Kitchen (exhibition,
MoMA), 400
Count Turf (horse), 299
Courtens, Jean-Paul, 139
Cowin, Dana, 211
cow shares, 388
cracker bakeries, 30, 31, 403
Craddock, Harry, 481
Craft (restaurant)
Chang at, 101, 393
doughnuts, 178
menu, 384
Craftbar, 495
craft breweries. *See* microbreweries and brewpubs
Craig Claiborne's Gourmet Diet (Claiborne and Franey), 225
Craig's Restaurant, 587
Craik, Cecile (Sheila Hibben), 417
Crain's New York Business
on foodtruck industry, 220
Lape and, 333
on Starbucks, 562
Crane, Clarence, 341
Crane, Stephen, 68, 433
Crane, Steven, 36
Crawford, Joan, 456
cream cheese, **148–50**
at Ben's Cheese Planet, 160
Jewish, 309
lox and, 353
Creamy and Crunchy (Krampner), 135
Creel, Henry, 125
crème brûlée, 336
Cries of New-York, The (Wood), **150–51**
Critical Topics in Food, 202, 646
Crockett, Albert Stevens, 79

Croly, Jane Cunningham, 646, 647
Cronut, **151**, 178, 538
Crossing Delancey (movie), 457
Croton Aqueduct, 269, 634
Crown Heights, 97. *See also* West Indian Day Parade
Crown's Grocery, 209
Crumbs bakery, 156
Crush Wine & Spirits (restaurant), 429
CSA. *See* community supported agriculture
Cuban, **151–52**
    food at Victor's Café, 621
Cuban-Chinese restaurants, 114, 152
Cucina and Co., 365
Cucina de Lidia, La (Bastianich and Jacobs), 36, 592, 593
Cucina della Fontana (restaurant), 249
Cue (magazine), 532
Cuisinart and Zabar's, 660
Cuisine (magazine), 42, **152–53**
Cuisine, La (Bernard), 242
Cuisine of Hungary (Lang), 332
Cuisine Rapide (Franey), 225
Cuisinier François (La Varenne), 416
Culinary Academy of Design, 143
Culinary Adventures of Baron Ambrosia, The (television show), 78
Culinary Arts Foundation. *See* James Beard Foundation
Culinary Careers (Smilow and McBride), 539
Culinary Hall of Fame
    Batali in, 37
    Flay inducted in, 211
    French Culinary Institute in, 229
Culinary Historians of New York, **153–54**, 271, 335, 370
Culinary Institute of America, 106
    Bourdain at, 63
    brewing curriculum, 83
    culinary science major, 392
    Moulton at, 393
culinary organizations, 370
Culinary Sabbatical Scholarship program, 10
culinary schools. *See* cooking schools
Culintro, **154**
Cullen, Michael J., **155**, 252, 302, 319–20, 578
Cumberland Packing Corporation, 582
Cumin, Albert, 39
Cummings, E.E., 379, 586–87
Cunningham, Laura Shane, 460
Cunningham, Marion
    Beard and, 42
    Jones, Judith, and, 313
    and Knopf imprint, 488
CUNY. *See* City University of New York
Cuomo, Andrew, 510, 579
Cuozzo, Steve, 498
cupcakes, **155–57**
Curbed.com, 187
"Curl Up and Diet" (Nash), 418
curry, 289, 552
Curry Hill, **157**, 315, 343
Curry in a Hurry (restaurant), 157
Curtis, Tony, 329
Cybele's (restaurant), 394
Czech and Slovak Bohemian Hall and Beer Garden, 47
Czechs in Yorkville, 656

D
D'Agostino, **159–60**, 318, 579
Daguin, Ariane, 20, 549
Dahl, Joseph Oliver, 505
Daily Advertiser, 177
Daily Burger, The (restaurant), 501, 561
Daily Graphic, The, 459
Daily News, 63
dairy foods. *See also* milk
    associated with Chanukah, 102
    English colonial, 193
    Erie Canal and, 195
dairy stores, **160**
Dale, Chester, 447–48
Dale, Maud, 447–48
Dallmayr (Munich deli), 163
D'Ambrosi, Andrew, 212
DanceAfrica Bazaar, 570–71
Daniel (restaurant), 63, 593
Danjo (restaurant), 325
Dankaert, Jasper, 181
Dan's Supreme Supermarkets, Inc., 318
Danube (restaurant), 62, 471
Darden sisters, 6
D'Artagnan, 549
Dave's Potbelly Stove (restaurant), 249
David, Elizabeth, 271, 362
David, Larry, 655
Davidson, Alan, 440
Dawat (restaurant), 552
Daza, Nora Villanueva, 207
db Bistro Moderne, 63, 259
DBGB Kitchen and Bar, 63
Dead Rabbit Grocery and Grog, 293
Dean, Joel, 160–61, 252
Dean & DeLuca, 105, **160–61**, 252
Death & Co., 391, 435
Death and Life of Great American Cities, The (Jacobs), 570, 641
De Blasio, Bill, 48, 462
De Chirico, Joe, 235
Decker Farm, 565
Decré, Fred, 265, 329, 337, 550
Deeliée, Felix, 264
deep-fried Twinkies, **161–62**
Deer Park, 636
De Gouy, Louis P., **162**
    on chowder, 371
    at *Gourmet*, 171, 241, 361, 362
    in haute cuisine, 264
DeGroff, Dale, 128, **162–63**, 391, 645
    consultant for Promenade Bar, 487
    Cosmopolitan, 147
    Saunders student of, 521
De Gustibus Cooking School, 144, 335, 365
Dehn, Adolf, 459
De honesta voluptate (Sacchi), 416
Delancey, Etienne, 225
Delatour's soda-water stand, 543
Del Corral, Víctor, 152, 621
Delgado, George, 645
delicatessens. *See also* delis, German; delis, Jewish
    in the Bronx, 77
    distinguished from appetizing stores, 14

delicatessens (*contintued*)
Dr. Brown's sodas in, 178, 179
in Jamaica, 302
Korean, 253
late twentieth century, 334
post-World War II, 467–68
slang and, 537–38
DeLillo, Don, 434
delis, German, **163–64**. *See also* Schaller & Weber
delis, Jewish, **164–65**, 311, 312. *See also* Katz's Delicatessen
in the Bronx, 77
Dr. Brown's sodas in, 179
Junior's, 313–14
knishes at, 322–23
Lower East Side, 351–52
pastrami, 452–53
Upper East Side, 612–13
Delmonico (dining car), 484
Delmonico, Charles, 347
Delmonico, Lorenzo, 166
Delmonico, Peter and John, 13, 369, 500
Delmonico Brothers, **165–66**
Delmonico's (restaurant), 105, **166–68**, 226, 369, 500
black cooks, 6
business lunches, 87, 469
during Civil War, 122
Thanksgiving dinner for the Union soldiers, 596–97
eggs Benedict, 190–91
elitism in, 238–39
first real restaurant, 382
in haute cuisine, 264
lobster Newberg, 347
Maccioni at, 336, 362
New York Strip Steak and, 421
opening, 13
during Prohibition, 501
Ranhofer at, 488
recipes in *The Epicurean*, 489
Tschirsky at, 607
women's clubs meeting at, 647
Del Posto (restaurant), 35, 36, 296
DeLuca, Giorgio, 160–61, 252
Demby, Eric, 541
Demetrious, George, 94
Demille, Cecil B., 109
Demillo, Ernabel, 592
Demon Rum (Pegram), 558
Dempsey, Jack, 299
Denino's Pizzeria, 464, 565–66
De Niro, Robert, 429
Department of Public Markets, Weights and Measures, 476
department stores. *See also* Macy's
restaurants, **168**
ice cream shops, 288
lunch in, 356–57
at Macy's, 364, 365
women in, 239
and victory gardens, 622
depression food, **168–70**
De re coquinaria (Apicius), 416
Derrydale Cook Book of Fish and Game, The (De Gouy), 162

Derrydale Press, 162
Der Schwarze Kolner (restaurant), 238
De Silva, Cara, 154
Despaña (food importer), 301
Dessert Circus (Torres), 604
Dessert Circus at Home (Torres), 604
Dessert Circus with Jacques Torres (PBS series), 604
Deutsch, Jonathan, 121, 135, 136
Devi (restaurant), 553
De Voe, Thomas Farrington, **170–71**, 475, 631–32
Diat, Anne Alajoinine, 171
Diat, Louis, **171**
chef at Ritz-Carlton, 506
creator of Vichyssoise, 620
Gourmet and, 362
in haute cuisine, 264
Diat, Lucien, 454
Dickens, Charles, 119, 441
Dickinson, Orville A., 205, 407
Dickson's Farmstand Meats, 88
Dictionary of Occupational Titles, 106
Dieterle, Harold, 212
Dietrich, Marlene, 339
diets. *See also* veganism; Weight Watchers
raw, 490
recommended by Macfadden, 364
Dietz and Watson, 164
Di Fara (pizzeria), 464
Di Laurentiis, Giada, 488
DiMaggio, Joe, 461
dimsum, **171–72**, 480
diners, **172–73**, 480
Greek, 245
lunches, 357–58
Park Slope, 450
Polish, 465
Diners Club, **173–74**
Diner's Dictionary, The (Ayto), 440
Dining at the Pavillon (Wechsberg), 418, 638
Dining Diary (radio show), 333
Dining In—Manhattan (Blass and Hauser), 141
"Dining with George Rector" (radio program), 492
Dinkins, David, 301
Dinner at Julia's (television show), 110
Dinner Lab, The, 466–67
Dinner with Demons (play, Reynolds), 599
Dione Lucas Book of French Cooking, The (Lucas), 354
Dione Lucas's Cooking Show, The (television show), 354, 591
DiPalo's (dairy store), 160, 345
Directions for Cookery (Leslie), 142
Dirt Candy (restaurant), 406
Dirty French, 352
distilleries, **174–75**, 564
in Manhattan, 369
in New Amsterdam, 557
rum, 509–10
Divine, Father, 6
Dizzy's (restaurant), 450
D.L. Clark Candy Co., 492, 493
"Doctor Love" (Greene), 246
Doctorow, E. L., 459

documentaries on New York food, 395–96
Doma na Rohu (restaurant), 233
Dominguez, Olga, 105
Dominican(s), **175–77**
  bodegas, 59
  in the Bronx, 77
  in Brooklyn, 97, 643
  Essex Street Market and, 196
  food trucks, 219
  in Manhattan, 97, 292, 630
  in New York City, 550
Dominick's (restaurant), 77
Dominick's Quality Hot Dogs, 220
Domino Sugar, 81, 334, 576, 577
Don Antonio by Starita, Co. (pizzeria), 464
Don Hill's (nightclub), 249
Donovan, Dennis, 356
"Don't Eat Before Reading This" (Bourain), 418
Dorgan, T. A., 276
Dorlon's (oyster bar), 441
Dorotan, Romy, 208
Dorrian's Red Hand Restaurant, 657
Dory, John, 278
Dosha Pops, 95
Doubleday, 323, 324
Dough (bakery), 43, 178
Doughnut Corporation of America, 178
Doughnut Plant, 178
doughnuts, **177–78**
  breadlines and, 169
  Irving on, 294
  during World War I, 517
Dover (restaurant), 566
Do What You Love: Building a Career in the Culinary Industry (Hamilton), 261
Downard, Georgia Chan, 427
Downing, Thomas, 5, 14, 98, 441
Downing Corporation, 299
Down to Earth Markets, 302
Dr. Brown's Soda, 145, **178–79**, 529
Draper, Dorothy, 398
Drink: A Social History (Barr), 126
drinking establishments, slang terms for, 536
Drinks (Straub), 83
Drink Up (television show), 217
Drouant, Charles, 336–37, 549
DUB Pies, 23
Ducasse, Alain, 593
Dufour, Hugue, 399
Dufresne, Wylie, **179–80**
  at French Culinary Institute, 228, 260
  at Gotham Bar and Grill, 241
  kimchi recipes, 319
  Lower East Side restaurants, 352
  modernist cuisine, 391–92
  patron of Kitchen Arts and Letters, 637
Dugdale, John, 153
Duis, Perry R., 516
Duke and Duchess of Windsor, 329, 330
Dumaine, Alexandre, 418
dumplings, 73
dumpster diving, **180–81**

Durante, Jimmy, 235
Durst Organization, 44
Dutch settlers. *See* Colonial Dutch
Dutch-style New Year's Day parties, **181–82**, 414
Dutch West India Company, 67, 133, 134, 587
Dvorak, Antonin, 355
Dwight, Mable, 460
Dyer, Ceil, 140
Dylan, Bob, 93, 248
Dylan's Candy Bar, 95, **182–83**
Dylan Thomas in America (Brinnin), 641

E
E. F. Hutton, 464
Eagle Street Rooftop Farm, 508, 615
Eamonn Doran's (pub), 293
Ear Inn, 556, 586
Early, Eleanor, 371
EarthFriends, 135
Earth Institute, The, 135, 508
Easter, **185–86**
  Dominican food for, 175–76
  Greek Orthodox, 245
  Polish food for, 465
Eastern Europeans
  in Brighton Beach, 72
  in the Bronx, 76
  in Yorkville, 657
East Hampton Star (newspaper), 199
East New York Farms, 615
East New York Food Co-op, 214
East of Paris (Bouley), 62
East Village, 351, 352. *See also* Kleindeutschland
E.A.T., 31, 613
Eataly, **186**, 294, 495
  Bastianich and, 36
  Batali and, 37
  lunches, 358
Eat! Drink! Italy! With Vic Rallo (television show), 593
Eat Drink Vote (Nestle), 409
Eater, **187**, 499
Eater.com, 464
Eating for Health and Strength (Macfadden), 364
Eating My Words (Sheraton), 532
Eating Your Words (Grimes, ed.), 249, 440
Eberhardt, Charles, 267
Ebinger's Blackout Cake, **187–88**
Ebling Brewing, 45, 70, 76
Ecce Panis, 68
Ecco Books, 64
Eckstein, Peter, 355
Eckstein brewery, 565
Economy Candy, 95, 352
Ecuadorians in the Bronx, 78
Eden, Trudy, 136
Edge, John T., 91
Edible, **188–89**
Edible (magazine), 410
Edible Communities, Inc., 188
Edmunds, Lowell, 372
Edna Lewis Cookbook, The (Lewis), 340

education. *See also* cooking schools; New York University
  AIWF and, 10
  apprenticeships *versus* culinary programs, 105–6
  in butchering, 88
  C-CAP, **96**
  food-related at CUNY, 121–22
  urban farming and opportunities, 615
Educational Alliance, 311
Edwards, Owen, 153
egg creams, **189–90**, 536, 544
  as Brooklyn invention, 81
  seltzer and, 529
eggs Benedict, **190–91**
  created for the Waldorf, 627
  in Easter celebrations, 185, 186
Egli, Konrad, 100
Egyptian, **191**
Ehert, George, 71
Eichler's (brewery), 76
Eight O'Clock Coffee, 2, 4
Eileen's Special Cheesecake, 104
Einhorn, Marilyn, 154
Eisenberg, Lee, 222
Eisenberg's, 189
Eisenstadt, Benjamin, 81, 582
Eisenstadt, Marvin, 582, 583
Eisland, Benjamin, 316
Eisner, Michael, 256
El Barrio. See Spanish Harlem
Eleven Madison Park (restaurant), 190, 305, 386, 412
Elk Candy, 656
Ellen's Stardust Diner, 602
Elliot, Peter, 363
Elliot, Virginia, 371
Ellis Island
  food (1892–1924), **192–93**
  Guastavino design for, 244
  Italian immigrants through, 295
El Malecon (restaurant), 630
Elmhurst
  Asians in, 480
  Filipinos in, 207
  Thai in, 596
Elmhurst Cream Company, 302
El Mofongo Café, 630
El Morocco, 430
El Neovo Caridad (restaurant), 97
Elpine Drinks, 601
Elsie Presents James Beard in "I Love to Eat," 41
Elvin, Ella, 75, 338
Elza Fancy Food, 73
Emde, Jori Jayne, 86
Emergency Food Assistance Program, 280–81, 282
Empellon (restaurant), 392
Empellon Cocina (restaurant), 566
Empire Diner, 173
Employees Only (restaurant), 566
employment. *See also* unions
  discrimination at A&P, 2
  fair labor practices in food co-ops, 213–14
Employment of Women, The (Penny), 30
Encyclopedia of Chicago, The (Duis), 516
Enduro's (sandwich shop), 314

Engeman, William A., 72, 345
English Bread and Yeast Cookery (David), 271
English colonial, **193–94**
Entenmann's, 177, 237
entertainment. *See also* nightclubs
  in beer gardens, 47
Ephron, Nora, 246, 660
Épicerie Boulud, 63
Epicurean, The (Ranhofer), 166–67, 489
  eggs Benedict, 190
  haute cuisine, 264
  lobster Newberg, 347
  on naming of baked Alaska, 29
Epicurean Delight (Jones), 313
Epstein, Jason, 488
Epstein, Samuel, 432
Erie Canal, **194–95**, 369, 442, 643
Ermisch, Auguste, 259–60
Errico, Vincenzo, 83
Esca (restaurant), 35, 36, 186, 296
Escoffier, Auguste, 105
  brigade system of kitchens, 106
  De Gouy's cooking for, 162
  Diat as soup chef under, 620
  in haute cuisine, 264
  influence on Grand Central Oyster Bar, 243
  quoted by Cannon, 96
  at Ritz-Carlton, 506
  on steak tartare, 566
Escoffier, Michel, 338
Escoffier, Pierre, 338
Esperienze Italiane, 36
Esposito, Rafaele, 461
Esposito's Pork Store, 269
Esquire (magazine)
  Grimes in, 249
  on power lunches, 87, 469
Ess-a-Pickle, 458
Essence (magazine), 340
Essential Cocktail, The (DeGroff), 147
Essential New York Times Cookbook, The (Hesser, ed.), 141, 216,
    272, 423
Essex House, 264, 329
Essex Street Market, **195–96**, 247, 352, 476, 574
  cheese at, 105
  Heritage Meat at, 88
  La Guardia in creation of, 230–31
Estela (restaurant), 566
ethnic bakeries, 68, 142
ethnic food
  in Astoria, 21
  cookbooks and, 140
  in early restaurants, 500
  food trucks and, 574
  in Sunset Park, 577
ethnic restaurants
  brunch at, 85
  slang and, 537
"European Perspectives: A Series in Social Thought and
    Cultural Criticism" series, 136
Evans, Mary Elizabeth, 94
Evans, Meryle, 202, 399
Everyday Exotic (television show), 217

"Everything You Always Wanted to Know About Ice Cream But Were Too Fat to Ask" (Greene), 246
Evetts, Deborah, 416
Exchange Buffet, 92, 93, 369, 500
   fast food, 204
Exchange Coffee Room, The (coffeehouse), 128, 129
Experimental Cuisine Collective, **197**, 392
"Eyewitness Gourmet, The" (television show), 333

F
F. A. O. Schweetz (candy store), 182
F. & M. Schaefer Brewing, 45, 46, 70–71, 85, 333
   sporting events and, 559
   at World Fair, 1939–1940, 650
F. X. Matt Brewery, 82
Fabricant, Florence, **199–200**
   on butcher shops, 88
   on Kalustyan's, 315
   at the New York Times, 423
   on yerba mate, 202
Fairchild, John, 330
Fair Housing Act (1968), 300
Fairhurst, Patricia, 457–58
Fairway Market, **200–201**, 251, 252, 578, 614
   cheese, 105
   kosher food, 312
falafel, 191, **201**, 346
Fales Library, **201–2**, 240
Family Circle (magazine), 28, 647
Family Living on $500 a Year (Corson), 146
Family Market, 308
Famous Fat Dave's five-borough eating tour, 630
Famous Vegetarians and Their Favorite Recipes (Berry), 49
Fancher, Ed, 623
Fancy Food Show, **202–3**
Fannie Farmer Cookbook, The, 313, 324
Fardart, Frank, 92
Far East, The (chop suey house), 275
"Farewell to a Renaissance Mensch" (Mautner), 212
Farinetti, Oscar, 186
Farley, Thomas, 496, 544
Farm & Fireside (magazine), 446
Farmerie, Brad, 434
farmers' markets, 575, 608. See also Greenmarkets; GrowNY
   Hesses on, 270–71
   Jamaica, 302
   late twentieth century, 335
   organic food at, 438
   SNAP and, 579
   suburbanization and, 476
Farm Fresh Food Access Program, 281
Farmigo, 563
farms. See also urban farming
   in early Brooklyn, 80
   hunger programs and, 281–82
Farm-to-Consumer Legal Defense Fund, 388
farm to table, 138, **203–4**
   Bay Ridge restaurants, 40
   Blue Hill Restaurant, 33
   at French Culinary Institute, 228
Fassio, Anthony, 407

fast food, **204–6**
   impact on diners, 173
   Jackson Heights, 301
   Japanese, 308
   late twentieth century, 334
   lunches, 358
   pizza, 463
   post-World War II expansion of, 467
Fast Food Forward movement, 206
fast-food workers strikes, **206**
Fatty 'Cue barbecue, 81
Fauci, Alexis, 471
Faulkner, William, 339
Faust's (lobster palace), 330
Fawcett, Edgar, 356
Feast (Jones), 440
Feast Made for Laughter, A (Claiborne), 124
Fedele, Joe, 229
Federal Food Board, 451
Federal Water Pollution Control Act (1948), 209
Federal Writers' Project, 8, 9, 344
Federer, "Fed," 530
Federman, Mark Russ, 324, 353, 511
Federman, Niki Russ, 511
Feeding America, 282
Feeding Desire: Design and the Tools of the Table, 1500–2005 (exhibition, Cooper-Hewitt), 144, 399–400
"Feeding the City" project, 9
Feeding the Lions (Case), 7
Feeding Web, The (Gussow), 135
Feeding Your Family on $99 a Week (television show), 217
Feed Your Pet Right (Nestle and Nesheim), 409
Fei Long, 577
Feingold, Michael, 624
Feldman, Zachary, 86
Felidia (restaurant), 35, 36, 296
Felker, Clay, 4, 419
Feltman, Charles, 81, **206–7**
   Handwerker working for, 405
Feltman-Sailhac, Arlene, 144, 365
Ferguson, Katie, 98
Ferguson, Max, 655
Ferguson, Priscilla Parkhurst, 135
Ferguson, Sarah, Duchess of York, 639
Fernald, Anya, 538
Fernery, The (tearoom), 590
Ferrara Pastry Shop, 344
Ferrara's (coffeehouse), 130
Fessaguet, Roger, 265, 329, 337, 550
Festa di Santa Rosalia, 49
Field, Anna C., 647
Field, Benjamin C., 484
Field, Michael, 144
Fields, Tanya, 78
Fifteen-Cent Dinners for Workingmen's Families (Corson), 146, 417
Fifth Avenue Hotel, 277, 411
Filipino, **207–8**
   fast food, 205
Filippini, Alessandro, 166, 432
films. See movies
Finback Brewery, 387
Finkel, Fyvush, 323, 655
Finkelstein, Izzy, 322

Finnegan's Wake (pub), 657
Fiori, Pamela, 363
Firebird (restaurant), 512
Firehouse Kitchen (television show), 593
Fireside Cookbook, The (Beard), 41
First Hungarian Literary Society, 280
Firtle, Bridget, 510
fish. *See also* Fulton Fish Market
    changing trends, 284
    and chips, 293
    gefilte fish, 164, 311
    markets on Arthur Avenue, 19
    smoked (*See* smoked fish)
Fish (Bittman), 53
Fisher, Andrew, 19
Fisher, Edwin, 19
Fisher, M. F. K.
    Beard and, 42
    Brillat Savarin translation, 324
    James Beard Award, 304
    in Les Dames d'Escoffier, 338
    on Lewis, 340
    writing for
        Gourmet, 241, 362, 468
        The New Yorker, 335
fishing, **208–9**
    English colonial, 193
Fishkill Farms, 240
FishTag (restaurant), 245
Fitch, Noël Riley, 324
Fitzgerald, Ella, 299
Fitzgerald, F. Scott, 79
Fitz Gerald, John J., 52, 536
Five Guys (restaurant), 259
Five Napkin Burger, 259
Five Points, **209–10**
    groggeries, 253
    Irish in, 292–93
Flagship Brewing Company, The, 387
Flandrin, Jean-Louis, 135
Flatbush, 80, 97
Flatbush Food Co-op, 213, 437
Flay, Bobby, **210–11**
    in Food & Wine Classic, 211
    in French Culinary Institute, 260
    mayonnaise promotion, 268
    and meal in *Omnium Gatherum*, 599
    Scribner's, 528
    show on the Cooking Channel, 591
    supplied by Kalustyan's, 315
    television shows, 217, 218
Flea, The, 358
Fleischmann, Louis, 67
Fleischmann's, 31
    breadline at, 68
    Model Vienna Bakery, 2
Fleisher's (butcher), 88
Fleur de Sel (restaurant), 265
Florent (restaurant), 249
Floridita (restaurant), 97
Flushing
    Asians in, 480
    Chinese New Year in, 412

Koreatown, 327
    Momo Crawl, 608
Flying Food International, 242–43
Fly Market, 230
Fodero Dining Car Company, 173
foie gras, 65, 549
Folk City, 248, 249
Fonda del Sol (restaurant), 39
fondue, 100
food. *See also* ethnic food; fusion food
    access to, 78–79
    in beer gardens, 47
    at coffee shops, 132
    at Columbia University, 135
    fair, 161–62
    foreign foods
        restaurants and, 501
        at World's Fair, 1939–1940, 650
    regulation of prices and commodity exchanges, 137
    vegetarian
        Indo-Caribbean, 289
        Korean, 325
    in vending machines, 619
Food: A Cultural History (Flandrin and Montanari, eds.), 135
Food and Beverage Book Awards, 304
Food and Drink with Time Out New York (television show), 593
Food and Drug Administration
    on Cel-Ray, 179
    Northeast Regional Laboratory, 302
Food and Faith in Christian Culture (Albala and Eden, eds.), 136
Food and Fuel Control Act (Lever Act), 175, 653
Food and Healing (Colbin), 406
Food & Wine (magazine), 37, **211–12**
    on Barber, 33
    and culinary scene, 370
    debut, 335
    on Dufresne, 180
    Hamilton in, 262
    on Hesser, 272
    Kump in, 328
    on Lewis, 340
    NYC Wine and Food Festival and, 416
Food & Wine Classic, 211
Food Arts (magazine), 37, **212–13**
    Arnold technology contributor at, 392
    debut, 335
    on Dufresne, 180
    on Dorothy Cann Hamilton, 261
    Wolf and, 646
Food Bank Association of New York State, 281
Food Bank for New York City, 280–82, 416
    Ansel and, 151
    Batali and, 37
    Key Food donations to, 317
    NYC Food Film Festival and, 434
    research and policy initiatives, 282
food banks. *See* food pantries
Food52 Cookbook, 216
food co-ops, **213–14**, 253
    in Bay Ridge, 40
    organic food at, 437
    in Park Slope, 449–50
Food Culture in Japan (Ashkenazi), 309

Food Curated (television show), 593
food deserts, **214–16**, 608. *See also* food insecurity;
       hunger programs
  in Harlem, 263
  Key Food and, 318
  online grocers and, 229
food design, 410
Food Dynasty, 317
Food52, **216**, 271, 272
Food for the Gods (Berry), 49–50
Food52 Genius Recipes, 216
FoodHacker, 563
Food Heaven, 73
food history, 415–16
foodie, emergence of, 607–8
food insecurity, 579. *See also* food deserts; hunger programs
  among CUNY students, 121–22
  dumpster diving and, 180
  food deserts and, 214–15
  Key Food and, 318
  late twentieth century, 333
food labels, 605
Food Lover's Companion, The (Jones), 313
Food Matters (Bittman), 53
food movement, 334–35, 425
Food Network, **216–18**, 591
  Bourdain's show on, 63
  at Chelsea Market, 108
  Cupcake Wars, 156
  "The Eyewitness Gourmet" and, 333
  farm to table and, 204
  Flay on, 210
  James Beard Awards on, 305
  Moulton and, 394
  NYC Wine and Food Festival and, 416
  Puerto Ricans on, 478
  Rachael Ray on, 491
  Reichl and, 493
  Schwartz on, 527
  supplied by Kalustyan's, 315
  Torres on, 604
Food Network Magazine, 217
Food on Foot, 630
food pantries, 281, 282, 334, 371
  late twentieth century, 333
  for students, 122
Food Pantry of West Harlem, 281
Food Policy Task Force, 214–15
Food Politics (Nestle), 408
Food Politics (Paarlberg), 440
food politics and urban farming, 615
Food Politics blog, 408
Food Republic (online magazine), 518
"food rescue," 370
food restrictions during World War I, 652
Food Retail Expansion to Support Health, 318
food riots during World War I, 652
food safety
  distilleries and, 174, 175
  dumpster diving and, 180
  La Guardia in, 331–32
  public markets and, 474–76
Food Secure NYC, 283

foodservice sanitation consultants, impact of letter grading
    on, 496
food shortages and rationing during World War II, 653, 654
Foods of New York, 629
food sourcing, 608
food stamps. *See* Supplemental Nutrition Assistance
    Program (SNAP)
food studies
  Nestle and, 408
  at the New School, 370, 410
  at New York University (*See* New York University)
Food Talk (television show), 217
Food Talk with Arthur Schwartz (radio show), 527
food tourism, 608
food trucks, **218–21**, 574
  fusion, 233
  hot dogs, 275
  ice cream sandwiches, 287
  ice cream shops, 288
  Jackson Heights, 301
  Korean taco, 326
  lunches, 358
  Papaya King, 449
  Park Slope, 450
  Polish, 465
  Puerto Rican, 478
  South and Central American food, 551
  vegan, 618
Food Universe, 317
Food Values and Economies Exhibition (American Museum of
    Natural History, 1917), 10
FoodWorks, 139
Forbes Magazine, 324, 497, 646, 649
Forcella Pizzeria, 462
Forest Hills, 479
  Russians in, 512
Forgione, Larry
  at Beard House, 306
  Citymeals-on-Wheels, 120
  on farm to table, 203
  at P. J. Clarke's, 445
Fork in the Road blog, 624
Forman, Sol, 457
Fornal, Justin, 78
Forster, E. M., 323
Fort Defiance (soda fountain), 547
fortified wine, 127
Forty Ate (restaurant), 466
$40 a Day (television show), 592
Forum of the Twelve Caesars, The (restaurant), 39, 370
  on *All Around the Town*, 140
  menu, 384
  part of Restaurant Associates, 494
Forverts (newspaper), 311
For You & Yours (radio show). *See Radio City Matinee*
Foster, Georg, 253
Foster, George, 209
Fountain Restaurant (Metropolitan Museum of Art), 398
Four Seasons, The (restaurant), **221–22**, 370, 498
  Baum and, 39, 501
  Brody in, 243
  business lunch at, 87
  Flying Food International and, 242

Four Seasons, The (restaurant) (*continued*)
  as gay bar, 236
  haute cuisine in, 265
  Lang in, 332
  made historic landmark, 235
  on *Mad Men*, 366
  Paddleford on, 446
  part of Restaurant Associates, 494
  power lunches, 358
Fourth of July, **222–24**
Fourth St. Co-op (Good Food Co-op), 213–14, 437
Fox, Herman and Ida, 81, 189
Foxfire Americana Library, 324
Fox's U-Bet syrups
  Chocolate Syrup, 81, 189
  seltzer and, 529
Francher, Ed, 641
Francis H. Leggett Co., 267
Franco-American Cookery Book, The (Déliée), 264
Franey, Pierre, **224–25**
  arrival from France, 227
  Claiborne and, 124, 468
  at Le Pavillon, 337, 549
  and *New York Times*, 423
  Pépin and, 454
Frankenthaler, Helen, 221
frankfurters, 164. *See also* hot dogs
"Frankfurt on the Hudson," 630
Frankie Cooks (television show), 593
Franklin, Aretha, 222
Frank's Market, 631
Franny's (restaurant), 450, 462, 464
Fraser, John, 466
Fraunces, Samuel, 4, 225
Fraunces Tavern, 35, 194, **225**, 369, 586
  catering by, 98
  Washington farewell luncheon at, 356
Frawley, James J., 353
Frazier, T. W., 376
Fred's (restaurant), 168
Freedenberg, Dave, 630
freeganism, 180
Freeman's (gastropub), 352
Free Training School for Women, 417
Freiman, Jane, 498
French, **225–27**
  bakeries, 67
  celebrations on Bastille Day, 571
  Gourmet on, 242
  haute cuisine, 264–65
  Ladies Who Lunch and, 331
  late twentieth century, 333, 334
  Lucas in, 354
  post-World War II, 467
French Chef, The (television show, Child), 110, 313, 591, 592
French Cooking for Americans (Diat), 171
French Culinary Institute, 144, **227–29**, 335, 370. *See also* International Culinary Center
  Arnold director of technology at, 392
  Barber at, 33
  Chang at, 101
  Flay at, 210
  Hamilton founder of, 260

  in haute cuisine, 265
  teachers
    Hazan, 267
    Pépin, 454
    Soltner, 65, 549
    Torres, 604
French Laundry, The (restaurant), 305
FreshDirect, **229–30**, 251, 253
Fresh Food Fast (television show), 217
Fresh Fruit and Vegetable Juices (Walker), 491
FRESH (Food Retail Expansion to Support Health) program, 215
Freson, Robert, 153
Friedman, Jonah, 160
Friedman, Ken, 56
Friend, Tad, 272
Friends of the High Line, 274, 380
Friends of the U.S. Pavilion, 261, 307
Frito-Lay, Inc., 456
frolickings, 118
From Farm to City: Staten Island 1661–2012 (exhibit, MCNY), 401
Frommer's NYC Free & Dirt Cheap (Wolff), 85–86
From My Mother's Kitchen (Sheraton), 532
Frugal Housewife, The (Carter), 177
Fruits of Tantalus (Berry), 50
Fuji Sushi, 307, 308
Fuku (restaurant), 101
Fulton Fish Market, **230–32**, 475
  Grand Central Oyster Bar and, 244
  at Hunts Point, 283–84
  Il Pesce supplied by, 186
  Passover and strike at, 451
Fulton Market, 370, 409
  in antebellum period, 11
  contribution to Thanksgiving dinner for Union soldiers, 597
Fulton Market Stalls, 409
fusion food, 106, **232–33**
  Asian, 172
  Korean, 327
  late twentieth century, 334
Fussell, Betty, 202, 313

G
G. & R. Waite (publisher), 177
Gabila's, 322
Gabriel's (restaurant), 614
Gage & Tollner (restaurant), 105, **235**
  black cooks at, 6
  Lewis at, 340
Gaige, Crosby, 170
Galaxy, The, 57
Galloping Gourmet, The (television show), 591
Gamber, Wendy, 59
Gambrinus Seafood Café, 73
Gansevoort Market, 379
Gansevoort Market Co-op, 380
Garavuso, Michael, 373
Garden and Greening Program, 215
Garden Cafeteria, 92, 312
garden communities in Jackson Heights, 300
Garden of Eden (grocery store), 253
gardens. *See* community gardening; rooftop gardens

Gardner, Gayle, 217
Garifuna, 78
Garlic and Sapphires (Reichl), 493
Garten, Ina, 488
Gaslight (restaurant), 249
Gastronom Arkadia, 73
Gastronomica, 421
Gastronomique (Allen), 8
Gastropolis (Hauck-Lawson and Deutsch, eds.), 135, 136
Gato (restaurant), 210
Gaugin (restaurant), 464
gay bars, **235–37**. *See also* Stonewall Inn
    Greenwich Village, 248
gay community
    in Hell's Kitchen, 269
    walkers, 330
gay liberation movement, 236
Gay Scene Guide Quarterly, 568
gefilte fish, 164, 311
Geiger, Lincoln, 139
Geiger, Michael, 153
gelato, 297
Gelb, Arthur, 533
Gelinaz! (culinary performance organization), 180
Geller, Max, 407
Gellis, Isaac, 163, 311
Gem Spa, 189
gender. *See also* women
    chefs and, 105, 106
General Baking Company, 31
General Foods, 267–68, 333
General Growth Properties, 409
General Slocum (steamship), 237
    Kleindeutschland and, 321
    picnickers on, 459
Gentilcore, David, 136
Genzlinger, Neil, 466
George B. Corsa Hotel Collection, 419
George Hecker & Company, 67
George Rector (restaurant), 64
George's Place (speakeasy), 556
German(s), **237–38**, 522–23. *See also* delis, German; Germans;
        Kleindeutschland
    distilleries, 174
    doughnuts, 178
    Easter egg trees, 186
    Ebinger's, 187–88
    Hamburg steak, 259–60
    in Harlem, 262
    in Hell's Kitchen, 269
    in Jamaica, 302
    at Lüchow's, 355
    pickles, 457–58
    pretzels, 471
    smoked fish and, 540
    in Washington Heights, 630
    during World War I, 652
    1820-World War I immigration, 163
    in Yorkville, 612, 656
German Cookbook, The (Sheraton), 532
Gersten-Vassilaros, Alexandra, 599
Getting Healthy (television show), 217
Giannone, Paul, 462

Gift of Southern Cooking, The (Lewis and Peacock), 340
"Gift of the Magi, The" (Henry), 293
Gilded Age, **238–40**, 278
Gill, Brendan, 153
Gilman, George F., 1, 154, 251, 588
Gilsey House (hotel restaurant), 278
Ginny's Supper Club, 518
Gino's Italian Ice, 297
Ginsberg, Allen, 25, 248
Girl and Her Greens, A (Bloomfield and Goode), 57
Girl and Her Pig, A (Bloomfield and Goode), 57
Girl from Rector's, The (G. Rector), 492
Girl from Rector's, The (play, Potter), 492
Girls (Red Buttons) (Marsh), 448
Giuliani, Rudolph, 44
    on Fulton Fish Market, 231
    at Le Cirque, 336
    on Les Dames d'Escoffier, 338
    at Patsy's, 461
    street vendors and, 574
"Giving Good Weight" (McPhee), 48, 418
glace au four, 29
Glaser, Milton
    Baum and, 39
    Brooklyn Brewery logo, 82
    co-founder of *New York* magazine, 4, 419
    graphics of Windows on the World, 645
    iconic ads by, 4
    on knishes and politics, 322
Glaser's Bake Shop, 54, 657
Glickberg, Cynthia, 200
Glickberg, Dan, 201
Glickberg, Howard, 200–201, 252
Glickberg, Leo, 200, 252
Glickberg, Nathan, 200, 252, 578, 614
Global Culinary Initiative, 339
Globe Hotel, 264
Gluck, Sandy, 427
Gnosis Chocolate, 563
goat meat, 284, 303
Godfather, The (movie), 299
    in Little Italy, 344
    Patsy's in, 461
Goelet, Robert W., 505
Goin, Suzanne, 324
Gold, Jonathan, 219
Gold, Rozanne, **240**, 487, 645
    Baum and, 39
    Fales Library donation, 202
Goldberg, Gary A., 410
Goldberger, Paul, 437
Gold Cook Book, The (De Gouy), 162
Golden, Harry, 316
Golden, Hyman, 541
Goldenberg, Feige, 345
Golden Girls, The (television show), 323
Golden-Krust (bakery/restaurant), 97
Golden Unicorn (restaurant), 172
Goldfarb, Will, 197, 392
Gold Label Deli, 73
Gold Medal Mayonnaise, 267
Goldstein, Darra, 154
Goldstein, Herbert, 202

Golumbeck, Karen, 342
Gomberg, Alex, 529
Gomberg, Kenny, 529
Gomberg, Mo, 529
Gomberg Seltzer Works, 528–29
Gomez, Cornelia, 98
Gompers, Samuel, 502
Goodby, Mary, 340
Good Dine Restaurant, The, 77
Goode, J. J., 57
Good Eggs, 229, 438
Good Housekeeping (magazine), 171, 648
    Allen as food editor r, 8
    Brock at, 74
    Greene and, 246
    Sheraton at, 532
Good Humor, 218–19, 288, 573
Goodman's (bakery), 451
Good Morning America, 333, 394
Gordon, Elizabeth, 221
Gordon, Waxy, 60–61
Gorilla Coffee, 564
Gorodinsky, Ben, 160
Goss, Roswell, 617
Gotham Bar and Grill, 180, **240–41**, 249
Gotham Greens, 508, 615, 642
Gothamist.com, 464
Gottfried, John, 243
Gottlieb, Robert, 417
Gouffé, Jules, 620
Goulash Avenue, 280
Goulash Row, 279
Gourmet (magazine), **241–42**
    credit card, 174
    and culinary scene, 370
    donation to Fales Library, 202, 240
    ending restaurant reviews, 499
    founded by MacAusland, 361
    on Lewis, 340
    Menus Classiques column, 171
    post-World War II influence, 468
    Reichl editor of, 493
    restaurant reviews, 497
    writers
        Beard, 42
        Claiborne, 124
        De Gouy, 162
        Diat, 171
        Elizabeth David, 362
        Moulton, 394
        Wechsberg, 638
Gourmet Cookbook, The (MacAusland), 362
Gourmet Cooking School, 144
Gourmet Cooking School Cookbook, The (Lucas), 354
Gourmet Garage, **242–43**, 253
gourmet grocers. *See* Balducci's; Dean & DeLuca; Zabar's
Gourmet's Almanac, The (MacDougall), 9
Gourmet Society, 170
Gouy, Louis de, 468
Goya Foods, 59
GQ (magazine), 262
Grace's Marketplace, 32
Gracie Mansion, 162, 240

Graff, Richard, 9
Graham, Anthony, 139
Graham, Sylvester, 67, 287, 617
Graham crackers, 142
Gramercy Tavern, 334, 386, 495, 501
Grand Central Oyster Bar, **243–44**, 441, 443
    in *Mad Men*, 366
Grand Central Palace, 411
Grand Central Station food court, 358
Grandfather Stories (Hopkins), 182
Grand Hotel menu, 382, 384
Grand Tasting Walk-Arounds, 416
Grand Tier Restaurant (Metropolitan Opera), 495
Grand Union (supermarket), 159, 250, 251, 578
Grange Hall (restaurant), 249
Grant, Jane, 417
granulated sugar, 576
Grausman, Richard, 96
Gray, Jim, 435
Gray's Papaya (restaurant), 249, 277
grazing craze, 240
Great American Cookbook (Paddleford), 506
Great American Tea Company, 1, 251, 588
Great Atlantic and Pacific Tea Company, 588. *See also* A&P
Great Atlantic Tea Company, 251
Great Chefs (television show), 218
Great Depression. *See also* Depression food
    African American food, 6
    automats, 619
    breadlines, 68–69
    in the Bronx, 77
    films about food struggles during, 394
    food provided by Salvation Army, 517
    gay bars, 236
    grocery stores, 252
        King Kullen, 319–20
    hamburgers, 259
    haute cuisine, 264
    impact on railroads, 485
    Junior's and, 314
    lunch counters, 357
    Nedick's, 407
    paintings of, 448
    Prohibition's repeal and, 474
    school lunch programs, 524
    street vendors, 573
    tea rooms, 590
Greater Jamaica Development Corporation, 302
Greater New York Cooking School, 143
Great Fire of 1835, 166, 633
Great Food Truck Race, The (television show), 220
Great Hall Balcony Bar (Metropolitan Museum of Art), 399
Great Migration (1910–1945) and southern foods, 6, 649
Great Performances, **244–45**
    Chalsty's Café (MCNY), 402
Great Waters of France, 636
Greco, David, 19
Greek(s), **245**
    in Astoria, 22
    in Bay Ridge, 40
    in the Bronx, 78
    coffee shops, 357–58, 467–68
    diners, 173

Easter celebrations, 185–86
halva in Lent, 258
hot dogs, 277
late twentieth century, 334
pushcart vendors, 572
in Washington Heights, 630
Green, Adolphus, 403, 404
Green, Les, 397
Green, Max, 322
Greenberg, Arnold, 541
Greenberg, Murray, 397. *See also* Murray's Cheese
Greenberg, William, 54
Green Cart program, 56, 79, 608
Green Door, The, 556
Greene, Gael, **245–46**, 498
    co-founder of Citymeals-on-Wheels, 119–20
    on Flay, 210
    on Four Seasons, 221
    at *New York* magazine, 420
Greenfield, Albert M., 349–50
Greengrass, Barney, 353. *See also* Barney Greengrass
Greengrass, Gary, 353
green grocer carts, 215
Green Hill Food Co-op, 214
Greenleaf, Cat, 434
Greenmarkets, **246–48**, 253, 575, 608
    Benepe cofounder of, 47
    in Brooklyn
        Bay Ridge, 40
        Park Slope, 450
    doughnuts, 177, 178
    GrowNYC and, 254–55
    Hess in, 270
    Jackson Heights, 301
    late twentieth century, 333, 335
    public markets and, 476
    sponsored by Council on the Environment, 48, 247
    before the 19th century, 251
    in Upper West Side, 614
Greenpoint cocktail, 83
green roof movement, 508
Green Tables Initiative, 339
GreenThumb program, 215, 615
Green Tulip (restaurant), 464
Greenwich Market, 273–74
Greenwich Village, **248–49**
    coffeehouses, 130–31
    gay bars, 236
    Italian restaurants, 295
    Little Italy in, 344
    tearooms in, 590
Greenwich Village Society for Historic Preservation, 380
Green Witch (tearoom), 590
Gregory, Hanson, 178
Grief, Edvard, 163
Grigson, Jane, 362
Grillin' and Chillin' (television show), 210
Grill It! with Bobby Flay (television show), 211
Grimes, William, **249–50**, 592
    on Aquavit, 15
    on Brady, 64
    on Café des Artistes, 332
    on Chalet Suisse, 100
    on Daniel, 63
    on museum food, 398
    at the *New York Times*, 423
Gristede, Charles, 250, 252, 578
Gristede, Diedrich, 250, 252, 578
Gristedes, **250–51**, 252, 578
Griswold, Darius, 635
groceries
    delivery of, 468
    Greek, 245
    Hungarian, 280
    Jackson Heights, 301
    Jamaica, 302
    Japanese, 308
    Jewish, 309
    Puerto Rican, 477
grocery stores, **251–53**. *See also* bodegas; food co-ops
    in antebellum period, 11–12
    Armenian, 315
    Caribbean specialties, 97
    Five Points, 209–10
    German, 321
    Gourmet Garage, 242–43
    impact of street vendors on, 573
    Key Food, 317–18
    Korean, 325
    in late twentieth century, 335
    Little Italy, 345
    Little Odessa, 346
    Manhattan, 370
    online, 229–30
    Syrian, 278–79
groggeries, **253–54**
    Five Points, 209–10
Groh, Trauger, 139
Grohusko, J. A., 83
Grooms, Red, 448
Grosz, George, 448
Ground Support (coffee shop), 129
Growing Older (Gussow), 135
GrowNYC, 48, 215, 247, **254–55**, 614
    New School and, 410
    SNAP and, 579
Grow To Lean NYC: The Citywide School Garden Initiative, 525
Grub Street blog, 563
GrubStreet.com, 464
Guarneschelli, Maria, 528
Guastavino, Rafael, 243–44
Guastavino's, 47
Guérard, Michel, 63, 124
Guidara, Will, 278
Guide Culinaire, Le (Escoffier), 620
Guinan, Texas, 556
Guinness beer, 293, 558–59
Guinness Book of Records, 259
Gulden, Charles, 255
Gulden's Mustard, 237, **255**
gum, **255–56**
gummy bears, 163
Gun Hill Brewery, 76, 387
Gunn, Thomas Butler, 58
Guss, Isidore, 457
Gussow, Joan Dye, 135

Guss' pickles, 457–58
Gustiamo (food importer), 267
Guth, Charles, 94, 349, 455
Guthrie, Woody, 379
Guys and Dolls short stories (Runyon), 510

H
H. Fox & Co., 189
Häagen-Dazs, **257–58**
Haandi (restaurant), 157
Habana Outpost, 81, 561
Habibi (restaurant), 201
Haechler, Werner, 83, 84
Haffen (brewery), 76
Hage, Randy, 655
Hagiwara, Brian, 153
Haigh, Ted, 79–80
halal food, 17, 219
Halal Guys, 17
Hall, Ilan, 212
Hallett, William, 22
Hallo Berlin (restaurant), 47, 238
Halsey, Stephen A., 22
halva, **258**
    Armenian, 18
    Jewish, 311
    in Little Syria, 346
halvah. *See* halva
halwah. *See* halva
Hamburger Heaven, 259
hamburgers, **258–59**
    adoption of word, 164
    called liberty steaks, 163
    fast food, 205
    Fourth of July, 223–24
    origin of, 224
hamburg steak, **259–60**
Hamill, Pete, 556
Hamilton, Dorothy Cann, 144, **260–61**, 370
    French Culinary Institute, 227–28, 335
    in James Beard Foundation, 306
Hamilton, Gabrielle, **261–62**, 593
Hamilton, Thomas, 427
Hammond, Maria Matilda Ericsson, 143
Hampton Chutney (restaurant), 553
Hand-Book of Practical Cookery (Blot), 57, 143
Handwerker, Murray, 405
Handwerker, Nathan, 205, 224, 277, 405
Hangwai (restaurant), 325
Hanover, Donna, 217
Hanscom's (bakery), 300
Hanson, Stephen, 501
Hanukah. *See* Chanukah
Harbor School, 209
Harcombe, James, 24, 618
Hardart, Frank, 24
Hardenbergh, Henry Janeway, 627
hardtack, 403
Hardy, Hugh, 39, 487, 645
Hardy, Renee Lawson, 642
Harlem, **262–64**
    bodegas in East Harlem, 59
    Caribbeans in, 97

Easter parade, 185
Fairway, 200
    as food desert, 214–15
    gay bars, 236
    Little Italy in, 344
    Mexicans in, 385
    Puerto Ricans in, 477–78
    soul food, 6
    street cries in, 3
    tearooms in, 591
Harlem Market, 12, 632
Harlem Renaissance, 262, 448
Harmatz, Jacob, 311
Harmonie Club, 125
Harper's (magazine), 146–47, 458
Harriman, Florence J., 134
Harrington, John Walker, 6
Harrington, Michael, 587, 624
Harris, Richard, 293
Harris, William, 505, 506
Harrison, Wallace K., 486
Hart-Agnew law, 345
Hart-Celler Immigration Bill, 22, 300, 346
Hartford, George H., 1, 2, 154, 251, 588
Hartford, George L., 3
Hartford, John, 2, 3
Hartley, Robert M., 174, 389, 593
"Hasty Pudding" (Barlow), 103
Hatsuhana (restaurant), 581
Hattie Carthan Community Farm, 615
Hauck-Lawson, Annie, 121, 135, 136
Hauser, Joan G., 141
haute cuisine, **264–65**
    late twentieth century, 334, 338
    Le Pavillon in launching, 336–37
    in lobster palaces, 348–49
Havemeyer & Elder, 575, 643
Havemeyer family, 238, **265–66**
Have You Eaten Yet? (exhibition, MOCA), 400
Hawaiian Room, The (restaurant), 39, 370, 467, 501
Hawaiian Tropical Drinks, 448–49
Haywood, Big Bill, 502
Hazan, Giuliano, 266
Hazan, Marcella, **266–67**, 296
    in Institute of Culinary Education, 290
    Judith Jones and, 313
    Knopf and, 324, 488
    Kump and, 327
    in Les Dames d'Escoffier, 338
Hazan, Victor, 266
health
    fast food and, 205–6
    fishing and pollution, 208–9
    food co-ops and, 213–14
    food deserts and, 214–15
    Korean food and, 325
    Perrier and, 456
    public health measures (*See* menu labels; soda "ban";
        trans fat elimination)
Health Bucks Program, 56
Healthy Bodega Initiative, 56
Healthy Hunger-Free Kids Act (2010), 525
Healthy Neighborhoods, 282

Healthy Soul (television show), 593
Healy's Golden Glades (lobster palace), 330
Hearst, Steve, 269–70
Hearst Corporation, 217
Hearst Ranch, 269–70
Heartland Brewery, 387
Heat (Buford), 37, 324
Hebrew Immigrant Aid Society, 193
Hecker's (bakery), 31
Hederer, Emil, 492
Hefner, Hugh, 38, 211
Heidelberg Restaurant, 238, 657
Heinz, 428, 650
Helen Way Whitney Collection, 420
Hell Gate Brewery, 45, 70
Hellmann, Richard, 267
Hellmann's Mayonnaise, 237, **267–68**
Hello, Dolly!, 599
Hell's Kitchen, **268–69**, 292. *See also* Ninth Avenue
          Food Fair
   Farm Project, 508
Helme Products, Inc., 527
Helstolsky, Carol, 462, 463
Hemstrought's (bakery), 54
Henderson, Fergus, 20
Henry, O., 293, 355
Herger, Erwin, 100
Heritage Foods USA, 86, 269, 538
Heritage Meat, 88, 352
Heritage Radio Network, 86, 261, **269–70**, 483, 507, 538
Hertfordshire nuts. *See* doughnuts
Herzog (Bellow), 433
Hess, John L., **270–71**, 423
   on farmer's markets, 254
Hess, Karen, **270–71**
   in *Cuisine*, 153
   Culinary Historians of New York, 154
   at first American conference on culinary history, 153
Hesser, Amanda, 141, **271–72**
   founder of Food52, 216
   at the *New York Times*, 423
   on Riingo, 518
Hester, Kate, 556
Hester Street, 351
Hester Street Fair, 571, 620
High Line, 108, **272–74**
   pop-up food court, 466
High Line Food, 274
High Line Park, 380
High Road with Mario Batali, The (television show), 37
Hill, Graham, 128
Hill Country (restaurant), 561
Hilton, Conrad, 628
HIM Ital Health Food, 490
Hindy, Steve, 81, 82, 564
Hirsch, Sylvia Balser, 104
Hirschfeld, Al, 556
Hirschfeld, Leo, 94, 603
Hirsheimer, Chris, 521
Hispanics
   in the Bronx, 77
   Jackson Heights, 301
   in Sunset Park, 577

Historic Richmondtown, 565
History of New York (Irving), 177, 294, 414
Hitler: Neither Vegetarian nor Animal Lover (Berry), 50
HIV/AIDS, 236
H-Mart (grocery store), 325
Hofbräu Bierhaus NYC, 238
Hoffman, April, 278
Hoffman, James, 641
Hoffman, Peter, 203, 204
Hoffman Hotel, 191
Hoffman House, 375, 606
hokey-pokey (ice cream), 288
Hokinson, Helen, 527
Holidays (television show, Wolf), 592
Holly Buddy, 587
Holmes & Coutts Bakery, 403
Holt, Jane, 552
Hom, Ken, 313
Home as Found (Cooper), 433, 458
Home Food Advantage, 561
Homer, Winslow, 458–59
Home to Harlem (McKay), 433
Hondurans in the Bronx, 78
Hone, Philip, 119, 411
honey. *See also* beekeeping
   seasonal, 44
honey-pokey men, 536
Hong Kong Supermarket chain, 114, 596
honor system at Exchange Buffet, 92
Hook, Line & Dinner (television show), 217
Hooker, George, 460
Hooters, 529
Hoover, Herbert, 474, 652
Hopkins, Samuel, 182
Hopper, Edward, 132, **274–75**, 448
Horace Harding Expressway, 18
Horn, Joseph, 24, 92
Horn & Hardart, 24, 92, 369, 601, 619
   automats, 204–5
   Bickford's competitor of, 51
   decline, 334
   Hopper at, 275
   Jackson Heights, 300
   lunches, 357
   post–World War II expansion, 467
   during World War II, 654
Hornby, Nick, 587
Horowitz, Jonathan, 618
Hors d'Oeuvre, Inc., 41
Hors d'Oeuvre and Canapés (Beard), 41, 362, 468
HoSang, Vincent and Jeanette, 77
hospitality
   in Arab restaurants, 17
   tea and, 588
hospitality companies. *See* restaurant groups
Hospoda (restaurant), 657
Hostess Brands, 161–62
Hostess Cupcakes, 156, 157
hot dogs, **275–77**, 537. *See also* Nathan's Famous
   eating contests, 224, 405, 406
   fast-food chains, 205
   Feltman and Coney Island, 206, 207
   Fourth of July, 223, 224

hot dogs (*continued*)
   origins
      Brooklyn, 81
      German, 237
   Papaya King, 448–49
   pretzels and, 471
   at sporting events, 559
   street vendors and, 573
Hotel and Restaurant Employees National Alliance, 502
Hotel Astor, 178
hotel bars, 34
Hotel Brunswick, 278
Hotel Employees and Restaurant Employees, 503
Hotel Management (magazine), 162
Hotel Pierre, 264
hotel restaurants, **277–78**, 382
   early, 499–500
   in Upper East Side, 613
Hot Off the Grill with Bobby Flay (television show), 210, 218
Houghton Mifflin, 312
Hourglass Tavern (restaurant), 499
House & Garden (magazine), 42, 340
House Beautiful (magazine), 340
"Housekeeper's Chat" (radio program), 483
Houseman, John, 137
House of Brews, The (restaurant), 499
House of Mirth (Wharton), 433
How America Eats (Paddleford), 446
Howard, Albert, 508
Howard Hughes Corporation, 231–32
Howard Johnson's, 224, 337, 454
Howarth, Duska, 354
"Howl" (Ginsberg), 25
How the Other Half Lives (Riis), 239, 343, 433, 535
How to Cook Everything (Bittman), 52–53, 423
How to Cook Everything Quickly (Bittman), 53
how-to cooking shows, 591–92
How to Eataly, 507
How to Eat Better for Less Money (Beard), 42
How to Mix Drinks, or The Bon-Vivant's Companion (Thomas). *See Bartender's Guide, T*
Hoy, Brandon, 507
Hudson, Henry, 133
Hudson, Jennifer, 639
Hudson Cafeteria, 93
Hudson Heights, 630–31
Hudson River Club (restaurant), 240, 370, 467, 501
Huey, Richard, 552
Hume, Rosemary, 354
Humm, Daniel, 278
hummus, 191, **278–79**
Hummus Place (restaurant), 279
Hunam (restaurant), 113, 548
Hungarian(s), **279–80**, 657
Hungarian Meat Market and Delicatessen, 280
Hunger Action Network of New York State, 280, 281, 282
Hunger Prevention Nutrition Assistance Program, 280
hunger programs, **280–83**. *See also* soup kitchens
   late twentieth century, 333, 334
Hunger Solutions New York, 280, 282, 283
Hunt, Thomas, 284

hunt lunch. *See* brunch
Hunts Point, 78, 137, **283–85**
   farmer's market, 254
   Fulton Fish Market move to, 231
   replacing Washington Market, 633
Hunts Point Cooperative Market, 281
Hupfel Breweries, 76
Hurricane Katrina, 305
Hurwitz, Michael, 48, 247–48
Hussey, Rowland, 364
Hutchins, John, 129
Huxtable, Ada Louise, 221
Huxtable, Garth, 221
Huynh, Hung, 212
Hydrox Biscuit Bonbons, 436
Hygeian Home Cook-Book, The (Trall), 617
Hygrade Provisions Company, 277

I
IBM, 291
Ibold, Mark, 356
iceboxes, 13
ice cream
   Fourth of July, 223
   makers, 5, 257
   sodas, 547
   trucks, 218–19
ice cream parlors. *See* ice cream shops
ice cream sandwich, **287–88**
   Tofutti Cuties, 603
ice cream shops, **288–89**
   in the Bronx, 76
   Jackson Heights, 300
ice industry, 13
Iceland Brothers Deli. *See* Katz's Delicatessen
Iceland & Katz. *See* Katz's Delicatessen
IKEA, 522
Ilili Box (restaurant), 201
Il Leopardo (restaurant), 614
"I Love Le Cirque, but Can I Be Trusted" (Greene), 246
Il Talismano della Felicita (The Talisman to Happiness) (Boni), 266
Imbibe! (Wondrich), 373
immigrants. *See also* Ellis Island food (1892–1924)
   in Bay Ridge, 40
   from Brazil, 65–66
   in the Bronx, 77
   Caribbean, 97
      in Bushwick, 85
   diner owners, 173
   and diversity of Manhattan's culinary offerings, 369
   Dominican, 175
   fishing by, 208
   in Five Points, 210
   fusion food and, 232
   German, 237
      and beer, 45
      beer gardens and, 46
      breweries, 70
      in the Bronx, 76
      in Kleindeutschland, 321
   Gilded Age, 238, 239
   Greek, 245

in Greenwich Village, 248
in Harlem, 262
Hungarian, 279–80
Indian, 342–43
Indo-Caribbean, 289
Irish, 292–93
in the Bronx, 75
Italian, 295
Jewish, 76
in Little Italy, 343–44
Jackson Heights, 300
Japanese, 307
Jewish, 309–10
in the Bronx, 76
Chanukah and, 102
delis and, 164–65
Passover and, 451
Korean, 326
late twentieth century, 334
Latin Americans
in Bushwick, 85
Lower East Side, 351
Polish, 465
post-World War II, 467–68
public markets and, 475
in Queens, 479
restaurants and, 13
specialty food shops catering to, 14
in Staten Island, 564–65
in twenty-first century, 607
in Yorkville, 656
Immigration Act (1924), 295
Immigration and Nationality Act (1965),
    207, 467
Improved Housewife, The (Webster), 142
Inday, 553
India Bengal Garden (restaurant), 552
Indian(s). *See also* South Asian
diners, 173
fast food, 205
goat meat in, 284
halva, 258
influence of on Jamaican, 303
Jackson Heights, 300–301
at Kalusyan's, 315
in Little India, 342–43
in Sunset Park, 577
Indian Food Made Easy (television show), 217
Indian Road Café, 292
India Prince (restaurant), 552
India Rajah (restaurant), 552
India Restaurant, 552
Indo-Caribbean, 97, **289–90**
Indochine (restaurant), 554
Industrial Workers of the World (Wobblies), 502
Industry City, 564
Ingber, Sandy, 244
INOV8 Beverage Company, 432
In Pursuit of Flavor (Lewis and Goodby), 340
Inquisitive Eater blog, 410
Insatiable (Greene), 246
Insatiable Critic, The (website), 246
Inserra Supermarkets Inc. (ShopRite), 318

Institute of Culinary Education, 144, **290–91**, 335, 370
Kump and, 328
Laiskonis creative director of, 392
Smilow and, 539
Institute of Modern and Practical Cooking, 162
Intercontinental Exchange, 137, 138
International Association of Culinary Professionals, 527
Kump in, 327–28
on Lewis, 340
International Association of Culinary Professionals Award
Food52, 216
French Culinary Institute, 228–29
Dorothy Cann Hamilton, 260–61
Hesser, 272
Institute of Culinary Education, 291
International Bagel Bakers Union, 27
International Culinary Center, 144, 227, 335, 370. *See also*
    French Culinary Institute
in French Culinary Institute, 260
Hazan scholarship, 267
New School and, 410
Alain Sailhac dean of culinary studies, 515
International Grocery, 245, 269
International Hotel Workers Union, 502
International Review of Food and Wine, The (magazine).
    See Food & Wine (magazine)
Interstate Bakeries, 161–62
Invisible Man (Ellison), 433
Inwood, 97, **291–92**
Ippudo Ramen, 309
I Quant NY blog, 562
Irish, **292–94**
in Astoria, 22
corned beef and, 145–46
distilleries, 174
in Harlem, 262
in Hell's Kitchen, 269
in Inwood, 292
Jackson Heights, 300
Little Italy's displacement of, 343
in Sunset Park, 577
in Washington Heights, 630
in Yorkville, 656
Irish Brigade (pub), 292
Irish Eyes (bar), 292
Iron Chef (television show), 217
Iron Chef America (television show), 57, 567
"Iron Chef Boyardee" (Sietsema), 624
Iron Palace (department store), 168
Irving, Washington, 119, **294**
on doughnuts, 177
on picnics, 458
and word cookie, 142
Isnard, Marius, 337
Isreal, Mark, 178
Italfari Health Food and Juice Bar, 490
Ital food, 490
Italian(s), **294–96**
bakeries, 31, 67
in Brooklyn, 40, 49, 81, 577, 643
dairy stores, 160
doughnuts, 178
Easter processions, 185

Italian(s) (*continued*)
  Eataly, 186
  Essex Street Market and, 195–96
  in Five Points, 210
  food
    in New York movies, 395
    at San Gennaro Feast, 519
  food trucks, 219
  late twentieth century, 334
  in Little Italy, 343, 344–45
  pushcart vendors, 573
  in Queens, 22, 300, 302
  on Staten Island, 565
Italian ices, 295, **296**
Italian Welfare League, 193
Ital Kitchen, 490
It Must Have Been Something I Ate (Steingarten),
  324, 567
Iuzzini, Johnny, 392
Ivan Ramen (restaurant), 309
Ives, Charles, 459

J
J. M. Kaplan Fund, 48, 247
J. Russ National Appetizing Store, 511
J. Walter Thompson, 171
Jabez Burns & Sons, 131
Jack & Charlie's (speakeasy), 556
Jack Dempsey's (restaurant), **299–300**
Jack's Manual (Grohusko), 83
Jackson, Charles R., 445
Jackson, Reginald Martinez "Reggie," 95, 492
Jackson Diner, 173, 301, 343
Jackson Heights, **300–301**, 479. *See also* Little India
  Asians, 480
  Filipinos, 207
  food trucks, 219
  Indian food, 552, 553
  Indians, 343
  Little Colombia, 132
  Mexicans, 385
  South and Central American food, 550, 551
  Thai, 596
Jackson Hole hamburger chain, 173
Jack the Ripper (restaurant), 249
Jacob, Dianne, 606
Jacob Hoffman Brewing, 45, 70
Jacobi, Abraham, 387
Jacob K. Javits Convention Center, 202
Jacob Ruppert Brewing Company, 45, 70, 333–34
Jacobs, Jane, 570
Jacobson, Anita, 594
Jacob's Pickles, 458
Jacos, Jay, 36
Jacques Torres Chocolates, 95
Jacques Torres' Year in Chocolate (Torres), 604
Jade Mountain (restaurant), 117
Jaffrey, Madhur, 144, 313, 324, 488
Jahn's Ice Cream Parlor, 76, 300
Jaine, Tom, 440
Jamaica (Queens), **301–3**
  Jamaicans in, 97
  King Kullen in, 319–20

Jamaican, **303–4**
James Beard Awards, **304–5**, 335
  Alinea, 305
  Batali, 37, 305
  Bouley (restaurant), 304
  Chang, 305
  Child, 305, 306
  Dufresne, 180
  Eleven Madison Park, 305
  first, 306
  Fisher, 304
  Flay, 210–11
  Food52, 216
  The French Laundry, 305
  Gold, 240
  Hamilton, 261–62
  Institute of Culinary Education, 291
  Jones, 313
  Keen's, 305
  Keller, 305
  Kump and, 327
  Le Cirque, 336
  Lewis, 340
  Lucky Peach, 356
  Pépin, 454
  Puck, 304
  Steingarten, 567
  Waters, 305
James Beard Cooking School, 42
James Beard Foundation, 42, **305–7**, 335
  on Babbo, 37
  Barber and, 33
  on Bouley (restaurant), 62
  celebrity chef star system, 106
  cookbooks donated by, 202
  on Danube (restaurant), 62
  on Hamilton, Dorothy Cann, 261
  Kump in, 327
  New School and, 410
James Beard House, 110, 307, 327
James Beard's Theory & Practice of Good Cooking, 313
Jammet, André, 329–30
Jammet, Rita, 329–30
Jams (restaurant), 203, 210
J&J Snack Foods, Corp., 471
J &T Adikes', 302
Japanese, **307–9**
  post–World War II, 468
Jayaraman, Sary, 497
jazz clubs
  black food and, 6
  Greenwich Village, 248
Jean-Georges (restaurant), 227, 334, 614, 624, 625
  Dufresne at, 180
  at Madison Square Garden, 561
  modernist cuisine pastry chef at, 392
Jeepney (restaurant), 208
Jeffers, J. Paul, 64
Jefferson Market, 475
Jelly Rings, 297
Jenkins, Nancy, 153
Jenkins, Steven, 105, 200
Jennings, Michael J., 445

jerk meats, 303
Jernmark, Marcus, 15
Jerome, Jeanette "Jennie," 373
Jessel, George, 55
Jewish holidays. *See* hanukah; Passover
Jewish Museum, 354
Jewish Week, The, 529
Jews and Jewish, **309–12**. *See also* appetizing stores; delis, Jewish; knish
  of Arab countries heritage, 16
  bakeries, 31, 67
  in Bensonhurst, 49
  in Brighton Beach, 72, 345–46
  in the Bronx, 77
  Cel-Ray as, 179
  dairy stores, 160
  doughnuts, 178
  egg creams, 189
  Ellis Island food, 193
  Essex Street Market and, 195–96
  falafel, 201
  in first wave Russian immigration, 511–12
  Gilded Age immigration, 239
  halva, 258
  in Harlem, 262
  hot dogs, 276–77
  hummus, 279
  Hungarians, 279–80
  Jackson Heights, 300
  in Jamaica, 302
  Lower East Side, 351–52
  in the Lower East Side, 351
  and origin of bagel, 27
  Passover, 450–52
  pastrami, 452
  pickles, 457–58
  pushcart vendors, 573
  smoked fish industry, 540
  soda water and, 544
  and Stella D'Oro cookies, 567
  in Upper East Side, 612–13
  in Washington Heights, 630
  in Williamsburg, 81, 643
  Zabar's and, 659
Jimmy Day's (restaurant), 249
Joe Allen Restaurant, 210, 499
Joe's Dairy, 160
Joe Tuna, 231
John Dory Oyster Bar, 56
John Eichler Brewing, 45, 70
John F. Trommer, 45, 70
John Murray's Roman Gardens (lobster palace), 348
John's (pizzeria), 248, 350, 461, 463, 464
Johnson, Harry, 374
Johnson, Howard, 337, 454
Johnson, Hugh, 153
Johnson, J. J., 6
Johnson, Ken, 618
Johnson, Lyndon, 342
Johnson, Philip, 221
Johnson, R. T., 407
JoJo (restaurant), 180, 334, 613, 625
Jolly Bee (fast-food chain), 205

Jolson, Al, 165, 243
Jonas Bronck Beer Company, 76
Jones, Charles, 578
Jones, Cyrus, 578
Jones, Frank, 578
Jones, Judith, 488
Jones, Judith and Evan, 110, **312–13**
  at Knopf, 323, 324
  Lewis and, 340
Jones, Robert, 371
Jones Brothers Tea Company, 251, 578
Joseph Rubin & Sons, 604
Joseph Schlitz Brewing, 46, 71, 85, 333
Journal of Health and Longevity, 617
Joyce Chen Cooks (television show), 591, 592
Joy of Cooking, The (Rombauer and Becker), 528
Joyva, 258, 643
  Chocolate Jelly Rings, 297
juice movement, 491
Julia Child and Company (television show), 110
Julia Child and Jacques Pépin Cooking at Home (television show), 110
Julia Child and More Company (television show), 394
Julius' Bar, 236
Jumble Shop, 591
Jungle, The (Sinclair), 535
Junior's Cheesecake Cookbook (Rosen and Allen), 104
Junior's Restaurant, **313–14**
  cheesecake, 80, 104
  food at Barclays Center arena, 81
Junoon (restaurant), 553
Just Born, 81, 94
Just Food, 139, 410

K
Kabab Café, 201
Kafka, Barbara
  Baum and, 39
  on Gotham Bar and Grill menu, 240
  in Les Dames d'Escoffier, 338
  menu of Windows on the World, 644
Kaldis at the Cedar Bar (George), 448
Kalens, Dorothy, 521
Kallem, Henry, 448
Kalustyan, K., 315
Kalustyan's, 18, 157, 191, **315**, 596
Kamman, Madeleine, 290
Kamp, David, 64
Kaplan, Jack, 247
Karl Ehmer's Butcher Shop, 656–57
Karmel, Elizabeth, 561
Kasper, Lynne Rossetto
  in *Cuisine,* 153
  host of *The Splendid Table,* 483
  Scribner's, 528
Kasperzak, Ron, 74
Katchkie Farm, 244–45
Katz's Delicatessen, 164, 165, 312, **315–17**, 352, 512
  corned beef sandwich, 145
  pastrami, 453
Kaufelt, Robert, 105, 398
Kauffmann, Stanley, 312–13
Kaufman, Alan, 458

Kaufman, Cathy, 154
Kawahara, Shigemi, 309
Kawkab America (newspaper), 346
Kaye, Sidney, 513
Kazin, Alfred, 460
    on Russian Jewish meals, 512
Keens (restaurant), 104, 105, 305
    in *Mad Men*, 366
Kee's Chocolates, 94
Kefi (restaurant), 245
Keller, Thomas, 614
    James Beard Award to, 305
    in James Beard Foundation, 306
    on *Mike Colameco's Food Show*, 593
Kellock, Katharine Amend, 8
Kelpe, Paul, 399
Kelso, 564, 643
Kennedy, Diana, 144
    in Institute of Culinary Education, 290
    Kump and, 327
Kennedy, Jacqueline, 329, 330
Kennedy, John F., 329, 337, 454
Kennedy, Joseph P., 329, 337, 549
Kennedy Fried Chicken, 205
Kennerly, Michael, 323
Kenny, Brian, 269–70
Kenny's Castaways (café), 248
Kentucky Fried Chicken, 205
Kenyon, Lindy and Robert, 211
Kerouac, Jack, 248
    at Bickford's, 25
    at Caffè Reggio, 93
    at White Horse Tavern, 640, 641
Kerr, Graham, 591
Kesté (pizzeria), 248, 464
Key Food Stores Cooperative, Inc., **317–18**
Key Fresh & Naturals, 317
Kieft, William, 174, 557
Killmeyer's Old Bavarian Inn, 565, 565
Kim, Hooni, 228
Kim, Peter, 401
Kimball, Andrew, 564
Kimball, Christopher, 153
kimchi, **318–19**, 324, 325, 458
    in Korean tacos, 326
Kimchi Taco Truck, 326
Kin, Hooni, 325
King, John, 302
King, Rufus, 302
King Kullen, 155, 250, 252, **319–20**, 578–79
    in Jamaica, 302
King's Arms, The (coffeehouse), 128, 129
Kings' Coffee (coffee shop), 129
King's College. *See* Columbia University
Kings County Distillery, 175, 564
Kingston, Steven, 339
Kips Bay Brewing, 45, 70
Kira, K. Y., 551
Kirby, Felice, 82
Kirby-Allen (tearoom), 591
Kirsch, Abigail, 99
Kirsch, Hyman, 432
Kirsch, Morris, 432

Kirsch Beverages, 432
Kirshenbaum, Kent, 197
Kirshenbaum & Bond, 542
Kitchen Arts and Letters, **320–21**, 637
Kitchen Confidential (Bourdain), 63, 212, 418
Kitchen Mysteries (This), 135, 136
Kitchen Ventures Incubator Program, 121
Kittredge, Mabel, 523
Kleeman, Elayne, 75, 338
Klein, Murray, 659
Klein, Stephen, 94
Kleindeutschland, 237, **321–22**, 351, 522
    delis, 163
    hot dogs, 275
    move of Germans to Yorkville, 656
Kleine Konditerei, 656
Klimavicius, Max, 520
Klopfer, Donald, 488
Kludt, Amanda, 187
Knead It, Punch It, Bake It! Make Your Own Bread (Jones and
    Jones), 313
Knickerbocker (restaurant), 249, 601
Knickerbocker, Diedrich, 294
Knickerbocker brewery, 559
Knickerbocker History of New York (Irving), 119
Knickerbocker Hotel, 375
Knights of Labor and first culinary unions, 502
knish, 311, **322–23**
    Jewish deli, 164
    in Little Odessa, 345
    at Shea stadium, 560
Knish Alley, 323
Knish Nosh, 322–23
Knopf, **323–24**, 488
    Judith Jones at, 312–13
    Lewis published by, 340
Kobayashi, Masa, 227
Koch, Ed, 120
    Gold chef for, 240
    at grand reopening of Rainbow Room, 486
    street vendors permits, 574
Kogi Korean BBQ (food truck), 220
Kogi Taco Truck, 319
Korean(s), **324–25**
    in the Bronx, 78
    delis run by, 467–68, 538
    diners, 173
    doughnuts, 177
    grocery stores, 252–53
    kimchi (*See* kimchi)
    late twentieth century, 334
Korean taco, **325–26**
Koreatowns, 325, **326–27**
Korea Way, 327
Korilla BBQ, 326
Kornbleuth, Norman, 74
kosher foods, 309, 310, 312
    chocolate, 350
    Jewish deli, 164–65
    late twentieth century, 334
    pickles, 458
    in Washington Heights, 630
kosher vegetarian restaurant, 92

Kossar's, 51, 512
Kossar's Bialys, 352
Kovi, Paul, 222
Kraft Foods, 242, 404, 568
Kramer, Joseph, 342
Kramer, William, 46
Krampner, Jon, 135
Kreindler, Jack, 609
Kresevich, Joseph and Angela, 567
Kretchmer, Jerome, 210
Kreuther, Gabriel, 399
Krim, Seymour, 623
Krispy Kreme, 178
Kroger (supermarket chain), 250, 578
    D'Agostino competition with, 159
    Murray's Cheese kiosks in, 398
    origins of, 251–52
Kroger, Bernard H., 251–52
Kroger Grocery & Baking Co., 319
Królewskie Jadło (restaurant), 465
Krondl, Michael, 154
Kulchinsky, Lina, 471
Kum Gang San (restaurant), 319
Kumin, Albert, 644
Kump, Peter Clark, 144, **327–28**. *See also* Peter Kump's New
        York Cooking School
    creation of celebrity chef star system, 106
    in James Beard Foundation, 306, 335
Kunjip (restaurant), 325
Kuntz's (brewery), 76
Kuo, Irene, 313
Kurlansky, Mark, 154
Kurti, Nicholas, 391
Kurumazushi (restaurant), 581

L
labor disputes. *See also* strikes
    at Café des Artistes, 332
    at Key Food, 318
    at Le Pavillon, 337
LA Bottleworks, 179
La Caravelle (restaurant), 227, **329–30**, 498
    Fessaguet at, 337, 550
    haute cuisine in, 265
    Ladies Who Lunch at, 331
La Condesa (restaurant), 263
La Côte Basque (restaurant), 227, 265, 337, 549
    Bouley at, 62
    closed, 330
    murals at, 329
Ladies Home Journal (magazine), 202, 340, 648
Ladies' Mile, 168, 357
    ice cream shops, 288
Ladies' Refreshment Lounge, 99
ladies' restaurants, 500
Ladies Who Lunch, **330–31**
LaFayette (restaurant), 232
Lafayette, The (restaurant), 226, 331
Lafayette Café, 621
La Finca dal Sur, 615
La Fonda Boricua (restaurant), 263, 478
La Fonda del Sol (restaurant), 66, 370, 467, 495, 501
    part of Restaurant Associates, 494

Lagasse, Emeril
    in Food & Wine Classic, 211
    on Food Network, 217–18
    supplied by Kalustyan's, 315
lager beer, 46, 70, 565
La Grenouille (restaurant), 227, 265, 331
La Guardia, Fiorello, **331–32**
    demolition of Central park Casino, 100
    in Greenmarkets, 247
    markets, 19, 573, 574
        Essex Street Market, 352
        Fulton Fish Market, 230–31
    meatless Tuesdays during World War II, 654
    modernization initiatives, 195
    at Patsy's, 461
    on public markets, 476
    removal of peddlers from streets, 3
Lahey, Jim, 462
Laiskonis, Michael, 392
Lakshmi, Padma, 212
La Lanterna (café), 248
Lam, Celia, 181
La Marina (restaurant), 291
lamb
    in Arab cuisine, 17
    for Passover, 451
Lambert, Phyllis, 221
lamingtons, 23
LaMotta, Richard, 115
Lance Company, 568
Lancieri, Carmela, 461
Lancieri, Pasquale, 461, 463
Landmark Tavern, 587
Landry, Paul, 342
Lane, John, 323
Lang, George, **332–33**
    Fales Library donation, 202
    in The Four Seasons, 221
La Nueva Bakery, 551
Lao food, 555
Lape, Bob, **333**
La Poinière (restaurant), 265
Last Supper, The (play, Schmidt), 599
Late Night with David Letterman (television show), 293
late twentieth century, **333–36**
Latin American food on Staten Island, 566
Latinos. *See also specific nationalities*
    in Bensonhurst, 49
    diners, 173
    Essex Street Market and, 196
    food trucks, 219–20
    fusion food, 233
    goat meat and, 284
    in Jamaica, 302
    Lower East Side, 352
latkes, 102
Lattanzi (restaurant), 499
Latticini Barese (dairy store), 160
La Tulipe (restaurant), 394, 427
Laudan, Rachel, 154
Lauder, Ronald, 332
Lauren, Dylan, 95, 182–83
Lauren, Ralph, 182

Lauria, Tony, 568
LaValva, Robert, 409
Lavezzo, Dan and John, 445
Lawrence, Cornelius W., 411
Lawrence, Jacob, 448
Lawrence, William, 148–49
Layover, The (television show), 63–64
Leach, Robin, 217
Leahey, Jim, 31
Le Bernardin (restaurant), 212, 232–33
    kimchi at, 319
    on *Mike Colameco's Food Show*, 593
    modernist cuisine pastry chef at, 392
Le Chantilly (restaurant), 265
Le Cirque 2000 (restaurant), 363
Le Cirque (restaurant), 227, **336**, 369, 467
    Bouley at, 62
    Boulud at, 63
    Flying Food International and, 242
    Greene on, 246
    haute cuisine in, 265
    opening, 362
    Sailhac executive chef at, 515
    Torres executive pastry chef at, 604
Le Cirque: A Table in Heaven (NBO documentary), 336, 363
L'École (restaurant), 228, 515
Le Cygne (restaurant), 227, 515
Lederhosen (restaurant), 238
Lee, Chang-Rae, 433–34
Lefebvre, Ludovic, 466
Leff, Jim, 219
LeFrieda, Pat, 88
"Legend of Sleepy Hollow" (Irving), 294
Legends Hospitality Management, 559
Leibowitz, Andrew, 457–58
Leifferts Community Food Co-op, 214
Leigh, Dougals, 4
Leigh, Janet, 329
Leisure League of America, 162
Le Manoir (restaurant), 515
Lemcke, Gesine, 143
Le Mistral (restaurant), 515
Lemon Ice King, 479
Lemon Ice King of Corona, 297
Lenape, 193, 442, 469–70
Lender's Bagels, 28
Lenny's Sandwich Shops, 205
Lent
    Dominican food for, 175–76
    fasting, 185, 186
    halva in, 258
    Polish foods for, 465
Lenzi, Philip, 288
Leo's Latticini, 479
Le Pavillon (restaurant), 124, 224, 227, **336–37**, 369, 501, 549, 650
    decline, 334
    haute cuisine, 264–65
    Ladies Who Lunch at, 330, 331
    menu, 384
    Pépin at, 454
    post-World War II popularity, 467
    during World War II, 654

Le Périgord (restaurant), 62, 265, 369
Le Perigord Park (restaurant), 329
Le Plaisir (restaurant), 227
Le Regence (restaurant), 63
Le Restaurant Français, 650
LeRoy, Jennifer Oz, 377
LeRoy, Warner, 377, 513, 514, 585
Les Amis d'Escoffier, 170, 338, 370
Les Dames d'Escoffier, 74, 75, 335, **338–39**, 370
    Fales Library donation, 202
    Hesser scholarship from, 271
    on Lewis, 340
Lesem, Jeanne, 154
Les Halles (restaurant), 566
Leslie, Eliza, 142, 155
Leslie, Frank, 389
Leslie's Illustrated Newspaper, 61, 174, 389
"Lessons in Humility and Chutzpah" (Greene), 246
Le Train Bleu (restaurant), 168, 486
Lettuce Entertain You Enterprises, 494
Leventhal, Ben, 187
Lever Act. *See* Food and Fuel Control Act (Lever Act)
Levine, Ed, 27
Levine, Jack, 448
Levitt, Adolph, 178
Levy, Paul, 246
Levy's, 309
Lewis, Bob, 47, 48, 270
    in Greenmarkets, 246–47
    in GrowNYC, 254
Lewis, Edna, 6, 91, **339–40**
    Citymeals-on-Wheels, 120
    at Gage & Tollner, 235
    Judith Jones and, 313
    published by Knopf, 324
Lewis, Jerry, 339
Lexington Candy Store, 189
Liddabit Sweets, 563, 564
Lidia Cooks from the Heart of Italy (Bastianich), 36
Lidia's Commonsense Italian Cooking (Bastianich), 36
Lidia's Family Table (Bastianich/television show), 36, 592
Lidia's Favorite Recipes (Bastianich), 36
Lidia's Italian-American Kitchen (Bastianich/television show), 36, 592
Lidia's Italian Table (Bastianich/television show), 36, 592
Lidia's Italy (Bastianich/television show), 36, 592
Lidia's Italy (restaurants), 35
Lidia's Italy in America (Bastianich/television show), 36
Lieblich, Gerald, 514
Liebling, A. J., **340–41**, 418
Liebmann, Philip, 71
Liebrandt, Paul, 429
Liederman, David, 659
"Life of Delicious Excess" (Greene), 246
Life Savers, 94, **341–42**
Lifestyles of the Rich and Famous (television show), 217
Liffy Bar II, 292
Li-Lac Chocolates, 94
Lin, Florence, 113
Lincoln Center, 244, 305, 613
Lincoln Ristorante, 614
Lindbergh, Charles, 226
Lindemann, Leo, 103, 342

Lindsay, John, 254, 499
Lindy's, 165, **342–43**, 601
  cheesecake, 103
  Runyon at, 510
Lindy's Food Products, 103
Linking Food and the Environment (LiFE), 135
Lion's Head (restaurant), 249
Lippert, Albert and Felice, 428, 638
Lippold, A. Richard, 221
"Literary Dinner, A" (Nabokov), 418
Little Armenia, 17
Little Brazil, 66, 550
Little Collins (coffee shop), 129
Little Colombia, 132
Little Egypt, 191
Little Germany. *See* Kleindeutschland
Little Guyana, 551
Little Hungary, 279–80
Little India, 157, **342–43**
  Jackson Heights, 301
Little Italy, 295, **343–45**. *See also* San Gennaro, Feast of
  of the Bronx, 18, 76
  coffeehouses, 130
  dairy stores, 160
  groceries in, 210
  in Harlem, 262
  Lombardi's, 350–51
  pizzerias, 463
Little Italy with David Ruggerio (television show), 592, 593
Little Mexico, 385
Little Norway, 40
  now Little Hong Kong, 522
Little Odessa, 72, **345–46**, 512, 611
Little Odessa (movie), 346
Little Rumania, 452
Little Sri Lanka, 566
Little Syria, 16, **346–47**, 584
  coffeehouses, 130
  hummus, 278–79
Little Trinidad, 97
Little Ukraine (Ukrainian Village), 611
living-food. *See* raw food
Livingston, Malcolm, 392
L.L. Bean Book of New England Cookery, The (Jones and Jones), 313
L.L. Bean Game and Fish Cookbook, The (Jones and Cameron), 313
lobster Newberg, **347**
  in automats, 619
  created by Oscar Tschirky, 628
lobster palaces, **347–49**, 537
  catering to theatergoers, 601
  in haute cuisine, 264
  origin of nightclubs, 430
  of Rector, 492
  Shanley and, 500
Lobster Place, The, 108
Local Finds Queens Food Tours, 629
locavorism. *See also* farm to table
  Bittman and, 53
  CSA and, 138
  New Oxford American Dictionary on locavore, 203
  in Park Slope, 450

Lockyear, Benjamin, 589
Locust Valley Market, 317
Loews Regency Hotel, 468
Loft, George W., 349
Loft, Thomas, 94
Loft, William, 349
Loft's candy stores, 94, **349–50**, 455, 544
Loisaida. *See* Lower East Side
LOLO Organics, 108
Lombardi, Genarro, 350, 461, 462, 463
Lombardi's (restaurant), 246, **350–51**, 461, 462–63, 464
Lombardy hotel, 83–84
Lomonaco, Michael, 336, 363, 645
Londel's (restaurant), 263
London, Morris, 322
London Terrace street fair, 571
Long Island City, 22, 173
Long Island Railroad, 302, 484
Longone, Jan, 154
Longstreet, Abby Buchanan, 411
Longstreet, Stephen, 241
Longworth, Nicholas, 645
Lopate, Leonard, 483
Lopez, Jennifer, 478
Lo Pinto, Maria, 140
Loreley (restaurant), 238
Los Paisanos (market), 301
Los Tacos No. 1, 108
Lost Weekend, The (Jackson), 445
Loubat, Alphonse, 645
Louise's Family Restaurant, 263
Louis Martin's (restaurant), 412
Love Me, Feed Me (Jones), 313, 324
Lower East Side, 344, **351–53**. *See also* Essex Street Market; Kleindeutschland
  Armenians, 17
  demographic change, 15
  dimsum eateries, 172
  Dufresne restaurant on, 180
  egg creams, 189, 190
  German delis, 163
  Hungarians in, 279
  Jews/Jewish, 311
    delis, 164
    food, 14, 312
  Kleindeutschland in, 237
  lox, 353
  pickle district, 457–58
  Poles, 465
  public markets, 475
  Puerto Ricans, 477
  sausages, 275
  street cries, 3–4
Lower East Side Pickle Festival, 458
Lower Manhattan, 169, 287
Lowery, Ellin, 590
lox, 165, **353–54**, 539
Lucali (pizzeria), 464
Lucas, Dione, 143–44, **354–55**, 370, 591
Luchetti, Emily, 228
Lüchow, August Guido, 237, **355**
Lüchow's (restaurant), 237
Lucky Peach (print quarterly/mobile app), 101, **355–56**, 393, 495

Lucky Strike (restaurant), 334
Lucy's Whey, 105
LudoBites (restaurant), 466
Luger, Carl, 237–38, 456
Luger, Frederick, 457
Luger, Peter, 237–38, 456
Luna Restaurant, 344
lunch, **356–58**, 464. *See also* business lunch; power
    breakfasts and power lunches; three-martini
    lunch
Lunch Hour NYC (exhibition, New York Public Library),
    87, 400
lunchrooms, 500
lunch wagons, 172, 218
Lundy's (restaurant), 443
Luongo, Pino, 296
Lupa (restaurant), 249, 296
Lupowitz's (restaurant), 311
Lusk, Graham, 10
Lutèce (restaurant), **358–59**, 369, 467, 498
    closing, 227, 330
    farm to table and, 203
    haute cuisine, 265
    Ladies Who Lunch at, 331
    Sheraton and, 533
    Soltner and, 548–49
Lutèce Cookbook, The (Soltner and Britchky), 65, 549
Lyle the Crocodile (Waber), 459
Lynch, James, 49
Lynch, Thomas, 635
Lyons, Bill, 466
Lyons, Mary, 75, 338

M
M. F. K. Fisher Award, 339
M. Shanken Communications, 212, 213
M. Wells Dinette, 399, 566
Maass, Robert, 209
MacAusland, Earle, 171, 241, **361–62**, 468
Maccioni, Sirio, 330, **362–63**, 369, 467
    in haute cuisine, 265
    Le Cirque, 336
MacDougall, Alice Foote, 394
MacDougall, Allan Ross, 9
MacDougall, Edward A., 300
Macfadden, Bernarr, 92, **363–64**, 388
Mack, Walter, 349
Mackay, Charles, 441
Mackey, John, 642
Macklowe, Harry, 513
Macweeney, Alen, 153
Macy's, 168, **364–65**
    fireworks display, 224
    Herald Square, 495
    Passover food at, 452
    Thanksgiving Day Parade, 597
    victory gardeners and, 622
    women in restaurant of, 239
Madden, Owney, 60, 61, 148, 430
Madison Square Eats, 608
Madison Square Garden, 561
Madison Square Park Conservancy, 531
Madison Square Park Shake Shack, 466

Mad Men (television series), 3, 5, **365–66**
    Manhattan cocktail on, 592
    P. J. Clarke's in, 587
    on three-martini lunches, 600
Maeff, Sasha, 513
"Mafia Guide to Dining Out, The" (Greene), 246
Maggie: A Girl of the Streets (Crane), 433
Magnolia Bakery, 156, **366–67**
    on *Sex and the City*, 530, 531, 592
Magnolia Bakery Cookbook, The (Torey and Appel), 366
Maharlika (restaurant), 208
Maher, Matthew, 378
Maialino (restaurant), 278
Mailer, Norman, 623
    at White Horse Tavern, 640, 641
Main St. Vegan Academy, 617
Maison Calondre (restaurant), 171
Maison Dorée (restaurant), 122, 488
Maison Kayser, 31
Major's Cabin Grill, 173
Makami, Tadeo, 62
MakerBot, 564
"Malassol Caviar and Beluga Caviar War of 1983," 660
Malaysian cuisine, 577
Malecon (restaurant), 97
Malgieri, Nick
    in Institute of Culinary Education, 290
    at Windows on the World, 644
Mallomars, 142, **367**, 404
Maloney & Porcelli, 178
Mama O's kimchi, 319
Mamdouh, Fekkak, 497
Mamoun's Falafel (restaurant), 201, 248–49
Manatus (restaurant), 249
M&G Diner, 263
Manhattan, **368–71**. *See also* Five Points; Greenwich Village;
    Harlem; High Line; Inwood; Kleindeutschland; Little
    Italy; Little Syria; Lower East Side; Upper East Side;
    Upper West Side; Washington Heights
    access to organic food, 438
    Australian restaurants, 23
    as brewing center, 45, 70
    consolidation of, 239
    Indian food, 552, 553
    Irish in, 292
    Koreatown, 326, 327
    microbreweries, 387
    Polish in, 465
    purchase of, 292
    sugar refining, 575
    walking culinary tours, 629
Manhattan Brewing Company, 46, 334, 386
Manhattan Clam Chowder, **371–72**
Manhattan Club, 373
Manhattan cocktail, **372–73**
    Brooklyn cocktail variation on, 83
    on *Mad Men*, 592
Manhattan Fruit Exchange, 108
Manhattan Refrigerating Company, 379
Manhattan Special, **373–74**
Manila Karihan Restaurant, 207
Manila Strip, 207
Manischewitz, 451

Manischewitz, Behr, 376
Mansion, The (speakeasy), 556
manuscripts, culinary, 420
Man Who Ate Everything, The (Steingarten), 567
Má Pêche, 101, 393
Mapplethorpe, Robert, 153
Marathon Enterprises, 277
Marble Palace (department store), 168
Marcella Says (Hazan), 266–67
March, Stephanie, 211
Marco Polo (restaurant), 235
Marcus Off Duty (Samuelsson), 518
Margie's Red Rose Diner, 263
Margittai, Tom, 222
Maria Carolina, Queen of Naples, 461
Marino's Italian Ice, 297
Marion Nestle Food Studies Collection, 201–2
Marisco Centro (restaurant), 630
Mari Vanna (restaurant), 512
Mark, The (restaurant), 278, 613
Market Assistant, The (De Voe), 170, 475
Market Book, The (De Voe), 170
marketing
    digital by Batali, 37
    to middle- and upper-class women by A&P, 2
    by Nathan's Famous, 405
markets. See also Greenmarkets; markets by name; public
        markets; Smorgasburg
    African Americans and early Sunday markets, 5
    in Brighton Beach, 73
    for pushcart vendors, 572, 574
Markets of New York City (Seiger), 247
Marqueta, La (market), 477
Marriott Marquis rotating restaurant, 602
Marryat, Frederick, 166
Marsh, Leonard, 541
Marsh, Reginald, 448, 460
Marshall Fields, 168
Marta (pizzeria), 462
Martha Stewart's Cooking School (television show), 593
Martha Stewart Show, The, 527
Martha Washington's Booke of Cookery and Booke of
        Sweetmeats (Hess), 271
Martín, Arturo, 622
Martin, Dean, 339, 461
Martin, Jean, 226
Martin, Jean-Baptiste, 348
Martin, Louis, 226, 348
Martinez, Daisy, 478
martini, 374–76
    Ladies Who Lunch and, 331
    silver bullet, 600
Martini, Straight Up (Edmunds), 372
Martini and Rossi, 372
Martini di Arma di Taggia, 375
Martinique, The (restaurant), 412
Martins, Patrick, 86
    founder of Slow Food USA, 538
    in Heritage Radio Network, 269–70
Martin's Café, 412
Martling's Tavern, 586
Mary Elizabeth Tearoom, 94, 591
Mary's Celtic Kitchen, 75

Mary Waldo's Restaurant Guide to New York City and
        Vicinity, 552
marzipan, 163
Masa (restaurant), 581
Mason, John L., 376
Mason, Sam, 180, 392
Mason jar, 376
Massimo Zanetti Beverage Group USA, 116
Masson, Charles, Sr., 265
Mast Brothers, 190, 563
Mastering the Art of French Cooking (Child, Bertholle, and
        Beck), 109, 488
    Beard and promotion of, 42
    Judith Jones and, 312–13
    Knopf and, 323
    publication, 110
Master Purveyors (butcher), 284
Mathews, John, 543, 546–47
Matsuhisa, Nobu, 232, 429
Mattachine Society, 236
Mattus, Lea, 257
Mattus, Reuben, 257
Mattus, Rose, 257
matzah, 376–77
    bakeries dedicated to making, 31
    Lower East Side, 351, 352
    for Passover, 451–52
Maurice Moore-Betty Cooking School, 144
Mautner, Julie, 212
Mavis Candies, 349
Max Brenner, 530
Maximin, Jacques, 604
Maxim's (lobster palace), 330
Maxl's (restaurant), 656
Maxwell, Larry, 154
Maxwell's Plum (restaurant), 127, 377, 429
Mayer's (brewery), 76
Mayes, Herbert, 648
McBride, Anne E., 539
McBride, Mary Margaret, 483
McCall's (magazine), 171, 647, 648
McCarthy, Jenny, 639
McClure, Joe and Bob, 563
McClure's Pickles, 563
McClure's Pickles, 458
McCourt, Frank, 294, 587
McDonald's, 205
    Jackson Heights, 301
    at Macy's, 365
    workers strikes, 206
McGarry, Jack, 293
McGee, Harold, 391
    at Astor Center, 20
    in Experimental Cuisine Collective, 197
    Scribner's, 528
McInnis, Jeff, 212
McKay, Claude, 433
McKim, Mead, and White
    Childs and, 111
    Columbia University campus, 135
McKitrick Hotel, 508
McNally, Brian, 554
McNally, Keith, 334, 518, 614

McNamara, Frank X., 173
McNamee, Thomas, 141
MCNY. *See* Museum of the City of New York
McPhee, John, 48, 418
McSorley, John, 378
  Mitchell on, 418
McSorley's Old Ale House, 293, **378–79**, 586–87
  admitting women, 35
  St. Patrick's Day and, 558
McSorley's Wonderful Saloon (Mitchell), 418
McSweeney's Publishing, 356
McWilliams, James, 136
meals. *See also* Citymeals-on-Wheels
  at boarding houses, 58–59
  free meals during Depression at Municipal Lodging House, 69
  for 9/11 relief workers, 62
  school free meals, 523
Meals for the Million (Corson), 146
Mean Streets (movie), 344
meat
  availability in antebellum period, 11
  in Depression food, 170
  DuPont and packaging, 88
  Erie Canal transportation, 195
  industry, 87–88
Meatball Shop, The (restaurant), 613
Meat Hook (butcher), 88
Meatpacking District, **379–80**
  gay bars, 236
  High Line in, 274
  in Jamaica, 302
Meatpaper (magazine), 353
Mecca (restaurant), 346
media companies at Chelsea market, 108
Mednyi Chainik (restaurant), 512
Meehan, Peter, 101
  founder of *Lucky Peach*, 355, 356, 393
  on Momofuku Noodle Bar, 392
  on the Shake Shack, 531
Megarel, Roy C., 455
Mehlbach, Oscar von, 355
Meier, Frank, 55
Meilak, Frank, 398
Melissa cupcakes, 156
Mells Candy Corporation, 603
Mencken, H. L., 164, 355
Mendelson, Anne, 154
  Culinary Historians of New York, 154
  on *Gourmet*, 362
"Men in the Storm, The" (Crane), 68
Mennin, Mark, 108
Menu: The Restaurant Guide of New York, 552
menu labels, **381–82**, 608
Menu Making for Professionals in Quantity Cookery (Dahl), 505
menus, **382–84**
  collections
    digitized on *What's on the Menu?*, 421
    at New-York Historical Society, 419
    at New York Public Library, 420–21, 601
  at Toffenetti, 602
  at the Waldorf, 607
Mercer, Johnny, 293, 445, 587
Mercer Kitchen, 101

Merchants, The (coffeehouse), 128, 129, 130
Merchants Exchange, 129, 137
Merchants Hotel, 92
Merkato 55 (restaurant), 518
Merman, Ethel, 293
Mesa Grill, 210
Méthode, La (Pépin), 454
Metropolitan Club, 125
Metropolitan Hotel, 264, 390, 600
Metropolitan Museum of Art, 398–99
Metropolitan Sanitary Fair, 122
Metzelthin, Pearl, 241, 361, 468
Mexican(s), **384–85**
  bakeries, 31
  in the Bronx, 19, 77
  in Brooklyn, 81, 577
  food on Staten Island, 566
  food trucks, 219
  in Inwood, 291, 292
  in New York City, 550
Mexican Cooking School, 144
Meyer, Adolph, 191
Meyer, Claus, 522
Meyer, Danny, 88, 249, 334, **385–86**, 495, 611. *See also* Union
    Square Hospitality Group
  on closing of Union Square Cafe, 612
  on expectation of cheap Indian food, 553
  in Food & Wine Classic, 211
  hamburger stand, 259
  influenced by Baum, 501
  at Maialino, 278
  MoMA and, 399
  pizza market by, 462
  Romano and, 265
  Shake Shack, 531, 560
  at Whitney Museum, 399
Meyzen, Robert, 265, 329, 337, 550
Michel Rostand, 33
Michel's Restaurant, 449
Mi Cin (restaurant), 326
microbreweries and brewpubs, 46, 72, **386–87**
Middle Eastern
  food
    halva, 258
    hummus, 278–79
  population, 22
Midtown Lunch website, 220
Midtown West. *See* Hell's Kitchen
Mies van der Rohe, Ludwig, 221
Migration of the Negro (Lawrence), 448
Mike Colameco's Food Show, 592, 593
Mike's Deli, 19, 560
Mike's Papaya (restaurant), 277
Milbert, M., 271
Milford Farms, 317
milk
  canned, 61
  Depression distribution, 169, 170
  in egg creams, 189–90
  impurity of in Gilded Age, 239
  raw, **387–88**
  swill, 61, 174, **388–89**, 593
Milk & Honey (neo-speasy), 83

Milk Bar (restaurant), 23, 168
Millares de Mantilla, Carmen, 151
Millau, Christian, 153
Miller, Bryan, 62
    on Brazilian restaurants, 66
    on Gotham Bar and Grill, 241
    at the *New York Times*, 423
Mimi's Hummus (restaurant), 279
Mind of a Chef, The (PBS series), 57, 101, 592
Minimalist column (Bittman), 53, 423
Mint Products Company of New York, 94, 341
Mintz, David, 602–3
Mintz's Buffet, 603
Minuit, Peter, 70, 292
Miracle Grill, 210
Miranda, Carmen, 65
Mirarchi, Carlo, 507
Miró, Joan, 221
Miss Frank E. Buttolph Menu Collection, 420–21
Mission Chinese (restaurant), 233
Miss Korea BBQ, 325
Miss Leslie's New Cook Book (Leslie), 142
Miss Lilly's (restaurant), 303
Miss Mamie's Spoonbread Too (restaurant), 6, 649
Miss Maude's Spoonbread Too (restaurant), 6, 263, 649
Miss Tipton's (tearoom), 590
Mitchell, Henry, 376
Mitchell, Jan, 355
Mitchell, Joseph, **389–90**, 418
Mi Tierra grocery store, 551
Mixer and Server, 481
mixology, **390–91**
    DeGroff and revival of, 162–63
Mmmmm: A Feastiary (Reichl), 493
Mobile Markets, 282
MOCA. *See* Museum of Chinese in America
Mocca (restaurant), 280
Modern, The (MoMA restaurant), 386, 399, 501
Modern Bartender's Guide (Byron), 373, 374
modernist cuisine, **391–92**
Modernist Cuisine (Myhrvold, Young, and Bilet), 391
Moeller, William M., 82
MOFA. *See* Museum of Food and Drink
mofongo, 291, 477
Molasses Act (1733), 509, 589
molecular gastronomy. *See* modernist cuisine
Molecular Gastronomy (This), 136
Molly's Shebeen (pub), 293
Molto Italiano (Batali), 37
MoMA. *See* Museum of Modern Art
Momofoku Noodle Bar, 501
Momofuku (Chang), 101
Momofuku Ko, 101, 393
Momofuku Milk Bar, 101, 393, 466
Momofuku Noodle Bar, 101, 392
Momofuku Restaurant Group, 325, **392–93**
    on Eater, 187
    kimchi in, 319
Momoguku Ssäm Bar, 101, 393
Mondavi, Robert, 9
Mondelez International, 404, 436
Moneta's (restaurant), 344
Montana, Joe, 466

Montanari, Massimo, 135
Montayne's Tavern, 586
Montrachet (restaurant), 62, 334, 429, 495
Moore, Clement Clarke, 119
Moore, William, 403
Moore Street public market, 476
Moran, Victoria, 617
More From Magnolia (Torey), 367
Morgan, Anne, 134
Morgan, J. P., 355
    De Gouy chef of, 162, 241
    patron at the Waldorf, 607
Morgenthau, Robert, 240
Morris, Edna K., 306
Morrison, Jim, 587
Mortimer's (restaurant), 331
Mosaic Table (Krasner), 448
Moses, Robert, 78
Moskin, Julia, 82
    at the *New York Times*, 424
    on pretzels, 471
    on Trader Joe's, 605
Moskowitz (restaurant), 311
Mostel, Zero, 513
Mostly True (O'Neill), 436
Mother-in-Law's Kimchi, 319
Motorino (pizzeria), 464
Motz, George, 434
Moulton, Sara, 335, 370, **393–94**
    cooking shows, 592
    founder of NYWCA, 426
Mountain Dew, 456
Mouquin's (restaurant), 384
"Moveable Feast, A: Fresh Produce and the NYC Green Cart
    Program" (exhibit, MCNY), 401
movies, **394–96**
    Annie Hall, 587
    Balls, 434
    Bronx Cocktail, The, 79
    Café Society, 536
    Devil's Own, The, 293
    Do the Right Thing, 43
    Finding Gaston, 434
    Gangs of New York, 292
    Gentlemen Prefer Blondes, 601
    Gotham Fish Tales, 209
    Head On: Shrimping in the Low Country (film, Motz), 434
    Hog on Hog, 434
    Julie & Julia, 110, 272
    Jungle Fever, 583
    knishes in, 323
    Lady for a Day, 536
    on Little Odessa, 346
    Lost Weekend, 587
    New York locations in
        Barney Greengrass, 34
        Caffè Reggio, 93
        Childs, 601
        Jack Dempsey's, 299
        Little Italy, 344, 345
        P. J. Clarke's, 445, 587
        Rizzoli, 507
        Schrafft's, 527

movies (*continued*)
    Tavern on the Green, 585
    Zabar's, 660
    State of Grace, 293
    Stork Club, The, 570
    Thin Man, The, 79
    Tootsie, 513
    Wall Street, 566
    Weekend at the Waldorf, 627
    Whatever Works, 323, 655
    When Harry Met Sally, 165, 315–16, 317
MP Taverna, 245
Mr. and Mrs. Chester Dale Dining Out (Pène Du Bois), 447–48
Mrs. Stahl's Knishes, 322, 345, **396–97**
Mrs Allen's Book of Wheat Substitutes (Allen), 8
Mueller, Eberhard, 203
Mulberry Park, 210
Mulhall, William F., 79, 373
Mullan-Gage Act (1921), 473
Mullin, Francis, 603
Multo Mario (television show), 592
Municipal Lodging House, 69
Municipal Lodging House (Kallem), 448
Munoz, Alina, 154
Murphy, Kevin, 32
Murphy, Marc, 336
Murray's Cheese, 105, **397–98**, 409
    Ben's cream cheese at, 160
    kimchi at, 319
Murray's Roman Gardens (lobster palace), 601
Musemeci, Charles, 450
museum food, **398–400**
    at the American Museum of Natural History, 10–11
    at MoSEX, 529
    at the Museum of Modern Art, 386
Museum of Arts and Design, The, 399
Museum of Chinese in America (MOCA), 399, **400–401**
Museum of Food and Drink (MOFAD), 392, **401**
Museum of Modern Art (MoMA)
    Counter Space: Design and the Modern Kitchen, 400
    restaurants, 386, 399
Museum of Sex (MoSEX), 529
Museum of the American Cocktail (New Orleans), 163
Museum of the City of New York (MCNY), **401–2**
museums. *See also* museum food; *museums by name*
    events catered in, 99
    exhibition on automats, 25
    food exhibitions, 399–400
    in Upper East Side, 612
"Mussel Hunter at Rock Harbor" (Plath), 418
Musto, Michael, 624
Myer, Danny, 213
My Fine Feathered Friend (Grimes), 249–50
Myhrvold, Nathan, 391
My Life in France (Child and Prud'homme), 313, 324
Myriad Restaurant Group, 334, 429, 495, 501
Mystery Chef, The (radio show), 483
My Times (Hess), 271

N
Nabisco, 108, 142, 333, **403–5**
    Animal Crackers, 142, 404
    creation, 30

    Graham crackers, 142
    High Line trains, 274
    Mallomars, 142, **367**, 404
    Oreos, **436–37**
    as trust, 238
Nabokov, Vladimir, 418
Naples at Table (Schwartz), 527
Nash, Ogden, 418
Nasrallah, Nawal, 154
Nasty Bits (Bourdain), 63
Nathan, Joan, 153, 324, 488
Nathan's Famous, 205, 277, **405–6**, 601
    at Barclays Center arena, 81
    hot dog eating contests, 224
National Association for Catering and Events, 99
National Biscuit Company. *See* Nabisco
National Dunking Association, 178
National Prohibition Act (1919), 473. *See also* Prohibition
National Restaurant, 73
National Restaurant Association
    and calorie labeling, 381
    on minimum wage, 504
National School Lunch Program, 524
Nation's Restaurant News, 39, **406**
Native Americans. *See also* Lenape
    agriculture and diet, 193
    bread before European arrival, 66
    fishing, 208
    in Park Slope, 449
    pre-Columbian, 469–70
    smoked fish, 353
Native Speaker (Lee), 433–34
Natural Gourmet, The (Colbin), 406
Natural Gourmet Cooking School, 144, 335, 370, 406
Natural Gourmet Institute for Health and Culinary Arts, **406–7**
Nature's Own (Nicholson and Graham), 617
Near East (restaurant), 346
Nedick's, **407–8**, 601
Nedick's Orange Juice Company, 205
Neely, Robert T., 205, 407
Negroes Burial Ground (African Burial Ground), 5
Neill-Reynolds Commission, 535
Nepali, 553
Nespresso (coffee shop), 129
Nestle, Marion, **408–9**, 425, 440
    Culinary Historians of New York, 154
    Food Studies Collection, 201–2
    at NYU, 426
Neumark, Liz, 244
Nevins, Bruce, 456
New Albion Brewing Company, 386
New American Cuisine, 208, 240–41
New American Table (Samuelsson), 518
New Amsterdam, 368
    Africans in, 5
    bakers, 29
    beer, 45
    bread, 67
        regulation of, 29–30, 133
    Broadway Shambles Market, 137
    celebration of Saint Nicholas's Day, 118
    commodity trading, 137
    doughnuts, 177

first brewery, 70
Jewish immigrants, 65
New Year's Day parties, 181–82
taverns, 585
wine, 645
New Amsterdam Market, 231–32, **409–10**
New and Improved Bartender's Manuel (Johnson), 374
Newari cuisine, 553
Newarker, The (restaurant), 39, 493
Newbold, Joanne, 182–83
New England Sampler (Early), 371
New Family Cookbook (Corson), 442
Newfoundland, tea at, 588
New Fulton Fish Market Cooperative, 231
New Haven Railroad, 484, 485
New James Beard, The (Beard), 42
New Kochbuch, Ein (Rumpolt), 416
New Leaf Restaurant & Bar, 631
Newman, Jacqueline, 153
New Netherland Research Center, 133
New Nordic Cuisine, 522
New Scandinavian Cooking (television show), 593
New School, 144, 335, 370, **410**, 622
Newsday, 498, 499
Newsweek, 270–71
New Year, Chinese, **412–14**
New Year's, **411–12**
    Dutch-style parties, 181–82
New Year's cakes, **414–15**
New York Academy of Medicine, **415–16**
New York American (newspaper), 8, 510
New York and Harlem Railroad, 484, 612
New York Association of Cooking Teachers, 328, 527
New York Biscuit Company, 238, 403
New York cheesecake, 31
New York City Beer Week, 46
New York City Brewers Guild, 46
New York City Child Nutrition Project, 524
New York City Coalition against Hunger, 280, 281–82, 334
    research and policy initiatives, 283
New York City Coalition Against Hunger, 370–71
New York City Department of Health and Mental
        Hygiene, 263
New York City Department of Markets, 196
New York City Economic Development Council, 196
New York City Food Truck Association, 220
New York City Green Cart initiative, 215
New York City Housing Authority Garden and Greening
        Program, 215
New York City Human Resource Administration Emergency
        Food Assistance Program, 280
New York City Hunger Free Communities Consortium, 280
New York City Marathon, 456
New York City Wine and Food Festival, **416–17**
New York Cocoa Exchange, 137, 138
New York Coffee, Sugar, and Cocoa Exchange, 137
New York Coffee Exchange, 137, 138
New York Commercial Association, 137
New York Communities for Change, 206
New York Condensed Milk Company, 61, 122
New York Cookbook (Lo Pinto), 140
New York Cookbook (O'Neill), 141, 342, 436
New York Cooking Academy, 57

New York Cooking School, 143, 146, 335, 370, **417**
New York Daily News, 74, 187
New York Daily Tribune, 185, 287
New York Distilling Company, 82–83, 175
New York Eater, 308
New Yorker, The (magazine), 335, **417–19**
    caricatures of Schrafft's customers, 527
    and culinary scene, 370
    on eggs Benedict creation, 190–91
    on Lucas, 354
    on Paddleford, 446
    Pascale D'Agostino profiled by, 159
    in post–World War II culinary revolution, 468
    on raw milk, 388
    on Shattuck, 525
    writers
        Gabrielle Hamilton, 262
        Liebling, 340–41
        Mitchell, 390
        Trillin, 606
        Wechsberg, 637
New Yorkers for Beverage Choices, 544
New York Gazette, 288
New York Healthy Food & Healthy Communities, 318
New York Herald
    on Easter intoxication, 185
    on Thanksgiving dinner for Union soldiers, 597
New York Herald Tribune
    on Lewis, 339
    Paddleford in, 445–46, 468
New-York Historical Society, 118, **419**
    Beer Here: Brewing New York's History (exhibition), 400
    estimate of number of speakeasies, 556
    market records of, 170
New York Journal, 129, 276
New York Kom Tang (restaurant), 325
New York Law Journal, 333
New York magazine, 335, **419–20**
    and culinary scene, 370
    on Dough, 43
    founders, 4
    on fusion, 232–33
    on Junior's cheesecake, 314
    on Ladies Who Lunch, 330
    on Lewis, 340
    review of Zagat survey, 661
    writers
        Greene, 245–46, 498
        Platt, 498
        Sheraton, 532
New York Mail and Express, 287
New York Mercantile Exchange, 137
New York Mercury, 558
New York Observer, 63
New York Post, 330, 498
New York Press, 219
New York Produce Exchange, 137
New York Public Library, **420–21**
    Buttolph Menu collection, 601
    Lunch Hour NYC (exhibition), 400
    on prison food, 472
New York Restaurant (Hopper), 274–75, 448
New York School Lunch Committee, 523

New York's Gay Pride Parade, 568
New York sirloin. *See* New York strip steak
New York State Restaurant Association (NYSRA)
    opposed to calorie labeling, 381
    opposed to elimination of trans fats, 605
New York Strip Steak, **421–22**
New York Temperance Society, 174, 593
New York Times, **422–24**. *See also* Claiborne, Craig
    on alcohol on New Year's Eve during Prohibition, 412
    on Blot, 57, 226
    on bootleggers, 60
    on Brazilian restaurants and cuisine, 66
    on Cambodians, 554
    on Central Park Casino, 99
    on Chanukah, 102
    Christmas menus, 119
    and culinary scene, 370
    on delicatessens, 163
    on Diat, 171
    Dining section, 335
    on doughnuts, 178
    on food trucks, 219, 220
    on Fulton Fish Market, 231
    on Hamburg steak, 259–60
    on Harlem gentrification, 263
    on Hazan, 267
    on Hell's Kitchen, 268
    on Indian food, 552
    on knishes, 322
    on Ladies Who Lunch, 330
    on Lewis, 340
    on Lindy's cheesecake, 342
    list of products traded at Produce Exchange, 137
    on martinis, 375
    on *Mastering the Art of French Cooking*, 312
    on Meatpacking District, 379, 380
    on Mexican restaurants in the Bronx, 77
    on Meyer, 385
    Minimalist column, 240
    on NYU Food Studies, 408
    obituary of Ida Bailey Allen, 8
    obituary of Mitchell, 390
    on Old-Fashioned, 435
    on Passover, 451–52
    on platishers, 648
    in post–World War II culinary revolution, 468
    on pretzels, 471
    on refreshments at railroad stations, 484
    on registered hives, 44
    restaurant coverage, 498
    restaurant reviews
        Aquavit, 15
        Arirang House, 326
        Bouley, 62
        Café des Artistes, 332
        Danube, 62
        Four Seasons, 221
        Gotham Bar and Grill, 241
        Gristedes, 250–51
        Jean-Georges, 625
        JoJo, 625
        Kalustyan's, 315
        Katz's Delicatessen, 165
        La Caravelle, 330
        Le Cirque, 336, 363
        Le Pavillon, 337
        Maxwell's Plum, 377
        Momofuky Noodle Bar, 392
        Montrachet, 62
        Roberta's, 507
        Schwartz, 527
        Union Square Cafe, 612
        wd-50, 179
    60-Minute Gourmet column, 225
    on sports fans and refreshments, 559
    standards of restaurant reviewing, 498
    on Starbucks, 562
    on Thanksgiving, 597
    on Trader Joe's, 605
    on victory gardens, 615, 622
    World War II recipes, 654
    writers
        Bittman, 53
        Bruni, 498
        Claiborne, 224–25, 498
        Fabricant, 199–200
        Franey, 225
        Gold, 240
        Grimes, 249–50
        Hazan, 266
        Hess, 270–71
        Hesser in, 271, 272
        Kump, 328
        Nickerson, 427
        Pépin, 454
        Reichl, 493
        Sheraton, 532
New York Times Cookbook, The (Claiborne), 141
New York Times Dessert Cookbook, The (Fabricant), 200
New York Times Guide to Dining Out in New York, 329
New York Times Guide to New York City Restaurants (Grimes), 249
New York Times Restaurant Cookbook, The (Fabricant), 200
New York Times Seafood Cookbook, The (Fabricant), 200
New York Tribune, 163–64
New York University, **424–26**. *See also* Experimental
        Cuisine Collective
    courses on victory gardening, 622
    Fales Library, 201–2
    food studies program, 335
    Humanities Initiative, 197
    Nutrition, Food Studies, and Public Health, 370, 408, 646
New York Woman, 340
New York Women's Culinary Alliance, 335, 370, 394, **426–27**
    Fales Library collection, 202
New York World (newspaper), 472
Next Iron Chef, The, 567
Niblo's Garden (restaurant), 128, **427**
Niccolini, Julian, 222
Nicholson, Asenath, 617
Nicholson, Johnny, 91, 339
Nickerson, Jane, 124, **427–28**
    on curry, 552
    on Diat, 171
    at the *New York Times*, 422, 468
Nidetch, Jean, **428–29**, 638, 639
Niels, Joseph, 566

Nieporent, Drew, 334, **429**
  Daily Burger at Madison Square Garden, 561
  founder of Myriad Restaurant Group, 495
  influenced by Baum, 501
  partner of Bouley, 62
Nigella Express (television show), 217
nightclubs, **429–31**
  in Brighton Beach, 73
  Harlem, 262
  integration of, 556
Nighthawks (Hopper), 132, 274, 275
Night They Raided Minsky's, The (movie), 323
9/11
  anti-Pakistani sentiment after, 343
  Bouley Bakery meals for relief workers, 62
  James Beard Award for recovery efforts, 305
Ninth Avenue Food Fair, **431–32**, 570
Ninth Street Espresso, 129
Nippon (restaurant), 307
Niraula, Tara, 553
Nitehawk Cinema, 643
Nivison, Josephine, 274
Noble, Edward, 94, 341
Noble Experiment, The, 510
Nobody Knows the Truffles I've Seen (Lang), 332
"Nobody Knows the Truffles I've Seen" (Greene), 246
Nobu Fifty Seven (restaurant), 429
Nobu New York City (restaurant), 232, 334, 429, 495, 501
Nobu Next Door (restaurant), 429
No-Cal Soda, **432**
Noilly Prat & Cie, 372
NoMad (restaurant), 278
Nom Wah Tea Parlor, 172
Nonna's Birthday Surprise (Bastianich), 36
Nonna Tell Me a Story (Bastianich), 36
noodle bars, 308–9
Nordic Delicacies, 40, 522
No Reservations (television program), 63, 629
Norman, Zohar, 279
Northern Spy Food Co. (soda fountain), 547
North Fork Satur Farms, 203
Northside (brewery), 76
NoshWalks, 629
Nougatine (restaurant), 614
nouvelle cuisine, 106. *See also* New American Cuisine
  Diat on, 171
  farm to table and, 203–4
  French, 227
  at Gotham Bar and Grill, 241
  haute cuisine replaced by, 265
  Vongerichten and, 624
novels, **432–34**
NRN.com, 406
Nuchas (food kiosk), 602
Nuevo Latino movement, 66
Nugent, Ted, 356
Num Pang (sandwich chain), 108, 554
Nunu Chocolate, 117
Nureyev, Rudolf, 513
Nya Carnegie, 83
NYC Food Film Festival, **434**
NYC Sustainable Farm to Restaurant Producer Summit, 539
NYC Vegetarian Food Festival, 618

NY FoodStory (journal), 154
NYHS. *See* New-York Historical Society
NYU Urban Farm Lab, 424, 426
NYWCA. *See* New York Women's Culinary Alliance

O
Oak Room Bar, 366
obesity
  food deserts and, 214–15
  sodas and, 544
Obraitis, Sarah, 399
Oceana (restaurant), 325
Ocean Wine and Liquor, 73
Oda House (restaurant), 512
Odd Couple, The, 601
Odell, Kat, 308
Odeon (restaurant), 334, 566
O'Donnell, Rosie, 647
Official Foodie Handbook, The (Greene), 246
O'Gorman, Pat, 217
O'Keefe, Michael "Buzzy," 203
Oktoberfest, 238
Old-Fashioned cocktail, **435**
Old Homestead Steakhouse, 104, 105, 249, 259
"Old Mr. Flood" (Mitchell), 390
Old Town Bar, 293, 587
Old Traditional Polish Cuisine (food truck), 465
Old Waldorf-Astoria Bar Book, The (Crockett), 79
Oldways Preservation & Exchange Trust, 408
Oliver, Garrett, 82, 334, 386
Oliver, Sandra, 154
Omnium Gatherum (play, Rebeck and Gersten-Vassilaros), 599
One Big Table, 435–36
One Big Table (O'Neill), 436
"One for My Baby" (song, Mercer), 587
Onegin (restaurant), 512
181 Club (bar), 236
167th Street Deli, 77
100 Summer and Winter Soups (Robbins), 371
O'Neill, Eugene, 226, 598–99
O'Neill, Molly, 342, **435–36**
  on back and whites, 54
  New York Cookbook, 141
  at the *New York Times*, 423
  on Nickerson, 427–28
  on Ninth Avenue Food Fair, 431
  on Titan Greek food store in Astoria, 22
1, 000 Foods to Eat Before You Die (Sheraton)
On Food and Cooking (McGee), 391
On Location Tours, 629
Ono, Tadashi, 330
On The Town in New York (Batterberry and Batterberry), 38, 127
Open Market BackPack Program, 282
Open Space Greening Program, 254
Opera (Scappi), 416
OralFix Aphrodisiac (restaurant), 529
Orange Julius, 601
Oreo Cookie, 404
Oreos, 142, **436–37**
Organic Farming & Gardening (magazine), 508
organic food, **437–38**
  at D'Agostino, 159
  at Key Food, 317

Organic Foods Production Act (1990), 437
Oriental Brewery, 45, 70
Original Papaya (restaurant), 277
Orsini's (restaurant), 331
Orteig, Raymond, 226
Oscar's American Brasserie (restaurant, Waldorf), 627, 628
Oscar's OlDelmonico's, 167
Osmani, Aziz, 315
Ottaway, Eric, 83
Ottaway, Robin, 83
Otto Enoteca (restaurant), 296
Our Daily Food (radio program), 483
Our Global Kitchen: Food, Nature, Culture (exhibition, American Museum of Natural History), 10, 400
Our Lady of Mount Carmel festival, 262
Overland Monthly (magazine), 191
Oxford Companion to American Food and Drink, The (Smith, ed.), 440
Oxford Companion to Beer (Oliver, ed.), 82, 440
Oxford Companion to Food, The (Jaine, ed.), 440
Oxford Companion to Italian Food (Riley, ed.), 440
Oxford Companion to Sugar and Sweets, The (Goldstein, ed.), 440
Oxford Companion to Wine, The (Robinson, ed.), 439
Oxford Encyclopedia of Food and Drink in America, The (Smith, ed.), 440
Oxford English Dictionary, 438
    definition of "appetizing," 14
    on eggs Benedict, 191
Oxford University Press, 335, **438–40**
oyster bars, **440–41**, 537
    Five Points, 209
    Grand Central (*See* Grand Central Oyster Bar)
    at the Plaza, 464
oyster cellars, 13–14, 440, 442, 537
oyster houses, 5, 369, 537
oystering
    African Americans and, 5
    end of, 443
    Staten Island, 565
oysters, 440, **441–44**
    English colonial, 193
    Fourth of July, 223
    harvesting, 208
    restaurants and, 13

P
P. J. Clarke's, 293, 366, **445**, 587
Pacino, Al, 93, 299
Paddleford, Clementine, **445–46**, 506
    on expresso machine at Caffè Reggio, 93
    at *Gourmet*, 242, 361, 468
    on hummus, 279
    on Lewis, 339
    on Lindy's cheesecake, 342
Paddy Reilly's Music Bar, 558
Paddy's Market, 572
Pagán, Mario, 478
Pagès, Jean, 329
Pagremanski, Hedy, 655
Pahlmann, William, 221
Pain Quotidien, 31
paintings, **446–48**. *See also* Hopper, Edward
    of picnics, 458–59, 460
Pakistanis, 78, 301, 343

Pakula, Alan J., 460
Palmer, Charlie, 203
pan-Latino restaurants, 478
Pan Pan (restaurant), 263
Pantell, Richard, 460
Paolucci's (restaurant), 246
Papalexis, Gregory, 277
Papaya King, 277, **448–49**
Paprika Roth (grocery), 280
Paprika Weiss (grocery), 280
Parachini, Chris, 507
parades. *See also* West Indian Day Parade
    Easter, 185
    Macy's Thanksgiving Day Parade, 365
    St. Patrick's Day, 657
    Steuben Parade, 238, 657
Paradié, Jean-Pierre, 227
Parasecoli, Favio, 410
Paris Baguette, 31
Parisi, Domenico, 93
Park, Joseph, 148
Park & Tilford, 148
Park Avenue Potluck (Fabricant), 200
Park Avenue Potluck Celebrations (Fabricant), 200
Park Avenue public market, 476
Parker, Dorothy, 7, 536
Park Slope, **449–50**
    deep-fried Twinkies invented in, 161, 162
    gay bars, 236
Park Slope Brewing Company, 387
Park Slope Food Coop, 214, 437, 449–50
Park Town Coffee Shop, 450
Parlor (club), 126
Parlor Coffee (coffee shop), 129
Parts Unknown (television program), 63
Pascal, Guy, 342
Pascarelli, Anne, 153
Passaro, Albert, 374
Passaro, Aurora and Louis, 373, 374
Passover, **450–52**
    halva in, 258
    horseradish in, 458
Pasta, La (restaurant), 186
pasta primavera, 336
Pasternak, David, 186, 560
Pastis (restaurant), 334
Pastosa, 566
pastrami, 145, 164, **452–53**
Patel Brothers (grocery), 301
Patina (restaurant), 120
Patronite, Rob, 246, 420
Patsy's Pizzeria, 262, 350, 461, 463, 464
Patterson, David, 636
Paulding, James Kirk, 458
Paulie Gee's (pizzeria), 462
Paul's Da Burger Joint, 189
Pay Dirt (Rodale), 508
Paymaster Building, 175
Payne, B. W., 376
PDT, 435
Peacock, Scott, 313, 340
Peacock Alley (restaurant, Waldorf), 627
Peacock Café, 249
Peapod (online grocer), 229

Pearl Diner, 173
Peculiar Pub, 248
peddlers. *See also* street vendors
    in antebellum period, 11
    Essex Street Market, 196
Pedestrian in the City (Benepe), 47
Peek Frean, 287
Peel, Mark, 377
Pegu Club, 163, 391, 435, 520, 521
Pekin, The (lobster palace), 348–49
Pelaccio, Zakary, 86
Pelgram, Thomas, 558
Pellegrino, Frank, 489
Pelzer's Pretzels, 471
Peng's (restaurant), 113
Pennsylvania Station, 243
Penny, Virginia, 30
penny candies, 94
penny restaurants, 92, 363
Penton Restaurant Group, 406
Pépin, Jacques, **454–55**
    asked to be White House chef, 329
    Baum and, 39
    Claiborne and, 468
    in Food & Wine Classic, 211
    Franey and, 224
    at French Culinary Institute, 228
    haute cuisine and, 265
    in James Beard Foundation, 335
    Jones and, 313
    Knopf and, 324
    at Le Pavillon, 337
    menu consultant for Restaurant Associates, 494
    teaching at cooking school of New School, 144
    walking out in protest from Le Pavillon, 549
pepper pot, 194
Pepsi-Cola, 279, 333, 349, **455–56**, 456, 544
    bottled water, 636
    electronic billboard ad, 4
Perigord, Le (restaurant), 227
Pero, Antonio Totonno, 461, 463
Perrier, **456**, 636
Per Se (restaurant), 579, 593, 614
Pesach. *See* Passover
Pesca (restaurant), 385
Pesce, Il (restaurant), 186
Peter Kump's New York Cooking School, 144, 290, 327–28,
        370. *See also* Institute of Culinary Education
    Moulton instructor at, 394
    Saunders at, 520
Peter Luger's Steakhouse, 105, 237–38, **456–57**, 643
    cheesecake, 104
    Master Purveyors and, 284
Peterson, Eigel, 104, 314
Pete's Tavern, 293, 587
Pet Food Politics (Nestle), 409
Petiot, Fernand (Pete), 55
Petit Cordon Bleu, Le (restaurant), 144
Petitpas (restaurant), 447
Petrini, Carlo, 136, 269
    founder of Slow Food, 538
    Rizzoli and, 242
Phenix Cheese Company, 103, 149
Philadelphia Cream Cheese, 28, 103, 149

Philippe, Claudius Charles, 95
Philip's Candy, 95
Physical Culture (magazine), 363
Physiology of New York Boarding-Houses, The (Gunn), 58
Physiology of Taste, The (Brillat-Savarin), 324
Piazza, La (food/drinks bar), 186
Picholine (restaurant), 614
Pickell, Len, 306
Pickle Guys, 458
pickles, 191, 351, **457–58**
pickle wars, 458
Pic-Nic (Cole), 447
Picnic Excursion (Homer), 458–59
"Picnic in the Station" (Wasserstein), 460
picnics, **458–60**, 614
Picnic Season, The (Tavernier), 459
Picon, Molly, 323
Piel Bros., 45, 46, 59, 70, 71
Pierre Franey's Low-Calorie Gourmet, 225
Pileggi, Nick, 420
Pillsbury Company, 257
Pintard, John, 118
Piper's Kilt (pub), 292
pistachios, 584
pizza, 294, 295, **460–62**
    at Eataly, 186
    Egyptian, 191
    falafel, 201
    Greenwich Village, 248
Pizza, La (restaurant), 186
Pizza Connection, 462
Pizza Principle, 462
pizzerias, **462–64**
    coal-fired, 461
    in Greenwich Village, 248
    Lombardi's, 350–51
Place in the Country, A (Cunningham), 460
Planck, Nina, 48
Planet Taco (Pilcher), 440
plantains, 176, 477
Plated, 563
Plate House (restaurant), 204
Plath, Sylvia, 418
Platner, Warren, 39
Platt, Adam, 246
    at *New York* magazine, 420, 498
    on Riingo, 518
Play. The Café/Den/Bar, 529
Plaza, The, **464**
    as gay bar, 236
    Great Performances at, 244
    power breakfasts, 469
Please Don't Tell (bar), 557
Pleasure of Your Company, The (O'Neill), 436
Pleasures of Chinese Cooking, The (Hazan), 266
Pleasures of Cooking for One, The (Jones), 313, 324
Plimpton, George, 211
Po (restaurant), 36
Pogash, Jeffrey, 55
Point, Fernand, 418, 638
Pokhlebkin, William, 512
Polesny, Evie, 233
Polesny, Michael, 233
Polini, Giuseppe, 266

Polish, **465**
  bakeries, 31
  doughnuts, 177
  on Staten Island, 566
  in Williamsburg, 643
Pollan, Michael, 270, 356, 592
Pollinger, Ben, 325
Pollock, Jackson, 221, 448
pollution and fishing, 208–9
Polo Grounds, 276
Polonias, 465
Pol's Trow's New York Directory, 590
Pomodoro! A History of the Tomato in Italy
      (Gentilcore), 136
Ponzek, Debra, 211
Popil, Barry, 536
pop-up restaurants, 181, **466–67**
Portale, Alfred, 180, 240–41, 599
Port Arthur (restaurant), 210
Porter, Cole, 627
Poseidon Bakery, 245, 269
Postum Cereal Company, 267
post-World War II (1945–1975), **467–68**
potato pancakes. *See* latkes
potato salad, 163, 223
Potter, Tom, 82
Pough, Richard, 48
Poulos, Birdie, 449
Poulos, Constantine, 277
Poulos, Gus, 448–49
Powell, Julie, 110
power breakfasts and power lunches, 87, 222, 358,
      468–69
Powerhouse, The (American Museum of Natural History),
      10–11
power lunch. *See* power breakfasts and power lunches
Pranzo—La Scuola di Eataly (restaurant), 186
Preacher's (restaurant), 249
pre-Columbian, **469–70**
Presley, Elvis, 93, 246
Pret-a-Manger, 205, 358
pretzels, 163, **471–72**
Prevention Magazine, 508
Prial, Frank, 423
Primorski Restaurant, 73
prison food, **472–73**
Progressive Era, 238, 476
Prohibition, **473–74**. *See also* bootleggers
  anti-German feeling and, 652–53
  and brewing industry in New York, 45
  "21" Club during, 609
  cocktail lounges during, 126
  Cotton Club during, 148
  development of soda fountains, 547
  diners in, 172, 173
  on distilleries, 174–75
  Ear Inn during, 586
  gay bars, 236
  Greenwich Village, 248
  Harlem in, 262
  haute cuisine and, 264
  in Hell's Kitchen, 269
  ice cream shops, 288
  impact on
      French restaurants, 167
      high-end restaurants, 500
      saloons, 516
  Italians in, 295
  lobster palaces and, 348, 349
  Lüchow's during, 355
  McSorley's during, 379
  mixology during, 390–91
  nightclubs during, 430
  Peter Luger's raided in, 456
  Pete's Tavern during, 587
  the Plaza bars during, 464
  Rector's and, 492
  restaurant rebound after, 170
  and rum popularity, 509
  Sardi's during, 520
  Sherry's and, 535
  Stork Club during, 569
  White Horse during, 641
Promenade Bar, 487
Prosperity Dumpling, 352
Proust, Marcel, 341
Providence Journal Company, 217
Provisions (online store), 216
Prud'homme, Alex, 313, 324
Prune (restaurant), 261, 566
Pruyn, Huybertie, 182
Psilakis, Michael, 245
public markets, 409, **474–77**. *See also* Arthur Avenue Retail
      Market; Chelsea Market; Essex Street Market; Fulton
      Market; Washington Market
  in antebellum period, 11
      corruption of city government and, 12
      deregulation, 12
  groceries as complement to, 253
  Lower East Side, 352
  in Manhattan, 370
publishers. *See also* Knopf; Oxford University Press; Random
      House
  late twentieth century, 335
  in Little Syria, 346
pubs. *See also* microbreweries and brewpubs
  Inwood, 292
  Irish, 292–93
Puck, Wolfgang, 232, 494
  at Beard House, 306
  at De Gustibus, 365
  James Beard Award to, 304
Puerto Rican(s), **477–78**
  bodegas, 59
  in the Bronx, 77
  in Brooklyn, 97
  Essex Street Market and, 196
  in Harlem, 262, 263
  in Hell's Kitchen, 269
  late twentieth century, 334
  on Lower East Side, 352
  in New York City, 550
  post-World War II, 467
  in Williamsburg, 643
Puerto Rican Day Parade, 478
Pulitzer, Joseph, 472

Pulixi, Carlo, 233
Pulixi, Michelle, 233
Pullman, George, 484
Pullman Diner, The, 172
Pullman dining cars, 484–85
Puncheon Grotto, 609
Pure Food & Wine (restaurant), 406, 618
Purity (coffee shop), 450
Purple Pup, The (tearoom), 590
Purple Yam (restaurant), 208
Purviance, Helen, 517
Pushcart Coffee (coffee shop), 129
Pushcart Commission, 572
pushcart vendors. *See also* street vendors
    Essex Street Market, 196
    licensing, 572
    regulation, 571

Q

Quagliata, Carmen, 612
Queen of the Night, 599
Queens, **479–81**. *See also* Astoria; Elmhurst; Flushing; Jackson
        Heights; Jamaica (Queens); Little India; Richmond
        Hill; Woodside
    Australian restaurants, 23
    Brazilians in, 66
    Caribbeans in, 97
    Central and South Americans in, 550
    Chinatown in, 114
    diners, 173
    distilleries, 175
    Filipinos in, 207
    food deserts, 214–15
    food trucks, 219, 220
    Indians in, 343
    Irish in, 292
    Koreatown, 326–27
    Mexicans in, 385
    microbreweries, 387
    Polish in, 465
    Russians in, 512
    walking culinary tours, 629
Queensboro Corporation, 300
Queens Cocktail, **481**
Queens Harvest Food Coop, 214
Queens Head (tavern), 225. *See also* Fraunces Tavern
Queens Rackshow, The (coffee shop), 129
Quiche and Pâté (Kump), 328
"Quick, Jammacher, My Stomacher!" (Nash), 418
quick food. *See also* fast food
    in Manhattan, 369
    slang and, 537
Quinby, Moses, 43
Quinzio, Jeri, 484
Quisisana (automat), 24
Quo Vadis (restaurant), 370, 467, 501

R

Raaka Chocolate, 117
race segregation among restaurant workers, 503
Rachael Ray (television show), 592
Rachael Ray's Tasty Travels (television show), 592
Rachael vs Guy: Celebrity Cook-Off (television show), 592

Racked.com, 187
Radically Simple (Gold), 240
radio, **483–84**. *See also* Heritage Radio Network
    culinary programs, 8
    National Public Radio, 270
Radio City Matinee, 41
Radutsky, Nathan, 258
Raft, George, 587
railroad dining, **484–86**
Rainbow Room (restaurant), 430, **486–88**
    Brody at, 243
    created by Baum, 39
    DeGroff at, 162–63
    Gold at, 240
    menu, 384
Raintree's (restaurant), 450
Raisfeld, Robin, 246, 420
Ralph's Famous Italian Ices, 295, 566
Rambourg, Patrick, 566
ramen noodles, 308–9
Rana Pasta, 108
Randall, Tony, 72
Randolph, Mary, 271
Random House, 323–24, **488**
Ranhofer, Charles, **488–89**
    coining of name baked Alaska, 29
    at Delmonico's, 166–67
    eggs Benedict recipe, 190
    haute cuisine, 264
    lobster Newberg, 347
Rao's (restaurant), 262, **489**, 533
Rapaport, Ruben, 603
Rasch, Albertina, 513
Rastafari, **489–90**
Rath, August, 163
rationing during World War II. *See* food shortages and rationing
        during World War II
Ratnam, Basu, 553
Ratner, Alex, 311
Ratner's dairy restaurant, 311
raw food, 50, 263, **490–91**
Raw Soul (restaurant), 263
Ray, Rachael, **491**, 592
Ray's (pizzeria), 248, 463
Ray's Candy Store, 189, 190
Rays Pizzerias, 462
Real Food Summer School (online show), 268
Rebeck, Theresa, 599
Rector, Charles E., 348, 491, **491–92**
Rector, George W., 348, **491–92**, 492
    on word brunch, 84
Rector Cook Book, The (G. Rector), 492
Rector's (lobster palace), 348, 412, 601
Rector's Oyster House (Chicago), 491
Red Apple (grocery stores), 250
Redbook (magazine), 340, 648
Redding, Carl, 6
Red Flame (coffee shop), 131
Redgrave, Lynn, 639
Red Head (speakeasy), 609
Red Hook, 201, 207, 219, 563
Red Hook cocktail, 83
Red Rooster (restaurant), 6, 263, 518, 649

Red Tulip (restaurant), 280
Redzepi, Rene, 355–56, 522
refrigeration
    ice cream shops and, 288
    meat and, 87, 88
Regan, Gaz, 391
Reggie! Bar, 95, **492–93**
regulations
    on bakeries, 67
    on bread, 29–30, 67, 133
    concerning honey bees, 44
    of sodas, 544, 545–46
    of street vendors (*See* street vendors, regulation of)
Reichl, Ruth, **493**
    on Babbo, 37
    on Daniel, 63
    as *Gourmet* editor, 242
    on James Beard Awards, 304
    at the *New York Times*, 249, 423, 498
    review of Aquavit restaurant, 15
Reiner, Rob, 165, 317
Reinhold, Ralph, 361
Reisenweber's Café (lobster palace), 348–49, 430
Religion, Food and Eating in North America (Zeller, et al.),
        136
Remande, Pierre, 260
Remembrance of Things Paris (Reichl, ed.), 638
Remembrance of Things Past (Proust), 341
Remnick, David, 417, 418
Renaud, Cyril, 265, 330
René, André, 487, 644
Renggli, Seppi, 221
rent parties, 6
Renynard (restaurant), 278
Requiem for a Heavyweight (movie), 299
Rescue Home for Fallen and Homeless Girls, 517
Resnick, Irv, 529
Restaurant Associates, 369–70, 399, **493–94**, 494, 501
    Baum executive of, 39
    Beard and, 42
    Brody and, 243
    Lang and, 332
    Lüchow's and, 355
    Metropolitan Museum of Art and, 398
    Sheraton consultant for, 532
    subsidiary of Compass Group North America, 495
    and Tavern on the Green, 585
    theme restaurants by, 467
restaurant criticism. *See* restaurant reviewing
Restaurant Daniel, 259
Restaurant Français, Le, 226–27
restaurant groups, **494–96**
restaurant letter grading, **496–97**
Restaurant Management (magazine), 162
Restaurant Opportunity Center (ROC) (Restaurant
        Opportunities Centers United), 206, **497**,
        503, 504
    New School and, 410
restaurant reviewing, **497–99**
    Claiborne and, 124, 422
    in Eater, 187
    by Greene, 245–46
    by Hess, 270–71

    by Lape, 333
    Schwartz and, 527
    standards, 423
Restaurant Row, **499**
restaurants, **499–501**. *See also* department store restaurants;
        diners; hotel restaurants; pop-up restaurants; table
        d'hôte restaurants
    African American, 6
    Albanian, 77
    in antebellum period, 13–14
    Armenian, 18
    on Arthur Avenue, 19
    Australian, 22–23
    in the Bronx, 76, 77, 78
    in Brooklyn
        Bay Ridge, 40
        Bedford-Stuyvesant, 43
        Bensonhurst, 49
        Brighton Beach, 73
        Bushwick, 86
        Park Slope, 449–50
        Sunset Park, 577–78
        Williamsburg, 643
    Caribbean, 97, 98
    Chinese, 112–13
    Diners Club in, 173–74
    Dominican, 77
    in early Arab community, 16
    in films, 396
    German, 237–38
    Ital, 490
    Japanese, 581
    Lebanese, 16
    in Manhattan, 369–70
        Five Points, 209
        Greenwich Village, 248–49
        Upper East Side, 613
        Upper West Side, 614
        Yorkville, 656
    penny restaurants, 92, 363
    post-World War II, 467
    Puerto Rican, 77, 477–78
    in Queens, 480
        Astoria, 22
        Jackson Heights, 300
        Jamaica, 302
    Syrian and Lebanese, 16, 584–85
    Thai, 596
    Ukrainian, 611
    vegan, 617–18
restaurant unions, **501–3**
restaurant workers, **503–4**
retail groceries, 632
Reuben, Arnold, 505
    cheesecake of, 103, 342
Reuben's (delicatessen), 165
Reuben sandwich, 145, 316–17, **505**
Reuge, Maria, 335, 370, 427
Revolutionary War
    Brooklyn, 80
    Fraunces Tavern, 225
    German food, 237
    tea boycott, 588

Revolution in Eating, A (McWilliams), 136
Revsin, Leslie, 105
Reyes, Jose, 511
Reynolds, Alvah Lewis, 149
Reynolds, Jonathan, 599
Rheingold (brewery), 46, 71–72, 81
    in German delis, 164
    sporting events and, 559–60
Rhode, Bill and Irma, 41
Richards, Dan T., 154
Richman, Alan, 228
Richmond Hill, 289, 551, 552
Ricketts, Sean, 520
Rickshaw Dumplings (kiosk), 602
Rider's New York City, 590
Ridley, Helen E., 171
Riese Brothers, 355
Riese Organization, 342, 408
Riingo (restaurant), 518
Riis, Jacob, 239, 343, 344, 433
    on effect of saloons in New York, 516
Rikers Island, 472
Rimmer, Leopold, 167, 489
Ringgold, Faith, 460
Rio de la Plata Panaderia and Confiteria, 551
Ripert, Eric
    on *Food Arts*, 212
    fusion food, 232–33
    kimchi recipes, 319
    on *Mike Colameco's Food Show*, 593
"Rip Van Winkle" (Irving), 294
Ritz, César, 505
Ritz Carleton, 412
Ritz-Carlton, **505–6**
    Diat at, 171
    haute cuisine, 264
    London, Palm Court, 243
    Ridley at, 171
    Torres Corporate Pastry Chef at, 604
Ritz-Carlton Battery Park, 506
River Café, 203
Riverkeeper group, 209
Riverpark, 495
Rivers, Larry, 377
Riviera Café, 249
Rivinius (brewery), 76
Rizzo, Salvatore, 365
Rizzoli, **506–7**
Rizzuto, Phil, 461
Robbins, Ann Roe, 371
Robbins, Irvine, 288
Robert (restaurant), 399
Roberta's (restaurant), 86, **507**
    pizza at, 462, 464
    studio of Heritage Radio Network at, 269, 483
Roberto's (restaurant), 19, 77
Robert's (restaurant), 329
Robins, Missy, 296
Robinson, Jackie, 115
Robinson, Jancis, 439
Robuchon, Joel, 62, 324, 488
Roche, Pierre, 260
Rockaway Brewing Company, 387

Rockefeller, David, 33
Rockefeller, Happy, 330
Rockefeller Center
    Ice Rink, 495
    Luncheon Club, 486
Rockwell, David, 554
Rodale, Jerome Irving, **507–8**
Roden, Claudia, 313, 324, 488
Rodizio restaurants, 66
Romagnoli, Franco, 296
Romano, Michael, 265, 386
    at La Caravelle, 330
    at Union Square Cafe, 611
rooftop gardens, **508–9**
    in Brooklyn, 82
    honey bees and, 44
Rookery (restaurant), 303
Room4Dessert, 392
room service, 278, 627
Roosevelt, Eleanor, 322, 339
Roosevelt, Franklin D., 474, 579
Roosevelt, Theodore
    Ellis Island food system, 192
    knishes, 322
    Little Hungary frequented by, 279
    at Lüchow's, 355
    patron of McSorley's, 586
Rose, Carl, 418
Rosemary's (restaurant), 508
Rosen, Alan, 313
Rosen, Harry, 104, 314
Rosen, Mike, 314
Rosenbaum, Ron, 314
Rosenbaum, Wayne, 449
Rosengarten, David, 217
Rosenthal, A. M., 407
Rosenzweig, Anna, 203, 259
Rose's Turn (restaurant), 249
Rosie (magazine), 647
Roslyn Holiday Farms, 317
Ross, Al, 419
Ross, Alice, 153
Ross, Harold, 7, 417
Roth, Henry, 323
Roth, Terry, 3
Rothstein, Arnold, 165
rotimobiles, 219
Rotunda (restaurant), 278
Roundtable of Women in Food Service, 202
Roxbury Farm, 139
Royal Box (speakeasy), 60
Royal Caribbean Bakery, 77, 97
Royal Cookery Book (Gouffé), 620
R.T. French Co., 304
R.T. French Tastemaker Awards, 304
Rubin, Jeff, 182
Rubin, Miriam, 427
Rubin Museum, 399
Rubinow, Ray, 247
Rubirosa (pizzeria), 464
Rubsam and Horrmann's, 565
Ruggerio, David, 265, 592, 593
Ruhlman, Michael, 528

rum, **509–10**
  in colonial period, 557
  distilleries, 174
  rum-running during Prohibition, 60
rum punch, 34
Run-Through (Houseman), 137
Runyon, Damon, **510–11**, 601
Rupert, 71
Rural & Migrant Ministry, 493
Russ, Joel, 511
Russ & Daughters, 316, 352, **511**, 512, 537
  bagel, lox, cream cheese at, 353
  dairy products, 160
  egg creams, 189, 190
  full-service café, 354
  at New Amsterdam Market, 409
  Polish-owned, 465
Russ & Daughters Cafe, 511
Russell, Lillian, 64, 243, 607
Russian(s), **511–13**
  in Brighton Beach, 81
  in the Bronx, 78
  Easter celebrations, 185–86
  halva, 258
  immigration waves, 511–12
  in Little Odessa, 345–46
  in Washington Heights, 631
Russian Tea Room, 500, 512, **513–14**, 646
Ruth's (restaurant), 263
Ryan, Meg, 165, 317
Ryder, Tracey, 188
rye whiskey, 509
Ryley, Alison, 154

S
S. Liebmann's Sons, 45, 70
Sabin, Pauline, 474
Sabra, 279
Sabrett (hot dog maker), 277
Sachs, Adam, 521
Sachs, Jeffery D., 135
Safe Food (Nestle), 408
Sahadi's (grocery), 191, 278–79, 584
Sahara East (restaurant), 191
Sailhac, Alain, 228, 265, 336, **515**
Sailhac, Arlene Feltman, 335
Sala, George, 29, 166, 411
salad bars. *See* buffet/salad bars
Salad Book, The (De Gouy), 162
salami, 164, 316
Salinger, J. D., 433
Salisbury, James H., 259
Salisbury steak, 259, 260
Salmagundi (periodical), 119, 142, 294, 458
saloons, 34–35, 127, **515–16**, 536
  Five Points, 209–10
  groggeries and, 253–54
  lunch in, 356
  oyster saloons, 440
  P. J. Clarke's, 445
  turned into ice cream shops, 288
Salt, Henry S., 617
Salty Road Taffy, 95

"Salute to Women in Gastronomy, A" (event), 338
Salvage Supperclub, 181
Salvation Army, 92, 178, **517**
Salvation Taco, 57
Sam and Raj (Indian goods store), 301
Sammy's Roumanian Steak House, 352
Samuelsson, Marcus, **517–19**, 649
  at Aquavit, 15, 522
  in Food & Wine Classic, 211
  Harlem restaurant, 263
  Red Rooster, 6
  Starbucks and, 562
Sanchez, Rosio, 392
S&S Cheesecake, 104
San Gennaro, Feast of, 49, 345, **519–20**, 571, 661
San Rasa (restaurant), 553
Santa Anna, Antonio López de, 255–56
Sante Fe Grill, 450
Sarabeth's Bakery, 108, 168, 399
Sara Moulton Cooks at Home (Moulton), 394
Sara Moulton's Everyday Family Dinners (Moulton), 394
Sara's Secrets (television show), 394, 592
Sara's Secrets for Weeknight Meals (Moulton), 394
Sara's Weeknight Meals (PBS), 394
Saravana Bhavan (restaurant), 553
Sardi, Vincent, Jr., 520
Sardi's (restaurant), **520**
  actors at, 601
  business lunch at, 87
  on *Mad Men*, 366
  during Prohibition, 500
Sargent, Ben, 217
Sartwell, Matt, 637
sashimi, 308, 581
Sass, Lorna, 316
Sasso, John, 461, 463
Saucier's Apprentice, The (Sokolov), 548
sauerkraut, 163, 321
Saunders, Audrey, 163, 391, **520–21**
sausages, 163, 164. *See also* hot dogs
Saveur (magazine), **521**
  on Astor Center, 20
  and culinary scene, 370
  debut of, 335
  Hamilton, Gabrielle, in, 262
Saveur.com, 216
Savor This (online quarterly), 9
Savoy (restaurant), 203
Savoy Cocktail Book, The (Craddock), 481
Savuvin, Georges, 166
Sax, Richard, 153
Saxelby Cheesemongers, 105, 352
Saxon, Lyle, 8
Sazón (restaurant), 478
Sbarro, 40
Scandinavian(s), **521–22**, 577
Schaap, Rosie, 423
Schaefer brewery. *See* F. & M. Schaefer Brewing
Schaeffers, Antoine, 260
Schaller & Weber, 163, **522–23**, 612, 657
Scherber, Amy, 31
Schiller's Liquor Bar, 352
Schimmel, Yonah, 311, 655

Schlitz beer, 164. *See also* Joseph Schlitz Brewing
Schlosser, Eric, 425
Schlüter, Dietmar, 100
Schmidt, Ed, 599
Schmulka Bernstein's (restaurant), 312
Schoneberger & Noble (drink company), 179
School Breakfast Program, 282
school food, **523–25**
    gardens, 254
    vending machines on school grounds, 619
School of Classic Italian Cooking, 266
Schrafft's, 500, **525–27**, 591
   in the Bronx, 76
   fast food, 204
   Jackson Heights, 300
   lunches, 357
   during World War II, 654
Schraft, William F., 525
Schrager, Lee Brian, 416
Schultz, Carl, 179
Schultz, Dutch, 60, 61
Schultze, Leonard, 627
Schwartz, Arthur, 483, **527**
Schwebel, Gussie, 322
Scicolone, Michele, 427
Science of Cheese, The (Tunick), 440
Scorsese, Martin, 292, 345
Scott's multiborough pizza bus tours, 629
SCRATCH bakery, 43
Screwdriver, 84
Scribner's, **528**
Scribner's Magazine, 528
Scripps Networks Interactive, 217, 218
Sea Colony (bar), 236
seafood. *See also* fish; Fulton Fish Market; smoked fish
    consumption guidelines, 208–9
    English colonial, 193
    at Gage & Tollner, 235
    Il Pesce, 186
    Italian, 295
    Jamaican, 303
    pre-Columbian, 469–70
    transportation, 195, 231
Seafood Cookbook, The (Franey), 225
Seagram Building, 221, 235
seasonality
    food availability and, 11
    of menu at Union Square Cafe, 611
Second Avenue Deli, 165, 189, 312
Secret Ingredients (Remnick, ed.), 418, 638
Seiger, Karen, 247
Seinfeld, black and whites in, 54, 142, 592
Seitsema, Robert, 356
self-service restaurants. *See* cafeterias
Sell, Christopher, 161
seltzer, **528–29**, 544. *See also* soda
    in egg creams, 189–90
    Jewish taste for, 311
Seltzer Works (PBS documentary), 529
Selznick, David O., 329
Senator Frozen Products Company, 257
Sendel, Jan, 518
Seneca Chief (boat), 194

Senegalese in Bedford-Stuyvant, 43
Sergeant Litschoe's tavern, 586
Serious Eats (online guide), 512
Serve It Forth (Fisher), 362
Service Employees International Union, 206, 504
Sette MoMA (restaurant), 399
Setting the Table (Meyer), 386
Sevan's Restaurant & Catering, 18
Seventeen (magazine), 532
71 Clinton Fresh Food (restaurant), 180, 352
Severo, Richard, 390
Severson, Kim, 423–24
Sevilla (restaurant), 499
sex and food, **529–30**
Sex and the City (television series), **530–31**
    Cosmopolitan on, 147
    cupcakes, 156
    Magnolia Bakery on, 366, 367, 592
    tour of eateries made famous by, 629
Sex on the Table Cooking School, 530
sexual harassment, 504
Seybert, Howard, 200
SFNYC Book & Film Club, 539
Shad Festival—Drums along the Hudson: A Native American Festival, 292
Shake Shack (restaurant), 88, 259, 386, 495, 501, **531–32**
    at Citi Field Park, 560
Shalom Japan (restaurant), 643
Shanghai Cafe, 113
Shanken, Marvin, 38
Shanley, Thomas, 348, 500
Shanley's (restaurant), 500
Shapiro, Beth, 120
Shapiro, Laura, 153, 154
Shaplen, Robert, 418
Share Our Strength's No Kid Hungry, 416
Shattuck, Frank, 204, 525
Shawn, William, 417
Shearith Israel (synagogue), 309, 451
Sheed, Wilfred, 211
Sheik, The (restaurant), 346
Sheldon, Margaret, 517
Shelley's (bakery), 300
Sheraton, Mimi, **532–33**
    on Baum, 494
    on bialys, 50
    on Brazilian restaurants, 66
    on Felker, 420
    on Gallic food, 331
    at the *New York Times*, 423, 498
    reviews
        Chalet Suisse, 100
        The Four Seasons, 221
        La Caravelle, 329
        Le Cygne, 515
        Les Trois Petits Cochons, 227
        Victor's Café, 621
    on school lunches, 524
    on SoHo as Brunchville, 85
    standards for restaurant criticism, 423
    on sushi, 581
Sherman Antitrust Act, 238
Sherri Cup Company, 128

Sherry, Louis, 500, 533, 534
lobster palaces, 348
papers in Fales Library, 202
Sherry, Marc, 259
Sherry's (restaurant), 500, **533–35**
horseback dinner at, 534
New York State Federation of Women's Clubs and
Societies, 647
Shinn, Everett, 447, 464
ship's biscuits, 30, 67
Shop Healthy Initiative, 215
Shopping Bag Annie, 231
shops. *See also* ice cream shops
in antebellum period, 12
on Arthur Avenue, 19
carrying Armenian food, 18
Shore Dinners, 207
Shultz, Howard, 561–62
Shun Lee Dynasty (restaurant), 113
Shun Lee West (restaurant), 614
SideTour, 629
Sietsema, Robert, 187, 462, 498, 624
Sifton, Sam
on Aquavit, 15
at the *New York Times*, 423
on Red Rooster, 518
on Roberta's, 507
Sigiri (restaurant), 553
Sigmund's (pretzel shop), 471
Silliman, Benjamin, 543, 546
Silver Palate, 99
Silver Spoon Award, 213
Claiborne, 213
Dufresne, 180
Dorothy Cann Hamilton, 261
Trotter, 213
Silverton, Nancy, 324, 377
Silvestro, Ralph, 297, 566
Simmons, Amelia, 119, 142
Simmons, Gail, 212
Simmons, Marie, 153
Simonds, Nina, 313
Simple Cuisine (Vongerichten), 625
Simply Ming (television show), 593
Simpson, Jessica, 639
Sinatra, Frank, 299, 445, 461
Sinclair, Upton, 523, **535–36**
Singer, Isaac Bashevis, 323
Singeron, Auguste Louis de, 93–94
SingleCut Beersmiths, 387
single-origin cacao. *See* chocolate, craft
Sintourel, Alain, 227
Sirio: The Story of My Life and Le Cirque (Maccioni and Elliot),
336, 363
Sismondo, Christine, 46
sixpenny houses, 13
Sixpoint Brewery, 387, 564, 643
Sixth Street Community Center, 139
SixtyFive (bar-lounge), 487
"60-Minute Gourmet" (column, Franey), 423
Sketch Book, The (Irving), 294
Skiles, Mark, 642
slang, **536–38**

Slaughterhouse Row, 283
slaves and slavery
and Caribbean migration to New York City, 96
foodways brought by, 194
Indo-Caribbeans in, 289
in New York State, 96
and supply of New York city food, 5
Sleeper, Cleveland, 371
Slice of Brooklyn, A, 629
Sloan, John, 447, 448
Arch Conspirators, 460
regular of McSorley's, 379
Sloane, Roy, 257
Slotkin, Samuel, 277
Slow Food, 269, 296, **538–39**
Slow Food (Petrini), 136
Slow Food Guide to New York City, The (Martins and
Watson), 538
Slow Food International, 538
Slow Food Nation (conference), 538
Slow Food NYC, 407, 538
Slow Food USA, 335, 538
Slow U., 538
slumming, 237, 239
Slur, The, 539
Small's (café), 248
Smilow, Rick, 290, 328, **539**
Smith, Adam, 509
Smith, Al, 473
Smith, Andrew F., 154
Smith, Heather, 353
smoked fish, **539–41**
in Brighton Beach, 73
Jewish deli, 164, 165, 311
lox, 353–54
sold in appetizing stores, 14
sturgeon sold by Barney Greengrass, 33
smoked meats, 73
smokehouses, 540
Smorgasburg, 358, **541**, 563, 608, 620, 643
pop-ups in, 466
Snail of Approval, 538
SNAP. *See* Supplemental Nutrition Assistance
Program
Snapple, 334, **541–43**
Sneddon, David, 200
"Snug and Warm Inside McSorley's" (Cummings),
586–87
Snyder, Jerome, 322
social class
cocktails and, 372
Gilded Age, 238–39
ice cream sandwiches and, 287
ice cream shops and, 288
Ladies Who Lunch, 330–31
Prohibition's effects by, 473–74
public markets and, 475
social media. *See also* Twitter
Batali and, 37
food trucks and, 220
street vendors and, 620
Société Culinaire Philanthropique, 106
Society for the Suppression of Vice, 236

Sockerbit (candy shop), 95
Socoloff, Harry, 319–20
soda, **543–45**. *See also* seltzer
    Dr. Brown's, 178–79
    Indo-Caribbean, 290
    Pepsi-Cola, 455–56
    regulation, 544–45
soda "ban," 56, 455, 544, **545–46**, 608
soda fountains, 536, 543, **546–47**, 593
    Dr. Brown's sodas in, 179
    egg creams, 189–90
    Jackson Heights, 300
    Loft's, 349
soda jerk, 547
soda machines, 619
Sodamat Company, 619
sodamats, 619
Soda Politics (Nestle), 409, 440
SodaStream, 529
SoFi awards (Specialty Outstanding Food Innovation),
    202, 203
Sofrito (restaurant), 478
Soho House, 126
Soil and Health Society, 508
Sokolov, Raymond, 324, 423, **548**
    on Liebling, 341
    on Victor's Café, 152
Solace of Food, The (Clark), 354
Soldier's Return (Levine), 448
Solomon, Elke, 599
Solomon, Sidney, 99
Solomon R. Guggenheim Museum, 399
Solon, Johnny, 79, 481
Solt, George, 419
Soltner, André, 369, 467, **548–49**
    at French Culinary Institute, 228
    in haute cuisine, 265
    at Lutèce, 358–59
Somalians, 258
Somebody Up There Likes Me (movie), 299
Sondheim, Stephen, 269, 330
Sonnenfeld, Albert, 135
Sons of Liberty, 589
Sophie's Choice (Styron), 459–60
Sosa, Angelo, 212
Sotomayor, Sonia, 478
Soulé, Henri, 124, 227, 501, **549–50**
    falling out with Joseph Kennedy, 329
    Franey and, 224
    in haute cuisine, 264–65
    at Le Pavillon, 337–38
    Wechsberg on, 638
soul food, 6, 649
    in Harlem, 263
    Lewis in, 339–40
Soul of a New Cuisine, The (Samuelsson), 518
Soup Bar (restaurant), 168
Soup Book, The (De Gouy), 162, 371
Soup Kitchen International, 592
soup kitchens, 280–81, 517, 536
soup lines, 536
Soups and Sauces (Elliot and Jones), 371
South and Central American, **550–51**. *See also specific countries*

South Asian(s), **551–54**
    in Jamaica, 302
South Beach (Sloan), 460
South Bronx Food Co-op, 214
South Bronx Mobile Market, 78
Southeast Asian, **554–55**
Southern Food and Beverage Museum, 305
Southern Foodways Alliance, 340
Southland Corporation, 250
Soyer, Isaac, 448
Spanish-American War, 207
Spanish Harlem, 262, 263
speakeasies, 35, 473–74, 536, **555–57**
    gay, 236
    Greenwich Village, 248
    Hell's Kitchen, 269
    P. J. Clarke's, 445
    started by Kreindler and Berns, 609
Speakeasies of 1932, The (Hirschfeld), 556
Specialty Food Association, 202
Speedy Romeo (pizzeria), 464
Spencer, Colin, 136
Sphere (magazine), 152
Spice Market (restaurant), 272
Spicer, Susan, 324
Spiegel's Hungarian Restaurant, 77
spirits, **557–58**. *See also* alcohol
Splendid Table, The (radio program), 483
Spotted Pig, The (restaurant), 56, 57, 249
Spring Gardens, 588
Spring in Central Park (Dehn), 459
Spur Tree Lounge (restaurant), 303–4
Sri Lankan on Staten Island, 566
St. George Food Co-op, 214
St. George's Melkite Church, 347
St. James (hotel), 278
St. Nicholas Hotel, 264, 277–78
St. Patrick's Day, **558–59**
    corned beef and, 145
    parade, 657
St. Regis Hotel, 55
Staat's Herberg, 585
stadium food, 276–77, **559–61**
Stage Deli, 165
Stahl, Fannie, 396
Stahlhut, Henry, 361
Stamp Act (1765), 509, 589
Standard Brands, 95, 492, 493
Stanton Social (restaurant), 352
Starbucks, 128–29, 131, 132, **561–62**
    in Inwood, 291
    Jackson Heights, 301
    at Macy's, 365
Starlight Café (American Museum of Natural
    History), 10
Starr, Stephen, 399, 419, 494
startups, **562–64**
Staten Island, **564–66**
    diners, 173
    distilleries, 174, 509
    Italian ices, 297
    microbreweries, 387
    oyster beds, 208

Statue of Liberty
in D'Agostino advertising, 159
reopening celebration, 244
steak tartare, **566–67**
steamships, 273
Steele, Alfred N., 456
Steele, Lockhart, 187
Steeplechase Coffee shop (coffee shop), 129
Stein, Marcia, 120
Stein, Robert, 648
Steingarten, Jeffrey, 324, **567**
Steinhardt School, 197
Steinway, William, 355
Stella D'Oro, 77, **567–68**
Stella 34 (restaurant), 168, 365
Sterling Investment Partners, 200–201
Stern, Henry, 48
Stern & Saalberg, 603
Steuben Parade, 238, 657
Steuben Society, 238
Stevens, Harry M., 276, 559
Stewart, Alexander Turney, 168
Stewart, Martha
baked Alaska recipe, 29
in City Meals on Wheels, 246
at Le Cirque, 336
published by Clarkson Potter, 488
SiriusXM channel dedicated to, 483
Stewart-Gordon, Faith, 513
Stockli, Albert, 221, 493
Stokes, Rose Pastor, 502
Stollwerck Brothers, 618
Stone, Edie, 615
Stone Barns, 33
Stoned Crow (restaurant), 249
Stonewall Inn, 35, 236, 248, **568–69**, 586
began as speakeasy, 556
Stork Club, 126, 430, **569–70**
Stork Club Bar Book, The (Beebee), 570
Stork Club Cookbook, The (Billingsley), 570
Story of Weight Watchers, The (Nidetch), 428
Straight Up or On the Rocks (Grimes), 249
Straub, Jacques, 83
Straus, Gladys Guggenheim, 361
Straus, Isidor and Nathan, 364–65
Straus, Nathan, 387
Strauss, Richard, 355
Strauss Group, 279
street cries, 3–4, 11, 574
street fairs, **570–71**
Streets International, 291
Street Vendor Project, **571–72**, 574
Vendy Awards and, 619
street vendors, 536, 570, **572–74**. *See also* food trucks;
hot dogs; pushcart vendors
of dimsum, 172
in Dominican Washington Heights, 630
Essex Street Market, 196
falafel, 201
Filipino, 208
"green carts," 575
hamburgers, 259
hot dog, 277
of ice cream, 288
Indo-Caribbean, 289
Italian, 295, 344
of Italian ices, 297
knish, 322
lunch and, 357
Mexican food, 385
pretzel, 471
public markets and, 475, 476
selling candy, 94
in Sunset Park, 577
at West Indian Day Parade, 640
street vendors, regulation of, 172, 571, **574–75**
food trucks and, 220
Street Vendor Project, **574–75**
Streit's, 376–77
Streit's Matzoh, 352, 451
Strength from Eating (Macfadden), 364
strikes, 502
bagel workers, 27
fast food workers, **206**
New Year's Eve 1912, 502
Stritch, Elaine, 330
Stubbs, Merrill, 216, 272
Stupak, Alex, 180, 392
Sturgeon Queens, The (documentary), 511
Sturgis, Julius, 471
Stuyvesant, Peter, 283
Styler, Christopher, 584
Styron, William, 459–60
Suarez, Phil, 179, 553
sugar
in Brooklyn, 81
cubes, 576
English colonial consumption, 193, 194
ice cream and, 288
during World War II, 455, 654
Sugar Act (1764), 509, 589
Sugar Cane (restaurant), 6
sugar refining, 265–66, **575–77**
in Jamaica, 303
late twentieth century, 334
in Manhattan, 369
trade with Cuba, 151–52
Sugar Trust, 238, 265–66, 575
Sugary Drink Portion Cap Rule. *See* soda "ban"
Sullivan, John Jeremiah, 356
Sullivan Bakery, 31
Sullivan Street, 68
Summer Food Service Program, 282
Summer Streets, 570
Sunset Park, **577–78**
Chinatown in, 81
Industry City, 564
Mexicans in, 385
Sun-sik, Hong, 326
supermarkets, **578–79**, 579. *See also* Fairway Market;
King Kullen
A&P and, 1
Gristedes, 250–51
independent grocers and, 252
Jewish, 312
late twentieth century, 335

post-World War II, 468
public markets replaced by, 476
Supplemental Nutrition Assistance Program (SNAP), 281, **580–81**
  Green Carts and, 215
  at Key Food, 318
  outreach and education, 281–82
Surmain, André, 42, 358, 548
sushi, 307–8, **581–82**
Sushi of Gari (restaurant), 499, 581
Sushi Seki (restaurant), 581
Sushi Yasuda (restaurant), 581
sustainability
  Bittman and, 53
  Center for Food and Environment and, 135
  dumpster diving and, 180
  food co-ops and, 213–14
sustainable. *See* farm to table
Sutter's Bakery, 76
Sutton, Ryan, 187
Sutton Place Gourmet, 32
Svensson, Johan, 518
Swahn, Håkan, 15
Swallow Restaurant (Berkeley), 493
Swedish, French, American Cooking School, 143
Sweeney, Dennis, 39
Sweeney's, 500
Sweeney's (restaurant), 13
Sweet and Low: A Family Story (Cohen), 583
Sweet Holy Beans, 175–76
Sweet'N Low, 81, **582–83**
sweets
  Colonial Dutch baked goods, 133
  sold in appetizing stores, 14
Sweet's (restaurant), 13, 500
Sweets Company of America, 603, 604
Sweet Smell of Success, The, 601
Swift & Co., 650
SwissAm Hospitality Business School, 291
Sylvia and Herbert Woods Scholarship, 584
Sylvia Center, The, 245
Sylvia's (restaurant), 6, 263, **583–84**, 649–50
  supportive of elimination of trans fats, 605
Sylvia's Family Soul Food Cookbook (Woods and Clark), 263, 584
Sylvia's Soul Food (Woods and Styler), 263, 584
Sylvia Woods Enterprises, 263
Syrian and Lebanese, 278–79, **584–85**

T
Tabla (restaurant), 386, 553
Table, The (Filippini), 166
Table at Le Cirque, A (Maccioni and Fiori), 363
table d'hôte restaurants, 239, 277–78, 279, 356
Taco Bell, 205, 206, 301
tacos
  food trucks, 219
  Korean, 325–26
Tailor (restaurant), 392
Taina Group, 495
Takashi (restaurant), 566
Takayama, Masayoshi, 581
Takeshi, Kaga, 218

Talde (restaurant), 233, 450
Talde, Dale, 212, 233, 466
tally-ho lunch. *See* brunch
Tamarind (restaurant), 553
Tamashii (restaurant), 308
Tanaka, Shigenori, 518
Tap'd NY, 636
taprooms, 34
Tar Beach (Ringgold), 460
Tarlow, Andrew, 278
Tarowsky, Harry, 316
Taste, The (cooking competition), 518
Taste America food festival, 307
TasteBooks, 488
Taste of America, The (Hess and Hess), 270–71
Taste of Country Cooking, The (Lewis), 340
Taste of Seafood (restaurant), 263
Tatiana Restaurant and Nightclub, 73, 80, 512
Tava-Indian, 553
Tavernier, Claude, 459
Tavern in the Field, 588
Tavern on the Green (restaurant), 370, 467, 501, **585**
  Clark at, 6–7
  Nieporent director at, 429
  part of Restaurant Associates, 494
taverns, **585–87**. *See also* Fraunces Tavern
  colonial era, 194, 277
  hotel restaurants compared with, 277
  in Jamaica, 302
  Jewish, 310
  lunch in, 356
Tavola, A: A Performance (play, Solomon), 599
Taylor's (restaurant), 13, 288, 382, 500
tea, 177, 194, **587–88**
Tea Act (1773), 589
Tea Cup, The (Pollock), 448
Tea Party, **589–90**
tearooms, 588, **590–91**
  as alternative to bars and taverns, 593
  in department stores, 168
tea stores, 588
Technique, La (Pépin), 454
Teikei, 139
Teit, Lillian, 659
Teitel's deli, 19
Telepan, Bill, 241, 336, 614
television, **591–92**. *See also* Cooking Channel; Food Network
  Bourdain, 63–64
  Franey, 225
  knishes, 323
  Lape, 333
  Lucas, 354
  Pépin, 454
  public, **592–93**
  Puerto Rican, 478
  Zabar's, 660
television programs
  Appetite City, 250
  of Batali, 37
  of Bobby Flay, 210–11, 217, 218
  on food trucks, 220
  Dorothy Cann Hamilton in, 261
  Italian food in, 296

television programs (*continued*)
  Magnolia Bakery mentioned on, 367
  restaurants in, 592
  Top Chef, 211–12
temperance movement, **593–94**
  diners in, 172
  groggeries and, 253
  New Year's Day and, 411
  public water fountains, 634
  supporting soda fountains, 543
"Ten Days in Blackwell's Island" (Bly), 472
Tender at the Bone (Reichl), 493
Tenement Museum, **594–95**, 608
tenements
  fusion food and, 232
  Gilded Age, 239
  Hell's Kitchen, 269
  Italian, 295
  kitchens in, 195–96
  in Little Italy, 343
  Lower East Side, 351
Tengelmann Group, 3
Tenth Muse, The (Jones), 313, 324
Terrace 5 (MoMA), 399, 501
Terrace (restaurant), 614
Thai, 577, **595–96**
Thanksgiving, **596–98**
  Macy's Thanksgiving Day Parade, 365
theater and food, **598–99**
  Gourmet on, 241–42
  Jewish, 311
  knishes, 323
  in Little Odessa, 345
  lobster palaces, 347–49
Thelawala (restaurant), 553
theme restaurants, 467, 501
Thiebe, Otto, 415
Third Helpings (Trillin), 606
Third Plate, The (Barber), 33
30 Minute Meals (television show), 592
This, Hervé, 135, 136, 197, 391
This Organic Life (Gussow), 135
This Week (magazine), 446
Thomas, Anna, 313
Thomas, Dylan, 293, 587, 623, 641, *641*
Thomas, George, 600
Thomas, Jerry, 34, 127, **599–600**
  first mixologist, 390
  influence on DeGroff, 162
Thomas Adams and Sons, 256
Thomas Adams Gum Company, 618
Thomaschevsky, Boris, 189
Thompson, Hunter S., 587, 640
Thompson, J. Walter, 30
Thompson Bagel machine, 28
Thompson's (ice cream shop), 288
Thompson's (restaurant), 13, 500
three-martini lunch, **600–601**
Three Strikes, The, 176
Throwdown with Bobby Flay (television show), 210, 218
Thurber, James, 418
Tibbett Diner, 173
Tic-Taco (food truck), 219

Tierney, Patrick, 172
Tiffin (restaurant), 553
Tiger Blossom (restaurant), 233
Tilford, John, 148
Tillie's Chicken Shack, 6
Time (magazine), 33, 446
Time Out New York (magazine), 335, 596
TimeOutNY.com, 464
TimesLedger, 75
Times Square, **601–2**
  gay bars, 236
  Italian restaurants, 295
  New Year's Eve and, 412
Times Square Brewery and Restaurant, 387
Times Square Business Improvement District, 499
Tim Hortons (fast-food chain), 205
Tin Pan Alley, 299
tips, 504
Tiro a Segno (club), 125
Tisch, Jonathan, 468–69
Tisch, Robert, 468–69
T.N.T. (restaurant), 590
Today Café on One (American Museum of Natural History), 10
Todd, Ruthann, 641
To Die Dreaming (beverage), 176
Toffenetti (restaurant), 384, 602
Toffenetti, Dario, **602**
Tofu on Pedestal in Gallery (Horowitz), 618
tofutti, **602–3**
Tokio, The (lobster palace), 348–49
Toklas, Alice B., 42
Tom and Jerry, 411
Tom Cat Bakery, 31, 68
Tong, Kee Ling, 94
Tong, Michael, 614
Tonic Restaurant, 521
Tontine, The (coffeehouse), 128, 130
  soda water outlet at, 543, 546
Tony n' Tina's Wedding, 599
Tootsie Roll, 94, **603–4**
Topalian, Carole, 188
Top Chef (television show), 211–12, 233, 246
Top Chef Masters (television show), 493, 518
Topping Rose House, 495
Topps Chewing Gum, 256
Torey, Allysa, 366
Torres, Jacques, **604**
  at French Culinary Institute, 228
  in haute cuisine, 265
  at Le Cirque, 336
  pop-ups by, 466
Torrisi Italian Specialties (restaurant), 296, 345
Tortilleria Nixtamal, 550
Tosi, Christina, 101
  in French Culinary Institute, 260
  in *Lucky Peach*, 356
  in Momofuku Restaurant Group, 393
To the Queen's Taste (television show), 354, 591
Totonno's (pizzeria), 350, 461, 463, 464
Tower Suite (restaurant), 39, 332
Towle, George Makepeace, 441
Townshend Acts, 589

trade cards, 4
Trader Joe's, 251, 253, **604–5**, 614
Trader Vic's, 464
trains. *See* railroad dining; Transcontinental Railroad
Trall, Russel Thacher, 617
Transcontinental Railroad, 251
trans fat elimination, 205–6, **605–6**
Trans Fat Help Center, 605
Transmitter Brewing, 387
transportation. *See also* Erie Canal
    farm to table and, 203
    food, 108
    of food to Washington Market, 273–74
    grocery stores and, 251
    High Line in, 272–74
    in late twentieth century, 334–35
    pre-Columbian, 469
    of seafood, 231
Trattoria (restaurant), 494
Treme (television show), 592
Trevino, Manuel, 212
Treviño, Roberto, 478
Tribeca Grill (restaurant), 62, 334, 429, 495, 501
Tricorne, Le (Picasso), 221
Trifles Make Perfection (Wechsberg), 638
Trillin, Calvin, 153, 418, **606**
Trinidadian food, 219
Trois Petits Cochons, Les (restaurant), 227
Trotter, Charlie, 213, 306
truck markets, 476
Tschirky, Oscar, **606–7**, 627
    De Gouy's friendship with, 162
    in haute cuisine, 264
    inventor of Waldorf salad, 628
Tsuji Culinary Institute, 62
Tucci, Oscar, 167
Tucciarone, Frank, 159
Tuck Shop, 23, 108
Tudda, Louis, 105, 397
Tulsi (restaurant), 553
Tummy Trilogy (Trillin), 606
Tupper, Joshua Russ, 511
Turf Restaurant, 103, 299, 505
Turgeon, Charlotte, 119, 362
Turkish food, 258, 315
Turner, Kathleen, 246
Turner, Ted, 217
Turnier, William Adelbert, 404
Tutt Café, 191
Twain, Mark, 226, 469
20th Century Limited, 485
Twenty-Eighth Street Group, 448
twenty-first century, **607–9**
Twenty-five Cent Dinners for Families of Six (Corson), 146
"21" Club, 391, **609**
    on *All Around the Town*, 140
    hamburgers, 259
    during Prohibition, 126
    Sailhac at, 515
Twitter
    Cronut and, 151
    food trucks and, 220, 358
    Vendy Awards and, 620

Two Boots (pizzeria), 248, 450
Two Little Red Hens Bakery, 104
Typhoon Brewery, The, 387

U
Ubangi Club, 236
Ukrainian Festival, 611
Ukranian(s), 186, 345–46, **611**
Ultimate Baseball Road-Trip, The (Pahigian and O'Connell), 560
Unadulterated Food Products, Inc., 334
Unadulterated Fruit Juices, 541, 542
Uncle Tai's Hunan Yuan, 113
Uncle Vanya Café, 512
Underbelly NYC (television show), 78
Underground Gourmet, The (Glaser and Snyder), 322
Underground Gourmet column, 4
Uneeda Biscuit, 404
Ungaro, Susan, 306–7
Union Club, 125, 191
Union League Club, 122, 125, 596–97
Union Market, 253
unions. *See also* restaurant unions; strikes
    International Bagel Bakers Union, 27
Union Square Cafe, 249, 334, 385, 495, **611–12**
    part of Union Square Hospitality Group, 501
    Romano in, 265
Union Square Cafe Cookbook (Meyer and Romano), 386
Union Square Events, 466
Union Square Greenmarket, 139, 178
Union Square Hospitality Group, 213, 334, 385, 386, 495, 501, 612
    Institute of Culinary Education courses, 290
    Shake Shack, 531
United Cigar Store, 341
United Hebrew Communities Charity, 451
United Pickle, 457–58
United States Baking Company, 403
University of California Press, 136
University of North Carolina Press, 136
Untitled (restaurant), 399
Up in the Old Hotel and Other Stories (Mitchell), 390
Upper East Side, **612–13**. *See also* Yorkville
    gay bars, 236
    Greenmarkets, 247
    Ladies Who Lunch and, 331
Upper West Side, **613–14**
    Cubans in, 152
    gay bars, 236
Upstairs (restaurant), 62
Uptown Brasserie (restaurant), 518
urban farming, 215, 608, **614–16**. *See also* rooftop gardens
    CUNY and, 121
Urban Foragers (radio show), 86
Urban Harvest, 538
Urban Justice Center, 571, 574
Urban Oyster, 608, 629
Urbanspoon, 499
Urvater, Michèle, 217

V
Valenti, Nick, 120
Valenti, Tom, 614

Valentine Loewer's Gambrinus Brewing, 45, 70
Valentine's Manual of Old New York (Brown, ed.), 373
Van Aken, Norman, 232
Van Alen, William, 111
Van Brunt Stillhouse, 510
Van der Donck, Adriaen, 133
Van En, Robyn, 139
Vanity Fair (magazine), 590
Van Rensselaer, Maria Sanders, 414
Varenichnaya (restaurant), 73
Vargas, Herman, 511
Vatel Club, 106
Vaux, Calvert, 99
Vauxhall Gardens, 588
Vegan Before 6 (Bittman), 53
Vegan Guide to New York City, The (Berry and Abreu-Suzuki), 50, 491, 617
veganism, 490, **617–18**
Vegan's Delight, 490
Vegan Shop-Up, 618
Vegemite, 23
vegetarian food. *See also* veganism
    Indo-Caribbean, 289
    Korean, 325
Vegetarian Guide to Diet & Salad, The (Walker), 491
Vegetarians, The (Berry), 49
Veggie Castle II, 490
Veggie Pride Parade, 618
Veggies Natural Juice Bar, 490
Vehling, Joseph Dommers, 502
vending machines, **618–19**
    post-World War II expansion of, 467
    in schools, 525
"Vendor Power!," 571
Vendy Awards, 571, 575, **619–20**
Venezuelans in Inwood, 291
Veniero's (pastry shop), 31
Verdon, René, 329, 468
Vergé, Roger, 62, 63
Vergnes, Jean, 369, 467, 468
Vermeire, Robert, 481
Vermillion Hound (tearoom), 590
vermouth's influence on cocktails, 372, 373
Verrazano-Narrows Bridge, 449
Veselka (restaurant), 189, 512, 611
Vichyssoise, 171, **620–21**
Victoria (hotel), 278
Victor's Café, 152, **621–22**
Victory Bread, 653
victory gardens, 615, **622–23**, 653, 653
Vietnamese in Sunset Park, 577
Views of a Near-Sighted Cannoneer (Krim), 623
Vigne, Jean, 45, 70
Village Gate (restaurant), 249
Village Vanguard, 248, 430
Village Voice, **623–24**
    on Junior's cheesecake, 314
    possibly conceived at the White Horse, 641
    restaurant criticism, 498
        by Sheraton, 532
        by Sietsema, 187
    on Thai restaurants, 596
Villa Secondo (restaurant), 36, 296

Vintage Food Corporation, 73
Virginia House-Wife, The (Randolph), 103, 271
"Visit from Saint Nicholas, A" (Moore), 119
Visser, Edward, 243
Vitelio's Marketplace, 317
Vogue (magazine), 567
Volks Garten, 46
Volna (restaurant), 73
Volpe, Joan, 350
Volstead Act (1919), 473. *See also* Prohibition
Vong (restaurant), 227, 232, 554
Vongerichten, Jean-Georges, 101, 227, 334, 553, 613, 614, **624–25**
    Dufresne partnership with, 179, 180
    on food at Madison Square Garden, 561
    fusion food, 232
    Hesser review of, 272
    hotel restaurants of, 278
    influenced by Baum, 501
    patron of Kitchen Arts and Letters, 637
Vourderis, Marinos, 297
Vox Media, 187

W
Waber, Bernard, 459
Wadi Halfa (restaurant), 584
Wagner, Robert, 240
Wakefield, Dan, 587
Waldorf, The, 105, **627–28**
    eggs Benedict, 190–91
    haute cuisine at, 264
    on *Mad Men*, 366
    paintings of, 448
    tearoom in Palm Room, 590
    Tschirsky at, 607
Waldorf Astoria
    catering departments, 99
    cocktails, 127
    De Gouy at, 162
    Franey at, 224
    haute cuisine at, 264
    Lang at, 332
    rooftop garden, 508
    women's clubs meeting at, 647
Waldorf salad, 627, **628–29**
Walker, James "Jimmy," 99
Walker, Kara, 81
Walker, Norman W., 491
Walker in the City, A (Kazin), 460
walking tours, culinary, 608, **629–30**
Wall, Caesar, 163
Wall Street Burger Shoppe, 259
Wall Street Journal, 548
Walouf, Waldy, 521
Ward, John, 182
Ward's Bakery, 31
Washington, George, 225, 356
Washington, Martha, 271
Washington Heights, **630–31**
    bodegas, 59
    Dominicans, 97, 175, 176
    as food desert, 214–15
    gay bars, 236

Washington Market, 370, 409, **631–33**
  in antebellum period, 11
  D'Agostino purchases from, 159
  De Voe at, 170
  diners, 173
  fish in, 230
  food transportation to, 273–74
Washington Square Arch, 460
Washington Square Park, 236, 248
Wasserstein, Rosanne, 460
wastED dinners, 466
water, **633–35**
  bottled, **635–36**
    Perrier, 456
  brought to Manhattan, 45
  free public water fountains, 593
  for tea, 588
Waterfront Ale House, 521, 605
Waters, Alice, 33
  on farm to table, 203
  on food systems, 340
  on Heritage Radio Network, 270
  James Beard Award to, 305
  organizer of Slow Food Nation, 538
  published by Random House, 488
  Roberta's and, 507
water supply systems, 634, 634–35
Watson, Ben, 538
Watson, Donald, 617
Waxman, Jonathan
  Citymeals-on-Wheels, 120
  on farm to table, 203
  Flay and, 210
  on Gotham Bar and Grill, 240
Waxman, Nach, 154, 320–21, **637**
Wayward Reporter (Sokolov), 341
wd-50 (restaurant), 179, 180, 319, 352, 391
Weaver, Robert, 419
Weaver, S. Fullerton, 627
Weaver, William Woys, 154, 414
Weber, Max, 448
Webster, A. L., 142
WebVan (online grocery), 229
Wechsberg, Joseph, 362, 418, 468, **637–38**
Week, Caleb, 302
"Weekend Food Talk" (radio show), 483
We Had a Picnic Sunday Last (Woodson), 460
Weight Watchers, **638–39**. *See also* Nidetch, Jean
Weiner, Matthew, 366
Weingast, Sam and Morris, 397
Welch Grape Juice Company, 247
Welcome Back, Kotter (television show), 323
Weller, Craig, 642
Wells, Patricia, 272, 528
Wells, Pete, 498
  on Blanca, 86
  at the *New York Times*, 423
  on Tavern on the Green, 585
Well Seasoned Appetite, A (O'Neill), 436
Wendy's (fast-food chain), 205, 206
Wertheim, Morris, 407
West, Mae, 235
West Africans, 43, 78

West India Company, 45, 193
West Indian Day Parade, 570, **639–40**
West Indians, 334, 538
Weston A. Price Foundation, 388
West Side Brewery, 387
West Side Cowboy, 273, 300
West Side Freight Line, 273. *See also* High Line
West Side Story (musical), 269
West Washington Market, 379, 631
What Are They Eating? (television show, Wolf), 592
What Happens When project, 466
What to Eat (Nestle), 409
What to Eat, and How to Cook It (Blot), 57
What We Eat and Why (television show, Wolf), 592
wheat, 193, 195
Wheaton, Barbara, 154
When You Entertain (Allen), 8
whiskey, 558
  distilleries, 174–75
  Irish, 293
  rye whiskey, 509
Whiskey Cocktail, 435
Whiskey War (1869), 174, 175
White, E. B., 418
White, Jasper, 528
White, Michael, 278, 365
White, Stanford, 134, 348, 534
White Castle (restaurant chain), 205, 224, 259
White Horse Tavern, 249, 293, 586, 587, **640–42**
  St. Patrick's Day and, 558
Whiteman, Michael, 39, 486, 644
White Mountain gum, 256
Whitney Museum of American Art, 379, 399
Whole Foods, 251, 253, 437, 438, **642–43**
  Indian food at, 553
  in Manhattan, 370, 614
  organic foods, 437
  Rooftop Greenhouse, 508
Whole World Loves Chicken Soup, The (Sheraton), 533
Who's Who of Cooking in America, 304
Who's Who of Food and Beverage in America, 200, 261
Whynot Coffee and Wine (coffee shop), 129
Whythe Hotel, 278
Why We Eat What We Eat (Sokolov), 548
Willan, Anne, 271
Williams, Karl Franz, 391
Williamsburg, **643–44**
  diners, 173
  gay bars, 236
  German restaurants, 237–38, 456–57
  Germans, 321
  Havemeyer factory, 265
  Jews, 81, 311
  pop-ups in, 466
  sugar refining, 575
Williamsburg Walks, 570
Williams Candy Shop, 95
WillPowder, 197, 392
Will Write for Food (Jacob), 606
Wilmerding, Enid, 590
Wilson, Margaret Barclay, 415, 416
Winchell, Walter, 316, 609

Windows on the World (restaurant), 370, 467, 486, **644–45**
  created by Baum, 39
  Glaser's design of logo, 4
  Gold at, 240
wine and winemaking, 165, **645–46**
wine education. *See* Astor Center
Wines Vines Analytics, 646
Wine with Food (Fabricant and Asimov), 200
Winfrey, Carey, 153
Wintour, Anna, 567
With the Grain (Sokolov), 548
Wm. Wrigley Jr. Company, 341
Wolf, Burt, 592
Wolf, Clark, **646**
  Fales Library collection, 202
  Nestle and, 408
  at NYU, 426
Wolf, Dan, 623, 641
Wolfe, Elsie de, 134
Wolfe, Thomas, 433
Wolfe, Tom, 433
Wolfert, Paula, 153, 338
Wolff, Ethan, 85
Wolfgang Puck Catering, 495
Wolfgang Puck Companies, 494
Wolfson, Alex, 655
Woman's Day (magazine), 42, 647
women
  admission
    at the Plaza, 464
    unescorted in bars, 236
    at the Waldorf Astoria, 607
  in catering, 244–45
  during Civil War, 122
  as confectioners or pie makers, 30
  dining in public
    at Café Martin, 226
    English colonial, 194
    Gilded Age, 239
  ice cream shops for, 288
  lunch and, 356–57
  McSorley's and, 379
  paintings of, 448
  restaurants catering to ladies, 13
  in saloons, 209
  as servers at Childs, 110–11
  smoking at Ritz-Carlton, 506
  soda fountains and, 547
  in speakeasies, 556
  suffrage movement, 239
  working at counters of New York bakeries, 30
Women, Infants, and Children Program (WIC), 281, 282, 580
Women's Auxiliary of the Church Temperance Society,
        172, 218
women's clubs, **646–48**
Women's Day (magazine), 2
Women's Educational and Industrial Society of New York, 417
women's magazines, **648–49**
Women's Organization for National Prohibition Reform, 474
Wonder Bread, 67
Wondrich, David, 373, 599
Wood, Samuel, 150
Woods, Herbert, 263

Woods, Sylvia, 6, 263, 583, **649–50**
Woodside, 479
  Filipinos, 207
  South and Central American food, 550
  Thai, 596
Woodside, Patrick, 91
Woodside Café, 553
Woodson, Jacqueline, 460
Woollcott, Alexander, 7, 536
Woolworth's, 300, 302, 357
Word of Mouth (Ferguson), 135
workingman's clubs, 209–10
Works Progress Administration, 207, 344, 448, 552
World Expo Milano, 307
World of Cheese, The (Jones), 313
World's Columbian Exposition (Chicago, 1893), 255
World's Fair (1939–1940), 170, *650*, **650–51**
  doughnuts, 178
  Franey in, 224
  Ladies Who Lunch and, 331
  La Guardia and, 332
  Miranda at, 65
  restaurants, 501
    of Amiel, 299
    Childs, 112
    French, 226–27
    haute cuisine, 264
    Le Restaurant du Pavillon de France, 549
    Toffenetti, 602
World's Fair (1964–1965), **651–52**
  Lang in, 332
  Le Pavillon in launching, 336–37
  Marino's Italian Ices in, 297
World Trade Center
  French restaurants closed after attacks, 330
  Little Syria replaced by, 347
  restaurants created by Baum's company, 39
  The Three Strikes served at, 176
World War I, **652–53**
  Allen's cookbooks and, 8
  backlash against German foods, 164
  De Gouy in, 162
  denouncing of distillers, 174–75
  doughnuts, 178, 517
  Food Values and Economies Exhibition, 10
  German restaurants closed in, 355, 456
  Greek immigrants after, 245
  impact on breweries, 45
  Perrier during, 636
World War II, **653–54**. *See also* victory gardens
  backlash against German foods in, 164
  curry, 552
  doughnuts in, 178
  Ellis Island detention center, 472
  Franey in, 224
  gay bars, 236
  German restaurants closed in, 456–57
  Gourmet during, 361–62
  haute cuisine in, 264–65
  impact on breweries, 45
  La Guardia in, 332
  Paddleford in, 446
  Passover in, 452

Pepsi-Cola in, 455
Perrier during, 636
poster encouraging victory gardens, 653
railroads during, 485
salamis shipped in, 316
sugar production, 576
Tootsie Rolls in ration kits, 604
urban farming during, 615
World Wide Cook Book, The (Metzelthin), 241, 361, 468
Worth, Helen, 144
Wright, Jonathan, 487
Wright, The (restaurant), 399
Wythe Diner, 173

Y
Yamada, Isao, 62
Yankee Clipper (dining car), 485
Yankee Stadium, food at, 559, 560, 561
Yeats, John Butler, 447
Yeats at Petitpas' (Sloan), 447
Yeganeh, Ali, 592
Yelp, 233, 472, 499, 553
Yes, Chef (Samuelsson), 518
Yiddish Family Cook Book, The (Braun), 311
Ying, Chris, 356
YMCA (Young Men's Christian Association), 69, 92, 622
Yonah Schimmel Knish Bakery, 311, 316, 352, **655**
    Ausubel on, 322
    egg creams, 189
Yorkville, 522–23, **655–57**
    Germans in, 163, 237–38, 321, 522, 540, 612
    Hungarians in, 279–80
Yorkville Brewery, 387
Yorkville Coffee Mill, 656
Yorkville Food Shoppe, 159
Yorkville Meat Emporium, 657
You Can't Go Home Again (Wolfe), 433

Young, Chris, 391
Your Brain on Food (Wenk), 440
YWCA (Young Women's Christian Association), 92

Z
Zabar, Eli, 31, 68, 659
Zabar's, 537, 614, **659–60**
    cheese, 105
    kimchi at, 319
    kosher food at, 312
Zabb Elee (restaurant), 555, 596
Zagat, Tim and Nina, 62, 498, **660–61**
Zagat Survey, 498, 499, 660–61
    on food trucks, 220
    on Thai restaurants, 596
    on Union Square Cafe, 612
Zaidi, Hasnaian, 553
Zakarian, Geoffrey, 336, 377
Zaldívar, Monica, 622
Zambetti, Phil, 567
Zantilaveevan, Pecko, 221
Zarela (restaurant), 384
Zaro's (bakery), 31
Zaytoon's (restaurant), 201
Zeller, Benjamin E., 136
zeppole, 178, 519, **661**. *See also* doughnuts
Zero Otto Nove (pizzeria), 19, 464
Zero Point Zero Production, 355–56
Zia Chu, Grace, 113
Zimmern, Andrew, 434, 629
Zip City/The Tap Room, 387
Zraly, Kevin, 645
Zum Brauhaus (speakeasy), 556
Zum Schneider, 47, 238
Zum-Zum (restaurant), 39, 370, 467, 494, 501
Zwerdling, Daniel, 153
Zysman, Jacob, 513